EGAN'S FUNDAMENTALS OF
RESPIRATORY CARE

EGAN'S FUNDAMENTALS OF
RESPIRATORY CARE

Senior Editor

CRAIG L. SCANLAN, EdD, RRT

Professor and Chairman
Department of Cardiopulmonary Sciences
School of Health Related Professions
University of Medicine and Dentistry of New Jersey
Newark, New Jersey

Contributing Editors

CHARLES B. SPEARMAN, BS, RRT

Assistant Professor
Department of Respiratory Therapy
School of Allied Health Professions
Loma Linda University
Loma Linda, California

RICHARD L. SHELDON, MD, FCCP, FACP

Professor of Medicine
Loma Linda University School of Medicine
Chief, Section of Pulmonary and Intensive Care Medicine
Veteran's Administration Hospital
Medical Director, Department of Respiratory Therapy
School of Allied Health Professions
Loma Linda University
Loma Linda, California

Previous Editions by

DONALD F. EGAN, MD

formerly Chief, Pulmonary Disease Section
Veteran's Administration Medical Center
Asheville, North Carolina

FIFTH EDITION

with **23** *contributors and* **850** *illustrations*

The C. V. Mosby Company

ST. LOUIS • BALTIMORE • PHILADELPHIA • TORONTO   1990

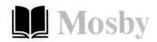

Publisher: David T. Culverwell
Developmental Editors: Maureen Slaten, Christi Mangold
Assistant Editor: Cynthia E. Lilly
Project Manager: Carol Sullivan Wiseman
Production Editor: Pat Joiner
Editing and Production: Cracom Corp.
Designer: Gail Morey Hudson

FIFTH EDITION

The C.V. Mosby Company
11830 Westline Industrial Drive, St. Louis, Missouri 63146

Library of Congress Cataloging-in-Publication Data
Egan's fundamentals of respiratory care.—5th ed. / senior editor,
    Craig L. Scanlan, contributing editors, Charles B. Spearman, Richard
    L. Sheldon; previous editions by Donald F. Egan; with 23
    contributors.
        p.   cm.
    Rev. ed. of: Egan's fundamentals of respiratory therapy / edited
and revised by Charles B. Spearman, Richard L. Sheldon. 4th ed.
1982.
    Includes bibliographical references.
    ISBN 0-8016-4737-1
    1. Respiratory therapy.   I. Egan, Donald F., 1916-   Fundamentals
of respiratory therapy.   II. Scanlan, Craig L., 1947-
III. Spearman, Charles B.   IV. Sheldon, Richard L.   V. Title:
Fundamentals of respiratory care.
    [DNLM: 1. Respiratory Therapy.   WB 342 E278]
RM161.E37   1990
615.8′36—dc20
DNLM/DLC
for Library of Congress   90-5408
                                                                CIP

C/VH/VH 9 8 7 6 5 4 3

Contributors

DAVID H. DAIL, MD

Department of Pathology
The Virginia Mason Clinic
Seattle, Washington

RICHARD D. DUNBAR, MD, FACP, FACR

Associate Professor of Radiology
Loma Linda University School of Medicine
Chief of Radiology
Loma Linda Community Hospital
Loma Linda, California

RAYMOND S. EDGE, EdD, RRT

Associate Dean, School of Allied Health
Ferris State University
Big Rapids, Michigan

HARRY ELIAS, MPH, RRT, RPFT

Assistant Professor
Department of Cardiopulmonary Sciences
School of Health Related Professions
University of Medicine and Dentistry of New Jersey
Newark, New Jersey

G. WOODWARD GROSS, BS, RRT

Clinical Assistant Professor and Program Director
Respiratory Therapy Program
Department of Cardiopulmonary Sciences
School of Health Related Professions
University of Medicine and Dentistry of New Jersey
Camden, New Jersey

TARSEM L. GUPTA, RPh, MD

Staff Physician, Clayton General Hospital
Riverdale, Georgia

ROBIN A. HARVAN, EdD

Assistant Professor and Program Director
Graduate Program in Health Professions Education
School of Health Related Professions
University of Medicine and Dentistry of New Jersey
Newark, New Jersey

BEAUFORT B. LONGEST, Jr., PhD

Director, Health Policy Institute
Graduate School of Public Health
University of Pittsburgh
Pittsburgh, Pennsylvania

PATRICK M. McDONALD, MA, RRT

Western Regional Director
Primedica, Inc.
Marietta, Georgia

BARBARA A. PETERS, AS, RRT

Department of Respiratory Care
St. Helena Hospital and Health Center
Deer Park, California

JAMES A. PETERS, MD, DHSc, MPH, RD, RRT

Preventive Medicine and Assistant Medical Director
Department of Respiratory Care
St. Helena Hospital and Health Center
Deer Park, California
Associate Professor
Department of Respiratory Therapy
School of Allied Health Professions
Loma Linda University
Loma Linda, California

FRANCES W. QUINLESS, PhD, RN, CCRN

Associate Professor and Chairman
Department of Nursing Education and Services
School of Health Related Professions
University of Medicine and Dentistry of New Jersey
Newark, New Jersey

ALAN M. REALEY, BA, RRT

Instructor, Department of Cardiopulmonary Sciences
School of Health Related Professions
University of Medicine and Dentistry of New Jersey
Camden, New Jersey

NORMAN C. SCHUSSLER, MS, RRT

Assistant Professor, Respiratory Therapy Program
Division of Allied Health, School of Medicine
University of Louisville
Louisville, Kentucky

KIM F. SIMMONS, MHS, RRT

Instructor and Director of Clinical Education
Department of Cardiopulmonary Science
School of Allied Health Professions
Louisiana State University Medical Center
New Orleans, Louisiana

HALCYON ST. HILL, MS, EdD, MT(ASCP)

Director, School of Medical Technology
Mountainside Hospital
Montclair, New Jersey

JOHN V. TESORIERO, PhD

Associate Professor and Director
Basic Science Education and Research
School of Health Related Professions
University of Medicine and Dentistry of New Jersey
Newark, New Jersey

F. ROBERT THALKEN, BS, RRT

Instructor and Director of Clinical Education
Respiratory Therapy Program
Department of Cardiopulmonary Sciences
School of Health Related Professions
University of Medicine and Dentistry of New Jersey
Camden, New Jersey

ANN W. TUCKER, DEd

Assistant Professor and Chairman
Department of Dental Auxiliaries Education
School of Health Related Professions
University of Medicine and Dentistry of New Jersey
Newark, New Jersey

ROBERT L. WILKINS, MA, RRT

Assistant Professor and Associate Chairman
Department of Respiratory Therapy
School of Allied Health Professions
Loma Linda University
Loma Linda, California

SHARON WILLIAMS-COLON, MA, RRT

Assistant Professor and Program Director
Respiratory Therapy Program
Department of Cardiopulmonary Sciences
School of Health Related Professions
University of Medicine and Dentistry of New Jersey
Newark, New Jersey

KENNETH A. WYKA, MS, RRT

Assistant Professor, Department of Cardiopulmonary Sciences
School of Health Related Professions
University of Medicine and Dentistry of New Jersey
Newark, New Jersey

JOHN W. YOUTSEY, PhD, RRT

Associate Professor and Chairman
Department of Cardiopulmonary Care Sciences
College of Health Sciences
Georgia State University
Atlanta, Georgia

Preface

It was with a profound sense of both humility and trepidation that I accepted responsibility to serve as senior editor for the fifth edition of *Egan's Fundamental of Respiratory Care*.

My sense of humility derived from the fact that "Egan" —as it is so fondly called—has become a classic in the field of respiratory care. Indeed, some twenty years after it first appeared, my tattered first edition still sits on the bookshelf, paying homage to the tens of thousands of students and practitioners for whom it has served as guide and mentor.

Unfortunately, the term "classic" denotes a certain degree of stability and reverence that no foundation text in the health sciences can long claim. Clearly, since publication of the fourth edition some eight years ago, the field of respiratory care has undergone dramatic changes. Of course, many of these changes have been technological in nature, as has been the case since the inception of the field. Thus, as would be expected, a primary goal in creating this new edition was to account for these changes by updating and expanding its technical contents.

In terms of updating, the reader familiar with the fourth edition will find that most of the prior content has been entirely rewritten, and is now based on the most contemporary reference sources available. Moreover, the technical content has been significantly expanded to include areas not previously addressed in earlier editions. These entirely new chapters include Terms, Symbols, and Units of Measure (Chapter 3), Physical Principles in Respiratory Care (Chapter 4), Principles of Infection Control (Chapter 14), Physical Assessment of the Patient (Chapter 16), Synopsis of Cardiopulmonary Diseases (Chapter 19), Airway Care (Chapter 21), Emergency Life Support (Chapter 22), Hyperinflation Therapy (Chapter 26), Chest Physical Therapy (Chapter 27), Respiratory Failure and the Need for Ventilatory Support (Chapter 28), Patient Management and Cardiopulmonary Monitoring (Chapter 31), Neonatal and Pediatric Intensive Care (Chapter 32), and Computer Applications in Respiratory Care (Chapter 36).

Although an ambitious undertaking in itself, this technical updating was not the source of my trepidation. As I approached the project, it became increasingly clear that the new edition would have to do more than simply update the knowledge base in respiratory care. In order to remain a "classic," the new Egan would have to reflect the ongoing maturation of the field, and—with it—the changing philosophy of respiratory care that has become so evident as we move into this new decade.

By changing philosophy, I mean the ongoing shift in the orientation of the field from the merely technical to the professional, from an equipment-centered focus to a more balanced perspective with the patient at the core, from a delimited concentration on curative acute care to a broader interpretation of the meaning of health, and with it a changing view on both the settings of practice and the types of care that can and should be provided.

In addressing these changes, the new edition attempts to provide a clear vision of both current and future directions in the field. To this end, Chapters 1 (Respiratory Care and the Health Care System) and 2 (Modern Respiratory Care Services) provide a broad orientation to the problems and prospects characterizing the current health care system, and the importance of both quality assurance *and* cost-effectiveness in the delivery of health care. Chapters 11 (Health Communication), 12 (Ethical and Legal Implications of Practice), and 13 (General Patient Care) lay the groundwork for a more patient-oriented approach to practice, while Chapters 33 (Health Education and Health Promotion), 34 (Cardiopulmonary Rehabilitation), and 35 (Respiratory Home Care) emphasize the new and expanding roles that respiratory care practitioners can and must assume outside the acute care setting.

Complementing the technical updating and shift in text orientation is a third major change. Unlike its predecessors, the fifth edition has been specifically written and organized to facilitate learning. Changes and refinements made in this area include a direly needed downward adjustment in reading difficulty (now approaching the 13th grade level); a greater emphasis on explanatory illustrations (three times as many as the fourth edition); the addition of learning objectives, key terms, and a content summary for each chapter; and provision of a comprehensive glossary of terms. Moreover, a student workbook and study guide (available separately and designed specifically to accompany the new edition) provides activities and exercises intended to encourage student participation in classroom, laboratory, and clinical assignments related to the text content.

Despite the scope of changes made in this edition, efforts have been made to assure that the text retains what have always been considered its major strengths. First and foremost, the new edition continues to emphasize theory and principles as the basis for intelligent and safe practice. In this regard, the previous strong focus on the basic and life sciences has been expanded and further strengthened. This emphasis on principles also extends into the realm of therapeutic and diagnostic equipment. Here, the approach taken is to explain and elaborate on the *underlying concepts,* purposefully leaving details on specific equipment design and operation to other texts designed exclusively for that purpose.

Also retained in this new edition is a rigorous and often highly critical approach to many of the therapeutic modalities used in respiratory care. This emphasis reflects the growing importance of disciplined scientific inquiry as the basis for determining the efficacy of our clinical interventions, and represents one of the most visible components in the ongoing professionalization of the field.

As we move into the 1990s, it becomes increasingly clear that no single resource can any longer hope to portray the full framework of knowledge in the field of respiratory care. This new edition of Egan is no exception. Nonetheless, I believe that the editors and contributing authors have created a wholly new *foundation* text in the field, providing—as its title conveys—a comprehensive overview of concepts "fundamental" to the safe and effective practice of respiratory care. It is upon this strong foundation that I hope others will build.

Craig L. Scanlan

Contents

SECTION VI
BASIC THERAPEUTICS

20 Pharmacology for Respiratory Care, 455

James A. Peters
Barbara A. Peters

21 Airway Care, 483

Kim F. Simmons

22 Emergency Life Support, 513

Craig L. Scanlan

23 Humidity and Aerosol Therapy, 557

Craig L. Scanlan

Foundations of Respiratory Care

1

Respiratory Care and the Health Care System

Beaufort B. Longest, Jr.
Craig L. Scanlan
Harry Elias

Because students and practitioners provide respiratory care daily, it is only natural that they focus their attention on the knowledge and skills required to effectively fulfill their professional roles and responsibilities. However, respiratory care is part of a larger, dynamic health care system in which the respiratory care professional plays an essential role. As a provider of health care, the practitioner is responsible for planning, implementing, and evaluating a variety of therapeutic and diagnostic services under medical supervision. When interacting with patients and other professionals, the practitioner's role as a provider is enhanced by the ability to understand and relate key organizational and operational elements of health care delivery.

OBJECTIVES

This chapter describes the organizational context of the U.S. health care system as it relates to the role and function of respiratory care practitioners. Specifically, on completion of this chapter, the reader will be able to:

1 Define the terms *health, health services,* and *health care system;*

2 List factors affecting the health status of the American population and the relative expenditures devoted to each;

3 Identify the primary resources supporting the U.S. health care delivery system;

4 List the organizations representing primary providers of health services and the role respiratory care plays in each;

5 List the organizations providing the resources necessary to support the health care system (secondary providers), including those directly involved in respiratory care;

6 List the public and private organizations that plan for or regulate the primary and secondary health service providers, with an emphasis on those overseeing respiratory care;

7 Identify the current role, expectations, and unmet needs of U.S. health care consumers; and

8 Identify and describe the major problems confronting the current U.S. health care system.

KEY TERMS

Most terms used in this chapter are defined in context. The following terms are introduced without explicit definition but may be found in the Glossary:

AARC	for-profit
academic health center	GNP
accreditation	JRCRTE
advocacy	length of stay
allocation	long-term care
beneficiary	NBRC
board certified	not-for-profit
BOMA	paradox
CON	physical plant
consumerism	politicization
convalescence	postbaccalaureate
croup	premium
determinant	prospective payment
diversification	recredentialing
DME company	R & D
DRG	rehabilitation
entitlement	

Adapted with permission from: Modern health services in an organized setting. In Longest BB Jr: Management practices for the health professional, ed 3, East Norwalk, Conn, 1984, Appleton & Lange.

HEALTH, HEALTH SERVICES, AND THE HEALTH CARE SYSTEM

Describing the modern health care system is a complex task. The scope of the subject is broad, and the system itself is constantly changing. As a useful starting point, we will define the meaning of the terms *health, health services,* and *health care system,* and then look at factors affecting the health status of the population.

Health and health status

Health has been defined by the World Health Organization as a state of "complete physical, mental, and social well-being and not merely the absence of disease." From this ideal, the World Health Organization has attempted to give meaning to the term *health* by setting as a goal "the attainment by all citizens of the world by the year 2000 of a level of health that will permit them to lead a socially and economically productive life."

Health or health status in a human being is a function of many factors, including basic biologic characteristics and processes composing human biology (some diseases are inherited); the conditions external to the body (some diseases are caused by or worsened by environmental conditions); and the behavior patterns constituting a person's lifestyle (some diseases result from the pattern or style of life). The World Health Organization's definition of health describes an ideal state—one that is impossible to measure; yet it represents a target that permits a definition of a second important term.

Health services

Dictionaries generally define *service* as "an act of helpful activity." Thus health services, in their simplest terms, are acts of helpful activity specifically intended to maintain or improve health.

Health services can be divided into three basic types:
1. Public health services. These are activities that must be conducted on a community basis such as communicable disease control and the collection and analysis of health statistics.
2. Environmental health services. These often overlap with public health services and include activities such as insect, rodent, and air pollution control.
3. Personal health services. These are activities directed at individuals and include promotion of health, prevention of illness, diagnosis, treatment (sometimes leading to a cure), and rehabilitation.

Activities as diverse as the emergency room treatment of a child with croup, the drainage of a swamp in Louisiana during mosquito season, the dietary counseling of an obese member of a health maintenance organization, and the separation of smokers and nonsmokers on a commercial airliner are examples of health services.

Of course, in fulfilling their professional role, respiratory care personnel traditionally function in the area of

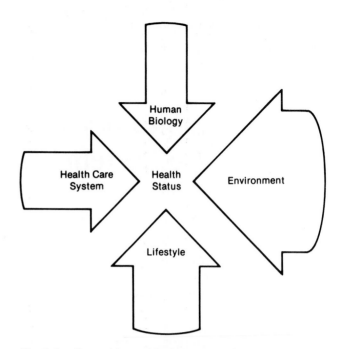

Fig. 1-1   Determinants of health status. (Redrawn from Blum HL: Planning for health: development and application of social change theory, New York, 1973, Human Sciences Press, p 3.)

personal health services, providing diagnostic testing and treatment for individuals with a variety of existing cardiopulmonary disorders. More recently, respiratory care practitioners are expanding their role in the delivery of personal health services by assuming greater responsibility for the promotion of health and the prevention of illness. Moreover, as both health professionals and members of society at large, respiratory care personnel are taking advocacy roles in public and environmental health services.

Health care system

Building on these definitions, it is possible to define the *health care system* as resources (money, people, physical plant, and technology) and the organizational configurations necessary to transform them into health services. It is the "act of helpful activity specifically intended to maintain or improve health" that forms the ultimate purpose of the health care system. Thus the accessibility, quality, appropriateness, and efficiency of these health services constitute the basis for fair and rational judgments about the system.

Factors affecting health status

The health care system and its services are only one of many factors affecting health status. Fig. 1-1 represents, through the relative size of the arrows, assumptions about the relative importance of these determinants of health status.[1] For example, the death from lung cancer of a person with a family history of (genetic tendency toward) cancer,

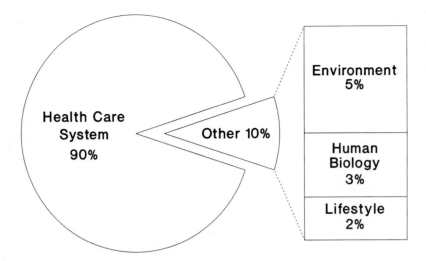

Fig. 1-2   Federal health expenditures by health determinant (estimated).   (Redrawn from Longest BB Jr: Management practices for the health professional, ed 3, East Norwalk, Conn, 1984, Appleton & Lange.)

and who smoked heavily, lived in a polluted urban environment, and consulted a physician long after symptoms emerged is not a fair and rational basis on which to judge the health care system inadequate. On the other hand, the death of an infant whose mother could not obtain good prenatal care (accessibility), unnecessary surgery performed by a less than fully qualified surgeon (appropriateness and quality), or a grossly inflated price for a diagnostic procedure because the machine needed to perform the procedure is owned by a hospital in a community where too many such machines exist (efficiency) are fairer and more rational bases on which to judge the system inadequate.

Ironically, expenditures on health services, especially at the federal level, are inconsistent with the view of the determinants of health status represented in Fig. 1-1. Fig. 1-2 depicts a rough estimate of the distribution of federal health expenditures by these determinants. This paradox between determinants of health and expenditures for health is unlikely to change dramatically in the next few years. The health care system absorbs the majority of dollars spent to affect health status, but its future positive effect on the status of health of the U.S. population appears to be limited.

This does not mean the health care system is unimportant to health status. It is, after all, the source of intervention when illness or disease occurs, even though their roots may lie in environmental, biologic, or behavioral determinants. In this sense the health care system can be viewed as a line of defense against untreated environmentally, biologically, and/or behaviorally caused illness and disease. Largely because preventive measures in these areas have been insufficient, the health care system is vital in maintaining and improving the health status of the population.

THE DYNAMICS OF THE HEALTH CARE SYSTEM

The resources—money, people, physical plant, and technology—and organizational configurations necessary to transform them into health services are described in the sections that follow. Also, we will consider the problems confronting the system as it attempts to provide high-quality, appropriate, efficiently produced, and accessible services. First, however, it is important to recognize the dynamic nature of the U.S. health care system.

The dynamic nature of the U.S. health care delivery system is nowhere more evident than in the amount of money spent for it. In 1990, total U.S. health expenditures will climb past $640 billion. This is a dramatic increase from the $250 billion spent in 1980 and only $75 billion in 1970.[2] Even when adjusted for inflation, real health care costs have nearly tripled over the last three decades.

To put this number in perspective, in the average time it takes to read this chapter, the United States will spend over $50 million on the provision of health care. During 1990, these health care expenditures will amount to about 12% of the total value of all goods and services (the gross national product [GNP]) produced during that year. As a nation, we spend more on health care than on defense, education, or housing. By the year 2000, these expenditures are expected to reach more than $1.5 trillion, representing about 15% of the GNP.[2] These dramatic increases reflect not only inflation and increased use of health care services but also growth and change in the system.

Factors contributing to the dynamic state of the health care system reflect social change, different priorities, new technology, more regulation of the system, changes in disease trends, new delivery methods, and new approaches to paying for health care. For example, there have been sig-

YEAR

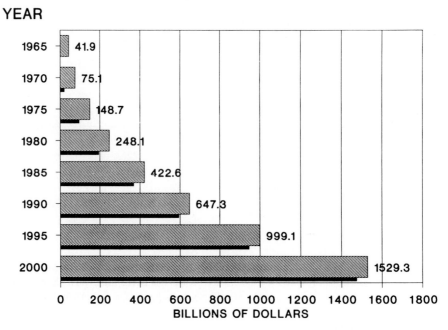

BILLIONS OF DOLLARS

Fig. 1-3 Growth in total U.S. expenditures for health care, 1965 to 2000. (From Health Care Financing Administration, Division of National Cost Estimates, Office of the Actuary.)

nificant increases in drug addiction (particularly alcoholism) and sexually transmitted disease in recent years. Because these problems are viewed as health issues rather than social or criminal problems, they create increased expectations that the health care system can or should provide solutions. In regard to technology, we "marvel at new drugs, devices and scientific research, and recognize the miracles they can produce. But these innovations are expensive, and third-party payers must help determine the proper distribution and financing of these technologies."[3] When the effects of these factors are considered, the dynamic nature of the health care system comes into focus.

RESOURCES IN THE HEALTH CARE SYSTEM

The U.S. health care system, ultimately devoted to the provision of health services, requires an enormous quantity and variety of resources, defined here as the basic "building blocks" of the system—money, people, physical plant, and technology.

Money

As already noted, the health care system requires total expenditures of over $600 billion annually and consumes about 12% of the GNP. Fig. 1-3 illustrates the trend of this growth in total expenditures while Fig. 1-4 illustrates the source of these funds and how they are currently distributed.[2] The majority of health expenditures are for provision of hospital care and physicians' services. These and other forms of personal health services are paid for in one of four basic ways:

1. Direct or "out-of-pocket" payment, in which individuals pay for their care directly from their own funds.
2. Private insurance, in which individuals or someone on their behalf, such as an employer, enters into a contractual arrangement with an insurer who agrees to pay for a specified set of services under specified conditions in return for premium payments; or in which a prepayment is made to a provider such as a health maintenance organization or an organization such as Blue Cross who then contracts with providers to provide services to subscribers.
3. Government programs, principally Medicare, in which the federal government pays for health care services provided to social security recipients over age 65, and Medicaid, in which federal funds are combined with state funds to pay for health care services received by welfare recipients and other people, as defined by state law, to be medically indigent. Payments under Medicare and Medicaid are made to providers of service on behalf of program beneficiaries.
4. Charitable contributions, endowment funds, or revenue generated by providers from other sources of income, such as hospital parking lots, although the amount of payment is decreasing.

All but the first of these mechanisms of payment are called "third-party payments" because the providers of

WHERE IT COMES FROM

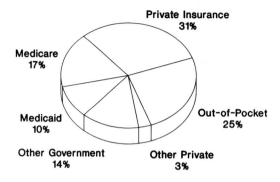

WHERE IT GOES

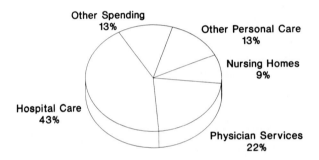

Fig. 1-4 The nation's health dollar: 1986. Almost three quarters of national health expenditures were channeled through third parties. Nearly two thirds were channeled through private hands. Bulk of that expenditure was for patient care, and remaining 12% was spent for research, construction, administration, and government public health activity. (Redrawn from Health Care Financing Review 8(4):3, 1987. Source: Health Care Financing Administration, Office of the Actuary. Data from the Division of National Cost Estimates.)

health care services receive payment from a source other than the individual who received the care. Although direct, out-of-pocket payment now accounts for approximately 25% of total health expenditures, all monies necessary to support the health care system, whether from direct payments, taxes, or job-related benefits, ultimately come from the public. The complex flow of funds for the payment for health care services in the U.S. is shown in Fig. 1-5.[4]

People

Another basic building block of the health care system is human resources. The U.S. Department of Labor lists more than 225 categories of workers employed primarily in the health care system, with a total of over 5 million employees. Approximately 1.6 million registered nurses,

over 1.2 million allied health personnel (including over 70,000 respiratory care practitioners), 560,000 licensed practical nurses, 534,000 active physicians, 160,000 pharmacists, and 143,000 dentists currently work in the U.S. health care system.[5]

Whereas in 1976 almost two thirds of all health personnel worked in hospitals, today only about 55% of the U.S. health care workforce is employed in this setting.[2] This trend toward employment of health professionals in alternative settings indicates a growing diversification of health services beyond the traditional boundaries of the acute care hospital.

Just as locales of employment are varied, so too are the settings in which health personnel are trained and educated. A large proportion of nurses and allied health professionals, including respiratory care personnel, undergo training in hospital-based programs or in the community college setting, whereas physicians and dentists are characteristically educated in universities or academic health centers.

Supplementing the entry and graduation requirements of these educational programs are extensive credentialing regulations designed to ensure the competence of health care workers. *Credentialing* refers to the recognition of individuals who have met certain predetermined standards attesting to their occupational skill or competence. There are two primary forms of credentialing in the health fields: licensure and certification.[6]

Licensure is the process whereby a government agency grants permission to an individual to practice a given occupation after verification that the applicant has demonstrated the minimum competency necessary to protect public health, safety, or welfare. Because licensure is one of the "police powers" delegated to the states, licensure laws are normally enacted by state legislatures and regulated by a specific state agency, such as a medical or nursing board. In states where licensure laws govern an occupation, practicing in that occupation without a license normally is considered a crime punishable by fines or even imprisonment. The exceptions to this rule are so-called "permissive" licensure regulations, which allow unlicensed individuals to maintain employment in particular occupations.

Certification is a voluntary process whereby a nongovernment or private agency or association grants recognition to an individual who has met certain predetermined qualifications, including graduation from an approved educational program, completion of a given amount of work experience, and acceptable performance on a qualifying examination or series of such examinations. The term *registration* is often used synonymously with certification but may simply imply an official listing of credentialed persons maintained by a private or public agency. As a voluntary process, certification standards can and often do exceed the minimum standards deemed necessary for entry-level competency. However, certification generally does

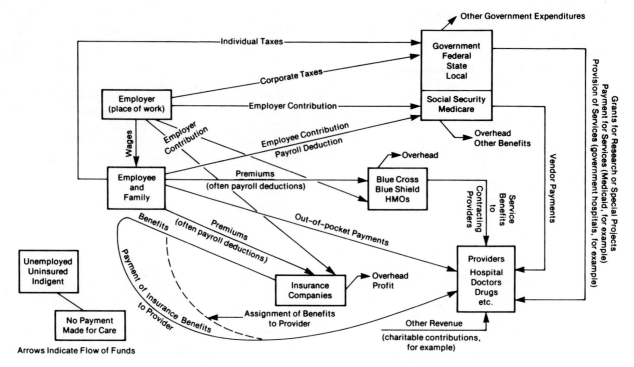

Fig. 1-5   Flow of funds for payment of health care services in the United States. (Redrawn from Wilson FA and Neuhauser D: Health services in the United States, 1974, Ballinger Publishing Co.)

not exclude others from working in that occupation, as do most forms of licensure.

Both credentialing mechanisms exist in respiratory care.[7] The primary mechanism of quality assurance operating in respiratory care is voluntary certification, as conducted by the National Board for Respiratory Care (NBRC). The NBRC is an independent national credentialing agency for individuals involved in the delivery of respiratory care and related services. The NBRC is collaboratively sponsored by the American Association for Respiratory Care (AARC), the American College of Chest Physicians (ACCP), the American Society of Anesthesiologists (ASA), the American Thoracic Society (ATS), and the National Society for Cardiopulmonary Technology (NSCPT). In combination, representatives from these organizations constitute the governing board of the NBRC, which assumes responsibility for all examination standards and policies through a standing committee structure.

The NBRC provides two levels of credentialing for respiratory care practitioners: the entry-level credential (Certified Respiratory Therapy Technician [CRTT]) and the advanced practitioner credential (Registered Respiratory Therapist [RRT]). As of 1987, there were approximately 43,000 CRTTs and 28,000 RRTs listed with the NBRC. In addition to certification and registration of respiratory therapy practitioners, the NBRC has recently developed a credentialing mechanism in the specialty of pulmonary function testing.

The NBRC also encourages continuing competency assurance of its certified and registered personnel through a voluntary program of recredentialing. Both CRTTs and RRTs can demonstrate ongoing professional competency by retaking examinations. Individuals passing these examinations are issued a certificate recognizing them as "recredentialed" practitioners.

Supplementing this private sector certification has been the recent development of state licensure laws to regulate the practice of respiratory care. As of 1988, approximately 20 states have developed licensure regulations for respiratory care, most of which are mandatory. Further discussion of licensure is provided in Chapter 12.

Ideally, certification and licensure ensure the availability of appropriate numbers of health care workers with acceptable levels of preparation. However, certification and licensure can restrict the supply of human resources for health care delivery and thus can increase the cost of this critical resource of the health care system.

Physical plant

Another building block of the health care system is the nation's investment in the "bricks and mortar" of physical facilities required to meet health care needs.

Approximately 6800 hospitals now operate in the U.S. health care system, with nearly 1.3 million beds. On any given day, about 880,000 people are patients in these facilities, and nearly 300 million outpatient visits occur annually.[8] Table 1-1 shows trends in hospitals, beds, and admissions for selected years. There is substantial variation in hospitals in terms of size, scope of service, ownership, and other characteristics.

Supplementing these hospital resources are approximately 20,000 nursing homes with nearly 2 million beds.[9] The federal government recognizes three categories of nursing homes based on the type of service they provide:

1. Skilled nursing facilities (SNF), which provide continuous nursing service on a 24-hour basis;
2. Intermediate care facilities (ICF); and
3. Residential facilities, commonly called rest homes.

During 1986, expenditures for nursing home care totaled $38 billion, or about 8% of the total spent on health care.[2]

Another major category of physical plant resources in the health care system includes facilities necessary for the office practices of the nation's physicians. Because a great deal of personal medical care is rendered in physicians' offices, these facilities represent a substantial investment in physical plant. Approximately 80% of physicians are engaged in direct care of patients as their primary activity. Of these, approximately 70% are engaged in office-based practices and 30% in hospital-based practices. Although the majority of office-based physicians are in solo practice (i.e., independent practice by a physician usually with individually owned facilities and equipment), many physicians are in group practices (three or more physicians formally organized to provide medical care, consultation, diagnosis, and/or treatment through the joint use of equipment and personnel and with income from the practice distributed in accordance with methods previously determined by members of the group). These groups may be organized as general practice, single specialty, or multispecialty groups.

Although all of the physical plant resources of the health care system are too numerous to mention here, some components worthy of mention include approximately 13,000 ambulance services and 2800 medical laboratories independent of those in physicians' offices and hospitals.

Technology

The technologic base of modern medicine is remarkable and must be viewed as one of the building blocks of the health care system, making organ transplants and microscopic surgery possible, eradicating many diseases, improving treatment for others, and making early diagnosis possible in many cases. These advances have had a marked effect on the health care system. Diseases that once were not even diagnosed are treated, societal expectations of the health care system have risen (often unrealistically) as technology has advanced, and the costs of health care have risen dramatically as expensive new technology has been adopted.

The paradox of technologic advance is that, even as people benefit from it (live longer), they need to use additional health services; the net effect is to drive up health care expenditures. This phenomenon becomes important, even critical, when there is limited money for these expenditures. The result is complex and frustrating. Indeed, "as technological advances continue, we will increasingly be confronted with difficult decisions related to coverage (payment for) new technology by insurers and the federal government. These decisions will become even more difficult as resources for health care become more limited, forcing trade-offs between providing primary health care services and providing new, potentially expensive but quality-enhancing technology."[10] Yet, this is precisely the problem that technology presents the health care system today. For this reason, decisions regarding the adoption of newly developed technologies increasingly will be viewed in terms of their relative cost compared to their projected benefits. This cost/benefit approach represents a new direction for the health care system.

It is clear that the health care delivery system requires vast sums of money, people with specialized training, an impressive investment in physical plant, and a growing technology. In the next section, we turn our attention to some of the organizations that these resources have been used to build and maintain and that, in turn, convert these resources into health services.

ORGANIZATIONS IN THE HEALTH CARE SYSTEM

Organizations within the health care system are its most visible component, with thousands of organizations giving form and substance to the system. The variety of these organizations defies easy categorization. Fig. 1-6, however, can serve as a starting point for description. The shortcomings of such a categorization become quickly apparent when it is considered, for example, that Blue Cross plans, which are essentially providers for a basic resource (payment for services rendered to its subscribers), sometimes require proof of the need for expansion of services, and Blue Cross plans typically have representatives on areawide planning boards. Such activities could qualify them

Table 1-1   Total U.S. Hospitals, Beds, and Admissions

Year	Number	Beds (000)	Admissions (000)
1950	6788	1456	18,483
1955	6956	1604	21,073
1960	6876	1658	25,027
1965	7123	1704	28,812
1970	7123	1616	31,759
1975	7156	1466	36,157
1980	6965	1365	38,892
1985	6872	1318	36,304
1986	6841	1290	35,219

Adapted from American Hospital Association: Hospital statistics data from the 1986 survey, Chicago, 1987, American Hospital Association.

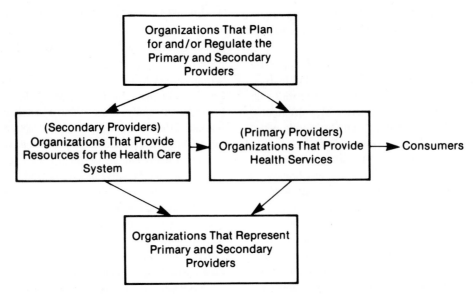

Fig. 1-6   Organizations in health care system.   (Redrawn from Longest BB Jr: Management practices for the health professional, ed 3, East Norwalk, Conn, 1984, Appleton & Lange.)

as planning and regulating organizations. Or consider the case of a hospital with the primary purpose of providing health care services but which also operates a school of nursing or is heavily involved in allied health education or a medical school that operates a hospital. It is not always easy to categorize organizations in the health care system.

Organizations that provide health services

Primary providers deliver health care services directly to consumers, whether the purpose of those services is curative, preventive, or rehabilitative. They include hospitals, nursing homes, physicians' offices, health maintenance organizations, home care programs, clinics, local health departments, and others.

Because most respiratory care practitioners work in a hospital setting, we will look at this type of institution first, followed by a short description of other primary providers where respiratory care services are used.

Hospitals. Hospitals are perhaps the most complex organization in the health care system. In general a hospital is "a health care institution with an organized medical and professional staff, and with permanent facilities that include inpatient beds, that provides medical, nursing, and other health related services to patients."[11]

There are two primary categories of hospitals: community and noncommunity.[8] *Community hospitals* include all nonfederal, short-term, general, and other special hospitals whose facilities and services are available to the public. *Noncommunity hospitals* include federal hospitals, long-term hospitals, hospital units of institutions, psychiatric hospitals, hospitals for tuberculosis and other respiratory diseases, chronic disease hospitals, institutions for the mentally retarded, and alcohol- and chemical-dependency hospitals.

Hospitals may be further categorized according to how they are controlled. The two primary types of hospital control are *governmental,* or publicly controlled, and *nongovernmental,* or privately controlled. Governmentally controlled hospitals may be further divided into those controlled by federal, state, or municipal governments. Likewise, nongovernmentally controlled hospitals may be organized as not-for-profit or investor-owned (for-profit) institutions.

The function of the general nongovernmental community hospital that serves the public has been described as follows[12]:

First, there are diagnostic and treatment services to inpatients. Within this broad function are many subdivisions of medical, surgical, obstetrical, pediatric, and other special forms of care. Psychiatric service and rehabilitation may be included. Involved in all of these inpatient services are various modalities, including nursing, dietetics, pharmaceutical skills, laboratory and x-ray services, and varying refinements of diagnosis and therapy. Second, there are services to outpatients, with an equally wide range of specialties and technical modalities. A third hospital function concerns professional and technical education, for many classes of health personnel must work in hospitals and thereby receive training. A fourth function is medical research, since the accumulation of patients in hospitals provides the basis for scientific investigation into the causes, diagnosis, and treatment of diseases. A fifth function concerns prevention of diseases or health promotion in the surrounding population; there are many ways that hospitals, as centers for technical skill, can offer services to people before they are sick or can protect patients from the hazards of disease beyond that for which they have come to the hospital.

The emphasis given to these functions will vary from hospital to hospital, depending largely on the basic objectives and goals of the hospital. For example, the large medical center may emphasize education and research to a much greater extent than the small, general hospital.

The hospital is a complex social system with substantial conflicts among the participants—patients, physicians, nurses, allied health professionals, trustees, administrative staff, and other personnel. The diversity of the organization can create major problems. More detail on the organizational structure of hospitals in general and of respiratory care services in particular is provided in Chapter 2.

Nursing homes. Since the enactment of the Social Security Act of 1935, which made public assistance funds available for the needy aged, the nursing home industry has flourished in the U.S. Several other factors have exacerbated the need for institutional care for the aged. Among them (and perhaps most important) are the increased numbers of people over age 65 in the population and the changes in the family structure.[13] For these reasons, expenditures for nursing home care are projected to be among the most rapidly expanding categories of health care costs, rising from their current level of some $38 billion to about $129 billion in the year 2000.[2]

The nursing home is an "institution with an organized professional staff and permanent facilities, including inpatient beds, that provides continuous nursing and other health-related, psychological, and personal services to patients who are not in an acute phase of illness but who primarily require continued care on an inpatient basis."[11]

The nursing home serves several basic health care functions, including the following[14]:

1. To provide continuing care for persons recovering from surgical or medical disorders;
2. To assist patients in reaching optimal physical and emotional health;
3. To provide for the total needs of patients—physical, emotional, and spiritual;
4. To assist the aging toward an active participation in life;
5. To provide for rehabilitative services when the need exists; and
6. To work cooperatively with other community and social agencies.

The typical organization pattern of the nursing home is similar to that given for the hospital; the main difference is that the nursing home offers a narrower range of services. A second major difference is the less complex medical staff organization in the nursing home, where medical staff are not as involved in day-to-day patient care.

Until recently, respiratory care practitioners had little involvement in the nursing home. However, with the increasing tendency for acute care hospitals to shorten patients' lengths of stay, many more individuals with severe, long-term illnesses are treated in nursing homes, particularly in those categorized as skilled nursing facilities. For this reason, respiratory care personnel are being called on more frequently to provide day-to-day patient care services in this setting.

Health maintenance organizations or HMOs. Although the hospital and the nursing home represent two of the most important traditional health service provider organizations, other types of organizations fit this category. Few subjects have aroused more interest or generated more discussion in the health care community during the past decade than health maintenance organizations, or as they are more commonly called, HMOs.

Over 700 HMO plans now operate in the U.S., with about 30 million subscribers. Projections indicate that HMO enrollment will top 48 million by 1992.[15]

There are five essential features of an HMO. Each single component or feature does not make the HMO special but, taken together, the five components make the HMO a unique form of health care delivery. An HMO is an organized system providing a comprehensive range of health care services to a voluntarily enrolled consumer population. In return for a prepaid, fixed fee, the enrollee is guaranteed a defined set of benefits. This fixed fee is usually the same for all members (enrollees) of the HMO regardless of the extent of services utilized. The prospective enrollee usually has a dual choice of joining either an HMO delivery system or another form of health insurance (e.g., Blue Cross/Blue Shield or commercial insurance policy). Enrollees join the HMO primarily on a year-to-year (contractual) basis and have the option of changing their choice once a year.[16]

Organizationally, there are four basic HMO models.[15] The *staff* model serves patients with mostly salaried physicians. The *independent practice association* (IPA) uses independent physicians who practice alone or in small, single-specialty groups. *Group* HMOs contract with independent, multispecialty physician group practices. These group practices, which are often physician partnerships, provide physicians to the HMO. *Network* HMOs contract for services with two or more large physician group practices. Currently, nearly two thirds of the nation's HMOs are organized under the IPA model, with a growing number of plans operating under multiple organizational designs.

In terms of ownership, just over half (52%) of the currently operating HMOs are owned and managed by private corporations. About one in four HMOs are owned by or affiliated with hospitals, with the remainder being independently owned and operated.[15] About two thirds of all HMOs are categorized as for-profit companies.

Although hospital-owned HMOs operate their own acute care facilities, it is more common for an HMO to contract with local hospitals to provide its inpatient services. In the former case a respiratory care practitioner would actually be an employee of the HMO whereas in the latter situation the practitioner would be considered an employee of the hospital. However, many HMOs operate their own clinic facilities or large group practices, in which some respiratory care personnel—especially those involved primarily in diagnostic testing—may be directly employed.

Home health care. Unlike the other primary provider organizations, home health care is more a concept than a discrete organizational structure. According to the *Discursive Dictionary of Health Care,* a document prepared for the Subcommittee on Health and Environment of the U.S. House of Representatives, home health care represents "the provision of health services rendered to an individual as needed in his/her home environment. Services are provided to aged, disabled, or sick or convalescent individuals who do not need institutional care."

Given this broad definition, it is not surprising that home health care currently is provided by a diverse group of organizations, including home health agencies, visiting nurse services, hospitals, outpatient facilities, durable medical equipment (DME) companies, charitable organizations, hospice groups, and other private organizations.

Although projections of total activity in this sector of health services are difficult to obtain, it is estimated that total expenditures for home health care range between $4 and $5 billion.[2] Between 1973 and 1984, expenditures for home health services increased annually by an average of about 31%. Recently, however, stricter federal regulations and reporting requirements have slowed this rapid annual growth rate to about 10%.

Although some aspects of home care are debatable with regard to efficacy, studies over the years have demonstrated that this type of health service can play an important role in improving a patient's quality of life, in increasing functional performance, and in reducing costs related to hospitalization.

Partly because of these important benefits, respiratory care is assuming a greater role as a component of home health services. The American Association for Respiratory Care (AARC) defines respiratory home care as "those specific forms of respiratory care provided in the patient's place of residence by personnel trained in respiratory therapy working under medical supervision."[17] Continuous oxygen therapy, long-term mechanical ventilation, and in-home continuation of planned pulmonary rehabilitation are among the key areas of respiratory care practitioner involvement in home care. More details regarding this relatively new organizational setting for respiratory care are provided in Chapter 35.

Organizations that provide resources for the health care system

Secondary providers include educational institutions, financing mechanisms, and drug and equipment suppliers, which furnish resources for the direct provision of health services.

Educational institutions. Medical and nursing schools are prominent examples of educational organizations supplying human resources to the health care system. After a brief review of medical and nursing education, we will de-

scribe educational programs that prepare personnel for entry into the field of respiratory care.

Medical education. Physicians receive their basic education in one of the nation's 126 medical schools or in a foreign medical school. Foreign medical graduates (FMGs) now represent about 20% of the total active physicians in the U.S.

Although there are variations in curriculum among U.S. medical schools, they generally provide 4 years of postbaccalaureate training, consisting of 2 years of preclinical or basic sciences work and 2 years of clinical and practical experience. After medical school a physician must pass a licensure examination, as set forth in each state's Medical Practice Act. Although this license permits the holder to practice medicine, physicians typically enter a period of postgraduate medical education called *residency.* Depending on the specialty chosen, this residency lasts from 2 to 7 years.

After specialty training a physician can apply for certification in that specialty by a specialty board. After meeting the requirements (which generally include completion of an approved residency, written and oral examination, and varying years of experience), the physician becomes a *board certified specialist.* For example, a board certified pulmonologist is a physician who has met the specialty requirements in this area, as prescribed by the American Board of Internal Medicine. Although licensure provides some minimal assurance of general medical competency, board certification indicates that the physician holds specialized knowledge and skills in a given area of practice.

Nursing education. Professionally licensed nurses, usually called registered nurses (RNs), are trained in three different types of organizational settings: (1) baccalaureate programs, which are 4- or 5-year university-based programs leading to a bachelor of science degree; (2) associate degree programs, which are 2-year programs usually based in junior or community colleges; and (3) diploma programs, which usually provide 3 years of training after high school and are based in hospital-operated schools of nursing. After completion of one of these approved programs, the nurse can become "registered" by passing a state licensure examination.

Nurses who desire to demonstrate competency beyond entry level may do so through specialty credentialing processes. For example, a certified critical care nurse (CCRN) has met the eligibility requirements and passed the certification examination in this specialty offered by the American Association of Critical Care Nurses.

Education in respiratory care. As in nursing, there is more than one route of entry into respiratory care. Two levels of educational preparation exist in this field: the *technician* or entry-level practitioner and the *therapist* or advanced level practitioner.[18]

Technician programs typically last 1 year and are sponsored primarily by postsecondary technical schools or 2-

year colleges. There are about 170 accredited technician programs in the U.S. In 1987 these programs graduated approximately 2600 entry level respiratory care practitioners.

There are approximately 260 accredited therapist programs in the U.S. These programs are sponsored mainly by 2-year colleges and typically lead to an associate degree. About 10% of the therapist programs are sponsored by 4-year colleges and universities and provide a baccalaureate degree on completion. In 1987 these therapist programs graduated almost 2700 advanced level respiratory care practitioners.

As with medical schools, the educational curriculum for respiratory care personnel typically consists of preclinical basic sciences coursework followed by or in combination with intensive classroom and laboratory study and clinical experience in the theory and application of respiratory care. Typically, basic sciences coursework and classroom and laboratory instruction are provided by the full-time faculty of the technical school or college, with the clinical experience occurring in hospitals affiliated with the sponsoring educational institution.[18] On completion of an accredited educational program of study, graduates are eligible for the applicable NBRC credentialing examination and, where pertinent, state licensure. More detail on the accreditation of educational programs in respiratory care is provided in a later section of this chapter.

Organizations that pay for care. A second important category of organizations providing resources for the health care system are those that pay for care. Except for "out-of-pocket" payments by individuals, health care in the U.S. is largely paid for through third parties. A maze of third parties has recently grown, largely in response to the rising cost of health care and the concurrent financial risk individuals run if they make no provision through insurance or prepayment for protection against potential health care costs. More than half of all third-party payments now comes from two sources—Blue Cross and the federal government (principally Medicare and Medicaid).

Blue Cross and Blue Shield. The Blue Cross organization began as a prepayment plan for hospital expenses for school teachers in Dallas, Texas, in 1929. The original plan provided 21 days of hospitalization for a prepayment of 50 cents a month. Blue Shield plans now provide for prepayment of physician fees in a similar manner. Today there are 77 Blue Cross and Blue Shield plans covering almost 78 million subscribers. These plans are members of the Blue Cross and Blue Shield Association.[19]

Medicare and Medicaid. On July 1, 1966, the federal government initiated two programs that had their bases in the 1965 amendments to the Social Security Act. These amendments (Title XVIII—Health Insurance for the Aged and Title XIX—Grants to the States for Medical Assistance Programs), more commonly known as Medicare and Medicaid, were the culmination of many years of national debate. Although substantial changes have been made in the Medicare and Medicaid programs in the intervening years, they were at their inception and still are insurance mechanisms to help pay for the health care needs of the elderly and the poor. Together, these programs account for nearly 40% of the revenues flowing into the nation's hospitals.

Medicare provides health care benefits to over 30 million aged and disabled enrollees and is the largest single purchaser of hospital and physician services in the country. The program consists of two parts: *Part A* is compulsory insurance for hospital care and related services for people over age 65; *Part B* is voluntary supplementary insurance to partially cover the costs of physician and surgeon fees, clinic visits, diagnostic and laboratory tests, and home health visits. Part A, constituting about two thirds of the total expenditures, is financed through Social Security payroll taxes. Part B, which accounts for the remaining outlay, is financed through premiums paid by enrollees and matching general revenues.

In 1983, under amendments to the Social Security Act, hospital reimbursement under Part A of the program underwent a dramatic change. Until that time, reimbursement to hospitals was based on the actual cost of providing services (cost-based reimbursement). Generally, under this original system, a hospital could expect to be reimbursed for what it spent on patient care.

The 1983 amendments switched the mechanism to a prospective payment system, based on diagnosis related groups (DRGs). A DRG is simply a predefined category of patient illness, as identified by the admitting diagnosis, nature of care (surgical versus nonsurgical), patient age, and presence or absence of complicating factors.

For each DRG, the Health Care Financing Administration (HCFA) of the U.S. Department of Health and Human Services has established a fixed rate of reimbursement. Because the DRG amount remains fixed for a given admitting diagnosis, hospitals that provide care for less than the fixed rate can keep the difference, thereby realizing a "profit." On the other hand, hospitals whose cost of care exceeds the fixed rate must absorb the cost difference, thereby taking a financial loss.[20]

By placing hospitals at risk financially, prospective reimbursement by DRGs has provided a powerful incentive for cost-efficiency in inpatient hospital services. Because the cost of a patient's care is directly related to the length of stay, most hospitals have focused their cost-containment efforts on minimizing the duration of inpatient care while simultaneously attempting to reduce or prevent "needless" admissions (i.e., cases that could be handled effectively on an ambulatory or outpatient basis). More details on the nature of this reimbursement system and its effect on the provision of respiratory care services are provided in Chapter 2.

Medicaid is a program through which the federal government provides a subsidy to the states, ranging from 50% to 85% of the total cost, to help provide health care to the poor. Each state administers its own Medicaid program under federal requirements. Certain basic services must be provided, including inpatient and outpatient hospital care, laboratory and x-ray services, skilled nursing services, home health care, physician services, and family planning services. Originally intended to provide medical services mainly to low-income women and children, Medicaid has evolved to be the largest third-party financier of long-term care in the U.S., with nearly a third of its total expenditures going to nursing home care.

Private insurance. Private insurance companies—often called "commercials"—represent another component of third-party payers. There are several hundred private insurance companies in the U.S., including Prudential, Equitable, Aetna, Metropolitan, and Connecticut General. These companies, through policies, provide "protection by written contract against the hazards (in whole or in part) of the happenings of specified fortuitous events."[21] Although private insurance companies were initially reluctant to enter the health insurance market, the market created by the large industrial unions that grew up during World War II provided sufficient stimulus for their entry, and by carefully experience-rating the various groups they serve, they have been successful.

Pharmaceutical and medical supply industries. A third category of resource-providing organizations is the pharmaceutical and medical supply industries. National expenditures for pharmaceutical and medical supplies represent nearly 10% of total health care costs, equivalent to about $40 billion in 1986.[2]

These high expenditures partly reflect research and development costs associated with the development of new drugs and medical equipment. With regard to pharmaceuticals in particular, these costs are large because of the complexity of the search for new, effective drugs and the nature of the process for obtaining approval from the Food and Drug Administration before a drug can be placed on the market.[22]

Organizations manufacturing and distributing medical supplies are as diverse as their products, which range from cotton balls to computerized axial tomography (CAT) scanners. There are over 1100 medical supply organizations in the U.S., ranging from large firms, such as the Baxter Healthcare Corp. (formerly the American Hospital Supply Corp.), to relatively small firms that specialize in a narrow range of products.

Until 1976, most medical devices, unlike prescription drugs, could be designed, marketed, and used in the U.S. without federal controls.[23] However, with implementation of the Medical Device Amendment Act of 1976, all medical devices fell under a comprehensive regulatory framework administered by the Food and Drug Administration.

ORGANIZATIONS THAT PLAN FOR OR REGULATE PRIMARY AND SECONDARY PROVIDERS

Although many components of the U.S. health care system are planned and regulated, no one entity plans for or regulates the system as a whole. A good deal of internal self-regulation and self-planning in health care organizations occurs, as when hospitals regulate their own performance through organizational policies and procedures. However, we shall look mainly at external regulation and planning (i.e., separate organizations that regulate the primary and secondary providers or plan for the provision of health services).

Voluntary regulating groups

Regulation of the components of the health care system has historically been on a voluntary basis. The voluntary regulatory process sets standards but does not carry the mandate of law. Voluntary regulating groups typically set standards for organizations such as health care agencies, educational institutions, or equipment manufacturers. We will briefly describe some key voluntary regulatory agencies affecting the delivery of respiratory care services.

Health care organizations. In terms of standard setting for health care organizations, the best example of a voluntary regulating group is the Joint Commission on Accreditation of Healthcare Organizations (JCAHO). The JCAHO, through established standards, accredits hospitals and nursing homes that voluntarily seek such accreditation, thus guiding and regulating operations of these providers. Originally developed in 1915 as an outgrowth of a project of the American College of Surgeons, JCAHO now has representation on its board from the American Medical Association, the American Hospital Association, the American College of Surgeons, the American College of Physicians, and, more recently, the American Association of Homes for the Aging and the American Nursing Home Association.

The JCAHO accrediting standards include requirements for health care organizations as a whole and each of their key service departments.[24] The importance of these standards as applied to respiratory care services is discussed in detail in Chapter 2.

Educational institutions. Voluntary regulation of organizations that educate health personnel is also extensive. As with health care organizations, this process is called *accreditation*. Educational accreditation represents the process whereby a private, nongovernment agency grants public recognition to an institution or specialized program of study meeting certain established educational standards.[25]

Programs for the education of respiratory care personnel are accredited by the Committee on Allied Health Education (CAHEA) in collaboration with the Joint Review Committee for Respiratory Therapy Education (JRCRTE).

CAHEA is a quasi-independent, broadly representative agency sponsored, in part, by the American Medical Association. In addition to respiratory care, CAHEA oversees the accreditation process for approximately 25 other allied health occupations through an umbrella review committee structure.[25]

The JRCRTE is responsible for assuring that respiratory therapy educational programs comply with the accrediting standards, or *Essentials,* adopted by the American Medical Association.[26] Representatives of the JRCRTE visit educational programs for respiratory care personnel to evaluate applications for accreditation and perform periodic reviews. In cooperation with CAHEA, the JRCRTE publishes an annual listing of accredited programs for the education of respiratory therapy technicians and respiratory therapists.

The JRCRTE is collaboratively sponsored by the American Association for Respiratory Care (AARC), the American College of Chest Physicians (ACCP), the American Society of Anesthesiologists (ASA), and the American Thoracic Society (ATS). Along with a public member, representatives from these organizations serve as members of the Committee, which, with the support of an executive office staff and many volunteer site visitors, assumes responsibility for reviewing accreditation applications, conducting on-site evaluations of programs, and making accreditation recommendations to CAHEA.[18]

Equipment manufacturers. Given the diversity of types of medical equipment, it is not surprising that voluntary regulation in this sector of the health care industry is not as well developed as that applicable to health care providers and educational institutions. The general lack of voluntary efforts in this area served as the basis for the Medical Device Amendment Act of 1976. Nonetheless, several key organizations are involved in voluntary efforts to establish standards related to medical devices and equipment. Among those of most importance to respiratory care are the Association for the Advancement of Medical Instrumentation (AAMI), the American National Standards Institute (ANSI), the National Committee for Clinical Laboratory Standards (NCCLS), and the Institute of Electrical and Electronic Engineers (IEEE).

Federal regulating efforts

Although the level of voluntary regulation in the health care system has been and continues to be extensive, government involvement in planning for and regulating the quality, cost, availability, and delivery of health care services in the U.S. has increased dramatically in the last 25 years, especially since enactment of the Medicare and Medicaid programs in the mid-1960s. In 1974, with the enactment of the National Health Planning and Resources Development Act (PL 93-641), government efforts to regulate the health care system reached their zenith.

This legislation created health systems agencies (HSAs),

which were intended to assume responsibility for health planning at the local level. Their responsibilities included forecasting demand and developing area-wide plans for services and facilities. In addition, PL 93-641 called for the establishment of state health planning and development agencies (SHPDAs), which were to develop statewide health plans. The single strongest element in this law was the requirement that all states enact certificate-of-need (CON) legislation that meets federal standards. This feature provided tighter regulation over high-cost capital expenditures for many existing health care providers and restricted duplication of expensive resources.

Although elements of this structure still exist, particularly the state health planning agencies and the CON requirements, the concept of the local HSA has generally failed. The general inability of HSAs to contain costs, the politicization of the process, and federal funding cutbacks have caused the failure of many of these local planning agencies.

More recently, the federal government has sought to decrease its regulation of the health care industry in hopes that increased competition among health care providers will help stem extraordinary increases in costs. This deregulation has been largely responsible for the increased number and diversity of health care providers in the health care system and the concomitant increase in the health care options available to the American public.

State regulating aspects

State government (and those aspects delegated to counties, cities, and towns) involvement in the health care system is made through a complexity of organizations and agencies that vary from state to state. Some of this involvement is focused in a department of public health but ranges from assurance of water quality to education of physicians in state-supported medical schools. State governments are also heavily involved in planning and regulating their health care systems. Regulatory involvement by the states includes licensing for many categories of health care workers and provider organizations and the establishment and enforcement of insurance laws and health and safety codes. A final and important example of state regulatory involvement is rate review, which already has been enacted in a number of states and is being seriously considered in others. Under these programs the rates charged by providers for health services are subject to review and approval by rate review agencies.

ORGANIZATIONS THAT REPRESENT PRIMARY AND SECONDARY PROVIDERS

Providers of health services or provider organizations are represented by associations that promote the interests of their members. These include national associations (e.g., the American Medical Association, the American

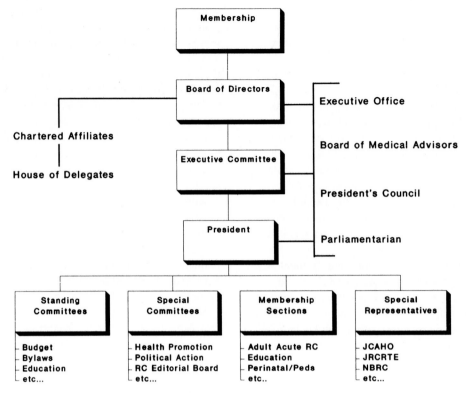

Fig. 1-7 Organizational chart of the American Association for Respiratory Care.

Hospital Association), state associations (e.g., the Illinois Hospital Association, the Kentucky Medical Association), and frequently local organizations (e.g., the Allegheny Medical Society, the Hospital Council of Western Pennsylvania).

The American Association for Respiratory Care (AARC) is an example of an organization representing individual professionals. With some 27,000 members nationwide, the AARC represents the profession of respiratory care. The AARC strives to facilitate cooperation between respiratory care personnel and the medical profession, hospitals, health care organizations, service companies, and government organizations. In addition, the AARC serves as a focal point for guidance and assistance to its members in the practice of respiratory care. This role is partly achieved through the provision of national and regional meetings and through periodical publications, which include the AARC official scientific journal, *Respiratory Care,* and the *AARC Times,* a monthly professional interest magazine. The AARC also acts as a center for communication with other health professions, institutions, and state and federal agencies.

As depicted in Fig. 1-7, the AARC functions under the direction of a voluntary board of directors elected by and accountable to the membership as a whole. An executive committee of the board, chaired by the president of the association, is responsible for overseeing the AARC central office, including its executive director. The executive director, in turn, oversees the day-to-day operations of the central office and its full-time staff. The AARC oversees medical affairs through its board of medical advisors (BOMA), a broadly representative group of physicians with expertise in the clinical, educational, or research aspects of pulmonary medicine.

According to its bylaws, decision making within the AARC occurs at two complementary levels. Major policy and budgetary decisions are normally made by the board of directors. Other elements of operation are under the control of the general membership, either by direct vote (as in the election of officers) or through the association's representative body, called the house of delegates. Representation in the AARC house of delegates is through affiliated state chapters of the association.

State chapters of the AARC share a purpose and structure similar to the national association, but limit their activities to respiratory care practitioners within their geographic locale. In some densely populated states, such as New York and California, the state society is broken into regional components, allowing better communication and coordination of services for local needs. In combination with the national AARC, these state affiliates provide a rich network of resources to promote and advance the practice of respiratory care.

CONSUMERS

Perhaps the largest and least organized component of the health care system is its consumers, who potentially include every person in the U.S.

Among the major problems facing consumers have been gaps in access to health care by certain segments of the population. Among the findings provided by two major national surveys conducted in the early 1980s were the following[27,28]:

- Some 28 million Americans had difficulty obtaining health care when they needed it, including:
  —1 in 4 poor people (9 million);
  —1 in 3 unemployed individuals (2.3 million);
  —1 in 5 Hispanics (2.6 million);
  —1 in 6 Blacks (2.5 million); and
  —1.5 million elderly.
- 6.5 million families included at least one member with a serious or chronic illness; of these families, about 1 in 4 reported that the chronic illness represented a "major" financial burden;
- Nearly 1 in 20 Americans who had a medical emergency had difficulty getting emergency care;
- Although 20% of adults believed the health care system worked "pretty well," nearly 1 in 3 believed the system "has so much wrong with it that we need to rebuild it completely."

In recent years these access problems have intensified, especially for some segments of society.[29] For example:

There are indications which suggest that obtaining necessary health care is becoming more difficult for the poor and uninsured. Several surveys have been funded by the Robert Wood Johnson Foundation in recent years to determine American satisfaction with and access to the health care system. Results of the 1986 survey indicate that 16 percent of the survey respondents (the equivalent of 38.8 million Americans) had difficulty obtaining needed health care. Over half of these reported that the reason for the difficulty was financial. The results also indicated that access to care (measured as the number of ambulatory visits during the prior 12 months) for the uninsured and the poor has declined since 1982. Despite their generally poorer health and greater likelihood of chronic disease or serious illness, between 1982 and 1986, the number of ambulatory visits for poor adults (ages 17 to 64) declined 30 percent. In addition, the number of ambulatory visits for the poor in fair or poor health declined almost eight percent between 1982 and 1986 (from 9.1 to 8.4 visits). In comparison, the number of visits for the nonpoor in fair or poor health increased 42 percent during the same period (from 9.1 visits to 11.5 visits). Differences between the uninsured and the insured in fair to poor health are also striking. In 1986, the uninsured in fair to poor health had only six visits annually, compared to 10 visits for the insured.[10]

Despite these trends, consumers tend to be satisfied with the quality of health care they personally receive. Indeed, over three fourths of Americans express satisfaction with

their personal health services. At the same time, there is a growing dissatisfaction with waiting time to see a physician and the amount of information provided in interactions with health care professionals. In addition, 70% of Americans believe that health care costs are going up too fast and are dissatisfied with this trend.[30] Moreover, the demand for a larger voice in decision making in the health care system—a phenomenon called consumerism—has never been stronger.

Perhaps the most obvious reason for the lack of active participation in health care decision making by consumers is the difficulty faced when relating to large, complex systems. For example, what effect does an individual have on the banking industry? Although critical questions remain about the knowledge and relative persuasive strength of consumers, few seriously question that the consumer, who directly or indirectly pays for the services provided by the health care system, is any longer willing to leave the decision-making power entirely in the hands of others.

PROBLEMS CONFRONTING THE HEALTH CARE SYSTEM

The health care system faces an array of problems, the more complex of which are not transitory and will not be solved soon or easily. Full enumeration of the set of problems is impossible because the list developed by one individual or group will differ frequently in content and almost always in priority from those developed by someone else.

One of the most encouraging signs of resolution is the considerable time and money devoted to identifying the system's problems and developing viable solutions. For example, one of the most comprehensive examinations of problems confronting the health care system today has come from a symposium of leading experts convened by the American Hospital Association with support from the National Center for Health Services Research. A book reporting the deliberations of this symposium and summarizing its results listed the following problems facing the U.S. health care system[31]:

1. Cost. How should society establish means for determining limits on the quantity of resources to be expended on health care services?
2. Entitlement. How should society establish a guaranteed minimum set of health care services available for all citizens?
3. Technology. How should society establish methods for evaluating the development and use of new medical technologies?
4. Decision making. How should society achieve better decision-making capabilities by individuals who are not providers of health care services in matters concerning the appropriate allocation, distribution, and use of these services?

5. Structure. How should society exert substantial pressures for the reorganization and restructuring of the health care, education, financing, and delivery system to make it more efficient, effective, and economical?

More recently, 172 organizations with varying perspectives on the problems confronting the health care system collaborated in developing a framework to address them. Called "The Health Policy Agenda for the American People," this consensus report includes 195 specific recommendations addressing such problems as[3]:

- The growing cost of health care in the U.S.;
- Inequities in access to needed health care among the population;
- The ethical and moral consequences raised by new technologies; and
- The lack of information needed by consumers to make informed choices among the many options in health care.

Concerns about cost reflect the staggering level of total health care expenditures and the continuing steep increases in these expenditures. However, the other problems also are important and demonstrate the complexity, breadth, and interrelatedness of problems facing the health care system. They will probably be solved in the future because they are so important, but, as solutions emerge, we can be sure that other equally difficult and important problems will replace them. This is the price of society's effort to achieve a goal so important and so elusive as "complete physical, mental, and social well-being."

SUMMARY

Respiratory care is part of a large and dynamic health care system. Within this system the respiratory care professional serves an essential role as a provider of health care services. Effectively fulfilling this role demands knowledge of the key structural and operational elements involved in the delivery of these services. Moreover, by understanding the complexity, breadth, and interrelatedness of these components, the practitioner can make a significant contribution toward solving the problems characterizing health care delivery in the U.S.

REFERENCES

1. Blum HL: Planning for health: generics for the eighties, ed 2, New York, 1981, Human Sciences Press, Inc.
2. Division of National Cost Estimates, Office of the Actuary, Health Care Financing Administration: National health expenditures, 1986-2000, Health Care Financing Rev 8(4):1-36, 1987.
3. Hirt EJ, editor: The health policy agenda for the American people: reference report, Chicago, 1987, The Health Policy Agenda for the American People.
4. Wilson FA and Neuhauser D: Health services in the United States, ed 2, Cambridge, Mass, 1982, Ballinger Publishing Co.
5. U.S. Department of Health and Human Services, Public Health Service, Health Resources and Services Administration: Report to Congress on the status of health personnel in the United States, DHHS Publication No. HRS-P-OD 84-4, Washington, DC, 1984, U.S. Department of Health and Human Services.
6. U.S. Department of Health, Education, and Welfare: Report on licensure and related health professional credentialing, HMS Publication No. 72-11, Washington, DC, 1971, U.S. Department of Health, Education, and Welfare.
7. Mishoe SC: Current and future credentialing in respiratory therapy, Respir Care 25:345, 1980.
8. American Hospital Association: Hospital statistics: data from the 1986 annual survey, Chicago, 1987, American Hospital Association.
9. American Health Care Association: Facts in brief on long term health care, Washington, DC, 1984, American Health Care Association.
10. Rubin RJ et al: Critical condition: America's health care in jeopardy, Washington, DC, 1988, Lewin.
11. American Hospital Association: Hospital administration terminology, Chicago, 1982, American Hospital Association.
12. Roemer MI and Friedman JW: Doctors in hospitals, Baltimore, 1971, The Johns Hopkins University Press.
13. Harrington C et al: Long-term care of the elderly: public policy issues, Beverly Hills, Calif, 1985, Sage Publications, Inc.
14. McQuillan FL: Fundamentals of nursing home administration, ed 2, Philadelphia, 1974, WB Saunders Co.
15. Donald E.L. Johnson and Associates: Marion managed care digest, HMO edition, Kansas City, Mo, 1988, Marion Laboratories, Inc.
16. U.S. Department of Health and Human Services: A student's guide to health maintenance organizations, Washington, DC, 1978, U.S. Department of Health and Human Services.
17. American Association for Respiratory Care: Standards for respiratory therapy home care: an official statement by the American Association for Respiratory Care, Respir Care 24:1080-1082, 1979.
18. DeKornfeld TJ and Scanlan CL: Education of respiratory care personnel. In Burton GG and Hodgkin JE, editors: Respiratory care: a guide to clinical practice, ed 2, Philadelphia, 1984, JB Lippincott Co.
19. Blue Cross and Blue Shield Association, Office of Communications, Chicago, Personal communication, 1988.
20. Scanlan CL: The prospective payment system: what you see is what you get, Pulmon Med Tech 1(5):19-34, 1984.
21. Health Insurance Institute: Source book of health insurance data, New York, 1988, Health Insurance Institute.
22. Goddard JL: The medical business, Scientific American, September 1973, pp. 161-166.
23. Goodwin GG: Governmental regulation of medical devices, Respir Care 33:251-257, 1988.
24. Joint Commission on Accreditation of Healthcare Organizations: Accreditation manual for hospitals, Chicago, 1988, Joint Commission on Accreditation of Healthcare Organizations.
25. American Medical Association: Allied health education directory, Chicago, 1988, American Medical Association.
26. Joint Review Committee for Respiratory Therapy Education: Essentials and guidelines of an accredited educational program for the respiratory therapy technician and respiratory therapist, Euless, Texas, 1986, Joint Review Committee for Respiratory Therapy Education.
27. Aday L, Andersen R, and Fleming GV: Health care in the US: equitable for whom? Beverly Hills, Calif, 1980, Sage Publications.
28. Center for Health Administration Studies, University of Chicago: Updated report on access to health care for the American people, Princeton, NJ, 1983, The Robert Wood Johnson Foundation.
29. The Robert Wood Johnson Foundation: Access to health care in the United States: results of a 1986 survey, Princeton, NJ, 1987, The Robert Wood Johnson Foundation.
30. Health Insurance Association of America: Health and health insurance: the public's view, Washington, DC, 1983, Health Insurance Association of America.
31. Phillips DF: The public policy issues facing hospitals in the 1980's. In Hospitals in the 1980's, Chicago, 1977, American Hospital Association.

2

Modern Respiratory Care Services

Patrick M. McDonald

The modern respiratory care service is a challenging and dynamic place in which to work. Technologic advances in the medical field have created an ever-changing environment, with significant and rewarding opportunities for respiratory care practitioners nationwide. Despite advancements in technology, one aspect of respiratory care remains unchanged—total commitment to the quality of patient care, to the profession, and to the service department. Advancements in technology cannot replace the dedicated, committed professional.

This chapter introduces the structure and function of the respiratory care practitioner's work unit. While by no means covering respiratory care services in detail, those common and essential to all are discussed.

Over the past several years, hospitals have faced an increasing load of patients with cardiopulmonary diseases. Technologic and educational advances continue to improve the quality of care rendered. The techniques that have evolved for the treatment of these patients require supervision of highly educated and skilled professionals whose degree of specialization is beyond the scope of the average attending physician or nurse. In response to this need, the technical specialty of respiratory care emerged within the hospital.

Historically, the predecessor of respiratory care was the hospital oxygen service. However, its highly specialized successor bears little resemblance to these beginnings. Today, respiratory care practitioners undergo intensive, medically supervised education and training, enabling them to provide skills and service of a very complex and sophisticated nature. The importance of the role played by respiratory care personnel in quality and cost-efficient care is evident in the use of these services. It is not unusual for a respiratory care service in a busy hospital to provide some form of therapy to 25% or more of all patients admitted.

OBJECTIVES

Although recent changes in health care delivery have created alternative organizational structures in which respiratory care personnel deliver vital services, the acute care setting still provides the primary foundation for service provision and is usually the point of entry for newly trained professionals. The purpose of this chapter is to introduce the reader to the organization and delivery of respiratory care services in the acute care setting.

On completion of this chapter, the reader will be able to:

1 Describe the general standards for organizing, staffing, and delivering hospital-based respiratory care services;

2 Delineate the scope of services and service coverage provided by a typical comprehensive, hospital-based respiratory care service;

3 Define the relationship of the respiratory care service to the overall administrative and medical organizational structure of a typical hospital;

4 Compare and contrast the roles and functions of key personnel constituting a respiratory care service;

5 Describe the importance of written policies and procedures in the operation of a respiratory care service;

6 Relate patient care priorities to personnel scheduling and work assignments in a respiratory care service;

7 Identify the mechanism by which personnel and material resource needs for a respiratory care service are determined; and

8 Define the goals and outline the major procedures underlying a respiratory care service quality assurance program.

KEY TERMS

Most terms used in this chapter are defined in context. The following terms are introduced without explicit definition but may be found in the text glossary:

AARC	JRCRTE
accreditation	liability
anesthesiology	MDC
biomedical instrumentation	morbidity
	mortality
CAHEA	NBRC
continuing education	neonatal
contraindication	obstetrics
CPFT	pediatrics
CRTT	preventative maintenance
disinfection	recycle
DRG	rehabilitation
echocardiography	RPFT
electrocardiography	RRT
gynecology	sterilization
hemodynamic monitoring	triage
in-service education	
JCAHO	

STANDARDS FOR RESPIRATORY CARE SERVICES

Respiratory care services are a vital component of comprehensive hospitalized care. Like other hospital operations, high standards apply to the operation of these services. Such standards provide a basis for organizing, staffing, and delivering quality and cost-efficient respiratory care that meets the needs of patients and medical and health-related professional staffs.

Each hospital establishes its own expectations about the scope of respiratory care services. However, minimum basic standards that apply to all hospitals are provided by the Joint Commission on the Accreditation of Healthcare Organizations (JCAHO).* The six general JCAHO standards that apply to respiratory care services are outlined in the box opposite. For each general standard, the JCAHO provides several "required characteristics" that define in more detail the minimum basic expectations necessary for quality respiratory care services.

The standards address the scope, organization, and direction of services; the preparation of respiratory care providers; the policies and procedures underlying departmental operations; necessary facilities and equipment; the initiation and documentation of services; and mechanisms for quality assurance. These key areas provide the organizational focus for the remainder of this chapter, which provides an overview of modern respiratory care services.

*Formerly the Joint Commission on Accreditation of Hospitals (JCAH).

SCOPE AND ORGANIZATION OF RESPIRATORY CARE SERVICES

Scope of services

The key services provided by a modern respiratory care department in a comprehensive acute care hospital are outlined in the box on p. 21. The remaining sections of this book provide detailed analyses of the scientific and clinical bases for these services. As is typical of a centralized, multipurpose department, these services often cut across established medical and administrative lines. This flexible approach to service organization and delivery is based on the fact that patients in need of respiratory care can span all age groups and diagnoses. The administrative implications of this organizational approach will be discussed later.

The listing of typical services in the box is neither static nor all-inclusive. Traditionally, the boundaries of respiratory care services have been flexible and responsive to changing needs and demands. Moreover, substantial variations in the number and type of services offered exist between hospitals. Indeed, in some hospitals, efforts to contain the ever-rising costs of hospitalized care have resulted in the clustering of once separate departments into a single administrative structure, often called "cardiopulmonary services." In addition to traditional respiratory therapy, a

---

JCAHO MAJOR STANDARDS FOR RESPIRATORY CARE SERVICES

1. Respiratory care services that meet the needs of patients, as determined by the medical staff, are available at all times; are well organized, properly directed, and appropriately integrated with other units and departments of the hospital; and are staffed in a manner commensurate with the scope of services offered.
2. Personnel are prepared for their responsibilities in the provision of respiratory care services through appropriate training and education programs.
3. Respiratory care services are guided by written policies and procedures.
4. The respiratory care department/service has equipment and facilities to assure the safe, effective, and timely provision of respiratory care services to patients.
5. Respiratory care services are provided to patients in accordance with a written prescription by the physician responsible for the patient and are documented in the patient's medical record.
6. As part of the hospital's quality assurance program, the quality and appropriateness of patient care provided by the respiratory care department/service are monitored and evaluated, and identified problems are resolved.

Joint Commission on Accreditation of Healthcare Organizations: Accreditation manual for hospitals, Chicago, 1988, Joint Commission on Accreditation of Healthcare Organizations.

TYPICAL SERVICES OFFERED BY A COMPREHENSIVE RESPIRATORY CARE DEPARTMENT

GENERAL THERAPEUTIC SERVICES

Therapeutic gas administration
Aerosols and humidity therapy
Inspiratory positive pressure breathing (IPPB)
Hyperinflation therapy (incentive spirometry)
Pulmonary physical therapy
Airway care

CRITICAL CARE SERVICES (ADULT, PEDIATRIC AND NEONATAL)

Mechanical ventilation
Continuous positive airway pressure (CPAP)
Physiologic and hemodynamic monitoring

PULMONARY REHABILITATION AND HOME CARE

Home care discharge planning and follow-up
Outpatient pulmonary rehabilitation
    Patient instruction
    Follow-up supervision

DIAGNOSTIC SERVICES

Pulmonary function testing
Arterial blood gas analysis
Pulmonary exercise testing
Sleep studies
Metabolic studies
Diagnostic bronchoscopy
Sputum induction

EMERGENCY SERVICES

Cardiopulmonary resuscitation
Endotracheal intubation
Patient transport

EDUCATIONAL SERVICES

Patient and family education
In-service education (staff, physicians, nurses, etc.)
Student clinical education (educational affiliation)
Community education

SUPPORT SERVICES

Equipment cleaning, disinfection, and sterilization
Biomedical equipment quality control and preventative
    maintenance

---

comprehensive cardiopulmonary service may provide therapeutic and diagnostic support in areas such as electrocardiography, echocardiography, cardiovascular catheterization, pulmonary function and stress testing, sleep disorders, and hemodynamic monitoring.

The rapidly changing face of health care delivery has resulted in many respiratory care services also engaging in more nontraditional services, including home care, outpatient rehabilitation, and health education. These new horizons in respiratory care are described in detail in the last section of this book.

Regardless of the scope of service provision, it is essential that all respiratory care departments are operated under a philosophy of flexibility and cooperation with other members of the health care team. Only in this manner can respiratory care effectively meet the needs and expectations of patients and providers.

Service coverage

Therapeutic services. Local hospital needs and available personnel are the determining factors in time coverage and scope of therapeutic services. Ideally, therapeutic services should be available at all times. Most routine therapeutic services are provided during the day and evening shifts. Nights and weekend coverage is usually less extensive, with priority given to critical and emergency care.

For this reason, attending physicians ideally should order therapy in advance so it can be scheduled at the start of each working day. Nonetheless, flexible staff scheduling and assignments must assure that emergency situations can always be accommodated, even under the heaviest workload.

Diagnostic services. Pulmonary function and blood gas evaluation facilities should be available where respiratory care is used to its maximum potential. Data obtained from these diagnostic services has become an important tool in determining the need for and appropriate use of therapeutic respiratory care modalities.

This is especially true where patients are maintained on mechanical ventilation. In such circumstances, it is mandatory that the physiologic status be monitored by frequent examination of blood for pH, carbon dioxide tension, and oxygenation. The experienced respiratory care practitioner uses these data with other criteria to adjust the ventilators. Because patients in ventilatory failure need close supervision at all times, facilities for blood gas monitoring must be available at all hours. The ease with which this can be accomplished is determined by available laboratory facilities and personnel. Ideally, the blood gas laboratory should provide continuous service. On the other hand, pulmonary function services, mainly elective in nature, generally need not be provided around the clock.

Administrative organization and personnel

A large, comprehensive respiratory care service normally includes some or all of the following personnel: medical director, technical director or manager, assistant technical director, shift supervisors, area supervisors, staff respiratory therapists and technicians, pulmonary function laboratory technicians, in-service and clinical instructors, equipment technicians, and clerical staff. In addition, some departments may have electrocardiographic and echocardiographic personnel, pulmonary rehabilitation and home care coordinators, and hemodynamic monitoring technicians. In teaching hospitals, some practitioners may also be involved in clinical research activities. The number and variety of these personnel will vary according to the size of the hospital and its scope of services.

Organizational structure. Effective coordination of the activities of these personnel requires some form of organizational structure. Fig. 2-1 shows an organizational chart of a typical respiratory care service department operating in a medium-to-large comprehensive acute care hospital that is privately owned.

Typically, overall policy-making responsibility is vested in a governing board of directors. Under the board of directors, and also typical of most hospitals, is a dual administrative and medical structure.

The administrative side of the institution is organized bureaucratically and oversees the traditional management functions of planning, supervising, controlling, and budgeting. The director of the respiratory care service typically reports to a higher administrative official, such as a vice-president, who is responsible for several related ancillary service areas.

The medical staff structure is more collegial in nature, is typically organized into specialty departments such as surgery, medicine, pediatrics, and obstetrics and gynecology, and is governed by an executive board or committee. The medical staff provides policy and administrative supervision over matters directly related to health care service provision. Under this side of the organizational structure, the respiratory care department is typically responsible to a medical director of the service. Details on the critical role of the medical director in the supervision of respiratory care services are provided in the following section.

In this particular organizational scheme, the departmental services are further divided into three major operational areas: clinical or therapeutic specialties, diagnostic services, and educational support. Variations in this structure are common and again depend on the size and scope of services offered.

Ideally, a respiratory care service department should be an independent administrative unit with a defined budget and managerial support stemming from the hospital administration. Thus, in administrative and fiscal matters, the director of the department works directly with the hospital administration.

The education services component of the department is particularly important in hospitals holding affiliations with respiratory therapy educational programs. Even in the absence of such a relationship, ongoing in-service education and training usually demand at least part-time supervision of the educational activities of the department. In-service and continuing education are essential elements of any progressive respiratory care department. Such in-service education normally extends beyond the bounds of the de-

partment staff and includes nurses, residents, and other professionals involved in respiratory care.

A medium-to-small community hospital will be primarily interested in the therapeutic and diagnostic functions of their respiratory care departments. A small hospital may be adequately served by a single medical director supervising both a service function and a modest pulmonary function laboratory.

In a respiratory care department where there is a larger demand, there may be an effective division of labor with two or more associate medical directors. Here the duties may be divided, with one director responsible for service functions, another for the laboratory, and perhaps another for critical care and clinical research projects.

In the largest hospitals, where the work load may be exceptionally heavy, administrative and professional relationships may be even more decentralized. In some instances it is practical to consider the service function of the respiratory care department, the pulmonary function laboratory, the training and educational facilities in respiratory care, and the respiratory rehabilitation program as components of a larger professional unit. Such a facility might have an overall administrative director, with the subdivisions of the department having their own section heads. In such a large and complex structure, ongoing professional cooperation and communication with physicians is necessary to ensure the highest quality and continuity of patient care.

Classification of personnel. Most hospital respiratory care services use officially recognized categories of personnel in the development of job titles and the assignment of clinical responsibilities. The current definitions operable in the field of respiratory care are provided in the box on p. 24.

Based on this classification, two major therapeutic personnel levels exist: the respiratory therapist and the respiratory therapy technician. Based on factors such as local institutional needs, geographic area, and personnel availability, the duties of the therapist and technician often overlap. However, differences in depth and scope of training, often lead respiratory therapists to assume responsibilities for supervision and management (particularly in specialty or critical care areas), patient assessment and respiratory care planning, clinical and in-service education, special projects and research, and physiologic monitoring. Respiratory therapy technicians, on the other hand, are more often responsible for general bedside respiratory care, while providing essential support in critical care and specialized diagnostic areas.

The functional relationship between therapist and technician is summarized in Table 2-1. Obviously, this format cannot and should not be applied dogmatically, for the job belongs to those who do it best. Also, education and experience are not the sole indicators of who shall be assigned therapist or technician duties; technical performance, atti-

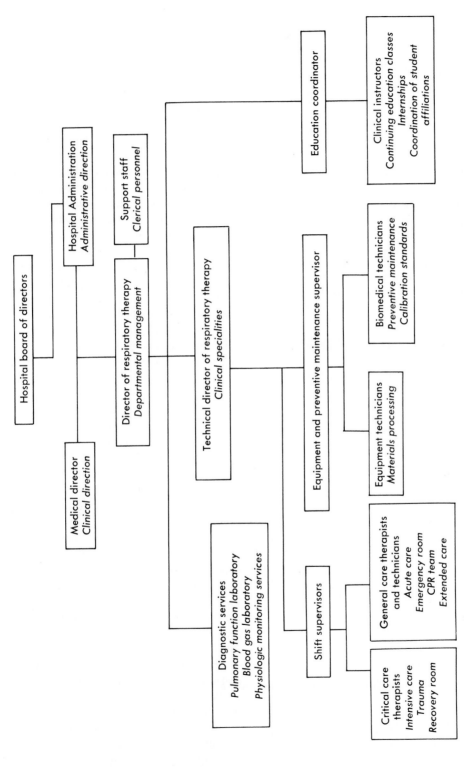

Fig. 2-1 Organizational outline for respiratory therapy service. (Modified from forms used by Donald N. Sharp Memorial Community Hospital, San Diego, Calif.)

CLASSIFICATION OF RESPIRATORY CARE PERSONNEL

RESPIRATORY THERAPIST

A graduate of a school accredited by the American Medical Association's Committee on Allied Health Education and Accreditation (CAHEA), in cooperation with the Joint Review Committee for Respiratory Therapy Education (JRCRTE) designed to qualify the graduate for the registry examination of the National Board for Respiratory Care (NBRC). Usually this means a 2- to 4-year college-based program, granting an associate or bachelor degree.

REGISTERED RESPIRATORY THERAPIST (RRT)

A respiratory therapist who has successfully completed the registry (therapist) examination of the NBRC.

RESPIRATORY THERAPY TECHNICIAN

A graduate of a CAHEA/JRCRTE approved school designed to qualify the graduate for the technician (entry-level) certification examination of the NBRC. Usually, this means a 1-year program combining a special curriculum of basic sciences with supervised clinical experience.

CERTIFIED RESPIRATORY THERAPY TECHNICIAN (CRTT)

A respiratory therapy technician who has successfully completed the technician (entry-level) certification examination of the NBRC.

CERTIFIED PULMONARY FUNCTION TECHNICIAN (CPFT)

An individual, qualified by education and/or experience, who has successfully completed the pulmonary function certification examination of the NBRC.

REGISTERED PULMONARY FUNCTION TECHNOLOGIST (RPFT)

An individual, qualified by education and/or experience, and previously certified in pulmonary function technology, who has successfully completed the pulmonary function registry examination of the NBRC.

RESPIRATORY THERAPY ASSISTANT

One who has received on-the-job training as part of employment in a respiratory care service. For such a program, there are no official guidelines or credentials. On-the-job training is being phased out in favor of one of the two formal therapist or technician programs.

RESPIRATORY THERAPY STUDENT

One who is enrolled in a program accredited by CAHEA/JRCRTE.

tude, and commitment to the profession are far more important than the label one carries after graduation.

Recognizing the differences and similarities among respiratory care personnel as well as trends in terminology, we will use the term "respiratory care practitioner" to refer to anyone involved in the provision of respiratory care services.

Key roles and functions. Based on the previous descriptions of departmental structure and formal personnel classifications, we will provide a general overview of the roles and functions of the key personnel normally involved in the provision of respiratory care services. The intent here is not to delineate job descriptions but rather to give the reader an indication of the important aspects of these roles. For the respiratory therapy student, these descriptions should help to clarify functional responsibilities within an affiliated service department and also demonstrate the opportunities for upward and lateral job mobility within the field.

Medical director. The quality and strength of a respiratory care service depends first on the commitment to active medical direction and leadership. The medical director must be a member of the medical staff who is interested in chest diseases and who has had extensive training and clinical experience in this area.

From a practical point of view, only two major departments lend themselves to affiliation with respiratory care—pulmonary medicine and anesthesiology. Historically, many departments of respiratory care have been organized under the direction of anesthesiologists for two primary reasons: (1) the common foundation of pulmonary physiology and technical nature of the duties underlying both anesthesiology and respiratory care and (2) the presence of anesthesiologists in the hospital for extended periods of time.

Anesthesiologists may be justly credited with much of the early development of respiratory care. The evolution of respiratory care, however, has evoked some subtle changes in its function that affect its relationship to anesthesiology. Whereas the respiratory care practitioner in the early days of the technology performed relatively simple tasks, under the direct guidance of the medical director, the contemporary practitioner is permitted a significant degree of independence in judgment and plays an important role in patient care and assessment.

Respiratory care, as it is now practiced, is primarily directed toward the diagnosis and treatment of diseases and medical complications of surgery or trauma. To realize their full potential, respiratory care practitioners must be well rounded in many aspects of clinical medicine. It is not sufficient for practitioners to be skilled merely in specific tasks, but they must understand cardiopulmonary physiology as well as changes in physiologic conditions caused by disease. Such a view implies a clinical and medical orientation in the teaching and direction of respiratory care, most realistically provided by a pulmonary physician trained in the physiologic and clinical aspects of chest diseases. Ideally, then, the department's medical direction would be provided by a pulmonary physician, with input welcome from the anesthesiology service.

Whether the designated hours are full or part time, being a medical director for a respiratory care service is a full-time responsibility. The medical director must be reasonably available for consultation and advice for the safe and effective supervision of the department, both to other physicians and to the respiratory care staff, on a 24-hour basis.

Unfortunately, there is still a shortage of clinicians able or willing to undertake the medical direction of a respiratory care department. However, greater emphasis on postgraduate training in chest disease provides hope for an improved supply in the future.

Although the choice of a medical director depends on available personnel and the objectives of respiratory care in the hospital, a general recommendation can be made. If the treatment of cardiopulmonary disease in a hospital is completely managed by each attending physician and respiratory personnel provide only a skilled technical service of limited scope, the supervision and quality control of such services can be performed by an anesthesiologist or an internist. If, however, respiratory care is to provide state-of-the-art capabilities, integrating diagnostic laboratory facilities, professional consultation, referral services, and outpatient and rehabilitation care, a clinically trained pulmonary physician is preferred as medical director.

The medical director of the respiratory care department is professionally responsible for the clinical function of the department. Because of this responsibility, the medical director should have considerable authority in establishing the professional policies and practices of respiratory care in the hospital. Of course, any major policy involving patient care or the relationships between the department and staff physicians must be approved by the hospital's executive medical board.

The major responsibilities of the medical director include the following: medical supervision of patients with respiratory diseases (including consultation and referral), general medical and respiratory intensive care, ambulatory care (including rehabilitation), pulmonary function evaluation, development and approval of departmental clinical policies and procedures, medical direction of respiratory care in-service training and education programs, education of medical and nursing staffs in pulmonary physiology and pathophysiology, input into the selection and promotion of technical staff, and input into the preparation of the departmental budget. The medical director's involvement in personnel and budgetary matters, while by no means extensive, provides the integration of medical and administrative thinking necessary within the hospital's dual organizational structure.

A challenge to the medical and technical leadership of respiratory care services is provision of an increasingly better quality of patient service at lower cost. This is the current philosophy of cost containment and cost-effectiveness. The need for administrative education for medical directors has long been recognized by those active in this work, but it has been given significant exposure only recently. Physicians who contemplate assuming medical directorships of respiratory care services must be willing and

Table 2-1 Functions of Respiratory Therapists and Respiratory Therapy Technicians

Therapist	Technician	Therapist	Technician
Management and supervision		Resuscitation, emergency	X
Diagnostic procedures		Teaching	
Arterial blood collection	X	Clinical	X
Blood gas analysis		Curriculum development	
Lung volume measurements		Special procedures	
Compliance studies		Therapy	
Spirometry, bedside	X	Aerosol/humidity	X⁄
Spirometry, laboratory		Gas	X
Equipment		Positive pressure breathing	X
Evaluation		Ventilation, mechanical	
Maintenance	X	Initiate	
Modification		Maintain	X
Chest physiotherapy		Patient assessment	
Breathing exercise	X	Therapeutic objectives of care	
Postural drainage	X	Fiberoptic bronchoscopy assistance	
Pulmonary rehabilitation		Critical care	
		Clinical research	

Modified from Egan DF: What is inhalation therapy? Clin Notes Respir Dis 11:3, 1972.

ready to accept administrative responsibilities. It is hoped that meaningful exposure to relevant aspects of hospital management and health care economics will some day be part of pulmonary education.

As a hospital service, the department provides care on the orders of all staff physicians. At the same time, the services provided are under the responsibility of the medical director of the department. Whereas care must be taken to minimize the risk of interference with the autonomy of the attending physician, appropriate assurances for the quality and appropriateness of respiratory care services must be provided by the medical director. To this end, the medical director must assume overall responsibility for the development and implementation of the respiratory care service's quality assurance activities, as described later in this chapter.

To carry out the responsibility for quality assurance, the medical director must be given the appropriate authority. Two administrative policies can be used to ensure appropriate authority of the medical director over the provision of respiratory care services. First, it can be established that the use of certain specified treatments requires prior official note consultation with the medical director, who will follow the patient's management with the attending physician. Alternatively, the medical director can be given the authority to observe closely all patients receiving the services of the department and to intervene in their management when professional judgment indicates that the best interests of the patient are not being served.

The degree of sophistication of the medical staff in the management of cardiopulmonary problems usually determines the type of medical supervisory program most suitable. Given the fact that respiratory care is still a growing field and the exact legal and moral responsibilities of a respiratory care medical director toward other physicians and their patients is not always clear, a variety of arrangements may be satisfactory. Nonetheless, the medical director must assume responsibility for both the actions of the staff under his or her jurisdiction and for the quality and appropriateness of the services offered by the department. To assume these responsibilities, the medical director must be given the appropriate level of authority.

Technical director. The efficiency of departmental operation depends on the quality of technical or managerial leadership. In most cases, the technical director of a respiratory care service must be well trained in all aspects of respiratory care and experienced in its clinical application. Such individuals must be thoroughly versed in the techniques of therapy and the function of equipment and possess leadership qualities and management ability.

Although the position probably has more prestige if the director is registered by the National Board for Respiratory Care, registration alone is insufficient, for there are many registered therapists who do not possess the necessary leadership and management skills to function effectively in

this key role. No guideline exists to indicate the depth of experience necessary for this position, but a technical director should probably have at least 3 years of practical experience in the field after completion of a formal educational program. Moreover, a technical director should ideally have demonstrated supervisory abilities, as acquired through 2 or more years in a supervisory role.

Whereas the medical director is responsible for the clinical policies and professional functioning of the department, the technical director is responsible for the daily operation and management of this service. The administrative authority of the position must be well understood and completely supported by the medical director because the technical director is an important link between the medical director and the technical staff.

Among the technical director's duties are assignment of staff according to departmental need; maintenance of payroll data on all personnel; development and enforcement of a system that accurately measures staff productivity; preparation of the departmental budget; development and implementation of special projects; generation of statistical data for reports of departmental activity, including justification of personnel needs; provision of advice and assistance to technical personnel; training and orientation of new practitioners; conduction of quality assurance audits; and major equipment evaluation.

Assistant technical director. Given the scope of duties for which the technical director is responsible, one or more assistant technical directors may be needed, especially in large service departments. The assistant should possess technical skills at least equal to those of the technical director but does not need as much administrative experience.

Typically, an assistant technical director serves a dual role. In the absence of the technical director, the assistant acts as the director of the department. On a daily basis, however, the assistant director commonly functions as the chief clinician and first-line supervisor. The assistant director may also supervise the service in the respiratory care or intensive care unit and consults with or advises staff practitioners in the management of difficult patients. The assistant director may also take an active role in the training and orientation of students and practitioners and the evaluation of new or recently repaired equipment. In teaching settings, the assistant director may also be involved in clinical research relevant to respiratory care.

With the increased emphasis on quality assurance in the provision of respiratory care services (covered later in this chapter), the assistant technical director may also serve as the coordinator for the departmental quality assurance plan.

Shift supervisor. Shift supervisors are responsible for the respiratory care service function during particular segments of the day. Generally, they are directly responsible for the staff on their shifts, although they may have the assistance of area supervisors or coordinators in large hospitals.

Specific duties of these key personnel vary considerably from place to place. In response to general patient loads and specific area needs, shift supervisors generally coordinate the work schedules of employees assigned to their shift and make daily assignments of duties. Typically, shift supervisors also coordinate responses to emergency resuscitation calls and assist in clinical training or student supervision. Shift supervisors may also assist staff personnel with common problems and participate in service provision as needed.

The difference in overall hospital activity between shifts also gives different responsibilities to the respective shift supervisors. For example, the day or evening supervisors might be primarily concerned with fulfilling requests for service, whereas the night shift supervisor might be responsible for overseeing clerical work requiring technical knowledge. These supervisors must be flexible and adaptable, as well as mature, experienced, and totally supportive of the department's philosophy and purpose.

Area supervisor. In areas of the hospital where there is a high concentration of specialized services, an area supervisor may be required. The area supervisor is a specialist with specific technical expertise in a particular area, in contrast with a shift supervisor with wider supervisory skills.

Quality and continuity of care can be better achieved in areas of heavy demand when an area supervisor assumes technical supervision of the specialized services. The most common need for this type of supervision is in areas such as intensive care (e.g., separated organized medical, surgical, respiratory, and cardiac care units), neonatal or pediatric intensive care units, recovery and emergency rooms, and rehabilitation clinics. Well-trained area supervisors often serve in these locations, overseeing the performance of staff practitioners assigned to them and participating in educational programs to teach new personnel to maintain proficiency of the regular staff.

Staff practitioners. The character of services provided by a respiratory care department depends on the quality of its staff practitioners. As the primary providers of bedside care, staff practitioners are expected to be technically proficient in the therapeutic modalities offered by the service, including a full knowledge of the indications, contraindications, and hazards associated with procedures. They must also know the basic maintenance procedures for equipment in the event of malfunction.

Because of close interaction with other health care professionals directly involved in the patient's care, staff practitioners must demonstrate an understanding of the anatomy and physiology of respiration and circulation, both normal and abnormal, as they apply to respiratory care and have knowledge of the pathophysiologic conditions of all diseases affecting the respiratory system.

However, technical proficiency and knowledge alone are not sufficient. Staff practitioners also must be ethically sensitive to those aspects of care with which they are directly or indirectly involved, including the values and beliefs of patients and other health care providers. Often these human-oriented skills are just as important in determining patient outcomes as are technical knowledge and proficiency.

Pulmonary function and arterial blood gas laboratory personnel. In most hospitals the pulmonary function and arterial blood gas laboratories operate under the respiratory care service department. Ideally, an experienced and well-trained respiratory care practitioner or cardiopulmonary technologist provides technical supervision of these diagnostic services.

The director of the pulmonary function laboratory should be certified or registered in this specialty area by NBRC (see box on p. 24). By education and experience, the director of the pulmonary function laboratory must have in-depth knowledge of all the diagnostic tests available and be able to train or orient students or new employees. The director supervises the quality of the work done by laboratory technologists, schedules assignments, and maintains laboratory records and an inventory of supplies. The director must be able to recognize equipment malfunctions and know the measures necessary for their repair. The director of the pulmonary function laboratory must also work closely with the manager of respiratory care services when coordinating diagnostic and therapeutic services.

In many institutions, pulmonary function laboratory personnel may also draw and analyze arterial blood gas samples. In small institutions, this duty may be broadly assigned to the respiratory care staff. In large centers, however, it is common for the pulmonary function and blood gas laboratory personnel to be specifically trained in the complexities of many of these tests. In addition, one group of pulmonary laboratory individuals is more desirable than a rotation of each staff person through this area because the group ensures quality control and more reproducible results.

The laboratory staff must be well versed in the technical aspects of the procedures. Like the therapeutic staff, diagnostic laboratory personnel must also possess good communication skills, including the ability to gather pertinent information by interview and the ability to effectively train patients in diagnostic procedures requiring cooperation.

Education coordinator. There should be a relevant educational program suitable for the size and sophistication of the hospital and its staff where respiratory care services are available. This program may vary from a series of periodic in-service or continuing education sessions to daily supervision of students enrolled in an accredited educational program for technicians or therapists.

In places where the primary focus is on staff development, the educational coordinator assumes responsibility for regularly scheduled in-service workshops for the respiratory care staff, for the orientation of new personnel, and for the development of educational programs to introduce new techniques and skills.

In hospitals where an affiliation with a formal educational program exists, educational staff support the full-time program faculty by assisting in the evaluation of students and making recommendations about the degree of independent responsibility a student may be expected to have.

Regardless of the focus, educational personnel must be well trained, experienced, and able to transmit their knowledge to others. Capable respiratory care practitioners should be given teaching roles if they are motivated to participate and are truly interested in providing quality educational experiences.

Equipment manager. In large departments, an equipment manager may be necessary to supervise the evaluation, selection, care, and maintenance of major therapeutic and diagnostic equipment. The equipment manager normally assumes responsibility for all new product evaluations and solicits input about specific needs and expectations from the medical director, technical director, assistant technical director, and other interested persons. The equipment manager also develops and implements a preventative maintenance program that ensures the safe and effective operation of life support and monitoring equipment. In addition, the equipment manager may supervise inventories of supply items essential to the daily operation of the department. Last, the equipment manager may be responsible for supervising the equipment-processing activities included in the departmental infection control program.

The equipment manager's position is extremely vital to the department because it calls for a high degree of communication, technical, mechanical, and supervisory ability. Although individuals with education and experience in respiratory care can and often do serve as equipment managers, those with backgrounds in biomedical instrumentation are equally well suited for this role. Indeed, because of the increasing sophistication of respiratory care equipment, in-depth knowledge of biomedical instrumentation (including electronics and computer technology) is essential.

Equipment aides. Although not officially recognized as a member of the respiratory care profession, most departments employ one or more equipment aides. These aides fulfill many important tasks that do not require technical knowledge.

Nontechnical personnel can be employed and trained to perform duties such as cleaning, disinfecting, sterilizing, and packaging of equipment; ordering, restocking, and delivering supplies; simple equipment repair and maintenance; and basic clerical work. The best results are found using students who are involved in their field and are

learning as well as enjoying that field during nonschool hours.

DEPARTMENTAL OPERATION

Effective operation of a respiratory care service department must be guided by written policies and procedures and a clear delineation of priorities given to various aspects of patient care. Written policies and procedures specify the scope and conduct of patient care services, including ways to respond to situations in which explicit instructions are lacking. Policy also must delineate the priority of services, according to patient need and medical staff expectations.

Policies and procedures

Of and by themselves, written policies and procedures provide no absolute assurance of quality. Obviously, policies and procedures must be carefully followed and executed by knowledgeable and dependable personnel. Nonetheless, without the foundation provided by clear and explicit policies and procedures, consistent and high-quality care cannot be expected.

The respiratory care service policy and procedure manual specifies the scope and conduct of patient care services, as approved and regularly updated by the staff, under the guidance of the department's technical and medical directors.

Regarding specific procedures, the manual must specify who may perform the designated procedure, under what circumstances, and with what degree of supervision. Moreover, each procedural description must indicate the steps to be taken in the event of adverse reactions. Last, the policy and procedure manual must establish protocols for responding to situations in which explicit instructions are lacking.

For staff and students, the department policy and procedure manual represents the primary technical and legal guide to service provision. On a technical basis, such policies and procedures should represent state-of-the-art approaches to the management of patients with respiratory-related disorders, thereby providing a ready resource for effective clinical practice.

On a legal basis, practitioners and students are obliged to carry out these procedures under the conditions of and according to the protocols specified. Failure to follow the specifications can result in personal liability, especially if harm to a patient results from oversight or neglect.

Service priorities

Although there is no general rule for classifying patients according to need for respiratory care, the basic principles of triage must apply in establishing service priorities. The box on p. 29 suggests a priority scale to help respiratory care, medical, and nursing personnel in scheduling priorities of work assignments for respiratory care services.

This grouping represents a common-sense classification of patients from those most in need of attention to those least in need. The objective of such a priority scale is not to restrict the application of respiratory care services but rather to enable the department to make maximum use of personnel. Proper assessment of the needs of patients determines the acuity of illness, such that the highest quality care can be given to those in greatest need.

Scheduling of assignments

The assistant director or shift supervisor designates the work and assigns patients to the staff practitioners or area supervisors at the beginning of the day. A "zone" system is usually the most effective, and with experience, most hospitals can be divided into areas according to the average work load density. One practitioner may be designated to circulate, helping in the busy areas, responding to emergencies, and performing such routine duties as monitoring oxygen concentrations, checking oxygen humidifiers, and examining other operating equipment. Arrangements are made to give priority service to intensive care units and the emergency room as needs dictate.

Throughout the day, all calls for services are submitted to the clerical staff in the assistant director's or supervisor's office. A written record should be kept to include date and time, nature of the request, and its disposition. The record is kept on file. The supervisor is responsible for expediting service during the day's operation and shifting personnel on assignments as needed, a critical task that requires skill, judgment, and knowledge of the hospital's daily functions and unique logistics.

RESOURCES

Because of the wide variation in hospital needs, opinions concerning the personnel, facility, and equipment resources necessary to start and maintain a quality respiratory care service must be general. Nonetheless, based on the experience of the author in a variety of settings, a few general observations will be made.

SUGGESTED PRIORITIES OF PATIENT CARE

1. Emergency care (including resuscitation)
2. Continuous mechanical ventilation
3. Other intensive care services
4. Postoperative care
5. Oxygen administration
6. Prescheduled inpatient basic therapeutics
7. Elective inpatient diagnostic studies
8. Outpatient and ambulatory services

Personnel requirements

In determining labor requirements, factors such as the average work load should be considered. Part-time and "on-call" help can supplement increases in the work load, whereas decreases below the average, if predicted or foreseen, will provide time for vacations, special projects, educational endeavors, or opportunities for progressive updating of the entire staff's skills.

The most effective way of determining labor requirements is to evaluate the work load over a period of several months using a standardized mechanism to convert common procedures into work units. Factors such as the number of hours in the period being monitored compared with the total hours spent doing actual work will yield the estimated number of employees needed to perform the work.

Facilities

Hospitals anticipating expansion should allow the respiratory care service extra space beyond its immediate needs because a growing department usually finds its existing facilities inadequate within 2 to 3 years. The general service area should be large enough to accommodate a sufficient work space for repair and preventive maintenance of equipment. A facility specifically designed to handle specialized equipment processing (including physically separate dirty and clean areas) is required, unless processing is provided by a centralized service. Bulk equipment storage space should be near the general departmental area. Office space for the medical director, technical director, clerical help, and a staff room for practitioners should also be provided.

Pulmonary function testing and arterial blood gas analysis facilities can be physically integrated or provided separately. If they are separate, the blood gas laboratory may be located close to the areas of highest demand, such as the intensive care areas. Regardless of location, the pulmonary function laboratory should provide ample privacy for testing procedures.

Often a special procedures room is associated with the medical director's office or the pulmonary function laboratory. This room provides facilities for elective bronchoscopy and other special procedures and should ideally have central compressed gas and suction outlets comparable to those provided in patient care areas. Moreover, applicable monitoring and emergency equipment should be available in this location.

Outpatient facilities, where provided, may be localized to the respiratory care department or integrated within the general ambulatory care clinic. If an outpatient rehabilitation program operates within the department, separate classroom and physical reconditioning facilities should be provided.

The difficulties of incorporating new facilities into existing buildings are well recognized, and makeshift arrangements often must be made. In new construction, however, every attempt should be made to locate the general services areas, laboratories, and offices together and in physical proximity to the intensive or respiratory care units.

Equipment

In past years there was a tremendous increase in the use of prepackaged, disposable respiratory care equipment. Such equipment was designed to provide greater patient protection as well as save labor costs associated with reusable equipment processing.

However, the rising costs of disposable plastics, with general hospital-wide efforts to contain supply expenditures, have resulted in a return to smaller inventories of recyclable items, especially humidifiers, nebulizers, and ventilator circuits. In this context, cost savings can be achieved with more efficient systems for cleaning, sterilizing, and packaging reusables.

However, disposables still must be used in those areas where infection control problems preclude equipment reuse, as with oxygen delivery systems. In addition, the labor costs and overhead of maintaining a large inventory of recyclable items may justify disposables under certain circumstances.

Of the major capital equipment, the largest and most expensive items are the mechanical ventilators. Because there is no "best" ventilator capable of serving all purposes, most departments select at least one primary general-duty system supplemented, as needed, by a smaller number of ventilators reserved for special duty, such as pediatric or neonatal application. This approach maintains consistency, lowers training costs, and reduces the likelihood of errors caused by unfamiliarity with equipment. Ultimately, however, the medical director, technical director, and equipment manager must determine whether it is in the best interest of the hospital to strive for maximum uniformity through the use of a limited variety of equipment or for greater flexibility with a wider variety of technical support.

The minimum equipment for the pulmonary function laboratory consists of a spirometry system capable of measuring all standard lung volumes, capacities, and flows. Substantial long-term cost savings can be realized if such equipment provides computerized computation and reporting. Likewise, automated blood gas analysis equipment, besides providing more consistent and repeatable results, saves time in calibration, error determination, and troubleshooting. In either case, personnel responsible for operating such devices must be well versed in the automated and manual techniques of testing. Only in this manner can they understand the limits of the technology and when and how to intercede in the event of equipment malfunction.

RECORDKEEPING

Good records are the hallmark of a quality respiratory care service. Two general categories of records are main-

tained by a hospital and respiratory care service: patient records and financial (accounting) records. Patient records document the initiation, provision, and outcome of the care provided by the respiratory care service, thereby providing a primary source of data for quality assurance monitoring (discussed in the next section). Financial records represent the business end of documentation, serving to ensure accurate patient billing and cost accounting for services rendered.

Until recently, these two categories of records generally were originated and processed separately. However, changes in the methods of reimbursement for hospital care have demanded at least a partial consolidation of patient care and financial information.

Patient records

The medical record. The medical record of a patient represents the comprehensive, cumulative, and legal documentation of the care provided to a patient throughout his or her course of stay. Typically, the medical record includes admitting data, history and physical information, physician's orders, physician's progress notes, nursing notes, and records of diagnostic and therapeutic interventions.

Diagnosis related groups. Under current methods of third-party hospital reimbursement for patient services, the admitting diagnosis of the patient is of critical importance. First, based on the admitting diagnosis, the patient is assigned to a specific diagnosis related group (DRG). There are over 470 DRGs grouped within about two dozen major diagnostic categories (MDCs). Table 2-2 lists DRGs that compose major diagnostic category 4, disorders of the respiratory system (including two recent additions).

For each DRG, the Health Care Financing Administration (HCFA) of the U.S. Department of Health and Human Services has established a fixed rate of hospital reimbursement and a mean length of stay (LOS). Based on complex formulas that take into account the mix of patients typically admitted to a given hospital and regional variations in labor costs, a hospital will be reimbursed a fixed amount for each patient, based on admitting DRGs.

Because the DRG amount remains fixed for a given admitting diagnosis, *regardless of the amount or intensity of services provided or the patient's length of stay,* hospitals that provide care for less than the fixed rate can keep the difference, thereby realizing a profit. On the other hand, hospitals whose cost of care exceeds the fixed rate must absorb the cost difference, thereby taking a financial loss.

By placing hospitals at risk financially, prospective reimbursement by DRGs provides a powerful incentive for cost efficiency in the provision of services. Because the cost of patient care is directly related to length of stay, most hospitals have focused cost containment efforts on minimizing the duration of inpatient care, while simultaneously attempting to reduce or prevent needless admis-

Table 2-2 Diagnosis Related Groups (DRGs) Major Diagnostic Category 4

DRG number	DRG title
75 (Sur)	Major chest procedures
76 (Sur)	Operating room procedure on respiratory system except major chest and complications/co-morbidity
77 (Sur)	Operating room procedure on respiratory system except major chest without complications/co-morbidity
78 (Med)	Pulmonary embolism
79 (Med)	Respiratory infections and inflammation, age >69, and/or complications/co-morbidity
80 (Med)	Respiratory infections and inflammations, age 18-69, without complications/co-morbidity
81 (Med)	Respiratory infections and inflammations, age 0-17
82 (Med)	Respiratory neoplasms
83 (Med)	Major chest trauma, age >69, and/or complications/co-morbidity
84 (Med)	Major chest trauma, age <70, without complications/co-morbidity
85 (Med)	Pleural effusion, age >69, and/or complications/co-morbidity
86 (Med)	Pleural effusion, age <70, without complications/co-morbidity
87 (Med)	Pulmonary edema and respiratory failure
88 (Med)	Chronic obstructive pulmonary disease
89 (Med)	Simple pneumonia and pleurisy, age >69, and/or complications/co-morbidity
90 (Med)	Simple pneumonia and pleurisy, age 18-69, without complications/co-morbidity
91 (Med)	Simple pneumonia and pleurisy, age 0-17
92 (Med)	Interstitial lung disease, age >69, and/or complications/co-morbidity
93 (Med)	Interstitial lung disease, age <70, without complications/co-morbidity
94 (Med)	Pneumothorax, age >69, and/or complications/co-morbidity
95 (Med)	Pneumothorax, age <70, without complications/co-morbidity
96 (Med)	Bronchitis and asthma, age >69, and/or complications/co-morbidity
97 (Med)	Bronchitis and asthma, age 18-69, without complications/co-morbidity
98 (Med)	Bronchitis and asthma, age 0-17
99 (Med)	Respiratory signs and symptoms, age >69, and/or complications/co-morbidity
100 (Med)	Respiratory signs and symptoms, age <70, without complications/co-morbidity
101 (Med)	Other respiratory diagnoses, age >69, and/or complications/co-morbidity
102 (Med)	Other respiratory diagnoses, age <70
474 (Sur)	Tracheostomy*
475 (Med)	Mechanical ventilation*

*Recent additions

sions (i.e., cases that could be handled effectively on an ambulatory care or outpatient basis).

For the respiratory care department, this change in reimbursement policy means that services must be rendered in the most cost-efficient manner possible. Specifically, respiratory care services must contribute to getting patients well as quickly as possible, thereby decreasing their lengths of stay. Typically, this new orientation has resulted in the provision of a greater intensity of services to patients over a shorter time. In addition, there is now greater emphasis on documenting the need for and results of respiratory care interventions.

Respiratory care records. When providing respiratory care services, the patient's medical record must document the origination of prescribed treatments, respiratory-related consultations, actual service, and evaluation of the results of intervention.

Origination of prescribed treatments. All respiratory care interventions must be by order of a member of the hospital's medical staff.

According to JCAHO standards, such prescriptions must specify the type, frequency, and duration of treatment, and, as appropriate, the type and dosage of medication, including the desired oxygen concentration, where applicable.

For purposes of both progress monitoring and quality assurance, the prescription should also specify the goals and objectives of the respiratory care intervention. Ideally, the goals and objectives of respiratory care should derive from a respiratory assessment of the patient conducted by the medical director or by appropriately trained staff practitioners. Further, these goals and objectives should provide the bases for a respiratory care plan, individualized according to patient needs.

Documentation of care. Whether provided separately or incorporated into the general progress notes, there must be ongoing documentation of respiratory care provided to patients. Such documentation must minimally include the type of therapy provided, the date and time of administration, the effects of the therapy, and any adverse reactions exhibited by the patient.

Evaluation. In consultation with the respiratory care staff, the physician must provide timely and pertinent evaluation of the clinical results of the respiratory care provided. Such evaluations help to determine the need to continue, modify, or terminate a therapeutic regimen. Moreover, evaluation of the clinical results of respiratory care can later be used in retrospective quality assurance audits.

Departmental records. Each respiratory care service maintains its own record and accounting system separate from the legal medical record of the patient. The departmental record system may be manually maintained or integrated with a hospital-wide computer information system.

The departmental record system normally serves two purposes. It provides a portable or "in-the-room" charting system whereby staff practitioners maintain an abbreviated record for each patient under care, and it provides the basis for departmental charges for patient services.

Typically, a departmental record system works in the following manner. In addition to the required entries in the patient's comprehensive medical record, the practitioner enters all treatments or services for a given day on the departmental record card or chart. At the end of the shift, charges for each service rendered are entered into the computer information system or submitted manually to the accounting office.

The departmental record system also provides the basis for communicating essential patient information between staff members and assisting in the transfer of patient responsibilities such as occurs at change of shift.

Accounting records

From the accumulated departmental records and charges, data are obtained for patient discharge billing and statistical accounting of the respiratory care service activities.

Statistical accounting of respiratory care service activities may involve periodic (daily, weekly, monthly, quarterly, and/or yearly) tabulation of the number and types of patients treated, the number of days patients have received treatment, the number of services, and patient charges according to the type of service provided.

More recently, statistical accounting of respiratory care service activities is providing comparative data by admit-

ting DRG. Such comparative data may include respiratory costs as a percentage of total costs for a given DRG, mean LOS as compared to national or regional norms, and even a comparison of DRG costs and mean LOS to other hospitals. Moreover, new computer information systems are providing the capability to compare DRG morbidity and mortality statistics within or among hospitals and according to the admitting physician or surgeon.

Although such statistical portrayals have limitations, the merger of patient and cost accounting data is becoming a reality for hospitals in general and respiratory care services in particular. Rather than perceiving such an orientation as a threat, progressive respiratory care services are using these data to improve cost efficiency and quality.

QUALITY ASSURANCE

Despite increased emphasis on cost containment, the provision of quality care remains the first goal of hospitals and respiratory care services. *Quality assurance* (QA) is an ongoing process designed to ensure the detection and correction of factors hindering the provision of optimum, appropriate, and cost-effective health care.

Organization of a quality assurance program. As depicted in Fig. 2-2, overall authority and responsibility for a hospital's quality assurance program is in the hands of its board of directors or trustees. Normally, the board delegates its authority to the medical and administrative staffs

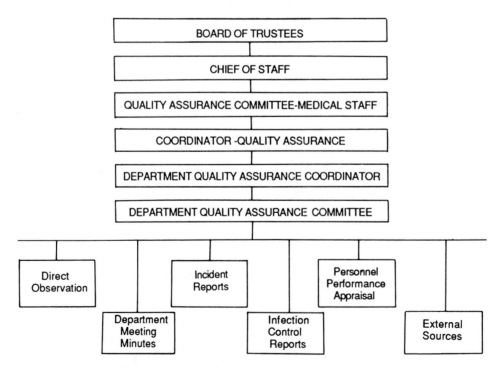

Fig. 2-2   Model respiratory care quality assurance plan: organizational chart for sources of problem identification and accountability. (Redrawn from Hastings D: The AARC's model quality assurance plan, AARC Times 12(2):25, 1988.)

through a hospital-wide quality assurance committee. This committee develops general policies and objectives for the overall quality assurance effort and, with the assistance of a coordinator, monitors and evaluates implementation within the institution's service departments. Each service department, in turn, develops a quality assurance program consistent with these general objectives. To implement these efforts at the department level, the identification of a departmental coordinator and the appointment of a departmental quality assurance committee is desirable.

Guidelines for respiratory care services. For the respiratory care service department, quality assurance activities must focus on the identification and resolution of problems related to patient care and clinical performance. The JCAHO guidelines for a respiratory care quality assurance program are summarized in the box below.

According to the American Association for Respiratory Care (AARC) Standards Committee, ultimate authority for the continued development and practice of quality assurance within a respiratory care service must lie with the medical director. Normally, the medical director of the service appoints a departmental coordinator for quality assurance and supervises a representative quality assurance departmental committee.

The departmental committee develops and implements a quality assurance plan. According to the AARC's Standards Committee, the goals of a respiratory care quality assurance plan should include at least the following:

1. To provide a method for monitoring both the quality and appropriateness of respiratory care;
2. To assure that respiratory care methods and procedures are *efficient* in terms of cost;

JCAHO RESPIRATORY CARE SERVICES QUALITY ASSURANCE STANDARDS

1. The quality and appropriateness of patient care will be reviewed and evaluated in accordance with the hospital's overall quality assurance plan.
2. The review and evaluation should, where applicable, involve the use of the medical record.
3. The review and evaluation will be based on preestablished criteria which will include:
   Indications for any procedure;
   Effectiveness of procedure;
   Adverse effects of procedure.
4. The review and evaluation will include input from the medical staff and personnel of the respiratory care services.
5. The review and evaluation will be done within the overall hospital quality assurance program.
6. Particular attention will be given to evaluation of those respiratory care services having the highest utilization rates.

---

3. To assure that respiratory care methods and procedures are *effective;*
4. To identify, rank, and resolve patient care–related problems;
5. To develop, implement, and monitor intervention strategies aimed at problem resolution; and
6. To evaluate the respiratory care quality assurance plan at least annually and to revise it as necessary.

Quality assurance procedures. As recommended by the AARC Standards Committee, nine key steps are necessary to systematically implement a quality assurance plan. As depicted in Fig. 2-3, these procedural steps include identifying problems, determining the causes of problems, ranking problems, developing strategies for problem resolution, developing appropriate measurement techniques, implementing problem resolution strategies, analyzing intervention results, reporting results, and continuously evaluating intervention outcomes.

Successful implementation of a QA plan demands that the respiratory care service develop criteria addressing the therapeutic goals, appropriateness, and means of evaluating the effectiveness of each specific high-utilization and high-risk procedure. The box on p. 34 provides an example of such criteria for oxygen therapy.

Identifying problems. Using the quality assurance process just described, various data sources, including the patient's medical record, would be used to determine the extent to which oxygen therapy services are appropriately used.

Normally, an objective problem indicator such as "90% of all patients receiving oxygen therapy will meet the appropriateness of care criteria" is helpful in problem identification. If the indicator is not met (e.g., if only 70% of the patients meet the appropriateness of therapy criteria), a problem exists.

Determining causes. Once a problem has been identified, its cause must be determined. For example, the fact that only 70% of patients receiving oxygen therapy meet the specified criteria may result from factors such as the ordering physicians' lack of knowledge of the criteria, their failure to follow known criteria, or their failure to discontinue therapy when indicated.

Resolving identified problems. Once the underlying cause is identified, a strategy to resolve the problem must be developed, implemented, and evaluated. For example, if the problem with oxygen therapy use is found to be based on the new medical residents' lack of knowledge of the appropriateness of care criteria, proper orientation and in-service education may be necessary. Once conducted, the effect of the selected strategy on the desired outcome should be assessed. Ideally, evaluation of the outcomes of intervention should be based on the initial problem indicator. For example, we would want to know whether the in-service education program for the medical residents increased the percentage of patients meeting the appropriateness of therapy criteria.

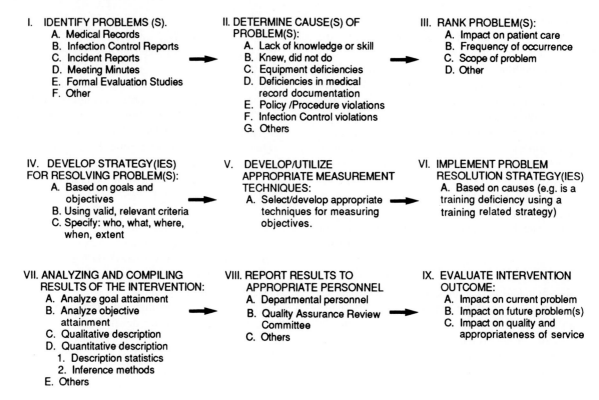

Fig. 2-3   Model respiratory care quality assurance plan flow chart. (Redrawn from Hastings D: The AARC's model quality assurance plan, AARC Times 12(2):25, 1988.)

QUALITY ASSURANCE CRITERIA FOR OXYGEN THERAPY

THERAPEUTIC GOALS

1. To prevent or reverse hypoxemia and tissue hypoxia;
2. To decrease myocardial work;
3. To decrease the work of breathing.

APPROPRIATENESS OF CARE

1. The patient must be diagnosed as having or being at risk of developing hypoxemia and/or tissue hypoxia; or
2. The patient must be diagnosed as having suffered a myocardial infarction within the previous 72 hours; and
3. Oxygen dosing and mode of therapy will follow the criteria specified in the Respiratory Care Service *Policy and Procedure Manual.*

EVALUATION OF THE EFFECTIVENESS OF THERAPY

The effectiveness of therapy will be evaluated by comparing the pretreatment and posttreatment status of the patient according to the following criteria *(at least one must apply):*

1. Increase in Pao_2 or in arterial saturation; or
2. Reversal or absence of cyanosis; or
3. Decrease in heart rate; or
4. Decrease in blood pressure; or
5. Decrease or absence of cardiac dysrhythmias; or
6. Decrease in respiratory rate; or
7. Increase in level of consciousness; or
8. Decrease in carboxyhemoglobin saturation; or
9. Relief of dyspnea.

Adapted from Larson K: The well-defined quality assurance plan, AARC Times 12(2):15-24, 1988.

Reporting and continuous monitoring. Problem identification and resolution activities, including the relative success of intervention strategies, must be documented and reported on a regular basis. Moreover, even successful interventions must be monitored over time to assure that a given problem does not recur. Only in this manner can the respiratory care service assume ongoing accountability for its quality assurance program and ensure that its services are appropriately used and effective.

SUMMARY

Respiratory care services play a vital role in the provision of comprehensive and acute hospital care. A quality respiratory care service is organized under medical and technical directorship to provide a broad range of services, according to patient and staff needs. To ensure that these services are efficiently delivered and effective in achieving desired patient outcomes, the service must have appropriate facilities, adequately trained personnel, and state-of-the-art equipment. Moreover, the operation of the service must be guided by clear and comprehensive policies and procedures. Last, the respiratory care service must be an active partner in hospital-wide efforts to assure optimum and cost-effective care.

Advancements in technology notwithstanding, the ability of a respiratory care service to meet the challenge of providing quality and cost-effective care depends on the dedication and commitment of its professional staff.

BIBLIOGRAPHY

Anderson EL and McPeck M: The modern respiratory care department. In Burton GG and Hodgkin JE, editors: Respiratory care: a guide to clinical practice, ed 2, Philadelphia, 1984, JB Lippincott Co.

Bartow SL: Quality assurance: a good management tool for respiratory care services, AARC Times 6(12):26-30, 1982.

Crockett RJ: Quality assurance: setting up department goals, AARC Times 6(12):20-22, 24-25, 1982.

Durren M: Strategies for quality assurance in the respiratory care department, Mich Soc Respir Therap J 17(1):3-6, 1983.

Egan DF: The stethoscope and the ledger, Chest 68:1, 1975.

Fink JB and Fink AK: The respiratory therapist as manager, Chicago, 1986, Year Book Medical Publishers.

Hastings D: The AARC's model quality assurance plan, AARC Times 12(2):26, 28-33, 1988.

Joint Commission on Accreditation of Healthcare Organizations: Accreditation manual for hospitals, Chicago, 1988, Joint Commission on Accreditation of Healthcare Organizations.

Larson K: The well-defined quality assurance plan, AARC Times 12(2):15-24, 1988.

McLaughlin AJ: Organization and management for respiratory therapists, St Louis, 1979, The CV Mosby Co.

Miller WF et al: Guidelines for organization and function of hospital respiratory care services: section on respiratory therapy, American College of Chest Physicians, Chest 78:1, 1980.

Rakich JS, Longest BB, and O'Donovan T: Managing health care organizations, Philadelphia, 1977, WB Saunders Co.

Scanlan CL: The prospective payment system: what you see is what you get, Pul Med Tech 1(5):19-34, 1984.

Yanda RL: The need for leadership in hospital respiratory services, Chest 68:81, 1975.

Scientific Bases for Respiratory Care

3

Terms, Symbols, and Units of Measure

Craig L. Scanlan

The clinical practice of respiratory care involves extensive observation and communication skills. Consistency in the use and application of these skills among health professionals requires a common frame of reference that is embodied in systems of clinical communication and measurement.

Like any branch of knowledge, medicine has its own language. This language, called medical terminology, represents a coherent system of word building with a few simple rules. Once these rules are mastered, the respiratory care practitioner can build and define thousands of new medical terms.

Medical terminology represents the language of medicine, and abbreviations and symbols are its "shorthand." Abbreviations are used mainly in charting and medical record keeping. Although there are some exceptions, the use of medical abbreviations is not as standardized as the use of medical terms. Fortunately, the abbreviations and symbols used in respiratory care and pulmonary physiology are an exception. Respiratory care practitioners must be well versed in the use of both general medical abbreviations and those used exclusively in pulmonary physiology.

Respiratory care practitioners also are engaged regularly in the measurement, description, and communication of physical events. These responsibilities require that the practitioner master a variety of measurement systems. In the U.S. there are three primary systems of scientific measurement used in the clinical setting. Until complete standardization in a single system occurs, respiratory care practitioners must be adept in working with all three measurement approaches.

OBJECTIVES

This chapter focuses on the use of terms, symbols, and units of measure in clinical practice. Specifically, after completion of this chapter, the reader will be able to:

1. Apply standard conventions of medical terminology to define and translate common medical terms;

2. Identify the common medical abbreviations used in written communication and medical record keeping;

3. Identify and apply the primary and secondary symbols used in pulmonary physiology and respiratory care;

4. Apply the concepts of scientific notation and Greek and Latin prefixes to clinical measurement;

5. Define the major units of measure used in the cgs, fps (British), and SI systems, and convert a given value between any two systems.

MEDICAL TERMINOLOGY

Medical terminology provides consistent meanings among diverse groups of health professionals, facilitating communication and interaction. Most medical terms are Greek or Latin derivatives and represent a blend of stem or root words in combination with suffixes and prefixes. Building a medical vocabulary begins with mastery of key root, suffix, and prefix terms. Once these key terms are learned, new words can be "translated" and applied by understanding their component parts.

Word roots and combining forms

Word roots represent "stem" or "building block" words. These roots provide the basis for describing most anatomic terms, medical and surgical procedures, and laboratory tests.

Word roots are seldom used alone. Often a prefix or suffix is added to the word root, or it is combined with another root to form a compound word. For this reason, each word root has a combining form, usually consisting of the word root with an added combining vowel, most frequently an "o."

Table 3-1 lists the most common word roots and their combining forms. The word root appears before the slash, with the combining vowel shown after the slash. For each root, a definition of its meaning and an example of its use is provided. For example, the root word "cardi" is derived from the Greek word *kardia,* meaning heart. The combining form of cardi is cardio-.

Many medical terms are built simply by combining root words. These combinations of root words are called compound words. As an example, the combination of "cardi/o" (meaning heart) with "pulmon/o" (from the Latin *pulmo,* meaning lung) yields the compound word "cardiopulmonary" (meaning heart and lungs), as in cardiopulmonary resuscitation. Combining "cost/o" (ribs) with "chondr/o" (cartilage) gives us the new term "costochondral," referring to the cartilaginous portion of the ribs.

A few basic rules apply to the use of roots and their combining forms. First, in building a compound word, one should always retain the combining vowel when the second word root begins with a consonant. Cardiopulmonary and costochondral are good examples. Second, even if the second root begins with a vowel, the combining vowel is usually retained, as in the following example:

Root	+	Root	+	Suffix	=	New word	Meaning
gastr/o (stomach)		enter/o (intestine)		itis (inflammation)		gastro-enteritis	inflammation of the stomach *and* intestines

In this example the two root words "gastr/o" and "enter/o" are combined to form a compound word meaning stomach and intestines. Although "enter/o" begins with a vowel, the combining "o" of "gastr/o" is not dropped. The suffix "itis" (meaning inflammation) completes the word building, giving us the new term, "gastroenteritis," which means inflammation of the stomach and intestines.

Suffixes

A suffix is a word element that, when placed at the end of a word, creates a new or modified meaning. Suffixes common in ordinary English include "less" (doubt<u>less</u>), "y" (dirt<u>y</u>), and "al" (person<u>al</u>).

As in English, adding a suffix to a medical word changes its meaning. In medical terminology there are two broad categories of suffixes: (1) those that simply modify the meaning of a noun, verb, or adjective; and (2) combining suffixes that actually give new meaning to root words.

Table 3-2 lists selected suffixes that modify the meaning of nouns, verbs, or adjectives. For example, by adding the suffix "al" to the noun root "neur/o" (meaning nerve), the new adjective "neural," meaning pertaining to the nerves, is formed. Other good examples of the use of the simple modifiers include immun<u>ize</u>, hepat<u>ic</u>, hypox<u>ia</u>, pneumat<u>ic</u>, and ven<u>ous</u>.

Table 3-1 Selected Wood Roots and Combining Forms

Word roots	Meaning	Example	Word roots	Meaning	Example
aden/o	gland	adenopathy	immun/o	safe, protected	immunoglobin
adren/o	adrenal gland	adrenergic	lapar/o	abdomen	laparotomy
arter/o	artery	arterial	later/o	side	lateromedial
atel/o	incomplete	atelectasis	leuk/o	white	leukocyte
brachi/o	arm	brachiocephalic	lob/o	lobe	lobectomy
bronch/o	bronchus	bronchitis	medi/o	middle	mediosternal
cardi/o	heart	cardiopulmonary	medull/o	medulla	medullary
cephal/o	head	cephalad	my/o	muscle	myopathy
cervic/o	neck	cervical	nephr/o	kidney	nephrectomy
chondr/o	cartilage	costochondral	neur/o	nerve	neuropathy
cost/o	ribs	costochondral	or/o	mouth	oral
crani/o	skull	craniotomy	ox/o	oxygen	hypoxia
cutane/o	skin	subcutaneous	oxy/o	oxygen	oxyhemoglobin
cyst/o	bladder	cystoscopy	pharyng/o	pharynx	glossopharyngeal
derm/o	skin	dermoid	phleb/o	vein	phlebotomy
dermat/o	skin	dermatotome	phren/o	diaphragm	phrenic
encephal/o	brain	encephalitis	pleur/o	pleura	pleurisy
enter/o	intestines	enteritis	pneum/o	lung, air	pneumotachygraph
epiglott/o	epiglottis	epiglottitis	pneumat/o	lung, air	pneumatocele
erythr/o	red	erythrocyte	poster/o	posterior	posterolateral
esophag/o	esophagus	esophageal	pulmon/o	lung	pulmonary
gastr/o	stomach	gastritis	rhin/o	nose	rhinoplasty
glomerul/o	glomerulus	glomerulonephritis	thorac/o	thorax	thoracotomy
gloss/o	tongue	glossopharyngeal	thromb/o	clot	thrombolysis
hem/o	blood	hemostasis	trache/o	trachea	tracheostomy
hemat/o	blood	hematocrit	vas/o	vessel	vasoconstrictor
hepat/o	liver	hepatomegaly	ven/o	vein	venous
histo/o	tissue	histocyte			

Actual new meanings also can be created with medical suffixes. Table 3-3 lists selected combining suffixes that give root words new or extended meanings. For example:

Root	Suffix	New word	Meaning
atel/o	ectasis	atelectasis	incomplete expansion
bronch/o	itis	bronchitis	inflammation of the bronchi
trache/o	malacia	tracheomalacia	softening of the trachea
cardi/o	megaly	cardiomegaly	enlargement of the heart
hem/o	ptysis	hemoptysis	spitting (coughing) blood

When a root word is combined with a suffix that begins with a vowel, as in "atelectasis" and "bronchitis," the combining vowel is usually dropped. However, the combining vowel is usually retained if the suffix begins with a consonant, as in "tracheomalacia," "cardiomegaly," and "hemoptysis."

Prefixes

A prefix is a word element that, when placed at the beginning of a word, creates a new or modified meaning. Prefixes common in ordinary English include "pre" (precooked), "bi" (bicycle), and "retro" (retroactive). As with suffixes, the addition of a prefix to a medical word changes its meaning. In medical terminology, prefixes most commonly occur in combination with a word root, but may also serve as a combining form.

Table 3-4 provides several examples of the most common prefixes used in medical terminology. A good example of a prefix in combination with a word root is "anoxia." Breaking this term down into its component parts demonstrates its derivation:

Prefix	Root	Suffix	Meaning
an (lack of)	ox/o (oxygen)	ia (condition)	a condition characterized by the lack of oxygen

Table 3-2 Selected Modifying Suffixes

Suffix	Use	Examples
ize, ate	add to nouns or adjectives to make verbs expressing to use and to act like, to subject to, make into	visual<u>ize</u> (able to see)
ist, or, er	add to verbs to make nouns expressing agent or person concerned or instrument	anesthet<u>ist</u> (one who practices the science of anesthesia)
ent	add to verbs to make adjectives or nouns of agency	recipi<u>ent</u> (one who receives)
sia, y, tion	add to verbs to make nouns expressing action, process, or condition	therap<u>y</u> (treatment) inhala<u>tion</u> (act of inhaling), anesthe<u>sia</u> (process or condition of not feeling)
ia, ity	add to adjectives or nouns to make nouns expressing quality or condition	septicem<u>ia</u> (poisoning of blood), acid<u>ity</u> (condition of excess acid), neural<u>gia</u> (pain in nerves)
ma, mata, men, mina, ment, ure	add to verbs to make nouns expressing result of action or object of action	trau<u>ma</u> (injury), fora<u>mina</u> (openings), liga<u>ment</u> (tough fibrous band holding bone or viscera together), fiss<u>ure</u> (groove)
ium, olus, olum, culus, culum, cule, cle	add to nouns to make diminutive nouns	bacter<u>ium</u>, alve<u>olus</u> (air sac), folli<u>cle</u> (little bag)
ible, ile	add to verbs to make adjectives expressing ability or capacity	contract<u>ile</u> (ability to contract), flex<u>ible</u> (capable of being bent)
al, c, ic ious, tic	add to nouns to make adjectives expressing relationship, concern, or pertaining to	neur<u>al</u> (referring to nerve), neoplas<u>tic</u> (referring to neoplasm), cardi<u>ac</u> (referring to the heart)
id	add to verbs or nouns to make adjectives expressing state or condition	flacc<u>id</u> (state of being weak or lax), flu<u>id</u> (state of being liquid)
tic	add to a verb to make an adjective showing relationship	caus<u>tic</u> (referring to burn) acous<u>tic</u> (referring to sound or hearing)
oid, form	add to nouns to make adjectives expressing resemblance	polyp<u>oid</u> (resembling polyp), plexi<u>form</u> (resembling a plexus), fusi<u>form</u> (resembling a fusion), muc<u>oid</u> (resembling mucus)
ous	add to nouns to make adjectives expressing material	fer<u>rous</u> (composed of iron) se<u>rous</u> (composed of serum)

On the other hand, a prefix may sometimes serve as the combining form itself, without a root word, as in "dyspnea":

Prefix	Root	Suffix	Meaning
dys (difficult)		pnea (breathing)	difficult breathing

Translating medical terms

Once the common root, suffix, and prefix terms are mastered, the learner can begin "translating" and applying new words encountered in reading, discussion, or presentations. This is accomplished by systematically breaking the term down into its constituent parts, using the following steps:

1. Identify and define the suffix.
2. Identify and define the prefix.
3. Define the middle part of the word.

If an unfamiliar root, prefix, or suffix is encountered, the learner should write it down and use a medical dictionary to define its meaning. Then one should practice with the new term, adding other familiar components to build new words. Simply memorizing a whole new term is discouraged. By always applying the rules of medical terminology, new terms can easily be understood and rote memorization avoided.

Throughout the remainder of this book, each chapter provides key terms useful in mastering the chapter content. To assist the reader in defining these terms, a comprehensive glossary is provided at the end of the book.

Pronunciation

All good medical dictionaries include pronunciation guides, which provide direction regarding oral usage of medical terms. However, several basic rules of pronunciation are useful in the early stages of building a medical vocabulary.

In general, the vowels and consonants of medical terms have ordinary English sounds. Exceptions to this generalization include the following:

- The letters c and g have a hard sound when they occur before other letters. Examples of this hard sound include cardiac (kaŕ-de-ak), cranial (krá-ne-al), and gastric (gaś-trik).
- The letters c and g carry the soft sounds of s and j, however, when they occur before the vowels e, i, and y. Examples of these soft sounds are cephalic (sef-aĺ-ik) and gynecology (jin-e-koĺ-o-je).
- The letter combination ch is sometimes pronounced like k. Examples of this sound include cholesterol (ko-leś-ter-ol) and chromatograph (kro-maŕ-o-graf).
- When ae or oe letter combinations are encountered, only the second vowel (e) is pronounced. Examples of this dropped vowel sound are pleurae (ploŕ-e) and coelom (sé-lom).
- When found at the end of a word, es is often pronounced as a separate syllable. Nares (naŕ-ez) is a good example.
- When i is used to form the Latin plural at the end of a word, it is pronounced as a long i. Examples are bronchi (brong̈-ki) and fungi (fuń-ji).
- When pn or ps occurs at the beginning of a word, the p is silent, as in pneumonectomy (nu-mo-nek̈-to-me) or psittacosis (sit-ah-kó-sis).

ABBREVIATIONS

Abbreviations, unlike medical terms, are used exclusively in written communication, especially in charting and medical record keeping. We will look first at medical abbreviations in general, followed by an analysis of those specific to respiratory care and pulmonary physiology.

General medical abbreviations

Many general abbreviations used in medicine, especially those associated with medical prescriptions, are simple

Table 3-3   Selected Combining Suffixes

Suffix	Meaning	Example
algesia	pain	analgesia
algia	pain	myalgia
asthenia	without strength	myasthenia
capnia	carbon dioxide	hypercapnia
cele	swelling	pneumatocele
crine	to secrete	endocrine
ectasis	expansion	atelectasis
esthesia	feeling	anaesthesia
globin	protein	hemoglobin
graph	recording instrument	electrocardiograph
itis	inflammation	bronchitis
malacia	softening	tracheomalacia
megaly	enlargement	hepatomegaly
oma	tumor	adenoma
paresis	partial paralysis	hemiparesis
pathy	disease	neuropathy
penia	decrease	leukocytopenia
phagia	swallowing	dysphagia
phylaxis	protection	anaphylaxis
plasia	growth	dysplasia
plegia	paralysis	hemiplegia
pnea	breathing	dyspnea
ptysis	spitting	hemoptysis
rrhea	discharge	rhinorrhea
sclerosis	hardening	atherosclerosis
scopy	visual exam	laryngoscopy
spasm	involuntary contraction	bronchospasm
stasis	standing still	hemostasis
stenosis	constriction	mitral stenosis
toxic	poison	cytotoxic
trophy	development	hypertrophy
tropin	stimulate	adrenocorticotropin
uria	urine	nocturia

Table 3-4   Selected Common Prefixes

Prefix	Meaning	Examples
a, an	without, lack of	apnea (without breath), anoxia (without oxygen)
ab	away from	abductor (leading away)
ad	to, toward	adductor (leading toward)
ante	before, forward	antecubital (before elbow)
anti	against, opposed	antisepsis (against infection)
bi	twice, double	bifurcation (two branches)
brady	slow	bradypnea (slow breathing)
cata	down, complete	catabolism (breaking down)
circum	around, about	circumflex (winding about)
contra	against, opposite	contraindicated (not indicated)
de	away from	decompensation (failure of compensation)
dia	through, across	diaphragm (wall across)
dis	reversal, apart from, separation	disinfection (apart from infection)
dys	difficult	dyspnea (difficult breathing)
e, ex	out, away from	eviscerate (take out viscera or bowels)
ec	out from	ectopic (out of place)
ecto	on outer side, situated on	ectoderm (outer skin)
em, en	in	empyema (pus in)
endo	within	endocardium (within heart)
epi	upon, on	epidural (upon dura)
eu	good, normal	eupnea (normal breathing)
exo	outside, on outer side, outer layer	exogenous (originating outside)
extra	outside	extrapleural (outside pleura)
hyper	over, above	hypertrophy (overgrowth)
hypo	under, below	hypotension (low blood pressure)
im, in	in, into	infiltration (act of filtering in)
im, in	not	involuntary (not voluntary)
infra	below	infraclavicular (below clavicle)
inter	between	interpleural (between the pleura)
intra	within	intraventricular (within ventricles)
intro	into, within	introversion (turning inward)
mal	bad, abnormal	malabsorption (bad absorption)
meta	beyond, after	metastasis (beyond original position)
micro	small	microelectrode (small electrode)
para	near	parathyroid (near the thyroid)
per	through	percutaneous (through the skin)
peri	around	peribronchial (around bronchus)
poly	many	polycythemia (many blood cells)
post	after, behind	postoperative (after operation)
pre	before, in front	premaxillary (in front of maxilla)
pro	before, in front	prognosis (foreknowledge)
re	back, again, contrary	regurgitation (backward flowing contrary to normal)
retro	backward, located behind	retrograde (going backward)
semi	half, partial	semipermeable (partially permeable)
sub	under	subarachnoid (under arachnoid)
super	above, upper, excessive	supernumerary (excessive number)
supra	above, upon	suprasternal (above sternum)
sym, syn	together, with	synapsis (joining together)
tachy	fast	tachycardia (fast heart rate)
trans	across, through	transection (cut across)
ultra	beyond, in excess	ultrasonic (sound waves beyond hearing)

shorthand for Latin words. A good example is bid (the abbreviation for the Latin *bis in die*), meaning twice a day. Many other medical abbreviations are acronyms. Acronyms are abbreviations formed from the initial letters of a series of words. COPD is a good example of an acronym, which is the abbreviation for <u>c</u>hronic <u>o</u>bstructive <u>p</u>ulmonary <u>d</u>isease. Usually, all letters in an acronym are capitalized.

Most of the abbreviations used in prescription writing are standardized. Unfortunately, most other medical abbreviations are not used as consistently. Variations in the use of these nonstandardized abbreviations occur between geographic regions, and even among hospitals within a given region. Nonetheless, there exists sufficient agreement on a number of medical abbreviations to include them here for review. Table 3-5 provides an alphabetical listing of these commonly accepted medical abbreviations along with their meanings.

Abbreviations used in respiratory care and pulmonary physiology

In the late 1940s the field of respiratory physiology experienced rapid growth. As in many new fields of study, the terms and abbreviations used by researchers were not standardized. This lack of standardization created substantial confusion and impeded effective communication in the scholarly publications and research articles that accompanied this emerging knowledge.

To minimize this confusion and achieve uniformity, a committee of researchers and scholars developed a set of standardized abbreviations to be used in respiratory physiology. Over the years, and with the cooperation of the American College of Chest Physicians and the American Thoracic Society, this set of standardized abbreviations or "pulmonary nomenclature" has undergone substantial modification and refinement, and is now generally well accepted as the basis for written communication in both pulmonary physiology and respiratory care.

There are four major categories of abbreviations in this system: (1) general abbreviations and usages, (2) abbreviations related to the gas phase, (3) abbreviations related to the blood phase, and (4) abbreviations used in assessing the mechanics of breathing.

General abbreviations. The following general abbreviations and usages are recognized:

P	pressure in general
V	volume in general
$\overline{X}$	dash above any symbol indicates a mean value, ie, $\overline{P}$ stands for the mean or average pressure
$\dot{X}$	dot above any symbol indicates a time derivative, ie, $\dot{V}$ stands for volume per unit of time, or flow
%X	percent sign preceding a symbol indicates percentage of the predicted normal value

X/Y%	percent sign following a symbol indicates a ratio function with the ratio expressed as a percentage; both components of the ratio must be designated, eg, $FEV_1/FEV\% = 100 \times FEV_1/FVC$
f	frequency of any event in time, eg, respiratory frequency = the number of breathing cycles per unit of time
t	time
anat	anatomic
max	maximum

Gas phase symbols. Gas phase abbreviations are divided into primary symbols and qualifying symbols. Primary symbols include the following:

V	gas volume in general; pressure, temperature, and percentage of saturation with water vapor must be stated
F	fractional concentration (usually in the dry gas phase)

Primary symbols are normally associated with a qualifying symbol, represented as either a small capital letter or a subscript. Qualifying symbols applicable to the gas phase include the following:

I	inspired
E	expired
A	alveolar
T	tidal
D	dead space
B	barometric
L	lung

Thus, P_B stands for barometric pressure (at a specified altitude); V_T is the accepted symbol for tidal volume; $\dot{V}_E$ the standard abbreviation for the volume of gas expired per minute; F_{IO_2} the proper term for the fractional concentration of inspired oxygen; and $\dot{V}_{CO_2}$ and $\dot{V}_{O_2}$ the appropriate symbols, respectively, for carbon dioxide production and oxygen consumption per minute.

Regarding the conditions of pressure, temperature, and humidity associated with gas phase measurements, the following standard abbreviations apply:

STPD	standard temperature and pressure, dry (These are the conditions of a volume of gas at 0°C at 760 mm Hg without water vapor.)
BTPS	body temperature (37°C), barometric pressure (at sea level = 760 mm Hg), and saturated with water vapor
ATPD	ambient temperature, pressure, dry
ATPS	ambient temperature and pressure, saturated with water vapor

By tradition, gas volumes in the lung are measured under BTPS conditions, whereas oxygen and carbon dioxide production per minute are measured at STPD. Methods used to convert from one condition of pressure, tempera-

Table 3-5   Common Medical Abbreviations

Abbreviation	Meaning	Abbreviation	Meaning
ABG	arterial blood gases	HCT, Hct	hematocrit
ac	before meals	Hg	mercury
ACTH	adrenocorticotropic hormone	HGB, Hgb, Hb	hemoglobin
ad lib	as desired	hs	at bedtime
ADH	antidiuretic hormone	ICF	intracellular fluid
AFB	acid-fast bacillus	I&D	incision and drainage
AP	anterior-posterior; anteroposterior	IM	intramuscular
ARDS	adult respiratory distress syndrome	IV	intravenously
ASD	atrial septal defect	kg	kilogram
ASHD	arteriosclerotic heart disease	L	liter
AV	atrioventricular	LAT, lat	lateral
BBB	bundle-branch block	lb	pound
BID, bid	twice a day	m	meter
BM	bowel movement	mcg	microgram
BMR	basal metabolic rate	MI	myocardial infarction
BP	blood pressure	ml	milliliter
BUN	blood urea nitrogen	mm	millimeter
bx	biopsy	NPO	nothing by mouth
C, °C	degrees Celsius, centigrade	od	once a day
c̄	with	OR	operating room
C-1	first cervical vertebra	os	mouth
CA, Ca	cancer	oz	ounce
CAD	coronary artery disease	PA	posteroanterior
CAT scan	computerized axial tomography	paren	parenterally
CBC	complete blood count	PAT	paroxysmal atrial tachycardia
CC	chief complaint	PC, pc	after meals
cc	cubic centimeter	PE	physical examination
CHF	congestive heart failure	PND	paroxysmal nocturnal dyspnea
cm	centimeter	PO, po	orally
CNS	central nervous system	prn	as required
COPD	chronic obstructive pulmonary disease	PT	prothrombin time
CPR	cardiopulmonary resuscitation	PVC	premature ventricular contraction
CSF	cerebrospinal fluid	q	every
CVA	cerebrovascular accident	qd	every day
CXR	chest x-ray; chest radiograph	qh	every hour
d	day (24 hours)	QID, qid	four times a day
/d	per day	qm	every morning
diff	white cell differential	qn	every night
Dx	diagnosis	RBC	red blood cell; red blood count
ECG, EKG	electrocardiogram	Rx	prescription
ECF	extracellular fluid	s̄	without
EEG	electroencephalogram	SOB	short(ness) of breath
EMG	electromyogram	Stat	immediately
ESR	erythrocyte sedimentation rate	subcu, SC	subcutaneous
F, °F	degrees Fahrenheit	T&A	tonsillectomy and adenoidectomy
FBS	fasting blood sugar	TB	tuberculosis
FEF	forced expiratory flow	TID, tid	three times a day
FEV	forced expiratory volume	top	topically
FHR	fetal heart rate	TPR	temperature, pulse, and respiration
FUO	fever of undetermined origin	UA	urinalysis
FVC	forced vital capacity	URI	upper respiratory infection
Fx	fracture	VC	vital capacity
GI	gastrointestinal	VSD	ventricular septal defect
Gm, gm	gram	WBC	white blood cell; white blood count
Gtt, gtt	drops	Wt	weight
GU	genitourinary	x	multiplied by
Gyn	gynecology		

ture, and humidity to another (eg, from BTPS to STPD) are discussed in the next chapter.

Blood phase symbols. Blood phase abbreviations also are divided into primary symbols and qualifying symbols. Primary symbols include the following:

Q	volume flow of blood
C	concentration in blood phase
S	saturation in blood phase

Unlike those used to describe the gas phase, qualifying symbols applicable to the blood phase are normally expressed as lower case letters. Blood phase qualifying symbols include the following:

b	blood in general (seldom used)
a	arterial (exact location to be specified in text when term is used)
v	venous (exact location to be specified in text when term is used)
$\bar{v}$	mixed venous (occurring after mixing in the heart)
c	capillary (exact location to be specified in text when term is used)
c′	pulmonary end-capillary
s	shunt

Thus, $C\bar{v}_{O_2}$ represents the concentration of oxygen in the mixed venous blood, Sa_{O_2} represents the saturation of hemoglobin with oxygen in the arterial blood, and $\dot{Q}c$ is the standard abbreviation for capillary blood flow per minute (location specified).

Combination of the general symbol for pressure (P) with the blood phase qualifying symbols is also common. For example:

Pa_{O_2}	arterial tension of oxygen, mm Hg
Pa_{CO_2}	arterial tension of carbon dioxide, mm Hg

Mechanics of breathing symbols. Most symbols used to represent measurements related to the mechanics of breathing are pressure terms, with the qualifying symbol designating the location of the pressure measurement. There are five basic locations for such pressure measurement:

P_{bs}	pressure at the body surface (equivalent to P_B)
P_{aw}	pressure at any point along the airways
P_{ao}	pressure at the airway opening, ie, mouth, nose, tracheal cannula
P_{pl}	pleural pressure: the pressure between the visceral and parietal pleura relative to atmospheric pressure
P_{alv}	pressure in the alveoli

These single measures may be combined to express a difference in pressure between two locations, as follows:

P_L	transpulmonary pressure, or the difference in pressure between the alveoli and pleural space ($P_L = P_{alv} - P_{pl}$)

P_W	transthoracic pressure, or the difference in pressure between the pleural space and the body surface ($P_W = P_{pl} - P_{bs}$)
P_{rs}	transrespiratory pressure, or the difference in pressure across the respiratory system ($P_{rs} = P_{alv} - P_{bs'}$ or $P_{rs} = P_L + P_W$)

SCIENTIFIC NOTATION AND MEASUREMENT PREFIXES

Scientific notation is a simple method of representing very large or very small numbers as powers of 10. This is accomplished by converting the number to an integer between 1 and 10 and then multiplying it by the appropriate power of 10.

To convert a number larger than 10 into scientific notation, the decimal is simply moved to the right of the first integer, and the new number is multiplied by 10 raised to the power equal to the number of places the decimal was moved. Zeros to the right of the last integer may be dropped. For example:

$$2655 = 2.655 \times 10^3$$
$$54,000 = 5.4 \times 10^4$$
$$301,010 = 3.0101 \times 10^5$$
$$866.67 = 8.6667 \times 10^2$$

To convert a number smaller than 1 into scientific notation, the decimal is moved to the right of the first integer, but the new number is multiplied by 10 raised to the negative power equal to the number of places the decimal was moved. For example:

$$0.454 = 4.54 \times 10^{-1}$$
$$0.00306 = 3.06 \times 10^{-3}$$
$$0.00000703 = 7.03 \times 10^{-6}$$
$$0.01010 = 1.01 \times 10^{-2}$$

Powers of 10 also are used in defining multiples and divisions of both measurement units in decimal-base systems. As depicted in Table 3-6, multiple prefixes are represented in Greek and fractional prefixes in Latin. The following examples of selected linear, volumetric, and mass measures demonstrate the use of these prefixes:

Linear measure	
kilometer (km)	$m \times 10^3$
meter (m)	
decimeter (dm)	$m \times 10^{-1}$
centimeter (cm)	$m \times 10^{-2}$
millimeter (mm)	$m \times 10^{-3}$
micrometer (μm)	$m \times 10^{-6}$
namometer (nm)	$m \times 10^{-9}$
Volume	
liter (L)	
deciliter (dL)	$L \times 10^{-1}$

Volume

milliliter (ml)	$L \times 10^{-3}$
microliter (μl)	$L \times 10^{-6}$
nanoliter (nl)	$L \times 10^{-9}$

Mass

kilogram (kg)	$g \times 10^{3}$
gram (g)	
milligram (mg)	$g \times 10^{-3}$
microgram (μg)	$g \times 10^{-6}$
nanogram (ng)	$g \times 10^{-9}$

UNITS OF MEASURE

Measurement represents a central component of both basic and applied science. Ideally, the same system should be used by both scientists and clinicians worldwide to measure, describe, and communicate physical events. Unfortunately, this ideal situation does not exist. Indeed, currently there are at least three primary systems of scientific measurement used in the clinical setting. If the apothecary and avoirdupois systems used in pharmacy were added, clinicians would have to master five different systems of measure!

Table 3-6 Standard Units Prefixes

Term	Abbreviation	Power of 10
deka	da	10^{1}
hecto	h	10^{2}
kilo	k	10^{3}
mega	M	10^{6}
giga	G	10^{9}
tera	T	10^{12}
deci	d	10^{-1}
centi	c	10^{-2}
milli	m	10^{-3}
micro	μ	10^{-6}
nano	n	10^{-9}
pico	p	10^{-12}
femto	f	10^{-15}
atto	a	10^{-18}

Measurement systems

Historically, two significantly different systems were developed separately in Great Britain and continental Europe. The British or Imperial system of measure—adopted early by the U.S.—is based on the foot (length), pound (mass), and second (time). For this reason, the British system is often referred to as the fps system. During the French revolution, a separate system of measure was developed on the continent. The basic units in this decimal-based system were the centimeter (length), gram (mass), and second (time). This system is often referred to as the cgs system.

In 1960, worldwide efforts were initiated to adopt a single standard, referred to as "Le Systeme International d'Unites" or SI system. SI units represent a simple modification of those used in the cgs system. Length is based on the meter instead of the centimeter, and mass is based on the kilogram instead of the gram. Seconds remain as the time standard, with electric current expressed in amperes, temperature in degrees Kelvin, and the chemical amount of substance designated in moles. Other SI units of measure are derived from the base units described. For example, the SI unit for force is the newton (N), and the unit for work or energy is the joule (J). Based on its primary units for length, mass, and time, the SI system is also known as the meter-kilogram-second or mks system. Table 3-7 compares the major units of measure used in the SI, cgs, and fps systems.

Since both systems are decimal-based, the changeover from the cgs to the SI system is relatively easy. However, given the nondecimal nature of the fps system, "metrification" generally has not fully succeeded in the U.S. For this reason the practitioner is still faced with the need to work with a variety of different units of measure in clinical practice. This skill often requires the clinician to convert units between these systems.

Unit conversions

The ability to convert units between these systems requires knowledge of several conversion factors. For exam-

Table 3-7 The Three Measurement Systems

Quantity	SI	cgs	fps
Length	meter (m)	centimeter (cm)	foot (ft)
Volume	cubic meter	cubic centimeter	cubic foot
Time	second (s)	second (s)	second (s)
Mass	kilogram (kg)	gram (g)	slug
Velocity	m/s	cm/s	ft/s
Acceleration	m/s^2	cm/s^2	ft/s^2
Force	newton (N) (kg·m/s^2)	dyne (gm·cm/s^2)	pound (lb) (slug·ft/s^2)
Pressure	pascal (Pa) (N/m^2)	dyne/cm^2	lb/ft^2
Work, energy	joule (J) (N·m)	erg (dyne·cm)	ft·lb
Power	watt (W) (joule/s)	erg/s	ft·lb/s

ple, the factor to convert inches (fps) to centimeters (cgs) is 2.54. Given a patient's height of 72 inches, conversion to centimeters is accomplished simply by multiplying the old unit times the conversion factor:

$$\text{old unit} \times \text{conversion factor} = \text{new unit}$$
$$72 \text{ in} \times 2.54 \text{ cm/in} = 182.88 \text{ cm}$$

The following sections provide factor tables useful in converting common measures of length, volume, mass, weight, force, pressure, work (and energy), and power between the three primary measurement systems used in clinical practice. Although not all table factors need be committed to memory, the respiratory care practitioner must be proficient in the use of selected conversions at the bedside. For this reason, these "must know" conversion factors are emphasized whenever appropriate.

Length. Table 3-8 provides the factors needed to convert common measures of length among the three measurement systems. To use the table, first identify the row for which the old unit equals "1." Using this row, find the conversion factor under the column for the new unit. Then use the above equation to make the conversion. For example, to convert 6 feet to centimeters, find the row where foot = 1 (the third row). Then find the conversion factor under the centimeter column in the third row (30.48). Then apply the above equation:

$$\text{old unit} \times \text{conversion factor} = \text{new unit}$$
$$6 \text{ feet} \times 30.48 \text{ cm/ft} = 182.88 \text{ cm}$$

The most common length conversions in clinical practice are between inches and centimeters. For this reason, practitioners should commit to memory the following two conversions:

$$\text{inches} \times 2.54 \text{ (cm/in)} = \text{centimeters}$$
$$\text{centimeters} \times 0.3937 \text{ (in/cm)} = \text{inches}$$

Volume. The standard units of volume in all systems are based on the cube of their length standards, that is, the cubic meter (m^3), cubic centimeter (cm^3 or cc), and cubic foot (ft^3). Related measures are the liter (L), the milliliter (ml), the cubic inch (in^3), and the gallon (US). Table 3-9 provides the factors needed to convert these common volumetric measures between measurement systems. Use this table as described above.

The most common volume conversions in clinical practice are between liters and milliliters (or cm^3), liters and cubic feet, cubic feet and gallons, and liters and gallons. For this reason, practitioners should commit to memory the following conversions:

$$\text{liters} \times 1000 \text{ (ml/L)} = \text{milliliters (or } cm^3)$$
$$\text{milliliters}/1000 \text{ (ml/L)} = \text{liters}$$
$$\text{cubic feet} \times 28.32 \text{ (L/ft}^3) = \text{liters}$$
$$\text{cubic feet} \times 7.48 \text{ (gallon/ft}^3) = \text{gallons}$$
$$\text{gallons} \times 3.785 \text{ (L/gallon)} = \text{liters}$$

Mass and weight. Mass and weight are the two most commonly confused concepts in scientific measurement. Mass represents an absolute quantity of matter. The standard unit of mass in the SI system is the kilogram (kg), with the gram (g) the accepted measure in the cgs system. In the fps system the standard unit of mass is the slug.

Weight, on the other hand, is a relative measure of mass times the acceleration due to gravity:

$$\text{weight} = \text{mass (M)} \times \text{acceleration due to gravity (G)}$$
$$\text{weight} = M \times G$$

Thus the mass of an object remains the same regardless of its position relative to the earth. However, the weight of the same object will change according to the nature of the gravitational field in which it is positioned. For example, although your mass on the earth is the same as on the

Table 3-8   Length Conversion Factors

Meter (m)	Centimeter (cm)	Foot (ft)	Inch (in)
1	100	3.28	39.37
.01	1	.0328	.3937
.3048	30.48	1	12
.0254	2.54	.0833	1

Table 3-9   Volume Conversion Factors

m^3	cm^3*	liter (L)	ft^3	in^3	gallons (US)
1	10^6	1000	35.315	61024	264.2
10^{-6}	1	.001	.000035	.0610	.00026
.001	1000	1	.0353	61.00	.2642
.0283	28,316	28.32	1	1728	7.481
.000016	16.387	.0164	.0006	1	.00433
.0038	3785	3.785	0.1337	231	1

*One cubic centimeter (cm^3) approximately equal to a milliliter (ml).

moon, your weight is approximately two thirds less on the moon because of its weaker gravitational field.

On the earth's surface, the acceleration due to gravity is a constant at any given altitude. For example, at sea level the acceleration due to gravity is measured as 9.807 m/s^2 (SI), 980.67 cm/s^2 (cgs), or 32.174 ft/s^2 (fps). Since the acceleration due to gravity is a constant at a given altitude, the weight and the mass of an object are directly proportional to each other. For this reason, it is common practice to interchange weight and mass units.

Table 3-10 compares the weights of common mass units at sea level, including the kilogram (SI) and gram (cgs). Although limited in use, the fps measure of mass (the slug) also is provided for completeness. The avoirdupois pound and ounce are also included here, although we shall see in the next section that these are actually measures of force. Application of this table is described above.

The most common weight conversions in clinical practice are between kilograms and grams, and pounds and kilograms. Practitioners should commit to memory the following weight conversions:

$$\text{kilograms} \times 1000 \text{ (g/kg)} = \text{grams}$$
$$\text{grams}/1000 \text{ (kg/g)} = \text{kilograms}$$
$$\text{pounds} \times 0.454 \text{ (kg/lb)} = \text{kilograms}$$
$$\text{kilograms} \times 2.205 \text{ (lb/kg)} = \text{pounds}$$

Force. Newton's second law of motion tells us that the acceleration of an object is directly proportional to the force exerted and inversely proportional to its mass:

$$\text{acceleration (A)} = \frac{\text{force (F)}}{\text{mass (M)}}$$

Rearranging the equation to solve for force (F):

$$\text{force (F)} = \text{mass (M)} \times \text{acceleration (A)}$$
$$F = M \times A$$

Thus force is a measure of mass times acceleration. In the SI system, the unit of force is the newton (N), where $1 \text{ N} = 1 \text{ kg} \times \text{m/s}^2$. The cgs unit of force is the dyne ($1 \text{ gm} \times \text{cm/s}^2$) whereas the fps unit of force is the pound (lb) (1

slug $\times \text{ft/s}^2$). Table 3-11 compares the common units of force in the SI, cgs, and fps systems. Use of this table is described in the preceding column.

As previously discussed, the pound is also commonly used as a measure of weight. This is because weight represents a special case of force, with the acceleration factor simply that due to gravity:

$$\text{force (F)} = \text{mass (M)} \times \text{acceleration (A)}$$
$$\text{weight} = \text{mass (M)} \times \text{acceleration due to gravity}$$

Pressure. Pressure is a measure of force per unit area, where area is the square of the length standard. Therefore pressure in the SI system is expressed as Newtons per square meter (N/m^2), a unit of measure called the pascal (Pa). The cgs unit of pressure is simply the dyne/cm^2. Although the standard fps unit of pressure is the lb/ft^2, it is more common to express pressure in this system as lb/in^2. Table 3-12 lists the factors needed to convert these common pressure units between measurement systems.

With one exception (lb/in^2), pressure measurements in clinical practice seldom use these units. Instead, pressure frequently is expressed in terms of the height of a column of fluid, such as centimeters of water (cm H_2O) or millimeters of mercury (mm Hg). More detail on this application of pressure measurement is provided in Chapter 4.

Work and energy. Mechanical work is a measure of the force exerted on an object over a given distance. Therefore the SI unit of work is the newton-meters (N $\times$ m), also called the joule (J). The cgs unit of work is the dyne-cm (dynes $\times$ cm) or erg. The standard fps unit of work is the foot-lb (lb $\times$ ft).

According to the first law of thermodynamics, the internal energy of an object must be equal to the work done on that object (externally) plus the heat transferred to that object (internally) by a substance existing at a higher temperature:

$$\text{internal energy} = \text{work done} + \text{heat energy transferred}$$

According to this formula, the same change in internal energy of an object could be achieved by either (1) perform-

Table 3-10   Weight Conversion Factors*

Kilogram (k)	Gram (g)	Slug†	Pound (lb)	Ounce (oz)
1	1000	.0685	2.205	35.28
.001	1	.00007	.0022	.0353
14.59	14594	1	32.174	514.78
.454	453.60	32.174	1	16
.0284	28.35	.0020	.063	1

*Where $g = 9.807 \text{ m/s}^2$ or 32.174 ft/s^2 (sea level).

†Although the slug is the standard unit of mass in the fps system, its use is no longer common. Instead, the pound is used as the measure of mass, weight (and force) in this system. At sea level ($g = 32.174 \text{ ft/s}^2$) 1 slug is equal to 32.174 lb.

ing work on the object or (2) heating the object. Thus, in physical terms, heat energy and work energy are synonymous terms. Therefore the same units of measure can be applied to both work and heat energy, that is the joule (SI), erg (cgs), or ft-lb (fps).

However, heat energy in the cgs and fps systems is not commonly expressed in these units. Instead, the cgs system uses the calorie (cal), and the fps system the British Thermal Unit or BTU. A calorie is defined as the quantity of heat required to raise the temperature of 1 g water from 14.5° to 15.5°C. A BTU is the amount of heat required to raise the temperature of 1 lb water 1°F. One BTU equals 252 calories. Table 3-13 provides the factors needed to convert both mechanical work and thermal energy units between the measurement systems.

Power. Power is a measure of the amount of work done over a period of time. Thus the SI unit of power is the joule per second (J/s), termed the watt (W). The cgs unit of power is the erg/s (dyne-cm/s), whereas the standard fps unit of power is the foot-lb/s. Table 3-14 provides the factors needed to convert between these units of power.

SUMMARY

As in most health professions, the clinical practice of respiratory care involves extensive observation and communication. Accurate and consistent observation and communication among health professionals requires a common frame of reference. This common frame of reference is embodied in various systems of clinical communication and measurement.

The language of medicine, or medical terminology, provides consistent meanings between diverse groups of health professionals, thereby facilitating communication and interaction. Complementing medical terminology is a system of abbreviations, used extensively in charting and medical record keeping. Unlike most abbreviations, those used in pulmonary physiology and respiratory care generally are well accepted and standardized. Effective clinical interaction demands that respiratory care practitioners master and apply these terms and symbols in consistent ways.

The purpose of a measurement system is to measure, describe, and communicate physical events. Unfortunately, at least three primary systems of scientific measurement are used in the clinical setting, namely, the Systeme International d'Unites (SI) system, the centimeter-gram-second (cgs) system, and the British foot-pound-second (fps) system. Until complete standardization on the SI systems occurs in the U.S., respiratory care practitioners must be adept in working with all three measurement approaches.

Table 3-11   Force Conversion Factors

Newton (N)	Dyne	Pound (lb)
1	100,000	.2249
.00001	1	.000045
4.45	445,000	1

Table 3-12   Pressure Conversion Factors

Pascal (Pa)	Dyne/cm^2	Lb/ft^2	Lb/in^2
1	10	.0209	.00015
0.1	1	.0021	.000015
47.88	478.80	1	.0609
6895	68950	144	1

Table 3-14   Power Conversion Factors

Watts	Erg/s	Ft-lb/s
1	10,000,000	.7376
.0000001	1	*
1.356	13,560,000	1

*Less than 10^{-7}.

Table 3-13   Work and Energy Conversion Factors

Joule (J)	Erg (dyne-cm)	Ft-lb	Calorie	BTU
1	10^7	.7376	.2389	.00095
10^{-7}	1	*	*	*
1.356	1.36×10^7	1	.3239	.0013
4.186	4.19×10^7	3.09	1	.00397
1055	1.06×10^9	778.68	252	1

*Less than 10^{-7}.

BIBLIOGRAPHY

Cotes JE: SI units in respiratory medicine, Am Rev Respir Dis 112:753-755, 1975.

Glanze WD, editor: Mosby's medical and nursing dictionary, ed 3, St Louis, 1986, The CV Mosby Co.

Gylys BA and Wedding ME: Medical terminology: a systems approach, ed 2, Philadelphia, 1988, FA Davis Co.

Nave CR and Nave BC: Physics for the health sciences, ed 3, Philadelphia, 1985, WB Saunders Co.

(Pappenheimer Committee) Standardization of definitions and symbols in respiratory physiology, Fed Proc 9:602, 1950.

Pulmonary terms and symbols: a report of the ACCP-ATS Joint Committee on Pulmonary Nomenclature, Chest 67:583, 1975.

Riggs JH: Respiratory facts, Philadelphia, 1989, FA Davis Co.

US Department of Commerce, National Bureau of Standards: The English and metric systems of measurement, Special Pub 304A, rev ed, 1970.

Vawter SM and DeForest RE: The international metric system and medicine, JAMA 218:723, 1971.

Young DS: Standardized reporting of laboratory data, N Engl J Med 290:368, 1974.

4

Physical Principles in Respiratory Care

Craig L. Scanlan

As a field of applied scientific and clinical study, respiratory care has a strong technologic base. Much of the technology involved in the delivery of respiratory care services is based on the application of basic physical principles. The branch of science involved in the study of the physical principles that govern the world around us is called physics.

Physics is further divided into several branches, including the properties of matter, thermodynamics (heat and energy), mechanics, sound, electricity, magnetism, and light. Although all these areas of physics affect the technology of respiratory care, an understanding of some key principles involving the properties of matter, thermodynamics, and mechanics is an essential prerequisite to further study.

OBJECTIVES

This chapter focuses on the application of selected physical principles in respiratory care. Specifically, on completion of this chapter, the reader will be able to:

1. Differentiate among the three primary states of matter, with special emphasis on the physical properties of fluids (liquids and gases);

2. Relate the concepts of heat transfer and change of state to the internal energy of matter and the measurement of temperature;

3. Relate the concept of vaporization to the presence of water vapor in gases and gas mixtures and its quantification as "humidity";

4. Apply the standard laws of gas behavior to explain changes in the temperature, pressure, volume, or mass of an ideal gas;

5. Explain how the behavior of gases deviates from ideal under extremes of pressure and temperature;

6. Relate the key principle of hydrodynamics to the behavior of fluids in motion and their application in respiratory care.

KEY TERMS

Most terms used in this chapter are defined in context. The following terms are introduced without explicit definition, but may be found in the text glossary.

aerosol	equilibrium
agitate	evacuate
ambient	homogenous
anesthetic	infrared
combustible	lateral
concave	orifice
concentric	plasma
constriction	vacuum
convex	

STATES OF MATTER

There are three primary states of matter: solid, liquid, and gas. Fig. 4-1 provides a schematic representation of the differences among these three states of matter.

The solid state is characterized by a high degree of internal order in which the positions of the atoms or molecules are more or less fixed. As depicted in Fig. 4-1, *A*, it is useful to consider the atoms of a solid as held together by a system of springs, their movement being restricted to back-and-forth motion about an equilibrium position. This structure is maintained by the presence of mutual attractive forces between the atoms, called van der Waals forces. These attractive forces in solids are strong enough to ensure that they will retain their shape and not readily conform to the shape of their surroundings.

Like the atoms or molecules of a solid, those in the *liquid* state also exhibit strong mutual attractive forces. These cohesive forces among liquid molecules are responsible for such phenomena as surface tension and viscosity (discussed later). However, unlike those characterizing solids, the attractive forces in liquids do not restrict molecular motion about an equilibrium point. Instead, the molecules of a liquid are free to move about relative to one another

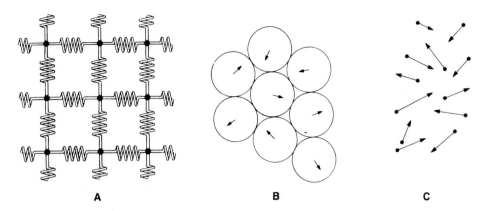

Fig. 4-1   Simplified models of the three states of matter. **A,** Solid. **B,** Liquid. **C,** Gas.   (From Nave CR and Nave BC: Physics for the health sciences, ed 3, Philadelphia, 1985, WB Saunders Co.)

(Fig. 4-1, *B*). This freedom of motion among liquid molecules explains why matter in this state flows readily and tends to take the shape of its container. Nonetheless, the molecules of both solids and liquids are quite dense and cannot be easily compressed.

The gas phase of matter invokes an impression of nothingness until we become aware of the tremendous activity of its components. In a gas, the attractive forces between atoms or molecules are negligible. Lacking restriction to their movement, these molecules exhibit rapid, random motion that is characterized by frequent collisions (Fig. 4-1, *C*). Thus, unlike a solid or liquid, a gas has no inherent boundaries and can be readily compressed and expanded. However, like liquids, gases are capable of flow. For this reason, both liquids and gases are considered fluids.

Internal energy of matter

All matter has energy. The energy inherent in matter is called internal energy. There are two primary forms of internal energy: (1) the energy of position, or potential energy, and (2) the energy of motion, or kinetic energy.

At ordinary temperatures the atoms or molecules of solids, liquids, and gases all exhibit continuous motion. Thus all matter exhibits some degree of kinetic energy. In both the solid and the liquid states, however, most of the internal energy of matter is in the form of potential energy. This potential energy is associated with the intermolecular forces of attraction that contribute the characteristics of rigidity to solids and of cohesiveness and viscosity to liquids. On the other hand, because the intermolecular forces of attraction among gas molecules are negligible, essentially all the internal energy of a gas is in the form of kinetic energy.

Internal energy and temperature

The temperature of a substance represents a measure of its internal energy. With essentially all of its internal energy expended in the maintenance of molecular motion, the temperature of a gas is a direct measure of its average kinetic energy.

Because of the potential energy associated with their intermolecular forces of attraction, the energy picture is more complicated in the case of solids and liquids. Although still a measure of average kinetic energy, the temperature of a solid or liquid represents only a portion of its total energy and is thus only indirectly proportional to its internal energy.

Absolute zero. In concept, there should exist a temperature at which all kinetic activity of matter ceases. This temperature, called absolute zero, is a theoretic value arrived at by projection and calculation. Although researchers have come close to approximating absolute zero, it has never been achieved.

Temperature scales. Obviously, the state of no kinetic activity provides a logical zero point on which to build a temperature scale. The SI units used to measure temperature are based on the Kelvin scale, which has a zero point equivalent to absolute zero ($0°K$). Because the Kelvin scale is calibrated to have $100°$ between the measured freezing and the measured boiling points of water, it is considered a centigrade (100-step) system of temperature measurement.

The cgs system for temperature measurement is based on Celsius units ($°C$). Like the Kelvin scale, the Celsius scale has $100°$ between the freezing and boiling points of water and is thus a centigrade scale. However, the zero point of the Celsius scale is not absolute zero; instead, it represents the freezing point of water ($0°C$).

In Celsius units, kinetic molecular activity stops at about $-273°C$. Thus $0°K = -273°C$ and $0°C = 273°K$. Conversion between Kelvin and Celsius units is therefore accomplished with the following simple formula:

$$°K = °C + 273$$

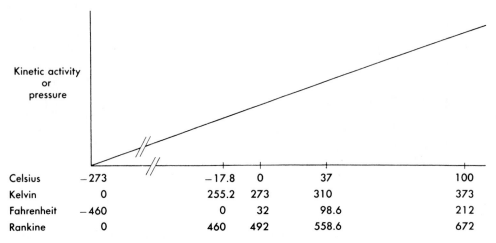

Fig. 4-2 Linear relationship between gas molecular activity, or pressure, and temperature. Comparable readings of the four scales are indicated for five temperature points.

To convert degrees Celsius to degrees Kelvin, one simply adds 273. For example:

$$25°C = 25 + 273 = 298°K$$
$$37°C = 37 + 273 = 310°K$$
$$-15°C = -15 + 273 = 258°K$$

To convert degrees Kelvin to degrees Celsius, one simply subtracts 273:

$$310°K = 310 - 273 = 37°C$$
$$373°K = 373 - 273 = 100°C$$
$$0°K = 0 - 273 = -273°C$$

In the fps or British system of measurement, either the Fahrenheit or the Rankine scale is used. Since it is neither an absolute nor a centigrade-based temperature system, the familiar Fahrenheit scale is used minimally in scientific measurement. Ironically, however, it still is retained in many U.S. hospitals as the primary system of temperature measurement. Absolute zero on the Fahrenheit scale is equivalent to −460°F.

The following formula is used to convert degrees Fahrenheit to degrees Celsius:

$$°C = \tfrac{5}{9}(°F - 32)$$

For example:

$$°F = 98.6$$
$$°C = \tfrac{5}{9}(98.6 - 32)$$
$$°C = \tfrac{5}{9}(66.6)$$
$$°C = 37$$

Obviously, in the conversion of degrees Celsius back to degrees Fahrenheit, the previous formula is reversed:

$$°F = (\tfrac{9}{5} \times °C) + 32$$

For example:

$$°C = 100$$
$$°F = (\tfrac{9}{5} \times 100) + 32$$
$$°F = (180) + 32$$
$$°F = 212$$

The Rankine scale is used frequently in engineering but rarely in medical science. Like the Kelvin scale, the Rankine scale has a zero point equivalent to absolute zero and is therefore considered an absolute scale of temperature measurement. However, the Rankine scale is based on Fahrenheit units. Thus 0°R = −460°F, and °R = °F + 460.

Fig. 4-2 provides a graphic portrayal of the relationship between the kinetic activity of matter and of temperature with all four temperature scales. For ease of reference, five key points are defined. These include the zero point of each scale (absolute zero for the Kelvin and Rankine scales), the freezing point of water (0°C), body temperature (37°C), and the boiling point of water (100°C).

Heat capacity and specific heat. Heat capacity refers to the number of calories required to raise the temperature of 1 g of a substance 1°C or 1 pound of a substance 1°F. By definition, the heat capacity of water is 1 calorie in the metric system and 1 BTU in the British fps system.

Specific heat represents a ratio between the amount of heat required to raise the temperature of 1 g of a substance 1°C or 1 pound of a substance 1°F at a specific temperature and the amount of heat required to raise the temperature of 1 g of water 1°C or 1 pound of water 1°F at the specified temperature. Numerically, specific heat is equal to heat capacity in either of the systems. However, because it is a ratio, it is a pure number with no inherent dimensions and has the same meaning in any system of units.

For example, the specific heat of hydrogen, measured at 1 atm and 21°C, is 3.41. This means that it takes 3.41

times as much heat to raise the gas temperature of hydrogen as that of water—3.41 calories for 1 g of gas as compared with 1 calorie for 1 g of water.

Because specific heat is among the data frequently provided for medical and commercial gases, special mention should be made of the two ways in which it can be measured. First, the specific heat can be calculated by heating a constant volume of a gas, in which case the heat energy applied is transformed into increasing molecular energy. Second, the heated gas may be kept at a constant pressure, as in a flexible container; in this instance, because the expanding gas performs work (uses up heat) in displacing the surrounding atmosphere, more energy is required to bring the gas to the specific temperature. Therefore, a gas has two specific heats—that of constant volume (C_V) and that of constant pressure (C_P), which is larger. In the previous example of hydrogen, the C_V is 2.40 whereas the C_P value is 3.41. When gases are stored in cylinders, the specific heat at a constant volume (C_V) is the measure most frequently used.

Heat and the first law of thermodynamics

The first law of thermodynamics, or the law of conservation of energy, states that in any physical process energy can be neither created nor destroyed but only transformed in nature. Thus the energy gained by a substance in a physical process must exactly equal the energy lost by its surroundings. Conversely, if a substance loses internal energy, this must be offset by a gain in the energy of its surroundings.

In mathematical terms, the first law of thermodynamics may be formulated as follows:

$$U = E + W$$

where U equals the internal energy of an object, E equals the energy transferred to (or taken away from) the object by a body existing at a different temperature, and W equals the external work done on the object. In this sense, the quantity E is equivalent to heat. Thus heating is the transfer of internal energy from a high-temperature object to a lower-temperature object.

According to this formula, the internal energy of an object may be increased by heating it, by performing work on it, or both. In any case, an increase in the internal energy of an object must be accompanied by either a loss of heat from the surroundings or the external application of work. Here we are interested in the first physical phenomenon, that is, the transfer of heat.

Heat transfer

When a temperature gradient exists between two objects, the first law of thermodynamics tells us that heat will tend to move from the object of high temperature to the object of low temperature until their temperatures are equal. Two objects that are at the same temperature are said to be in thermal equilibrium.

This transfer of internal energy may occur by one or more of three primary mechanisms: (1) conduction, (2) convection, or (3) radiation. Heat transfer may also occur through the process of evaporation and condensation.

Conduction. Conduction is the primary means by which heat transfer occurs in solids. Conduction is defined as the transfer of heat by the direct interaction of atoms or molecules in a hot area that contact atoms or molecules in a cooler area. The efficiency of heat transfer by conduction depends on the number of collisions between the atoms or molecules per unit of time and the amount of energy transferred during each collision.

The efficiency of heat transfer between objects is quantified by a measure called thermal conductivity. In cgs units, thermal conductivity is measured in (cal/s)/(cm^2 × °C/cm). As evident in Table 4-1, solids, particularly metals, exhibit the highest coefficients of thermal conductivity. This is the reason metals feel cold to the touch, even at room temperature. In this case, their high thermal conductivity quickly draws heat away from the skin and creates a feeling of "cold." On the other hand, gases tend to be poor heat conductors. This is due mainly to the smaller number of molecular collisions per unit of time that occur in the gaseous state.

Convection. Convection represents the primary means by which heat transfer occurs in fluids, both liquids and gases. Heat transfer by convection involves the mixing of fluid molecules at different temperature states. For example, although air is a poor heat conductor, it can be used to efficiently transfer heat by convection if it is first warmed

Table 4-1   Thermal Conductivities in (cal×s)/(cm^2°C/cm)

Material	Thermal conductivity (k)
Silver	1.01
Copper	0.99
Aluminum	0.50
Iron	0.163
Lead	0.083
Ice	0.005
Glass, ordinary	0.0025
Concrete	0.002
Water at 20°C	0.0014
Asbestos	0.0004
Hydrogen at 0°C	0.0004
Helium at 0°C	0.0003
Snow (dry)	0.00026
Fiberglass	0.00015
Cork board	0.00011
Wool felt	0.0001
Air at 0°C	0.000057

From Nave CR and Nave BC: Physics for the health sciences, ed 3, Philadelphia, 1985, WB Saunders Co.

in one location and then circulated to carry the heat elsewhere. This is the principle that underlies forced-air heating in houses and convection heating in infant incubators. The movements of fluids that carry heat energy are called convection currents.

Radiation. The transfer of heat by radiation occurs in a manner substantially different from that characterizing either conduction or convection. In both conduction and convection, energy transfer can occur only by direct contact between atoms or molecules. Radiant heat transfer, however, occurs without direct contact between the warmer and cooler substances. Indeed, heat transfer by radiation can occur even in a vacuum, as evident in the radiant warming of the earth by the sun.

Thus radiant energy is similar in concept to light energy. Radiant energy given off by objects at room temperature is mainly in the infrared frequency range, whereas such objects as an electric burner on a stove or a kerosene heater radiate some of their energy in the form of visible light. Radiant warmers are used commonly to maintain the body temperature of newborn infants in the nursery.

The radiant heat loss or gain of an object in a given time period may be quantified according to the following formula:

$$\frac{E}{t} = ekA(T_2 - T_1)$$

where E is the heat loss or gain; t is the time period; e is the relative effectiveness of the object as a radiator, referred to as its "emissivity"; k is a constant related to mass and surface area (the Stefan-Boltzman constant); A is the area radiating; and T_1 and T_2 equal, respectively, the temperature of the environment and the temperature of the object. In simple terms, for an object with a given emissivity, the larger the radiating surface area and the lower the surrounding environmental temperature (relative to the object's temperature), the greater will be the radiant heat loss per unit of time.

Vaporization. Vaporization is the process whereby matter in its liquid form is changed into a gas. To effect this change of state, heat energy is needed. According to the first law of thermodynamics, this heat energy must be supplied externally from the surroundings. In one form of vaporization, called evaporation, this heat is taken from the air immediately adjacent to the liquid, thereby cooling the surrounding air. In warm weather or during strenuous exercise, the body takes advantage of this "evaporation cooling" effect by producing sweat, which, on evaporation, cools the skin.

The opposite process, whereby the gaseous or vaporous form of a substance is changed back into its liquid state, is called condensation. Whereas vaporization causes heat to be taken from the air immediately adjacent to the liquid, condensation results in heat being "given back" to the surroundings. More details on change of state in general and on vaporization and condensation in particular are provided in the next section.

CHANGE OF STATE

All matter can change from a solid to a liquid to a gas. This process is called a change of state. In respiratory care, we deal mainly with the so-called "permanent" gases because, under normal ambient conditions, they exist solely in the gaseous state. Nonetheless, depending on the pressures or temperatures to which they are exposed, these same gases can also be in the liquid or solid forms. Indeed, as we shall see, for ease of transportation and storage, it is often convenient to transform these permanent gases into their liquid state. Thus it is important that respiratory care practitioners understand the basic physical processes involved in matter's change of state. Moreover, as each phase change is described, we will focus on a few essential characteristics of each state of matter.

Liquid-solid phase changes (melting and freezing)

The application of heat to a solid body increases the kinetic energy of its atoms or molecules. This added internal energy causes more agitated vibrations of the atoms or molecules. If enough heat is added, the molecular activity will eventually be sufficient to weaken the mutually attractive forces between the molecules, free them from their relatively rigid structure, and convert the substance into a liquid.

Melting. The breakdown of this rigid structure corresponds to melting. A solid will convert to its liquid form at a given temperature known as its melting point. The range of melting points is considerable. For example, water (ice) has a melting point of 0°C, carbon more than 3500°C, and helium less than −272.2°C.

Fig. 4-3 depicts the phase change caused by the application of heat (in calories) to water, beginning on the left at the origin of −50°C, where water exists as a solid (ice). As heat energy is applied to the ice, there occurs a simultaneous rise in its temperature. At 0°C, the change in state from solid ice to liquid water begins. At melting point, however, additional heat energy does *not* immediately change the water temperature.

The additional heat energy needed to effect the changeover from solid to liquid is referred to as the latent heat of fusion. In the cgs system, the latent heat of fusion is defined as the calories required to change 1 g of the substance from the solid to the liquid state without changing its temperature. The term latent means that the heat energy is used solely to melt the substance, without changing its temperature. To give some idea of the diversity of energy needed for this change in state, the latent heat of fusion of ice is 80 cal/g, calcium chloride is 54 cal/g, and oxygen is 3.3 cal/g. As compared to the process of simply raising the temperature of the solid, this change of phase requires a large amount of internal energy.

Freezing. Freezing is the reverse of melting. Because considerable external energy is used in transforming a solid into a liquid, this energy must be reclaimed by the surroundings during the process of freezing. Thus freezing

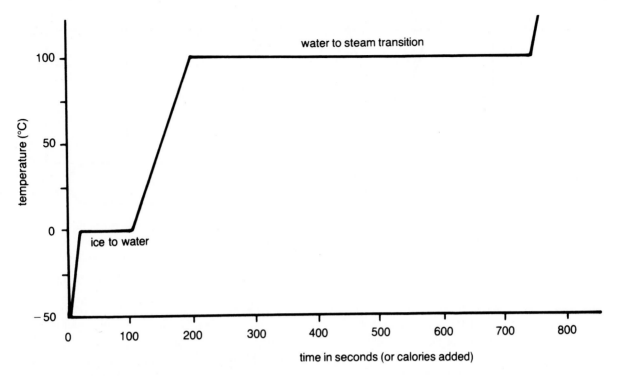

Fig. 4-3   Temperature as a function of time for 1 g of water to which heat is added at the rate of 1 cal/s. (From Nave CR and Nave BC: Physics for the health sciences, ed 3, Philadelphia, 1985, WB Saunders Co.)

represents the transfer of heat energy from a liquid back to the environment, usually by exposure to cold. As the kinetic energy of the substance decreases, its molecules begin to regain the stable configuration of a solid mass. According to the first law of thermodynamics, the energy required to effect this freezing process must be the same as that needed to cause melting. Thus the freezing and melting points of a substance are the same.

Properties of liquids

As discussed previously, because of the weakening of the intermolecular attractive forces caused by melting, liquids exhibit the properties of a fluid. Specifically, liquids can flow and tend to take the shape of their containers. Because a liquid takes the shape of its container but cannot be easily compressed, it will tend to exert a supporting force on the liquid above it. Because of this effect, liquids exert both pressure and buoyant force.

Although the intermolecular forces of attraction are weakened in the changeover from the solid to the liquid phase, liquid molecules still are attracted to one another. The relative strength of these cohesive forces among liquid molecules explain such phenomena as viscosity, capillary action, and surface tension.

Pressure in liquids. The pressure exerted by a liquid is directly proportional to the depth of the liquid and its density. Mathematically, this relationship may be expressed in the following equation:

$$P_l = dgh$$

where P_l is the static pressure exerted by the liquid, d is the density of the liquid, g is the acceleration due to gravity, and h is the height of the liquid column.

Density (d) is a measure of the mass per unit volume of a substance. Given the proportionality between mass and weight at a given distance from the earth's surface (refer to Chapter 3), density is usually expressed as weight per unit volume, called weight density or d_w. Since, under most clinical conditions, $d_w = d \times g$, use of weight density allows simplification of the above equation to the following:

$$P_l = d_w \times h$$

In the cgs system, weight density is most often measured in grams per cubic centimeter (g/cm^3) for solids and liquids and in grams per liter (g/L) for gases. As an example, the pressure exerted by water at the bottom of a 33.9 foot (1034 cm) column would be calculated as:

$$
\begin{aligned}
P_l &= d_w \times h \\
&= (1\ g/cm^3) \times 1034\ cm \\
&= 1034\ g/cm^2
\end{aligned}
$$

As will be demonstrated later, this pressure is equivalent to 1 atmosphere (atm), or about 14.7 pounds per square inch (psi). Of course, this pressure does not take into account the additional atmospheric pressure (P_B) acting on the top of the liquid. Thus, the total pressure at the bottom of the column must equal the sum of the atmospheric pressure and the liquid pressure. In this case, the total pressure

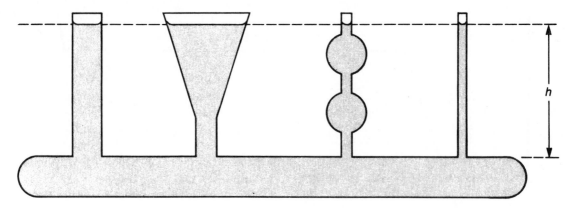

Fig. 4-4 The pressure is dependent only on the height *(h)* and not on the shape of the vessel or the total volume of water. (From Nave CR and Nave BC: Physics for the health sciences, ed 3, Philadelphia, 1985, WB Saunders Co.)

would be 2068 g/cm^2, equal to 29.4 psi, or 2 atmospheres.

It is important to note that the pressure in a liquid is dependent on the depth and density of the liquid only and not on the shape of the vessel. As illustrated in Fig. 4-4, the pressure exerted by a liquid at a depth h is the same, regardless of the shape of the container holding the water. This is because the pressure in a static liquid acts equally in all directions. This concept, known as Pascal's principle, also tells us that any change of pressure in an enclosed fluid will be transmitted undiminished to all parts of the fluid.

Buoyancy. Thousands of years ago, Archimedes demonstrated that an object submerged in a liquid such as water appeared to weigh less than it did in air. This effect, called buoyancy, is responsible for the flotation of certain objects in water and is often referred to as Archimedes' principle.

The buoyant force of a liquid is attributable to the difference in pressure exerted above and below the submerged object. Since the liquid pressure at the bottom of the object (relative to gravity) will always be greater than that at the top, an upward or supporting force is created. According to this phenomenon, if the upward buoyant force supporting a submerged object is greater than its weight, the object will float. On the other hand, if the weight of the object exceeds the buoyant force, the object will sink.

According to Archimedes' principle, the buoyant force exerted on an object is equal to the weight of the fluid displaced by the object. Since the weight of fluid displaced by an object equals its weight density times its volume ($d_w \times V$), the buoyant force ($F_{buoyant}$) may be calculated as follows:

$$F_{buoyant} = d_w \times V$$

Thus, if the average weight density of a submerged object is less than that of water (1 g/cm^3), then it will dis-place a weight of water greater than its own weight. In this case, the upward buoyant force will exceed the downward force on the object caused by gravity, and the object will float. On the other hand, if the weight density of a submerged object is greater than that of water, the downward force attributable to gravity will exceed the upward buoyant force, and the object will sink.

Clinically, Archimedes' principle is used to measure the specific gravity of certain liquids, such as urine. Specific gravity is a variation of the weight density measurement, whereby the density of a substance is calibrated against the density of water. (The specific gravity of gases can also be measured, with oxygen or hydrogen as the standard.)

The device used to measure specific gravity in the clinical setting is called the hydrometer. Fig. 4-5 depicts the use of a hydrometer to measure the specific gravity of a urine sample. The resulting value of 1.025 indicates that the sample has a weight density 1.025 times greater than that of water.

Another common application of Archimedes' principle is the use of the buoyancy concept to determine the volume and density of an irregularly shaped object. By measuring the volume of water displaced by such an object, and the difference between its weight in air and its weight in water, one may calculate its weight density. The following formula applies to this computation:

$$d_w = \frac{W_{air} - W_{water}}{V}$$

where d_w equals the weight density of the object, W_{air} and W_{water} represent, respectively, the object's weight in air and water, and V is the volume of the object as measured by the amount of water displaced.

Gases also can exert buoyant force, albeit less than that provided by higher-density liquids. The buoyant force exerted by gases plays an important role in maintaining par-

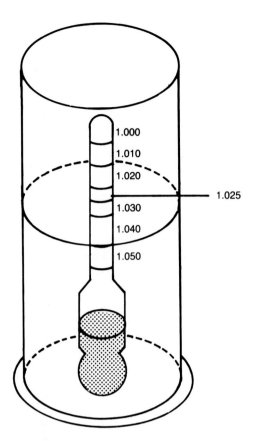

Fig. 4-5 A hydrometer used to measure the specific gravity of a urine specimen. The narrow tubing is calibrated so that the specific gravity 1.025 can be read from the tube. (From Nave CR and Nave BC: Physics for the health sciences, ed 3, Philadelphia, 1985, WB Saunders Co.)

ticulate matter in gaseous suspensions. These suspensions, called aerosols, play an extremely important role in respiratory care and will be discussed in detail in Chapter 23.

Viscosity. Viscosity may be thought of as an internal force that opposes the flow of a fluid, either liquid and gas. Viscosity in fluids is thus equivalent to the frictional forces opposing the movement of solid substances over one another.

The viscosity of a fluid is directly proportional to the strength of the cohesive forces between its fluid molecules. The stronger these cohesive forces, the greater will be the viscosity of the fluid. The greater the viscosity of the fluid, in turn, the greater its resistance to deformation and the greater its opposition to flow.

Viscosity is an important property of liquids, mainly under conditions of laminar flow. In laminar flow, the gas moves in discrete cylindrical layers called laminae (layers), or streamlines. Because of frictional forces between the streamlines and the wall of the tube, movement of the outer layer (closest to the tube wall) is minimal. As we move toward the center of the tube, each layer impedes the next inner layer but does so less and less. Thus, as de-

picted in Fig. 4-6, gas moving in a laminar pattern consists of concentric layers flowing parallel to the tube wall at linear velocities that increase toward the center.

The difference in the velocity among these concentric layers is called the shear rate. The shear rate is simply a measure of how easily the laminae separate, and that, in turn, depends on two factors: the force per unit area (pressure) applied to drive the fluid, called the shear stress, and the viscosity of the fluid. Shear rate is directly proportional to shear stress and inversely proportional to viscosity:

$$\text{shear rate} \propto \frac{\text{shear stress}}{\text{viscosity}}$$

Rearranging the equation to solve for viscosity:

$$\text{viscosity} \propto \frac{\text{shear stress}}{\text{shear rate}}$$

In cgs units, the viscosity of a fluid is measured in a unit called a poise. A poise equals the force of 1 dyne over an area of 1 cm^2 for a period of 1 second (dynes-sec/cm^2). It should be apparent that viscosity of liquids is greater than that of gases, and the values for both are small enough that they are expressed as fractions of poises. Viscosity of liquids is usually recorded as centipoises (10^{-2} poises) and that of gases as micropoises (10^{-6} poises). A few examples in Table 4-2 illustrate the ranges of these values. The SI unit for viscosity is the pascal-second (Pa-s), with 1 Pa-s equal to 10 poises.

In homogenous fluids such as water, the ratio of shear stress to shear rate remains constant. Thus the viscosity of a homogenous fluid is essentially constant, varying only with changes in temperature. Since an increase in temperature weakens the cohesive forces between the fluid molecules, viscosity in such fluids decreases with increasing temperature.

In complex fluids, such as blood, the ratio of shear stress to shear rate varies, so that viscosity increases with a decrease in the shear rate. Thus in the venous side of the circulation, where the driving pressure (shear stress) and the shear rate are low, the viscosity of blood rises. On the other hand, where the driving pressure and the shear rate are high, as on the arterial side of the circulation, the vis-

Table 4-2   Examples of Viscosity Measurements

	Substance	°C	Poises
Liquids	Water	20	1.005×10^{-2}
	Alcohol, ethyl	20	1.2×10^{-2}
	Glycerine	20	1490×10^{-2}
	Oil, castor	10	2420×10^{-2}
Gases	Air	18	182.7×10^{-6}
	Carbon dioxide	20	148×10^{-6}
	Oxygen	19	201.8×10^{-6}
	Helium	20	194.1×10^{-6}

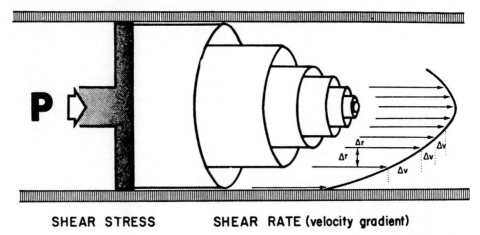

SHEAR STRESS   **SHEAR RATE (velocity gradient)**

Fig. 4-6   The effects of shear stress or pressure *(P)* on shear rate (velocity gradient) in a newtonian fluid. (Redrawn from Winters WL and Brest AN, editors: The microcirculation, Springfield, Ill, 1969, Charles C Thomas, Publisher.)

cosity of the blood will tend to drop. In either case, the viscosity of blood is still some five times greater than that of water, meaning that the heart must perform more work to pump this fluid than would be needed to circulate a simple solution of plasma.

Cohesion and adhesion. Cohesive forces represent attraction between like molecules. Attractive forces between *unlike* molecules are called adhesive forces.

The relationship between cohesive and adhesive forces is clearly demonstrated in the formation of the curved surface or *meniscus* that one observes when a liquid is placed in a tube of small diameter. As illustrated in Fig. 4-7, *A,* a water meniscus is concave because the water molecules at the edge adhere to the glass wall more strongly than they cohere to each other. In contrast, a mercury meniscus is convex because the cohesive forces between the like atoms of mercury are greater than the adhesive forces that tend to attract the mercury to the container wall (Fig. 4-7, *B*).

Surface tension. Surface tension may be defined as the force exerted by like molecules at the surface of a liquid. All liquids display surface tension to some degree. It commonly occurs at the interface or junction between a liquid and a gas and is best illustrated in a relatively small drop of fluid. Molecules within the liquid are subjected to balanced cohesive forces from all directions. Molecules on the surface, however, are attracted only inwardly. This imbalance in cohesive forces at the surface causes the surface film to contract into the smallest possible area, usually a sphere or curve (meniscus).

Fig. 4-8 illustrates this concept. Molecules at the fluid-air interface have no molecules distally to attract them but are pulled only centrally. This tension over the surface of a drop of liquid is responsible for the spherical shape of liquid droplets and for their ability to maintain this shape when placed in an aerosol suspension (refer to Chapter 23).

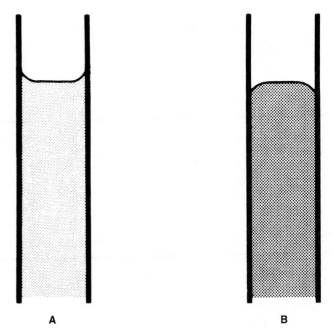

A   **B**

Fig. 4-7   The shape of the meniscus depends on the relative strengths of adhesion and cohesion. **A,** Water; adhesion stronger than cohesion. **B,** Mercury; cohesion stronger than adhesion. (From Nave CR and Nave BC: Physics for the health sciences, ed 3, Philadelphia, 1985, WB Saunders Co.)

In cgs units, surface tension is measured in dynes per centimeter across the fluid surface and may be visualized as the force necessary to produce a "tear" 1 cm long in the surface layer of a liquid. Surface tension is a demonstrable phenomenon that permits an insect to walk on the surface of a pond and enables a needle to float in a glass of water. Surface tensions vary widely among substances and, for the same substance, vary inversely with temperature. Ta-

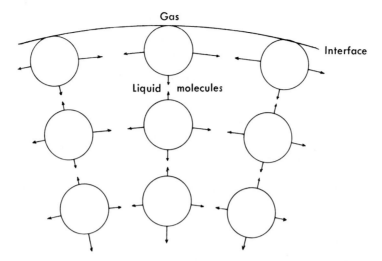

Fig. 4-8 The force of surface tension in a drop of liquid is shown by the action of its fluid molecules. Those molecules within the substance of the drop are mutually attracted to one another *(arrows)* and can move about randomly in a state of balance. Mass attraction can pull the molecules of the outermost layer inward only, creating a centrally directed force, called surface tension, which tends to contract the liquid into a sphere. Pressure within the drop is raised above atmospheric pressure and is expressed by the formula of Laplace, described in text.

ble 4-3 lists some examples of surface tension values for common substances.

The force of surface tension, like a fist compressing a ball, produces an increase in pressure within a drop of liquid above the ambient. Thus a pressure gradient, or difference in pressure (ΔP), exists across the surface of the drop.

According to the Laplace formula, the pressure within a drop due to surface tension depends on the specific surface tension of the liquid and the radius of the drop:

$$P = 2 \times \frac{ST}{r}$$

where *P* is the pressure within the drop in dynes per square centimeter, *ST* is the surface tension in dynes per centimeter, and *r* is the radius of the drop in centimeters. For example, in a drop with a radius of 2 mm (0.2 cm), consisting of a liquid with a surface tension of 60 dynes per cen-

timeter, we would calculate the pressure within the drop as follows:

$$P = 2 \times \frac{60}{0.2} = \frac{120}{0.2} = 600 \text{ dynes/cm}^2$$

The principle regulating internal pressure of a drop applies equally to a gas bubble in a liquid mass. The gas in the bubble is subject to the same pressure as the center of a drop of the same radius if the substance forming the drop has the same surface tension as the liquid surrounding the bubble.

The effect of surface tension on a liquid bubble is somewhat different. As depicted in Fig. 4-9, a liquid bubble is essentially a spherical volume of gas enclosed in a thin film of fluid. The thin film contains a finite amount of liquid called the hypophase. As is evident, the hypophase has two surfaces, one exposed to the external gas and one enclosing the gas inside the bubble. Since a liquid bubble has two gas-fluid interfaces, the compression force of surface tension on the enclosed gas is twice that exerted by a spherical drop of the same size and substance. Thus the surface tensions of the two surfaces act together to compress the gas bubble. The pressure gradient across a bubble wall can also be expressed by the Laplace formula, modified as follows:

$$P = 4 \times \frac{ST}{r}$$

Regardless of whether there are one or two liquid-gas interfaces, the smaller the drop or bubble, the greater the pressure due to surface tension. When inflating a balloon, we must use maximum force to start the inflation, to overcome the initial resistance, and then progressively less up

Table 4-3 Examples of Surface Tension

Substance	°C	ST in dynes/cm
Water	20	73
Water	37	70
Tissue fluid	37	50
Whole blood	37	58
Plasma	37	73
Ethyl alcohol	20	22
Mercury	17	547

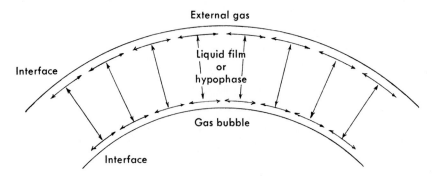

Fig. 4-9   A bubble is a volume of gas enclosed by a thin film of fluid, which has two surfaces. Thus, the forces of surface tension on both surfaces produce a pressure within the bubble twice that in a liquid drop of the same substance and radius.

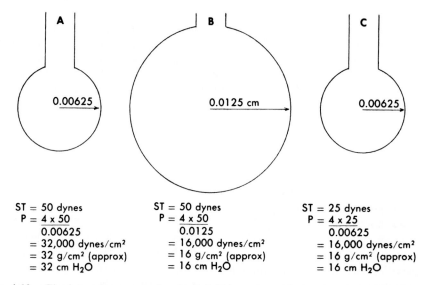

Fig. 4-10   The internal pressure of a single bubble varies with the size of the bubble and the surface tension of its liquid film. An increase in radius from **A** to **B** drops the pressure, but **C** shows that the same pressure drop can accompany a reduction in surface tension without changing bubble size.

to the capacity of the balloon. Similarly, it would require more pressure to inflate a small bubble than a large one because of the greater surface tension exerted on the small bubble.

Fig. 4-10 illustrates changes in pressure in an isolated bubble accompanying changes in size and in surface tension. As the size of the bubble increases from A to B, the pressure drops, as predicted by the Laplace formula. The bubble at C demonstrates that the pressure can remain unchanged if the surface tension is somehow lowered. Viewed differently, if two bubbles of different sizes are allowed to communicate, the smaller will empty into the larger because of the greater pressure in the former (Fig. 4-11).

Bubbles massed together as a foam behave differently than when individually isolated. Fig. 4-12 shows that bubbles in clumps lose their outer air-fluid surfaces and retain only single interfaces, resembling bubbles in a volume of liquid. As a consequence, the internal pressure in grouped bubbles is proportional to twice the surface tension of the surrounding liquid rather than four times the surface tension.

Given that the alveoli in the lungs are essentially clumped bubbles, surface tension forces play a significant role in the normal mechanics of ventilation, as described in Chapter 8. Moreover, alterations in the surface tension forces in the lung are responsible, in part, for certain abnormal conditions, such as respiratory distress syndrome of the newborn. The role of surface tension forces in disease is addressed in Chapters 28 and 32.

Capillary action. Capillary action is a phenomenon whereby a liquid in a small tube tends to move upward, against the force of gravity. Capillary action occurs as a result of both adhesive and surface tension forces. As il-

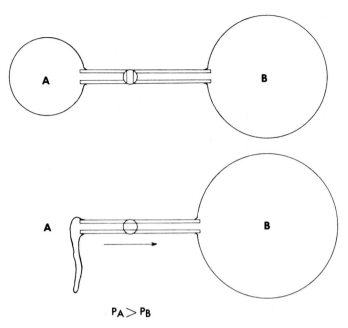

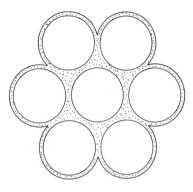

Fig. 4-12   The bubble in the center of the sketch illustrates that while an isolated bubble suspended in air can have two air-fluid interfaces, when it is clumped in a mass of foam it retains only its inner interface. (See text for the significance of this.)

$P_A > P_B$

Fig. 4-11   When two bubbles of different sizes, **A** and **B,** but with the same surface tension, are allowed to communicate, the greater pressure in the smaller causes it to empty into the larger.

lustrated in Fig. 4-13 *A*, the adhesion of water molecules to the walls of a thin tube will cause an upward force on the edges of the liquid and result in a concave meniscus.

Since surface tension forces act to maintain the smallest possible area of liquid-gas interface, instead of just the edges of the liquid moving up, the whole liquid surface is pulled upward. The force with which this occurs is proportional to the length of the liquid edge in contact with the tube surface. Because a small capillary tube creates a more concave meniscus and thus a greater area of contact between the liquid and the tube wall, liquid will rise higher in tubes with smaller cross-sectional areas (Fig. 4-13, *B*).

The principle of capillary action is applied in obtaining "capillary stick" blood samples. Absorbent "wicks" used in some humidification devices are also an application of this principle, as are certain types of surgical dressings.

Liquid-vapor phase changes (vaporization and condensation)

Returning to Fig. 4-3, only after the change of state from solid to liquid has taken place does continued heat elevate the temperature of the newly formed liquid. As the temperature of the liquid water reaches 100°C, a new change of state begins, in this case from the liquid to the vapor phase. This change of state is called vaporization.

Actually, there are two different forms of vaporization: boiling and evaporation. In boiling, the liquid molecules must be given enough kinetic energy to force them into the surrounding atmosphere, against its opposing pressure. In evaporation, random fluctuations in kinetic energy are suf-

ficient to allow some liquid molecules to escape into the surrounding atmosphere.

Boiling.   Boiling occurs at the boiling point, a temperature at which the vapor pressure of a liquid equals the pressure exerted on the liquid by the surrounding atmosphere. Since the weight of the surrounding air molecules retards the escape of vapor molecules, the boiling point of a liquid varies with the pressure exerted on its surface by the atmosphere. The greater the ambient pressure, the greater must be the kinetic energy of the liquid molecules to escape against that pressure. On the other hand, lower ambient pressures allow molecules to escape more easily, and boiling can occur at much lower temperatures.

Although we are accustomed to associating the phenomenon of boiling with high temperatures, such as that of water (100°C), the boiling points of the liquid state of substances we call gases have exceedingly low values. For example, at a normal atmospheric pressure of 760 mm Hg, oxygen boils at −183°C.

Just as energy is needed to liquefy a solid, energy is also required to vaporize a liquid. The energy required to vaporize a liquid is called the latent heat of vaporization. In cgs units, the latent heat of vaporization is defined as the calories required to vaporize 1 g of a liquid at its normal boiling point (standard pressure at sea level, or 760 mm Hg).

As previously discussed, the solid-to-liquid phase change reduces the intermolecular forces of attraction but does not abolish them. Indeed, the liquid-to-gas phase change requires enough energy to completely overcome these attractive forces and thus convert essentially all the internal energy of the substance into the kinetic energy of motion. This transition requires substantially more energy than the solid-liquid transition. As evident in Fig. 4-3, it takes nearly seven times as much energy to convert water to steam (540 cal/g) as is necessary to change ice to liquid water. The latent heats of fusion and vaporization of some common substances are given in Table 4-4.

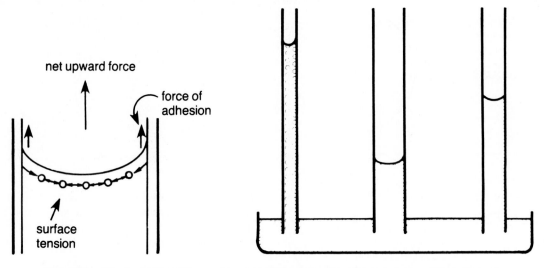

Fig. 4-13 The basis of capillary action. *Left,* Adhesion and surface tension contribute to capillarity. *Right,* The liquid rises highest in the smallest tube. (From Nave CR and Nave BC: Physics for the health sciences, ed 3, Philadelphia, 1985, WB Saunders Co.)

Evaporation, vapor pressure, and humidity. Although the change in state from a liquid to a gas is most often associated with boiling, this phase transition can and does occur below the boiling point. The change in state of a substance from its liquid to its gaseous form that occurs below the boiling point is a special form of vaporization called evaporation. Evaporation occurs at a liquid-gas interface because some of the liquid molecules have greater than average kinetic energy, thereby allowing them to escape from the liquid surface. The phase transition of water below its boiling point is a good example of evaporation.

Invisible moisture, called humidity, is present in the atmosphere in the form of water vapor. In its vapor form, water assumes the state and characteristics of a gas and is sometimes referred to as "molecular water" to distinguish it from visible gross "particulate water," such as mist. Molecular water is subjected to the same kinetic activity as other gases and, like them, exerts a pressure, called water vapor pressure. Atmospheric conditions vary the amount of water vapor in the air, but molecular water is constantly entering the air whenever air is exposed to a water surface.

Below its boiling point, water enters the atmosphere by evaporation. As in the gas phase, the molecules of liquid water are in a state of constant motion. Although less intense than in the gaseous state, the kinetic energy of some molecules near the surface causes them to escape into the surrounding air, as depicted in Fig. 4-14, *A.*

The concept of latent heat of vaporization tells us that heat is required to produce this change in state. In the evaporation of water, this heat is taken from the air immediately adjacent to the water surface, thereby cooling the air. This is the principle underlying the cooling effect of evaporation, as described previously.

However, if a cover is placed over a volume of water, air trapped over the surface and below the cover will be filled with all the water vapor molecules it can hold and

Table 4-4 Normal Melting and Boiling Points and Latent Heats of Fusion and Vaporization of Some Common Substances

	Melting point (°C)	Heat of fusion (cal/g)	Boiling point* (°C)	Heat of vaporization (cal/g)
Water	0	80	100	540
Ammonia	−75	108	−33	327
Ethyl alcohol	−114	26	78	204
Nitrogen	−210	6.2	−196	48
Oxygen	−219	3.3	−183	51
Lead	327	5.9	1620	208
Mercury	−39	2.7	357	68

*At standard atmospheric pressure of 760 mm Hg.

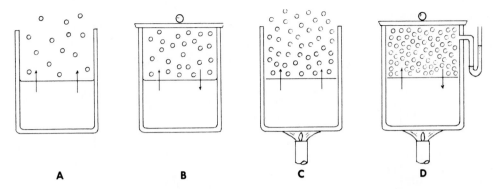

A   B   C   D

Fig. 4-14   The factors influencing vaporization of water are shown in these four sketches. **A,** The kinetic activity of molecules at the surface carries the molecules into the surrounding air, and evaporation gradually reduces the reservoir. **B,** If the container is covered, vaporization does not stop, but a state of equilibrium is reached when the air trapped in the container becomes saturated. At this point, water molecules leave and return to the reservoir in equal numbers. **C,** If the open container is heated, the increased molecular activity speeds the rate of vaporization. **D,** When the container is both covered and heated, more vapor will crowd into the trapped air, raising the vapor pressure as indicated by the attached manometer.

will become *saturated* with water vapor (Fig. 4-14, *B*). At this point, vaporization does not stop, but a state of equilibrium is established. For every molecule that escapes from the water, another molecule returns to the reservoir from the overlying saturated air.

Influence of temperature. The primary factor influencing evaporation is temperature. The rate of evaporation is directly related to temperature in two ways. First, the warmer the air, the more vapor it can hold. In other words, the capacity of air to hold water vapor increases with temperature. Therefore, if warm air is in contact with a water surface, the air's greater capacity will permit an increased escape of molecules from the water per unit of time, and evaporation will be faster.

Second, if heat is applied to the water, the increased kinetic energy of the liquid will allow more molecules to escape the surface per unit of time (Fig. 4-14, *C*). If a cover is placed over a surface of heated water, the increased kinetic energy of the escaping molecules will force more of them into the trapped air, increasing the saturation of the air and increasing the vapor pressure (Fig. 4-14, *D*). Therefore, the water content and the degree of saturation of air or any gas are a function of temperature.

Actual measurements of water vapor pressure in saturated air have been made over a wide range of temperatures. Fig. 4-15 plots the water vapor pressure (in both millimeters of mercury and kilopascals) of saturated air at normal atmospheric pressure on the left vertical axis against temperatures between 0 and 60°C (on the x-axis). As is evident, the saturated water vapor pressure (indicated by bold black dots) increases with increasing temperature. The specific values for water vapor pressure in saturated air in the clinical range of temperatures (20° to 37°C) are provided in Table 4-5.

Whereas water vapor pressure is a measure of the kinetic activity of water molecules, water vapor content is a measure of the actual amount, or weight, of the water molecules in a volume of gas. The actual content or weight of water present in a given volume of air is called the *absolute humidity.*

Absolute humidity is expressed either in grams of water vapor per cubic meter (g/m^3) or in milligrams per liter (mg/L). The absolute humidity of a known volume of air can be measured by physically extracting the water vapor with an absorbing agent and then weighing the water thus removed. Alternatively, absolute humidity may be computed by meteorologic data according to the techniques of the U.S. Weather Bureau. These data, expressed in milligrams of water per liter of saturated air at normal atmospheric pressure, are plotted on the *right* vertical axis of Fig. 4-15 with x hash marks. The specific values of absolute humidity for saturated air at normal atmospheric pressure between 20° and 37°C are provided in Table 4-5.

Obviously, a gas need not be fully saturated with water vapor. For example, if a gas is only half-saturated with water vapor, its water vapor pressure and water vapor content (absolute humidity) would be only half that of the fully saturated state. As an example, air saturated with water vapor at 37°C and 760 mm Hg has a water vapor pressure of 47 mm Hg and an absolute humidity of 43.8 mg/L (Table 4-5). However, if the same volume of air were only 50% saturated with water vapor, its water vapor pressure would be 0.50 × 47, or 23.5 mm Hg, and its absolute humidity would be 0.5 × 43.8, or 21.9 mg/L.

When a volume of gas is less than fully saturated with water vapor, it is useful to express the amount of water vapor present in relative terms. For this purpose, we apply a third measure of water vapor content, called *relative hu-*

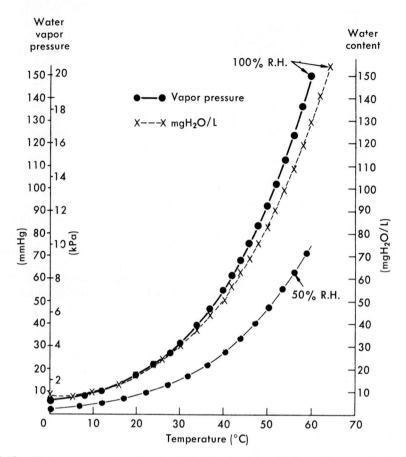

Fig. 4-15   Water vapor pressure (P_{H_2O}) and absolute humidity (H_2O mg/L) curves for gas that is fully saturated (RH = 100%) and gas that is half saturated (RH = 50%).   (From Sykes MK, McNicol MW, and Campbell EJM: Respiratory failure, ed 2, Oxford, England, 1976, Blackwell Scientific Publications.)

Table 4-5   Water Vapor Pressures and Contents at Selected Temperatures

Temperature (°C)	Vapor pressure (mm Hg)	Water vapor content (mg/L)	ATPS to BTPS correction factor*
20	17.50	17.30	1.102
21	18.62	18.35	1.096
22	19.80	19.42	1.091
23	21.10	20.58	1.085
24	22.40	21.78	1.080
25	23.80	23.04	1.075
26	25.20	24.36	1.068
27	26.70	25.75	1.063
28	28.30	27.22	1.057
29	30.00	28.75	1.051
30	31.80	30.35	1.045
31	33.70	32.01	1.039
32	35.70	33.76	1.032
33	37.70	35.61	1.026
34	39.90	37.57	1.020
35	42.20	39.60	1.014
36	44.60	41.70	1.007
37	47.00	43.80	1.000

*Correction factors based on atmospheric pressure of 760 mm Hg.

midity. Relative humidity is defined as the ratio of actual water vapor present in a gas to the capacity of the gas to hold the vapor at a given temperature. Relative humidity (RH) is expressed as a percentage and can be derived by means of the following simple formula:

$$\%RH = \text{content (absolute humidity)}/\text{saturated capacity} \times 100$$

For example, at an average room temperature of 20°C, air has the capacity to hold about 17.3 mg/L water vapor. If the absolute humidity is measured as 12 mg/L, then the relative humidity is calculated as:

$$\%RH = \frac{\text{content (absolute humidity)}}{\text{saturated capacity}} \times 100$$

$$\%RH = \frac{12}{17.3} \times 100$$

$$\%RH = 69$$

In reality, it is not necessary to measure the actual content of water vapor to derive the relative humidity. Instruments called hygrometers allow direct and simple measurement of relative humidity without the necessity of extracting and weighing the water content of air samples.

Obviously, when the water vapor content of a volume of gas equals its capacity, the relative humidity is 100% (fully saturated). Even slight cooling of a gas saturated with water vapor will result in condensation. Condensation reverses the process of vaporization, causing the vapor or gaseous form of the substance to change back to its liquid form. The concept of latent heat of vaporization tells us that heat is given up during condensation. In the condensation of water, this heat is given up to the air immediately adjacent to the water surface, thereby warming the air. This is exactly the opposite of the previously described principle of the cooling effect of evaporation.

Let us consider the example of air with a relative humidity of 90%. Should the air temperature drop, the capacity of the air to hold water vapor lessens. Eventually, a temperature will be reached at which the water content fully saturates the air (i.e., a relative humidity of 100%). At this point, excess water vapor begins to condense as visible droplets. This temperature at which water vapor condenses to back to its liquid form is known as the *dew point.* This condensation occurs on whatever surface is available, such as on the sides of a container, on the walls of tubing, or on liquid or solid particles suspended in the gas. As this condensation process occurs, heat is given off to the surrounding air.

For evaluation of humidity in clinical practice, the term *percent body humidity* (%BH) is sometimes used. It refers to the amount of water vapor in a volume of gas as the percentage of the water in gas saturated at body temperature (37°C).

$$\%BH = \frac{\text{content (absolute humidity)}}{\text{capacity at 37°C}} \times 100$$

or

$$\%BH = \frac{\text{content (absolute humidity)}}{43.8 \text{ mg/L}} \times 100$$

For example, saturated air at a room temperature of 20°C contains about 17.3 mg/L water vapor, whereas saturated air at body temperature contains 43.8 mg/L. In this case, the room air could be said to provide about 40% (17.3/43.8 × 100) body humidity.

Influence of pressure. Whereas higher temperatures increase the rate of vaporization, higher pressures impede this process. It is convenient to visualize evaporation as the escape of water molecules from the surface against the opposition of adjacent air molecules. As the surrounding air pressure increases, the rate of vaporization will decrease. On the other hand, decreased ambient pressures are associated with an increased rate of vaporization.

Influence of surface area. Logically, the greater the surface area available for evaporation, the greater will be the opportunity for liquid molecules to escape into the surrounding gas. Thus, the rate of evaporation of a liquid is directly proportional to the surface area available for vaporization.

Properties of gases

As fluids, gases share many of the previously described properties of liquids. Specifically, gases exert pressure, are capable of flow, and exhibit the property of viscosity. Unlike liquids, however, gases can be readily compressed and expanded, and they tend to fill the space available to them by rapid diffusion.

Kinetic activity of gases. As previously discussed, since the intermolecular forces of attraction among gas molecules are negligible, essentially all the internal energy of a gas is in the form of the kinetic energy of motion. Although gas molecules are extremely small (ranging in size from 10^{-8} to 10^{-7} cm in diameter, with weights varying from 10^{-23} to 10^{-20} g), kinetic theory tells us that these particles are in constant rapid motion, following completely random paths at phenomenally high speeds. For example, the average velocity of hydrogen molecules at 0°C is about 1.84×10^5 cm/s (greater than 1 mile/s), and oxygen molecules under the same conditions move at approximately 4.6×10^4 cm/s (⅓ mile/s).

During this intense activity, the particles collide with one another and with the surface of enclosing containers. On average, a single hydrogen molecule will undergo about 1×10^{10} collisions per second, an oxygen molecule approximately 4.6×10^9 collisions per second, and a carbon dioxide molecule about 6.2×10^9 collisions per second. The mean free path of gas molecules is a term used to describe the average distance traveled by the molecules between collisions. This distance is 1.66×10^{-5} cm for hydrogen, 8.8×10^{-6} cm for oxygen, and 5.8×10^{-6} cm for carbon dioxide.

Gas particle velocity is not constant, however, but is directly related to gas temperature. As temperature rises, the kinetic activity increases, molecular collisions increase, and the pressure of the gas rises. Conversely, when temperatures drop, molecular activity declines, particle velocity and collision frequency drop, and pressure is lowered.

The intensity of this kinetic activity becomes apparent when very fine particles such as those in smoke are suspended in gas and viewed under a microscope. Under such circumstances, one observes these particles moving about in a rapid and erratic random manner. This phenomenon is called *Brownian movement* and is produced by the kinetic activity of the gas molecules striking the suspended material.

Molar volume and gas density. One of the major principles of physics and chemistry is Avogadro's law, named after Italian chemist and physicist Count Amadeo Avogadro (1776-1856). This principle tells us that 1 g atomic weight (gaw), 1 g molecular weight (gmw), or 1 g formula weight (gfw) of a substance contains exactly the same number of particles, that is, 6.023×10^{23} atoms, molecules, or ions. This quantity of matter is known as Avogadro's number. Each of these quantities (1 gaw, 1 gmw, or 1 gfw) is technically known as a *mole*. In SI units, a mole is any quantity of matter that contains 6.023×10^{23} atoms, molecules, or ions.

Molar volume. As applied to gases, Avogadro's law tells us that equal volumes of gases at the same temperature and pressure contain the same number of molecules or, conversely, that at constant temperature and pressure, equal numbers of molecules of all gases occupy the same volume. The volume occupied by 1 mole of gas is termed the molar volume. According to this principle, under standard conditions of temperature and pressure (0°C and 760 mm Hg), 1 mole of any gas should occupy 22.4 L. This constant allows us to calculate densities of gases and gas mixtures and to convert values for dissolved gases from volumes percent to moles per liter, a topic that is considered in detail later.

In reality, we find that the natural intermolecular behavior of each gas causes its molar volume to deviate slightly from that predicted by Avogadro's law. Table 4-6 compares the molar volumes of several gases measured directly under standard conditions. As is evident, the molar volumes of most gases of clinical importance—oxygen, nitrogen, and carbon monoxide—are very close to the predicted value of 22.4 L/mole. The one exception is carbon dioxide. Carbon dioxide has a molar volume of approximately 22.3 L/mole. Thus, in this text, the standard molar volume of 22.4 L/mole will be used for all respired gases except carbon dioxide, for which we will use 22.3 L/mole.

Density. As previously described, density represents the amount of mass per unit volume of a body, and is thus equivalent to the concentration of atomic particles in a substance. In most clinical applications, we substitute weight for mass and thereby actually measure weight density, symbolized as d_w. In this context, d_w is the weight of a body per unit volume. In cgs units, the weight density of solids and liquids is most often described in grams per cubic centimeter. For gases, it is more common to use units of grams per liter.

Since weight density equals weight divided by volume, the density of any gas at STPD can readily be calculated by dividing its gram molecular weight by the universal molar volume of 22.4 L (22.3 for carbon dioxide). The quotient is expressed as grams per liter. Examples of simple gas density calculations are shown in Table 4-7.

Densities of gas mixtures are easily calculated if the percentage composition of the mixture is known. For example, to calculate the density of air at STPD, we first need to know the proportion of gases constituting this mixture:

Gas	Percent (%)	Fraction (F)
oxygen	21	0.21
nitrogen	79	0.79

Using the gram molecular weights of these gases (Table 4-7), we set up a proportionality as follows:

Table 4-6 Molar Volume of Selected Gases Under Standard Conditions

Gas	Symbol	Molar volume (L)
"Ideal gas"		22.414
Ammonia	NH_3	22.094
Carbon dioxide	CO_2	22.262
Carbon monoxide	CO	22.402
Chlorine	Cl_2	22.063
Helium	He	22.426
Hydrogen	H_2	22.430
Hydrogen chloride	HCl	22.248
Nitrogen	N_2	22.402
Oxygen	O_2	22.393
Sulfur dioxide	SO_2	21.888

Modified from Pimental GC, editor: Chemistry, an experimental science, San Francisco, 1963, WH Freeman & Co, Publishers.

Table 4-7 Examples of Gas Densities (D) Under Standard Conditions

$$D\ O_2 = \frac{gmw}{22.4} = \frac{32}{22.4} = 1.43\ g/L \qquad D\ He = \frac{gmw}{22.4} = \frac{4}{22.4} = 0.1785\ g/L$$

$$D\ N_2 = \frac{gmw}{22.4} = \frac{28}{22.4} = 1.25\ g/L \qquad D\ CO_2 = \frac{gmw}{22.3} = \frac{44}{22.3} = 1.973\ g/L$$

$$\text{Density of mixture } (d_w) = \frac{(F_1 \times gmw_1) + (F_2 \times gmw_2) + etc}{22.4}$$

where F_1 equals the fractional concentration of gas No. 1, gmw_1 equals the gram molecular weight of gas No. 1, F_2 equals the fractional concentration of gas No. 2, gmw_2 equals the gram molecular weight of gas No. 2, and so on, according to the number of gases in the mixture.

We thus compute the weight density of air as follows:

$$d_w \text{ air} = \frac{(FN_2 \times gmwN_2) + (FO_2 \times gmwO_2)}{22.4}$$

$$d_w \text{ air} = \frac{(0.79 \times 28) + (0.21 \times 32)}{22.4}$$

$$d_w \text{ air} = 1.29 \text{ g/L}$$

Gaseous diffusion. Diffusion is the physical process whereby atoms or molecules tend to move from an area of higher concentration or pressure to an area of lower concentration or pressure. The energy that drives this net transfer of atoms or molecules is their random kinetic energy. For this reason, diffusion occurs most rapidly in gases, although it also occurs in liquids and can even occur in solids.

Diffusion in the gas phase is described by Graham's law, according to which the rate of diffusion of a gas (D) in the gas phase is inversely proportional to the square root of its density (or gram molecular weight):

$$D \propto \frac{1}{\sqrt{gmw}}$$

The rate of diffusion of a gas (D) is expressed in standardized terms as a diffusion coefficient. In cgs units, the diffusion coefficient is defined as the number of milliliters of a gas at 1 atmosphere of pressure that will diffuse a distance of 1 μm over a 1 cm^2 surface area per minute of time.

Since diffusion results from the motion of molecules, anything that increases the activity of molecules or atoms will increase their rate of diffusion. Thus, heating and mechanical agitation will hasten the diffusion process of both gases and liquids.

Gas pressure. All gases exert pressure, whether they are free in the atmosphere, enclosed in a container, or dissolved in a liquid such as blood. The amount of pressure exerted by a gas depends on the number of particles present and the frequency of their collisions. The frequency of gas particle collisions is directly related to their average velocity, since the greater their velocity, the greater the number of collisions per unit of time, and the greater the energy of these collisions. In physiology, this pressure is frequently referred to as the tension of a gas. In addition, the force of the earth's gravity affects gas pressure or tension. Although the kinetic activity of gas molecules is random, the pressure exerted by a gas is always higher near the earth's surface. This is because the density and the frequency of collisions are aided by gravity.

As we learned in Chapter 3, pressure is defined as the force exerted over a given area. Thus, the units of pressure are those of force divided by area. The SI unit is the newton per square meter, called the pascal (Pa). In cgs units the dyne per square centimeter is used. In the British system, the basic unit would be pounds per square foot (lb/ft^2), but pounds per square inch (lb/in^2 or psi) is the more commonly used unit. Also in common use are pressure units based on the height of liquid columns, since such columns are often used for pressure measurements. This approach is used most often in measuring atmospheric pressure.

Measurement of atmospheric pressure. If we visualize the atmospheric mantle surrounding the earth, we can understand that the molecular activity of atmospheric gases will exert a force against the surface of the earth. Many miles of atmosphere rest on the earth, exerting force on its surface.

Atmospheric pressure is measured indirectly by means of a barometer. A barometer consists of an evacuated glass tube approximately 37 inches tall with an inside diameter of 0.25 inch, closed at the top and with its lower end immersed in a reservoir of mercury (Fig. 4-16). The pressure of the atmosphere on the mercury reservoir forces the mercury up the vacuum tube a distance equivalent to the force exerted. Thus the atmospheric pressure is measured in

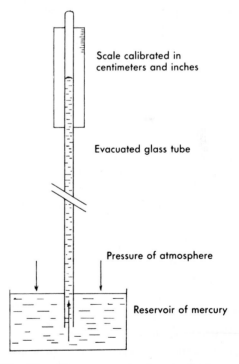

Scale calibrated in centimeters and inches

Evacuated glass tube

Pressure of atmosphere

Reservoir of mercury

Fig. 4-16 The major components of a mercury barometer include a mercury reservoir, into which is inverted the open end of an evacuated glass tube, and a scale, by which the height of the mercury column can be read in inches and centimeters above the surface of the reservoir. The atmospheric pressure, acting on the surface of the mercury reservoir, is balanced by the weight of the column of mercury in the tube.

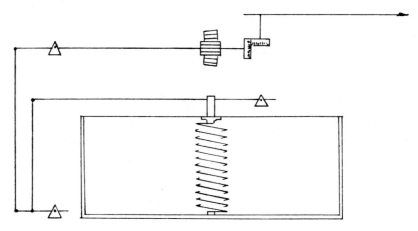

Fig. 4-17   Aneroid barometer. (See text for description.)

terms of the height of the column of mercury, in inches (fps system) or in centimeters or millimeters (cgs). This procedure balances the pressure of the atmosphere against a column of mercury in a vacuum, and if the weight per surface area of the mercury can be calculated, this value will equal the pressure of the air.

As previously described, the pressure exerted by a liquid is directly proportional to the depth of the liquid times its density. Therefore:

$$\text{Pressure } (P) \text{ in g/cm}^2 = \text{height in cm} \times \text{density in g/cm}^3$$
$$P = \text{cm} \times \text{g/cm}^3$$
$$P = \text{g/cm}^2$$

or

$$\text{Pressure } (P) \text{ in lb/in}^2 = \text{height in inches} \times \text{density in lb/in}^3$$
$$P = \text{inches} \times \text{lb/in}^3$$
$$P = \text{lb/in}^2$$

At sea level the average atmospheric pressure will support a column of mercury 76 cm (760 mm) or 29.9 inches high. If we also know that mercury has a density of 13.6 g/cm^3 (ie, is 13.6 times as heavy as water) or 0.491 lb/in^3, then we can calculate the atmospheric pressure (P$_B$) by the formulas just given:

$$P \text{ in g/cm}^2 = 76 \times 13.6 = 1034 \text{ g/cm}^2$$
$$P \text{ in lb/in}^2 = 29.9 \times 0.491 = 14.7 \text{ lb/in}^2$$

These two values, 1034 g/cm^2 and 14.7 lb/in^2, are used as standards and are called 1 atmosphere of pressure (1 atm). It is not necessary, however, in recording air pressure to calculate the actual grams per square centimeter or pounds per square inch; it is sufficient to record only the height of the mercury column. Pressure might be reported as 77.2 cm (772 mm) or 30.4 inches of mercury (Hg). This means that the atmospheric pressure is of such a magnitude that it is able to hold up a column of mercury 772 mm or 30.4 inches high. This translates to actual force per surface area values of 1050 g/cm^2 or 14.9 lb/in^2.

Mercury is used as the agent for measuring atmospheric pressure because its density is such that at ordinary pressures it assumes a height that is easy and convenient to read. It would be possible, although not practical, to construct a barometer of water. At 1 atm (76 cm Hg or 29.9 inches Hg), water, which is 13.6 times lighter than mercury, would rise to a height of 33.9 feet!

A device called an aneroid barometer is frequently used because of its convenient small size. It consists of a sealed evacuated metal box with a flexible, spring-supported top that responds to changes in pressure (Fig. 4-17). Motion of its top is magnified by levers to activate a geared pointer, which indicates the pressure on a scale calibrated against a mercury barometer. Less precise than a mercury instrument, the aneroid barometer is practical for nonscientific or domestic use.

Correction of barometric readings. Like any solid material, a barometer housing reacts to ambient temperature changes by expanding and contracting. Even more important, the mercury column barometer behaves like a large thermometer and is even more affected by temperature changes than the aneroid type. Therefore, when we read a mercury barometer, we see the effects of both pressure and temperature. For accuracy, we must correct our observed reading for changes in the mercury column caused by temperature.

The U.S. Weather Bureau provides a table of factors for correcting barometric readings at any given temperature. These factors, reproduced in part in Appendix 1, are based on expansion coefficients of brass and mercury at various temperatures. The pertinent value in the table is subtracted from the observed reading. For example, at 30°C an observed barometric reading of 750 mm Hg would be corrected for temperature by subtraction of 3.66 from 750 for a corrected reading of 746.34 (usually rounded off to 746.3 or just 746). For P$_B$ values between those listed in the table, simple linear interpolation is used.

From a practical point of view, the only temperature variations that affect barometric readings are those of the

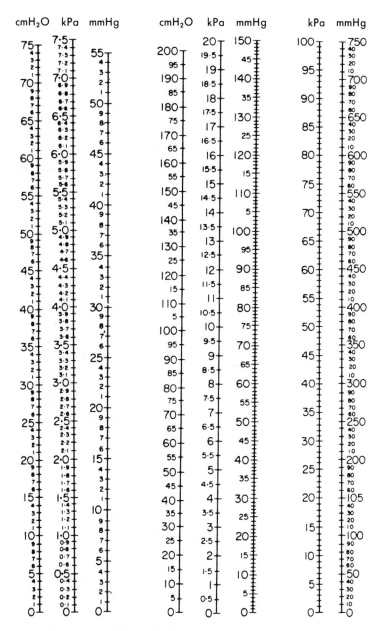

Fig. 4-18 Chart for converting the more traditional units of pressure of cm H_2O and mm Hg to SI units: kPa. (From Sykes MK, McNichol MW, and Campbell EJM: Respiratory failure, ed 2, London, 1976, Blackwell Scientific Publications.)

room housing the barometer. Since it is unlikely that the temperature of the average laboratory would exceed seasonal changes of 16° to 27°C (60° to 80°F), or the P_B range of 740 to 780 mm Hg, the correction factors would usually range between 1.9 and 3.4.

Clinical gas pressure measurements. In clinical practice, liquid and gas pressures are commonly expressed in either millimeters of mercury or centimeters of water. More recently, efforts have been made to encourage adoption of the SI standard for pressure, the pascal. However, the pascal is a very small unit of pressure. Because 1 Pa is so small, the kilopascal is typically used for physiologic measurements when SI units are used. Fig. 4-18 is an

alignment nomogram designed to facilitate conversion among these three different pressure units. To use the nomogram, one simply finds the pressure being converted and places a straightedge at right angles to the vertical scale at the point selected. The equivalent pressure is then read from the parallel scale corresponding to the units desired. Alternatively, the following table of conversion factors may be used:

cm H_2O	kPa	mm Hg
10.197	1	7.501
1.359	0.133	1
1	0.098	0.736

Partial pressures (Dalton's law). The pressure exerted by a mixture of gases, such as air, represents the sum of the kinetic activity of all the constituent gases. In cardiopulmonary physiology, the pressure exerted by a single gas in a gas mixture is called the partial pressure.

The relationship among the partial pressures and the total pressure exerted by a gas mixture is expressed in Dalton's law, which states that the total pressure of a gas mixture is equal to the sum of the partial pressures of the constituent gases. A corollary to this principle is that the partial pressure of any single gas in a gas mixture is equal to the pressure it would exert if it alone occupied the entire gas volume. Therefore, each gas contributes its share of the total pressure of a mixture in proportion to its percentage of the mixture. Thus a gas that represents 25% of a mixture of gases would exert a partial pressure equivalent to 25% of the total pressure.

As an example, dry air may be considered to consist of only two major gases, O_2 at 21% and N_2 at 79%. Assuming a normal atmospheric pressure of 760 mm Hg, we can calculate the individual partial pressures as follows:

$$P_B \text{ (dry)} = 760 \text{ mm Hg}$$
$$P_{O_2} = 760 \times 0.21 = 160 \text{ mm Hg}$$
$$P_{N_2} = 760 \times 0.79 = \frac{600 \text{ mm Hg}}{760 \text{ mm Hg}}$$

Since we are ultimately interested in the amount of oxygen available to the body cells and will soon study the relationship between the availability and the pressure of oxygen partial pressure, let us consider the effect of changing atmospheric pressure on oxygen partial pressure. We assume a concentration of oxygen in dry air of 20.95% (this is expressed as the F_{IO_2}, or fractional concentration of inspired oxygen). At a P_B of 760 mm Hg, the $P_{O_2} = 760 \times 0.2095 = 159$ mm Hg. Although the F_{IO_2} of air at 25,000 feet is still 0.2095, the P_B is only 282 mm Hg and the P_{O_2} is thus 59 mm Hg. Although the F_{IO_2} at sea level and at 25,000 feet is the same, the kinetic activity of oxygen at the high altitude is equivalent to that of a mixture containing only 7.8% oxygen on the ground! In contrast, at a depth of 66 feet into the sea, the weight of water exerts a pressure equal to 3 atm, or 2280 mm Hg. Air breathed by a diver at this depth would also be subjected to this same pressure, and its P_{O_2} would be 20.95% of 2280, or 477 mm Hg.

Solubility of gases in liquids. Gases are capable of dissolving in liquids. Carbonated water and soda pop are good examples of a gas, in this case carbon dioxide, dissolved in a liquid (water).

How much of a given gas can dissolve in a given liquid is described by Henry's law. Henry's law states that the volume of a gas dissolving in a liquid at a given temperature is equivalent to its solubility coefficient times the partial pressure of the gas above the liquid:

$$V_{\text{dissolved gas}} \cong \alpha \times P_{\text{gas}}$$

where α is the solubility coefficient of the gas in the given liquid and P_{gas} is the partial pressure of the gas above the liquid. The solubility coefficient of a gas is defined as the volume of that gas that can be dissolved in 1 ml of a given liquid at standard pressure and specified temperature. For example, the solubility coefficient of oxygen in plasma, at a temperature of 37°C and a pressure of 760 mm Hg, is 0.023 ml; for carbon dioxide, it is 0.510 ml.

An increase in temperature decreases the amount of gas that can dissolve in a liquid at any given pressure. This effect is due to the increase in kinetic activity that occurs with increased liquid temperatures. As the temperature of the liquid increases, the tendency for the dissolved gas molecules to escape back into the surrounding gas increases, thereby decreasing the amount left in solution. This phenomenon is the reverse of that observed for solids dissolved in liquids as described in Chapter 5.

Solid-vapor phase changes (sublimation)

Our analysis of changes in the states of matter would not be complete without a discussion of the direct transition between the solid and vapor phases. Solid matter, as well as liquid, can vaporize, and at any given temperature solids can exert vapor pressures. The strong odor given off by naphthalene (mothballs) is evidence of the escape of vapor from a solid. The direct transition from the solid to the gaseous state is called *sublimation*, and, because a change of state is involved, energy is transferred. The heat, in calories per gram required to convert 1 g of a solid into a vapor, is called the heat of sublimation.

Sublimation resembles boiling because it occurs when the vapor pressure of the solid equals that of the opposing ambient pressure. Also, as with boiling, increasing and decreasing the ambient pressure directly displaces the temperature at which sublimation will occur, called its "subliming point." For example, at exactly 0°C, the vapor pressure over ice is 4.6 mm Hg; if a vacuum is applied to the ice, the ice will sublime directly into water vapor. Even though the direct transformation from solid to vapor eliminates the liquid phase, the same total energy is required, and the heat of sublimation is therefore equal to the sum of the heats of fusion and vaporization.

Carbon dioxide is an interesting example of sublimation. If the gas is cooled to −57° C at a pressure of 5.1 atm, it will freeze and the vapor will equilibrate with the solid. When solid carbon dioxide is exposed to normal atmospheric pressure, the drop in pressure from 5.1 to 1 atm causes the solid state to sublime directly into vapor. Most people are familiar with the behavior of commercially prepared solid carbon dioxide, called "dry ice," as it gradually disappears when exposed to ambient conditions, leaving no trace of moisture. On the other hand, if solid carbon dioxide is subjected to pressures in excess of 5.1 atm and allowed to warm above −57°C, it will melt into a liquid without boiling.

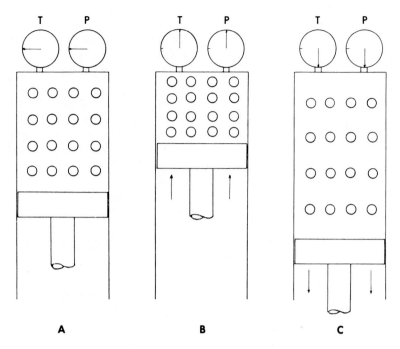

Fig. 4-19 A mass of gas in the resting state exerts a given pressure at a given temperature, in cylinder A. In B, as the piston compresses the gas, the molecules are crowded closer together, and the increased energy of molecular collisions is reflected in a rise of both temperature and pressure. Conversely, retraction of the piston in C allows the gas to expand, and temperature and pressure drop as molecular interaction decreases.

GAS BEHAVIOR UNDER CHANGING CONDITIONS

Because of the relatively great distances between their molecules, gases possess the quality of compressibility. When pressure is exerted on a gas, the molecules are pushed closer together, and their intervening spaces are narrowed. On the other hand, if the container of a volume of gas enlarges, the gas expands to accommodate the new volume, and its molecules spread farther apart.

Fig. 4-19 illustrates the relationship between compression and expansion of a given mass of gas molecules and corresponding temperatures and pressure changes. Because the tremendous energy of molecular collision is expended as heat, compression of a gas produces heat as well as a buildup of pressure among the molecules (Fig. 4-19, *B*). As compression brings the molecules closer together, the frequency of collisions increases, and both heat and pressure increase. Conversely, the expansion of a gas produces a drop in temperature as molecular collision frequency decreases (Fig. 4-19, *C*).

The relationships among the pressure, temperature, mass, and volume of gases are expressed in the gas laws. These laws allow us to explain and quantitatively predict the behavior of gases under a variety of conditions. Underlying all these laws are three basic assumptions: (1) that collisions between molecules are perfectly elastic (meaning that no energy is lost during collisions), (2) that the

volume actually occupied by the gas molecules is negligibly small, and (3) that no forces of mutual attraction exist between the molecules. These three assumptions describe an "ideal gas." As we shall see, no gas is truly ideal. Variations in the behavior of gases from this ideal do occur, especially at the extremes of pressure and temperature. Under normal conditions, however, most gas behavior is consistent with the conception of an ideal gas.

Constant temperature processes (Boyle's law). During the 1600s, Robert Boyle, the eminent British physicist and chemist, observed that if the temperature and the mass of a gas remain constant, its volume (V) would vary inversely with its pressure (P). Mathematically, this inverse relationship can be expressed as follows:

$$PV = k$$

where *P* is the pressure of the gas, *V* is its volume, and *k* is a constant of proportionality. As described in this relationship, if a given mass of a gas is maintained at a constant temperature, increasing its pressure will decrease its volume. On the other hand, decreasing the pressure of a given mass of gas at a constant temperature will result in an increase in its volume.

To calculate the change in volume that occurs when a gas is subject to a change in pressure, one simply establishes an equality between the conditions of pressure and volume before (condition 1) and after (condition 2) the change, as follows:

$$P_1V_1 \;=\; P_2V_2$$

or, rearranging the equation to solve for the new volume (V_2),

$$V_2 \;=\; V_1 \times \frac{P_1}{P_2}$$

As an example, suppose we have a 2 L of a gas (V_1) existing at 1 atm, or 760 mm Hg of pressure (P_1). What would be the new volume of the gas (V_2) if we were to increase its pressure to 1520 mm Hg (P_2)? Using the above equation:

$$V_2 = V_1 \times P_1/P_2$$
$$V_2 = 2 \text{ L} \times 760 \text{ mm Hg}/1520 \text{ mm Hg}$$
$$V_2 = 2 \text{ L} \times 0.5$$
$$V_2 = 1 \text{ L}$$

Thus, by doubling the pressure on the gas, we observe a halving of its original volume.

Boyle's law describes the behavior of a gas under conditions of no temperature change. Processes of compression or expansion in which the gas temperature remains constant are referred to as *isothermal* processes. In order to maintain a constant gas temperature during the compression or expansion of a gas, the first law of thermodynamics dictates that heat energy must be either added (during expansion) or taken away (during compression) to maintain the energy equilibrium.

During isothermal expansion in which no external work is performed (as when a gas is allowed to escape from a high-pressure cylinder into the atmosphere), the temperature of a gas should not change. However, this is not the case. In fact, the rapid expansion of a gas without the application of external work causes a substantial drop in the temperature of the gas. This phenomenon, called the Joule-Thompson effect, is based on the fact that during rapid expansion of a gas, the forces of mutual attraction (van der Waals forces) between gas molecules must be entirely broken. The energy for accomplishing this internal work must come from the gas itself, resulting in a decrease in the gas temperature. Depending on the pressure drop that occurs, this decrease in temperature can be large enough to actually liquefy the gas. This is the primary method used to liquefy air for the production of oxygen, as described in Chapter 24.

Adiabatic processes, on the other hand, are those in which no heat energy is added to or taken away from the gas during compression or expansion. Thus that portion of a gas's internal energy that is attributable to kinetic or heat energy will vary according to changes in its pressure or volume. Rapid adiabatic compression can thus result in a dramatic rise in the kinetic energy of a gas, as manifested by a rapid increase in its temperature. A diesel engine uses this principle of adiabatic compression to ignite the fuel mixture without a spark. Adiabatic compression can also occur in medical gas delivery systems whenever a gas undergoes a rapid rise in pressure within a fixed container. Under such circumstances, the rise in temperature may be sufficient to ignite any combustible material in the system. It is for this reason that respiratory care practitioners must take care to ensure that any combustible particulate matter is cleared from high-pressure gas delivery before pressurization.

Constant pressure processes (Charles' Law). About a century after Boyle's discovery, the French physicist and chemist, Jacques Alexandre Cesar Charles (1746-1823), observed that if the pressure and mass of a gas were kept constant, its volume would vary directly with changes in its absolute temperature. Mathematically, this direct relationship can be expressed as follows:

$$\frac{V}{T} = k$$

where T is the temperature of the gas (in degrees Kelvin), V is its volume, and k is a constant of proportionality. As described in Charles' law, if a given mass of a gas is maintained at a constant pressure, an increase in its absolute temperature will result in an increase in its volume. On the other hand, decreasing the temperature of a given mass of gas at a constant pressure will result in a decrease in its volume.

To calculate the change in volume that occurs when a gas is subject to a change in temperature, we establish another simple equality:

$$\frac{V_1}{T_1} = \frac{V_2}{T_2}$$

or, rearranging the equation to solve for the new volume (V_2),

$$V_2 = V_1 \times \frac{T_2}{T_1}$$

As an example, suppose we have 8 L of a gas (V_1) existing at 0°C or 273°K (T_1). To compute the new volume of the gas (V_2), if we were to decrease its temperature to 200°K (-73°C), we simply apply the above equation:

$$V_2 = V_1 \times T_2/T_1$$
$$V_2 = 8 \text{ L} \times 200° \text{ K}/273°\text{K}$$
$$V_2 = 8 \text{ L} \times 0.73$$
$$V_2 = 5.84 \text{ L}$$

Obviously, the mass of gas cannot be cooled into nothingness, and at a certain point the ideal behavior ceases and other factors come into play.

Constant volume processes (Gay-Lussac's law). As a corollary to Boyle's and Charles' laws, the French chemist and physicist, Joseph Louis Gay-Lussac (1778-1850), observed that if the volume and mass of a gas remained fixed, the pressure exerted by the gas would vary directly with its absolute temperature. Mathematically, this relationship can be expressed as follows:

$$\frac{P}{T} = k$$

where T is the temperature of the gas (in degrees Kelvin), P is its pressure, and k is a constant of proportionality. As described in this relationship, if a given mass of a gas is maintained at a constant volume, an increase in its absolute temperature will result in an increase in its pressure. On the other hand, decreasing the temperature of a given mass of gas at a constant volume will result in a decrease in its pressure.

To calculate the change in pressure that occurs when a gas is subject to a change in temperature, we establish another simple equality:

$$\frac{P_1}{T_1} = \frac{P_2}{T_2}$$

or, rearranging the equation to solve for the new pressure (P_2),

$$P_2 = P_1 \times \frac{T_2}{T_1}$$

As an example, suppose we have a volume of gas in a cylinder of fixed size existing at 2200 psi (P_1) and at a room temperature of 20°C or 293°K (T_1). To compute the new pressure of the gas (P_2), if the temperature were to increase to 323°K, or 50°C (T_2), we simply apply the above equation:

$$P_2 = P_1 \times T_2/T_1$$
$$P_2 = 2200 \text{ psi} \times 323°K/293°K$$
$$P_2 = 2200 \text{ psi} \times 1.102$$
$$P_2 = 2425 \text{ psi}$$

Combined gas law. In reality, seldom is any one of the four primary properties of gases (pressure, volume, temperature, and mass) actually held constant. For this reason, it is useful to treat all four properties as variables and combine them into a single equation, called the combined gas law:

$$PV = nRT$$

where P is the pressure of the gas, V is its volume, n is its mass, T is its temperature, and R is a combined constant of proportionality, often called the gas constant. The gas constant varies only according to the measurement system used. For example, if liters is used as the measure of volume and atmospheres as the measure of pressure, $R = 0.082$ L-atm/°K/mole; on the other hand, in pure SI units (with volume in cubic meters and pressure in pascals), $R = 8314$ joules/°K/kmole.

In pulmonary physiology and in clinical practice, we are interested mainly in how changes among pressure, volume, and temperature affect each other. Because the gas constant (R) does not change under changing conditions of pressure, volume, and temperature, it need not be included in our calculations. Moreover, since the total mass of a gas will not be affected, the quantity n (mass) can be eliminated from the computations. We can thus establish a simple equality relationship between the three primary variables of clinical concern, namely, pressure, volume, and temperature:

$$\frac{P_1V_1}{T_1} = \frac{P_2V_2}{T_2}$$

This equation represents the "working form" of the combined gas law under conditions of constant mass. Using rearrangements of this equation, one may determine the combined effect of changes in any two variables on the third. For example, to solve for V_2 under conditions of changing temperature and pressure, we rearrange the equation as follows:

$$V_2 = V_1 \times P_1 \times \frac{T_2}{P_2} \times T_1$$

Thus, to calculate the new volume (V_2) of 3 L of gas existing at 273°K (T_1) and 760 mm Hg (P_1) when heated to 300°K (T_2) and subject to 1520 mm Hg (P_1) pressure:

$$V_2 = V_1 \times P_1 \times \frac{T_2}{P_2} \times T_1$$
$$V_2 = 3 \text{ L} \times 760 \text{ mm Hg} \times 300°K/1520 \text{ mm Hg} \times 273°K$$
$$V_2 = 1.65 \text{ L}$$

Correcting for the presence of water vapor. Most calculations of physiologic gas volume involve gases saturated with water vapor. Since water vapor occupies space in a mixture of gases, its removal from a gas volume will shrink the volume, and its addition will increase the volume. Therefore, whenever a volume of gas saturated with water vapor must be treated as if in the dry state, its dry volume at a constant pressure and temperature will be smaller than its saturated volume. The opposite must also be true. Correcting from the dry state to the saturated state will yield a larger volume.

At a fixed temperature, if a gas sample is in a container that permits it to respond to ambient pressure, it reaches a static volume where the pressure it exerts exactly balances ambient pressure. Water vapor, if added to dry gas at ambient pressure, will thus have two effects. First, the increased number of molecules will enlarge the volume until the total molecular kinetic activity again equilibrates with ambient pressure. Second, because water vapor exerts a pressure that is dependent only on temperature and relative humidity and is independent of other gases with which it mixes, the partial pressures of the other gases will be reduced to maintain parity with the ambient pressure.

Corrected pressure computations. The pressure of the other gases in a mixture must therefore be corrected for the presence of water vapor. The corrected pressure of a gas in the presence of water vapor can be calculated as follows:

$$P_C = F_{gas} (P_T - P_{H_2O})$$

where P_C is the corrected gas pressure, F_{gas} is the fractional concentration of the gas in the gas mixture, P_T is the total gas pressure of the mixture, and P_{H_2O} is the water vapor pressure at the given temperature, as listed in Table 4-5. If only a single gas is present, then F_{gas} equals 1, and the above formula can be simplified:

$$P_C = (P_T - P_{H_2O})$$

For example, if we are dealing with gas saturated with water vapor, Boyle's law would be modified as follows:

$$V_2 = V_1 \times \frac{(P_1 - P_{H_2O} \text{ at } T_1)}{(P_2 - P_{H_2O} \text{ at } T_2)}$$

$$= V_1 \times \frac{P_{C_1}}{P_{C_2}}$$

Use of correction factors. Instead of doing the individual arithmetic for each calculation, correction factors may be used. In gas volume determinations, three frequently encountered computations are (1) correction from ATPS to BTPS, (2) correction from ATPS to STPD, and (3) correction from STPD to BTPS.

Factors to correct volumes from ATPS to BTPS. The values in the third column of Table 4-5, when multiplied by V_1, will correct a gas volume from ATPS to BTPS. Because these factors are based on a PB of 760 mm Hg, they provide only a close approximation of the corrected gas volume at other atmospheric pressures. At sea level, however, this discrepancy will usually be of little clinical significance. For example, to correct a saturated gas volume at 25°C and 760 mm Hg to BTPS conditions at the same pressure, the correction factor would equal 1.075. If, on the other hand, P_1 were 752 mm Hg and P_2 were 758 mm Hg, the value by which V_1 would be multiplied would be 1.066.

For example, to convert a saturated gas volume of 3.0 L at an atmospheric pressure of 760 mm Hg and a room temperature of 20°C to its equivalent saturated volume at 37°C, one simply finds the appropriate factor (in this case, 1.102). Therefore:

$$V_{BTPS} = V_{ATPS} \times \text{conversion factor}$$
$$V_{BTPS} = 3.0 \text{ L} \times 1.102$$
$$V_{BTPS} = 3.306 \text{ L}$$

Factors to correct volumes from ATPS to STPD. Factors in Appendix 2, when multiplied by V_1, will correct V_1 from ATPS to STPD. Since these factors already account for the appropriate temperature correction of the barometric reading, one simply uses the uncorrected barometric value to obtain the appropriate factor.

For example, to correct a saturated gas volume of 2.0 L at an observed PB of 770 mm Hg and a room temperature of 20°C to its equivalent dry gas volume at 760 mm Hg and 0°C (STPD), one simply finds the appropriate factor (in this case, 0.919). Therefore:

$$V_{STPD} = V_{ATPS} \times \text{conversion factor}$$
$$V_{STPD} = 2.0 \text{ L} \times 0.919$$
$$V_{STPD} = 1.838 \text{ L}$$

Factors to correct volumes from STPD to BTPS. Factors for this conversion are given in Appendix 3. As is evident, in this conversion ambient pressure is the only variable.

For example, to convert a dry gas volume of 4.0 L at a standard pressure of 760 mm Hg to its equivalent saturated volume at 37°C and a PB of 740 mm Hg, one again uses the table to identify the appropriate factor (in this case, 1.245). Therefore:

$$V_{BTPS} = V_{STPD} \times \text{conversion factor}$$
$$V_{BTPS} = 4.0 \text{ L} \times 1.245$$
$$V_{BTPS} = 4.98 \text{ L}$$

Properties of gases at extremes of temperature and pressure

To this point, only the theoretic responses of an ideal gas to changes in pressure, volume, and temperature have been discussed. Now we will consider variations from the ideal state, in which gases are subjected to extremes of temperatures and pressure. Only under such circumstances do gases begin to deviate substantially from "ideal" behavior. Understanding the unique behavior of matter under these circumstances will help prepare the reader to work effectively with commercially prepared medical gases, as discussed in Chapter 24.

As previously discussed, the weak attractive forces between the molecules of a gas tend to oppose their kinetic activity. Although independent of temperature, the impact of these van der Waals forces is related to both temperature and pressure. For example, at high temperatures, the increased kinetic molecular activity of a gas far overshadows these forces of attraction, rendering them relatively unimportant. At very low temperatures, however, the resulting decrease in kinetic action makes the molecules much more responsive to mutual attraction. Likewise, low pressures exerted on a gas permit the molecules to move freely about with little mutual attraction. In contrast, at high pressures the molecules become crowded together, thereby increasing the influence of the van der Waals forces.

In addition to the attractive force between gas molecules, another factor that influences the relationship between pressure and volume is attributed to the space occupied by the molecules themselves. When moderate to low pressures are exerted on a given container full of gas, the total mass of matter is a negligible fraction of the total volume of the gas. However, as the volume is reduced by the application of high pressure, the resulting molecular density, which is not compressible, comprises a proportionately larger amount of the overall gas volume, disturbing the volume response to pressure predicted by the ideal gas law.

These observations can be summarized by the generalization that, at very low temperatures or very high pressures, gases deviate from their ideal behavior. These deviations are due to both the influence of the van der Waals intermolecular attractive forces and the volume occupied by the compressed gas molecules. For those scientists and technicians whose work requires maximum precision, there is available a modification of the combined gas law that includes correction for the van der Waals effect and the density of molecules. Handbooks of chemistry and physics also contain prepared tables of constants to facilitate such calculations for a wide variety of gases. The interest here, however, is in the effects of excessive temperatures and pressures on the state of gases, since those we use may be in liquid or solid as well as gaseous forms. We will again use water as our example of these effects.

Triple point

If the three states of a given substance, such as water, were drawn on a graph that includes combinations of temperature, in degrees Celsius, and pressure, in atmospheres, three dividing lines would emerge (Fig. 4-20). Line *A-B* represents the boiling points of water at various pressures and also indicates the saturated vapor pressure at different temperatures. This emphasizes the relationship between increasing pressure and increasing boiling points of water. Line *A-B* terminates at the so-called critical point (described later). Line *A-D* represents conditions for water to sublimate from ice to a vapor or from a vapor to ice. Line *A-C* indicates the transition points between ice and liquid water (the melting or freezing point). The steepness of line *A-C* indicates the relatively small effect exerted by pressure on melting or freezing points.

These three lines intersect at point *A,* called the triple point. The triple point represents the only combination of temperature and pressure that allows the solid, liquid, and vapor forms of a given substance to exist in equilibrium with one another. Every substance has its own triple point.

At any plot of pressure and temperature that falls within the confines of the points *CAB,* water can exist only as a liquid. At points below *DAB,* pressures are too low for water to be anything other than gaseous. However, if the temperature is above the triple point, an elevation of pressure would transform the vapor into a liquid and, if below this point, directly into ice. The points *DAC* delineate the pressure-temperature condition necessary for the formation of ice. Therefore, at all points along each line, two phases of matter exist in complete equilibrium, but only at the triple point do all three equilibrate simultaneously.

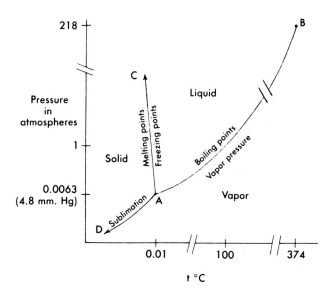

Fig. 4-20   The intersection of the three lines at *A* represents the *triple point* of water. Thus, at a temperature of 0.01°C and a pressure of 4.8 mm Hg, the three states of water (solid, liquid, and vapor) exist in equilibrium. The graphs show the pressure-temperature relationships of boiling, freezing, and sublimation of water.

If the pressure on a volume of water is reduced from 1 atm (760 mm Hg) to 0.0063 atm (4.8 mm Hg), the boiling point of water will drop from 100°C to almost 0°C. However, because the reduced pressure slightly alters the melting point of ice, the lines intersect at 0.01°C. Therefore, at a pressure of 4.8 mm Hg and a temperature of 0.01°C, ice, water, and water vapor coexist in equilibrium, not in a static state but actively, as molecules of the substance transform themselves from one form to the other forms. To appreciate the wide variation in range of triple points, note that the value for Freon-14 is −184°C and 0.88 mm Hg, whereas that of krypton is −157°C and 548 mm Hg.

The reader should keep in mind that changes in state are always made at the expense of energy. This energy is supplied by heat that is either given or taken by the matter undergoing change.

Critical temperature and pressure

For every liquid there is a temperature above which the kinetic energy of the molecules is so great that the attractive forces cannot maintain them in a liquid state. This temperature is called the *critical temperature.* Because there is no pressure able to maintain the molecules of the matter in a liquid state above this temperature, the critical temperature is the highest temperature at which a substance can exist as a liquid.

If an evacuated sealed tube partially filled with liquid is heated, vapor will escape into the vacuum. The density of the vapor will steadily increase as that of the liquid substance decreases, and when the critical temperature of the liquid is reached, the densities of both vapor and the remaining liquid will be equal and the two phases of matter will become identical without a line of demarcation between them. Further elevation of the temperature will transform the entire mass into vapor. The pressure exerted by the vapor within the evacuated tube at the critical temperature is the *critical pressure,* and on a plotted vapor pressure-temperature curve, the two values identify what is known as the critical point. Each substance has its own critical point at which the gas phase is in equilibrium with the liquid phase and the two are not visibly separated.

Point *B* in Fig. 4-20 represents the critical point of water at a pressure of 218 atm and a temperature of 374°C. Here the densities of the liquid and vapor phases are not distinguishable; the two are in equilibrium, and beyond this temperature no pressure can revert the mass to liquid. Compare the high values for water with the critical values of the gases in Table 4-8.

The terms *gas* and *vapor* are often erroneously used interchangeably, but the concept of critical temperature will help to differentiate them. A gas is a substance with a critical temperature so low that at usual ambient conditions of temperature and pressure it cannot exist as a liquid with a surface exposed to the atmosphere. If the temperature of a gas is above its critical value, it cannot be compressed into a liquid by a pressure of any magnitude. Such substances are referred to as permanent gases. On the other hand, vapor is the gaseous state of a substance that also exists simultaneously in a liquid or a solid state. Oxygen, therefore, is a permanent gas, since it has no solid or liquid phase under ambient conditions. Water is both a liquid and a gas at room temperature and 1 atm of pressure, and therefore its gaseous phase is a vapor. Appendix 4 lists the critical temperatures of several gaseous and vaporous substances.

Although we have described the critical points of matter in terms of the stability of liquids, they apply as readily to the transition of gas to liquid. To effect a change of state from gas to liquid, we must cool the gas below its critical temperature and then compress it. Theoretically, it is possible to liquefy a gas by cooling alone, dropping its temperature below the substance's boiling point, but under no circumstances is it possible to liquefy it by pressure alone if its temperature is above its critical point. The farther below its critical temperature a gas can be cooled, the less pressure is needed to liquefy it.

Therefore, any gas whose critical temperature is above ambient can be liquefied by pressure alone, because allowing the gas to equilibrate with ambient temperature actually keeps it below its critical temperature. Carbon dioxide has a critical temperature slightly above normal room temperature (31°C), with a corresponding critical pressure of 73 atm, but at a room temperature of 21.5°C less than 60 atm of pressure is needed to convert the gas to liquid.

Only those gases whose critical temperatures are above ambient can be kept in the liquid state for everyday use at room temperature, and they must be under pressure in strong storage cylinders. The anesthetic gases cyclopropane and nitrous oxide, along with carbon dioxide, are commercially supplied as tanked liquids, and Table 4-9 compares their critical points with the approximate pressures at which they are kept at room temperature to maintain their liquid state. There are many industrial gases that are converted to the liquid state for ease of mass transportation; with critical temperatures above ambient, they need only be kept under sufficient pressure to ensure their liquid form. With release of pressure, the liquid reverts immediately to gas.

Oxygen presents a more complicated problem. However, because of its widespread medical and industrial use, moving and storage are made easier by keeping it in the liquid state. In contrast to the three gases illustrated here, oxygen has a low critical temperature of −118.8°C (−181.1°F), and we know that no pressure will be able to keep it in liquid form above that value.

In the manufacture of oxygen, large quantities of filtered air are subjected to tremendous pressures of up to 200 atm. This produces a great deal of heat, and the compressed gas is passed through heat exchangers and then subjected to a rapid pressure drop down to 5 atm. This rapid reduction in pressure causes a rapid expansion of the gas and, according to the Joule-Thompson effect, a significant reduction in the temperature of the gas. Thus the oxygen in the air is

Table 4-8 Critical Points of Three Gases

	°C	°F	atm
Helium	−267.9	−450.2	2.3
Oxygen	−118.8	−181.1	49.7
Carbon dioxide	31.1	87.9	73

Table 4-9 Pressures Needed to Maintain Liquid State of Gases at Room Temperature

Gas	Critical temperature		Critical pressure		Approximate pressure in commercial cylinder at room temperature	
	°C	°F	atm	psi	atm	psi
Cyclopropane	125	257	54.2	797	5.4	79
Nitrous oxide	36.5	97.7	71.8	1054	50.6	745
Carbon dioxide	31.1	87.9	73.0	1071	57.0	838

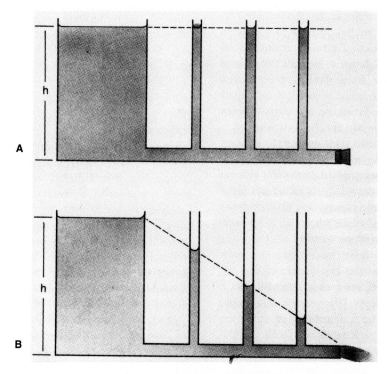

Fig. 4-21   A, The pressure is the same at all points along the horizontal tube when there is no flow. **B,** A uniform pressure drop occurs when there is smooth flow through a uniform tube. (From Nave CR and Nave BC: Physics for the health sciences, ed 3, Philadelphia, 1985, WB Saunders Co.)

brought below its boiling point of $-183°C$ ($-297°F$), and it liquefies. If oxygen can be kept in an insulated container so that its temperature does not exceed its boiling point, it will remain liquid at atmospheric pressure. Should higher temperatures be necessary, higher pressures must be used, but at no time can oxygen be allowed to exceed the critical temperature of $-118.8°C$, because it then converts immediately to gas.

FLUID DYNAMICS

Our analysis of the physical principles underlying the behavior of liquids and gases so far has been limited mainly to static conditions. However, both liquids and gases exhibit the *dynamic* characteristic of flow, or the ability for bulk movement (as opposed to random diffusion) through space.

The branch of fluid physics involved in the study of fluids in motion is called hydrodynamics. Since many aspects of hydrodynamics are directly applicable to the practice of respiratory care, a careful analysis of its underlying principles is essential to further study.

Pressures in flowing fluids

In contrast to a static liquid, in which the pressure depends solely on the depth and density of the fluid and the externally applied pressure, the pressure exerted by a

flowing liquid is dictated by the nature of the flow itself.

As depicted in Fig. 4-21, *A,* the pressure exerted by a static fluid at all points in the horizontal tube is the same, depending only on the height of the liquid column *(h).* However, when the fluid is allowed to flow out through the bottom tube, we observe a continuous drop in pressure (as indicated by the liquid height in the vertical tubes) from the reservoir on the left to the exit point on the right (Fig. 4-21, *B*).

We also observe that the relative pressure drop between the equally spaced vertical tubes is the same. That is, the drop in pressure along each successive unit length in a flowing fluid is equal. Thus, for our uniform-diameter horizontal tube, as long as a perfectly uniform pattern of flow is maintained, we can expect the drop in pressure to be the same at all points in the tube.

These drops in pressure during flow represent a loss of energy, as predicted by the second law of thermodynamics. In simple terms, the second law of thermodynamics states that in any naturally occurring mechanical process there will always be a decrease in the total energy available to do work. This decrease in available work energy is due mainly to frictional resistance against flow, both within the fluid itself (viscosity) and between the fluid and the tube wall. In general, the greater the viscosity of the fluid and the smaller the cross-sectional area of the tube, the greater will be the drop in pressure along the tube.

For any given tube length, this resistance to flow may be quantified as a ratio of the difference in pressure between the two points along the tube length to the volumetric flow of the fluid per unit of time:

$$R = \frac{P_1 - P_2}{\dot{V}}$$

where R is the total resistance to fluid flow, P_1 is the pressure at the upstream point (point 1), P_2 is the pressure at the downstream point (point 2), and $\dot{V}$ is the volumetric flow per unit of time (volume/time).

The pressure difference accompanying fluid flow through a tube also varies according to the characteristics of the flow itself. There are three primary patterns of flow through tubes.

Patterns of flow

The three primary patterns of fluid flow through tubes are laminar, turbulent, and transitional. The concept of laminar flow, where gas moves in discrete cylindrical layers called laminae (layers) or streamlines, was described earlier in our discussion of viscosity.

Laminar flow. Under conditions of laminar flow through a smooth, unbranched tube of fixed dimensions, the difference in pressure required to move a volume of gas through a tube per unit of time (flow) is defined by Poiseuille's law:

$$\Delta P = n8l\dot{V}/\pi r^4$$

where ΔP is the driving pressure gradient in dynes per square centimeter, n is the viscosity of the gas in poises, l is the tube length in centimeters, $\dot{V}$ is the gas flow in cubic centimeters per second, r is the tube radius in centimeters, and π and 8 are constants.

According to this formula, the pressure difference necessary to drive a fluid flowing in a laminar pattern through a tube is directly proportional to the viscosity of the fluid, the length of the tube, and the rate of flow and inversely proportional to the fourth power of the tube radius. Therefore we can expect the pressure difference to rise whenever there is an increase in the fluid viscosity, the length of the tube, or the rate of flow. Likewise, we can predict that the pressure difference also will rise if the radius of the tube decreases.

Turbulent flow. Under certain conditions, the characteristics of gas flow through a tube undergo a significant change. The orderly pattern of concentric layers is no longer maintained. Molecular movement becomes chaotic, with the formation of irregular eddy currents. This pattern is called turbulent flow.

When flow becomes turbulent, Poiseuille's law no longer applies. Instead, the difference in pressure required to move a volume of gas through a tube per unit of time (flow) is defined by the following equation:

$$\Delta P = fl\dot{V}^2/4\ \pi^2 r^5$$

where ΔP is the driving pressure gradient, f is a friction factor that incorporates gas density, gas viscosity, and the roughness of the tube wall, l is the tube length, $\dot{V}$ is the gas flow, and r is the tube radius.

The major difference between this formula and Poiseuille's law is the relationship between ΔP and $\dot{V}$. Whereas in Poiseuille's law the driving pressure is linearly proportional to the flow, under conditions of turbulent flow driving pressure is proportional to the square of the flow.

Transitional flow. A mixture of laminar and turbulent flow is termed transitional flow. Quantitatively, the relationship between pressure and flow during conditions of transitional flow depends on the relative influence of the laminar and turbulent components. To the extent that flow is mainly laminar, the driving pressure will vary linearly with the flow. On the other hand, when flow is mainly turbulent, the driving pressure will vary exponentially with the flow. Moreover, if laminar flow is the major influence, pressure and flow changes will be affected mainly by the viscosity of the fluid. On the other hand, if turbulent flow predominates, pressure and flow changes will be affected most by the density of the fluid.

Flow, velocity, and cross-sectional area

As we have seen, fluid flow is measured in terms of the bulk movement of a volume per unit of time. Clinically, the units of flow most commonly used are liters/minute (L/min) or liters per second (L/sec). Velocity, on the other hand, is a measure of linear distance traveled by the fluid per unit of time. Centimeters per second (cm/s) is a common velocity unit used in pulmonary physiology.

The important relationship between fluid flow, velocity, and the cross-sectional area of a conducting tube are depicted in Fig. 4-22. In this case, the fluid is flowing at a constant rate of 5 L/min. At point A the cross-sectional area is 5.08 cm^2, and the velocity of the fluid is calculated as 16.4 cm/s. As the fluid approaches point B, the cross-sectional area is halved to 2.54 cm^2. At this point the velocity of the fluid doubles to 32.8 cm/s. Finally, as we move toward point C, the tube divides into eight smaller conduits. Although each of these tubes by itself is smaller than its parent tube, together they result in a 10-fold increase in the total cross-sectional area available for flow, as compared to point B. Here the velocity of the fluid decreases proportionately, from 32.8 cm/s to 3.28 cm/s.

On the basis of these observations, we may state that the velocity of a fluid flowing through a tube at a constant rate of flow varies inversely with the available cross-sectional area. Mathematically, this relationship, is expressed as follows:

$$(A_1 \times v_1) + (A_2 \times v_2) + (A_n \times v_n) = k$$

where A equals the cross-sectional area of the tube; v equals the velocity of the fluid; 1, 2, and n represent different points in the conduit; and k equals a constant value.

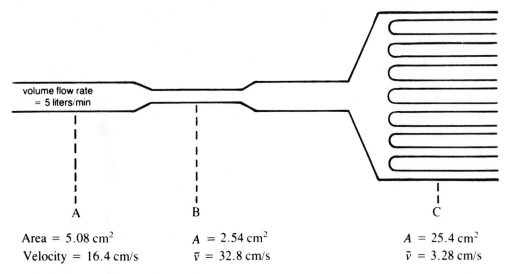

Area = 5.08 cm^2 A = 2.54 cm^2 A = 25.4 cm^2

Velocity = 16.4 cm/s $\bar{v}$ = 32.8 cm/s $\bar{v}$ = 3.28 cm/s

Fig. 4-22   The flow rate is maintained at a constant value by varying the velocity of the fluid. (From Nave CR and Nave BC: Physics for the health sciences, ed 3, Philadelphia, 1985, WB Saunders Co.)

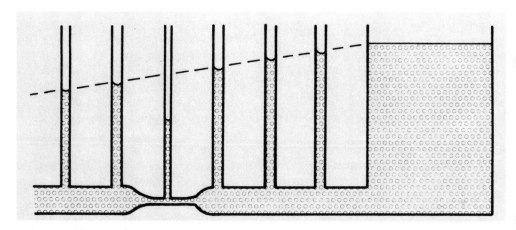

Fig. 4-23   The Bernoulli effect. (From Nave CR and Nave BC: Physics for the health sciences, ed 3, Philadelphia, 1985, WB Saunders Co.)

This strict proportionality between fluid velocity and cross-sectional area, often referred to as the *law of continuity*, holds true only for the flow of incompressible liquids, but the qualitative features are similar for gas flow. This principle also underlies the application of nozzles or "jets" in fluid streams. Nozzles and jets are simply narrow passages in a tube designed to increase the velocity of the fluid flowing through them.

The Bernoulli effect

As previously described, when a fluid flows through a tube of uniform diameter, there occurs a progressive drop in pressure over the length of the tube. This progressive pressure drop is illustrated by the first three water columns in Fig. 4-23.

However, as indicated by the fourth water column in Fig. 4-23, when the fluid encounters a constriction in the

tube the pressure drop is much greater. Daniel Bernoulli (1700-1782) was the first to carefully study this effect, which now bears his name. On the basis of his analysis, Bernoulli formulated a theorem that explains the interaction of variables causing this drop in pressure.

According to the Bernoulli theorem, the energy per unit volume for a flowing fluid consists of three components:

1. The kinetic energy imparted by the velocity of moving fluid, representing the amount of work performed by matter in motion against a resistive force.
2. The potential energy resulting from the force of gravity acting on the fluid volume elevated above its plane of horizontal flow.
3. The pressure energy, or the radial force exerted by the moving fluid.

According to the first law of thermodynamics, if the volumetric flow through a tube is constant, the sum of the

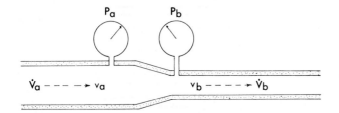

Fig. 4-24 The Bernoulli effect demonstrates that the *pressure* exerted by a steady flow of gas or liquid in a conducting tube varies *inversely* as the *velocity* of the fluid. With an abrupt narrowing of the passage since the volume of fluid per unit of time leaving ($\dot{V}_b$) must equal the time-volume entering the tube ($\dot{V}_a$), the linear motion of the fluid per unit of time (velocity, v) must increase as it traverses the structure ($v_b > v_a$). Thus there is a pressure drop distal to the restriction ($P_b < P_a$).

kinetic, potential, and pressure energies at any given point in a fluid stream must equal the sum of these energies at any other point.

Symbolically, these relationships may be expressed in the following equation:

$$\frac{E}{V} = \tfrac{1}{2}dv^2 + dgh + P$$

where E/V is the energy per unit volume of the fluid in motion, d is the density of the fluid, v is the velocity of the fluid, g is the acceleration due to gravity, h is the height of the fluid column, and P is the dynamic pressure exerted by the fluid because of its motion. The expression $\tfrac{1}{2}dv^2$ is equivalent to the kinetic energy of the moving fluid, whereas dgh, as previously discussed, is the static pressure exerted by the liquid, equivalent to its potential energy of position. Since, in a level tube, the static pressure exerted by the liquid remains constant, the potential energy term in the above equation can be deleted:

$$\frac{E}{V} \cong \tfrac{1}{2}dv^2 + P$$

Under conditions of constant flow, E and V are constant, and the sum of the kinetic energy ($\tfrac{1}{2}dv^2$) and pressure energy (P) at any given point in a fluid stream must equal the sum of these energies at any other point:

$$\tfrac{1}{2}dv_a^2 + P_a \cong \tfrac{1}{2}dv_b^2 + P_b$$

Where a and b are different points in the fluid stream.

If we assume that we are dealing with a single fluid, density will also be a constant and can be eliminated from the equation, giving the following proportional expression:

$$v_a^2 + P_a \cong v_b^2 + P_b$$

Fig. 4-24 applies this proportionality to a fluid flowing through a constriction. As dictated by the law of continuity, the velocity of the fluid at point b, after the constriction, must be greater than at point a, before the tube narrowing. According to the foregoing proportionality, since the velocity at point b is greater than at point a, the pressure at b must be less than the pressure at a. Thus, as a fluid flows through a stricture, its velocity increases and its lateral pressure decreases. Moreover, the magnitude of this pressure drop across the constriction is proportional to the increase in the square of the velocity. Simply stated, the additional energy expended by the increased velocity reduces the amount of energy available to exert pressure.

Fluid entrainment

According to the Bernoulli theorem, the drop in fluid pressure at a constriction in a tubing conduit is directly related to the increase in the velocity of the fluid. If the tube is narrowed sufficiently, the large increase in fluid velocity will result in a negative lateral fluid pressure relative to atmospheric pressure.

As depicted in Fig. 4-25, if we place an open tube distal to such a constriction, the negative pressure difference between the tube and the atmosphere will literally "push" another fluid into the tube of flow. The use of the Bernoulli effect to draw a second fluid into the stream of flow is called *entrainment*.

In this example, the entrained fluid is air. This application is common in the home, where "aerators" attached to faucets mix air into the water stream. In the laboratory setting, the negative pressure generated at a constriction in a water faucet can also be used as a source of negative pressure. This application is called the water aspirator.

Of course, any fluid (liquid or gas) may provide the primary flow source, and any fluid (liquid or gas) may be entrained into the stream of flow. In respiratory care, the most common application of the Bernoulli effect is the air injector, a device designed to increase the available flow in a gas stream. In this case, a pressurized gas, usually oxygen, serves as the primary flow source. This pressurized gas is passed through a constricted nozzle or jet, distal to which is an air-entrainment port. The negative pressure created distal to the jet causes the air to be entrained into the primary gas stream, thereby increasing the total flow output of the system. As depicted in Figs. 4-26 and 4-27, the amount of air entrained depends on both the size of the jet orifice and the size of the air-entrainment ports.

The Venturi tube

A modification of the Bernoulli principle, called the Venturi tube, was developed some 200 years ago by Giovanni Venturi (1746-1822). As illustrated in Fig. 4-28, the Venturi tube includes a dilation of the gas passage just distal to the tube narrowing. Venturi demonstrated that if the angulation of the dilation was not more than 15 degrees, the fluid pressure would be restored nearly to its prerestriction level.

This smooth tapering helps to prevent turbulence and make it possible to transform much of the kinetic energy generated at the jet back into pressure energy. When the

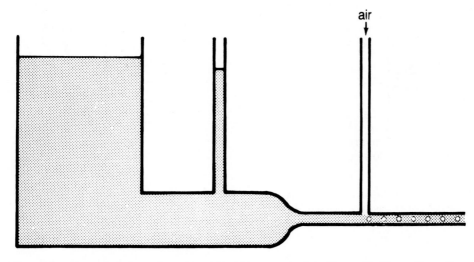

Fig. 4-25   The entrainment of gas into a liquid by means of the Bernoulli effect. (From Nave CR and Nave BC: Physics for the health sciences, ed 3, Philadelphia, 1985, WB Saunders Co.)

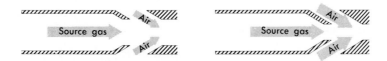

Fig. 4-26   Smaller restriction (right) causes greater increase in forward velocity of gas, resulting in lower lateral pressure and larger quantity of air entrained through ports. (From McPherson SP: Respiratory therapy equipment, ed 4, St Louis, 1989, The CV Mosby Co.)

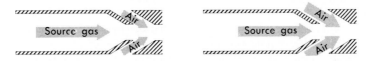

Fig. 4-27   Same orifice size in jet provides (1) same forward velocity, (2) same lateral subatmospheric pressure, and therefore (3) same pressure gradient (atmospheric to subatmospheric) for air entrainment. Entrainment-port size on right is larger; therefore more air will be entrained at set pressure gradient. (From McPherson SP: Respiratory therapy equipment, ed 4, St Louis, 1989, The CV Mosby Co.)

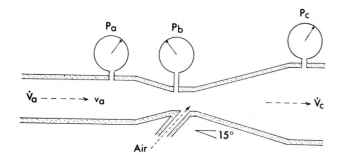

Fig. 4-28   The venturi principle states that the pressure drop distal to a restriction can be closely restored to the prerestriction pressure if there is a dilation of the passage immediately distal to the stenosis, with an angle of divergence not exceeding 15 degrees. Thus P_c approximately equals P_a. The venturi is a widely used device to entrain a second gas to mix with the main-flow gas. The subambient pressure distal to the restriction draws in the second gas just past the restriction, and the increased outflow ($\dot{V}_c > \dot{V}_a$) is accommodated by the widened distal passage.

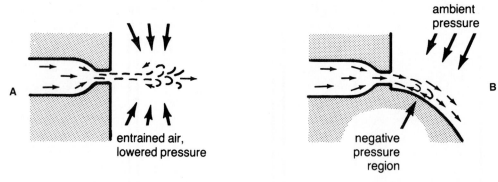

Fig. 4-29   The Coanda wall effect. **A,** Entrainment into the driving airstream. **B,** Wall attachment initiated by negative pressure near wall. (From Nave CR and Nave BC: Physics for the health sciences, ed 3, Philadelphia, 1985, WB Saunders Co.)

pressure energy is restored toward its prerestriction levels, the pressure gradient necessary to maintain flow is also restored, thereby making it possible to entrain larger volumes of gas. Moreover, restoration of the pressure energy through a Venturi tube helps keep the percentage of entrained gas constant, even when the total flow varies. Reference will be made in subsequent chapters to both the Bernoulli phenomenon and the Venturi tube during discussions of equipment.

Fluidics and the Coanda effect

Fluidics is a branch of engineering in which hydrodynamic principles are incorporated into flow circuits for such purposes as switching, pressure and flow sensing, and amplification. Since such devices use only the driving force of the fluid and its interaction with precisely contoured passageways, no moving parts are required. Without moving parts to fail or wear out, fluidic devices are very dependable and require a minimum of maintenance.

The physical principle underlying most fluidic circuitry is a phenomenon called the "wall attachment" or Coanda effect, which is observed primarily when a fluid flows through a small orifice or jet that has properly contoured downstream surfaces.

According to the Bernoulli theorem, if a fluid is driven through a constriction, negative pressure distal to the constriction will cause entrainment of surrounding fluid, such as air, into the primary flow stream (Fig. 4-29, *A*). If a carefully contoured curved wall is added on one side of the orifice, as shown in Fig. 4-29, *B,* the confinement of the wall causes the pressure near the wall to become more negative relative to atmospheric pressure. Thus the atmospheric pressure on the other side of the gas stream "pushes" the stream against the wall, where it remains "locked" until interrupted by some counterforce. Using this principle, Coanda demonstrated that a fluid stream could be deflected through a full 180-degree turn by careful extension of the wall contour.

As applied to respiratory care equipment, fluidic

switches, pressure- and flow-sensing devices, and flow amplifiers are often combined into an integrated fluidic logic circuit, which functions much like an electronic circuit board. This fluidic logic circuit can provide overall control of most equipment function without electrical power. Details on fluidic applications in ventilatory support equipment are provided in Chapter 30.

SUMMARY

Much of the technology involved in the provision of respiratory care services is based on the application of basic physical principles. Although all areas of physics have an impact on the technology of respiratory care, the properties of matter, thermodynamics, and mechanics represent fundamental areas of knowledge for the practitioner.

In regard to the properties of matter, we recognize three primary states: solid, liquid, and gas. The solid state is characterized by a high degree of internal order, in which the positions of the atoms or molecules are more or less fixed by strong mutual attractive forces. Because of the weakening of the intermolecular attractive forces caused by melting, liquids can flow and tend to take the shape of their container. Liquids also exert pressure and buoyant force and exhibit the properties of viscosity, capillary action, and surface tension. In the gas phase, the attractive forces between atoms or molecules are negligible. Lacking restriction to their movement, these molecules exhibit rapid, random motion, characterized by frequent collisions. Thus, unlike a solid or a liquid, a gas has no inherent boundaries and can readily be compressed and expanded. Like liquids, however, gases are capable of flow. For this reason, both liquids and gases are considered *fluids.*

In both the solid and the liquid states, most of the internal energy of matter is in the form of potential energy. On the other hand, because the intermolecular forces of attraction among gas molecules are negligible, essentially all the internal energy of a gas is in the form of kinetic energy.

With essentially all of its internal energy expended in maintaining molecular motion, the temperature of a gas is a direct measure of its average kinetic energy.

The first law of thermodynamics tells us that heat will tend to move from an object of high temperature to an object of low temperature until their temperatures are equal. This transfer of internal energy may occur by one or more of three primary mechanisms: (1) conduction, (2) convection, or (3) radiation. Heat transfer may also occur through the process of evaporation.

Heat transfer provides the basis for matter's change of state. The additional heat energy needed to effect the changeover from solid to liquid is referred to as the latent heat of fusion. The heat energy required to vaporize a liquid into a gas is called the latent heat of vaporization. There are two different forms of vaporization: boiling and evaporation. In boiling, the liquid molecules must be given enough kinetic energy to force them into the surrounding atmosphere, against its opposing pressure. In evaporation, random fluctuations in kinetic energy are sufficient to allow some liquid molecules to escape into the surrounding atmosphere.

The relationships among the pressure, temperature, mass, and volume of gases are expressed in the gas laws. These laws allow us to explain and quantitatively predict the behavior of gases under a variety of conditions. Underlying all these laws are three basic assumptions: (1) that collisions between molecules are perfectly elastic, (2) that the volume occupied by the gas molecules is negligibly small, and (3) that no forces of mutual attraction exist between the molecules. These three assumptions describe an "ideal gas." Variations in the behavior of gases from this ideal do occur, especially at the extremes of pressure and temperature. Under normal conditions, however, most gas behavior is consistent with the conception of an ideal gas.

In contrast to a static liquid, in which the pressure depends solely on the depth and the density of the fluid and the externally applied pressure, the pressure exerted by a flowing liquid varies according to the characteristics of the flow itself. The three primary patterns of fluid flow through tubes are laminar, turbulent, and transitional. Under conditions of laminar flow through a smooth, unbranched tube of fixed dimensions, the difference in pressure required to move a volume of gas through a tube per unit of time (flow) is defined by Poiseuille's law.

The velocity of a fluid flowing through a tube at a constant rate of flow varies inversely with the available cross-sectional area. Moreover, as a fluid flows through a stricture, its velocity increases and its lateral pressure decreases. If a tube is narrowed sufficiently, the large increase in fluid velocity will result in a negative lateral fluid pressure relative to atmospheric pressure, which allows additional fluids to be entrained. Design variations on this principle of negative lateral pressure allow restoration of downstream pressures, as in the venturi tube, or direction of the fluid stream along a wall, as in the Coanda effect.

BIBLIOGRAPHY

Barker JA and Henderson D: The fluid phases of matter, Sci Am, 130, Nov 1981.

Epstein II: Basic physics in anesthesiology, Chicago, 1976, Year Book Medical.

Flitter HH: An introduction to physics in nursing, ed 7, St Louis, 1976, The CV Mosby Co.

Green JF: Mechanical concepts in cardiovascular and pulmonary physiology, Philadelphia, 1977, Lea & Febiger.

Hill DW: Physics applied to anesthesia, London, 1976, Butterworth.

List RJ, editor: Smithsonian meteorological tables, Washington, DC, 1958, The Smithsonian Institute.

Nave CR and Nave BC: Physics for the health sciences, ed 3, Philadelphia, 1985, WB Saunders Co.

Parbrook GD: Basic physics and measurement in anesthesia, ed 2, Baltimore, 1986, Appleton-Lange Publishing Co.

Quagliano JV: Chemistry, Englewood Cliffs, NJ, 1964, Prentice-Hall, Inc.

Richardson IW: Physics for biology and medicine, New York, 1972, John Wiley & Sons.

Smith RK: Respiratory care applications for fluidics, Respir Ther 3:29, 1973.

Weast RC, editor: Handbook of chemistry and physics, ed 69, Cleveland, 1988, Chemical Rubber Co Publishing.

Whitaker S: Introduction to fluid mechanics, Englewood Cliffs, NJ, 1968, Prentice-Hall, Inc.

Williams AL, et al: Introduction to chemistry, Reading, Mass, 1973, Addison-Wesley Publishing Co, Inc.

5

Solutions, Body Fluids, and Electrolytes

Craig L. Scanlan

The humble beginnings of life on earth probably began as a series of complex organic chemical reactions occurring in a solution of salt water. Billions of years later, mankind still depends on these primitive beginnings, with the body being mainly a watery medium in which large numbers of organic and inorganic chemicals interact in solution or suspension.

In health, the amount and distribution of body water and the concentration of these various substances are carefully regulated to maintain an ideal medium in which the biochemical life processes continually proceed. Imbalances in the amount of water or the concentration of organic and inorganic chemicals in the body may be either the cause or the result of a variety of disease processes. An understanding of these abnormalities requires a sound foundation in physiologic chemistry and the nature and importance of body fluids and electrolytes.

OBJECTIVES

After completion of this chapter, the reader should be able to:

1. Differentiate among the characteristics of colloids, suspensions, and true solutions;
2. Differentiate among the three primary types of physiologic solutions according to their relative electrolytic activity;
3. Quantify and calculate both the solute content and the chemical activity of any standard solution or solution dilution;
4. Differentiate among the ionic characteristics of acids, bases, and salts;
5. Apply the concept of ionization constant to the designation of the acidity or alkalinity of solutions;
6. Compare and contrast the nanomolar (nmol) and pH scales for measurement of hydrogen ion concentrations;
7. Compare and contrast the distribution of water and dissolved solutes among the various fluid compartments of the body;

8. Describe the basic physiologic mechanisms regulating fluid and solute transport between body fluid compartments and the control of water loss and gain;
9. Differentiate among the roles played by the major body fluid electrolytes in health and disease.

KEY TERMS

Most terms used in this chapter are defined in context. The following terms are introduced without explicit definition but may be found in the text glossary:

acetazolamide	ileus
acromegaly	interstitium
Addison's disease	lassitude
aldosterone	metastases
ascites	oliguria
catabolism	orthostatic
chelating agent	pancreatitis
diuretic	peritoneal dialysis
extrasystole	sarcoidosis
hypothyroidism	titration

SOLUTIONS

Definition of a solution

The body is mainly a watery medium in which large numbers of chemical substances and particles exist in solution or suspension. There are three primary ways in which these chemical substances or particles exist in combination with water: as colloids, as suspensions, or as true solutions.

Colloids (sometimes called dispersions or gels) consist of large molecules, or clumps of molecules, that are able to attract and hold large numbers of water molecules. Typically, these molecules become uniformly distributed throughout the dispersion and tend not to settle out. Egg white, gelatin, and intracellular protoplasm are common examples of colloids.

Suspensions, of which red blood cells in plasma are an example, consist of large particles that are merely suspended in a liquid vehicle without the normal relationship between solvent and solute found in true solutions. Dispersion of these suspended particles depends on physical agitation, and when the mixture is allowed to stand the particles settle out.

A true solution, on the other hand, is a stable mixture of two substances, with one evenly dispersed throughout the other. The substance dissolved or going into solution is called the solute, and the medium in which it is dissolved is called the solvent.

The ease with which a solute mixes with a solvent is a measure of its solubility. Four primary factors influence solubility:

1. The nature of the solute. The degree to which all substances go into solution in a given solvent is a physical characteristic of matter, with wide variability.
2. The nature of the solvent. As with solutes, solvents vary widely in their ability to incorporate substances into solutions.
3. Temperature. In general, the solubility of most solid solutes increases with temperature; the solubility of gases, however, varies inversely with temperature.
4. Pressure. Solubility of gases in liquids varies directly with pressure.

Concentration of solutions

A solution is described as dilute if it has a relatively small amount of solute in proportion to solvent. Fig. 5-1 shows three different states of a solution. In Fig. 5-1, *A,* the solution is considered dilute because it has relatively few solute particles.

A saturated solution is one with the maximum amount of solute that can be held by a given volume of a solvent at a constant temperature in the presence of an excess of solute. In such a mixture the dissolved solute is in equilibrium with the undissolved solute. Saturated solutions are usually prepared by the addition of a known excess of solute to the solvent, allowing the excess to remain in contact with the solution. Fig. 5-1, *B* is a saturated solution, and the excess solute is depicted as an undissolved mass at the bottom of the container. Although there is more solute in contact with solvent than the latter can accommodate at a fixed temperature, the excess must not be thought of as completely inert. Particles of solute precipitate into the solid state at the same rate that new molecules leave the supply of solute and go into solution. This is the state of equilibrium that characterizes a saturated solution.

A solution is said to be supersaturated when it contains more solute in solution than does a saturated solution at the same temperature and pressure. If a saturated solution is heated, upsetting the solute equilibrium and allowing more solute to go into solution, and the remaining undissolved solute is filtered and the solution is allowed to cool gently, then the solution will contain an excess of dissolved solute. Solution *C* in Fig. 5-1 can be considered the

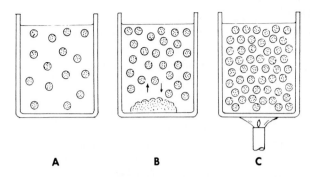

Fig. 5-1   In the dilute solution, **A,** the solute particles are relatively few in number, whereas in the saturated solution, **B,** the solvent contains all the solute it can hold in the presence of an excess of solute. Heating the solution, **C,** dissolves more solute particles, which may remain in solution if gently cooled, creating a state of supersaturation.

result of applying heat to solution *B,* driving the remainder of the excess solute into solution. The additional dissolved particles may remain in solution, even after cooling to the temperature of the original saturated state, if extreme care is taken. Such a supersaturated solution is unstable, and the excess of dissolved solute may be precipitated out of solution by such physical stimuli as shaking or vibrating or by addition to the solution of a small amount of the solid solute.

Characteristics of solutions

Most of the solutions of physiologic importance in the body are dilute, and solutes in dilute solution demonstrate many of the properties of gases. This behavior is a result of the relatively large distances between the molecules of solute in dilute concentrations. The four major characteristics of solutions are vapor pressure depression, boiling point elevation, freezing point depression, and osmotic pressure.

Vapor pressure depression. The vapor pressure of a solution is less than that of the pure solvent, in direct proportion to the concentration of the solute. This is attributed to interference with the escape of solvent molecules by solute molecules at the liquid surface.

Boiling point elevation. The boiling point of a solution is higher than that of the pure solvent, and its elevation is directly proportional to the concentration of the solute in a given weight of solvent.

Freezing point depression. The freezing point of a solution is lower than that of a pure solvent, and its depression is directly proportional to the concentration of the solute in a given weight of solvent.

Osmotic pressure. Physiologically, the most important characteristic of solutions is their ability to exert *osmotic* pressure. Osmotic pressure is a measurable force produced by mobility of the solvent particles under certain conditions. Imagine a thin porous sheet constructed so as to permit the passage through it of molecules of solvent but not of solute. Such a structure is called a *semipermeable membrane*. Should such a membrane be placed so as to divide a solution into two compartments, molecules of solvent would pass freely through it from one side to the other (Fig. 5-2, *A*). However, probability theory dictates that the number of molecules that pass (or diffuse) in one direction must be equaled by the number passing in the opposite direction to maintain an equal ratio between solute and solvent particles (which determines the concentration of the solution) on both sides of the membrane.

If a solution is put on one side of the semipermeable membrane and pure solvent on the other, probability theory dictates that more solvent molecules will move through the membrane in the direction of the solution than will move in the direction of the pure solvent. The force driving the solvent molecules through the membrane is termed *osmotic pressure* and can be measured by connecting the expanding column of the solution to a manometer (Fig. 5-2, *B* and *C*). This pressure can be considered a force that tries to distribute solvent molecules so that there will be the same ratio between solute and solvent particles and thus the same concentration on both sides of the membrane.

Osmotic pressure can also be visualized as the attractive force of solute particles in a concentrated solution. If the conditions include placement of a 50% solution on one side of the membrane and a 30% solution on the other, again the solvent molecules will penetrate the barrier from the dilute side to the concentrated side (Fig. 5-2, *D* and *E*). The greater number of solute particles per solvent molecules in the concentrated solution "attract" solvent molecules away from the smaller concentration of solute particles in the dilute solution until a condition of equilibrium is reached. An equilibrium condition is one in which an equal ratio of solute/solvent particles exists in both compartments, in this case an equal concentration of 40%. At this point, solvent particles move equally in both directions.

Osmotic pressure is dependent on the number of actual particles in solution, irrespective of any charge they may carry. Thus a 2% solution will have twice the osmotic pressure of a 1% solution. Moreover, for a given amount of solute, the osmotic pressure is inversely proportional to the volume of solvent. Also, osmotic pressure varies directly with temperature, increasing 1/273 for each 1° C.

Body cell walls are semipermeable membranes and, through the action of osmotic pressure, the distribution of water throughout the body is kept within physiologic ranges. The term *tonicity* refers to the relative degree of osmotic pressure exerted by a solution. The average body cellular fluid has a tonicity equal to that of a 0.9% solution of sodium chloride, often referred to as physiologic saline. For comparative purposes, any other solution with similar tonicity is called isotonic, one with greater tonicity is

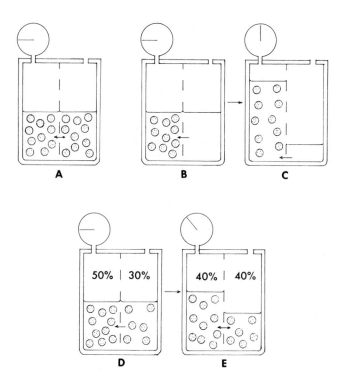

Fig. 5-2   Osmotic pressure is illustrated by the solutions in the above five containers. The containers are divided into two compartments by semipermeable membranes that permit the passage through them of solvent molecules but not solute *(dotted circles)*. The numbers of solute particles represent relative concentrations of the solutions; since they are fixed in number and are confined by the membranes, volume changes are a function of the diffusible solvent, movements of which are indicated by the arrows through the membranes. The arrows between containers **B** and **C** and **D** and **E** indicate progressive sequences of osmotic pressure. (See text for further description.)

called hypertonic, and one with less is called hypotonic. Some cell walls have selective permeability, allowing the passage not only of water but of specific solutes; through this mechanism, nutrients and physiologically active substances are distributed throughout the body.

Types of physiologic solution

With water serving as the primary solvent for body fluids, there are three basic types of physiologic solution. Depending on the nature of the solute, these solutions are called ionic or electrovalent solutions, polar covalent solutions, and nonpolar covalent solutions.

The distinguishing characteristic of ionic and polar covalent solutions is the tendency of all or some of the solute to ionize or dissociate into separate particles known as ions. If electrodes carrying a weak charge are placed in an electrolyte solution, the positive ions will migrate to the negative electrode and are consequently called cations. The negative ions migrate to the positive electrode and are called anions. Compounds that behave in this manner are known as electrolytes.

In nonpolar covalent solutions, on the other hand, the molecules of the solute remain intact and thus do not carry an electrical charge. For this reason, they are often referred to as nonelectrolytes.

In reality, all three types of solution coexist in the body. Moreover, these various solutions also serve as the medium in which the colloids and simple suspensions that constitute the various body fluids are dispersed.

Ionic (electrovalent) solutions. Lacking true molecular structure, ionic compounds such as potassium or sodium chloride exist as orderly arrangements of ions in masses called crystals. Ions are present in such compounds, even in the dry undissolved state. For this reason, solutions in which ionic compounds serve as the solute are often referred to clinically as crystalloids.

The process of dissolving ionic compounds consists of separation of their crystals into individual ions. The ions are freed from their mutual bonds and immediately distribute themselves uniformly throughout the solvent. This phenomenon is referred to as ionic dissociation, or just dissociation.

A common example of ionic or electrovalent dissociation in aqueous solution is that of sodium chloride (NaCl), shown as follows:

$$NaCl \rightarrow Na^+ + Cl^-$$

Solutions of sodium chloride contain equal numbers of sodium and chloride ions to maintain electrical equilibrium. Calcium chloride ($CaCl_2$), in contrast, produces twice as many anions as cations, but the total charges remain equal:

$$CaCl_2 \rightarrow Ca^{++} + Cl^- + Cl^-$$

It was originally thought that the role of water as a solvent for ionic compounds was purely passive, providing a uniform medium in which electrolytic dissociation could spontaneously occur. The dipole water molecule is now recognized as being critically important in this phenomenon, participating in solute dissociation and regulating the degree to which ions are produced.

Fig. 5-3 represents the dissociation of sodium chloride in water. A crystalline mass of sodium and chloride ions rests on the bottom of the container. Water molecular dipoles are separating the crystalline ions through the electrical attraction of their polar charges. Negative oxygen poles of water molecules draw the positive sodium ions away from the crystal, while positive hydrogen poles relate similarly to chloride ions. As the ions diffuse throughout the solvent, each is loosely held by several water molecules surrounding it and facing it with oppositely charged poles. The number of water dipoles associated with a particular ion depends on the size and charge of the ion, and Fig. 5-3 is not intended to be quantitatively accurate. An ion associated with water dipoles is said to be *hydrated*. Hydration

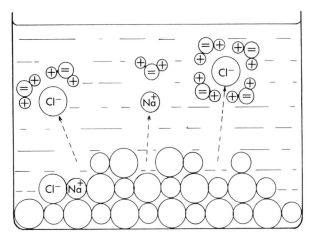

Fig. 5-3 Sodium chloride is shown as a crystalline mass of ions being dissociated by the attraction of water dipoles. (See text for a more detailed description.)

is a kinetic state, as water molecules continually interchange from ion to ion and between ions and the solvent mass.

Generally, ionic compounds are strong electrolytes, strength being a function of the degree of electrical conductivity. Conductivity, in turn, depends on the number of ions formed; the larger the concentration of ions made available by a solute, the stronger the electrolyte is.

Polar covalent solutions. Molecular covalent compounds have no ions of their own. In solution, however, through action similar to that described for the dissociation of sodium chloride, water dipoles can break the covalent bonds of polarized molecules and produce ions. In this circumstance, ions are made from molecules in water where none existed before; such a phenomenon is called ionization, as differentiated from dissociation.

Ionization of a strong polar covalent electrolyte. Hydrogen chloride is a good example of a strong covalent electrolyte. In the pure liquid state, or when dissolved in an organic nonpolar covalent solvent such as benzene, hydrogen chloride does not conduct electricity, thus demonstrating a lack of ionic structure. However, when hydrogen chloride is dissolved in water, it becomes an active electrolyte. The dramatic change in properties after hydrogen chloride dissolves is attributed to a function of the water solvent molecules. Fig. 5-4 illustrates the fundamental reaction between hydrogen chloride molecules and water dipoles. Fig. 5-4, *A* shows the negative pole of a water molecule reacting with the positive pole of a hydrogen chloride molecule. The effect is seen in Fig. 5-4, *B*, where the water dipole, through electrical attraction, has pulled the hydrogen from the chloride atom, leaving the chloride with the shared electrons, creating a chloride anion and a hydrogen cation. Ionization has been accomplished.

Hydrogen ions, however, cannot exist alone in solution

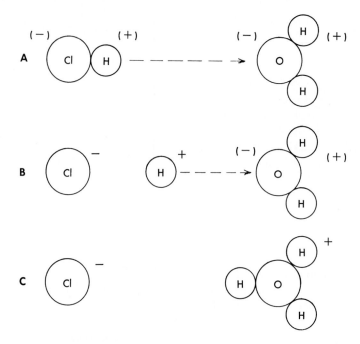

Fig. 5-4 Ionization of hydrogen chloride molecule by a water dipole. The hydrogen atom is separated from the chloride by the negative pole of a water molecule. (See text for details.)

but only in combination with a dipole water molecule, as shown in Fig. 5-4, *C*. The hydrated hydrogen ion becomes a group of three atoms with an overall net electrical charge of +1. It is called a hydronium ion. In terms of chemical action, the hydronium ion is the hydrogen ion with the same meaning as the notation H^+. For convenience, the latter is more commonly used in chemical equations involving hydrogen ions, and it is used almost exclusively in the remainder of this book.

The reader should understand that the process of ionization changes the nature of the substance ionized. Hydrogen chloride, as a solute in a nonpolar solvent, is transformed into hydrochloric acid when ionized in an aqueous solution. It then acquires properties characteristic of acids.

Ionization of a weak polar covalent electrolyte. Many of the organic compounds of the body are weak electrolytes. These weak electrolytes play important roles in maintaining homeostasis, particularly as related to acid-base balance.

Acetic acid (CH_3COOH) is an example of a weak electrolyte. Under normal conditions, acetic acid dissociates into a hydrogen ion, H^+, and an acetate ion, CH_3COO^-. Acetic acid is characterized as a weak electrolyte because it has some, but not much, molecular polarity and a strong covalent bond that is difficult for the water dipole to break. Its ionizing equation is

$$CH_3COOH \rightleftharpoons H^+ + CH_3COO^-$$

The use of the double arrows in this equation indicates that the reaction can go in both directions simultaneously and is reversible. While molecules of acetic acid are breaking down into ions (movement to the right), some of the ions are recombining into molecules (movement to the left). The arrows represent a state of equilibrium in which the number of molecules ionizing is equaled by the number re-formed from ions.

Weak polar covalent electrolytes such as acetic acid exist in aqueous solution mostly as molecules, with only a few ions. Fig. 5-5 compares the relative ionization of acetic acid with that of hydrochloric acid, which is almost completely ionized.

Ionization of water. Water is one of the weakest electrolytes. Nonetheless, the ionization of water provides the foundation for both physiologic acid-base balance and our system of recording it.

Attraction between a pair of water dipoles can develop a bond that unites the oxygen of one and a hydrogen of the other that is stronger than the internal covalent bond of the second molecule. Fig. 5-6 illustrates the union of two water molecules and then their separation into hydronium and hydroxide ions according to the following reaction:

$$H_2O + H_2O \rightleftharpoons H_3O^+ + OH^-$$

or more simply

$$HOH \rightleftharpoons H^+ + OH^-$$

The hydronium ion formed is exactly like that generated in the ionization of hydrogen chloride. The formula H_2O indicates that a molecule consists of two hydrogen atoms linked to one oxygen atom; HOH indicates the same thing

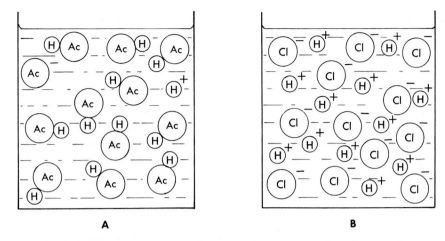

Fig. 5-5   A, The weak electrolyte, acetic acid (CH₃COOH), exists almost entirely as intact molecules, with only one cation and one anion each illustrated. **B,** In contrast, the strong electrolyte, hydrogen chloride, is completely ionized.

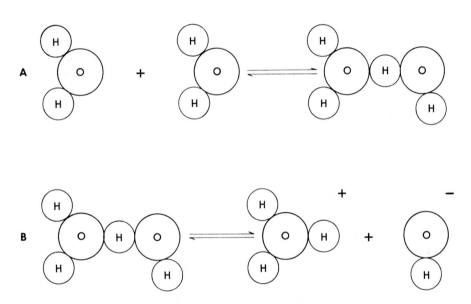

Fig. 5-6   Ionization of water. A, A rare union of the oxygen of one water dipole with a hydrogen atom of another. **B,** The two dipoles separate into hydronium and hydroxide ions. (See text for description of ion formation.)

but, in addition, emphasizes the two ions that are derived from some of the molecules. The latter is the preferred notation, especially in an ionization equation.

The ionization equation, with its unequal arrows, indicates the weakness of water as an electrolyte. Nonetheless, because some ionization does occur, water may be thought of as a very dilute aqueous solution of hydrogen and hydroxide ions.

Nonpolar covalent solutions. An even distribution of charges gives to nonpolar covalent compounds an electrical symmetry that prevents polarity. It creates strong internal molecular bonding that resists the attraction of water solvent dipoles. A nonpolarized molecule may be imagined as presenting a defensive perimeter on which any

given point is electrically neutral because of surrounding balanced charges. Glucose is a good example of a nonpolar covalent substance. Solutions of nonpolar covalent substances such as glucose produce no ions, conduct no electrical current, and are therefore considered nonelectrolytes.

Quantifying solute content and activity

There are two primary ways to quantify the amount of solute in a solution: (1) by actual weight (grams or milligrams) or (2) by chemical combining power. Although the weight of a solute is relatively easy to measure and specify, it does not necessarily gives us an indication of its chemical combining power. For example, the sodium ion (Na⁺) has a gram ionic weight of 23, whereas the bicarbonate ion (HCO_3^-) has a gram ionic weight of 61. However, since the gram atomic (or formula) weight of every substance has the same number of particles (6.023×10^{23}), these ions have the same chemical combining power in solution and are therefore chemically equivalent. Thus, the number of chemically reactive units present in the body is more meaningful than their bulk weight.

Equivalent weights. For this reason, it has become customary in medicine to refer quantitatively to certain essential substances that are physiologically active in the body in terms of their chemical combining power, as expressed by a measure called equivalent weight. Equivalent weights are quantitative amounts of reacting substances that have equal chemical combining power. Therefore, when A reacts chemically with B, one equivalent weight of A will react exactly with one equivalent weight of B, and there will be no excess of reactants remaining.

There are two magnitudes of equivalent weight measurements used in quantifying chemical combining power: the gram equivalent weight (gEq) and the milligram equivalent weight or milliequivalent (mEq). A gram equivalent weight is related to a milligram equivalent weight as a gram is related to a milligram. Thus 1 g equivalent weight equals 1000 mEq.

Gram equivalent weights. In general, the gram equivalent weight of a substance normally is calculated as its gram atomic (or formula) weight divided by its valence, with no regard for the valence sign:

$$gEq = \frac{gram\ atomic\ (formula)\ weight}{valence}$$

For example, the gram equivalent weight of sodium (Na^+), with a valence of $+1$, is equal to its gram atomic weight of 23 g. On the other hand, the gram equivalent weight of calcium (Ca^{++}) is its atomic weight divided by 2, or 20 g. The gram equivalent weight of ferric iron (Fe^{+++}) is its atomic weight divided by 3, or about 18.6 g.

For a radical such as sulfate (SO_4^{--}), the formula for sulfuric acid (H_2SO_4) shows us that one sulfate group combines with two atoms of hydrogen. Therefore, 0.5 mole of sulfate is the equivalent of 1 mole of hydrogen atoms. The equivalent weight of SO_4^{--} is therefore one half its gram formula weight, or 48 g. If an element or a radical has more than one valence, the valence must either be specified or apparent from the element's observed chemical combining properties.

Gram equivalent weight of an acid. The gram equivalent weight of an acid is the weight in grams of the acid that contains 1 mole of replaceable hydrogen. As a general rule, the gram equivalent weight of an acid can be calculated by division of its gram formula weight by the number of hydrogen atoms in its formula.

For example, in the reaction $HCl + Na^+ \rightarrow NaCl + H^+$, the single hydrogen atom of hydrochloric acid is replaced by sodium. Thus, 1 mole of hydrochloric acid has 1 mole

of replaceable hydrogen and, by definition, the gram equivalent weight of hydrochloric acid must be the same as its gram formula weight, or 36.5 g. On the other hand, the two hydrogen atoms of sulfuric acid (H_2SO_4) are both considered replaceable. Therefore 1 mole of sulfuric acid contains 2 moles of replaceable hydrogen. The gram equivalent weight of sulfuric acid is therefore one half its gram formula weight, or 49 g.

Exceptions to this rule are those acids in which hydrogen atoms are not completely replaceable or those in which hydrogen replacement varies according to specific reactions. Carbonic acid (H_2CO_3) and phosphoric acid (H_3PO_4) are good physiologic examples of these exceptions. Equivalent weights of both are determined by the conditions of their chemical reactions.

For instance, carbonic acid (H_2CO_3) has two hydrogen atoms, but in reactions occurring under physiologic conditions only one is considered replaceable. This is illustrated in the following important reaction:

$$H_2CO_3 + Na^+ \rightarrow NaHCO_3 + H^+$$

Here, only one hydrogen atom is released and the other remains bound. Despite the presence of two hydrogen atoms, under these conditions, 1 mole of carbonic acid contains only 1 mole of replaceable hydrogen, and the gram equivalent weight of carbonic acid is the same as its gram formula weight, or 62 g.

Gram equivalent weight of a base. The equivalent weight of a base is the weight of the base in grams that contains 1 mole of replaceable hydroxyl (OH^-) ions. Like the acids just described, the gram equivalent weight of a base is calculated by dividing its gram formula weight by the number of OH groups in its formula.

Conversion of gram weight to equivalent weight. To determine the number (or fraction) of gram equivalent weights in a given substance, the gram weight of the substance is divided by its calculated equivalent weight. Therefore 58.5 g of NaCl divided by its gram equivalent weight of 58.5 g equals 1 gEq, whereas 29.25 g of NaCl divided by 58.5 g equals 0.5 gEq.

Milligram equivalent weights. Since the concentrations of most body chemicals, such as Na^+, Cl^-, K^+, and HCO_3^-, are very small, the term milligram equivalent weight or milliequivalent is preferred. A milliequivalent is simply 0.001 of a gram equivalent weight:

$$mEq = \frac{gEq}{1000}$$

Conversely, there are 1000 milliequivalents in 1 gram equivalent weight:

$$gEq = mEq \times 1000$$

For example, the normal concentration of potassium (K^+) in the plasma ranges between 0.0035 and 0.005 gram equivalent weights per liter. Rather than using such small numbers, we convert these values to milliequivalent weights by multiplying by a factor of 1000. Thus the normal concentration of potassium in the plasma ranges between 3.5 and 5.0 mEq/L.

Solute content by weight. Although in the quantification of solutions the number of chemically active units is physiologically more meaningful than their weight, the measurement of most electrolytes in the clinical laboratory is based on actual weight and not on milliequivalents. Typically, this weight, as measured in a sample of blood or body fluid, is expressed as milligrams per 100 ml of fluid, customarily referred to as milligrams percent (mg%) or milligrams per deciliter (mg/dL). This text uses the modern designation of milligrams per deciliter.

These values are then converted into the corresponding equivalent weights and reported as milliequivalents per liter of fluid (mEq/L). Transposition between mEq/L and mg/dL is performed as follows:

$$\text{mEq} = \text{mg weight/equivalent weight} \qquad (1)$$

$$\text{mEq/L} = \text{mg/dL} \times 10/\text{equivalent weight}$$

$$\text{mg} = \text{mEq} \times \text{equivalent weight} \qquad (2)$$

$$\text{mg/dL} = \text{mEq/L} \times \text{equivalent weight}/10$$

For example, to convert a measure of serum value of 322 mg/dL of sodium to mEq/L:

$$\text{mEq/L} = \text{mg/dL} \times 10/\text{equivalent weight}$$
$$= 322 \times 10/23$$
$$= 140 \text{ mEq/L}$$

In hospital practice, electrolyte replacement is commonplace therapy. This is accomplished by the intravenous infusion of solutions in which the electrolyte content often is stated in milligrams per 100 ml of solution and as milliequivalents per liter. A typical example is a solution known as lactated Ringer's injection, the label of which lists its ingredients as shown in Table 5-1.

Table 5-2 lists the equivalents of electrolytes more accurately, as calculated from milligram percentage according to the above formula for conversion to milliequivalents per liter.

Calculating solute content

In addition to the use of gram equivalent weights, milligram equivalent weights, and simple weight measures (such as milligrams per deciliter), there are several other ways to classify solute content. A knowledge of these various common chemical standards is essential in the computation of solute contents and in the dilution of solutions.

Quantitative classification of solutions. There are six methods whereby the amount of solute in a solution may be quantified. These include the ratio solution, the weight per volume (w/v) solution, the percent solution, the molal solution, the molar solution, and the normal solution.

1. Ratio solution. The relationship of the solute to the solvent is expressed as a proportion (eg, 1:100, parts per thousand, etc). This is used frequently in describing concentrations of pharmaceuticals.

2. Weight per volume solution. Often erroneously referred to as a "percent solution," the weight per volume solution is the one most commonly used in pharmacy and medicine for solids dissolved in liquids. It is calibrated in weight of solute per volume of solution as grams of solute per 100 ml of solution. Therefore, 5 g of glucose dissolved in 100 ml of solution is properly called a 5% (weight per volume) solution. In contrast, a liquid dissolved in a liquid is measured as volumes of solute to volumes of solution.

3. Percent solution. Used in chemistry, a percent solution is calibrated as weight of solute per weight of solution. Five grams of glucose dissolved in 95 g of water is a true percent solution since the glucose is 5% of the total solution weight of 100 g.

4. Molal solution. Less frequently used in physiologic chemistry than are the molar solution and the normal solution, a molal solution contains 1 mole of solute per kilogram of solvent (or 1 mmol per gram of solvent).

Table 5-1 Concentrations of Ingredients Listed on Label of Ringer's Solution Container

	mg/dL		Approximate mEq/L
NaCl	600	Na	130
$NaC_3H_5O_3$ (Na lactate)	310	Cl	109
KCl	30	$C_3H_5O_3$	28
$CaCl_2$	20	K	4
		Ca	3

Table 5-2 Calculated Milliequivalents (mEq) of Ingredients of Lactated Ringer's Solution

	Na	Cl	Lactate	K	Ca
NaCl	102.6	102.6			
NaLac	27.7		27.7		
KCl		4.0		4.0	
$CaCl_2$		3.6			3.6
TOTAL mEq/L	130.3	110.2	27.7	4.0	3.6

With its solvent measured in weight, the concentration of a molal solution is independent of temperature.

5. Molar solution. Physiologically, the molar solution and the normal solution are the most important of all solutions. A molar solution has 1 mol of solute per liter of solution (or 1 mmol/ml solution). A 1 mol/L solution of sodium chloride contains 58.5 g (1 gfw) per liter of solution, a 0.5 mol/L solution has 29.25 g/L of solution, a 2 mol/L solution has 117 g/L of solution, and so on. The solute is measured into a container, and the solvent is added to the total solution volume desired. The molar solution is chemically important because equal volumes of solutions of equal molarity contain the same number or fractions of solute moles.

6. Normal solution. Widely used in chemistry and biochemistry, the normal solution has 1 gram equivalent weight of solute per liter of solution (or 1 mEq/ml of solution). Accordingly, 1 mol of hydrochloric acid or 0.5 mole of sulfuric acid, each dissolved in 1 L of solution, make 1 N solutions of the respective solutes. For all monovalent solutes, normal and molar solutions are the same because the equivalent weights of such solutes equal their gram formula weights. Equal volumes of solutions of the same normality contain chemically equivalent amounts of their solutes. If the solutes react chemically with one another, then equal volumes of the solutions will react completely and neither substance will remain in excess. Solutions of known normality are often used as standard solutions in an analytic process known as titration for determining the concentrations of other solutions.

Dilution calculations. It is often necessary to make a dilute solution from a stock preparation. This can be done accurately if the concepts of solution concentrations are understood. Such dilution problems usually involve medications and are based on the pharmacologic weight per unit volume (w/v) percent principle defined earlier.

Diluting a solution increases its volume without changing the amount of solute it contains but reduces its concentration. Therefore the amount of solute in a given sample after dilution is the same as was present in the smaller original volume. The amount of solute present in a sample of a solution can be expressed as volume times concentration. For example, the amount of solute in 50 ml of a 10% w/v solution (10 g/dL) is $50 \times 0.1 = 5$ g. In dilution of a solution, then, the initial volume times the initial concentration equals the final volume times the final concentration. This can be simplified with the following formula:

$$V_1C_1 = V_2C_2$$

and when three of the data are known, the fourth can be calculated.

1. Given 10 ml of a 2% solution, dilute to a concentration of 0.5%.

   This requires finding the new volume:

$$V_1C_1 = V_2C_2$$
$$V_2 = V_1C_1/C_2$$
$$V_2 = 10 \times 2/0.5$$
$$V_2 = 40 \text{ ml}$$

Thus the addition of 30 ml to 10 ml of 2% solution makes 40 ml of 0.5% solution.

2. If 50 ml of water is added to 150 ml of a 3% solution, calculate the new concentration.

$$V_1C_1 = V_2C_2$$
$$C_2 = V_1C_1/V_2$$
$$C_2 = 150 \times 3/200$$
$$C_2 = 2.25\%$$

3. Given 50 ml of a 0.33 N solution, dilute it to a 0.1 N concentration. Here, concentration is given as normality, but it can be used as well as percent.

$$V_1C_1 = V_2C_2$$
$$V_2 = V_1C_1/C_2$$
$$V_2 = 50 \times 0.33/0.1$$
$$V_2 = 167 \text{ ml}$$

ELECTROLYTIC ACTIVITY AND ACID-BASE BALANCE

Acid-base homeostasis ultimately depends on the relative concentration and activity of certain electrolytic solutes in the body fluids. Clinical application of acid-base homeostasis is covered in detail in Chapter 10. A sound understanding of the clinical applications of acid-base balance depends first and foremost on mastery of some basic physiologic chemistry. To that end, this section will explore the basic concepts of physiologic chemistry relevant to acid-base balance. We will look first at the ionic characteristics of acids, bases, and salts, followed by discussions of electrolytic activity and the designation of acidity and alkalinity.

Ionic characteristics of acids, bases, and salts

Acids. Traditionally, an acid is a compound that yields hydrogen ions when placed into an aqueous solution. Typically, such substances consist of a hydrogen atom or atoms covalently bonded to a negative-valence nonmetal or radical, such as hydrochloric acid.

A more modern conception of an acid is the Brönsted-Lowry definition, which states that an acid is any compound that is a proton donor. According to the Brönsted-Lowry definition, many substances other than traditional acids are included. For example, the ammonium ion (NH_4^+) qualifies as an acid since it can release a proton (H^+) in the following reaction:

$$NH_4Cl + NaOH \rightarrow NH_3 + NaCl + HOH$$

In this reaction, the sodium and chloride ions are essentially "spectator" ions because they are not involved in the proton transfer. By eliminating these nonparticipating ions, we can write the equation ionically and demonstrate the acidity of the ammonium ion:

$$NH_4^+ + OH^- \rightarrow NH_3 + HOH$$

The ammonium ion donates a hydrogen ion (proton) to the reaction, which combines with the hydroxide ion (OH^-), converting the former into ammonia gas and the latter into water.

Acids with single ionizable hydrogen. Simple compounds such as the following ionize into one cation and one anion each:

$$HCl \rightarrow H^+ + Cl^-$$
$$HBr \rightarrow H^+ + Br^-$$
$$HNO_3 \rightarrow H^+ + NO_3^-$$

Acids with multiple ionizable hydrogens. All of the potential hydrogen ions in an acid may not be made available at once but in stages. The degree of ionization tends to increase as an electrolyte solution becomes more dilute. Concentrated sulfuric acid ionizes only one of its two hydrogen atoms per molecule:

$$H_2SO_4 \rightarrow H^+ + HSO_4^-$$

With further dilution, second-stage ionization occurs:

$$H_2SO_4 \rightarrow H^+ + H^+ + SO_4^{--}$$

Bases. Traditionally, a base is a compound that yields hydroxyl ions when placed into an aqueous solution and is capable of inactivating acids. These compounds, called hydroxides, typically consist of a metal, or the metal-equivalent ammonium cation (NH_4^+), ionically bound to a hydroxide ion or ions. A good example of a base under this traditional definition is sodium hydroxide (NaOH).

According to the Brönsted-Lowry definition, a base is any compound that accepts a proton, including many substances other than hydroxides. Nonhydroxide bases include ammonia, the carbonates, and certain proteins.

Hydroxide bases. In aqueous solution the following are typical dissociations of hydroxide bases:

$$Na^+OH^- \rightarrow Na^+ + OH^-$$
$$K^+OH^- \rightarrow K^+ + OH^-$$
$$Ca^+(OH^-)_2 \rightarrow Ca^{++} + 2(OH^-)$$

Inactivation of an acid, as part of the definition of a base, is accomplished by OH^- reacting with H^+ (proton acceptance by the base), forming water:

$$NaOH + HCl \rightarrow NaCl + HOH$$

Nonhydroxide bases. Ammonia and the carbonates are good examples of nonhydroxide bases. Physiologically,

proteins can also serve as nonhydroxide bases by virtue of their amino groups.

Ammonia. In the description of acids it was demonstrated how an ammonium ion can be called an acid when it donates a proton and becomes ammonia. Ammonia also qualifies as a base by reacting with water to produce OH^-

$$NH_3 + HOH \rightarrow NH_4^+ + OH^-$$

and by neutralizing H^+ directly

$$NH_3 + H^+ \rightarrow NH_4^+$$

In both instances NH_3 accepts a proton to become NH_4^+. This "acidification" of ammonia plays a crucial role in renal excretion of acid, as discussed subsequently in Chapter 10.

Carbonates. The reactions of this group, of which sodium carbonate is an example, are very relevant to pulmonary physiology. The carbonate ion, CO_3^{--}, can react with water to produce OH^-. First,

$$Na_2CO_3 \rightleftharpoons 2Na^+ + CO_3^{--}$$

then

$$CO_3^{--} + HOH \rightleftharpoons HCO_3^- + OH^-$$

In this reaction, the carbonate ion accepted a proton from water, becoming the bicarbonate ion, while simultaneously producing a hydroxide ion. The carbonate ion can also directly react with H^+ to inactivate it as follows:

$$CO_3^{--} + H^+ \rightleftharpoons HCO_3^-$$

Proteins as bases. Proteins are composed of amino acids bound together by peptide linkages. Since physiologic reactions in the body tend to occur in a mildly alkaline environment, cell and blood proteins tend to act as anionic proton receptors, or bases. Cell and blood proteins acting as bases are symbolized as "prot$^-$," indicating their role as anionic proton receptors.

It is the imidiazole group of the amino acid histidine that serves as the primary proton acceptor on protein molecules, as depicted in Fig. 5-7. Imidiazole groups constitute the major portion of the strong buffering power of hemoglobin, each molecule of which contains 38 histidine residues. Since the oxygen-carrying component (heme group) of hemoglobin is attached to a histidine residue, its ability to accept hydrogen ions is influenced by the state of oxygenation of the molecule. Specifically, when it is in the deoxygenated state, the hemoglobin molecule is a stronger base (better proton acceptor) than when it is in the oxygenated state. This change accounts, in part, for the ability of deoxygenated hemoglobin to "inactivate" more acid than oxygenated hemoglobin, as described further in Chapter 10. Because the plasma proteins contain less histidine, their buffering power is somewhat less than that of hemoglobin.

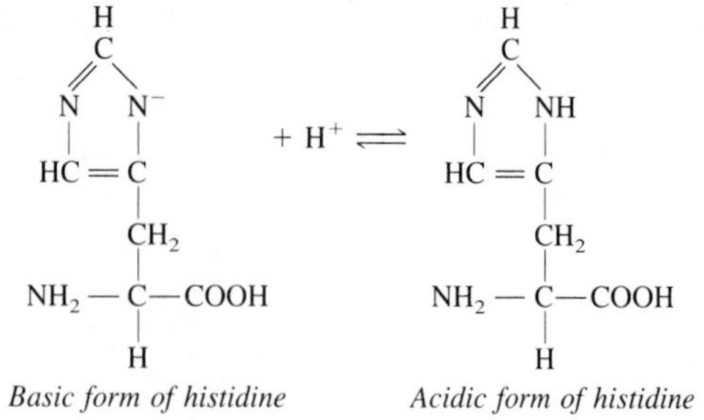

Basic form of histidine   *Acidic form of histidine*

Fig. 5-7 Histidine portion of protein molecule serving as a proton acceptor (base).

Salts. The most common of compounds, salts are composed of metal or ammonium ions electrovalently joined to anions other than the hydroxyl. There are many ways of producing salts, but the simplest is by the reaction between an acid and a base, as noted in the descriptions of these last two compounds:

$$HCl + NaOH \rightarrow NaCl + HOH$$

There are three classifications of salts, which depend on the degree of hydrogen and hydroxyl replacement from the parent acids and bases.

Normal salt. A normal salt is a compound formed by the complete replacement of hydrogen ions from its acid as follows:

$$H^+Cl^- + Na^+OH^- \rightarrow Na^+Cl^- + H^+OH^-$$
$$H^+NO_3^- + K^+OH^- \rightarrow K^+NO_3^- + H^+OH^-$$

Acid salt. An acid salt results from only partial replacement of hydrogen ions from the related acid, leaving some "acidity" (hydrogen ion or ions) in the salt:

$$H_2^{+}{}^+CO_3^{--} + Na^+OH^- \rightarrow Na^+HCO_3^- + H^+OH^-$$

Sodium bicarbonate can also be called sodium acid carbonate because of its hydrogen atom. Both hydrogen atoms in H_2CO_3 may ionize under proper conditions, but in the physiologic environment of the human body the single hydrogen ionization is the only reaction possible. To underscore the ions involved, carbonic acid can be rewritten to show it composed of only one hydrogen ion and the univalent bicarbonate ion, HCO_3^-. The reaction would look like this:

$$H^+ + HCO_3^- + Na^+OH^- \rightarrow Na^+HCO_3^- + H^+OH^-$$

Basic salt. A basic salt contains an unreplaced hydroxide ion from the base generating it, such as:

$$Ca^{++}(OH^-)_2 + H^+Cl^- \rightarrow Ca^{++}(OH^-)Cl^- + H^+OH^-$$

Measurement of electrolytic activity

The physiologically active chemical compounds of the body are, for the most part, weakly electrolytic covalent substances, and their ionic behavior can be summarized as follows:

1. A proportion of the molecules in an aqueous solution of a weak covalent electrolyte ionize, and the remainder of the molecules persist intact. At a given temperature and concentration, equilibrium is maintained between the ions and the un-ionized molecules.
2. After the establishment of ionic equilibrium, the product of the molar concentration (moles per liter) of the ions divided by the molar concentration of the un-ionized molecules is a constant value at a given concentration of solution and temperature. This is a special type of equilibrium constant called an ionization constant, or K. It cannot be emphasized too strongly that such a relationship exists only with aqueous solutions of weak electrolytes.

Degree of dissociation or ionization. As pointed out earlier, the strength of an electrolyte depends on the percentage of its solute that dissociates (true electrovalent or ionic compounds) or ionizes (polar covalent compounds). In evaluating the electrolytic strength of a substance, it is important to know its percent of ion production. Handbooks of chemistry and other sources provide this information, always specifying the molar concentrations of the solutions and the temperature at which the values are valid. Table 5-3 lists the percentages of three strong and three weak electrolytes that produce ions in 0.1 mol solutions at a temperature of 25°C. Sodium hydroxide (NaOH) is the only electrovalent compound in the group; 90% dissociates into sodium and hydroxide ions. With hydrochloric acid, 90% of its molecules ionize into hydrogen and chloride ions. In contrast, only 0.01% of the molecules of boric acid (H_3BO_3) ionize.

As an example, if a quantitative comparison is made between a 0.1 mol/L solution of hydrochloric acid with 90% ionization and a 0.1 mol/L solution of carbonic acid with 0.207% ionization, 1 L of each solution will contain 0.1 mole, or 0.1 gmw, of its respective acid solute. Ninety percent of the hydrochloric acid molecules, or 0.90 of 0.1 mole, 0.09 mole, dissociate into ions; 0.01 mole or gmw remains as intact molecules. Since each dissociating molecule produces one cation and one anion, the concentration or number per liter of each is the same as the concentration of the dissociating molecules. The ionic and molecular concentrations of the 0.1 mol/L hydrochloric acid solutions would be as follows:

$$\text{concentration of } H^+ \text{ ions} = 0.09 \text{ mol/L}$$
$$\text{concentration of } Cl^- \text{ ions} = 0.09 \text{ mol/L}$$
$$\text{concentration of HCl molecules} = 0.01 \text{ mol/L}$$

Table 5-3 Percent Ion Formation of 0.1 M Solutions at 25°C

NaOH	90%	CH$_3$COOH	1.33%
HCl	90%	H$_2$CO$_3$	0.207%
HNO$_3$	90%	H$_3$BO$_3$	0.0076%

Of the 0.1 mol/L solution of carbonic acid, which dissociates into hydrogen (H^+) and bicarbonate (HCO_3^-) ions, 0.00207 of 0.1 mole, or 0.000207 mole of the acid, dissociates into ions; 0.9979 of 0.1 mole, or 0.09979 mole, remains undissociated. Therefore:

$$\text{concentration of } H^+ \text{ ions} = 0.000207 \text{ mol/L}$$

$$\text{concentration of } HCO_3^- \text{ ions} = 0.000207 \text{ mol/L}$$

$$\text{concentration of } H_2CO_3 \text{ molecules} = 0.09979 \text{ mol/L}$$

Furthermore, a 0.1 mol/L solution contains $6.02 \times 10^{23} \times 0.1$, or 6.02×10^{22} molecules per liter. Therefore, on the basis of the known percentage of molecules that ionize, the actual number of ions and molecules per liter can be computed as shown in Table 5-4.

Examples of ionization can be expressed in one equation. This relationship holds only for weak electrolytes. The numerators of the following equations are in molar concentrations of ions, and the denominators are in molar concentrations (moles or gram molecular weights per liter) of un-ionized molecules of solute.

Brackets indicate concentrations of ions as well as of molecules and undissociated solute. Unless otherwise specified, the concentration implied is moles per liter. Thus $[H^+]$ means moles per liter of hydrogen ions, $[HCO_3^-]$ means mole per liter of bicarbonate ions, and $[H_2CO_3]$ signifies moles per liter of un-ionized, intact carbonic acid molecules.

(1) Symbolic representation of an acid, HA:

$$\frac{[H^+][A^-]}{[HA]} = K$$

(2) Symbolic representation of a base, BOH:

$$\frac{[B^+][OH^-]}{[BOH]} = K$$

(3) Acetic acid:

$$\frac{[H^+][CH_3COO^-]}{[CH_3COOH]} = 1.8 \times 10^{-5}$$

(4) Carbonic acid:

$$\frac{[H^+][HCO_3^-]}{[H_2CO_3]} = 4.3 \times 10^{-7}$$

Calculation of ionization (equilibrium) constant. The following is an actual calculation of an ionization constant involving acetic acid (CH_3COOH). At 25°C, 1.33% of a 0.1 mol/L solution of the acid undergoes ionization, and

therefore 98.76% of the molecules do not ionize. Ionization of acetic acid is represented as

$$CH_3COOH \rightleftharpoons H^+ + CH_3COO^-$$

1. Since 0.1 mol/L solution of acetic acid contains 0.1 gmw of acid per liter, of which 1.33% ionizes, then 0.1×0.0133 or 0.00133 mole of acid per liter produces ions and 0.1×0.9867 or 0.0987 mole per liter remains un-ionized.
2. Each molecule that ionizes produces two ions, H^+ and CH_3COO^- (acetate ion), and the concentration of each is the same as that of the ionizing molecules, 0.00133 mole of ions per liter. Accordingly, the concentration of un-ionized molecules is 0.09867 mole of ions per liter.
3. By definition, K is equal to the ratio between the product of the molar ion concentrations and the molar concentration of the un-ionized molecules, or

$$\frac{[H^+][CH_3COO^-]}{[CH_3COOH]} = K$$

$$\frac{0.00133 \times 0.00133}{0.09867} = K$$

$$K = 1.8 \times 10^{-5}$$

Ionization constant of water. The ionization of water is the basis for a system of calibrating acidity and alkalinity that is discussed below. Pure water produces the two ions H^+ and OH^-, and although its degree of ionization is small, it has an important ionization constant. In a sense, water consists of an aqueous solution of H^+ and OH^-. Its ion/molecule ratio can be expressed as:

$$\frac{[H^+][OH^-]}{[HOH]} = K$$

However, the degree of ionization of water is so small and the concentration of un-ionized molecules is proportionately so large that any small change in the degree of ionization would not produce a detectable reciprocal change in the concentration of the un-ionized molecules. Therefore the molar concentration of molecular water does not change significantly and can be considered as another constant in the ratio. The ratio can be rewritten as

$$\frac{[H^+][OH^-]}{K_2} = K_1$$

and

$$[H^+][OH^-] = K_1K_2 = K_w$$

Table 5-4 Concentrations of Ions and Molecules in 0.1 mol Hydrochloric Acid and 0.1 mol Carbonic Acid

	H^+ per liter	Anions per liter	Undissociated molecules per liter
0.1 M HCl	5.418×10^{22}	5.418×10^{22}	6.02×10^{21}
0.1 M H_2CO_3	1.246×10^{20}	1.246×10^{20}	6.0074×10^{22}

The dissociation constant of water, K_w, has been determined to be 1×10^{-14}. Therefore if

$$[H^+][OH^-] = 10^{-14}$$

then, because there is one H^+ for each OH^-, the concentration of each ion must be 10^{-7} mol/L. Thus pure water is as much acid as it is base, and it is therefore neutral in action.

Designation of acidity and alkalinity

When pure water is used as a reference point, it can be stated that any solution that has either a greater hydrogen ion concentration or a lesser hydroxide ion concentration than that of water is acid in its reactions. Conversely, a solution that has either a lesser hydrogen ion concentration or a greater hydroxide ion concentration than that of water is alkaline or basic in its reactions.

By agreement, the hydrogen ion concentration of pure water has been adopted as the standard by which to compare reactions of other solutions. Electrochemical techniques are used to measure the hydrogen ion concentration of unknown solutions, with their degree of acidity or alkalinity determined by variation of their $[H^+]$ above or below 1×10^{-7}. For example, a solution with an $[H^+]$ of 89.2×10^{-4} has a higher $[H^+]$ than water and is therefore acidic; one with a $[H^+]$ of 3.6×10^{-8} has fewer hydrogen ions than water and is thus alkaline.

There are two related techniques for recording acidity and alkalinity of solutions that use the hydrogen ion concentration of water as the neutral standard: (1) the actual measured molar concentration of hydrogen ions in nanomoles per liter and (2) the logarithmic pH scale.

Nanomolar concentrations. The first method of recording acidity and alkalinity of solutions reports the actual measured molar concentration of hydrogen ions, which is then compared with that of water. The $[H^+]$ of water is 1×10^{-7} mol/L or 0.0000001 (one ten millionth of a mole). Since one ten millionth equals 100 billionths, and since the prefix for billionths is "nano," the hydrogen ion concentration of water can be designated as 100 nanomoles per liter, or 100 nmol/L.

With this as a reference, any solution that has a $[H^+]$ of 100 nmol/L is neutral; greater than 100 nmol/L, acid; and less than 100 nmol/L, alkaline. Thus the degree of acidity or alkalinity is proportional to the distance of a given $[H^+]$ from the 100 nmol/L reference.

This system of recording is limited in its use because of the tremendous range of possible $[H^+]$, from the very acid to the very alkaline. However, this system is applicable to the needs of clinical medicine, because the physiologic range of hydrogen ion concentrations is very narrow, usually between 20 and 100 nmol/L.

pH scale. To simplify acid-base comparisons, the principle of pH was developed. pH is defined as the negative logarithm of the hydrogen ion concentration. It is derived

by conversion of the value for $[H^+]$ to a single negative exponent of 10 by calculation of its logarithm.

For example, the $[H^+]$ of water is 1×10^{-7} mol/L and, since the negative log of 1×10^{-7} is 7, the pH of water is 7. Other examples include the following:

$[H^+]$ of 8.2×10^{-4} mol/L: (1)

$$pH = -\log (8.2 \times 10^{-4})$$
$$pH = -\log 8.2 + -\log 10^{-4}$$
$$pH = -\log 8.2 + \log 10^4$$
$$pH = -0.914 + 4$$
$$pH = 3.09$$

$[H^+]$ of 4.0×10^{-8} mol/L: (2)

$$pH = -\log (4.0 \times 10^{-8})$$
$$pH = -\log 4.0 + -\log 10^{-8}$$
$$pH = -\log 4.0 + \log 10^8$$
$$pH = -0.602 + 8$$
$$pH = 7.40$$

$[H^+]$ of 6.7×10^{-11} mol/L: (3)

$$pH = -\log (6.7 \times 10^{-11})$$
$$pH = -\log 6.7 + -\log 10^{-11}$$
$$pH = -\log 6.7 + \log 10^{11}$$
$$pH = -0.826 + 11$$
$$pH = 10.17$$

Under this scheme, any solution with a pH of 7 is neutral, corresponding to the $[H^+]$ of pure water. As the pH value decreases below 7, the $[H^+]$ increases logarithmically, becoming more acid. Conversely, as the pH value increases above 7, the $[H^+]$ decreases logarithmically, becoming more alkaline.

Fig. 5-8 compares the pH and nanomole scales over a physiologic range. By comparison, a pH of 7.0 is equivalent to a $[H^+]$ concentration of 100 nmol, a pH of 7.4 is equivalent to a $[H^+]$ concentration of 40 nmol, and a pH of 8.0 is equivalent to a $[H^+]$ concentration of 10 nmol. Thus it becomes clear that a one-unit change in pH is equivalent to a ten-fold change in $[H^+]$.

BODY FLUIDS AND ELECTROLYTES
Body fluids

As we already know, water is the major component of the body, constituting between 45% and 80% of a person's body weight. The percentage of total body water depends on a person's weight, sex, and age. Leanness is associated with a higher body water content, whereas obese persons tend to have a lower percentage of body water, since fat is essentially free of water. Indeed, an obese person may have as much as 30% less water than a lean person of the same weight. This lack of fluid reserve is a primary factor in making the fat person a poorer surgical risk.

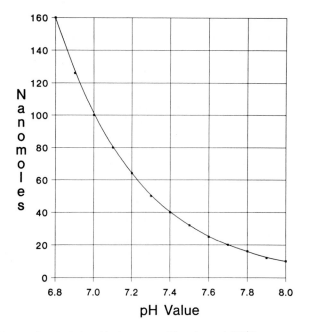

Fig. 5-8 Relationship between pH and nmol [H^+] concentrations.

The total body water of the average male is approximately 60% of his body weight and that of the average female is 50%. The lower percentage in females correlates with the larger amount of subcutaneous fat tissue that they have.

The percentage of weight attributable to water in infants and children is substantially greater than that in adults. In the newborn, water accounts for 80% of the total weight. There is a rapid decline in the proportion of body water to body weight during the first 6 months of life. This proportion then remains constant until puberty, when differences occur between boys and girls, and as age increases there is a steady decrease in total body water content.

Distribution. Total body water is divided into two major compartments: (1) the intracellular water (water within the cells) and (2) the extracellular water (water outside the cells). Intracellular water, or ICW, represents about two thirds of the total body water, or about 45% of body weight. The remaining one third of body water is extracellular. Extracellular water, or ECW, is further divided into two subcompartments: (1) intravascular water (water within the blood vessels, or plasma), comprising approximately one fourth of the ECW, or 5% of body weight, and (2) interstitial water (water in the tissues between the cells and vascular spaces), comprising about three fourths of the ECW, or approximately 15% of body weight.

Table 5-5 delineates the relative percentage of water in these compartments, depending on sex and age. Note that whereas the infant has more body water than the adult, most of this water lies in the extracellular compartment, which is approximately two times greater than that of the adult.

Composition. As depicted in Fig. 5-9, the composition of solutes in the intracellular and extracellular fluid compartments differs markedly. The predominantly extracellular electrolytes are sodium, chloride, and bicarbonate, whereas potassium, magnesium, phosphate, sulfate, and protein ($prot^-$) constitute the main intracellular electrolytes. Although intravascular water and interstitial fluid have similar electrolyte compositions, plasma contains substantially more protein than interstitial fluid. The plasma proteins, chiefly albumin, account for the high colloid osmotic pressure of plasma, which is an important determinant of the distribution of fluid between vascular and interstitial compartments (as discussed subsequently).

Regulation. Although the movement of certain ions and proteins between the various body fluid compartments is restricted, water is freely diffusible. Control of total body water occurs through regulation of water intake (thirst) and water excretion (urine volume, insensible loss, and stool water), with the kidneys being the chief regulator. If water intake is low, the kidneys can reduce urine volume and raise urine solute concentration some four times above that in the plasma. If, on the other hand, water intake is high, the kidneys can excrete large volumes of dilute urine.

The kidneys maintain the volume and composition of body fluids constant by two related mechanisms: (1) filtration and reabsorption of sodium, which adjust urinary sodium excretion to match changes in dietary intake, and (2) regulation of water excretion in response to changes in secretion of antidiuretic hormone (ADH). These two mechanisms allow the kidneys to maintain the volume and concentration of body fluid constant within a few percentage points despite wide variations in the intake of salt and water. For this reason, analysis of the composition and volume of the urine usually provides valuable clues in the diagnosis of disorders involving body fluid volume.

Water losses. As indicated in Table 5-6, water may be lost from the body through the skin, lungs, kidneys, and gastrointestinal tract. Normally, these losses are necessary to maintain normal body function. These obligatory losses can be subdivided into those that are *insensible* (nonvisible), such as the vaporization of water from the skin and lungs, and *sensible* losses (discerned by visible means) from the urine and the gastrointestinal tract.

Table 5-5 Distribution of Body Fluids

	Adult male (% body wt)	Adult female (% body wt)	Infant (% body wt)
Total body water	60±15	50±15	80
Intracellular	45	40	50
Extracellular	15-20	15-20	30
Interstitial	11-15	11-15	24
Intravascular	4.5	4.5	5

Electrolyte composition

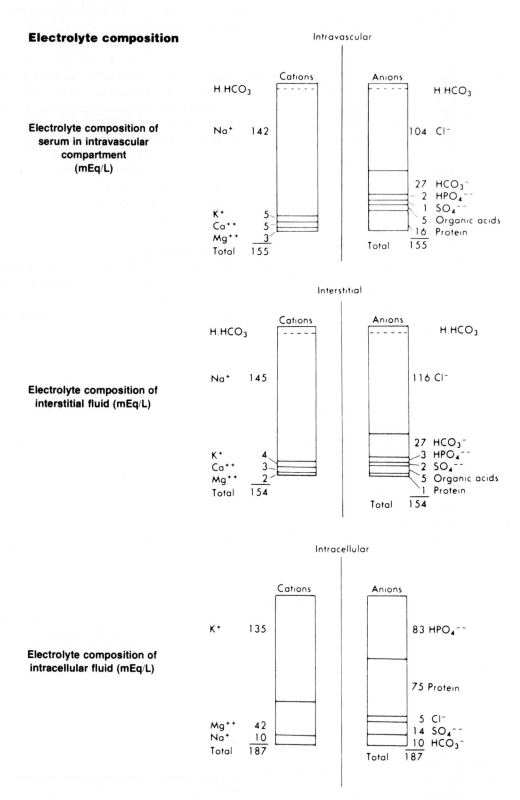

Electrolyte composition of serum in intravascular compartment (mEq/L)

Electrolyte composition of interstitial fluid (mEq/L)

Electrolyte composition of intracellular fluid (mEq/L)

Fig. 5-9   Electrolyte concentrations in the body fluid compartments.   (From Weldy NJ: Body fluids and electrolytes: a programmed presentation, ed 5, St Louis, 1988, The CV Mosby Co.)

Insensible loss accounts for about 900 ml/day, with 500 to 700 ml lost through insensible skin vaporization in the body regulation of heat and 200 ml from moisture in the expired air from the lungs.

Sensible losses amount to approximately 1200 ml of water per day. It takes 30 ml of water for 1 g of nitrogen to be excreted by the kidneys; since the average person produces approximately 15 g of nitrogenous waste in 24 hours, the minimum urine output required is about 450 ml per day. The average urine output in the normal adult is between 1000 and 1200 ml per day. On average, daily stool contains approximately 200 ml of water.

There may be other fluid losses from the body. These are called *additive* losses, as they are not essential for body function. Such losses may occur in vomiting, diarrhea, sweating, suctioning from intestinal tubes, etc. Other additive losses—often overlooked by clinicians—include sweating, which can constitute a 1000 to 2000 ml water loss per 24 hours, and fever. A rule of thumb is that for each degree of temperature above 99°F that persists for 24 hours, an additional 1000 ml of fluid will be lost. Whereas there is no salt in lung water, perspiration does contain dilute concentrations of sodium chloride, so that the normal adult excretes between 10 and 70 mEq of sodium chloride per liter of perspiration.

The gastrointestinal tract manufactures some 8000 to 10,000 ml of fluid per day but normally reclaims more than 98% of this volume. However, in patients who are vomiting or have diarrhea or intestinal drainage, water losses through the gastrointestinal tract can be considerable. Also, persons with open wounds can lose large quantities of water (in both plasma and lymph fluid).

Additional causes of abnormal fluid loss include some renal and respiratory disorders. Patients with certain renal diseases will have to excrete larger quantities of urine in order to get rid of the extra nitrogenous wastes. Patients with increased ventilation will also have increased water losses as a result of increased evaporation from the respiratory tract. Patients with artificial airways whose inspired air is not adequately humidified are particularly prone to evaporative water loss. In these cases, because the normal heat and water exchange processes of the nose are bypassed, the lower airway must make up the difference between the low humidity content of the inspired air and the normal BTPS conditions in the lung. This difference, called the humidity deficit, can result in large evaporative water losses. For example, a patient with a tracheostomy who is not provided with adequate airway humidification may lose as much as 700 ml of additional water per day. Of course, this water loss can be minimized if adequate humidification is provided to the inspired air (as discussed in Chapter 23).

As mentioned before, the infant has a greater amount of body water, particularly in the extracellular compartment. The water loss of an infant is double that of the adult for two reasons. First, the infant has a proportionately greater body surface area, and thus a basal heat production that is twice as high as an adult's. Second, an infant's greater metabolic rate results in greater production of waste products, which necessitates a greater urinary excretion. Thus, the daily turnover of water in the infant is approximately one half of the extracellular fluid volume, as compared with about one seventh in the adult. With fluid loss or lack of intake, the infant depletes his extracellular fluid much more rapidly.

Water replacement. As indicated in Table 5-6, water is replenished in two major ways: by ingestion and by metabolism.

Ingestion. The most obvious mechanism for water replacement by ingestion is through the consumption of liquids. However, solids, such as meat and vegetables, contain as much as 60% to 90% water. The average adult drinks 1500 to 2000 ml of water per day and gains another 500 to 600 ml of water from solid food.

Metabolism. Water also is gained endogenously from the oxidation of fats, carbohydrates, and proteins in the body and from the release of water from the destruction of cells. In total starvation, it is estimated that 2000 ml of endogenous water is produced daily by the metabolism of 1 kg of fat. Early surgical convalescence is equivalent to starvation. During this period, it is estimated that approximately 0.5 kg of protein and a similar amount of fat are metabolized, yielding approximately 1 L of endogenous water daily.

Transport between compartments. Proper homeostasis depends not only on the total quantity of body fluids but also on the transport of these fluids and solutes between and among the different body compartments and into and out of the cells. Some insight into these transport mechanisms may be obtained from an examination of the

Table 5-6   Daily Water Exchange

	Average daily volume	Maximum daily volume
WATER LOSSES		
Insensible		
Skin	700 ml	1500 ml
Lung	200 ml	
Sensible		
Urine	1000-1200 ml	2000+ ml/hr
Intestinal	200 ml	8000 ml
Sweat	0 ml	2000+ ml/hr
WATER GAIN		
Ingestion		
Fluids	1500-2000 ml	1500 ml/hr
Solids	500-600 ml	1500 ml/hr
Body metabolism	250 ml	1000 ml

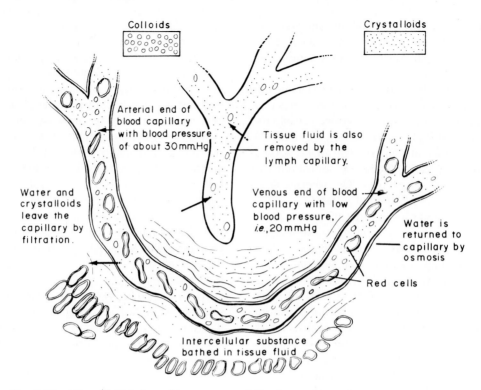

Fig. 5-10   Tissue fluid is formed by a process of filtration at the arterial end of the blood capillary, where blood pressure exceeds colloidal osmotic pressure. The fluid is absorbed by the blood capillaries and lymphatic vessels. It will return to the venous end of the capillary when colloidal osmotic pressure exceeds blood pressure. Fluid is absorbed into the lymphatic capillary when interstitial fluid pressure is greater than pressure within the lymphatic capillary. Normally, little colloid escapes from the blood capillary. Colloid that does escape is returned to the blood circulation by the lymphatic vessels. (From Burke SR: The composition and function of body fluids, ed 3, St Louis, 1980, The CV Mosby Co.)

movement of fluids from the capillaries into the interstitial fluid and then into the cells.

The first stage of this process, the exchange of fluids between the systemic capillaries and the interstitial fluid, proceeds by passive diffusion. The capillary wall is completely permeable to all the crystalline electrolytes, so that 100% equilibrium between the two extracellular compartments occurs very quickly. The plasma, with the exception of its very large protein molecules, is also capable of moving through the capillary walls into the tissue spaces.

At the systemic capillary level, this movement of fluid and solutes from the blood to the interstitial space is enhanced by the difference in hydrostatic pressure between these compartments. This hydrostatic pressure difference, in turn, depends on the blood pressure, the volume of intravascular fluid (blood), and the distance of the capillary from the heart (relative to gravity).

Opposing this hydrostatic force is a difference in osmotic pressure between the interstitial and the intravascular compartments. Given the relatively equal concentrations of crystalline electrolytes in these two compartments, this osmotic pressure difference is mainly a function of the

proteins, particularly albumin, that exist in colloidal suspension in the plasma. Being too large to be filtered through the pores of the capillary, these proteins normally remain in the intravascular compartment, where they tend to draw water and small solute molecules back into the capillaries.

Fig. 5-10 depicts these events in a typical systemic capillary region. In this example, the mean arterial blood pressure is assumed to be 100 mm Hg, resulting in a capillary blood pressure of about 30 mm Hg at the arteriolar end and about 20 mm Hg at the venular end. The colloidal osmotic pressure of the intravascular fluid remains at a constant level of about 25 mm Hg. Clearly, the hydrostatic pressure along the capillary continually decreases, so that by the time the blood reaches the venous end, the hydrostatic pressure is less than the osmotic pressure. On the venular side of the capillary, the colloidal osmotic pressure is sufficient to overcome the hydrostatic forces and water returns into the vascular compartment.

Normally, the outflow of water and electrolytes from the capillary on the arteriolar end is not completely balanced by the return on the venular end, there being a slight outward excess. This slight outward excess is balanced by fluid return via the lymphatic circulation.

The return of tissue fluid via the lymphatic channels is also dependent on pressure differences. The amount of pressure in the interstitial space is determined by the quantity of interstitial fluid and the electrolyte content of this fluid. The interstitial fluid in this instance moves from a region of greater pressure (in the interstitial space) to a region of lower pressure (in the lymphatic channels). From there this "lymph" moves on into larger and larger lymphatic vessels, where the pressure is continuously decreasing, until it is ultimately returned to the innominate vein in the chest, where the pressure is very low. The return of lymph to the central circulation, like venous flow, is enhanced by skeletal muscle activity.

Quantitatively, these relationships are expressed in the Starling equilibrium equation:

$$Q_f = K_1(P_{ch} - P_{ih}) - K_2(P_{co} - P_{io})$$

where Q_f is the bulk flow of fluid between the intravascular and interstitial compartments, P_{ch} is the capillary hydrostatic pressure, P_{ih} is the interstitial fluid hydrostatic pressure, P_{co} is the capillary osmotic pressure and P_{io} is the interstitial osmotic pressure. The K values represent permeability coefficients, with K_1 being a measure of capillary permeability to fluids and electrolytes, and K_2 quantifying capillary permeability to proteins. Three good examples of the importance of the forces expressed in this equation are fluid return from gravity-dependent areas of the body, fluid exchange in the lung, and tissue edema.

Because of the hydrostatic effects, capillary hydrostatic pressure in the feet can be as high as 100 mm Hg in a person who is standing erect. How can the reabsorption of tissue fluid be accomplished when the hydrostatic pressure so greatly exceeds the colloidal osmotic pressure? There are three factors that favor fluid reabsorption under these circumstances. First, the high intravascular hydrostatic pressure is somewhat balanced by a proportionately greater interstitial pressure. Second, the "pumping" action of the skeletal muscles surrounding leg veins lowers venous pressures below what would otherwise exist in this area. Finally, by a similar mechanism, the flow of lymph back to the thorax is enhanced, thereby facilitating the clearance of excess interstitial fluid.

The lung presents a somewhat different problem. Unlike the systemic tissues, where a constant exchange of interstitial fluid is essential, the alveolar region must be kept relatively "dry." This is because large amounts of interstitial fluid in the alveolar-capillary region could impede gaseous diffusion between the lung and blood. Since the colloidal osmotic pressure of the blood in the pulmonary circulation is the same as that in the systemic circulation, the only way to ensure minimum filtration of fluids in the alveolar-capillary region is to keep the hydrostatic pressure difference low. Indeed, the pulmonary circulation has been "de-

signed" as a low-pressure system, with mean pressures some one sixth of those in the systemic circulation. Thus, the colloidal osmotic pressure tending to draw fluid back into the pulmonary circulation tends to exceed the hydrostatic forces throughout the length of the capillary, keeping the region relatively free of excess interstitial water.

Obviously, should the hydrostatic pressures in the pulmonary circulation rise, this balance can be upset, causing fluid movement into the alveolar-capillary interstitium. This excess fluid in the interstitial space is called edema. In the lungs, edema caused by increased hydrostatic pressure usually is due to a "back-up" of pressure from a failing heart.

Of course, edema can be caused by other factors. Inspection of the Starling equilibrium equation reveals that, in addition to increased hydrostatic pressures, edema also can be caused by either a decrease in the colloidal osmotic pressure of the blood or an increase in the permeability of the capillary membrane. For example, if a person loses albumin from the blood, then the balance of forces is upset, favoring increased movement of fluid into the interstitium. Likewise, with all else constant, an increase in the permeability of the capillary membrane will result in more fluid leaving the capillaries. Indeed, increased capillary permeability is a major factor in certain types of acute lung injury, as described in Chapter 28.

As compared with the capillary region, the exchange of fluid and solute between the interstitium and the body cells is more complex. Like the capillary membrane, the cell membrane is permeable to water. Thus water can diffuse very rapidly into and out of the cells. Some water also enters and leaves the cells by osmosis; this is due to the slight osmotic pressure gradient on the two sides of the cell membrane.

Of course, osmosis is usually limited to those processes in which the solvent, in this case water, is transported across the membrane. Many cells have membranes that are permeable to several other types of molecule. For example, certain membranes in the body are permeable to glucose, urea, and other small organic molecules. Such membranes are considered selectively permeable. This process, involving the diffusion of several types of molecule through a selectively permeable membrane, is referred to as dialysis.

Osmosis and dialysis are basically diffusion processes in which the membrane plays a passive role. The membrane controls the rate of diffusion of a given substance by its permeability, supplying no energy to facilitate the transport process. However, when the cellular concentrations of some types of solute are examined, it becomes clear that these passive transport mechanisms alone cannot explain the often substantial differences between the constituency of the intercellular and extracellular fluids.

Unequal concentrations of certain substances, particularly potassium, chloride, and phosphate, are maintained across cell walls without appreciable hydrostatic pressure differences between these compartments. Indeed, some molecules are transported across membranes in the direction opposite that dictated by diffusion probability. Such transport requires that energy be supplied to the molecules by the membrane, since they are being moved "uphill" against the normal osmosis or dialysis gradient. This process, referred to as active transport, can be accomplished only by living membranes that have a source of energy.

Electrolytes

The electrolytes in the various body fluid compartments are not passive solutes. These substances are essential to life itself and serve a variety of important roles in maintaining the internal environment and making possible key chemical and physiologic events. We will explore the role played by six of these major electrolytes, including sodium, chloride, bicarbonate, potassium, calcium, and phosphorus (phosphate).

Sodium. Regulation of the sodium concentration in plasma and urine is intimately associated with regulation of total body water. Half of the total body stores of sodium are extracellular, with the remainder being found in the bone (40%) and within the cells (10%). The normal serum concentration of sodium ranges from 135 to 145 mEq/L. Within the cells, the sodium concentration is much lower, averaging only 4.5 mEq/L.

The average adult ingests and excretes about 100 mEq of sodium every 24 hours. A child exchanges about half this amount, and an infant typically exchanges 20 mEq of sodium per day. Most sodium is reabsorbed through the kidney. Some 80% of the body's sodium is reclaimed passively in the proximal tubules, with the remainder being actively reabsorbed in the distal tubules. Sodium reabsorption in the kidneys is governed mainly by the level of the hormone aldosterone, as secreted by the adrenal cortex. Since sodium reabsorption in the distal tubules of the kidney always occurs in exchange for another cation, sodium balance is also involved in acid-base homeostasis (exchange for H^+) and the regulation of potassium (K^+).

Abnormal losses of sodium (hyponatremia) may be due to gastrointestinal losses, excessive sweat or fever, prolonged use of certain diuretics (e.g., acetazolamide), and in certain diseases, such as Addison's disease, ascites, congestive heart failure, and renal failure. Moreover, serum sodium levels may be seriously decreased when sodium shifts from the intravascular to the interstitial fluid compartment, as occurs with serious burns. Clinical symptoms of hyponatremia include weakness, lassitude, apathy, and headache. In the presence of a decrease in intravascular volume, orthostatic hypotension and tachycardia may also be present.

Hypernatremia is almost always associated with an excess accumulation of body water. Intrinsic factors that cause hypernatremia are an increase in aldosterone produc-

tion and a decrease in its inactivation, as in certain liver diseases. Administration of steroids can also cause hypernatremia.

Chloride. Chloride is the most prominent anion in the body. Two thirds of the body stores of chloride are extracellular, with the remainder being in solution within the cells. Intracellular chloride is present in significant amounts only in red and white blood cells and in those cells with an external excretory function such as the gastrointestinal mucosa.

Normal serum levels of chloride range between 96 and 105 mEq/L. In general, the concentration of chloride in the extracellular compartment is inversely proportionate to that of the other major anion, bicarbonate. Chloride concentrations are regulated by the kidney in much the same manner as sodium (80% reabsorbed in the proximal tubules, 20% in the distal tubules). Because chloride is usually excreted with potassium in the form of potassium chloride, a deficiency of one of these electrolytes is usually associated with a deficiency in the other, and replacement therapy usually includes both. The stomach (with its hydrochloride-rich gastric juices) and the small bowel also affect the balance of this anion. Insensible perspiration and sweat contain hypotonic quantities of chloride.

The most common cause of low serum chloride levels (hypochloremia) is gastrointestinal losses. Hypochloremia is also caused by certain diuretics, such as furosemide (Lasix) and ethacrynic acid. Since loss of chloride is equivalent to a gain in bicarbonate (a base), hypochloremia is usually associated with metabolic alkalosis (see Chapter 10). Clinically, hypochloremia may cause muscle spasm and, if severe, coma.

Hyperchloremia can occur in dehydration, metabolic acidosis, respiratory alkalosis, and with the administration of excessive amounts of $K+$ and NaCl.

Bicarbonate. Next to chloride, bicarbonate (HCO_3^-) is the second most important body fluid anion. Bicarbonate plays a key role in acid-base homeostasis, representing the strong base in the bicarbonate/carbonic acid buffer pair (refer to Chapter 10). Moreover, bicarbonate represents the primary vehicle in the hydration and subsequent elimination of carbon dioxide through the lungs.

Body stores of bicarbonate are evenly divided between the intracellular and extracellular fluid compartments. Normal serum bicarbonate levels range from 22 to 26 mEq/L, and, under normal conditions, the ratio of this base to carbonic acid is maintained in a precise 20:1 ratio, resulting a normal pH of 7.4.

More than 80% of the blood bicarbonate is reabsorbed in the proximal tubules of the kidney, with the remainder being reclaimed in the distal tubules. A reciprocal relationship exists between chloride and bicarbonate ion concentrations, so that bicarbonate retention is associated with chloride excretion, and vice versa. Details on the role of this important electrolyte and buffer base in acid-base homeostasis is provided in Chapter 10.

Potassium. Potassium is the main cation of the intracellular compartment. In fact, some 98% of the body's potassium is found within the cells. Active transport of potassium into cells occurs through an ionic pump mechanism. An electrical differential across the cell membrane also facilitates potassium movement into the cell. However, for every three potassium ions that enter the cell, two sodium ions and one hydrogen ion must leave, thus maintaining electrical neutrality within the cell.

This significant difference in potassium distribution is evident when K^+ concentrations between fluid compartments are compared. Whereas the intracellular K^+ concentration is approximately 150 mEq/L, the serum potassium K^+ concentration normally ranges between only 3.5 and 5.0 mEq/L. Thus the serum K^+ is only an indirect indicator of the total body potassium. For this reason, analysis of serum potassium is usually combined with assessment of both its intake and its excretion.

The average patient excretes 40 to 75 mEq of potassium in the urine per 24 hours and 10 mEq in the stool. Average dietary intake of potassium is 50 to 85 mEq per day. The patient who is undergoing stress from surgery, trauma, or disease will have greater potassium losses and consequently will need additional K^+ replacement (an average of 100 to 120 mEq per day).

The serum potassium concentration is determined primarily by the pH of extracellular fluid and the size of the intracellular K^+ pool. With extracellular acidosis, a large proportion of the excess hydrogen ions are exchanged for intracellular K^+. This movement of K^+ from the intracellular to the extracellular compartments may produce a dangerous level of hyperkalemia. Alkalosis has an opposite effect: as the pH rises, K^+ moves into cells. In the absence of an acid-base disturbance, serum K^+ reflects the total body pool of potassium. With excessive external losses of potassium, such as from the gastrointestinal tract, the serum K^+ level falls. On average, a 10% loss of total body K^+ drops the serum K^+ level about 1 mEq/L.

Renal excretion of potassium is controlled by aldosterone levels. Aldosterone inhibits the enzymatic potassium carrier within the distal renal tubular cells of the kidney. Metabolic acidosis also inhibits the carrier system and thus permits sodium ions and hydrogen ions to enter the cell at the expense of an increased potassium excretion. Alkalosis, on the other hand, has the reverse effect, stimulating the cellular retention of potassium. Renal failure, particularly acute oliguric renal failure, results in potassium retention and hyperkalemia.

Hypokalemia due to excessive renal excretion may follow administration of diuretics or adrenal steroids and is associated with certain renal tubular disorders. Other causes of hypokalemia include gastrointestinal losses (vomiting, diarrhea, fistulas), malnutrition, and trauma (crush injuries, burns, etc). Severe trauma releases large quantities of K^+ into the extracellular fluid. Unlike many electrolytes, the kidney does not have the capability to conserve potassium. Therefore, despite body depletion, the loss of K^+ can continue.

Hypokalemia causes disturbances in cellular function which affect a number of organ systems, primarily the gastrointestinal, neuromuscular, renal, and cardiovascular systems. Muscle weakness and paralysis are common. Electrocardiographic findings, such as a depressed ST segment, prolonged QT and PR intervals, and supraventricular arrhythmias, are found only in about 50% of all cases (refer to Chapter 22). Extrasystoles, circulatory failure, and cardiac arrest can develop when potassium stores are diminished. Hypokalemia may also lead to decreased motility of the gastrointestinal tract, thereby causing ileus and distention.

The clinical management of hypokalemia involves both replacement of potassium losses and treatment of the underlying disorder. To replace the associated chloride deficit, potassium is given with chloride. Caution must be exercised when large quantities of potassium are administered intravenously, because the heart muscle is very sensitive to extracellular concentrations of this electrolyte.

An excess of potassium (hyperkalemia) is most common in cases of renal insufficiency. Patients with chronic renal disease cannot adequately excrete potassium. Other causes of hyperkalemia include conditions that increase the extracellular potassium level, such as hemorrhage or tissue necrosis. The clinical manifestations of potassium excess are similar to those of hypokalemia, with a greater effect on the heart muscle. The diagnosis of hyperkalemia is made by serum determinations and electrocardiographic changes. With severe potassium intoxication, irregular ventricular rhythms may develop, resulting in eventual cardiac arrest.

The first step in the treatment of hyperkalemia is restriction of all potassium intake. Ultimately, the underlying processes that precipitated the hyperkalemia must be controlled. Temporary measures useful in reducing serum potassium level include the administration of insulin, calcium gluconate, sodium salts, and large volumes of hypertonic glucose. Cation exchange resins may be given orally or rectally. If these measures fail, peritoneal or renal dialysis can aid in potassium removal.

Calcium. Calcium is an important mediator of neuromuscular function and cellular enzyme processes. The usual dietary intake of calcium is 1 to 3 g per day, most of which is excreted unabsorbed in the feces. Urine excretion of calcium averages 150 mg/day. Most of the body's calcium is contained in the bones.

The normal serum calcium concentration (4.25 to 5.25 mEq/L) is maintained by humoral factors, mainly vitamin D, parathyroid hormone, calcitonin, and thyrocalcitonin. The calcium in blood is present in three forms: ionized, protein bound, and complex. The relative proportion of these calcium fractions is affected by the pH of the blood, the concentration of plasma proteins, and the presence of calcium-combining anions such as bicarbonate and phosphate. Approximately one half of the serum calcium is nonionized and bound to plasma protein, chiefly albumin. Five percent is in the form of a calcium anion complex, leaving the remaining 45% as ionized calcium. It is the ionized calcium that is physiologically active in such processes as enzyme activity, blood clotting, neuromuscular irritability, and bone calcification. Acidemia increases and alkalemia decreases the concentration of ionized calcium in the serum.

Hypocalcemia occurs in hypoparathyroidism, severe pancreatitis, chronic or acute renal failure, and severe trauma. The clinical manifestations of hypocalcemia are mainly neuromuscular and include hyperactive tendon reflexes, muscular twitching and spasm, muscle and abdominal cramps, and, rarely, convulsions. Hypocalcemia is reflected in the electrocardiogram by a prolonged Q-T interval (refer to Chapter 7). Treatment consists of correction of the underlying cause and replacement of this ion, either orally or intravenously.

Hypercalcemia most frequently is caused by hyperthyroidism, hyperparathyroidism, cancer with metastases to the bones, ectopic production of parathyroid hormone, vitamin D or A intoxication, sarcoidosis, milk-alkali syndrome, or prolonged immobilization. Hypercalcemia is also a rare complication of administration of thiazide diuretics. The symptoms of hypercalcemia are fatigue, depression, muscle weakness, anorexia, nausea, vomiting, and constipation. With severe hypercalcemia, stupor and coma may occur.

Acute hypercalcemia should be treated on an emergency basis, as death may quickly occur when the serum calcium level rises above 8.5 mEq/L. In such cases, there is usually an associated deficit of extracellular fluid so that volume replacement will tend to lower the serum calcium by dilution. Steroids and chelating agents (EDTA) are sometimes helpful in lowering serum calcium.

Phosphorus. About four fifths of the body phosphorus is contained in the bones and teeth. Half of the remaining 20% is combined with proteins, carbohydrates, and lipids in muscle tissue and in the blood, with the last portion being incorporated into a variety of complex organic compounds. Organic phosphate (HPO_4^{--}) is the principle organic anion within the cells. Inorganic phosphate plays a primary role in cellular energy metabolism, being the source from which adenosine triphosphate is synthesized. In acid-base homeostasis, phosphate is the primary urinary buffer for titratable acid excretion (refer to Chapter 10).

Like potassium levels, serum phosphate levels (1.2 to 2.3 mEq/L) are only approximate indicators of total body phosphorus. Serum phosphate levels are influenced by a number of factors, including the serum calcium concentration and the pH of blood.

Hyperphosphatemia, or high serum phosphorus level, is associated with certain endocrine disorders, such as hypoparathyroidism and acromegaly. Phosphorus excesses may also occur in chronic renal insufficiency and acute renal failure. Catabolic states and tissue destruction may also cause hyperphosphatemia, especially in the presence of renal insufficiency. A high serum phosphorus level is also associated with hypocalcemia. Treatment is directed at the underlying disorder. Dialysis can be used to reduce an acutely elevated serum phosphate level.

Hypophosphatemia, or a low serum phosphorus level, may be due to a diminished supply, as in starvation, or poor absorption, as when the small bowel is bypassed. Increased loss of phosphorus may occur in hyperparathyroidism, hyperthyroidism, certain renal tubular defects, and uncontrolled diabetes mellitus. Hypophosphatemia is also associated with hypercalcemia and respiratory alkalosis. Treatment involves either intravenous administration of a potassium phosphate buffer mixture or oral phosphate salts, with careful ongoing assessment of renal sufficiency and serum calcium levels.

SUMMARY

The body is mainly a watery medium in which large numbers of chemical substances and particles exist in solution or suspension. The four major characteristics of solutions are vapor pressure depression, boiling point elevation, freezing point depression, and osmotic pressure. Body cell walls are semipermeable membranes and, through the action of osmotic pressure, the distribution of water throughout the body is kept within physiologic ranges.

With water serving as the primary solvent for body fluids, there are three basic types of physiologic solution. Depending on the nature of the solute, these solutions are called ionic or electrovalent solutions, polar covalent solutions, and nonpolar covalent solutions. The distinguishing characteristic of ionic and polar covalent solutions is the tendency of all or some of the solute to ionize or dissociate into separate particles known as ions. Compounds that behave in this manner are known as electrolytes. The electrolytes in the body fluids are essential to life itself, serving a variety of important roles in maintaining the internal environment and making possible key chemical and physiologic events.

There are two primary ways to quantify the concentration of electrolytes in a solution: (1) by actual weight (grams or milligrams) or (2) by chemical combining power. Although the weight of a solute is relatively easy to measure and specify, it does not necessarily gives us an indication of its chemical combining power. For this reason, it has become customary in medicine to measure electrolyte concentrations in the body in terms of their chemical combining power, using either gram equivalent weights or milliequivalents. In addition to the use of simple weight measures and equivalent weights, there are several other ways to classify solute content. A knowledge of these various common chemical standards is an essential prerequisite in the computation of solute contents and in the dilution of solutions.

The physiologically active chemical compounds of the body are, for the most part, weakly electrolytic covalent substances. In aqueous solution only a proportion of the molecules of these substances ionize, with the remainder staying intact. At a given temperature and concentration, equilibrium is maintained between the ions and the unionized molecules, as quantified by the ionization constant, K.

The ionization constant of water is used as the basis for quantifying the relative strengths of acids (proton donors) and bases (proton receptors). Electrochemical techniques are used to measure the hydrogen ion concentration of unknown solutions, with their degree of acidity or alkalinity determined by variation of their $[H^+]$ above or below 1×10^{-7} mol/L. There are two related techniques for recording acidity and alkalinity of solutions, with the hydrogen ion concentration of water as the neutral standard: (1) the actual measured molar concentration of hydrogen ions in nanomoles per liter and (2) the logarithmic pH scale.

Water is the major component of the body, constituting between 45% and 80% of a person's body weight. The percentage of total body water depends on a person's weight, sex, and age. Total body water is divided into two major compartments: the intracellular water and the extracellular water. Extracellular water is further divided into two subcompartments: intravascular water and interstitial water.

The composition of solutes in the intracellular and extracellular fluid compartments differs markedly. The predominantly extracellular electrolytes are sodium, chloride, and bicarbonate, whereas potassium, magnesium, phosphate, sulfate, and protein ($prot^-$) constitute the main intracellular electrolytes. Although intravascular water and interstitial fluid have similar electrolyte compositions, plasma contains substantially more protein than interstitial fluid. The plasma proteins (chiefly albumin) account for the high colloid osmotic pressure of plasma, which is an important determinant of the distribution of fluid between vascular and interstitial compartments.

Control of total body water occurs through regulation of water intake (thirst) and water excretion (urine volume, insensible loss, and stool water), with the kidneys being the chief regulator. The kidneys keep the volume and composition of body fluids constant by two related mechanisms: (1) filtration and reabsorption of sodium, which adjust urinary sodium excretion to match changes in dietary intake, and (2) regulation of water excretion in response to changes in secretion of antidiuretic hormone.

BIBLIOGRAPHY

Burgess A: The nurse's guide to fluid and electrolyte balance, ed 2, New York, 1979, McGraw-Hill Book Co.

Burke SR: The composition and function of body fluids, ed 3, St Louis, 1980, The CV Mosby Co.

Carrol HJ and Oh MS: Water, electrolyte, and acid-base metabolism, Philadelphia, 1978, JB Lippincott Co.

Chenevey B: Overview of fluids and electrolytes, Nurs Clin North Am 22:749-759, 1987.

Collins RD: Illustrated manual of fluid and electrolyte disorders, New York, 1976, Harper & Row.

Humes HD: Pathophysiology of electrolyte and renal disorders, New York, 1985, Churchill-Livingstone.

Keyes JL: Fluid electrolyte and acid-base regulation: physiology and pathophysiology, New York, 1985, Jones & Bartlett.

Kruck F: Endocrine regulation of electrolyte balance, New York, 1986, Springer-Verlag.

Masiak MJ: Fluids and electrolytes through the life cycle, New York, 1985, Appleton & Lange.

Maxwell MH and Kleeman CR, editors: Clinical disorders of fluid and electrolyte metabolism, ed 3, New York, 1980, McGraw-Hill Book Co.

Metheny NM: Fluid and electrolyte balance: nursing considerations, ed 3, Philadelphia, 1987, JB Lippincott Co.

Mishoe SC: A review of the physiology, measurement, and clinical significance of colloid osmotic pressure, Respir Care 28:1129-1142, 1983.

Pestana C: Fluids and electrolytes in the surgical patient, ed 3, Baltimore, 1985, Williams & Wilkins.

Puschett JB: Disorders of fluid and electrolyte balance: diagnosis and management, New York, 1985, Churchill-Livingstone.

Reed GM: Regulation of fluid and electrolyte balance: a programmed instruction in clinical physiology, ed 2, Philadelphia, 1977, WB Saunders Co.

Rooth G: Acid-base and electrolyte balance, Chicago, 1975, Year Book Medical Publishers, Inc.

Rose BD: Clinical physiology of acid-base and electrolyte disorders, New York, 1977, McGraw-Hill Book Co.

Schrier RW: Renal and electrolyte disorders, Boston, 1976, Little, Brown & Co.

Stroot VR, Lee CAB, and Barrett CA: Fluids and electrolytes: a practical approach, ed 3, Philadelphia, 1984, FA Davis Co.

Weldy NJ: Body fluids and electrolytes: a programmed presentation, ed 5, St Louis, 1988, The CV Mosby Co.

Willatts SM: Lecture notes on fluid and electrolyte balance, St Louis, 1982, The CV Mosby Co.

York K: The lung and fluid-electrolyte and acid-base imbalances, Nurs Clin North Am 22:805-814, 1987.

SECTION III

Applied Life Science

6

Functional Anatomy of the Respiratory System

John V. Tesoriero
David H. Dail

Like all organ systems of the body, the respiratory system represents a complex integration of cells, tissues, and organ structures designed to sustain the living organism under both normal and stressful conditions. Working in close cooperation with the cardiovascular system, the respiratory system functions primarily to exchange gaseous metabolites between the atmosphere and the cells of the body.

Although simple in concept, this process of respiration involves a host of specialized structures designed to fulfill a series of complex functions. The system must protect itself against the onslaught of animate and inanimate contaminants; it must properly condition atmospheric air and move it in and out of the system with a minimum of work; it must expose gases to blood in a manner that facilitates rapid and efficient exchange; and it must possess reserves sufficient to respond and adapt to changing internal and external circumstances. The provision of effective respiratory care clearly is founded upon both an appreciation for and rigorous understanding of these anatomic and physiologic relationships in health and disease.

OBJECTIVES

This chapter focuses on the development of and interrelationship between the major structures of the respiratory system. Specifically, after completion of this chapter, the reader should be able to:

1. Differentiate between the major events characterizing the prenatal, perinatal, and postnatal periods of lung growth and development;

2. Identify and describe the gross structures of the thorax and their functions;

3. Characterize the actions of the primary and secondary muscles of ventilation during various levels of activity in health and disease;

4. Identify and describe the origin and action of the somatic and autonomic pathways innervating the lung and thoracic musculature;

5. Compare and contrast the form and function of the pulmonary and bronchial circulations;

6. Distinguish between and describe the roles and major structures constituting the upper and lower portions of the respiratory tract;

7. Delineate the segmental anatomy of the lungs and tracheobronchial tree;

8. Compare and contrast the cellular structure and function of the large airways, small airways, and respiratory zones of the lung.

KEY TERMS

Most terms used in this chapter are defined in context. The following terms are introduced without explicit definition, but may be found in the text glossary:

abduct	dyspnea
adduct	edema
alveolarization	effusion
anastomose	elastin
anomoly	electromyography
anteroposterior	embolization
aponeurosis	embryogenesis
axilla	endothelium
bronchoconstriction	endotracheal
bronchoscopy	epithelium
cartilagenous	extrauterine
catheterization	gastrointestinal
cephalad	hyperplastic
cervical	hyperpnea
collagen	hypertrophic
cuboidal	hypoxia

interstitial
intrauterine
intubation
laryngoscopy
lumen
medial
mesothelium
morphometry
mucosa
neurologic
neuromuscular

parietal
patency
pathologic
pathophysiology
perfuse
pericardium
perinatal
ramus
tracheoesophageal
tracheostomy

DEVELOPMENT OF THE RESPIRATORY SYSTEM

Understanding how the respiratory system develops prior to and after birth is of critical importance to students of respiratory care. Such knowledge provides important insights into pulmonary function in health and disease and helps explain certain developmental anomalies encountered in clinical practice. Moreover, understanding prenatal and postnatal changes in respiratory structure and function is an essential element in the delivery of effective pediatric and neonatal respiratory care (see Chapter 32). Of more intrinsic value, this knowledge helps one appreciate the wondrous ability of the respiratory system to assume, within minutes after birth, the complete role of providing adequate gas exchange for the newborn infant.

Overview

Unlike the other major organs that begin functioning early in fetal life and increase their capacities throughout gestation, the lungs are not afforded any practice for their role. The process of embryogenesis must therefore prepare the respiratory system to respond to the immediate demands inherent in the transition from fetal to postnatal life.

The growth and development of the respiratory system is an ongoing process that begins in the embryo and extends throughout a large portion of postnatal life. Table 6-1 summarizes the timelines for the major events characterizing intrauterine development of the respiratory system. Table 6-2 compares newborn lung structure and function to that typical of an 8- to 10-year-old child and the fully developed adult, demonstrating the substantial changes that occur after birth.

Three major periods are useful in describing these complex developmental processes. The first or *prenatal period* results in embryologic formation of the major airway and lung structures. Abnormalities during this period often manifest themselves at birth as congenital anatomic anomalies. The second phase of development is termed the *perinatal period*, during which the respiratory system must prepare itself for its extrauterine function of gas exchange. Many of the respiratory problems exhibited by preterm infants are associated with the failure to complete this critical

stage of development. The third or *postnatal period* occurs after birth and is associated with both an increase in number (hyperplastic growth) and an increase in size (hypertrophic growth) of important respiratory structures.[1] Like the growth of the body as a whole, postnatal lung development is influenced by a variety of physiologic, anatomic, and environmental factors, any one of which can impede the process and thereby limit normal adult lung function.

Table 6-1   Summary of Respiratory Tract Development

Approximate time of occurrence	Developmental event
24 days	Laryngotracheal groove develops
26-28 days	Bronchial buds form
2 weeks	Intraembryonic coeloms form
3 weeks	Diaphragm development begins
4 weeks	Primitive nasal cavities
	Tongue development
	Pharynx formation begins
	Pulmonary artery development
	Pulmonary vein development
	Phrenic nerves originate
5 weeks	Pseudoglandular phase begins
6 weeks	Arytenoid swellings (lead to formation of larynx)
	Lung bud migration into pleural canals
7 weeks	Oropharynx
	Tracheal cartilage development begins
	Smooth muscle cells of bronchi develop
8 weeks	Bronchial arteries develop
10 weeks	Secondary palate
	Vocal cords
	Ciliary development
	Cartilaginous rings of trachea
11 weeks	Lymphatic tissue appears
12 weeks	Mucous glands appear
13 weeks	Goblet cells appear
15 weeks	Pseudoglandular phase ends
16 weeks	Canalicular phase begins
22 weeks	Methyltransferase system for lecithin synthesis
	Lecithin appears
24 weeks	Alveolar phase begins
	Respiratory bronchioles
	Alveoli develop
26-28 weeks	Alveolar-capillary surface area of respiratory system developed sufficiently to support extrauterine life
35 weeks	Phosphocholine transferase system for lecithin synthesis

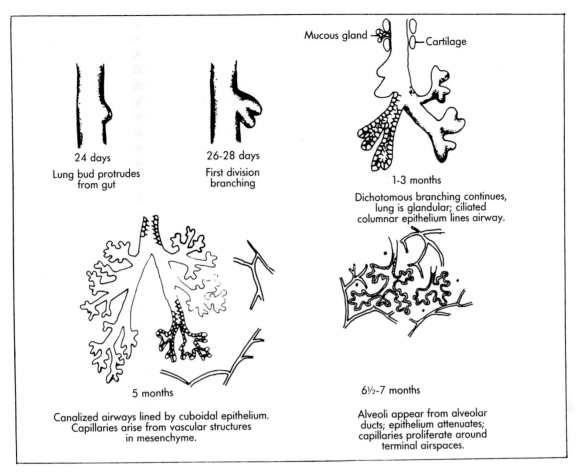

Mucous gland — Cartilage

24 days
Lung bud protrudes
from gut

26-28 days
First division
branching

1-3 months
Dichotomous branching continues,
lung is glandular; ciliated
columnar epithelium lines airway.

5 months
Canalized airways lined by cuboidal epithelium.
Capillaries arise from vascular structures
in mesenchyme.

6½-7 months
Alveoli appear from alveolar
ducts; epithelium attenuates;
capillaries proliferate around
terminal airspaces.

Fig. 6-1   Diagram of the major prenatal stages of lung development. (Redrawn from WB Saunders Co.)

Table 6-2   Postnatal Development of Lung Structure and Function

	Newborn	8-10 yrs	Adult
Lung weight, g	50	350	800
Lung tissue, % total	28	15	9
Number of alveoli, $\times 10^6$	20	300	300
Diameter of alveoli, μm	50	150	300
Surface area, m^2	3	32	70
Generations of airways	23	23	23
Number of respiratory airways, $\times 10^6$	1.5	14	14
Total lung capacity, L		3.0	6.0
Vital capacity, L	0.15	2.2	4.5
P_{tp} at 80% TLC, cm H$_2$O	8	10	15
Anatomic dead space, ml	7	50	150
$\dot{V}_{max_{50\%}}$, FVC/s ↑	1.5-2.2	0.8-1.2	0.8-1.2

Data courtesy of EK Motoyama. From Fishman AP: Assessment of pulmonary function, New York, 1980, McGraw-Hill Book Co.
Note: P_{tp} = transpulmonary pressure at 80% of total lung capacity (TLC);

$\dot{V}_{max_{50\%}}$ = maximum expiratory flow rate at 50% of forced vital capacity (FVC).

Prenatal development

Development of the respiratory system in utero traditionally is divided into four stages: the embryologic, the pseudoglandular, the canalicular, and the alveolar.[2] These prenatal developmental stages are pictorially represented in Fig. 6-1.

In early embryologic development, one central tube is formed from an inpouching of the surface of the spherical embryo. This tube forms the mainstream of the gastrointestinal tract and its derivatives. Between 3 and 4 weeks into gestation, a laryngotracheal groove develops, followed by the formation of a bronchial bud. This event marks the beginning of the pseudoglandular stage of prenatal lung development, during which the bud divides, grows distally, and evolves into the major airways and accompanying blood vessels and nerves. By 12 weeks the lobes of the lung are identifiable, and by 16 weeks formation of the bronchial tree is complete. Partial residual connections in the form of tracheoesophageal fistulas may occur during this time.

At about the same time as formation of the bronchial bud, the palate forms from the maxillary bones of the skull. This divides the intake end of this primitive tube into a nasal passage and an oral cavity. Simultaneous with the appearance of these primitive nasal cavities, the embryonic tongue and pharynx are developing, followed soon thereafter by the larynx, oropharynx, and vocal cords.

Also around 3 to 4 weeks gestation, the diaphragm begins a gradual process of development, to be completed during the seventh week of embryonic life.[2] Abnormalities in the development of the diaphragm can result in a persistent opening between the abdominal and thoracic cavities, known as a congenital diaphragmatic hernia. Because of displacement of the abdominal contents into the thorax, this condition may impede lung growth and development on the affected side.

Interestingly, the diaphragm begins development in the cervical region of the neck, being pushed downward by the developing heart and lungs. As it migrates downward, it carries with it the paired phrenic nerves from the neck region. Toward the end of fetal development, these phrenic nerves span the entire length of the thoracic cavity, from their cervical origins to the diaphragm. For this reason, postnatal conditions that irritate the diaphragm often cause pain in the lower neck or shoulder region. Such pain, occurring at a site distal to its origin, is called *referred pain*. The referred pain associated with irritation of the diaphragm is thus explained by the embryologic development of this muscle and its accompanying phrenic nerves.

By the end of the pseudoglandular stage at 15 weeks gestation, all upper airway structures are recognizable, cartilaginous support structures are developing, the cellular structure of the respiratory mucosa has begun its differentiation, and the mediastinum, pleural cavities, and diaphragm have been formed.

The 16th through 24th weeks of gestation define the canalicular stage of prenatal lung development, during which distal vascularization of the lung progresses rapidly, and the conducting airways begin their differentiation into respiratory bronchioles. At the cellular level, this stage is marked by fusing of the respiratory epithelial and capillary endothelial basement membranes into a primitive gas exchange surface. Toward the end of the canalicular stage, precursors to specialized alveolar cells begin to develop and start synthesis of pulmonary surfactant, a surface-active substance containing a phospholipid called lecithin.

At about 24 weeks gestation, the fetal lung begins its final alveolar stage of prenatal lung development. This stage involves the differentiation of epithelial saccules into primitive alveolar pouches and the maturation of the surfactant producing type II alveolar cells. With the maturation of these type II cells at approximately 35 weeks gestation comes the development of a stable pathway for production of surfactant. At this point, the fetal lung normally is fully prepared to take on its extrauterine role of gas exchange.

Perinatal development

The perinatal period is marked by the rapid and complex transition of the lung from a nonaerated, fluid-filled, and poorly perfused structure to a remarkably efficient organ of extrauterine gas exchange. At birth, the fetal lung fluid must be removed and replaced by air, the lung inflated, and the cardiac and pulmonary circulations altered to redirect blood flow from the placenta to the lung.

Successful accomplishment of this changeover involves a host of interrelated anatomic, physiologic, and mechanical factors. The success of this remarkable transition depends, in part, on both the maturation of the lung itself and the satisfactory development of a central nervous system mechanism for ventilatory control.

Toward the end of normal gestation the respiratory units of the fetal lung consist of three generations of respiratory bronchioles, a generation of alveolar ducts, and terminal clusters of alveolar saccules and primitive alveoli. Thinning of the intrasaccular septa, begun in the alveolar stage, is by now sufficient to provide adequate gas exchange. In utero, the fetus increasingly is demonstrating a variety of respiratory movements, including gasps or deep breaths, small rapid breaths, and coughing. Moreover, prior to birth, the normal fetal nervous system has developed appropriate responses to maternal changes in blood oxygen and carbon dioxide. In combination, these normal developmental activities ensure that the remarkable transition from placental dependence to independent extrauterine life proceeds quickly and uneventfully. The changes necessary for the fetal cardiopulmonary system to assume extrauterine gas exchange are described in more detail in Chapter 32.

Postnatal restructuring

In the newborn infant, airway branching is complete, but alveolarization is not. The gas exchange portions of the newborn lung consist mainly of thick-walled saccules or pouches. True alveoli are relatively small in size and number, and the ratio of the lung's surface area to its weight is relatively low (see Table 6-2).

Postnatal maturation of the respiratory system involves two major stages.[1] During the first 8 to 10 years of life, alveolar development is intense, with the number of these gas exchange units and the resultant surface area increasing some 10- to 15-fold (see Table 6-2). This alveolarization appears to occur through two related mechanisms. In the first, additional alveolar buds form from the large saccules, dividing these pouches into multiple, smaller compartments. In the second, out-pouching of alveoli occurs from the walls of the terminal bronchioles, forming additional alveolar ducts and respiratory bronchioles. The second major stage of postnatal restructuring begins at 8 to 10 years of life and continues throughout adolescence and young adulthood. Development during this final stage of postnatal growth involves enlargement of all structures within the lung (hypertrophic growth), with little or no further new alveolar formation (hyperplastic growth). Connective tissue synthesis also continues, and the collagen content of the lung increases, but tissue mass increases less than total volume. The overall size of the lung increases some threefold, and the average size of alveoli double.[3]

By the end of adolescence, all respiratory structures have completed their development, providing the adult with a full functional basis for both normal respiration and the reserves necessary to meet the challenges imposed by the increased demands of exercise or acute illness. The remainder of this chapter will focus on the form and function of the adult respiratory system as a whole, including its remarkable abilities to respond to changing internal and external conditions.

THE THORAX

Our study of the functional anatomy of the adult respiratory system will begin with a focus on the thorax. Besides containing the major organs of respiration and circulation, the thorax functions as the mechanical "bellows" responsible for movement of gas into and out of the lungs. Therefore a working knowledge of its gross structure and important role in ventilation is essential for effective provision of respiratory care.

Overview

The thorax is that area of the body formed by the rib cage, thoracic vertebrae and sternum, and containing the esophagus, trachea, lungs, heart, and great vessels (Fig. 6-2). Shaped somewhat like a cone, the thorax has a wide base bounded by the diaphragm below and a narrow opening at the top called the operculum. The operculum is bounded by the first ribs and the upper portion of the sternum.

Conceptually, the thorax consists of three "compartments" or potential spaces, although in reality these are filled by the major organs just described. The centrally located mediastinum contains the trachea, esophagus, heart, and great vessels of the circulatory system, while the left and right pleural cavities contain the lungs.

The "cage" surrounding these thoracic compartments serves two primary purposes. First, its bony structures provide protection for the vital organs inside. Second, the interaction of thoracic bones and muscles varies its volume, thereby generating the pressure differences necessary to create cyclical gas flow.

Gross structure and function

The mediastinum. The mediastinum is the central compartment of the chest, dividing the thorax vertically and separating the left and right pleural cavities. The mediastinum is bounded laterally by the parietal pleura along the medial aspects of both lungs; anteriorly by the sternum; posteriorly by the thoracic vertebrae; inferiorly by the diaphragm; and superiorly by the thoracic inlet.

Functionally, the mediastinum is divided into three subcompartments.[4] The anterior compartment, between the sternum and pericardium, contains the thymus gland and the anterior mediastinal lymph nodes. The middle compartment contains the pericardium and heart, great vessels, phrenic and upper portions of the vagus nerves, the trachea and mainstem bronchi, and their associated lymph nodes. The posterior compartment lies between the pericardium and the vertebral column and contains the thoracic aorta, esophagus, thoracic duct, sympathetic chains and lower portions of the vagus nerve, and the posterior mediastinal lymph nodes.

The lungs and pleura. The lungs are paired conical-shaped organs lying in the pleural cavities, and separated by the mediastinum. Although the adult lungs average 800 g in weight, by volume they consist of nearly 90% air and only 10% tissue. Because of the protrusion of the heart and mediastinum to the left, forming a concavity called the *cardiac notch,* the left lung is somewhat narrower than the right. However, due to the placement of the liver and resultant elevation of the right hemidiaphragm, the right is somewhat shorter than the left.

The lungs extend from the diaphragm below to a point approximately 1 to 2 cm above the clavicles, forming their apices. The lung surfaces lying against the ribs form the curved costal margins, with the medial surface being adjacent to the mediastinum. This mediastinal surface contains a vertical opening called the hilum, through which the major airways, blood vessels, lymphatics, and nerves enter and exit. This grouping of pathways, bound together by connective tissue, is often referred to as the root of the lung.

Each lung is further divided into smaller anatomic units called lobes, separated by one or more fissures (see Fig. 6-2). The right lung has an upper, middle, and lower lobe. The upper and middle lobes of the right lung are separated by a horizontal fissure; its middle and lower lobes are set apart by an oblique fissure. The left lung has only an upper and lower lobe, separated by a single oblique fissure. The lobes further divide into segments according to the branchings of the tracheobronchial tree, and ultimately into secondary lobules, the smallest gross anatomic units of lung tissue set apart by true connective tissue septa (Fig. 6-3). Secondary lobules correspond to clusters of from three to five terminal bronchioles and can be observed from the external and cut surface of the lung (Fig. 6-4). They are polygonal in shape and range in size from 1 to 2.5 cm on a side.[5] Localized infection, hemorrhage, or aspiration initially are contained by the boundaries between these lobules.

The surface of the lungs, portions of the major interlobular fissues, the inside of the chest walls composing the

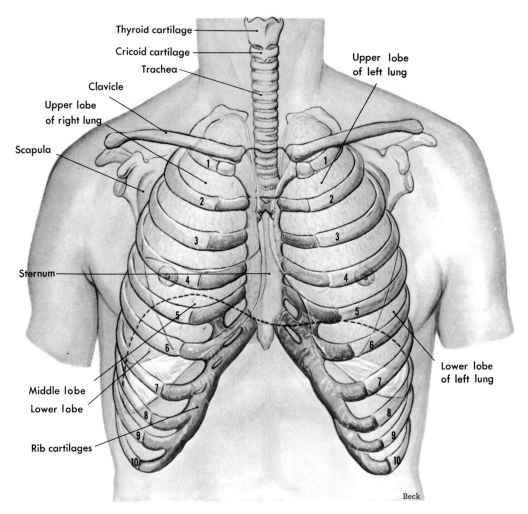

Fig. 6-2   Projection of the lungs and trachea in relation to the rib cage and clavicles. Dotted line indicates location of the dome-shaped diaphragm at the end of expiration and before inspiration. Note that apex of each lung projects above the clavicle. Ribs 11 and 12 are not visible in this view. (From Anthony CP and Thibodeau GA: Textbook of anatomy and physiology, ed 12, St Louis, 1987, The CV Mosby Co.)

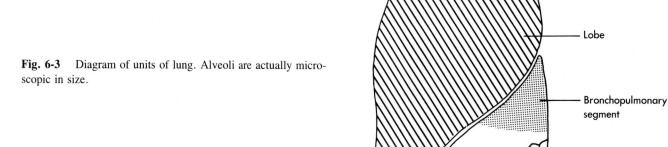

Fig. 6-3   Diagram of units of lung. Alveoli are actually microscopic in size.

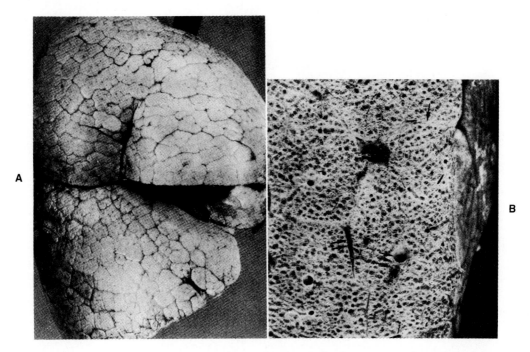

Fig. 6-4   Outer surface (**A**) and cut surface (**B**) of lung. **B,** One arrow marks an interlobular septum, two arrows mark small veins in these septa, and three arrows point to a pulmonary artery and bronchiole near center of secondary lobule. (From Heitzman ER: The lung: radiologic-pathologic correlations, St Louis, 1973, The CV Mosby Co.)

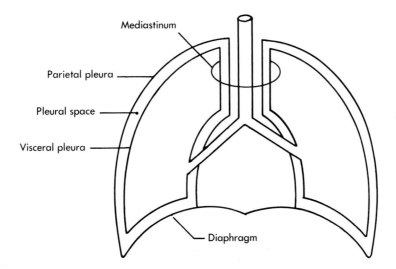

Fig. 6-5   This diagram shows overall relationship of chest organs, cavities, and investments. The mediastinum occupies space between lungs. Each lung sits within its chest cavity. This cavity is lined by parietal pleura, which covers chest cage, diaphragm, and lateral mediastinum, and by visceral pleura, which covers lungs.

chest cavities, the diaphragm, and the lateral portions of the mediastinum are covered by a thin mesothelial layer called the pleura. That portion covering the lungs and extending onto the hilar bronchi and vessels and into the major fissures is called the *visceral pleura*. The deeper portions of the visceral pleura contain elastic and fibrous fibers, small venules, and lymphatics. The interlobular septa

are continuous with this layer; the veins and lymphatics course along these septa, starting as fine caliber vessels in the pleura.

The portion of the pleura covering the inner surface of the chest wall and the mediastinum is called the *parietal pleura* (Fig. 6-5). Portions of the parietal pleura are named according to the structures which they contact. Thus the

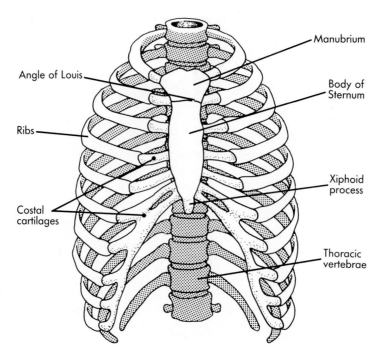

Fig. 6-6 Chest cage. Ribs arch around from vertebral column joining sternum through cartilaginous extensions.

costal pleura lines the inner surface of the rib cage, the mediastinal pleura covers the mediastinum, and the diaphragmatic pleura covers the diaphragm. The acute angle where the costal pleura joins the diaphragmatic pleura is known as the costophrenic angle. This area contains no lung tissue and is clearly visible on chest radiography. Moreover, any excess fluids in the pleural space have a tendency to gather here first, especially in the standing position. This causes the angle to appear blunted or flattened on the chest radiogram.

The upper dome of the parietal pleura extends above the first rib and encloses the thoracic inlet. This area, called the cupula, is strengthened by a layer of connective tissue known as the suprapleural membrane or Sibson's fascia. At the root of the lung, the parietal pleura becomes continuous with the viseral pleura as it passes onto the surface of the lung. Thus, although the two portions of the pleura are described by different names, they are really one continuous lining.

Between the viseral and parietal pleura is the pleural cavity, a potential space normally occupied by a serous fluid thought to be produced by the single-layered cells lining the parietal pleura. This fluid forms a thin film of uniform thickness that couples the viseral and parietal pleural surfaces, allowing them to slip easily over one other, and provides ready transmission of chest wall forces to the lungs. If air, blood, or other fluids are introduced into this area, the two pleural surfaces can separate. Under such circumstances, the parietal pleura stays relatively fixed against the inner wall of the thorax, but the lung and the

visceral pleura are displaced away from the chest wall.

The lung itself has elastic properties. This elasticity is a result of both surface tension forces in the alveoli, and tissue forces associated with the presence of elastin fibers in the alveolar walls and surrounding the small airways and pulmonary capillaries.[3] Collagen fibers probably contribute little to the elastic properties of the lungs, acting primarily to limit expansion at high lung volumes.[6]

Because of these elastic properties, the lung always tends to recoil to a lower volume. These elastic properties are demonstrated clearly when a lung is removed from the chest cavity and quickly collapses into a smaller size, or when air or fluid is introduced into the pleural space. This tendency of the lung to contract is important in the development of negative intrapleural pressure (see Chapter 8). In addition to collapse of an entire lung, it is possible for a portion, such as a lobe, to collapse. The most common cause of a lobar collapse is obstruction of its bronchus.

Bones of the thoracic cage

Key thoracic bony structures include the thoracic vertebrae, the sternum, and the ribs and costal cartilages (Fig. 6-6). These bony structures provide support and protection to the thoracic viscera and serve as points of origin and insertion for the respiratory muscles.

Vertebrae. The 12 thoracic vertebrae share a common structure with those of the vertebral column as a whole, having a body with pedicles, laminae, and a spinous and transverse process. In distinction to their cervical and lumbar counterparts, the bodies and transverse processes of the thoracic vertebrae have distinctive facets that serve as points of articulation for the head of each rib and the tubercle of its neck. The orientation of these facets, in combination with a rounded vertebral foramen, provides for the rotation and elevation characterizing rib movement.

Sternum. The sternum is a dagger-shaped bony structure situated in the median line of the front of the chest. Besides providing protection for the underlying organs, it serves as the point of attachment for the costal cartilages and numerous muscles. In the adult, the sternum averages 7 in. in length and consists of three portions: the upper triangular-shaped *manubrium,* the long and narrower *body,* and the pointed lower *xiphoid process.*

The manubrium articulates with the first and second ribs and the clavicle. Between its connections with the clavicles, the upper surface of the manubrium forms an easily palpable depression called the suprasternal notch. The manubrium affords a point of attachment for portions of the pectoralis major muscle and serves as the sternal origin of the sternomastoid muscle.

At a level equivalent to the intervertebral disk separating the fourth and fifth thoracic vertebrae, the manubrium articulates with the body of the sternum and second costal cartilages (second ribs), forming a slightly oblique angle called the *angle of Louis,* or sternal angle. An important external landmark, the angle of Louis demarcates the point at which the trachea divides into left and right mainstem bronchi, and the top of the heart and pericardium.

The body of the sternum, or corpus sterni, begins as a cartilaginous structure in early fetal life. Even in childhood the body consists of four or more bony sections separated by cartilage. By adulthood, the corpus sterni is fully ossified and fused into a single bone, articulating with the second through seventh ribs via the costal cartilages.

Unlike the body of the sternum, the xiphoid process remains cartilaginous through most of adulthood. Located at approximately the level of the tenth thoracic vertebrae, the xiphoid process is the smallest portion of the sternum and is variable in shape. It articulates with the seventh rib pair and serves as a point of attachment for some of the fibers of the diaphragm and the aponeuroses of the abdominal muscles.

Ribs. Corresponding to the 12 thoracic vertebrae are 12 pairs of ribs. The first seven pairs, or *vertebrosternal* ribs, connect directly to the sternum via bars of hyaline cartilage called the costal cartilages. The 8th through 10th pairs, or *vertebrochondral* ribs, connect to the ribs above and, through the costal cartilages, indirectly to the sternum. This cartilage is soft and moderately flexible in younger individuals. These qualities are lost as the individual ages and cartilages usually become calcified. The rib cage then becomes less flexible. This can be noted during external cardiac compression in different age groups. The 11th and 12th rib pairs have no connection to the other rib pairs or sternum, and, for this reason, are often referred to

as "floating ribs." The floating ribs terminate in cartilaginous free ends in the wall of the abdomen.

In a small number of individuals, extra or supernumerary ribs exist. A nonarticulated rib, attached to the transverse process of the seventh cervical vertebra is sometimes found. The presence of this "cervical" rib has been associated in some patients with vascular and neurologic symptoms in the arm or hand. Less common is the finding of a supernumerary rib articulated with the first lumbar vertebra. This so-called "gorilla" rib rarely manifests its presence by symptoms and is generally discovered only upon radiographic examination.

Each rib consists of a *head,* a *neck,* and a *body* or shaft (Fig. 6-7). With the exception of ribs 10-12, the rounded head has two facets for articulation with corresponding facets located on the bodies of the thoracic vertebrae. The flattened neck is about 1 in long and extends outward from the head, providing a point of attachment for the costo-transverse ligaments. On the posterior surface of the neck, near its attachment to the shaft, is a tubercle, most prominent in the upper ribs. A portion of the tubercle articulates with the transverse process of the lower of the two vertebrae to which the head of the rib is connected. The rib shaft is thin and curved, punctuated by numerous ridges and grooves. The irregular ridges serve as points of origin or attachment for muscles; the costal groove on the underside of each rib (Fig. 6-8; see Fig. 6-7) contains an intercostal artery, vein, and nerve. Because of the placement of these vital structures, puncture of the intercostal space via needles or tubes must always occur at the superior rib margin.

Rib movements. The first rib moves about the axis of its neck, raising and lowering the sternum. Although the motion is slight, it produces some increase in the anteroposterior (AP) diameter of the chest. During quiet breathing this action is not utilized, but it becomes important under conditions of stress.

The remaining six vertebrosternal ribs play an important role in ventilation. In contrast to the first rib, these move simultaneously about the axis of the rib neck and the axis between the angle of the rib and its sternal junction (Fig. 6-9). As they rotate about the axes of their necks (Fig. 6-9, *A*), their sternal ends rise and fall, thus increasing the AP thoracic diameter. This action is referred to as the "pump handle motion." The simultaneous movement about the longer axes from the rib angles to the sternum (Fig. 6-9, *B*) leads to an up-and-down motion of the middle segments of the ribs. This "bucket handle" motion produces an increase and decrease in the transverse diameter of the chest. Thus the compound action of these ribs increases and decreases both AP and transverse diameters smoothly and synchronously.

The vertebrochondral ribs have rotation patterns similar to the vertebrosternal group. However, elevation of the anterior ends of these ribs produces a backward movement of

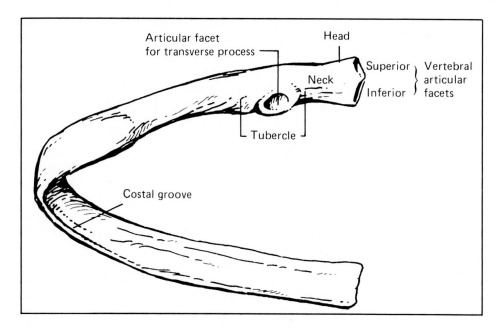

Fig. 6-7   A typical middle rib, from the left side of the body, viewed posteriorly (from the back). The head end (and tubercle) articulate with the vertebral column, while the shaft articulates with the sternum. (From Martin DE and Youtsey JW: Respiratory anatomy and physiology, St Louis, 1988, The CV Mosby Co.)

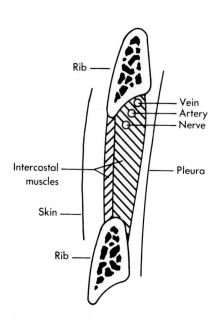

Fig. 6-8   Intercostal muscles fill spaces between ribs. An intercostal artery, veins, and nerve run in groove just beneath lower edge of each rib.

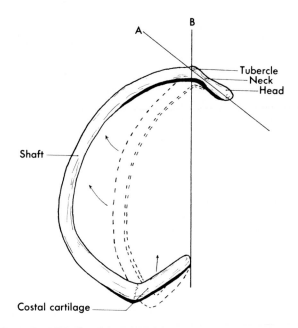

Fig. 6-9   The two axes about which the vertebrosternal ribs rotate during ventilation are indicated by lines *A* and *B*. The former passes through the length of the rib head and neck; the latter follows an AP direction from the tip of the costal cartilage to the tubercle. The rib undergoes a compound movement from its starting position *(dotted outline)*, the shaft swinging upward and laterally about axis *B*, and the anterior end moving upward about axis *A*.

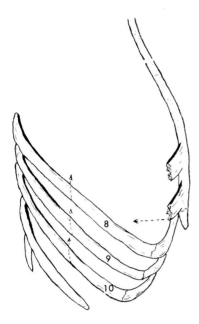

Fig. 6-10 The vertebrochondral ribs, *8* to *10,* have laterosuperior movement, but elevation of their anterior ends retracts the lower end of the sternum, shortening the AP diameter of the thorax in that plane.

the lower end of the sternum, with a reduction in thoracic AP diameter (Fig. 6-10). Like the motion described for the vertebrosternal ribs, outward rotation of the middle portions of the ribs increases the transverse diameter of the thoracic cage.

Some do not believe the ribs rotate about their neck axes but rather abduct by sliding motion. Ribs eleven and twelve are not included in any of the three categories mentioned, since they do not participate in changing the contour of the chest but act as muscular insertion points.

Muscle action

Various muscles of the thorax and abdomen contribute to the cyclical movement of gas into and out of the respiratory tract. Traditionally these muscles are divided into two groups: the primary and accessory muscles of ventilation. The primary muscles of ventilation are active during both normal quiet breathing and exercise and are represented by the diaphragm and intercostal muscles. The accessory muscles of ventilation primarily serve other purposes but assist the diaphragm and intercostals under conditions of increased ventilatory demand. Although any muscles attached to the ribs or sternum may be considered accessory muscles of ventilation, the scalenes, sternomastoids, abdominals, and pectoralis major best represent this latter group. Discussion will focus on these muscles in order of their relative contributions to ventilation.

Diaphragm. This large transverse muscle arises from the lumbar vertebrae, the costal margin, and the xiphoid process, with its fibers converging to interlace into a broad connective tissue sheet called the central tendon. This muscle configuration is that of a tent or a dome, dividing the chest from the abdomen. Although the diaphragm is a single anatomic structure, the union of its central tendon with the fibrous pericardium functionally divides its dome into two "leaves." For convenience these are often referred to as the right and left hemidiaphragms. Because of the presence of the liver immediately below it, the position of the right hemidiaphragm at the end of exhalation is normally about 1 cm higher than the left. Movements of the left and right hemidiaphragms are usually synchronous. However, dual innervation by separate phrenic nerves indicates that one hemidiaphragm can function independently of the other.

The diaphragm probably accounts for some 75% of the normal changes in thoracic volumes during quiet inspiration. At rest, the normal tidal movement of the diaphragm is approximately 1.5 cm, and during deep breathing, some 6 to 10 cm. In the normal adult, each centimeter of vertical movement moves approximately 350 ml of air.

With quiet breathing, the excursions of both leaves of the diaphragm are about equal, but with a deep inspiration the right diaphragm may move more than the left. In the supine position the total diaphragmatic movement is the same as in the erect position. In a head-down, 45-degree supine tilt, however, the resting level of the diaphragm rises about 6 cm, causing a reduction of the functional residual capacity and the expiratory reserve volume. When the subject lies in a lateral position, the lower diaphragm tends to rise into the chest.[7]

The diaphragm takes no active part in exhalation and returns to its inspiratory resting position during the passive recoil of the thorax. During forced exhalation, as against resistance, the diaphragm acts as a passive piston, expelling gas from the lung as it is pushed upward by intraabdominal pressure generated by contracting abdominal muscles.

The mechanical action of the diaphragm is twofold. First, contraction draws the central tendon down, flattening its contour, increasing the volume of the thorax, and lowering intrapleural pressure. As the diaphragm descends, intraabdominal pressure increases and the muscles of the abdominal wall relax, allowing the upper abdomen to balloon outward. Splinting or rigidity of the abdominal wall interferes with diaphragmatic descent during inspiration.

The second mechanical action of the diaphragm is achieved through contraction of its costal fibers, raising and everting the lateral costal margins. Increasing abdominal pressure during inspiration acts as a fulcrum against which continued contraction of the diaphragmatic fibers pull up and out on the costal margin (Fig. 6-11).

In Fig. 6-11, *A,* the descending diaphragm is opposed

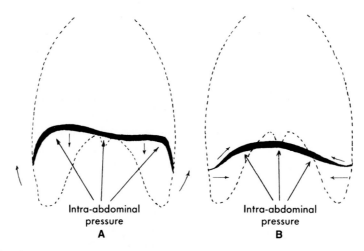

Intra-abdominal
pressure
A

Intra-abdominal
pressure
B

Fig. 6-11   A, As the normal diaphragm contracts, it descends, gradually building up pressure in the abdomen until the intraabdominal pressure acts as a fulcrum against which continued contraction everts the costal margin, enlarging the thorax further. **B,** Contraction of the diaphragm, which is abnormally low at the start of inspiration, can only pull in the costal margin, reducing the lower thoracic diameters.

by increasing intraabdominal pressure. This pressure finally stabilizes the central portion of the diaphragm so that the force of continued contraction is expended as traction on the costal attachments of the diaphragm. Because of the spring-like tension of the ribs and the contour of the thorax at this level, the costal margin is pulled upward and outward, increasing the lateral diameter of the chest.

This combined vertical and transverse action of the diaphragm is easily disturbed in pulmonary disease. As an example, in some types of advanced emphysema, the diaphragm is in an abnormally low and flat position. Under such circumstances, not only will there be a diminished vertical excursion, but contraction of the costal fibers may well pull in the lower chest boundary and narrow rather than expand the lateral dimensions of the thorax. Fig. 6-11, *B,* shows an abnormal diaphragm, low in position and relatively flat in contour. Because of its starting position, it can descend little on contraction, and with loss of its domed shape, contraction tends to pull its fibers centrally on a horizontal plane. This pulls in the costal margin and reduces the diameter of the chest.

Although the diaphragm is the principal ventilatory muscle, it is not essential for survival; adequate ventilation is possible even when the diaphragm is completely paralyzed. Affected by paralysis, the diaphragm (either or both leaves) tends to stay at the normal level at rest. During deep inhalation, however, it rises as other ventilatory muscles or one normal hemidiaphragm produce a fall in intrapleural pressure. In quiet breathing the paralyzed leaf may remain immobile or move in either direction. The inspiratory balance of pressure above and below the diaphragm tends to make the paralyzed leaf rise, whereas outward movement of the lower ribs tends to stretch and flatten it;

its final course is the result of these two forces.

Finally, the diaphragm performs important functions other than ventilation. Because it is able to aid in generating high intraabdominal pressure by remaining fixed while the abdominal muscles contract, the diaphragm greatly facilitates defecation, vomiting, coughing, sneezing, and parturition.

Intercostal muscles. The intercostal muscles consist of two sets of fibers located between each rib pair (Fig. 6-12). The external intercostal muscles arise from the inferior edge of each rib from the rib tubercle to its costochondral junction. The fibers pass inferiorly and anteriorly to insert into the superior edge of the rib below. These muscles are thicker posteriorly than anteriorly and are thicker than the internal intercostals.

The internal intercostal muscles are located beneath the external intercostals and arise from the inferior edge of each rib from the anterior end of the intercostal space to the rib angles. The fibers pass inferiorly and posteriorly to insert into the superior edge of the rib below. This muscle group is divided into two functional parts: (1) an interosseous portion located between the sloping parts of the ribs, and (2) an intercartilaginous portion located where the costal cartilages slope superiorly and anteriorly.

Although there is considerable controversy regarding intercostal muscle function, electromyographic studies indicate that the most active groups during breathing are the external intercostals and the intercartilaginous portion of the internal intercostals. Contraction of these muscles during inhalation would tend to elevate the ribs and thereby increase thoracic volume, a function documented by noting its absence during periods of paralysis. In addition, these muscles probably stabilize the chest wall and prevent

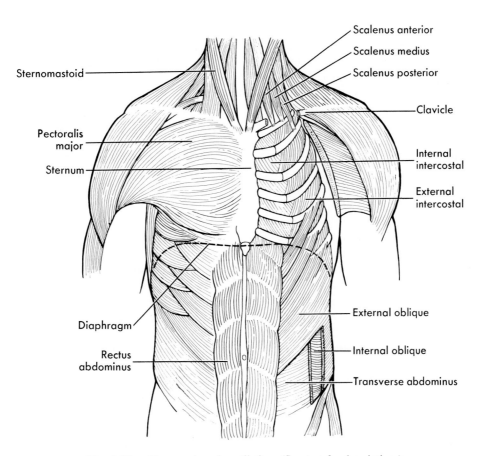

Fig. 6-12   The muscles of ventilation. (See text for description.)

intercostal bulging or retraction during large intrapleural pressure changes.

Interestingly, myographic studies also reveal intercostal activity continuing during quiet breathing into early exhalation. This initial expiratory activity may help to retard high airflows and facilitate a smoother and less turbulent exhalation. However, with flows in excess of 50 L/min or during maximum voluntary exhalation, the intercostals of the lower spaces also contract toward the end of exhalation. This action presumably gives stability to the chest in the presence of powerful abdominal contraction.

Scalene muscles. The anterior, medial, and posterior scalene muscles, although individual structures, are considered as a functional unit (see Fig. 6-12). Primarily skeletal muscles of the neck, they are also accessory muscles of ventilation and play an important role in breathing. The scalenes arise from the transverse processes of the lower five cervical vertebrae and insert into the upper surface of the first rib (anterior and medial scalenes) and the second rib (posterior scalene).

Although the scalenes give support to the neck, we are interested in their ventilatory action. Basically, they elevate and fix firmly the first and second ribs. Their most important function aids inhalation under conditions of stress when the diaphragm and intercostal muscles are in-

adequate to fulfill respiratory needs; this may occur in normal subjects undergoing severe exertion or in patients with pulmonary disease. In a normal subject, static inspiratory efforts (against a closed glottis or other obstruction, with no movement or air) bring the scalenes into play as intraalveolar pressure drops; and when this pressure reaches -10 cm H_2O, scalenes are active in all subjects. During expiratory efforts the scalene muscles are inactive until intraalveolar pressure reaches 40 cm H_2O, at which point they contract. It is thought that the expiratory function of the scalene muscles is to fix the ribs against the contraction of the abdominal muscles and to prevent herniation of the apex of the lung during coughing.

Sternomastoid muscles. The sternomastoids are another important accessory muscle group (see Fig. 6-12). Designed to rotate the head and support it, they arise bilaterally by two heads from the manubrium of the sternum and the medial end of the clavicle. The heads fuse into a single body that courses superiorly and slightly posteriorly to insert into the mastoid process and occipital bone of the skull. This muscle is usually prominent on each side of the neck of subjects and is especially noticeable with rotary movements of the head.

When functioning to mobilize the head, the sternomastoids pull from their sternoclavicular origin, rotating the head to the opposite side and turning it slightly upward. However, when the subject fixes the head and neck with other skeletal muscles, the sternomastoids, as a ventilatory muscle, pull from their skull insertions and elevate the sternum, increasing the AP diameter of the chest. In all subjects it contracts when intraalveolar pressures reach -10 cm H_2O but has no action during exhalation. In the supine position during normal free breathing, most subjects can attain a volume of 2.5 L and a flow of 60 L/min without use of the sternomastoids. An interesting discrepancy should be noted. During natural, free breathing, normal subjects can move about 2.5 L of air at intraalveolar pressures varying from -25 to -50 cm H_2O with the diaphragm and intercostals alone, and yet when attempting to inhale against an obstructed airway, an intraalveolar pressure of -10 cm H_2O brings the sternomastoids into play. Why this happens is not clearly understood.

In chronic pulmonary disease, the sternomastoids become active in inhalation when the thorax becomes so inflated (elevated resting level) that the low diaphragm loses its efficiency. As the sternomastoids contract and pull up on the sternum, the ribs rotate about their neck axes but not about the rib angle–sternal junction axes. This produces an up-and-down motion with little side expansion. In extreme cases, AP expansion of the thorax may cause the lower ribs to become indrawn, partially negating the increase in chest volume.

Pectoralis major muscle. The third most important accessory muscle of ventilation is the pectoralis major, a powerful bilateral anterior chest muscle with the primary function of pulling the upper arms into the body in a hugging motion (see Fig. 6-12). It is a large, fan-shaped muscle arising from the medial half of the clavicle, the anterior surface of the sternum and the first six costal cartilages, and a fibrous sheath enclosing muscles of the abdominal wall. The muscle fibers converge into a thick tendon that inserts into the upper part of the humerus. The pectoralis major forms the anterior fold of the axilla, and in a muscular individual its outlines are plainly visible beneath the skin.

Like the other accessory ventilatory muscles, the pectoralis pulls in a direction opposite to that of its primary function. If the arms and shoulders are fixed, as by leaning on the elbows or firmly grasping a table, the pectoralis muscle can use its insertion as an origin and pull with great force on the anterior chest, lifting up ribs and sternum and increasing thoracic AP diameter. The respiratory care practitioner soon becomes accustomed to seeing patients with chronic pulmonary disease assume characteristic poses for maximum use of the pectoralis. In advanced cases most of the air moved may be the result of the action of this powerful muscle. It aids inhalation only, taking no part in exhalation.

Abdominal muscles. Several muscles make up the abdominal wall, with the obvious purpose of providing support and safety to the abdominal contents (see Fig. 6-12). However, four abdominal muscle groups play an indirect but important role in ventilation and can thus be considered as accessory muscles of ventilation. These include the external and internal obliques, the transverse abdominal, and the rectus abdominis groups.

The external oblique muscle arises from the lower eight ribs. Its posterior fibers insert into the iliac crest, and the rest course obliquely down and forward to insert into a fibrous sheath or aponeurosis with their counterparts from the other side. The lower edge of the external oblique forms the inguinal ligament. The internal oblique arises from the iliac crest and the inguinal ligament. Its posterior fibers pass upward to insert onto the last three ribs. The remainder slope upward and forward to a fibrous aponeurosis.

The transverse abdominus or transversalis muscle arises from the costal cartilages of the lower ribs, iliac crest, and lateral part of the inguinal ligament; it courses horizontally forward to an aponeurosis. The rectus abdominus arises from the pubic bones, passes upward in a sheath formed

Table 6-3   Summary of Respiratory Muscle Action

Level	Inspiration	Expiration
Quiet ventilation	Diaphragm in all subjects Intercostals in most subjects Scalenes in some subjects	Some persistence of inspiratory muscle contraction in expiration
Modest increase in ventilation (< 50 L/min)	Diaphragm in all subjects Intercostal in most subjects Scalenes in some subjects	Some persistence of inspiratory muscle contraction in expiration
Moderate increase in ventilation (50-100 L/min)	Diaphragm in all subjects Intercostals in most subjects Scalenes in most subjects Sternomastoid action toward end of inspiration	Some persistence of inspiratory muscle contraction Abdominal and intercostals toward end of expiration
Significant increase in ventilation (> 100 L/min)	All inspiratory accessories active	Abdominals active throughout inspiration

by the aponeuroses described above, and inserts into costal cartilages five through seven; it is often well defined in a muscular individual.

As accessory muscles of ventilation, the abdominals function mainly to aid in forced expiratory activity. This action is achieved by both increasing intraabdominal pressure and by drawing the lower ribs down and medially. In both the relaxed supine and standing positions, these muscles are normally inactive during quiet breathing. They come into play only when the normal elastic recoil of the thorax provides insufficient force to achieve the needed expiration. Such conditions occur when: (1) expiratory flows reach or exceed 40 L/min, (2) significant resistance impedes exhalation, or (3) gas is forcibly exhaled below the resting expiratory level. In such circumstances, contraction of the powerful abdominals builds up strong intraabdominal pressure and drives the diaphragm, like a piston, into exhalation. Contraction of these muscles also occurs at the end of voluntary maximum inhalation and is a factor limiting the extent of inhalation. In chronic pulmonary disease, especially in the presence of airway obstruction, effective use of the abdominals is often lost, and without these powerful generators of force to push the diaphragm into expiratory action, the patient is at a great disadvantage.

Actions of the primary and secondary muscles of ventilation are summarized in Table 6-3.

INNERVATION OF THE LUNG AND THORACIC MUSCULATURE

As depicted in Fig. 6-13, the lung is innervated by elements of both the autonomic and somatic divisions of the nervous system. The autonomic system provides both motor and sensory pathways to the lung; the somatic system provides only motor innervation to the respiratory muscles.[8]

Somatic innervation

Somatic innervation of the respiratory system is mainly by way of efferent motor stimulation of the primary muscles of ventilation, the diaphragm and intercostals.

The diaphragm is innervated by paired phrenic nerves. The phrenic nerves originate as deep (muscular) branches of spinal nerves C3–C5 in the cervical plexuses. They enter the chest in front of the subclavian arteries and lateral to the carotid arteries, running on each side of the mediastinum anterior to the hilar structures. The left phrenic nerve travels a longer course than the right, as it extends around the left projection of the heart. Injury of the

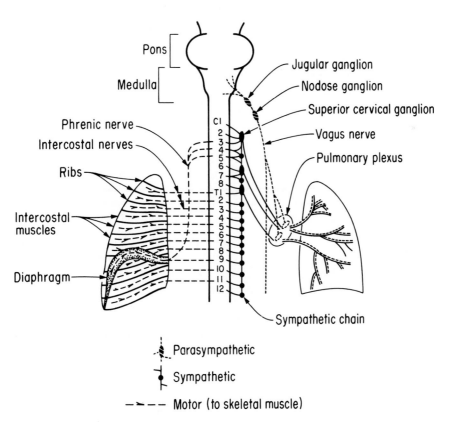

Fig. 6-13   Schema of the autonomic innervation (motor and sensory) of the lung and the somatic (motor) nerve supply to the intercostal muscles and diaphragm. (Redrawn from Murray JF: The normal lung, ed 2, Philadelphia, 1986, WB Saunders Co.)

phrenic nerves, as can occur in neck trauma, may result in paralysis of the diaphragm.

The intercostal muscles receive their motor innervation via the intercostal nerves. Like the rest of the spinal nerves, the intercostals (T2–T11) leave the vertebral column from the intervertebral foramina between adjacent vertebrae. However, unlike their counterparts, the intercostals do not form plexuses, but are distributed directly to the structures they innervate. It is the ventral rami of the intercostal nerves that provide the motor innervation to the intercostal muscles. The dorsal rami innervate mainly the muscles and skin of the back.

Intercostal nerve T2 supplies muscles of the second intercostal space and portions of the skin of the axilla and arm. Intercostal nerves T3–T6 pass in the costal grooves of the ribs, innervating the adjacent muscles and skin of the anterior and lateral thoracic wall. Intercostal nerves T7–T11 are also distributed to the adjoining intercostal muscles, additionally innervating selected abdominal muscles and skin.[9]

Autonomic innervation

Autonomic innervation is via branches of the paired vagus nerves and the upper four or five thoracic sympathetic ganglia.[10] Both contribute fibers to the anterior and posterior pulmonary plexuses at the roots of the lung.

Efferent pathways. On their entry into the chest, each vagus nerve sends off a branch that curves back up to the larynx called the recurrent laryngeal nerve. The left recurrent laryngeal nerve leaves the vagus at the level of the aortic arch, loops around the arch, and follows the trachea and esophagus upward through the mediastinum to the larynx. The right recurrent laryngeal nerve originates at the

level of the subclavian artery, looping deep toward that vessel before heading cephalad toward the larynx.

High in the neck, each vagus nerve also gives off a branch called the superior laryngeal nerve. The external branch of this nerve separately supplies the cricothyroid muscle, while the internal branch provides sensory fibers to the larynx. The recurrent laryngeal nerves are the primary source of motor innervation to the larynx. Depending on which branches are involved, damage to the laryngeal nerves can cause unilateral or bilateral paralysis of the vocal cords, resulting in hoarseness, loss of voice, and an ineffective cough. The most common causes of laryngeal nerve damage are trauma and thoracic or mediastinal tumors.

As the bronchi, arteries, and veins enter the lung at the hilum, autonomic nerve fibers subdivide with the airways, with the largest branches accompanying the bronchi and the smallest paralleling the pulmonary veins.[11] Although efferent fibers from both the sympathetic and parasympathetic systems innervate the smooth muscle and glands of the airways, anatomic and physiologic evidence indicates that the influence of the parasympathetic system predominates.[6] In combination, however, autonomic motor fibers influence the caliber of the conducting airways, the volume of the terminal respiratory units, the activity of the bronchial glands, and the tone and diameter of the pulmonary blood vessels.[12]

Afferent pathways. Virtually all afferent nerve fibers from the lung to the central nervous system are vagal in origin. The most important of these sensory paths are associated with a variety of well-defined receptor sites in both the airways and lung parenchyma. The three best understood of these vagal sensory sites are the bronchopul-

Table 6-4   Characteristics of the Three Pulmonary Vagal Sensory Reflexes

Receptor	Location	Fiber type	Stimulus	Responses
Pulmonary stretch, slowly adapting	Associated with smooth muscle of intrapulmonary airways	Medullated	Lung inflation Increased transpulmonary pressure	Hering-Breuer inflation reflex Bronchodilatation Increased heart rate Decreased peripheral vascular resistance
Irritant, rapidly adapting	Epithelium of (mainly) extrapulmonary airways	Medullated	Irritants Mechanical stimulation Anaphylaxis Pneumothorax Hyperpnea Pulmonary congestion	Bronchoconstriction Hyperpnea Expiratory constriction of larynx Cough
Type J	Alveolar wall	Nonmedullated	Increased interstitial volume (congestion) Chemical injury Microembolism	Rapid shallow breathing Severe expiratory constriction of larynx Hypotension, bradycardia Spinal reflex inhibition

From Murray JF: The normal lung, ed 2, Philadelphia, 1986, WB Saunders Co.

monary stretch receptors, the irritant receptors, and the J receptors. Two additional categories of receptors located outside the lung, the muscle proprioceptors and the peripheral chemoreceptors, are involved in the sensory control of ventilation and respiration. The proprioceptors and chemoreceptors, and their relationship to the regulation of breathing, will be discussed in Chapter 10.

A summary of the characteristics of the pulmonary vagal receptors appears in Table 6-4.[6] The stretch receptors are located primarily in the bronchi and bronchioles and are associated with their smooth muscle. They progressively discharge nerve impulses during inflation of the lung up to the end of inspiration. Traditionally, this inflation reflex (a component of the Hering-Breuer reflex) was thought to modulate the depth of inspiration. However, recent experimentation in animals indicates that these receptors mainly influence the duration of the expiratory pause occurring between breaths, not their depth.[13] It now appears that the inflation reflex is weak or absent during normal quiet breathing in healthy adults. The only evidence of a strong inflation reflex in humans is among newborn infants.[6,12]

A special reflex thought to be associated with the sensory stimulation of the stretch receptors is Head's paradoxical reflex, which stimulates a deeper breath instead of inhibiting further inspiration. This reflex may be the basis for the occasional deep breath or sigh that punctuates normal breathing, thereby preventing alveolar collapse or microatelectasis. It may also be responsible for the successive gasping exhibited by newborn infants as they progressively inflate their lungs at birth.[12,14]

The irritant or mechanoreceptors of the lung are located in the subepithelia tissues of the larger airways, mainly in the posterior wall of the trachea, and at the bifurcations of the larger bronchi. Not active during normal breathing, these receptors respond to a variety of mechanical, chemical, and physiologic stimuli, including physical manipulation or irritation, inhalation of noxious gases, histamine-induced bronchoconstriction, asphyxia, and microembolization of the pulmonary arteries.[10-12]

Stimulation of the irritant receptors can result in bronchoconstriction, hyperpnea, reflex closure of the glottis, cough, and a reflex slowing of the heart (bradycardia). When caused by mechanical stimulation, as during procedures such as tracheobronchial aspiration, intubation, or bronchoscopy, this response often is referred to as the *vago-vagal reflex*. The vago-vagal reflex can be mitigated by the application of local anesthetics.

J receptors are so named because they have been primarily found in "juxtaposition" to the pulmonary capillaries. These receptors originally were considered part of a deflation reflex. Recent research indicates that the primary role of the J receptors is in response to increases in pulmonary capillary pressures such as that occurring in congestive heart failure.[10-12] Stimulation of the J receptors results in rapid, shallow breathing and can cause bradycardia, hypotension, and expiratory narrowing of the glottis. J receptor stimulation also may contribute to the sensation of dyspnea accompanying such conditions as pulmonary edema, pulmonary embolism, and pneumonia.[6]

VASCULAR SUPPLY

The vascular supply of the lungs is composed of two separate systems, the pulmonary and bronchial circulations. Also involved in fluid transport from the lung is a rich network of lymphatics. The pulmonary circulation conducts venous blood coming from the tissues to the lungs for purposes of restoring its oxygen contents and removing the gaseous product of metabolism, carbon dioxide. The bronchial circulation provides freshly arterialized blood back to the lungs to meet its own metabolic requirements. The lymphatic system gathers interstitial fluid from the lung parenchyma and pleural space for return to the systemic circulation.

Pulmonary circulation

Pulmonary circulation originates on the right side of the heart, and, via the main pulmonary artery, delivers unoxygenated blood to the lungs. The main pulmonary artery and aorta exit from the heart and pass superiorly (Fig. 6-14). Just below the point of tracheal division into the right and left mainstem bronchi (the carina), the main pulmonary artery divides into corresponding right and left pulmonary arteries, which accompany respective bronchi. This companionship continues through all the divisions into the distal air spaces. The branches of the pulmonary artery are always adjacent to the bronchi and bronchioles.

Pulmonary arterioles eventually reach the terminal respiratory units and subdivide into a rich alveolar capillary plexus, providing a large blood surface area to facilitate exchange of oxygen and carbon dioxide with the lungs.[15,16] Freshly arterialized blood leaves the alveolar region in pulmonary venules, which combine into larger veins. Four to five major pulmonary veins eventually direct the blood back to the left atrium of the heart, for distribution to the systemic circulation.

Pressure in the normal pulmonary circulation averages about one sixth of that in the systemic circulation.[15-17] Given that blood flow at any given time is normally equal in both systems, it is apparent that the pulmonary circulation offers substantially less resistance to flow than its systemic counterpart. This difference is essential in maintaining the delicate fluid balance at the alveolar-capillary region. Increases in pressure in the pulmonary circulation, such as occur in congestive heart failure, can disrupt this delicate balance and cause fluid transudation into the alveoli, thereby impairing gas exchange.

However, because the pulmonary circulation is a low pressure system, blood flow throughout the lung is highly

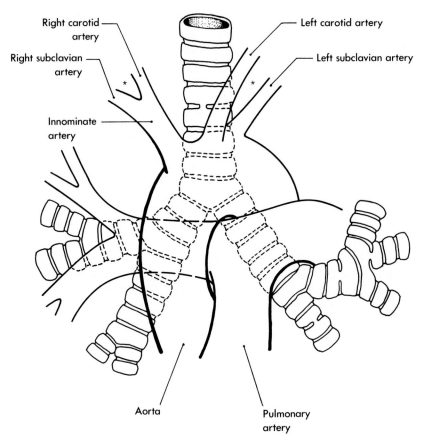

Right carotid
artery

Right subclavian
artery

Innominate
artery

Left carotid artery

Left subclavian artery

Aorta

Pulmonary
artery

Fig. 6-14   Diagram of relationship between main pulmonary artery and aorta, with their main branches, as they leave right and left ventricles of heart. Trachea is in background. The aorta arches over main pulmonary artery, which divides into right and left branches that enter the lungs. The aorta supplies oxygenated blood to remainder of body. The asterisk (*) on each side indicates the course of phrenic and vagus nerves as they enter thorax.

dependent on gravity. In the upright lung, hydrostatic pressures in the pulmonary circulation decrease about 1 cm H_2O for every cm distance from the lung base to its apex.[16] Thus, toward the apex of the upright lung, blood flow is very low. As one moves down the lung, perfusion increases linearly in proportion to the hydrostatic pressure, so that the lung bases receive nearly twenty times as much blood flow as the apices.[16]

These gravity-related effects also occur in recumbent positions, but are less pronounced. In any case, hydrostatic pressure differences in the pulmonary circulation always result in the dependent portions of the lungs receiving the greatest proportion of blood flow. The significance of this fact, as it relates to pulmonary gas exchange, is discussed in Chapter 9.

Bronchial circulation

Since blood coming through the pulmonary arteries lacks sufficient oxygen for the metabolism of the lung tissues, a separate arterial supply, called the bronchial circulation, also accompanies the bronchi.[18] Because the meta-

bolic needs of the lung are comparatively low, and because much of the lung parenchyma is oxygenated via direct contact with inspired gas, blood flow through the bronchial circulation normally amounts to only 1% to 2% of the total cardiac output.

Bronchial arteries vary in number and origin.[19] Usually a single artery on the right arises from an upper intercostal artery or the right subclavian or internal mammary artery. Two bronchial arteries normally supply the left lung and commonly arise as direct branches of the upper thoracic aorta. These bronchial arteries follow their respective bronchi, with two to three branches accompanying each subdivision of the conducting airway. Near the end of the terminal bronchioles, the bronchial arterial circulation terminates in a plexus of capillaries that anastomose extensively with the capillary bed of the alveoli.

Return flow of the bronchial circulation to the right heart (bronchial venous blood) takes one of at least two courses (Fig. 6-15). According to animal studies, some 25% to 33% of bronchial flow returns to the heart through true bronchial veins emptying into the azygos, hemizygos,

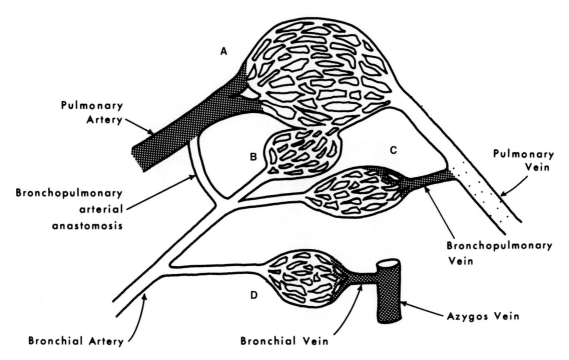

Fig. 6-15   Schema of the relationships between the bronchial and pulmonary circulations. The pulmonary artery supplies the pulmonary capillary network, **A.** The bronchial artery supplies capillary networks **B, C,** and **D.** Network **B** represents the bronchial capillary supply to bronchioles that anastomoses with pulmonary capillaries and drains through pulmonary veins. Network **C** represents the bronchial capillary supply to most bronchi; these vessels form bronchopulmonary veins that empty into pulmonary veins. Network **D** represents the bronchial capillary supply to lobar and segmental bronchi; these vessels form true bronchial veins that drain into the azygos, hemiazygos, or intercostal veins. (From Murray JF: The normal lung, ed 2, Philadelphia, WB Saunders Co.)

or intercostal veins. The remaining two thirds to three fourths of the bronchial flow courses through "bronchopulmonary veins" that originate from the bronchial capillaries and empty into the pulmonary veins. Direct vascular connections between the bronchial and pulmonary arteries, known as bronchopulmonary arterial anastomoses, may also exist and represent a third path for return to the heart.

The bronchial and pulmonary circulations appear to share an important reciprocal relationship in abnormal states that can compensate for impairment of either.[6] Decreases in perfusing pressures of the pulmonary arterial circulation, like that occurring with embolization, tend to cause an increase in bronchial artery blood flow to the affected area, thereby minimizing the likelihood of pulmonary infarction. Conversely, loss of bronchial circulation, as occurs with lung transplantation, can be partially offset by increases in pulmonary arterial perfusion. When circumstances prevent such collateral pathways from developing, tissue necrosis of the affected area usually ensues.

Lymphatics

The lymphatic system of the body consists of a network of lymphatic vessels, numerous lymph nodes, the tonsils, thymus gland, and spleen. It functions primarily to clear protein-containing fluid from the interstitial spaces of tissue. The lymphatic system also plays an important role in the body's immune system, removing bacteria, foreign material, and cell debris from the lymph fluid and producing lymphocytes and plasma cells to aid in defense. Both roles are essential for maintaining normal function of the respiratory system.

The pulmonary lymphatic system consists of two sets of vessels: superficial and deep.[20] The superficial or pleural network drains mainly the lung surface and pleura; the deep or peribronchovascular network serves mainly the lung parenchyma. Both originate as dead-end lymphatic capillaries in their respective regions. Although not extending to the level of the alveolar-capillary membrane, deep lymph vessels are closely associated with the terminal respiratory units of the lung. Here the lymphatic system works together with phagocytic cells in the alveoli to provide a final line of defense against foreign material able to penetrate this deeply.[21]

Lymph fluid returns to the circulatory system primarily through lymphatic channels that course toward the hilum. These channels freely join with each other in the pleura

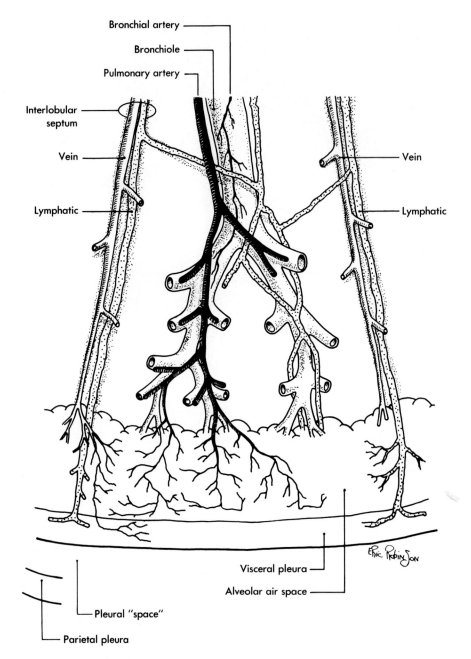

Bronchial artery

Bronchiole

Pulmonary artery

Interlobular septum

Vein

Vein

Lymphatic

Lymphatic

Visceral pleura

Alveolar air space

Pleural "space"

Parietal pleura

Fig. 6-16 Diagram of distal pulmonary arteries, bronchioles, and air spaces with their associated bronchial arteries. Pulmonary veins lie in fibrous tissue septa between these paired pulmonary arteries and airways. Note that lymphatic channels travel with both sets of structures.

and travel toward the hilar region, both in the septa accompanying veins and about the bronchopulmonary artery complexes (Fig. 6-16 and 6-17). The lymph flow is directed through one or more lymph nodes clustered about each hilus. From there lymph travels through the mediastinum to rejoin the general circulation via either the right lymphatic or thoracic duct.

Lymphatic channels generally are not detectable on standard chest roentgenograms unless they are distended or thickened by disease (see Chapter 18). Kerley "A" lines on

chest roentgenography represent distention and thickening of the connections between lymph vessels accompanying the pulmonary veins and arteries. Kerley "B" lines are the radiologic manifestation of distended lymph vessels in the interlobular septa.[22] Pulmonary edema and pleural effusion become evident on radiologic examination only when the lymphatic system no longer can provide adequate clearance of excessive fluid buildup in these regions of the lung.

Now that the gross structure of the thorax has been dis-

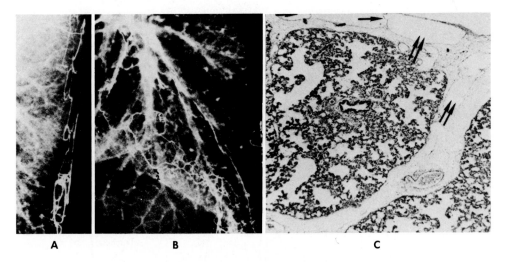

Fig. 6-17   Radiographs of lymphatic channels following their injection with contrast material. The pleural lymphatics are seen in profile in **A.** One lymphatic channel marked with an arrow in **B** is following a pulmonary vein. Tissue section, **C,** shows pleural lymphatics marked with one arrow, and septal lymphatics marked with two arrows. (From Heitzman ER: The lung: radiologic-pathologic correlations, St Louis, 1973, The CV Mosby Co.).

cussed, attention will be focused on the form and function of that portion of the respiratory system responsible for conditioning, conducting, and exchanging gases with the circulatory system.

ANATOMY OF THE RESPIRATORY TRACT

According to function, the respiratory tract conventionally is divided into an upper and lower portion (Fig. 6-18). The upper portion includes the oral and nasal cavities, the pharynx, and the larynx. As components of the upper respiratory tract, the distinguishing feature of these structures is their multiplicity of functions.

The lower respiratory tract traditionally begins at the inferior border of the larynx at the cricoid cartilage and extends through the numerous airway divisions to the level of the alveoli. Unlike the structures of the upper respiratory tract, those of the lower respiratory tract are devoted almost exclusively to conduction and gas exchange.

Upper respiratory tract

The upper respiratory tract consists of the nasal and oral cavities, the pharynx, and larynx (see Fig. 6-18). It serves four important respiratory functions. The nose, pharynx, and larynx conduct respiratory gases to and from the lungs. But first and foremost, these structures serve as key frontline defense mechanisms for the lungs.[23] In addition, the nasal passageways humidify inspired air and function as a heat exchange mechanism for the respiratory system and body as a whole.

The nose. Adults normally breathe through the nose. Exceptions to this observation are obstructive conditions such as nasal polyps, mucosal edema, and periods of high ventilatory rates and flows, as during strenuous exercise. This latter phenomenon is due to the comparatively higher resistance to gas flow through the nasal passages as compared to the mouth. This airflow resistance is attributable to the specialized structures necessary for the nose to fulfill its respiratory functions.

The external nose is formed by the frontal process of the maxilla, two nasal bones, cartilage, and fatty connective tissue (Fig. 6-19). Two flexible, flared entryways called wings, or *alae,* enclose a space on each side called the *vestibule.* The vestibules are lined by squamous epithelium and have large hairs that serve a gross filtration function. Posterior to the vestibules are the paired openings to the internal nose called the *anterior nares.* This point represents the smallest cross-sectional area in the adult respiratory tract.[24]

The main internal nasal passages begin at this point, separated in the midline by a septum formed anteriorly by cartilage and posteriorly by the vomer bone and the perpendicular plate of the ethmoid bone. Although normally in the midline, the septum is frequently deviated to one side or the other. Three bony shelves formed by downward and medial projections of the superior, middle, and inferior conchae extend out of the lateral wall and project into the nasal cavity. These turbinates divide the nasal cavities into three convoluted passageways: a superior, middle, and inferior meatus. The olfactory receptors of the nose lie above the superior turbinates bilaterally.

The turbinates are lined by highly vascularized tissue consisting of pseudostratified, ciliated, columnar epithelium interspersed with mucus-secreting goblet cells. In

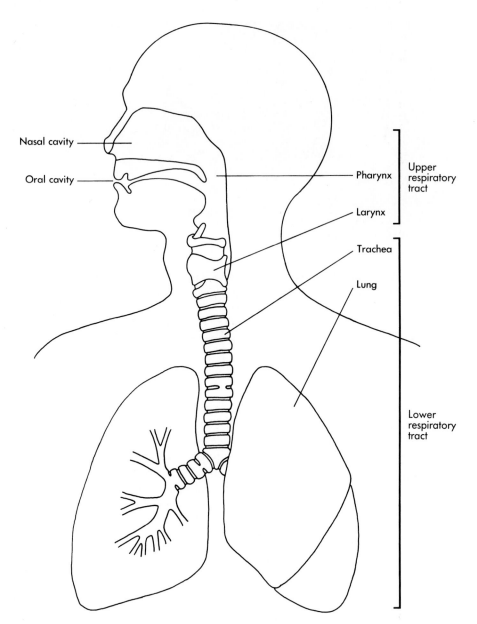

Fig. 6-18   The respiratory tract consists of the nasal cavity, oral cavity, pharynx, larynx, trachea, and lung. The larynx divides the system into the upper and lower respiratory tract.

combination, these structures present a large surface area for heat and water exchange with the incoming and outgoing airstream.

The normal nose warms the inspired air close to body temperature and saturates it with water vapor before the stream arrives at the nasopharynx.[24,25] Moreover, on expiration, condensation of water vapor retains both heat and moisture for subsequent modification of inspired gas. Contrary to popular belief, even under the driest environmental air conditions, the nasal mucosa functions unimpaired.[24] However, bypassing this efficient heat and water exchanger, as occurs with endotracheal intubation or trache-

ostomy, can severely compromise the respiratory system's ability to respond to extremes of ambient temperature and humidity.

The defense function of the nose involves both physical and physiologic mechanisms. As noted above, the large hairs of the vestibule provide a gross filtration function. This function is augmented by the nature and pattern of airflow within the nasal cavity. During nasal breathing, inspired gas is first accelerated to a high velocity through the anterior nares, making a sharp directional change as it enters the internal nasal cavity. By this action alone, large particles of foreign matter (those greater than a few mi-

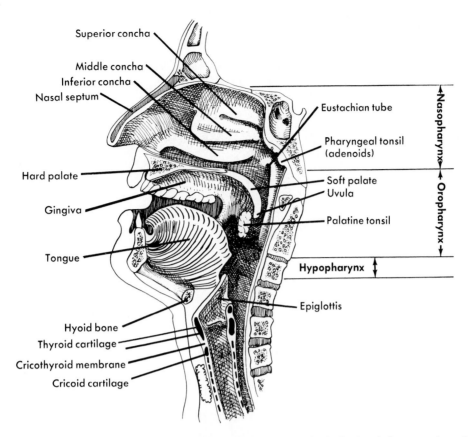

Fig. 6-19 Structures of upper airway and oral cavity. Larynx is the landmark for separation of upper and lower airway. (From Ellis PD and Billings DM: Cardiopulmonary resuscitation: procedures for basic and advanced life support, St Louis, 1980, The CV Mosby Co.)

crometers in size) readily impact on the nasal mucosa. Such matter normally is cleared either by ciliary action or nose blowing.

As inspired gas enters the main passageways of the nasal cavity beyond the external nares, the cross-sectional area increases, resulting in a relative decrease in linear velocity. However, because of the narrow width and convoluted nature of the meati, the pattern of flow tends to remain turbulent. In combination, the relative low velocity and turbulence of the airstream in this region ensure that most foreign particles that escaped earlier trapping will be effectively removed here by further impaction, sedimentation, or diffusion.

Surface fluids originating from the goblet cells and submucosal glands of the nasal cavity and paranasal sinuses have mild antibacterial properties. Moreover, mucosal fluids are responsible for removal of water-soluble, irritant gases such as sulfur dioxide. Ciliary activity normally transports surface fluids backward to the nasopharynx at a rate of about 6 mm/min, where foreign matter can be cleared by swallowing. Together, these defense and clearance mechanisms ensure that inspired air reaching the

lungs is essentially free of both inanimate and bacterial contamination and common air pollutants.

Paranasal sinuses. Connected with the nasal cavities are empty spaces in the facial and skull bones technically called the paranasal sinuses (Fig. 6-20). The paranasal sinuses are symmetrically paired structures, most of which open into the nasal cavity, usually between the turbinates (Fig. 6-20, *A*). The frontal and maxillary sinuses are the most accessible of the paranasal sinuses (see Fig. 6-20, *A* and *B*). The more anterior ethmoid and more posterior sphenoid sinuses are near the midline above and just behind the nasal cavities (see Fig. 6-20, *A* and *B*). All are named for the bones in which they occur. Although the exact purpose of the sinuses is unclear, it has been suggested that they may function to provide temperature insulation, to strengthen the skull without additional weight, and to enhance voice resonance.[14] Many problems can develop when the drainage of the paranasal sinuses becomes impaired. Foremost among these problems are chronic sinus infections and the role they can play as a source for aspiration of contaminated material into the lower respiratory tract.

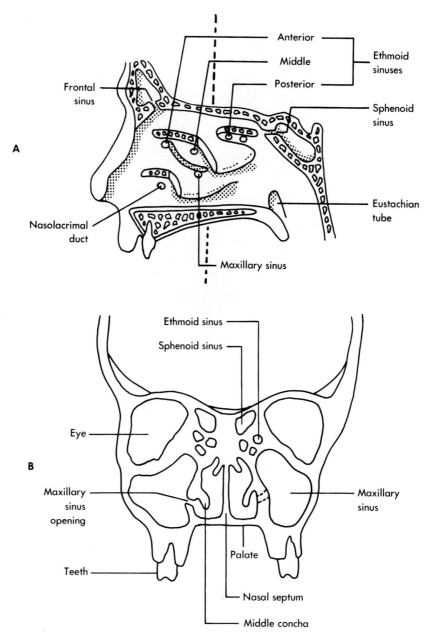

Fig. 6-20   The nasal sinuses are named for bones in which they occur. **A,** In lateral view (as in Fig. 3-2) but with conchae cut away. Note entrances into nasal cavity of various sinuses and their location within these cavities. **B,** Frontal view of face taken at level of dotted line in **A.** Note position of maxillary sinuses in each cheekbone. Sphenoid sinuses are behind ethmoid sinuses, although they appear to be at same level in this frontal view.

Oral cavity. Whereas the nasal cavity serves a predominantly respiratory function, the oral cavity serves multiple purposes, being involved in digestion as well as speech and respiration. For this reason, the oral cavity should be considered an accessory respiratory passage. Mouth breathing in adults is used mainly during speech, strenuous exercise, or when the nose is obstructed by upper respiratory tract infections or foreign materials.

Separating the nasal cavity from the oral cavity is the roof of the mouth, the *palate* (Fig. 6-21). The anterior two thirds has a bony skeleton that accounts for its designation, hard palate, whereas the posterior one third is without such support and is therefore called the soft palate. From the midline portion of the soft palate at the back of the mouth extends the soft, fleshy *uvula,* which points in the direction of the lower respiratory tract (see Fig. 6-21). Its pur-

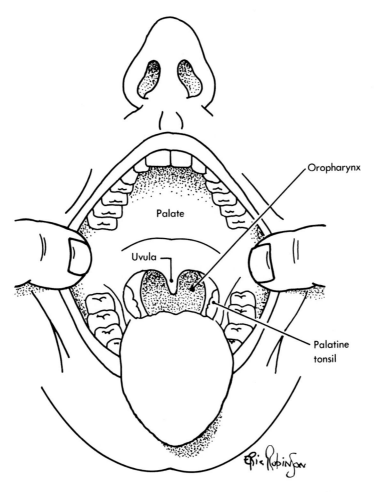

Fig. 6-21 View into opened mouth. Soft midline uvula is seen hanging from fleshy palatine pillars. Pharynx is seen at back of mouth.

pose, in coordination with the surrounding walls, is to control flow in eating, drinking, sneezing, coughing, and vomiting.

The lips, teeth, tongue, jaw muscles, and spontaneous reflexes help protect the mouth from injury or unwanted intrusion. The tongue is a strong, muscular mass involved in mechanical digestion, taste, and phonation. The posterior surface of the tongue is supplied with many sensory nerve endings that originate a protective vagal gag reflex when manipulated. This reflex is protective in nature and must be considered when passing fingers, tubes, instruments, or other objects through the mouth in the conscious or semiconscious patient. At the very base of the tongue are found paired lymphatic structures called *lingual tonsils*.

The mucosal surfaces of the oral cavity also provide wetting and warming qualities for incoming air, although less efficiently than those provided by the nose. Saliva is produced by major and minor salivary glands and provides some moisture for inhaled air. However, saliva functions primarily as both a wetting and digestive agent for food.

The oral cavity ends where double webs on each side, the *palatine folds,* arch up toward the midline, fleshy uvula (see Fig. 6-21). Between these folds and on each side sit paired, cryptic structures called the *palatine tonsils*. Similar in structure to the other highly vascularized, lymphoidal tissues of the upper airway, the palatine tonsils seem to play an immunologic role, especially in childhood.

The normal protective reflexes and coordinated functions of the mouth, pharynx, and larynx during swallowing generally protect the lower respiratory tract from entry of foreign material. However, these functions can be severely compromised during periods of anesthesia or unconsciousness. Moreover, poor oral hygiene can result in unnecessary exposure of the lower respiratory tract to pathogenic bacteria and the increased possibility of respiratory tract infection.

Pharynx. The space behind the nasal cavities and mouth is called the pharynx, from the Greek word for "throat." The pharynx extends from the rear of the nasal cavity to the point where the airway (at the larynx) and the digestive tract, esophagus, separate. Anatomically, it is di-

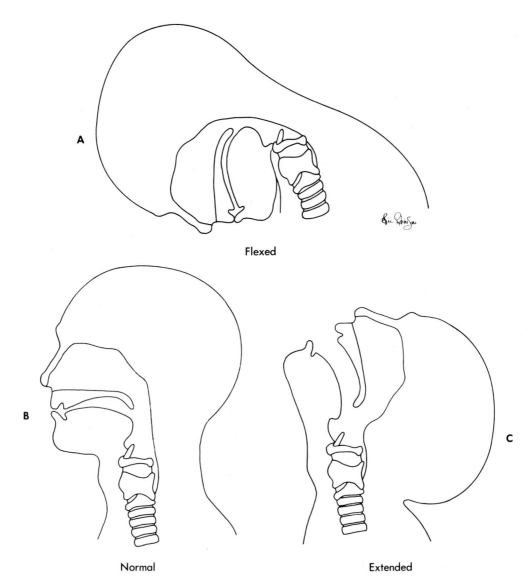

A

Flexed

B

Normal

C

Extended

Fig. 6-22   The position of head affects patency of airway. **A,** With head flexed, airway may be kinked, making breathing or intubation difficult. **B,** Normal upright relationship of head and neck to chest. **C,** Extension of head straightens airway, making breathing, clearance of material, or intubation easier.

vided into three contiguous portions: the nasopharynx, the oropharynx, and the hypopharynx or laryngopharynx (see Fig. 6-19). Histologically, the three portions of the pharynx are lined with stratified squamous epithelium.

The portion behind the nasal cavities is called the nasopharynx. Palatal muscles completely occlude the nasopharynx during swallowing and coughing. The eustachian, or auditory, tubes open into the lateral nasopharynx walls and connect the nasopharynx with the middle portion of each ear and with the mastoid sinuses. On the superior posterior wall is the other major lymphoid mass of the upper respiratory tract, the pharyngeal or adenoid tonsil, commonly called the *adenoids*. The palatine, lingual, and adenoid tonsils comprise the major components of Waldeyer's ring, the so-called guardian ring of lymphoid

material surrounding the entries of the respiratory and gastrointestinal tracts.

The portion of the pharynx at the back of the oral cavity is called the oropharynx. This extends from the uvula above to the epiglottis and base of the tongue below. Nasotracheal and nasogastric tubes passed through the nose must turn inferiorly at the nasopharynx and continue in that direction through the oropharynx if they are to reach the trachea, lungs, or stomach.

The inferior portion of the pharynx lying between the epiglottis and final entries into the larynx and esophagus is called the hypopharynx (or laryngopharynx). This is a short segment extending into the neck. It corresponds to the height of the epiglottis and is a critical dividing point in separating the digestive and respiratory tracts. The hy-

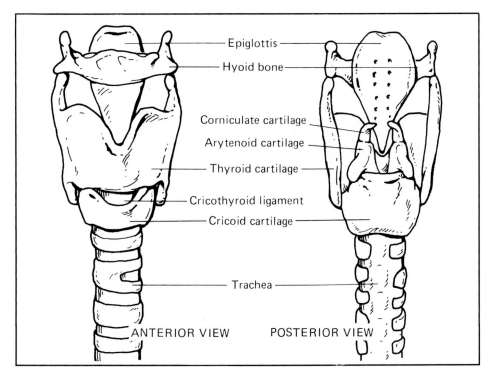

Epiglottis

Hyoid bone

Corniculate cartilage

Arytenoid cartilage

Thyroid cartilage

Cricothyroid ligament

Cricoid cartilage

Trachea

ANTERIOR VIEW   POSTERIOR VIEW

Fig. 6-23   Anterior and posterior views of the laryngeal cartilages and trachea.   (From Martin DE and Youtsey JW: Respiratory anatomy and physiology, St Louis, 1988, The CV Mosby Co.)

popharynx is capable of substantial changes in shape, especially during swallowing and speech.

The relative position of the oral cavity, pharynx, and larynx are critically important determinants of upper airway patency, particularly in unconscious individuals. In the upright position, the head and neck tend to form a roughly 90-degree angle with the pharynx-larynx axis (Fig. 6-22, *B*). With loss of consciousness, the head often droops downward, decreasing this angle (Fig. 6-22, *A*). This positional change can partially or completely obstruct the upper airway. Extension of the head and lower jaw helps alleviate this obstruction (Fig. 6-22, *C*). In addition to creating a better alignment of the upper airway structures, such an action displaces the flaccid tongue away from the rear of the pharynx. This technique is used both to maintain the normal airway in an unconscious patient and to facilitate introduction of artificial airways.

Larynx. The larynx is an extremely complex structure located immediately below the pharynx. "Hung" from the hyoid bone at the base of the tongue, the larynx is readily palpable at the thyroid cartilage prominence or "Adam's apple." Anatomically, it consists of nine cartilages and numerous muscles and ligaments (Fig. 6-23). In combination, these structures serve to protect the lower airway during breathing and swallowing, and to occlude it during certain specialized respiratory maneuvers.[26] Its major function in sound production is also notable.

The *epiglottis* is a platelike cartilage that extends from the base of the tongue backward and upward (see Fig. 6-19 and 6-23). It is attached by ligaments to the hyoid bone anteriorly and by its pointed stalk to the thyroid cartilage below. In adults it is 2 to 4 cm long and 2 to 3 cm wide. It is only 2 to 5 mm thick. During oral examination, this structure is not readily seen in adults, but, because of its higher position, can be seen easily in small children, especially crying babies. The positioning of the larynx in infants also explains in part why they are obligatory nose breathers and how they are able to breathe and suckle simultaneously.

Contrary to popular belief, the epiglottis does not close off the airway during swallowing. During this complex maneuver, it is pushed downward and backward by the tongue and rising larynx, simply facilitating the diversion of a bolus of food toward the piriform sinuses and into the esophagus.[26] Indeed, surgical removal of the epiglottis normally does not impair the act of swallowing at all.

The inlet to the larynx lies below and behind the base of the tongue. Fig. 6-24 portrays the view of the larynx inlet as observed during laryngoscopic examination. The posterior base of the tongue is attached to the epiglottis of the larynx by three folds that form a small space between the tongue and the epiglottis called the *vallecula,* a key landmark in oral intubation.

Above the true vocal cords are vestibular folds com-

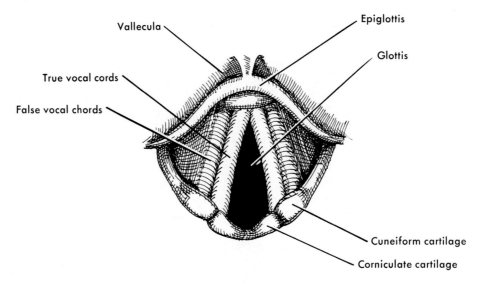

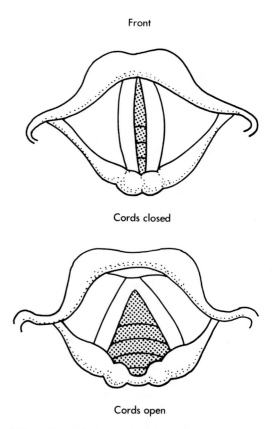

Fig. 6-24   Interior of larynx. (From Ellis PD and Billings DM: Cardiopulmonary resuscitation: procedures for basic and advanced life support, St Louis, 1980, The CV Mosby Co.)

monly known as the *false vocal cords*. These folds are not as highly developed as the true cords, but can act together with them to close off the lower airway. This latter action is essential in the compressive stage of a cough and explains why patients with artificial airways cannot produce an effective expulsion. The false cords also can completely adduct and totally obscure the view of the true cords and glottis during spasmodic or reflex contraction of the larynx muscles.

The true vocal cords appear as white bordered veils, separated by the space known as the rima glottidis or simply *glottis*. The vocal cords are composed of muscle, ligament, submucosal soft tissue, and a mucous membrane covering. Loose tissue below this mucous membrane represents potential space readily subject to fluid accumulation. Since the lymphatic drainage to this area is sparse, cord swelling resulting from such fluid accumulation resolves slowly.

The vocal cords project from the paired *arytenoid cartilages* to insert on the posterior surface of the thyroid cartilage. The distance between the vocal cords is altered by adduction or abduction of the arytenoids about their articulation with the cricoid ring. These movements of the arytenoids changes the tension on the vocal cords, thereby producing phonation and allowing sphincter control.

Sound is produced by vibration of the cords in the airstream. By varying cord tension, one may change the pitch of sound made. By varying the volumes of air passing the cords, one may vary the intensity of the sounds. Some fluttering of the cords in the airstream is also observed during normal breathing. They appear to be drawn apart in inspiration by active muscular contraction, and relax toward the midline during expiration (Fig. 6-25).

The lower border of the larynx is formed by a circular, cartilaginous ring called the *cricoid cartilage* (see Fig. 6-

Fig. 6-25   View into larynx from back of mouth to the front. Vocal cords vary in tension, length, and relationship to one another. Note open inspiratory position versus expiratory or resting closed position. Inside of trachea with its cartilaginous rings is seen through opening between vocal cords.

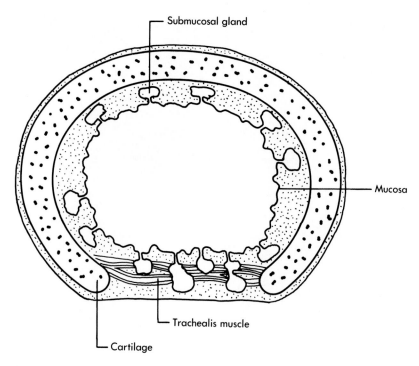

Submucosal gland

Mucosa

Trachealis muscle

Cartilage

Fig. 6-26 Trachea is composed of C-shaped cartilaginous rings connected posteriorly by membrane covering thin trachealis muscle. This arrangement allows variation in tracheal caliber. Note mucosal and submucosal glands lining airway.

23). As the only rigid structure of the upper respiratory tract that completely encircles the airway, the inner diameter of the cricoid sets the upper limit for the size of endotracheal tubes passed through the larynx. This relationship is particularly important in infants, where the cricoid ring (as opposed to the anterior nares in adults) represents the narrowest portion of the airway as a whole.

If the finger is allowed to slide down the midline of the neck from the thyroid cartilage into the groove immediately between it and the cricoid, a membranous space can be palpated. This space is the *cricothyroid ligament* (see Fig. 6-23). It is here that an emergency procedure for opening the airway, a cricothyrotomy, is performed. Also, catheters for removal of secretions (transtracheal aspiration), for provision of supplementary oxygen (transtracheal oxygenation), or for actual ventilation (high-frequency jet ventilation) can be inserted through the cricothyroid ligament. However, because of the proximity of the laryngeal nerves and vocal cords to this area, extreme caution must be exercised in such procedures. Indeed, this is why true surgical tracheostomy is usually placed 1 to 3 cm below the cricoid cartilage.

Lower respiratory tract

The lower respiratory tract begins where the upper respiratory tract ends, at the inferior border of the cricoid cartilage. The structures of the lower respiratory tract are designed to serve two primary functions: the conduction of respiratory gases and their exchange with the blood. These key functions of respiration are accomplished via a system of airway branchings leading to an enormous surface area where blood and respired gases can be placed in intimate contact with each other. For clarity, we will describe these structures in the sequence in which they are encountered as one progresses deeper into the lungs.

Trachea. The trachea marks the beginning of the conducting system of the lungs, often called the tracheobronchial tree. The trachea is a tubular structure that begins at the cricoid cartilage and extends through the neck into the mediastinum to a point behind the articulation between the manubrium and body of the sternum (angle of Louis). At this point it divides into the two mainstem bronchi.

The adult trachea is about 2.0 to 2.5 cm in diameter and 10 to 12 cm long. It contains 16 to 20 C-shaped, cartilaginous rings that give it structural support. Each tracheal cartilage is 4 to 5 mm high and not easily felt externally, except in very thin individuals. Posteriorly, a thin muscle, the *trachealis,* extends between the open ends of the cartilages (Fig. 6-26). This combined muscular-cartilaginous structure provides support yet allows some variation in diameter. The intrathoracic portion of the trachea is particularly affected by pressure differences across its walls, being dramatically compressed during coughing.[26]

The trachea can be seen on a roentgenogram as an air-filled structure in contrast to the blood vessels and other structures that have a water density appearance (Fig. 6-27). Therefore, on the usual negative x-ray film, it and

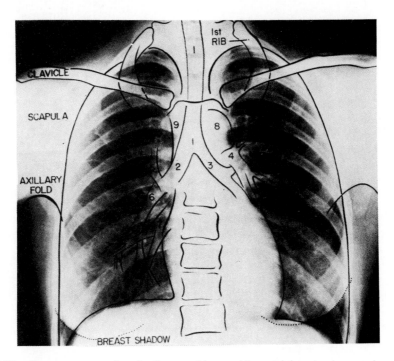

Fig. 6-27 Roentgenogram of mediastinum and lungs. Air-containing structures such as trachea and lungs are dark on this negative. The mediastinum is the central structure between lungs. Note air-filled trachea within this structure *(1)*. Hilus of each lung is its connection with the mediastinum. It contains mainstem and first division airways *(2 and 3)* as well as the major pulmonary blood vessels *(4, 5, 6, and 7)*. (From Fraser RG and Paré JA: Structure and function of the lung with emphasis on roentgenology, Philadelphia, 1971, WB Saunders Co.)

other air spaces, including most of the lungs, appear black compared with the grayer or whiter soft tissues (see Chapter 18).

The trachea is almost midline in the neck, but in the superior mediastinum it deviates slightly to the right, allowing room for the aorta to pass by on the left (see Fig. 6-14). At the point of tracheal bifurcation in the chest, a sharply dividing cartilage, the *carina,* extends up in midline to help demarcate flow into the right or left side. The right mainstem bronchus angles off at 20 to 30 degrees from the midline, whereas the left angles off more sharply at 45 to 55 degrees (Fig. 6-28). Therefore, aspirated solid objects and fluids have a tendency to follow the straighter course of the right mainstem bronchus. This tendency to follow the straightest course continues throughout the airways in a predictable manner that helps to determine the path aspirated materials will follow (Fig. 6-29).

Airway divisions and segmental anatomy. Each mainstem bronchus divides into branches supplying each lobe of the lung. At a point about 3 cm from the carina, the right mainstem bronchus gives rise to the upper lobe bronchus. The remaining major airway is called the intermediate bronchus. It continues for 3 to 4 cm and then divides into the middle and lower lobe bronchi.

The left mainstem bronchus proceeds for about 5 cm, before dividing into a left upper and lower lobe bronchi.

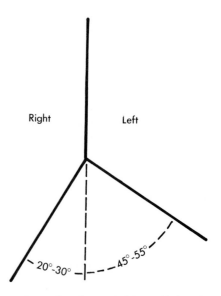

Fig. 6-28 Course of trachea and right and left main stem bronchi. Notice that right mainstem bronchus continues on straighter course from midline than left mainstem bronchus.

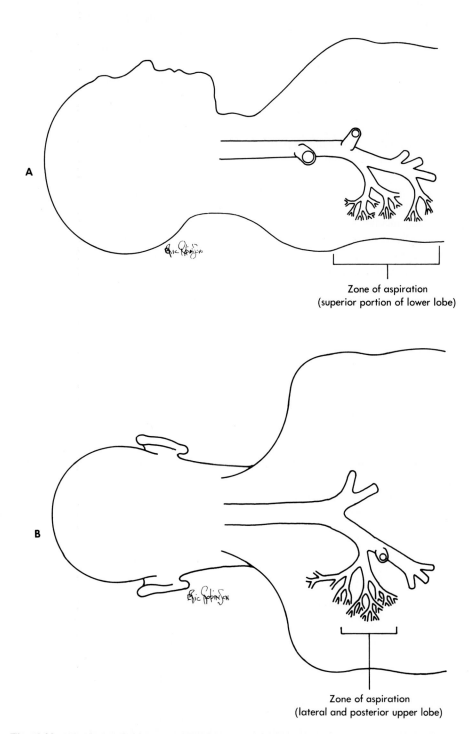

Zone of aspiration
(superior portion of lower lobe)

Zone of aspiration
(lateral and posterior upper lobe)

Fig. 6-29   Aspirated fluid can be spread about in many portions of lung, but some regions appear most frequently involved out to their most dependent position. If patient is in upright position, such material goes to basal portions of lungs. **A,** When patient is supine, this material involves predominantly the superior portions, especially the superior segment of the lower lobes. **B,** When patient is on one side or the other, this material involves lateral and posterior portions of upper lobe.

Although the left lung lacks a middle lobe, a division of the left upper lobe, called the *lingula,* corresponds developmentally to the right middle lobe. Its bronchus arises from the left upper lobe bronchus. There is no intermediate bronchus on the left.

The lobes divide further into fairly uniform anatomic units called bronchopulmonary *segments.* There are normally ten segments in the right lung and eight segments in the left (Table 6-5 and Fig. 6-30). Detailed knowledge of this segmental anatomy is essential in conducting a physical assessment of the thorax and in the effective provision of pulmonary physical therapy.

Fortunately, the segmental structure of the right and left lungs are similar, except as noted in Table 6-5 and Fig. 6-30. Moreover, a standardized naming system, developed by Jackson and Huber, is used widely in North America.[27] This numbering system helps show which segments on the left correspond to those on the right. Since the right middle lobe and lingular portion of the left upper lobe differ slightly, they are given names describing their segmental relationships. In the left lung, some units are combined to form a single segment.

Divisions of the bronchi continue to multiply the airway into smaller and more numerous conducting passages.[28] As delineated in Table 6-6, each branch gives rise to two lower "generations" or divisions. Lobar bronchi beget segmental bronchi; segmental bronchi divide into subsegmental bronchi, and so on until tiny conducting airways called *bronchioles* arise. Bronchioles, typically 1 to 2 mm in diameter, begin at a point anywhere from 5 to 14 generations below the segmental bronchi, and number in the tens of thousands. They are among the smallest purely conducting airways of the lower respiratory tract, and are anatom-ically distinguished from their larger counterparts by a distinct lack of cartilaginous support.

As further divisions occur in the airway system, the total number of airways increases tremendously, as does the total cross-sectional area of the conducting system (Fig. 6-31). For example, by the time the terminal bronchioles are reached, the cross-sectional area for airflow is at least ten times greater than what it was at the trachea. According to the laws of fluid physics, this increase in cross-sectional area should result in a decrease in the average velocity of gas flow during inspiration. It has been estimated that by the time inspired gas reaches the alveoli, its average velocity is not much greater than its rate of diffusion.[29]

This low velocity in the smaller airways and gas exchange units of the lung is necessary for two reasons. First, by maintaining conditions necessary for a laminar pattern of flow, it minimizes resistance to airflow in the small airways, thereby decreasing the work associated with inspiration. Second, low gas velocities in the periphery of the lung facilitate rapid mixing of respired gases, providing a relatively stable environment for gas exchange.

Histology of the conducting airways. The walls of the conducting airways of the lungs share a similar gross structure, but vary considerably in the number and type of certain cellular elements (Fig. 6-32).

All conducting airways have three major tissue layers: a mucosa, a submucosa, and an enveloping connective tissue sheath called the *adventitia.*[30] The mucosa is composed of an epithelial lining, a basement membrane, and a layer of loose connective tissue known as the lamina propria. The primary cell type constituting the mucosa of the larger airways is a pseudostratified, ciliated, columnar ep-

Table 6-5   Bronchopulmonary Segments*

Segment	Number	Segment	Number
Upper lobe		Left upper lobe	
Apical	1	Upper division	
Posterior	2	Apical-posterior	1 and 2†
Anterior	3	Anterior	3
Right middle lobe		Lower (lingular) division	
Lateral	4	Superior lingula	4
Medial	5	Inferior lingula	5
Right lower lobe		Left lower lobe	
Superior	6	Superior	6
Medial basal	7	Anteromedial	7 and 8†
Anterior basal	8	Lateral basal	9
Lateral basal	9	Posterior basal	10
Posterior basal	10		

*The subdivisions of the lung and bronchial tree are fairly constant. Slight variations between the right and left sides are noted by combined names and numbers.
†*Editor's note:* Some authors feel that the left lung should be numbered such that there are eight segments, where the apical-posterior is numbered 1 and anteromedial is numbered 6.

ithelium. Sandwiched between these ciliated cells are mucous-secreting *goblet cells*. Basal cells may also be observed on the basement membrane beneath these primary cell types. Basal cells are thought to replenish the ciliated and goblet cells in the normal process of growth and differentiation, and also are involved in mucosal repair.[31]

The cilia of the mucosal layer play a critical role in clearance and defense of the respiratory tract. Each ciliated cell has about 200 of these delicate filaments, with an estimated 1 to 2 billion per square centimeter of mucosa.[30] Individual cilia are about 6 to 7 μm in length, and they tend to beat in a synchronous manner at about 20 "strokes"

per second. Fig. 6-33 portrays this sequential motion of the cilia, termed a *metachronal wave*. The metachronal wave, about 20 μm in length, propels surface material in a specific direction of flow. This "ciliary escalator" function is found in the nose (propelling material back to the pharynx) and continuously from the bronchioles up to the larynx (propelling material up to the pharynx).

The effectiveness of this action depends, in part, on the fluid constituency of the respiratory epithelium.[32] In principle, particulate material is carried on a mucous blanket atop the cilia; the cilia beats in a less viscous layer below (see Fig. 6-33). Drying of the respiratory tract mucosa has

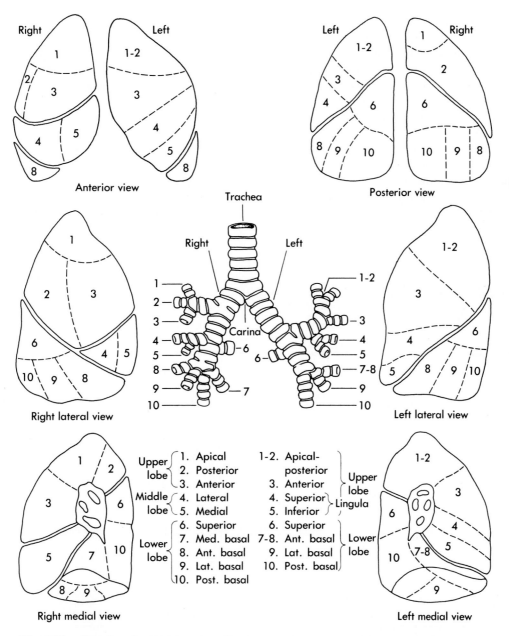

Fig. 6-30 Bronchopulmonary segments diagrammed. Again note similarities, with minor variations, between right and left lungs. (See editor's note for Table 6-5.)

a marked inhibitory effect on ciliary action, as does an excessive production of mucus. Drugs also may affect ciliary activity. Atropine is known to slow the rate of movement of the mucous blanket, but this may result more from its inhibiting effect on the production of secretion. Drugs causing parasympathetic stimulation may, however, stimulate ciliary activity.

Beneath the lamina propria of the conducting airways is the submucosa (see Fig. 6-32). The submucosa of larger airways contains the bronchial glands, a capillary network, and some smooth muscle and elastic tissue fibers. The bronchial glands vary in size up to a millimeter or so in length, and are connected to the bronchial surface by long, narrow ducts. These glands are the major source of respiratory tract secretions in the normal lung, and their number increases substantially in conditions such as chronic bronchitis. Also found in the submucosa are *mast cells,* which are responsible, in part, for the release of a potent, vasoactive substance called histamine. Histamine, released in certain hypersensitivity reactions such as asthma, causes vasodilation and bronchoconstriction via direct action on the respiratory tract smooth muscle.

The smooth muscle of the conducting airways varies in location and structure. In the large airways, such as the trachea and mainstem bronchi, smooth muscle is bundled in a posterior sheet. In smaller airways the smooth muscle forms a helical pattern, with fibers crisscrossing and spiral-

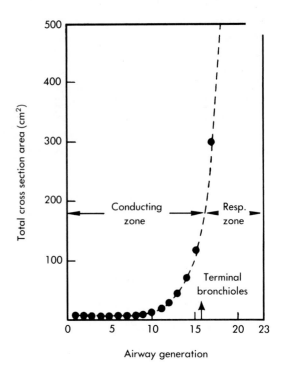

Fig. 6-31   Since no gas exchange takes place in the conducting zone, this region is called the anatomic dead space (see Chapter 8). The gas exchange surface increases markedly at the level of the terminal bronchiole. (From West J: Respiratory physiology—the essentials, Baltimore, 1974, Williams & Wilkins.)

Table 6-6   Bronchial and Bronchiolar Division

Structure	Generation from Trachea	Generation from Segmental bronchus	Generation from Terminal bronchiole	Number	Diameter of individual structures	Total cross-sectional area	
Trachea	0			1	2.5 cm	5.0 cm^2	
Main bronchi	1			2	11-19 mm	3.2 cm^2	
Lobar bronchi	2-3			5	4.5-13.5	2.7 cm^2	Cartilaginous conducting structures
Segmental	3-6	0		19	4.5-6.5 mm	3.2 cm^2	
Subsegmental bronchi	4-7	1		38	3-6 mm	6.6 cm^2	
Bronchi		2-6		Variable	Variable	Variable	
Terminal bronchi		3-7		1,000	1.0 mm	7.9 cm^2	
Bronchioles		5-14		Variable	Variable	Variable	
Terminal bronchioles		6-15	0	35,000	0.65 mm	116 cm^2	
Respiratory bronchioles			1-8	Variable	Variable	Variable	
Terminal respiratory bronchioles			2-9	630,000	0.45 mm	1,000 cm^2	No cartilage in walls
Alveolar ducts and sacs			4-12	14 × 10^6	0.40 mm	1.71 m^2	
Alveoli				300 × 10^6	0.25-0.30 mm	70 m^2	

Note marked increase in numbers of subunits and in cross-sectional surface area as bronchi divide. Bronchi contain cartilage in their walls, whereas bronchioles are smaller and do not have cartilage. (Adapted slightly from Bates DV, Macklem PT, and Christie RV: Respiratory function in disease, Philadelphia, 1971, WB Saunders Co.)

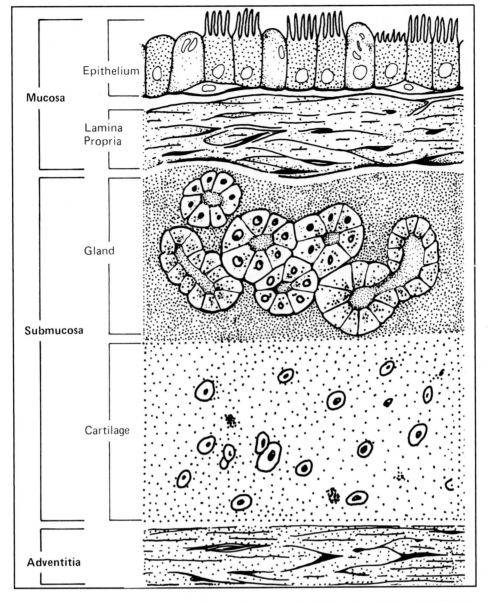

Fig. 6-32   Various tissue layers in the trachea, illustrating not only the epithelium but also the underlying lamina propria of the mucosa. Submucosal glands below this, whose ducts reach the tracheal lumen, allow secretory contribution to the mucus layer. Incomplete cartilaginous rings ensure a noncollapsible tube for airflow. (From Martin DE and Youtsey JW: Respiratory anatomy and physiology, St Louis, 1988, The CV Mosby Co.)

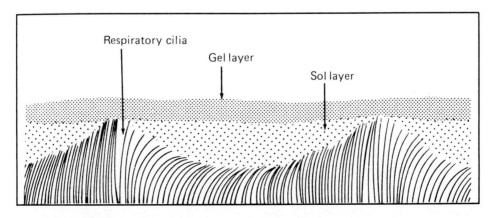

Fig. 6-33   Respiratory cilia are bathed in the sol portion of the mucus layer above them. Their power strokes allow mucus movement by contacting the viscous gel layer, always in the same direction. (From Martin DE and Youtsey JW: Respiratory anatomy and physiology, St Louis, 1988, The CV Mosby Co.)

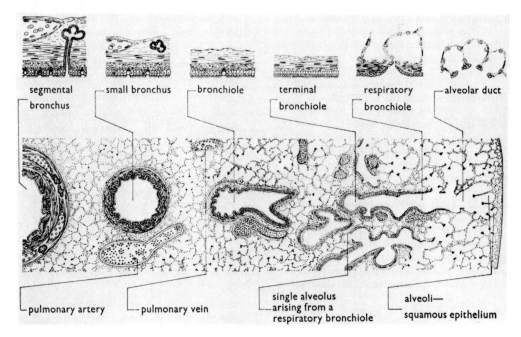

Fig. 6-34   Histologic diagram of airways from segmental bronchus to alveolus. (From Freeman WH and Bracegirdle B: An atlas of histology, London, 1966, Heinemann Educational Books Ltd.)

ing around the airway walls. This orientation tends to cause both a reduction in caliber and shortening of the airway on contraction. Spirals of smooth muscle continue into the terminal respiratory units of the lung, having been observed as far as the opening of the alveolar ducts.[5]

Between the submucosa and the adventitia of the larger airways are incomplete rings or plates of cartilage (see Fig. 6-32). This cartilage provides structural support to the larger airways; smaller airways must depend on transmural pressure gradients and the "traction" of surrounding elastic tissue to maintain their patency. During forced expiration, pressure differences across the walls of these smaller airways overcome the opposing forces of the surrounding elastic tissues, resulting in their collapse. Cartilaginous support in the larger airways prevents their collapse during such maneuvers.

Lastly, the enveloping connective tissue sheath of the conducting airways consists of loose connective tissue interspersed with bronchial arteries, veins, nerves, lymph vessels, and adipose tissue.

Fig. 6-35   The airways that only conduct gases back and forth are designated the conducting zone of lung. These include approximately the first 17 divisions of the tracheobronchial tree. The unit where gas exchange occurs, from respiratory bronchiole to alveolar space, is called the respiratory zone. *BR* = bronchus, *BL* = bronchiole, *TBL* = terminal bronchiole, *RBL* = respiratory bronchiole, *AD* = alveolar duct, *AS* = alveolar space, *Z* = order of airway division. (From Weibel ER: Morphometry of the human lung, Heidelberg, 1963, Springer-Verlag.)

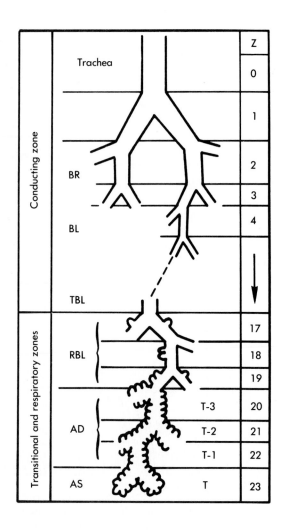

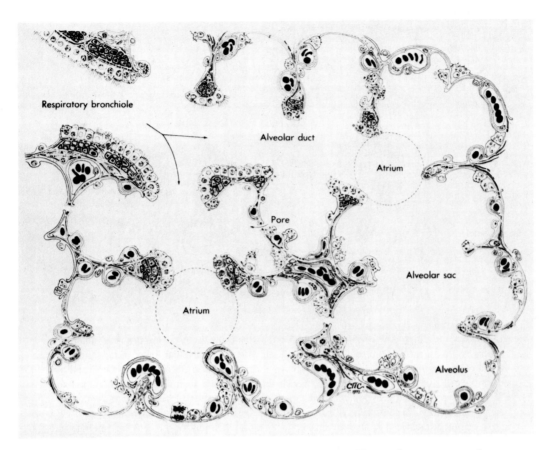

Respiratory bronchiole

Alveolar duct

Atrium

Pore

Alveolar sac

Atrium

Alveolus

Fig. 6-36 Diagram of microscopic view of terminal airways. These units compose respiratory zone of lung. (From Sorokin SP: The respiratory system. In Greep RO and Weiss L, editors: Histology, New York, 1973, McGraw-Hill Book Co. Used with permission of McGraw-Hill Book Co.)

As depicted in Fig. 6-34, the cellular constituency of the respiratory tract mucosa changes as one progresses into the smaller conducting airways. Besides a general decrease in the wall thickness of the conducting airways, bronchial glands become fewer in number. Approaching the bronchiolar level, the number of ciliated cells decreases, and a simple columnar to cuboidal epithelial layer begins to predominate, interspersed with occasional goblet cells. Also present at this level are plump, nonciliated Clara cells, believed to have secretory functions.

Transitional and respiratory zones. At a point about 17 generations beyond the trachea, at the terminal bronchiole level, a subtle transition takes place. All previous portions of the respiratory tract served only to condition and/or conduct gases. At this point, however, the smallest, strictly conducting airways, called terminal bronchioles, beget a series of unique passageways called *respiratory bronchioles* (Figs. 6-35 and 6-36).

Respiratory bronchioles are unique in their dual function. Like conducting airways, they move gas forward toward the true respiratory zones of the lung. But alveolar outpouchings on their surfaces also allow them to partici-

pate in actual gas exchange. For this reason, respiratory bronchioles are said to constitute the *transitional zone* of the lung, ie, that portion between the zones dedicated purely to conduction and purely to gas exchange.

The primary function of the lung, gas exchange, takes place in the *terminal respiratory unit,* also called the primary lobule or acinus.[6] The terminal respiratory unit begins at approximately the 17th division of bronchi, thereby consisting of all structures distal to a terminal bronchiole (see Fig. 6-35). Typically a terminal respiratory unit consists of two to five orders of respiratory bronchioles, followed by a similar number of generations of *alveolar ducts.* Alveolar ducts, about as long as they are wide, typically terminate in clusters of 10 to 16 alveoli.

The *alveolus* is the final anatomic unit in this system, and the primary site of gas exchange. There are some 300 million such terminal air spaces in the adult lung. The surface area for gas exchange provided by these spaces is gigantic, in the range of 40 to 100 m^2, the average being 70 m^2. This means that the lung has 35 times the surface area of the skin in the average person. The highly magnified architecture of an alveolar region is depicted schematically

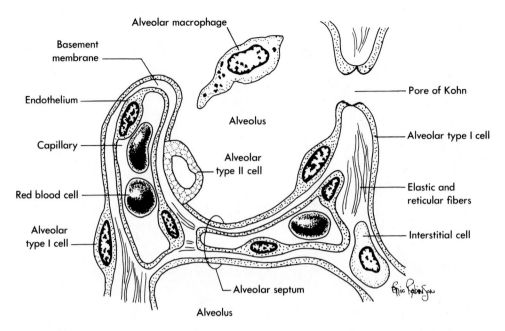

Fig. 6-37   Very high-power view of alveolus. Alveolar walls or septae are occupied mainly by capillaries. Basement membrane of capillary is fused with that of alveolar lining. Interstitium contains a few interstitial fibers, composed mostly of reticular support fibers, elastic fibers, and one interstitial cell. An incomplete portion of alveolar septum called a pore of Kohn is shown (see also Fig. 6-5). Type I lining cells are very flat. Small distance between blood and air makes gas exchange remarkably efficient. Type II cells are much less numerous than type I cells. Type II cells are source of surfactant. The alveolar macrophages are mobile phagocytic cells that migrate into alveoli from the bloodstream.

in Fig. 6-37. It is essentially a pocket of air extensively surrounded by a thin membrane containing an extensive network of capillaries.

Scanning electron microscopy of the alveolar region provides a detailed view of the various structures (Fig. 6-38). The two principal cells found here are the type I alveolar cells, or squamous pneumocytes, and the type II alveolar cells, or granular pneumocytes. The type I cells are the thin, flat cells that line the alveoli. Spaces between these type I cells, called *pores of Kohn,* provide intercommunication between adjacent alveoli. The more cuboidal cells, type II cells, which are also called septal cells, are more numerous than type I cells but, owing to their shape, occupy less than 5% of the alveolar surface area. These cells are thought to be the source of the surface-active substance called *pulmonary surfactant.*[33] Type II cells are also known to proliferate in cases of injury and may also give rise to new type I cells. A third cell type, the alveolar macrophage (sometimes called the type III cell), is a phagocytic cell chiefly responsible for clearance of bacteria and other particulate material that makes its way to the alveolar region. Evidence indicates that, unlike the type I and II cells, alveolar macrophages do not originate in the lung but are produced from stem cell precursors in the bone marrow and are transported to the lung by way of the circulatory system.[6]

The space between the alveolar air and capillary blood is called the alveolar septum or *alveolar-capillary membrane.* Fig. 6-39 depicts both a facial view and a magnified cross-section of this alveolar-capillary region. Note first the density of the capillary network in the facial view (Fig. 6-39, *A*). The short length and multiple branchings, characterizing the capillaries surrounding an alveolus, present a sheet-like surface of blood flow for gas exchange. This network is so well structured that the 100 to 300 ml of blood in the capillaries is spread over some 70 m^2 of surface. Considered another way, roughly a teaspoon of blood is spread over every m^2 of surface, a remarkable feat.

Although the surface area for gas exchange is large, the distance between alveolar gas and blood is small. The cross-section in Fig. 6-39, *B,* demonstrates this extremely small distance, ranging from 0.35 to 2.5 μm, separating the blood in the capillaries from the air in the alveoli. The enlarged view (Fig. 6-39, *C*) further identifies the tissue and fluid layers that must be transversed during gas exchange.

Since gas transfer in the lung depends soley on diffusion gradients across this membrane, and since blood typically spends less than a second in transit across the pulmonary capillaries, these short distances are essential for efficient and rapid respiratory exchange. In fact, the efficiency of

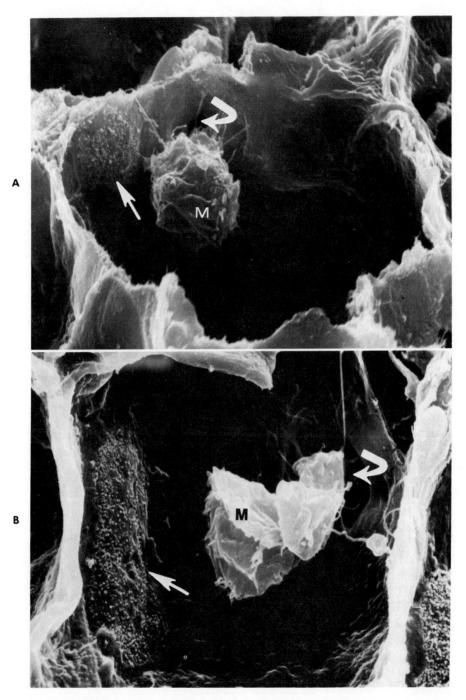

Fig. 6-38   Scanning electron micrographs of alveolar air spaces. **A,** Note thin partitions or septa between adjacent alveoli. The thin platelike type I cells compose most of these. Type II cells have projections off their surfaces that appear dotted or hairy *(straight arrow)*. Alveolar macrophage *(M)* is seen at back partially covering pore of Kohn *(upper curved arrow)*. **B,** Similar view with two or three macrophages passing through pore of Kohn. (Grateful appreciation is given to Mr. Mike Wagner, of San Diego, Calif, for use of the electron micrographs.)

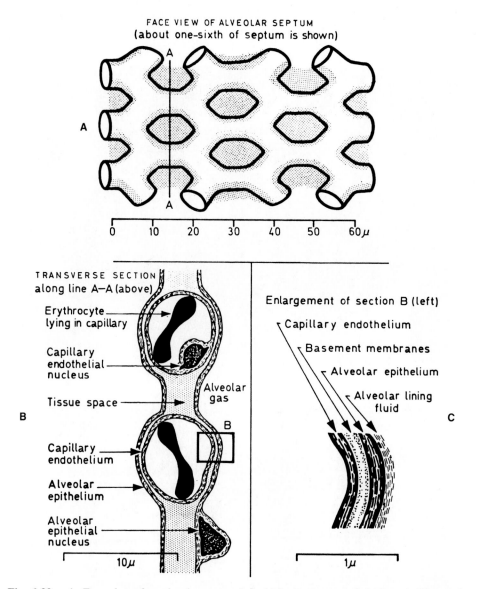

FACE VIEW OF ALVEOLAR SEPTUM
(about one-sixth of septum is shown)

0   10   20   30   40   50   60μ

TRANSVERSE SECTION
along line A–A (above)

Erythrocyte lying in capillary

Capillary endothelial nucleus

Tissue space

Alveolar gas

Capillary endothelium

Alveolar epithelium

Alveolar epithelial nucleus

B

10μ

Enlargement of section B (left)

Capillary endothelium
Basement membranes
Alveolar epithelium
Alveolar lining fluid

C

1μ

Fig. 6-39   A, Face view of an alveolar septum (of which about one sixth is shown). The capillary network is dense, with the spaces between the capillaries being rather less than the diameter of the capillaries. **B,** Section *(A–A)* through two capillaries, demonstrating the very thin membrane through which gas exchange takes place. **C,** Enlargement of **B.** (From Nunn JF: Applied respiratory physiology, ed 2, London, 1977, Butterworth & Co.)

this process is so good in the normal lung that gas exchange is essentially complete well before the blood reaches the end of the capillary. These reserves are important for normal exercise and in disease states.

Intercommunicating channels. Contrary to what was once believed, functional units of the lungs are not "dead-end" passages. Several forms of intercommunicating channels exist in the lung (Fig. 6-40). Recent evidence indicates such channels may be found at the alveolar level, between bronchioles and alveoli, and among bronchioles.[34]

Alveolar septa were at one time thought to be entirely intact, but now it is well known that communication chan-

nels, called pores of Kohn, exist between them (see Figs. 6-36 to 6-38). These pores range from 5 to 15 μm in diameter, presumably varying their size during breathing. In principle, they allow collateral drift between adjacent alveoli.

Alveolar pores are not present during the perinatal and early postnatal phases of lung development. They increase in number and size throughout life, although the mechanism for such development is unknown. However, it has been observed that their numbers increase in certain diseases affecting the lung parenchyma.

A second type of intercommunicating channel between

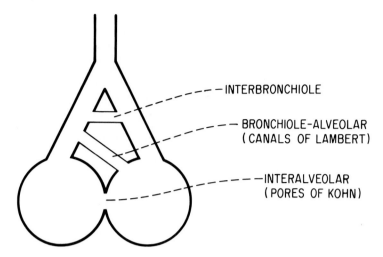

Fig. 6-40 Pathways for collateral ventilation. (Redrawn from Menkes and Traystman, Am Rev Respir Dis 116:297, 1977.)

terminal bronchioles has been described. These bronchiole-alveolar channels, or *canals of Lambert,* are approximately 30 μm in size and appear to remain open even when bronchiolar smooth muscle is in a contractile state. Whereas alveolar pores permit collateral ventilation only between adjacent alveoli, the canals of Lambert provide for gas movement between primary lobules.

A third, larger pathway for collateral ventilation may also exist. These *interbronchiolar channels,* although confirmed only in animal models, are as large as 120 μm in size and may represent a major source for collateral exchange of respiratory gases.

In combination, these intercommunicating channels probably facilitate a more even distribution of ventilation during normal breathing and contribute to the lung's ability to respond to alterations in structure accompanying certain lung diseases. This ability to maintain relatively normal function despite anatomic or physiologic disturbances is an important capacity of all organ systems.

OTHER FUNCTIONS OF THE LUNG

Although the lung functions primarily to exchange gases between the atmosphere and the cells of the body, it performs other functions vital to body homeostasis. Such functions involve both anatomic and metabolic roles.

Anatomically, the pulmonary circulation serves as a blood reservoir for the left ventricle. This reservoir function helps maintain stable left ventricular volumes despite minor fluctuations in cardiac output. Moreover, should inflow to the right heart dramatically decrease or momentarily stop, the pulmonary blood volume (about 600 ml) is sufficient to maintain normal left ventricle outflow for several cardiac cycles.

The pulmonary circulation also serves as a filter for the systemic circulation, trapping particulate matter before it

enters areas where blockages would be life-threatening, such as the coronary and cerebral circulations. Potentially harmful particulate matter that is filtered by the pulmonary circulation includes fibrin and blood clots, fat cells, platelet aggregates, and particulate debris found in stored blood or intravenous fluids.

Lastly, the lung plays an active role in body metabolism, being responsible for the synthesis, activation, inactivation, and detoxification of many bioactive substances. Heparin, histamine, bradykinin, serotonin, and certain prostaglandins are stored or synthesized in the lung and released in response to physiologic or immunologic challenges. Angiotensin I is converted by the lung to its active form, angiotensin II. Adenosine triphosphate (ATP) and norepinephrine (along with bradykinin and serotonin) are partially removed from the blood and inactivated by the lungs.

SUMMARY

The respiratory system fulfills its primary purpose of gas exchange by integrating its form and functions. Structures that develop during the prenatal and postnatal periods eventually assume a variety of roles in supporting these functions. The thorax not only houses and protects the lungs, but acts as the mechanical bellows that makes ventilation possible. Networks of motor and sensory nerves innervate the muscles of ventilation and provide reflex feedback mechanisms useful in responding to changing internal and external conditions. Dual circulatory systems sustain the lung and provide a vast capillary network for gas exchange. The upper respiratory tract modifies inspired air and protects the lungs against the unwanted intrusion of foreign substances. The lower respiratory tract efficiently conducts respired gases between the atmosphere and the respiratory zones of the lung and participates in clearance and defense. Finally, the respiratory zones of the lung provide a huge diffusing surface that facilitates the key process of external respiration.

In health, these structures continuously perform their roles with maximum efficiency throughout the lifespan. In addition, reserve capacities of the respiratory system provide the body with the ability to respond to a variety of changing circumstances. Alterations in structure or function can compromise this ability and threaten survival of the organism. The basis for all respiratory care is to alleviate such threats and to maintain or restore normal function.

REFERENCES

1. Thyurlbeck WM: Postnatal growth and development of the lung, Am Rev Respir Dis 111:803, 1975.
2. Sadler TW: Langman's medical embryology, ed 5, Philadelphia, 1985, Williams & Wilkins.
3. Fishman AP: Assessment of pulmonary function, New York, 1980, McGraw-Hill Book Co.
4. Fraser RG and Paré JA: Structure and function of the lung with emphasis on roentgenology, Philadelphia, 1971, WB Saunders Co.
5. von Hayek H: The human lung, New York, 1960, Hafner Publishers.
6. Murray JF: The normal lung: the basis for diagnosis and treatment of pulmonary disease, ed 2, Philadelphia, 1986, WB Saunders Co.
7. Wade OL and Gilson JC: The effect of posture on diaphragmatic movement and vital capacity in normal subjects, Thorax 6:103, 1951.
8. Richardson JB: Nerve supply to the lung, Am Rev Respir Dis 119:785, 1979.
9. Tortora GJ and Anagnostakos NP: Principles of anatomy and physiology, ed 4, New York, 1984, Harper & Row.
10. Widdicombe JG and Sterling GM: The autonomic nervous system and breathing, Arch Intern Med 126:311, 1970.
11. Spencer H and Leof D: The innervation of the human lung, J Anat 98:599, 1964.
12. Coleridge HM and Coleridge JCG: Reflexes evoked from the tracheobronchial tree and lungs. In Fishman AF et al, editors: Handbook of physiology, Sect 3, The respiratory system, vol 2, Control of breathing, Bethesda, Md, 1986, American Physiological Society.
13. Fishman NH, Phillipson EA, and Nadel JA: Effect of differential vagal cold blockade on breathing patterns in conscious dogs, J Appl Physiol 34:754, 1973.
14. Crofton J and Douglas A: Respiratory diseases, ed 3, Oxford, England, 1981, Blackwell Scientific Publications.
15. Harris P and Heath D: The human pulmonary circulation, Edinburgh, 1962, E & S Livingstone.
16. Green JF: The pulmonary circulation. In Zelis R: The peripheral circulation, New York, 1975, Grune & Stratton.
17. Milnor WR: Pulmonary hemodynamics. In Bergel DH, editor: Cardiovascular fluid dynamics, vol 2, New York, 1972, Academic Press.
18. Daly I and Hebb CO: Pulmonary and bronchial vascular systems, Baltimore, 1967, Williams & Wilkins.
19. Charan NB: The bronchial circulatory system: structure, function and importance, Respir Care 29:1226, 1984.
20. Nagaishi C: Functional anatomy and histology of the lung, Baltimore, 1972, University Park Press.
21. Lauweryns JM and Baert JH: Alveolar clearance and the role of the pulmonary lymphatics, Am Rev Respir Dis 115:625, 1977.
22. Heitzman ER: The lung: radiologic-pathologic correlations, St Louis, 1973, The CV Mosby Co.
23. Johanson WG: Lung defense mechanisms, Basics of RD, 6 (2): November 1977.
24. Proctor DF: The upper airways. Part I. Nasal physiology and defense of the lung, Am Rev Respir Dis 115:97, 1977.
25. Lough ML, Boat T, and Doershuk CF: The nose, Respir Care 20:286, 1975.
26. Proctor DF: The upper airways. Part II. The larynx and trachea, Am Rev Respir Dis 115:315, 1977.
27. Boyden EA: Segmental anatomy of the lungs, New York, 1955, McGraw-Hill Book Co.
28. Weibel ER: Morphometry of the human lung, New York, 1962, Academic Press.
29. Foster RE, et al: The lung: physiologic basis of pulmonary function tests, ed 3, Chicago, 1986, Year Book Medical Publishers.
30. Rhodin JAG: Ultrastructure and function of the human tracheal mucosa, Am Rev Respir Dis 93 (suppl 1): 1966.
31. Breeze RG and Wheeldon EB: The cells of the pulmonary airways, Am Rev Respir Dis 116:705, 1977.
32. Widdicombe JG: Control of secretions of tracheobronchial mucus, Br Med Bull 34:57, 1978.
33. Clements JA et al: Pulmonary surface tension and alveolar stability, J Appl Physiol 16:444, 1972.
34. Menkes HA and Traysman RJ: Collateral ventilation, Am Rev Respir Dis 116:287, 1977.

7

The Cardiovascular System

Craig L. Scanlan

The cardiovascular system provides the vital link between the processes of external respiration, or pulmonary gas exchange, and internal respiration at the cellular level. The approximately 100 trillion cells of the body, each a living entity, depend on the cardiovascular system to provide needed oxygen and nutrients and to remove metabolic waste products moment to moment throughout a lifetime. By keeping the blood and body fluids in constant motion, and ensuring their appropriate distribution throughout the tissues, the cardiovascular system maintains what Claude Bernard long ago called *le milieu interieur*, or the balanced internal environment of the body.[1]

Maintenance of these homeostatic conditions requires that the heart and vascular system work closely together to ensure that each area of the body receives adequate blood flow or perfusion according to its ever-changing needs. Moreover, the system must have reserves sufficient to accommodate both normal stresses such as exercise and abnormal conditions such as blood loss.

For the respiratory care practitioner, a working knowledge of the cardiovascular system in both health and disease is essential. Certainly the two organ systems are related in terms of structure and function. Of equal importance is the fact that clinical disorders occurring in one system are often closely associated with dysfunction of the other. Terms such as "shock lung," "cor pulmonale," and "pulmonary vascular hypertension" remind us that in the real world of clinical practice, artificial dichotomies between organ systems are a barrier to comprehensive care. Respiratory care practitioners find they must deal not with just the patient's lung, heart, or vasculature, but with a single integrated cardiopulmonary organ system. It is the intent of this chapter to develop the knowledge necessary to apply this integrated perspective in practice.

OBJECTIVES

To meet this goal, this chapter provides an overview of cardiovascular structure and function, with an emphasis on the mechanical and electrophysiologic properties of the heart and its coordinated interaction with the vascular system. Specifically, after completion of this chapter, the reader should be able to:

1. Relate the gross structure and microanatomy of the heart and vascular system to their functions;
2. Differentiate among the key functional properties of cardiac tissue;
3. Delineate the various factors responsible for local and central control of the heart and vasculature;
4. Describe how the cardiovascular system coordinates its functions under normal and abnormal conditions;
5. Explain the normal mechanisms responsible for conduction of electrical impulses and their electrocardiographic representation;
6. Relate the mechanical and electrical events occurring during a normal cardiac cycle.

KEY TERMS

Most terms used in this chapter are defined in context. The following terms are introduced without explicit definition, but may be found in the glossary:

adrenergic	myoneural
arteriole	parasympathetic
bradycardia	phonocardiography
catecholamine	pons
cholinergic	sequela
cor pulmonale	stenosis
cystoscopy	sympathetic
hemodynamic	tachycardia
hemorrhage	thoracotomy
humoral	transudation
hypertension	vasoconstriction
ischemia	vasodilation
isovolumic	vasomotor
medulla	venule
millivolt (mV)	

FUNCTIONAL ANATOMY

The heart

Gross anatomy. The heart is a hollow, muscular organ about the size of a fist and positioned obliquely in the middle compartment of the mediastinum just behind the ster-

153

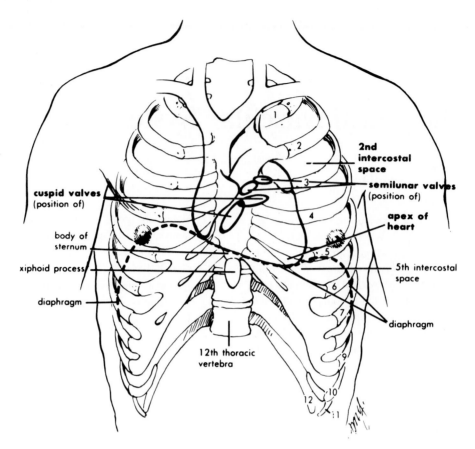

Fig. 7-1   Anterior view of the thorax showing the position of the heart in relationship to the ribs, sternum, diaphragm, and the position of the heart valves. (From Crouch JE: Functional human anatomy, ed 4, Philadelphia, 1985, Lea & Febiger.)

num (Fig. 7-1). About two thirds of the heart is to the left of the sternum's midline. Its pointed end, or apex, is formed by the tip of the left ventricle and lies just above the diaphragm at a level corresponding to the fifth intercostal space. The base of the heart is formed by the atria, projects to the right, and lies just below the second rib. Surface grooves or *sulci* mark the boundaries between atria and ventricles (the coronary sulcus), and between ventricles (the anterior and posterior longitudinal sulci).

The heart is enclosed in a loose, membranous sac called the parietal *pericardium*. The outer fibrous layer consists of tough connective tissue. The inner serous layer is thinner and more delicate, being continuous with a similar visceral layer (the visceral pericardium) on the outer surface of the heart and great vessels. Pericardial fluid separates these serous layers, minimizing the friction or viscous resistance to heart movement. Inflammation of these serous layers can result in a clinical condition called *pericarditis*.

The heart walls consist of three tissue layers: the external visceral pericardium or *epicardium*, the middle *myocardium*, and the inner *endocardium*. The endocardium is a thin layer of endothelial tissue continuous with the inner layer of the blood vessels. The myocardial tissue consists

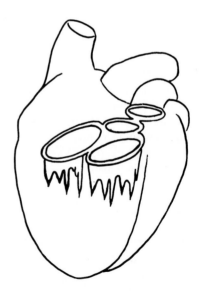

Fig. 7-2   Four rings that form anulus fibrosus with cusps hanging curtain-like from edges. (From McLaughlin AJ Jr: Essentials of physiology for advanced respiratory therapy, St Louis, 1977, The CV Mosby Co.)

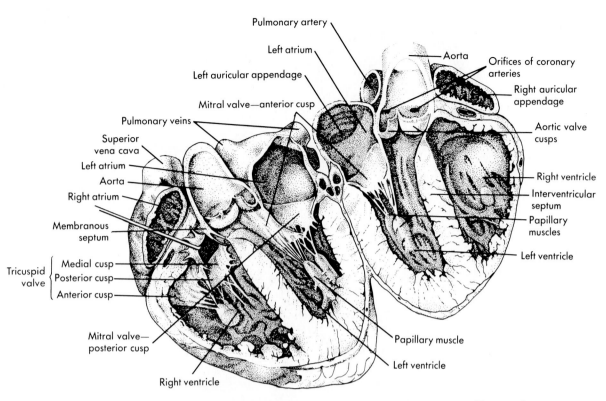

Fig. 7-3 Drawing of a heart split perpendicular to the interventricular septum to illustrate the anatomic relationships of the leaflets of the AV and aortic valves. (From Berne RM and Levy MN: Cardiovascular physiology, ed 5, St Louis, 1986, The CV Mosby Co.)

of involuntary striated muscle fibers and constitutes the bulk of the cardiac mass. These muscle fibers provide the heart with the ability to change the size of its chambers during contraction and relaxation, creating a pumplike action.

Four rings of dense connective tissue, or *annuli fibrosi,* join to form a fibrous "skeleton" for the heart, often called the AV ring (Fig. 7-2). Arising from this supporting structure are four interior chambers and four valves (Fig. 7-3). The two atrial chambers at the base of the heart are thin-walled "cups" of myocardial tissue separated by a partition called the interatrial septum. An oval depression of the surface of the right side of the interatrial septum, the *fossa ovalis,* represents the remnants of the fetal foramen ovale. Each atrium has an appendage, or auricle, the function of which is unknown.

The two lower chambers, or ventricles, constitute the bulk of the cardiac musculature and provide the major force for circulation of the blood. The myocardium of the left ventricle is two thirds thicker than that of the right, and, in AP cross-section, is spherical in shape. The right ventricle is thin-walled and oblong in shape, forming a pocket-like attachment to the left ventricular wall. Because of this arrangement, contraction of the left myocardium actually pulls the right ventricular wall in, facilitating its

contraction (Fig. 7-4). This supplemental effect of the left ventricle on the right is termed *left ventricular aid.* The left ventricular aid effect helps explain why some acute clinical disorders of the right ventricle have a less deleterious effect than would otherwise be expected.[2]

Like the atria, the right and left ventricles are separated by a muscle wall, the interventricular septum (see Fig. 7-3). Unlike those in the atria, the muscle fibers of the ventricles are arranged in a complex, overlapping spiral fashion, often compared with the wrappings of a turban. This orientation results in a wringing-like action during contraction that does not completely empty the chambers.

The valves of the heart are flaps of fibrous tissue firmly anchored to the annuli fibrosi (see Fig. 7-2). The atrioventricular, or AV, valves lie between the atria and ventricles and function to close off the ventricles during systole, thereby providing a critical period of isovolumic contraction, during which chamber pressures quickly rise without blood being ejected. The free ends of the AV valves are anchored to papillary muscles of the endocardium via chordae tendineae (see Fig. 7-3). During systole, contraction of the papillary muscles prevents the AV valves from swinging upward into the atria. Damage to the chordae tendineae or papillary muscles can severely compromise the function of the AV valves and thereby impair cardiac performance.

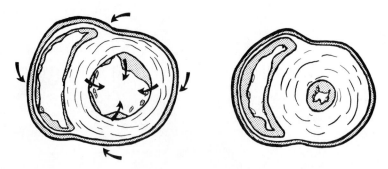

Fig. 7-4 Cross section of ventricles showing changes in size of left and right ventricles during contraction. (Adapted from Guyton AC: Textbook of medical physiology, ed 4, Philadelphia, 1971, WB Saunders Co. From McLaughlin AJ Jr: Essentials of physiology for advanced respiratory therapy, St Louis, 1977, The CV Mosby Co.)

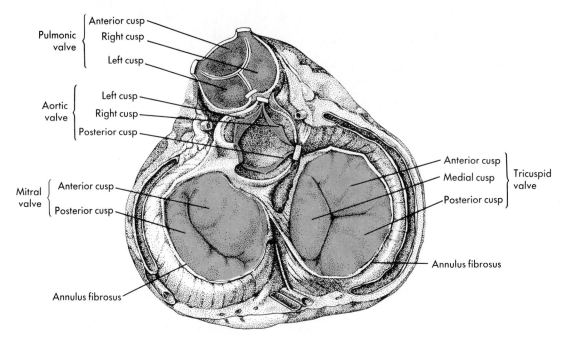

Fig. 7-5 Four cardiac valves as viewed from the base of the heart. Note how the leaflets overlap in the closed valves. (From Berne RM and Levy MN: Cardiovascular physiology, ed 5, St Louis, 1986, The CV Mosby Co.)

The AV valve between the right atrium and the right ventricle is called the *tricuspid valve*. This three-leafed valve directs blood flow from the atrium to the ventricle without allowing backflow to occur when the ventricle contracts. The bicuspid or *mitral valve* separates the left atrium from the left ventricle. When the left ventricle contracts, the mitral valve prevents backflow to the left atrium. Narrowing of these valves, a condition known as *stenosis,* increases downstream resistance to blood flow, thereby increasing upstream pressures. The more common mitral stenosis can create high upstream pulmonary vascular pressures and result in fluid transudation into the alveolar septal region.

The *semilunar valves* separate the ventricles from their arterial outflow tracts, preventing backflow during diastole

(Fig. 7-5). They both consist of three half moon—or crescent-shaped cusps attached by their convex margins to the arterial wall. The pulmonary valve is at the outflow tract of the right ventricle. During systole, it allows blood to flow from the ventricle into the pulmonary artery. The aortic valve is located at the outflow tract of the left ventricle at the beginning of the aorta. During systole, opening of the aortic valve allows blood to be ejected from the left ventricle into the systemic circulation. Stenosis of these valves also can occur, demanding that the affected ventricle create a higher pressure to eject its blood volume.

Like the lung, the heart has its own circulatory system, called the *coronary circulation*. Unlike the lung, however, the heart has an extremely high metabolic rate and requires substantially more perfusion per gram of tissue than most

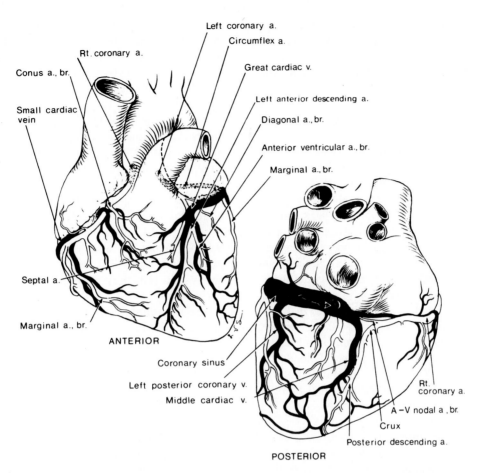

Left coronary a.
Circumflex a.
Rt. coronary a.
Conus a., br.
Great cardiac v.
Small cardiac vein
Left anterior descending a.
Diagonal a., br.
Anterior ventricular a., br.
Marginal a., br.
Septal a.
Marginal a., br.
ANTERIOR
Coronary sinus
Left posterior coronary v.
Middle cardiac v.
Rt. coronary a.
A–V nodal a., br.
Crux
Posterior descending a.
POSTERIOR

Fig. 7-6   Arteries and veins of the heart. Veins are black; arteries are clear-colored. Major vessels are described in the text. Note how the major cardiac veins parallel the coronary arteries. The direction of flow of blood in the coronary sinus is indicated by the arrow, whose tip is at the site of the coronary sinus ostium.   (From Sanderson RG: The cardiac patient: a comprehensive approach, ed 2, Philadelphia, 1983, WB Saunders Co.)

any other organ except the kidney.[3] To ensure that this special need is met, the coronary circulation provides an extensive network of branches to all myocardial tissues (Fig. 7-6).

Two main coronary arteries arise from sinuses at the root of the aorta immediately distal to the aortic valve (Fig. 7-6). This placement ensures that the coronary circulation receives the full head of pressure generated by the left ventricle during contraction. Beyond these two coronary arteries, substantial individual variations may exist in the branching of this important vascular system. In general, however, the left and right arteries are responsible for perfusion of their respective sides of the heart.

At a point between the pulmonary artery and the tip of the left atrial appendage, the left coronary artery divides into an anterior descending branch, which courses down the anterior sulcus to the apex, and a circumflex branch, which travels along the coronary sulcus posteriorly around the left atrial appendage (see Fig. 7-6). The circumflex branch further divides into smaller branches that course down the posterior surface posterior of the left ventricle.

Together these branches of the left coronary artery normally supply most of the left ventricle, the left atrium, the anterior two thirds of the interventricular septum, the lower half of the interatrial septum, and part of the right atrium.

After originating at the aorta, the right coronary artery immediately courses diagonally to the right across the coronary sulcus, giving off many small branches to the right ventricle as it moves posteriorly. The right coronary artery ends in its posterior descending branch, which descends within the posterior interventricular groove (see Fig. 7-6). In some 20% of individuals, this posterior descending branch arises from the terminal portions of the (left) circumflex artery, in which cases the person is said to have a predominant left coronary system.[4] Together the branches of the right coronary artery normally supply the anterior and posterior portions of the right ventricular myocardium, the right atrium, the sinus node, the posterior third of the interventricular septum, and a portion of the base of the left ventricle.

The coronary veins closely parallel the arterial circulation (see Fig. 7-6). The great cardiac vein follows the anterior descending artery in the anterior interventricular groove. The small cardiac vein accompanies the right coronary artery in the coronary sulcus. The left posterior coronary vein follows a branch of the circumflex artery, and the middle cardiac vein parallels the posterior descending artery. These veins gather into a large confluence called the *coronary sinus,* which passes from left to right across the posterior surface of the myocardium. The coronary sinus empties into the right atrium between the opening of the inferior vena cava and the tricuspid valve.

In addition to these major routes for return flow, some coronary venous blood flows back into the heart through the *Thebesian veins,* which empty directly into all heart chambers. That portion of the venous drainage that returns to the left chambers of the heart via the Thebesian veins mixes with the arterialized blood coming from the lungs, thereby lowering its oxygen content by a small but measurable amount. Because the blood from the Thebesian venous drainage effectively bypasses or "shunts" around the pulmonary circulation, the resultant mixing of deoxygenated venous blood with freshly oxygenated blood from the lungs is called an *anatomic shunt.* In conjunction with a similar bypass occurring in the bronchial circulation (see Chapter 6), this normal anatomic shunt totals some 1% to 2% of the total cardiac output.

Properties of cardiac muscle. The effectiveness of the heart as a pump depends on its ability to originate and conduct electrical impulses and to synchronously contract its muscle fibers quickly and efficiently. These actions are possible only because myocardial tissue possesses four key characteristics: excitability, inherent rhythmicity, conductivity, and contractility.[5,6]

The myocardial property of excitability, shared with other muscle and nerve tissue, represents a responsiveness to stimulation caused by electrical, chemical, or mechanical factors in the cell, or in its surrounding environment. In the clinical setting, factors such as acidosis and hypoxia can initially cause increased excitability of the myocardium, resulting in aberrations in electrical conduction and/or mechanical action.

The unique ability of cardiac muscle to spontaneously originate an electrical impulse is called inherent rhythmicity or automaticity. Although such impulses can originate in any cardiac tissue, this ability is particularly developed in specialized areas called pacemaker or nodal tissues. The sinoatrial (SA) and atrioventricular (AV) nodes are good examples of specialized tissues designed to originate electrical impulses. Origination of an electrical impulse from an area other than a normal pacemaker is considered abnormal and represents a major cause of abnormalities of electrical conduction called *cardiac arrhythmias.*

The cardiac property of conductivity represents the ability of myocardial tissue to propagate electrical impulses. This characteristic, similar to that of smooth muscle, al-

lows the myocardium to function without the direct neural innervation needed by skeletal muscle. The rate at which myocardial tissues conduct electrical impulses varies substantially, from the typically slow nodal areas (5 cm/s) to the extremely fast specialized fibers of the Purkinje system (300 to 400 cm/s).[2] These variations in conduction velocity are essential in maintaining synchronous contraction of the cardiac chambers. Aberrations in myocardial conductivity can affect the timing of mechanical events and, therefore, the efficiency of cardiac function.

The functional characteristic of contractility in response to an electrical impulse is the primary function of the myocardium, a function shared with other muscle tissue. However, unlike other muscle tissue, cardiac muscle contraction cannot be sustained or tetanized. This unique property is a result of the relatively long period of inexcitability (the refractory period) of myocardial tissue after contraction.[2]

Microanatomy. The ability of cardiac muscle to contract and the relationship between contractile force and myocardial structure are revealed best at the cellular level. Under the microscope the myocardium consists of an arrangement of striated, cylindrically shaped muscle fibers averaging 10 to 15 μm wide and 30 to 60 μm long. Individual fibers are enclosed in a membrane called the sarcolemma, surrounded by a rich capillary network (Fig. 7-7). These fibers branch and are separated by an irregular transverse thickening of the sarcolemma called the intercalated disk. These disks provide structural support while facilitating electrical conduction between fibers.[7]

Each muscle fiber consists of smaller, longitudinal subunits called myofibrils, which run the length of the fiber. Myofibrils are composed of repeated structures 1.5 to 2.5 μm long called sarcomeres. Sarcomeres contain myofilaments, which represent the actual contractile proteins responsible for shortening of the myocardium during systole.[7,8] Myofilaments are of two types: the thick myofilaments composed mainly of the protein actin, and the thin myofilaments consisting mostly of myosin.

According to the sliding filament theory, myocardial cells contract when actin and myosin combine to form reversible cross-bridges between these thick and thin filaments. Like the oars of a boat, these cross-bridges cause the filaments to slide over one another, shortening the sarcomere, and thus the myofibrils and muscle fiber as a whole.[7]

In principle, the tension developed during contraction of the myocardial fibers is directly proportional to the number of cross-bridges between the actin and myosin filaments. The number of cross-bridges, in turn, is directly proportional to the length of the sarcomere. This principle forms the basis for Starling's classic law of the heart, also known as the *Frank-Starling relationship.* Simply stated, as the length of a cardiac fiber is increased by stretching, the greater will be the tension it generates when electrically

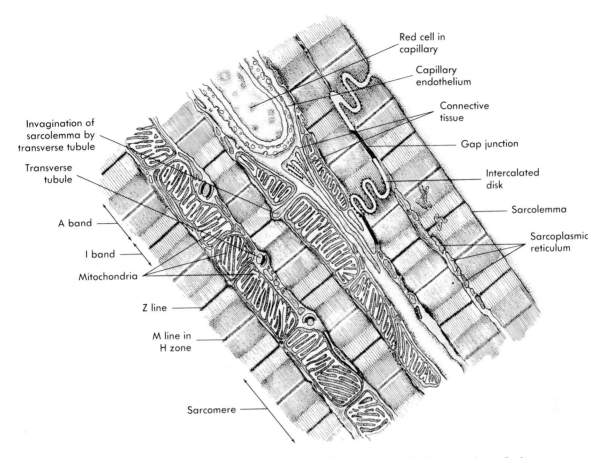

Red cell in
capillary

Capillary
endothelium

Connective
tissue

Gap junction

Intercalated
disk

Sarcolemma

Sarcoplasmic
reticulum

Invagination of
sarcolemma by
transverse tubule

Transverse
tubule

A band

I band

Mitochondria

Z line

M line in
H zone

Sarcomere

Fig. 7-7   Diagram of an electron micrograph of cardiac muscle showing large numbers of mitochondria and the intercalated disks with nexi (gap junctions), transverse tubules, and longitudinal tubules. (From Berne RM and Levy MN: Cardiovascular physiology, ed 5, St Louis, 1986, The CV Mosby Co.)

stimulated. This relationship is graphically depicted in Fig. 7-8. Note that the relationship holds only up to a certain point of stretch, equivalent to a sarcomere length of about 2.2 μm. Beyond this point, the actin and myosin filaments become partially disengaged, less cross-bridges can be formed, and the resultant force of contraction actually decreases. This relationship is of major clinical significance and will be explored later in discussion of the heart as a pump.

The vascular system

Plan of circulation. Fig. 7-9 represents the basic plan of blood flow to and from the heart. Venous, or "deoxygenated", blood from the head and upper extremities enters the right atrium from the superior vena cava while blood from the lower body and extremities enters from the inferior vena cava. From there, blood flows through the tricuspid valve into the right ventricle. The right ventricle pumps blood through the pulmonary valve, into the pulmonary arteries, and to the lungs. Oxygenated blood returns to the left atrium through the pulmonary veins. The

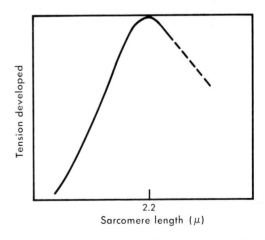

Tension developed

2.2
Sarcomere length (μ)

Fig. 7-8   The ultrastructural basis for the Frank-Starling curve, showing that peak tension development occurs at a sarcomere length of 2.2 μm; whether a downslope of the curve after peak tension exists is not known. (From Schroeder JS and Daily EK: Techniques in bedside hemodynamic monitoring, St Louis, 1976, The CV Mosby Co.)

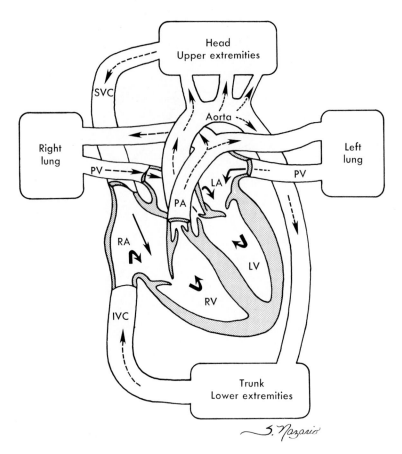

Fig. 7-9   Schematic of plan of circulation. *RA*, right atrium; *RV*, right ventricle; *LA*, left atrium; *LV*, left ventricle; *IVC*, inferior vena cava; *SVC*, superior vena cava; *PA*, pulmonary artery; *PV*, pulmonary vein.

left atrium pumps blood through the mitral valve into the left ventricle, where it is pumped through the aortic valve and into the aorta. From the aorta, the blood flows out to the tissues of the upper and lower body and extremities. From the capillary networks of the various body tissues, venous blood returns to the vena cava.

Although a single organ, the heart functions as two separate but synchronous pumps. The right side of the heart provides the pressures necessary to drive blood through the low resistance, low pressure pulmonary circulation; the left side generates the force needed to distend the highly elastic aorta and propel blood through the higher pressure systemic circulation. This distinction is most evident in the clinical setting when either the left or right heart can fail independently.

Components of the systemic vasculature. Having already described the pulmonary vascular system (see Chapter 6), our emphasis here will be on the systemic components of the circulatory system. The systemic vascular system as a whole is divided into three major subcomponents: the arterial system, the capillary system, and the venous system. All three components are responsible for circulating the blood to and from the tissues and lungs; however, the various blood vessels act as more than just passive

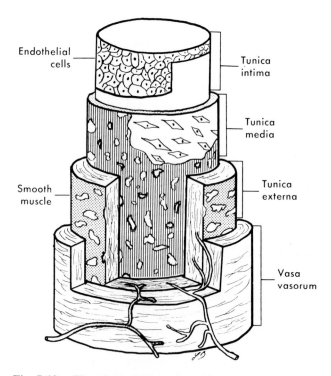

Fig. 7-10   Three layers of an artery with vasa vasorum. (From McLaughlin AJ Jr: Essentials of physiology for advanced respiratory therapy, St Louis, 1977, The CV Mosby Co.)

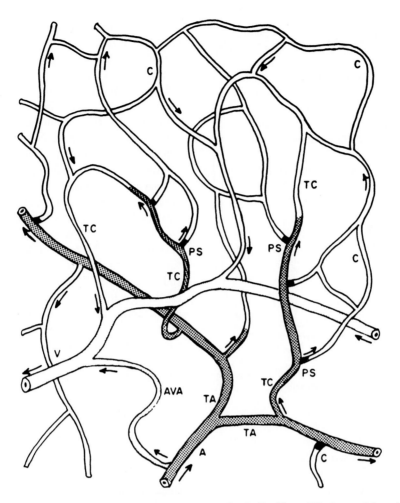

Fig. 7-11   Components of a microcirculatory network. *C,* Capillary; *TC,* thoroughfare channel; *V,* venule; *PS,* precapillary sphincter; *AVA,* arteriolovenous anastomosis; *A,* arteriole; *TA,* terminal arteriole. (From Zweifach BW: The microcirculation of the blood, January 1959, pp. 54-60. Copyright © 1959 by Scientific American, Inc. All rights reserved.)

conduits. Instead, they are active partners with the heart, regulating not only the amount of blood flow per minute (cardiac output) but also its distribution to the body.[2] To achieve this partnership, each component has a unique structure and serves a different role in the circulatory system as a whole.[9]

The arterial system consists of large, highly elastic, low resistance arteries and small, muscular, variable resistance arterioles. Because of their highly elastic composition, large arteries play a critical role in transmitting and maintaining the head of perfusion pressure generated by the heart, and are referred to as *conductance vessels.*[5,9] Arterioles act as variable resistors in controlling the flow of blood into the capillary beds much like a faucet regulates the flow of water into a sink. For this reason, arterioles are often referred to as *resistance vessels.*[5,9]

As depicted in Fig. 7-10, arteries are composed of three primary tissue layers: a thin tunica intima composed of endothelial cells attached to a basement membrane; a thick middle tunica media composed of mainly smooth muscle

and elastic tissue; and an outer tunica externa, or adventitia, consisting of fibrous connective tissue.[10] An external system of arteries and veins, the vasa vasorum, provides nutrient circulation to all but the tunica intima. The tunica media of large arteries has predominantly more elastic than muscle fibers; the reverse is true in smaller arteries and arterioles.

The vast capillary system or *microcirculation* is responsible for maintaining a constant internal environment for the body's cells and tissues via the transport and exchange of carbon dioxide, oxygen, nutrients, and waste products; therefore, these capillaries are commonly referred to as *exchange vessels.*[5,9]

The basic structure of a typical capillary network is depicted in Fig. 7-11.[11] Blood flows into the network via an arteriole, *A,* and out through a venule, *(V).* A direct connection between these vessels, termed an arteriolovenous anastomosis or *AVA,* is also evident. When open, the AVA allows arterial blood to shunt around the capillary bed and flow directly to the venous side of the network.

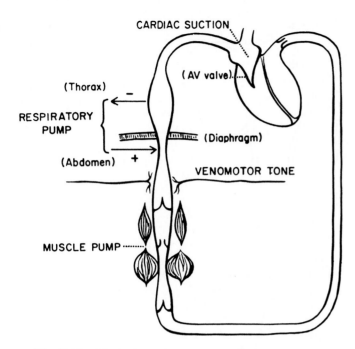

CARDIAC SUCTION

(AV valve)

(Thorax)

RESPIRATORY PUMP

(Diaphragm)

(Abdomen)

VENOMOTOR TONE

MUSCLE PUMP

Fig. 7-12   Mechanisms that assist venous flow from the extremities. See text for details. (From Richardson DR: Basic circulatory physiology, Boston, 1976, Little, Brown & Co.)

Downstream from the AVA, the arteriole divides into terminal arterioles, *(TA),* which branch further into thoroughfare channels, *(TC),* and true capillaries, *(C).* Thoroughfare channels have smooth muscle bands at their proximal ends and are like AVAs except that they give rise to some capillaries. Capillaries also have smooth muscle rings at their proximal ends, called precapillary sphincters, *(PS).* In combination, this complex of channels, sphincters, and bypasses allows substantial variation in the direction and amount of perfusion a given area of tissue will receive.

The venous system consists of small distensible venules and veins, and larger more elastic veins. Together these vessels serve as a volume reservoir for the systemic circulation, holding an average of three fourths of the total blood volume at any given time. The venous system also is capable of quickly altering its holding capacity to match the volume of blood needed to maintain adequate systemic perfusion; thus, the vessels of this system, particularly the small distensible venules and veins, are termed *capacitance vessels.*[5,9]

As the component of the vasculature having the lowest pressures, the venous system must contend with the force of gravity in returning blood to the heart. As depicted in Fig. 7-12, four interrelated mechanisms combine to assure adequate return flow even in the fully upright position.[2] Mechanisms facilitating venous return and preventing blood pooling in the peripheral vasculature include the following: (1) sympathetic venomotor tone, (2) skeletal muscle activity in conjunction with the venous valve system, (3) cardiac suction, and (4) thoracic pressure differences

associated with respiratory movements. This last mechanism, often referred to as the "thoracic pump," is of particular relevance in that positive pressure ventilation reverses thoracic pressure gradients and therefore impedes, rather than assists, venous return. Fortunately, as long as blood volume, cardiac function, and vasomotor tone are adequate, the thoracic pressure changes associated with positive pressure ventilation have a minimal effect on venous return. If this were not the case, positive pressure ventilatory support would be impossible.

Vascular resistance. Like any fluid, the movement of blood through the various components of the vascular system is opposed; this opposition is called the *total peripheral vascular resistance.* Using the concept of resistance developed in Chapter 4, total peripheral resistance must equal the difference in pressure between the beginning and end of the conduit divided by the flow. Beginning pressure for the systemic circulation is equivalent to the average, or mean, aortic pressure; ending pressure equals the mean right atrial pressure. Flow for the systemic circulation is equal to the cardiac output. The total peripheral resistance, or *afterload,* against which the left heart must pump may be calculated using the following formula[12]:

$$\text{total peripheral resistance} = \frac{\text{mean aortic pressure} - \text{right atrial pressure}}{\text{cardiac output}}$$

Since the vast majority of resistance to outflow from the left ventricle is associated with the arterial vessels, and since, in the absence of right heart disease, right atrial pressure approaches zero, the above equation can be simplified by deleting the right atrial pressure measurement.

The same concept can be applied to computing the pulmonary vascular resistance, or afterload, for the right heart. Simple substitution of mean pulmonary artery pressure for aortic and left atrial for right atrial pressure provides an approximation of afterload on the right ventricle.

$$\text{pulmonary vascular resistance} = \frac{\text{mean pulmonary artery pressure} - \text{left atrial pressure}}{\text{cardiac output}}$$

Since the total blood flow per minute through the pulmonary and systemic circulations is equal, and since mean pulmonary artery pressure (15 mm Hg) is about one sixth that of the aorta (90 mm Hg), it is evident that the pulmonary vascular resistance must be substantially less than that of the systemic circulation. The pulmonary vasculature is characterized as a low pressure, low resistance circulation.[12]

Determinants of blood pressure. Adequate perfusion to body tissues depends on the maintenance of a head of pressure sufficient to propel blood throughout the vascular system. The cardiovascular system's first priority is to maintain this perfusion pressure within narrow limits under a variety of changing conditions.[2] The average perfusion pressure for either the systemic or pulmonary circulation is equivalent to the mean pressure in their primary outflow vessels, that is, the aorta or pulmonary artery. By rearranging the above equations to solve for mean arterial pressure and eliminating the normally negligible atrial pressures it can be seen that the average blood pressure in the systemic or pulmonary circulation is directly related to both the cardiac output and the resistance of the vasculature.

$$\text{mean arterial pressure} = \text{cardiac output} \times \text{vascular resistance}$$

With a constant rate and force of cardiac contractions, cardiac output is essentially equivalent to the volume of blood in the circulatory system. Under similar conditions, vascular resistance is inversely related to the size of the system's blood vessels, that is, the *capacity* of the vascular system. All else being constant, mean arterial pressure is directly related to the volume of blood in the vascular system and is inversely related to its capacity[2]:

$$\text{mean arterial pressure} = \frac{\text{volume}}{\text{capacity}}$$

Based on this relationship, it can be seen that mean arterial pressure can be regulated by: (1) changing the volume of blood that is circulating, (2) changing the capacity of the vascular system, or (3) both. Volume changes can reflect absolute changes in total blood volume such as with shock or transfusion, or relative changes such as occur with variations in cardiac output. Changes in capacity of the vascular system occur with variations in the state of contractility of the smooth muscle in the walls of the blood vessels, particularly the capacitance vessels of the venous system.

To maintain adequate perfusion pressures under changing conditions, the cardiovascular system balances these two factors. In exercise, for example, the circulating blood volume undergoes a relative increase. Blood pressure is maintained near normal because the vascular beds in skeletal muscle dilate, dramatically increasing the capacity of the system. However, with the large blood loss associated with hemorrhage, the capacity of the system is decreased by constriction of the venous vessels. Perfusing pressures, therefore, can be kept near normal until the volume loss overwhelms the system.

Of course, the regulation of blood flow and pressure is more complex than indicated in these simplified equations and examples. Control of the cardiovascular system is accomplished via a complex array of integrated functions.

CONTROL OF THE CARDIOVASCULAR SYSTEM

As the body system responsible for transporting metabolites to and from the tissues under a wide variety of conditions and demands, the cardiovascular system must act in a highly coordinated fashion. This coordination is accomplished by integrating the functions of the heart and vascular system, with a final goal of maintaining adequate perfusion to all tissues according to their needs.

Contrary to common understanding, the heart plays a secondary role in adjusting tissue perfusion according to need. The cardiovascular system regulates perfusion mainly by altering the capacity of the vasculature and the volume of blood it contains. In essence, the vascular system tells the heart how much blood it needs, rather than the heart dictating what volume it will receive.[2]

This complex integration of function involves both local and central control mechanisms. Local or *intrinsic* mechanisms work independently of centralized nervous control, altering perfusion under normal conditions to meet metabolic needs. Central or *extrinsic* control involves both the central nervous system and circulating humoral agents and has the primary responsibility of maintaining a basal level of vascular tone. However, central control mechanisms will take over when the competing needs of local vascular beds must be coordinated.

A useful analogy is Richardson's comparison of the cardiovascular system to a factory.[2] As long as the supply of raw materials equals the rate of production in all the manufacturing areas, materials keep flowing smoothly. However, should production rates begin to vary among areas, the "head office" must intercede and alter materials flow to restore a coordinated function. Otherwise, raw materials will needlessly build up or the productivity of dependent areas will drop.

Keeping this analogy of local and centralized control in mind, we will explore vascular regulatory mechanisms, followed by an analysis of factors controlling cardiac output. Finally, these perspectives will be combined to demonstrate the full integration of the cardiovascular system under both normal and abnormal conditions.

Regulation of the vascular system

A basal level of vascular tone normally is maintained in the vascular system at all times.[2,3,5,7] Basal tone must be present for effective regulation to occur. If blood vessels were maintained in a completely relaxed or flaccid state, further dilation would be impossible, and local increases in perfusion could not occur.

Local vascular tone is maintained by the smooth muscle of the precapillary sphincters and thoroughfare channels of the microcirculation, and it can function independent of neural control. Central control of vasomotor tone involves direct neural innervation and indirect humoral influence on the musculature of the resistance and capacitance vessels of the system, mainly the arterioles and veins.[5]

Local control. Local control, or *autoregulation*, of blood flow in the tissues probably involves at least two related mechanisms. *Myogenic control* is based on the fact that the tone of vascular smooth muscle is directly related to perfusing pressures. Increased perfusing pressures increase and decreased perfusing pressures decrease the tone

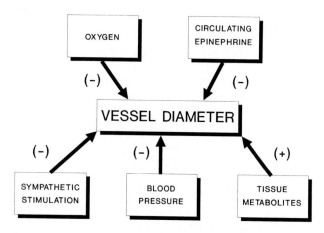

Fig. 7-13 Factors influencing vessel diameter in the microcirculation; (+) indicates dilation, (−) indicates constriction. Note that a variety of constrictor influences of circulating blood or neurogenic origin are balanced by dilatory influences related to local tissue metabolism. (Redrawn from Richardson DR: Basic circulatory physiology, Boston, 1976, Little, Brown & Co.)

of vascular smooth muscle. This form of autoregulation ensures relatively constant flows to capillary beds despite local changes in perfusion pressures.[13]

Local vascular tone also depends on the level of cellular metabolites present around the smooth muscle. This *metabolic control* is based on the fact that high amounts of carbon dioxide or lactic acid, low levels of pH, or low partial pressure of oxygen all cause dilation of the smooth muscle, thereby increasing perfusion to the affected area. This form of autoregulation provides tissue flow according to metabolic demand.[14]

As depicted in Fig. 7-13, the local regulatory mechanisms probably work in tandem;[15] however, their influence appears to vary according to the organ system involved. The brain, for example, exhibits powerful responses to changes in the levels of local metabolites, particularly carbon dioxide and pH. The heart, however, shows a strong response to both myogenic and metabolic factors.

Central control. The autonomic nervous system, particularly its sympathetic division, has primary responsibility for maintaining central control.[16] As with local control, the level of central control varies substantially among organs and tissues. The brain is minimally regulated by this mechanism.[17] However, skeletal muscle and skin are regulated mainly by central control.

Contraction and increased resistance to flow result primarily from adrenergic stimulation via release of norepinephrine at the myoneural junctions of smooth muscle in the vascular system.[18,19] Smooth muscle relaxation and vessel dilation, however, are evoked by either cholinergic stimulation (releasing acetylcholine) or the selective response of specialized adrenergic beta receptors. Whereas

the contractile response appears distributed throughout the entire vascular system, the centrally evoked dilation response is limited to the smooth muscle of the precapillary vessels.[5]

Regulation of cardiac output

Like the vascular system, the heart is regulated by both intrinsic and extrinsic factors. These local and central mechanisms act together with vascular controlling factors to ensure that the output of the normal heart matches the varying needs of the tissues.[20]

The total amount of blood pumped by the heart per minute, or *cardiac output,* is simply the product of the heart rate multiplied by the volume ejected by the left ventricle on each contraction, or stroke volume.

$$\text{cardiac output} = \text{rate} \times \text{stroke volume}$$

Substituting normal values for rate (70 to 75 contractions per minute) and stroke volume (70 ml per contraction), we calculate a normal resting cardiac output of between 4,900 and 5,250 ml per minute. Of course, this is a hypothetical average used for illustrative purposes only. Actual cardiac output varies considerably both in health and disease.

Whether in health or disease, a change in cardiac performance involves a change in stroke volume, a change in the rate of contractions, or both. Stroke volume is affected primarily by intrinsic control of three factors: preload, afterload, and contractility. The rate of cardiac contractions is affected primarily by extrinsic or central control mechanisms.

Changes in stroke volume. Stroke volume is the difference between the end diastolic volume (EDV) and the end systolic volume (ESV) of the ventricles. A change in stroke volume occurs only when the difference between EDV and ESV changes. When either EDV increases or ESV decreases relative to normal, an increase in stroke volume occurs. Likewise, when EDV decreases or ESV increases as compared to normal, a decrease in stroke volume results.

The ability of the myocardium to change stroke volume solely according to changes in EDV is an intrinsic regulatory mechanism based on the Frank-Starling relationship.[20] Since EDV represents the initial stretch or tension placed on the myocardium, the greater the EDV (up to a point), the greater will be the tension developed on contraction, and vice versa. This intrinsic control mechanism is called *heterometric autoregulation,* meaning regulation caused by a difference in size (filling) of the ventricles.[2]

In clinical practice, this initial stretch is called *preload,* and the tension of contraction is equivalent to ventricular stroke volume. Fig. 7-14 applies the Frank-Starling relationship to ventricular function as a whole, plotting ventricular stretch against stroke volume. Because the stretch of the myocardium is directly proportional to its EDV, and

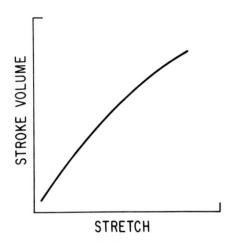

Fig. 7-14   The Frank-Starling relationship—stroke volume as a function of ventricular end diastolic stretch. An increase in the stretch of the ventricles immediately before contraction (end diastole) results in an increase in stroke volume. Note that ventricular end diastolic stretch is synonymous with the concept of preload. (From Green JF: Fundamental cardiovascular and pulmonary physiology, ed 2, Philadelphia, 1987, Lea & Febiger.)

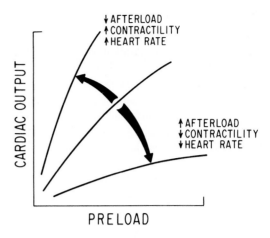

Fig. 7-15   Effects of preload, afterload, contractility, and heart rate on cardiac output function curve. (From Green JF: Fundamental cardiovascular and pulmonary physiology, ed 2, Philadelphia, 1987, Lea & Febiger.)

because EDV is directly related to the pressure difference across the wall of the ventricle, preload is usually measured indirectly as the ventricle end diastolic pressure.[5]

The second major factor affecting stroke volume is the force against which the heart must pump, or *afterload*. In clinical practice, the force against which the heart must pump to eject blood into the systemic circulation is equivalent to the total peripheral resistance to blood flow out of the left ventricle. Thus the greater the afterload on the ventricles, the less effective they will be in ejecting their blood volume. Specifically, for a given EDV, an increase in afterload will result in an increased ESV, thereby decreasing stroke volume. Normally, however, the heart muscle intrinsically responds to an increase in afterload by altering a third factor responsible for its performance, that is, its contractility.

Cardiac contractility is a relative term best defined as the amount of force or work exerted for a given amount of stretch or preload.[2] In concept, changes in contractility of the myocardium affect the slope of the ventricular function curve (see Fig. 7-14) such that for a given amount of stretch or EDV, a lower ESV will result, thereby increasing stroke volume. Greater stroke volumes for a given preload indicate a state of increased contractility, or a state of *positive inotropism*. Lesser stroke volumes for a given preload are indicative of a decreased state of contractility, a *negative inotropic effect*.

Contractility of the heart is affected mainly by local mechanisms, although neural control, circulating humoral factors, and certain drugs can and do exert an influence.[20,21] Whether local or central in origin, these factors all work at the cellular level to influence the activity of the contractile proteins, mostly by affecting the metabolism of calcium in the sarcomere. In general, sympathetic stimulation, whether directly evoked or mediated by drugs, has a positive inotropic effect on the myocardium. Parasympathetic stimulation, on the other hand, exerts a negative inotropic effect.[21] Profound hypoxia or acidosis impair myocardial metabolism, thereby decreasing cardiac contractility.

Changes in rate.   The last factor influencing cardiac performance is its rate of contraction. Unlike the factors controlling stroke volume, those influencing cardiac rate are mainly central in origin, that is, neural or humoral.[20,21] All else being equal, cardiac output is directly proportional to changes in cardiac rate. The normal rapid filling and emptying of the ventricles during diastole and systole ensure that this relationship can be maintained over a wide range of cardiac rates. However, at the upper end of this range (approximately 180 beats per minute), ventricular filling can be incomplete, resulting in an actual drop in stroke volume and a resultant drop in total cardiac output.[22]

The combined effects of preload, afterload, contractility, and cardiac rate in determining overall cardiac performance is graphically portrayed in Fig. 7-15. The middle ventricular function curve represents a normal state of affairs in which simple changes in preload cause corresponding changes in cardiac output. The upper, steeper, ventricular function curve is that of a hypereffective heart, in which, for a given preload, the cardiac output is greater than normal. Alone or in combination, a decreased afterload, increased contractility, or increased cardiac rate will exert this effect. The bottom curve has less slope than normal, indicating a hypoeffective heart. Factors contributing to this state include an increased afterload, a decreased state of contractility, or a decreased cardiac rate.[5]

Coordination of functions

The control of the cardiovascular system is accomplished by a complex integration of local and central regulatory mechanisms affecting both the heart and peripheral vasculature. The underlying goal is to ensure that all tissues receive perfusion sufficient to meet their metabolic needs at all times. Under normal resting conditions, this goal is achieved primarily through local regulation of the heart and vasculature, as monitored by the "head office."[2,5] Under states of increased demand, such as during intense exercise, or during abnormal states, such as massive hemorrhage, central mechanisms must take over primary control.[5]

Central control and coordination of cardiovascular function occurs via the interaction of brainstem centers with a variety of peripheral receptors. Second to second, the brainstem receives measurements from these peripheral receptors regarding the pressure, volume, and chemical status of the blood. The brainstem also receives input from higher brain centers such as the hypothalamus and cerebral cortex. These inputs are integrated with those arising from the heart and vasculature to maintain blood flow and pressures within optimum limits under all but the most abnormal conditions.[16,21]

The cardiovascular centers. A simplified diagram of the cardiovascular centers and their interconnections with each other, with higher brain centers, and with the various peripheral sensors appears in Fig. 7-16. Excitatory and depressor interactions are depicted by plus (+) and minus (−) signs, respectively.

These "centers" are actually four diffuse areas of neural tissue located in the reticular formations of the pons and medulla.[5] A vasoconstrictor area, labeled VC, evokes a pressor effect when stimulated, mainly via increased efferent output to adrenergic receptors in the vascular smooth muscle. A vasodepressor area, labeled VD, appears to exert its effect mainly by inhibition (−) of the vasoconstrictor center output. Closely associated with the vasoconstrictor center is a cardioaccelerator area, labeled CA. Stimulation of the cardioaccelerator center increases the heart rate (+) by increasing sympathetic discharge to the nodal tissues of the right atrium and AV junction. Closely associated with the vasodepressor center is a cardioinhibitory area, labeled CI. Stimulation of the cardioinhibitory center decreases heart rate (−) by increasing parasympathetic discharge to the heart via efferent fibers of the Xth cranial (vagus) nerve.

The two vascular and two cardiac centers interact together in mutually logical ways. Stimulation of the vasoconstrictor area tends to stimulate (+) the cardioaccelerator center, resulting in both elevation of blood pressure and an increase in cardiac rate. Stimulation of the vasodepressor area, however, tends to simultaneously inhibit (−) both the vasoconstrictor and cardioinhibitory areas, resulting in vasodilation and an increase in cardiac rate.

All these cardiovascular centers receive input from

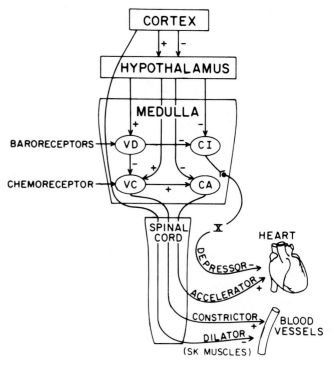

Fig. 7-16   Schematic summarizing major known neural pathways involved in central regulation of cardiovascular function. This design is oversimplified to illustrate the major relationships between excitatory (+) and depressor (−) fibers. *VD*, Vasodepressor area; *VC*, vasoconstrictor area; *CA*, cardioaccelerator area; *CI*, cardioinhibitory area. (From Green JF: Fundamental cardiovascular and pulmonary physiology, ed 2, Philadelphia, 1987, Lea & Febiger.)

higher portions of the brain. Signals received from the cerebral cortex, such as those arising in response to exercise, pain, or anxiety, pass directly via cholinergic fibers to the vascular smooth muscle, causing vasodilation. Signals from the hypothalamus, particularly its anterior heat-regulating areas, indirectly affect heart rate and vasomotor tone via stimulation or inhibition of the cardiovascular centers.[5]

The cardiovascular centers are also influenced by local environmental changes in blood or cerebrospinal fluid chemistry.[23] For example, a local decrease in the partial pressure of carbon dioxide can cause a marked fall in blood pressure due to overall inhibition of the centers and the resultant loss of vascular tone. However, decreased partial pressures of oxygen increase the rate of sympathetic discharge of the cardiovascular centers, thereby elevating blood pressure.

Peripheral receptors. Higher level and local inputs to the cardiovascular centers are balanced with signals coming from the peripheral sensory receptors.[23,24] In conjunction with the cardiovascular centers, peripheral receptors form a negative feedback control mechanism. In this type of regulation, stimulation of a receptor evokes an opposite response from an effector mechanism, so that a balance in a parameter can be maintained. For example, in a negative feedback loop a decrease in blood pressure will decrease the rate of discharge of the sensor. This decreased rate of afferent impulse formation increases the rate of efferent pressor signal activity, thereby stimulating a vasoconstrictor response. As the blood pressure is restored to normal limits, the sensor increases its rate of impulse formation, lessening vasoconstrictor action, and, in effect, bringing the system back in balance.

These receptors are of two general types: those responding mainly to changes in pressure or stretch are called *baroreceptors*.[24] Those responding to changes in the chemical contents of the blood are termed *chemoreceptors*.[23] Cardiovascular baroreceptors may be divided into two categories: (1) the low-pressure sensors in the walls of the atria and the large thoracic and pulmonary veins, and (2) the high-pressure sensors in the aortic arch and carotid sinuses.[2,24] The low-pressure sensors mainly respond to changes in vascular volumes, whereas the high-pressure sensors are sensitive mostly to the head of perfusion pressure established by the left ventricle.

The output of both types of baroreceptors depends on the degree of stretch of their chamber or vessel walls.[2,24] An increase in stretch (due to greater volume or pressure) increases their discharge rate, thereby inhibiting the vasoconstrictor center and decreasing efferent sympathetic activity. This decreased sympathetic discharge will relax the resistance and capacitance vessels of the vascular system and decrease heart rate and contractility. Decreased baroreceptor stretch will have the opposite effect.

The low-pressure sensors also appear to influence long-term volume regulation via affecting the release of antidiuretic hormone (ADH) and aldosterone.[2] Plasma levels of both these hormones are inversely related to the discharge rates of the low-pressure baroreceptors such that decreased thoracic blood volume increases their secretion. Increased levels of ADH promote the conservation of water in the renal tubules, and increased levels of aldosterone stimulate sodium (and, thus, water) retention, thereby increasing body fluid and vascular volumes.

As previously stated, chemoreceptors are small, highly vascularized tissues located in proximity to the high-pressure sensors in the aortic arch and carotid sinus area. Whereas baroreceptors respond to pressure changes, the chemoreceptors respond to variations in the chemical composition of the blood. They are strongly stimulated by a decrease in Po_2, although lowering of the pH or an increase in Pco_2 can also evoke an increase in their rate of discharge.[23] The major cardiovascular effects of increased chemoreceptor stimulation are peripheral vasoconstriction and an increase in heart rate. Since these changes occur only when the cardiopulmonary system is severely overtaxed, the chemoreceptors probably have little influence on cardiovascular performance under normal conditions.[22] However, because their influence on respiration is clinically important, the peripheral chemoreceptors will be covered in more depth in Chapter 10.

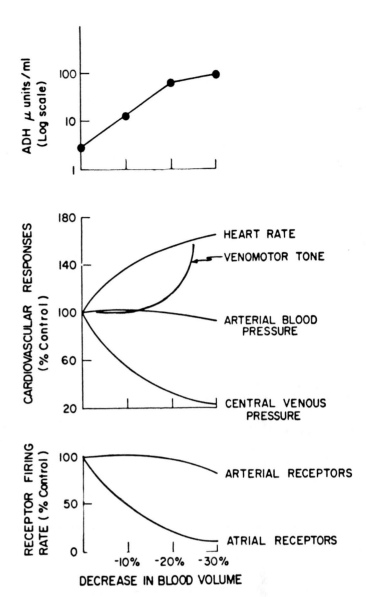

Fig. 7-17   Plasma levels of antidiuretic hormone *(ADH)*, cardiovascular responses, and receptor firing rates in response to graded hemorrhage in the dog. See text for details. (From Richardson DR: Basic circulatory physiology, Boston, 1976, Little, Brown & Co. Venomotor tone data are those of WJ Sears as cited in Gauer OH, Henry JP, and Behn C: The regulation of extracellular fluid volume, Annu Rev Physiol 32:547-595, 1970. All other data are from Henry JP et al: The role of afferents from the low-pressure system in the release of antidiuretic hormone during nonhypotensive hemorrhage, Can J Physiol Pharmacol 46:287-295, 1968.)

Response to changes in volume. The overall coordination of cardiovascular function is best demonstrated during abnormal conditions. Among the most common clinical conditions in which all key regulatory mechanisms come into play is the large blood loss that occurs with hemorrhage. Fig. 7-17 portrays changes in these key factors during progressive blood loss in an animal model.[2]

With a 10% blood loss, the immediate drop in the central venous pressure causes a 50% decrease in the rate of firing of the low-pressure (atrial) baroreceptors, with little change in the activity of the high-pressure (arterial) receptors. The initial response of the cardiovascular system, mediated through the brainstem centers, is an increase in sympathetic discharge to the sinus node and a resultant increase in cardiac rate. Also observed at this time is an increase in the plasma levels of antidiuretic hormone (ADH), apparently resulting from stimulation of the pituitary. These initial changes are sufficient to maintain arterial pressure at normal levels.

As the blood loss becomes more severe (20%), atrial receptor activity decreases further, resulting in an increased intensity of sympathetic discharge from the cardiovascular centers. Plasma ADH and heart rate continue to climb, as does the tone of the peripheral vasculature. This increase in vascular tone occurs mainly through constriction of the capacitance vessels in the venous system, thereby slowing the drop in central venous pressure.

Not until blood loss approaches 30% does the arterial pressure start to drop. At this point, arterial receptor activity begins to decrease, resulting in a marked rise in systemic vascular tone. Despite the magnitude of blood loss, central venous pressure levels off. As long as no further hemorrhage occurs, blood pressure and, therefore, tissue perfusion can be maintained at adequate levels.

Should blood loss continue, central control mechanisms begin drastic action. Massive vasoconstriction occurs in the resistance vessels, shunting blood away from skeletal muscle in an attempt to maintain cerebral and coronary perfusion pressures.[5,22] Rising levels of local metabolites in these critical vascular beds, especially carbon dioxide and other acids, overrides central sympathetic influences and causes further vessel dilation, thereby further increasing needed perfusion.[17,25] Unfortunately, as these byproducts of metabolism continue to concentrate, and as the tissues begin to suffer from inadequate oxygenation (hypoxia), cardiac function becomes impaired and a generalized vasodilation occurs throughout the body, signaling the onset of a state of irreversible shock, after which death quickly ensues.[22,26]

ELECTROPHYSIOLOGY OF THE HEART

Although loss of perfusing pressures resulting from blood loss is a common clinical occurrence, respiratory care practitioners will observe many other causes of cardiovascular insufficiency or failure. Among the most frequent of these conditions are disturbances in electrical conduction of the myocardial tissues. Called *arrhythmias,* these abnormalities can severely impair cardiac function and therefore compromise both blood flow and tissue perfusion. Understanding the origin of these arrhythmias, their clinical manifestations, and their treatment requires that the reader develop a sound understanding of normal cardiac electrophysiology.

Electrical potentials and depolarization

As with other muscles, contraction of myocardial fibers is an electrical phenomenon consisting of the buildup, discharge, and conduction of minute electrical currents. The electrical activity of the myocardium is generated at the level of its individual muscle fibers.[27] Because of differences in the concentration of electrolytes across the membrane of cardiac fibers, a difference in charge, or negative electrical potential, exists between the inside and outside of the cell. This *resting potential* primarily depends on the concentration differences of potassium and sodium ions across the cell membrane which average −90 mV in ventricular tissue. As depicted in Fig. 7-18, this resting potential can be altered by electrical stimulation. The resulting action potential is caused by a change in the membrane permeability for sodium ions, which rapidly diffuse into the cell, reversing its charge. This process, called *depolarization,* releases calcium ions into the myofibrils and activates the contractile process previously described. During most of the depolarization stage of the action potential, the muscle fiber cannot respond to additional electrical stimulation. This portion of the action potential is called the *refractory period.* As compared with other types of muscle, cardiac fibers exhibit a substantially longer action potential, and therefore a longer refractory period. In fact, the refractory period of cardiac fibers actually outlasts the peak of contraction, thereby making it impossible for the heart to go into a tetanic or sustained contraction.[2]

Repolarization is achieved by slowing the influx of sodium and increasing the permeability of the membrane so that potassium can readily diffuse outward (phases three and four of action potential in Fig. 7-18). As repolarization is completed, an active sodium-potassium exchange occurs across the cell membrane, reestablishing the prior ionic balance and fully restoring the resting potential.

The action potential of pacemaker tissue differs from that depicted in Fig. 7-18. Instead of maintaining a relatively stable voltage difference during the resting state, a slow influx of sodium ions causes a progressive decay in the membrane potential, eventually reaching −40 mV. This voltage difference represents the *threshold potential* for pacemaker tissue, equivalent to the point at which spontaneous depolarization occurs. The speed with which the resting potential of pacemaker tissue decays toward its threshold potential determines its rate of depolarization, and thus the rate of impulse formation in the tissue as a whole. As discussed earlier, all myocardial tissue has the potential to spontaneously originate such electrical impulses; such "latent" pacemakers or *ectopic foci* only take command when their excitability is increased, when normal nodal tissues are depressed, or when conducting pathways are blocked.[5,27]

Anatomy of the conducting system

Under normal resting conditions, the adult heart contracts rhythmically at a rate of 50 to 90 beats a minute. Ef-

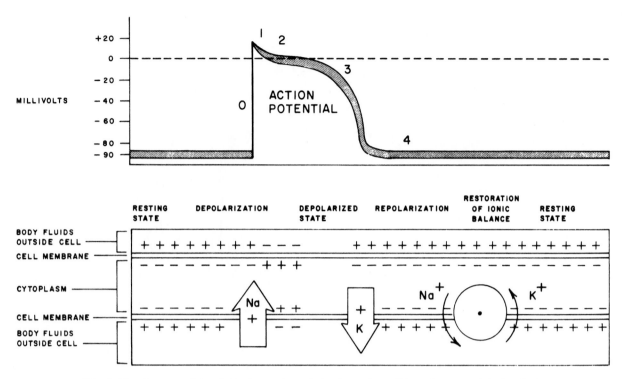

Fig. 7-18   Process of depolarization and repolarization. *Above:* The action potential of a single myocardial cell. Phase 0 is the rapid depolarization of the cell from a negative charge to a slightly positive charge. Phases 1, 2, and 3 represent repolarization; during this time the cell is refractory to a second depolarization. Phases 1 and 2 are periods of absolute refractoriness; during phase 3 the cell is relatively refractory. Phase 4 is the resting phase; repolarization is complete and the cell can be depolarized by another impulse. *Below:* The ionic shifts that occur with depolarization and repolarization. Sodium ions rapidly enter the cell with depolarization; as the cell repolarizes, potassium ions leave the cell, restoring the net negative electrical charge. Ionic balance is then restored by a sodium-potassium exchange across the cell membrane. (From Sanderson RG: The cardiac patient: a comprehensive approach, ed 2, Philadelphia, 1983, WB Saunders Co. After Netter FH: The CIBA collection of medical illustrations, Heart, vol 5, Ciba, 1969.)

fective function demands that the electrical and mechanical events of this cardiac cycle be highly synchronized. Synchronization is achieved by virtue of a specialized system of tissues specifically designed for conducting electrical impulses throughout the myocardium. Collectively, these modified cardiac muscle fibers represent the conducting system of the heart. They include the sinoatrial node, the atrioventricular node, the atrioventricular bundles, and the bundle branches and Purkinje fibers (Fig. 7-19).[27,28]

Sinoatrial node (sinus node). The sinus node is the dominant pacemaker of the heart. It is a small nodule of conducting tissue, about 1.5 cm long, located in the muscle of the right atrium just in front of the opening of the superior vena cava. Impulses initiated at the sinus node radiate from it like circular ripples from a stone dropped into water. Traveling at a rate of 80 to 100 cm/s through the atria, these impulses depolarize the atrial myocardium, causing the chambers to contract simultaneously.

The discharge rate of the sinus node is modified by nervous control, which is increased by the sympathetic stimulation and inhibited by the parasympathetic (vagal) action.[21] Circulating humoral agents or drugs that enhance or depress the effects of these components of the autonomic nervous system have a comparable action. This effect is termed *chronotropism*. A positive chronotropic effect increases discharge rate; a negative chronotropic effect decreases the rate of impulse formation. For example, sympathomimetic or adrenergic drugs like the catecholamine isoproterenol have a positive chronotropic effect, increasing the rate of sinus node discharge. A similar effect can be observed with administration of a parasympatholytic agent like atropine. On the other hand, antiadrenergic drugs like propranolol and parasympathetic stimulators such as edrophonium bromide have a negative chronotropic effect, decreasing the rate of impulse formation. Also, strong parasympathetic stimulation caused by the action of certain vagal reflexes can actually block sinus impulse formation, causing an abrupt and potentially lethal cessation of the cardiac cycle. All these effects are of considerable clinical importance.

Atrioventricular node (AV node). Because the atria and ventricles are separated by a fibrous skeleton of non-

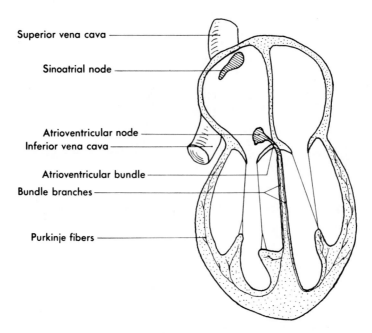

Superior vena cava

Sinoatrial node

Atrioventricular node
Inferior vena cava

Atrioventricular bundle
Bundle branches

Purkinje fibers

Fig. 7-19   Conduction system of the heart. (See text for description.)

conductive connective tissue, depolarization cannot proceed directly between them. Instead, the depolarization wave is routed through a specialized pickup and relay station called the atrioventricular or AV node. Similar in structure to the sinus node, the AV node is located in the right atrium on the lower part of the interatrial septum just above the septal tricuspid valve leaf and near the orifice of the coronary sinus.

With no structural connection to the sinus node, the AV node is stimulated by the radiating sinus impulses, which it relays on toward the ventricles after a short time delay. The delay at the AV node is a result of its comparatively slow velocity of impulse propagation (about 5cm/s). The purpose of this delay is to ensure that the atria have sufficient time to empty their contents into the ventricles before they contract. The AV node also functions as a backup pacemaker. Should the sinus node fail to function because of disease, the AV node can assume its duties, but at substantially slower rates (40 to 60 beats per minute).

Atrioventricular bundle (bundle of His). A well-defined bundle of modified muscle tissue approximately 12 mm in length originates at the AV node and runs horizontally forward over the septal tricuspid valve leaf to the upper part of the interventricular septum. The sinus impulse received by the AV node is transmitted through the bundle and is thus carried to the myocardium of the ventricular chambers. This is the only conduction link between atria and ventricles, and when it is damaged or destroyed by disease, a condition of *block* is said to exist, a cardiac condition commonly encountered in clinical medicine.

Bundle branches and Purkinje fibers. On the upper part of the interventricular septum, the AV bundle termi-

nates by dividing into two bundle branches, right and left, each going to its respective ventricle. The bundles pass down the septum, beneath the endocardium, giving off branches to the papillary muscles, and then continue into the ventricles, where they divide into innumerable fine filaments and form a network (Purkinje fibers) interlacing the depths of the ventricular muscle. The impulse, originating in the sinus node, is carried at a rate of some 5000 mm/s to every portion of the ventricles, in effect stimulating all myocardial fibers simultaneously for uniform contraction of both ventricles.

Electrocardiography

Electrocardiography is the measurement of the electrical events of the cardiac cycle. Electrocardiography is used clinically to diagnose abnormalities in myocardial impulse formation or conduction, and to monitor such activity, especially in the critically ill.[27] Our objective is to emphasize the basic concepts of normal electrocardiography. This knowledge will be applied later to develop the skill in recognizing common disturbances in the heart's electrical conduction (see Chapter 22).

The principles of electrocardiography are simple.[2] First, the heart is centrally located in a large conducting medium of body tissues and electrolytic fluid. Second, depolarization and repolarization of the heart generate a flow of current in the myocardium and in the conducting medium surrounding it. Third, sensitive electrodes placed on the surface of the body will detect this flow of current.

Because the strength of the current generated by the heart varies from point to point on the body's surface, two electrodes placed at different locations will record a differ-

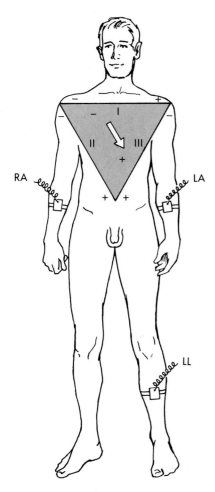

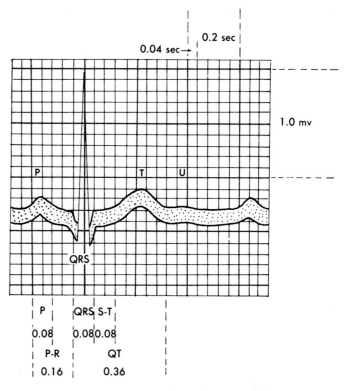

Fig. 7-21 A normal electrocardiographic pattern. (See text for description.)

Fig. 7-20 Einthoven triangle, illustrating the galvanometer connections for standard limb leads I, II, and III. (From Berne RM and Levy MN: Cardiovascular physiology, ed 5, St Louis, 1986, The CV Mosby Co.)

ence in electrical potential during both depolarization and repolarization. If these differences in electrical potential are recorded over a period of time, we will obtain a graphic representation of the electrical events of the cardiac cycle, called an electrocardiogram or ECG.

Although electrodes could be placed on the body in an infinite number of positions, in clinical practice electrode or lead positions are highly standardized. The simplest lead positions are the three bipolar limb leads, which, in combination, are referred to as Einthoven's triangle (Fig. 7-20). This configuration is established by placement of electrodes on both arms and the left leg.

The limb leads are wired so that a wave of depolarization progressing toward a positive electrode will create a positive (upward) deflection on a graph of voltage versus time, with a wave of repolarization having the opposite effect. With the net direction, or axis, of cardiac depolarization being from base to apex (as indicated by the arrow going down and to the left in Fig. 7-20), the bipolar limb

lead between the right arm (−) and the left leg (+), or lead II, should record a positive deflection during depolarization. Moreover, since the magnitude of electrical activity of the heart is directly related to the mass of cardiac tissue involved, we would expect that depolarization of the ventricles would produce the greatest change in recorded voltage.

Fig. 7-21, a segment of a typical lead II normal electrocardiographic recording, confirms these relationships. The bold vertical lines represent time intervals of 0.2 sec subdivided into increments of 0.04 sec. Bold horizontal lines are 1 cm apart, measuring the amplitude of 0.5 millivolt (mV), with each interval representing 0.1 mV. Key normal values of amplitude and duration are indicated in the illustration.

The major electrical events of the cardiac cycle appear as distinctive waveforms. The small, positive P wave records the electrical activity of atrial depolarization, whereas the large, positive QRS complex represents ventricular depolarization. Because atrial repolarization is simultaneous with the beginning of ventricular activity, its effect is masked by the larger QRS complex. Ventricular repolarization is then manifested by a positive T wave. Interestingly, given that current flows during repolarization are opposite those of depolarization, we would expect the T wave to record a negative, not positive, deflection. The lead II T wave is, in fact, positive because ventricular re-

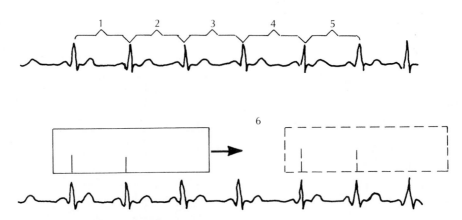

Fig. 7-22   To determine regularity of heartbeat, measure the distance between consecutive R waves *(1 through 5)* using calipers. If calipers are unavailable, mark the distance of one set of consecutive R waves and compare it to consecutive sets *(6)*.

polarization progresses in the opposite direction as depolarization; that is, the last ventricular tissue to depolarize is the first to repolarize. The T wave is sometimes followed by a small U deflection, thought to be caused by ventricular after potentials.

Intervals or time segments between these waves are used to indicate certain conduction events or electrical states of the heart. The PR interval (actually, the P-QRS interval) corresponds to the length of time taken by the atrial impulse to transverse the AV node and reach the ventricles. The duration of the QRS complex is equivalent to the time period for ventricular depolarization. The isoelectric ST segment represents the activated state of the ventricles immediately after depolarization, during which they are totally refractory to additional electrical stimulation. The QT segment corresponds to the time required for complete electrical excitation and recovery of the ventricles and is often referred to as electrical systole, as opposed to mechanical systole.

Comprehensive examination of an ECG rhythm strip proceeds through four systematic steps. First, the heart rate is calculated using the number of RR intervals in a given time span, usually at least 6 sec (Fig. 7-22). Then, again using the RR interval, the regularity of the rhythm is determined. Next, the presence or absence of P waves, their shape, and the duration of the PR interval are determined. Lastly, the QRS complex is inspected and its duration measured.

Within the range of normal cardiac rates (60 to 100 beats per minute), the regular occurrence of the P, QRS, and T waveforms according to preestablished time intervals indicates a *normal sinus rhythm*.[27,28] Any variations in the occurrence, duration, or pattern of these waveforms is called an arrhythmia. Arrhythmia recognition is addressed in Chapter 22.

EVENTS OF THE CARDIAC CYCLE

We have focused on the electrical and mechanical activities of the heart as if they were separate events. In fact, these events are highly integrated and interdependent. Given the critical role of respiratory care practitioners in dealing with abnormalities of the cardiovascular system, a rigorous knowledge of how these events relate in health and disease is essential.

Fig. 7-23 portrays the events of the cardiac cycle using a modification of the classical Wigger's diagram. From top to bottom, a fast-time axis, scaled in tenths of a second, appears first. Hemodynamic pressure events in the left heart and aorta appear next, with timing bars for ventricular systole, diastole, and phonocardiographic heart sounds immediately below. Right heart and pulmonary artery pressure curves are depicted next, followed by hemodynamic flow measurements in the aorta and pulmonary artery. At the bottom of Fig. 7-23 is the standard electrocardiographic portrayal of atrial and ventricular depolarization and repolarization.

Viewing from left to right, we will start at the beginning of the P wave of the ECG, equivalent to late diastole. Prior to this period, the ventricles have been passively filling with blood through the open AV valves. The P wave signals the beginning of atrial depolarization. Within 0.1 sec, atrial contraction commences, causing a slight rise in both atrial and ventricular pressures. The "a" wave on the left and right heart pressure graphs marks this hemodynamic event, corresponding to an increase of some 20% in end diastolic ventricular volumes. The occurrence of this "a" wave seems to vary with heart rate, disappearing at high rates.

Toward the end of diastole, the electrical impulses from the atria reach the SA node and bundle branches, beginning ventricular depolarization, as evidenced by the QRS complex. Within a few hundredths of a second after depo-

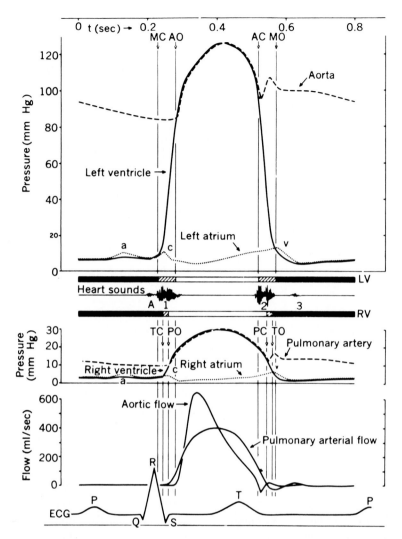

Fig. 7-23   Schematic of the hemodynamic events that occur during the cardiac cycle. *From the top downward:* pressure in the aorta, left ventricle, and left atrium; duration of left ventricular diastole (heavy shading), isovolumic periods (diagonal lines), and systole; pressure in the pulmonary artery, right ventricle, and right atrium; blood flow in the aorta and pulmonary artery; and electrocardiogram. Aortic valve opening and closure are indicated by AO and AC, respectively; MO and MC for the mitral valve; PO and PC for the pulmonic valve; and TO and TC for the tricuspid valve. (From Milnor WR: The heart as a pump. In Mountcastle VB, editor: Medical physiology, ed 14, vol 2, St Louis, 1980, The CV Mosby Co.)

larization the ventricles begin their contraction. At the point where ventricular pressures exceed atrial pressures, the AV valves close, indicated by the vertical lines marked MC and TC. Marking the end of ventricular diastole, AV closure is recorded by the phonocardiogram as the first heart sound, the characteristic "lub" heard on auscultation.

Immediately following AV closure, the ventricles become closed chambers. During this short period of time, called the isovolumic phase of contraction (marked by the diagonal hatching on the timing bars), pressures rise extremely rapidly as the ventricles contract around the incompressible blood in their chambers. Upward bulging of the AV valves during the isovolumic phase causes a slight

upswing in atrial pressures, indicated by the small "c" waves on the pressure graphs. Within 0.05 sec, ventricular pressures rise to equal the outflow pressures in the aorta and pulmonary artery, causing opening of their semilunar valves (the vertical AO and PO markers), and marking the beginning of ventricular systole.

As indicated in the flow curves, at the beginning of systole, outflow from the ventricles is extremely rapid, causing pressures to rise quickly in both the aorta and pulmonary artery. Moreover, because of the minimal resistance offered by the semilunar valves, ventricular and arterial pressures remain essentially equal throughout the 0.3 sec systolic period.

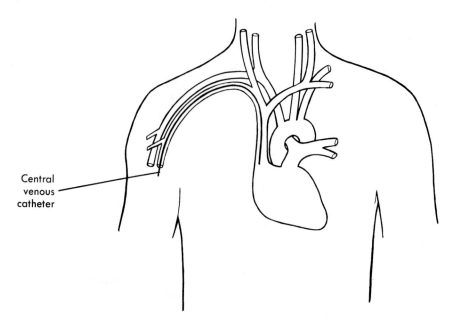

Fig. 7-24   Placement of central venous catheter.

Toward the end of systole, as repolarization starts (indicated by the T wave), the ventricles begin to relax. As a result, arterial pressures begin to drop rapidly. When the arterial pressures exceed those in the relaxing ventricles, the semilunar valves close, a point marked by the vertical AC and PC markers. Closure of the semilunar valves generates the familiar "dub," or second heart sound.

Rather than immediately dropping off, aortic and pulmonary pressures rise again after semilunar valve closure. More dramatic in the aorta than in the pulmonary artery, this incisura or *dichrotic notch* is caused by the elastic recoil of the arteries after valve closure. This extra "push" after ventricular ejection helps maintain the head of perfusion pressure established by cardiac contraction, ensuring its effective transmission downstream.

During this short period of the cycle, the ventricles are again fully closed off, undergoing an isovolumic relaxation phase. As the pressures in their chambers drop below those in the filling atria, the AV valves reopen. At this point (the vertical MO and TO lines) a phase of rapid ventricular filling begins as the blood collected in the atria during systole rushes to fill the lower chambers. Pressures that had built up in the atria now rapidly fall off, a point marked by the "v" wave. Finally, the rate of ventricular filling slows dramatically toward the end of diastole, just prior to the next electrical discharge of the SA node and the beginning of a new cycle.

These normal hemodynamic events provide the basis for understanding many of the diagnostic and monitoring procedures employed in the care of patients with cardiopulmonary disorders. In the cardiac catheterization laboratory, pressure measurements in the heart chambers and across the heart valves are used to diagnose both congenital and acquired structural abnormalities such as mitral stenosis. Of more direct relevance to respiratory care practitioners are the many invasive bedside procedures now used to monitor cardiovascular performance. Among the most common of these are the measurement of central venous pressure or CVP (Fig. 7-24), balloon-directed pulmonary artery or Swan-Ganz catheterization (Fig. 7-25), and direct arterial pressure monitoring.

Despite the "widening" effect of its fast time scale, Fig. 7-23 provides a useful point of reference for each of these clinical procedures. Normal CVP pressures correspond to those portrayed for the right atrium, including the characteristic a-c-v wave sequence. An indwelling pulmonary artery catheter connected to a pressure transducer will obviously produce a waveform similar to that depicted in Fig. 7-23 for the pulmonary artery. Direct arterial pressure measurement will likewise resemble the aortic waveform, although this pattern changes with increased distance from the heart.

SUMMARY

The goal of the cardiovascular system is to continually distribute and regulate the flow of blood in the body, thereby maintaining homeostatic conditions for its tissues and cells. The cardiovascular system consists of a highly specialized and efficient pump, the heart, and a complex and responsive vascular network.

The heart provides the driving force necessary to propel blood throughout the vascular network. Special mechanical and electrophysiologic properties of cardiac tissue,

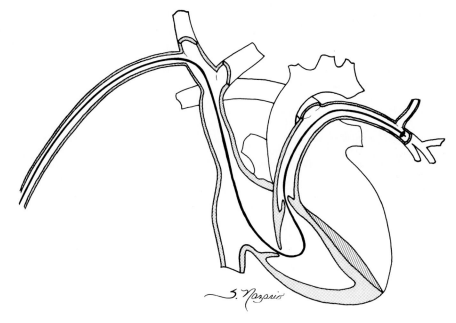

Fig. 7-25   Balloon-tipped flotation catheter in wedge position in pulmonary artery.

combined with intrinsic and extrinsic control mechanisms, provide the basis for coordinated cardiac function under a wide range of circumstances.

The vascular system also exhibits specialized structure and function in its various regions, and, like the heart, is regulated by both local and central control mechanisms. Rather than passively receiving blood from the heart, the vascular network assumes the role of active partner in the control and distribution of the cardiac output.

Normally, these two components of the cardiovascular system work together in a coordinated fashion to ensure that the body tissues are perfused in accordance with their metabolic needs. Under conditions of increased demand, or with dysfunction of one or the other component, reserve capacities or special compensatory mechanisms are called on to maintain stable conditions. Failure of these mechanisms often requires the intervention of respiratory care practitioners to help restore and maintain normal function.

REFERENCES

1. Bernard C: Lecons sur les phenomenes de la vie communes aux animaux et aux vegetaux, Paris, 1879, B Bailliere et Fils.
2. Richardson DR: Basic circulatory physiology, Boston, 1976, Little, Brown & Co.
3. Detweiler DK: Circulation. In Brobeck JR, editor: Best and Taylor's physiologic basis of medical practice, ed 9, Baltimore, 1973, Williams & Wilkins.
4. Sanderson RG: The cardiac patient: a comprehensive approach, Philadelphia, 1972, WB Saunders Co.
5. Green JF: Fundamental cardiovascular and pulmonary physiology, ed 2, Philadelphia, 1987, Lea & Febiger.
6. Brady AJ: Mechanical properties of cardiac fibers. In Berne SR, Sperelakis N, and Geiger SR: Handbook of physiology, Sect 2, The cardiovascular system, vol 1, The heart, Bethesda, Md, 1979, American Physiological Society.
7. Berne RM and Levy MN: Cardiovascular physiology, ed 4, St Louis, 1981, The CV Mosby Co.
8. Tortora GJ and Anagnostakos NP: Principles of anatomy and physiology, ed 4, New York, 1984, Harper & Row.
9. Mellander S and Johansson B: Control of resistance, exchange, and capacitance functions in the peripheral circulation, Pharmacol Rev 20:117, 1968.
10. Rhondin JAG: Architecture of the vessel wall. In Bohr DF, Somlyo AP, and Sparks HV: Handbook of physiology, Sect 2, The cardiovascular system, vol 2, Vascular smooth muscle, Bethesda, Md, 1980, American Physiological Society.
11. Wiedeman MP: Microcirculation, Stroudsburg, Penna, 1974, Dowdwn, Hutchingson & Ross.
12. Green JF: Mechanical concepts in cardiovascular and pulmonary physiology, Philadelphia, 1977, Lea & Febiger.
13. Johnson PC: The myogenic response. In Bohr DF, Somlyo AP, and Sparks HV: Handbook of physiology, Sect 2, The cardiovascular system, vol 2, Vascular smooth muscle, Bethesda, Md, 1980, American Physiological Society.
14. Sparks HV Jr: Effect of local metabolic factors on vascular smooth muscle. In Bohr DF, Somlyo AP, and Sparks HV: Handbook of physiology, Sect 2, The cardiovascular system, vol 2, Vascular smooth muscle, Bethesda, Md, 1980, American Physiological Society.
15. Johnson PL: The microcirculation and local and humoral control of the circulation. In Guyton AC, and Jones CE, editors: Cardiovascular physiology, Baltimore, 1974, University Park Press.
16. Korner PI: Central nervous control of autonomic cardiovascular function. In Berne SR, Sperelakis N, and Geiger SR: Handbook of physiology, Sect 2, The cardiovascular system, vol 1, The heart, Bethesda, Md, 1979, American Physiological Society.
17. Scheinberg P: The cerebral circulation. In Zelis R: The peripheral circulation, New York, 1975, Grune & Stratton.
18. Bevan JA, Bevan RD, and Duckles SP: Adrenergic regulation of smooth muscle. In Bohr DF, Somlyo AP, and Sparks HV: Handbook of physiology, Sect 2, The cardiovascular system, vol 2, Vascular smooth muscle, Bethesda, Md, 1980, American Physiological Society.
19. Rothe CF: Reflex control of veins and vascular capacitance, Physiol Rev 63:1281, 1983.

20. Guyton AC, Jones CE, and Coleman TC: Circulatory physiology: cardiac output and its regulation, Philadelphia, 1973, WB Saunders Co.
21. Levy MN, and Martin PJ: Neural control of the heart. In Berne SR, Sperelakis N, and Geiger SR: Handbook of physiology, Sect 2, The cardiovascular system, vol 1, The heart, Bethesda, Md, 1979, American Physiological Society.
22. Rushmer RF: Structure and function of the cardiovascular system, ed 2, Philadelphia, 1976, WB Saunders Co.
23. Coleridge JCG and Coleridge HM: Chemoreflex regulation of the heart. In Berne SR, Sperelakis N, and Geiger SR: Handbook of physiology, Sect 2, The cardiovascular system, vol 2, The heart, Bethesda, Md, 1979, American Physiological Society.
24. Downing SE: Baroreceptor regulation of the heart. In Berne SR, Sperelakis N, and Geiger SR: Handbook of physiology, Sect 2, The cardiovascular system, vol 1, The heart, Bethesda, Md, 1979, American Physiological Society.
25. Mark AL and Abboud FM: Myocardial blood flow: neuro-humoral determinants. In Zelis R: The peripheral circulation, New York, 1975, Grune & Stratton.
26. Bordicks KJ: Patterns of shock, New York, 1965, The Macmillan Co.
27. Goldberger AL and Goldberger E: Clinical electrocardiography, ed 2, St Louis, 1981, The CV Mosby Co.
28. Phillips RE and Feeney MK: The cardiac rhythms: a systematic approach to interpretation, Philadelphia, 1973, WB Saunders Co.

8

Ventilation

Craig L. Scanlan

The primary function of the lung is to supply the body with oxygen and to remove the waste product of metabolism, carbon dioxide. To fulfill this function, the lung must be adequately ventilated. Whereas respiration as a whole involves many complex chemical and physiologic events, ventilation is defined simply as the mechanical movement of air into and out of the lungs.

In health, ventilation is efficiently regulated to meet body needs under a wide variety of circumstances. In disease, this normal process can be disrupted, resulting in inadequate ventilation, inefficient ventilation, or an excessive work of breathing. Respiratory care can help restore adequate and efficient ventilation in such circumstances, reduce the work of breathing, and even provide artificial ventilation when necessary.

The effective provision of respiratory care demands in-depth knowledge of both the normal mechanical processes underlying ventilation and how various abnormalities affect these processes.

OBJECTIVES

After completion of this chapter, the reader will be able to:

1. Describe the events of a normal breathing cycle in terms of changes in pressure, flow, and volume;

2. Apply functional definitions to differentiate between and interrelate the various lung volumes and capacities;

3. Compare and contrast the elastic and frictional forces opposing inflation of the lung;

4. Explain the factors contributing to expiratory flow limitations in both health and disease;

5. Differentiate between the mechanical and metabolic work (oxygen cost) involved in ventilation and their significance in health and disease;

6. Relate the mechanical properties of the lung to regional and local differences in the distribution of ventilation during inspiration;

7. Differentiate between the efficiency and effectiveness of ventilation as related to alveolar ventilation and carbon dioxide excretion.

KEY TERMS

Most terms used in this chapter are defined in context. The following terms are introduced without explicit definition, but may be found in the text glossary:

ankylosing spondylitis	intrapleural
ascites	intrapulmonary
cartilaginous	intubation
collagen	kyphoscoliosis
distensibility	phospholipid
endotracheal	plethysmograph
impedance	pneumotachygraph
interphase	spirometer
intraalveolar	thoracotomy

MECHANICS OF VENTILATION

Normal resting ventilation is a cyclic activity consisting of two components: an inward flow of air, called inhalation or inspiration, and an outward flow, called exhalation or expiration. During each cycle, a volume of gas is moved into and out of the respiratory tract. This cyclical volume, measured during either inspiration or expiration, is called the tidal volume, abbreviated as V_T.

Whereas tidal volume exchange satisfies normal resting metabolic needs, sufficient lung reserves must exist to meet special demands, such as those occurring during exercise. A standard system of nomenclature is used to identify these additional lung volumes and capacities.

Lung volumes and capacities

Fig. 8-1 illustrates the various divisions of lung volume.[1] The lower dashed line identifies the end-expiratory resting level and the upper dashed line, the tidal volume at end-inspiration.

Four lung volumes constitute the total lung capacity, or TLC. These include the tidal volume (already described), the inspiratory reserve volume, the expiratory reserve volume, and the residual volume.

The inspiratory reserve volume, or IRV, is the maximum volume of air that can be inhaled following a normal, quiet inspiration. The expiratory reserve volume, or ERV, is the total amount of gas that can be exhaled from the lung following a quiet exhalation. The residual vol-

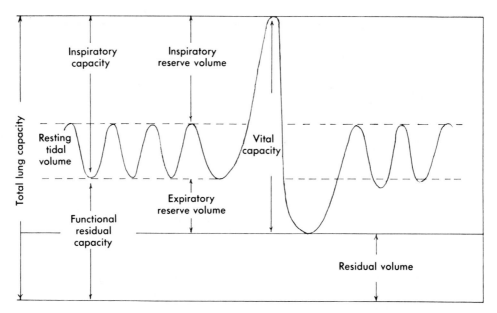

Fig. 8-1 Lung capacities and volumes. Volumetric divisions of the total gas capacity of the lungs. A capacity consists of two or more volumes. (See text for description.)

ume, or RV, is the volume of gas remaining in the lungs after a complete exhalation.

By definition, a lung capacity consists of two or more lung volumes. Traditionally, four lung capacities are so defined: the total lung capacity (TLC), the functional residual capacity (FRC), the inspiratory capacity (IC), and the vital capacity (VC).

As we have already seen, the TLC is the sum of all four lung volumes. Functionally, the TLC is defined as the total amount of gas in the lungs after a maximum inspiration.

The FRC is the sum of the residual volume and the expiratory reserve volume (RV + ERV). Functionally, the FRC is defined as the total amount of gas left in the lungs after a resting expiration. As we will see later, this resting expiratory level is maintained by the opposing forces of the chest wall and lungs.

The VC is the sum of the inspiratory reserve volume, the tidal volume, and the expiratory reserve volume (IRV + V_T + ERV). Functionally, the VC is defined as the total amount of air that can be exhaled after a maximum inspiration.

Lastly, the IC is the sum of the tidal volume and inspiratory reserve volume (V_T + IRV). Functionally, the IC represents the maximum amount of air that can be inhaled from the resting end-expiratory level, or FRC.

Chapter 17 reviews these lung volumes and capacities in more detail and provides additional information on their clinical measurement and use in diagnosis.

Pressure differences during breathing

Changes in lung volume occur in response to pressure gradients created by thoracic expansion and contraction.[2]

Fig. 8-2 portrays the key pressures and pressure gradients involved in ventilation. By convention, these pressures are measured in centimeters of water (cm H_2O) and expressed in units relative to atmospheric pressure. Thus a respiratory pressure of "0" is equivalent to 1034 cm H_2O or 760 mm Hg.

Mouth pressure, or pressure at the airway opening, is abbreviated by the term P_{ao}. Unless positive pressure is applied to the airway, P_{ao} is always zero. Pressure at the body surface (P_{bs}), equivalent to atmospheric pressure, also is normally zero. The primary exception to this generalization is negative pressure ventilation. Alveolar pressure (P_{alv}), often referred to as intrapulmonary pressure, varies throughout the breathing cycle. Pleural pressure (P_{pl}), which is normally negative during quiet breathing, also varies throughout the breathing cycle.

A difference between any two of these four primary pressure measurements is called a *pressure gradient*. Three key pressure gradients are involved in ventilation: the transrespiratory pressure gradient, the transpulmonary pressure gradient, and the transthoracic pressure.[3]

The transrespiratory pressure gradient (P_{rs}) represents the difference in pressure between the atmosphere (body surface) and the alveoli:

$$P_{rs} = P_{alv} - P_{bs}$$

In a spontaneously breathing person, both the pressure at the body surface and the pressure at the airway opening are equal to atmospheric pressure. Therefore, we can substitute P_{ao} for P_{bs}:

$$P_{rs} = P_{alv} - P_{ao}$$

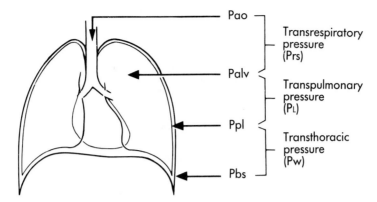

Fig. 8-2 Pressures involved in ventilation. Pao = pressure at the airway opening (mouth pressure); Palv = pressure in the alveoli (intrapulmonary pressure); Ppl = pressure in the pleural space (intrapleural pressure); Pbs = pressure at the body surface. Transrespiratory pressure gradient (Prs = Palv − Pao) is responsible for gas flow into and out of lungs. Transpulmonary pressure gradient (P_L = Palv − Ppl) is responsible for degree of alveolar inflation. Transthoracic pressure gradient (Pw = Ppl − Pbs) is difference in pressure across chest wall, or total pressure necessary to expand or contract lungs and chest wall together. (From Martin L: Pulmonary physiology in clinical practice: the essentials for patient care and evaluation, St Louis, 1987, The CV Mosby Co.)

The transrespiratory pressure gradient is responsible for the actual flow of gas into and out of the alveoli during breathing.[2]

The transpulmonary pressure gradient or pressure across the lung (abbreviated as P_L) represents the difference in pressure between the alveoli and the pleural space:

$$P_L = P_{alv} - P_{pl}$$

The transpulmonary pressure gradient represents the pressure difference responsible for maintaining alveolar inflation. Moreover, changes in the transpulmonary pressure gradient during active breathing are associated with the corresponding changes in alveolar volume.[4]

The transthoracic pressure gradient (Pw) represents the difference in pressure between the pleural space and the body surface:

$$P_W = P_{pl} - P_{bs}$$

As the pressure difference across the chest wall, the transthoracic pressure gradient represents the total pressure necessary to expand or contract the lungs and chest wall together.[3]

Fig. 8-3 portrays the key pressure, flow, and volume events occurring during a normal breathing cycle, in which the glottis is maintained in an open position.[2] Since P_{bs} and P_{ao} remain at zero throughout the cycle, only P_{alv} and P_{pl} are measured.

Prior to the beginning of inspiration, pleural pressure is about −5 cm H_2O and alveolar pressure is 0 cm H_2O. Thus, a transpulmonary pressure gradient of about −5 cm H_2O exists in the resting state. This normal resting, transpulmonary pressure gradient maintains the lung and alveoli at their resting inflation volume, that is, the functional residual capacity. With both alveolar pressure and the pressure at the airway opening being zero, the transrespiratory pressure gradient at this point is zero, and no gas moves into or out of the respiratory tract.

As inspiration begins, muscular effort expands the thorax. Thoracic expansion increases the transthoracic pressure gradient by causing a decrease in pleural pressure. As the pleural pressure drops, the transpulmonary pressure gradient widens, thereby causing the alveoli to expand. As the alveoli expand, alveolar pressures drop below the pressure at the airway opening. This negative transrespiratory pressure gradient causes air to move from the airway opening to the alveoli, increasing their volume.

As pleural pressures continue to decrease toward the end of inspiration, alveolar pressures begin to equilibrate with the atmosphere, alveolar filling slows, and inspiratory flow decreases to zero. At this point, called end-inspiration, alveolar pressure returns to zero. At end-inspiration, the transpulmonary pressure gradient reaches its maximum value (about −10 cm H_2O), corresponding to the tidal inflation volume.

As expiration begins, the thorax contracts, and pleural pressure starts to rise. As the pleural pressure rises, the transpulmonary pressure gradient narrows, and the alveoli begin to deflate. As the alveoli become smaller, alveolar pressure begins to exceed that at the airway opening. This positive transrespiratory pressure gradient now causes air to move out from alveoli to the airway opening, to be exhaled to the atmosphere. As alveolar pressure again equilibrates with the atmosphere, flow ceases, and a new cycle begins.

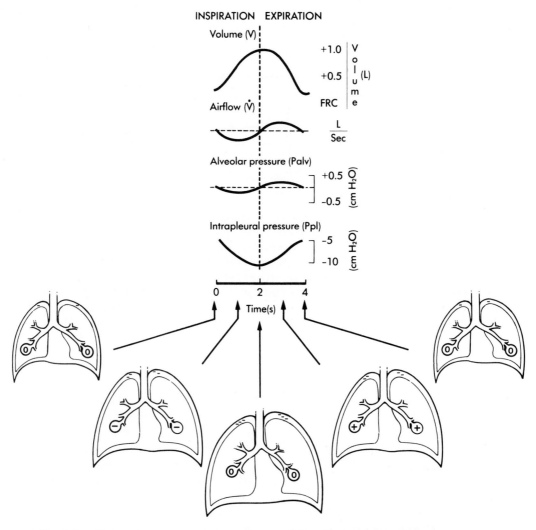

Fig. 8-3   Changes in pressure, volume, and flow during a single breath. (From Martin L: Pulmonary physiology in clinical practice: the essentials for patient care and evaluation, St Louis, 1987, The CV Mosby Co.)

Although these pressure events represent those occurring during normal tidal volume excursions, similar pressure changes occur during deeper inspiration and expiration. Of course, the magnitude of the pressure changes is greater with deeper breathing. During forced expiration pleural pressure may actually rise above atmospheric pressure. Before looking at these special circumstances, however, we will consider the forces opposing inflation of the lung.

Forces opposing inflation of the lung

Generation of the pressure differences necessary to move gas into the lungs requires that several opposing forces be overcome. Whereas forces must be overcome during inspiration, normal (unforced) expiration is accomplished passively, using energy stored during inspiration to move gas out of the lungs.[5] Forced exhalation, on the

other hand, represents a special case, which we will consider separately.

The forces opposing lung inflation may be grouped into two major categories: elastic forces and frictional forces.[6] Elastic forces represent static opposition to expansion of the lungs and thorax. Frictional forces represent dynamic opposition to the movement of gas and tissues during active breathing.

Elastic opposition to ventilation. Because of the presence of elastic and collagen fibers in its parenchyma, the lung possesses the property of *elasticity*. Elasticity is the physical tendency of a structure to offer resistance to a stretching force.[7] When stretched, an elastic body tends to return to its original shape.

Hooke's law. Elastic behavior is defined according to Hooke's law. This law states that the tension developed when an elastic structure is stretched is proportional to the

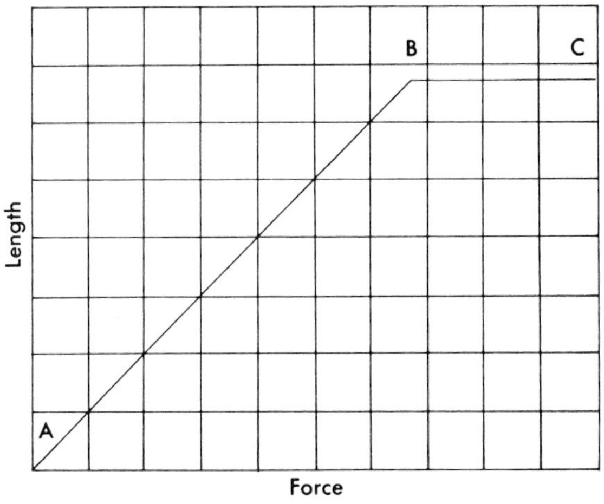

Fig. 8-4 Graphic demonstration of compliance of a simple spring (increase in length/increase in force). With increasing force, the spring lengthens in a linear manner, from *A* to *B*, but at the point of maximum stretch, further force produces no additional increase in length, *B* to *C*.

degree of deformation produced.[5] When applied to a longitudinal element such as a wire or spring, Hooke's law is expressed mathematically by the following equation:

$$F/A = E \times \left[\frac{L - L_o}{L_o}\right]$$

where *F/A* is the applied force per unit area or tension (in dynes/cm^2), L_o is the resting or "unstressed" length of the wire or spring, *L* is the stretched length, and *E* is the elastance of the element being stretched.

Fig. 8-4 provides a graphic example of Hooke's law as applied to a spring. As indicated in the above equation, with increasing tension or force the spring lengthens in a linear manner. However, the ability of the spring to stretch is limited. Once the point of maximum stretch is reached, additional tension produces little additional increase in length. Further tension actually may break the spring.

As applied to the lung, stretching is equivalent to volumetric inflation, which is opposed by elastic forces. To increase lung volume, pressure (F/A) must be applied. We therefore may rewrite Hooke's law as follows:

$$\Delta P = E \times \left[\frac{V - V_o}{V_o}\right]$$

where ΔP is the change in pressure applied to the lung, V_o is the resting volume, *V* is the inflated volume, and *E* is the elastance of the lung.

Rearranging the equation to solve for elastance *(E)*:

$$E = \frac{\Delta P}{\left[\frac{V - V_o}{V_o}\right]}$$

or

$$E = \frac{\Delta P}{\Delta V}$$

This property of elastance is best demonstrated by subjecting an excised lung to different degrees of force (pressure) and measuring its stretch (inflation volume). Fig. 8-5 depicts a simple experiment designed to demonstrate the elastic properties of an excised lung.

To simulate the pressure events of breathing, the lung is placed in a sealed jar. Inflation force is provided by an external pump, which varies the pressure around the lung inside the jar, in a manner similar to thoracic expansion and contraction. The amount of stretch is measured as volume by a spirometer. As was done with the spring, changes in volume for a given pressure on a graph are plotted.

During inflation (inspiration), as predicted by Hooke's law, greater and greater negative pressures are required to stretch the lung to a larger volume. Moreover, as the lung is stretched to its maximum, the inflation "curve" flattens, indicating increasing opposition to expansion.

As with a spring under tension, deflation, or expiration, occurs passively as pressure in the jar is raised toward atmospheric. However, deflation does not follow the inflation curve, as Hooke's law would predict. During deflation, the lung volume at any given pressure is greater than during inflation, signifying a change in elastance. This difference between the inflation and deflation curves is called *hysteresis*.[8] Clearly, lung inflation and deflation must be affected by factors other than simple elastic tissue forces.

Surface tension forces. The hysteresis exhibited by the lung is attributable, in part, to the presence of surface tension forces in the alveoli.[9] The role of surface tension forces in lung inflation and deflation was first demonstrated by von Neergaard in 1929.[10]

As depicted in Fig. 8-6, von Neergaard compared the volume-pressure curves of a lung filled with saline to those obtained when the lung was filled with air. Compared to the air-filled lung, less pressure was required to inflate the saline-filled lung to a given volume. Moreover, only when filled with air did the lung exhibit hysteresis.

In combination, these two observations lead to the conclusion that the presence of a gas-fluid interphase in the air-filled lung (not present in the fluid-filled lung) altered its inflation-deflation characteristics. First, the presence of the gas-fluid interphase increased the elastic recoil of the lung, making it harder to inflate. Second, the presence of the gas-fluid interphase altered the elasticity of the lung according to its volume.

We now know that a lung filled with air is harder to inflate than one filled with saline because of surface tension forces acting at the gas-fluid interphase of the alveoli. As described in Chapter 4, the microscopic structure of the lung has millions of alveoli, each in intimate contact with a thin film of fluid. The presence of this gas-fluid interphase subjects these "alveolar bubbles" to surface tension forces, which, according to Laplace's law, tend to contract the alveoli and compress the gas inside them.

Thus the elastic properties of the lung are a result of

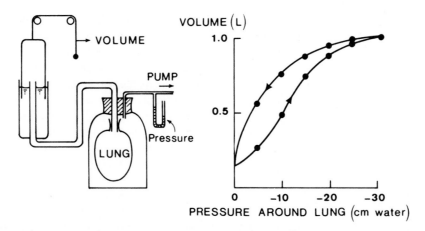

Fig. 8-5   Measurement of the pressure-volume curve of an excised lung. The lung is held at each pressure for a few seconds while its volume is measured. The curve is nonlinear and flattens at high expanding pressures. Note that the inflation and deflation curves are not the same; this difference is called *hysteresis*. (From West JB: Respiratory physiology: the essentials, ed 3, Baltimore, 1985, Williams & Wilkins Co.)

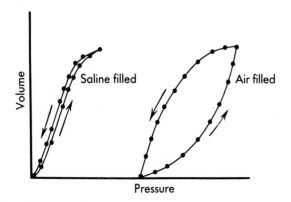

Fig. 8-6   Static pressure-volume curves of saline-filled and air-filled excised lungs, demonstrating the effects of elastic forces (left) and elastic plus surface tension forces (right) on static compliance of the lung. (From Slonim NB and Hamilton LH: Respiratory physiology, ed 5, St Louis, 1987, The CV Mosby Co.)

both the inherent elasticity of its tissues and the action of surface tension forces in the alveoli. Furthermore, the fact that surface tension forces tend to cause alveolar collapse explains, in part, why the inflation and deflation curves of the lung are so different. During inflation, additional pressure is needed at a given volume to open alveoli collapsed by surface tension forces. During early deflation from maximum lung volume, all alveoli are open, and less pressure is required to maintain a given volume.

However, both the inflation and deflation pressures of the lung are less than would be predicted according to Laplace's law.[8] Although some alveoli collapse during deflation, the inherent instability expected in a lung consisting of some 300 million bubbles of different sizes simply does not occur.

These findings suggest that the surface tension forces in the lung are lower than would normally occur at a simple water-gas interface. If this was not a fact, small alveoli would become highly unstable, deflation would result in massive alveolar collapse, and each inflation would require extraordinary pressures to reopen these collapsed alveoli.[11]

Surface tension forces in the lung are lowered by the presence of a remarkable substance called pulmonary surfactant. Pulmonary surfactant, believed to be produced by the type II alveolar cells, consists mainly of the phospholipid dipalmitoyl lecithin synthesized from fatty acids.[9]

Like any surface-active agent, pulmonary surfactant has the ability to lower surface tension. For example, a physiologic saline solution exhibits a surface tension of about 70 dynes/cm. Lung extract, on the other hand, exhibits an average surface tension of about 25 dynes/cm.[8] This characteristic alone increases the ease with which alveoli can be inflated, thereby decreasing the pressure differences (and work) necessary to achieve a given lung volume.[12]

However, unlike typical surface-active detergents, pulmonary surfactant has the unique ability to vary surface tension according to its area of exposure.[8] As the area of exposure increases, the ability of pulmonary surfactant to lower surface tension decreases. On the other hand, as the area of exposure decreases, the ability of pulmonary surfactant to lower surface tension increases.

In the lungs, this unique property of pulmonary surfactant is critical in maintaining alveolar stability. In small alveoli (with small surface areas), pulmonary surfactant exerts its maximum effect, dramatically lowering their surface tension and increasing their stability. Surface tension in larger alveoli is less affected. This variable effect tends to equalize deflation pressures, thereby preventing smaller alveoli from collapsing into larger ones.[11-13]

Moreover, the ability of pulmonary surfactant to vary its

surface tension according to area of exposure helps explain inflation-deflation hysteresis. As the lung inflates, surfactant exerts less effect, and surface tension increases; as the lung deflates, surfactant exerts more influence, and surface tension decreases. This lowering of surface tension during deflation prevents the recurrent closure of alveoli and ensures that the next inflation does not have to occur from a collapsed state.

The half-life of pulmonary surfactant is measured in hours, and if its natural replacement is impaired or it is destroyed faster than it can be replaced, alveolar collapse (atelectasis) rapidly develops.[11] Were it not for the action of pulmonary surfactant, inflating partially collapsed alveoli would require great physical effort, and inhalation would be seriously handicapped. Indeed, in diseased states characterized by absence of surfactant, the work of breathing is at times insurmountable. The best clinical example of the effects of surfactant deficiency is newborn respiratory distress syndrome, described in detail in Chapter 32.

Lung compliance. In combination, tissue elastic forces and surface tension impede inflation of the lung. This total impedance could be quantified according to Hooke's law as the elastance of the lung. According to this formula, a lung with high elastance would be harder to inflate than normal; a lung with low elastance would be easier to inflate than normal.

However, pulmonary physiology traditionally uses a measure called *compliance* to measure the opposition of the lung to inflation. Whereas elastance is the tendency of a structure to resist deformation, compliance represents the relative ease with which a body stretches, or its relative "distensibility." Compliance is thus the reciprocal of elastance:

$$\text{Compliance} = \frac{1}{\text{Elastance}}$$

Or, using Hooke's law:

$$\text{Compliance} = \frac{1}{[\Delta P/\Delta V]}$$

$$\text{Compliance} = \frac{\Delta V}{\Delta P}$$

Therefore, compliance of the lung (C_L) is defined as the volume change per unit of pressure change and is traditionally measured in liters per centimeter of water:

$$C_L = \frac{\Delta V \text{ (liters)}}{\Delta P \text{ (cm H}_2\text{O)}}$$

The volume component of the compliance equation is measured simply as the inhaled volume at any given pressure change. The pressure component represents the difference between the alveolar and pleural pressures, the transpulmonary pressure gradient.[1] Normal adult lung compliance ranges from 0.1 to 0.4 L/cm H_2O, with an average value of 0.2 L/cm H_2O.

To eliminate factors such as airflow resistance from contributing to this pressure gradient, compliance must be measured under *static* conditions, or conditions of no airflow. When there is no airflow, alveolar pressure equals zero. Therefore the transpulmonary pressure gradient under static conditions equals the intrapleural pressure, and compliance of the lung (C_L) equals:

$$C_L = \frac{\Delta V \text{ (liters)}}{\Delta P_{pl} \text{ (cm H}_2\text{O)}}$$

In spontaneously breathing subjects, measurement of compliance requires placement of a balloon in the esophagus.[1] During short breath holds at various volumes, the intrapleural pressure is measured by the esophageal balloon. The resulting graph of change in lung volume versus change in intrapleural pressure (Fig. 8-7, *A*) is the compliance curve of the lung.

Fig. 8-7, *B*, compares a normal compliance curve to that typically observed in emphysema and pulmonary fibrosis. As compared to normal, the curve of the patient with emphysema has a steeper slope, indicating a greater change in volume for a given pressure change, that is, an *increased* compliance. This finding is consistent with the loss of elastic fibers that occurs in some forms of emphysema, thereby causing an increase in distensibility of the lungs.

On the other hand, the curve of the patient with fibrosis has less slope than the normal curve. This indicates a lesser change in volume for a given pressure change, that is, a *decreased* compliance. This observation is consistent with the increase in connective tissue characterizing interstitial fibrosis and the resultant stiffening of the lungs.

Chest wall compliance. Of course, the lungs do not operate in isolation. Inflation and deflation of the lungs occur with, and by virtue of, changes in the dimensions of the chest wall.

The relationship between the lungs and chest wall is best illustrated when they are separated. Fig. 8-8 compares the intact lung-thorax relationship to that observed when the "seal" between them is broken, as would occur during surgical opening of the chest (a thoracotomy).

In Fig. 8-8, *A*, the intact lungs and thorax are at the resting level, or FRC. Fig. 8-8, *B*, depicts the results of exposing the pleural space to atmospheric pressure by opening the thorax. With pleural pressure now being atmospheric (instead of negative), the transpulmonary pressure gradient is lost, and the lungs collapse down to a smaller volume, called the minimal air volume. No longer drawn in by the contracting tendency of the lungs, the chest wall actually expands upward to its unopposed resting position.

Fig. 8-8, *C*, plots the volumes of the lungs and thorax relative to vital capacity (VC). As is evident, the normal lung-thorax resting position is about 30% of the VC. However, with disruption of the normal lung-thorax relationship, the lung collapses down to about 40% of the RV,

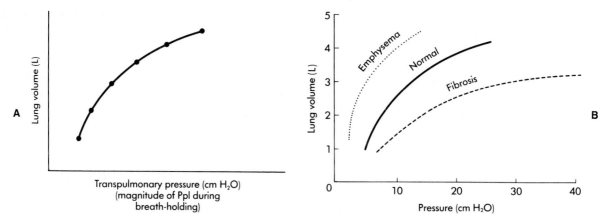

Fig. 8-7   A, Compliance measurement. After swallowing an esophageal tube, the patient inhales to a specified lung volume and holds his breath with the glottis open, assuring an alveolar pressure of zero. The amount of air inhaled (change in volume) divided by the change in esophageal pressure (read from a pressure meter) is the compliance at that point. Measurements are recorded at several different lung volumes, generating a compliance curve. **B,** Compliance curves. Normal lung compliance is approximately 0.2 L/cm H_2O. Compliance is high in emphysema and low in pulmonary fibrosis. (From Martin L: Pulmonary physiology in clinical practice: the essentials for patient care and evaluation, St Louis, 1987, The CV Mosby Co.)

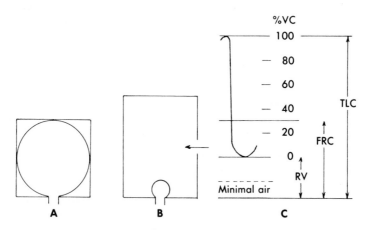

Fig. 8-8   The resting levels of the intact lung-thorax and the separated lung and thorax are plotted against the total lung capacity. **A,** The intact system at its resting level contains the *FRC* and is expanded to about 30% of the *VC*. **B,** The arrow indicates a break in the thoracic wall, exposing the lung to atmosphere and destroying the lung-thorax seal. The lung, containing the *minimal air*, collapses to a new resting level, which is about 40% of the *RV,* and the thorax expands to its own unopposed level of about 70% of the *VC.*

while the thorax expands to a level equivalent to about 70% of the VC.

These observations confirm that the chest wall, like the lungs, has elastic properties. The elastic properties of the chest wall are a result of the configuration of its bones and musculature, as described in Chapter 6. However, as we now know, the lungs tend only to collapse. The chest wall, on the other hand, may recoil either inward or outward. Which direction the chest wall tends to move depends on its initial volume, which, in turn, depends on its relationship to lung inflation.

To better understand how these two systems of elastic energy relate to one another, consider the lung-thorax complex as consisting of one set of bowed, flat springs (the chest wall) tending to expand, tied to a stretched, coiled spring (lungs) tending to contract (Fig. 8-9). Expansion and contraction of the coiled spring representing the lungs causes an increase and decrease, respectively, in lung volume.

At the resting level, the forces of the chest wall and lungs are in balance; the expansion tendency of the chest wall is offset by the contractile force of the lungs. It is this

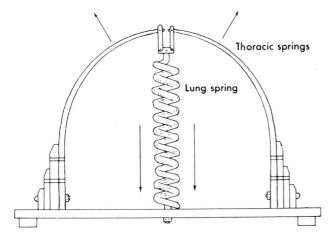

Thoracic springs

Lung spring

Fig. 8-9   The counteracting forces of the lungs and thorax are schematically represented by two sets of springs. In the resting position, the bowed flat *thoracic springs* are shown as held under bent tension by the coiled *lung spring,* itself partially stretched by the action. *Arrows* indicate the direction each spring tends to move to reach its own position of rest. From the lung-thorax resting position, the thorax can expand or contract, depending on the action of the ventilatory muscles. These muscles can assist the *thoracic springs* to overcome the restraint of the *lung spring,* or they can compress the *thoracic springs* and assist the recoil of the *lung spring.*

balance in forces that determines the resting lung volume, or FRC. The opposing forces between the chest wall and lungs are responsible, in part, for developing the negative pressure that normally exists in the intrapleural space.

Inhalation can occur only when the balance between the forces of the lung and chest wall is broken by the muscular energy needed to overcome the contractile force of the lungs.[5] During early inhalation, expansion of the lungs is facilitated by the tendency of the chest wall to expand toward its natural resting level. However, as lung expansion approaches its maximum (about 70% of the vital capacity) the chest wall reaches its equilibrium point, above which it will resist further expansion. Muscular effort must then overcome the contractile tendency of both the lungs and chest wall.

During normal exhalation, the potential energy "stored" in the stretched lungs (and chest wall at high volumes) is sufficient to cause deflation back to the resting level without muscular effort. However, exhalation below the resting level requires active muscular effort to overcome the tendency of the chest wall to expand. As described in Chapter 6, this energy is provided by the expiratory muscles.

Compliance of the chest wall, like that of the lungs, is a measure of its ease of expansion or distensibility. In fact, the normal compliance of the chest wall is approximately equal to that of the lungs, about 0.2 L/cm H_2O. Clinically, disorders such as severe obesity, kyphoscoliosis, and ankylosing spondylitis affect the elastic properties of the chest wall and limit lung expansion. However, to under-

stand the compliance of the respiratory system as a whole, we must consider the elastic behavior of both the lungs and chest wall in tandem.

Total compliance. The total compliance of the respiratory system as a whole, or lung-thorax compliance, represents the interaction between the compliance of the lung (C_L) and the compliance of the thorax (C_T). Because lung and thoracic compliance work in parallel, the total compliance of the lung-thorax system is less than that of either the lung or the thorax alone. As with electrical resistors in a parallel circuit, total lung-thorax compliance (C_{LT}) is calculated as follows:

$$\frac{1}{C_{LT}} = \frac{1}{C_L} + \frac{1}{C_T}$$

Lung-thorax compliance can be measured in one of three general ways. In the first method, depicted in Fig. 8-10, a completely relaxed or anesthetized subject is placed in a body respirator. Ventilation is controlled by the application of negative pressure to the surface of the body. By holding the negative pressure at various values and correlating these values with the volume of air, the subject subsequently exhales into a spirometer, the overall distensibility of the lung-thorax system can be calculated. C_{LT} of normal subjects measured by this method is about 0.1 L/cm H_2O.

In the second method, an anesthetized subject is intubated with a cuffed endotracheal tube. By holding the lungs at various levels of positive pressure, and measuring the corresponding volumes, similar compliance data can be obtained. This method is equivalent to the bedside method of measuring compliance of a patient receiving mechanical ventilation, as described in Chapter 31. C_{LT} of normal subjects measured by this method is also about 0.1 L/cm H_2O.

The third method requires construction of a relaxation pressure curve. With a small, pressure-transmitting plastic tube attached to a recording device and placed in the nose, the subject inhales a measured amount of air from a spirometer. Then, with tightly closed nose and mouth, the subject relaxes the ventilatory muscles; the elastic recoil of lung and thorax produces an alveolar pressure recorded by the nasal tube. Repeated at different tidal volume levels, a curve is produced. Compliance by this method is a bit higher than by the other methods, about 0.12 L/cm H_2O.

Obviously, the total compliance of the respiratory system can be altered from normal by disorders that affect the compliance of the lungs alone, the compliance of the thorax alone, or both simultaneously.

Frictional (nonelastic) opposition to ventilation. Additional opposition to ventilation is provided by frictional forces. Whereas compliance represents a measure of the static impedance to lung inflation caused by elastic forces, frictional opposition is unrelated to the elastic properties of the lungs and thorax. Moreover, frictional opposition to ventilation occurs only in the *dynamic* state, when the sys-

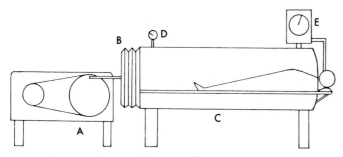

Fig. 8-10   This is a schematic representation of a subject in a body respirator. The motor, *A*, operates bellows, *B*, to create a rhythmic subatmospheric pressure in the cylindrical respirator, *C*, which is recorded by gauge, *D*. As the subject is ventilated by negative pressure applied to his or her body, exhaled air is collected and measured in a meter, *E*. Volume change of the lung-thorax per unit of pressure applied can be determined.

tem is in motion. Frictional opposition to ventilation has two major components: tissue viscous resistance and airway resistance.[14]

Tissue viscous resistance. Tissue viscous resistance represents the impedance to motion caused by displacement of tissues during inspiration and expiration.[14] These tissues include the lungs themselves, the rib cage, the diaphragm, and the abdominal organs. The energy required to displace these structures during inspiration corresponds to the retarding effect of friction in any dynamic system. Normally, tissue viscous resistance accounts for about 20% of the total frictional resistance to lung inflation. Conditions such as obesity, fibrosis, and ascites can increase tissue viscous resistance, thereby increasing the total impedance to ventilation.[5]

Airway resistance. Frictional resistance to ventilation is also caused by the movement of gas through the airways. The impedance to ventilation caused by this movement of gas is called airway resistance, which normally accounts for about 80% of the frictional resistance to ventilation.

Airway resistance (Raw) is defined simply as the ratio between the driving pressure responsible for gas movement and the flow of the gas:

$$Raw = \frac{\Delta P}{\dot{V}}$$

For the lung as a whole, the driving pressure, ΔP, is equivalent to the difference in pressure between the alveoli and the airway opening, the transrespiratory pressure gradient ($P_{alv} - P_{ao}$). Substituting the transrespiratory pressure gradient for ΔP, we derive the following formula for calculating total airway resistance:

$$Raw = \frac{P_{rs}}{\dot{V}}$$

or

$$Raw = \frac{P_{alv} - P_{ao}}{\dot{V}}$$

Traditionally, the transrespiratory pressure gradient is measured in centimeters of water and the flow in liters per second. The units of airway resistance are thus centimeters of water per liter per second. Normal airway resistance ranges from 0.5 to 2.5 cm H_2O/L/s, measured at a standard flow rate of 0.5 L/s.[2]

Measurement. Airway resistance is measured in specialized pulmonary function laboratories.[1] Flows are measured with a sensitive apparatus called a pneumotachometer. Precise alveolar pressures are best determined by a body plethysmograph, an airtight box in which the subject sits. As the subject breathes, the pressure changes in the alveoli are reciprocated in the surrounding box and relayed to a suitable recorder. Details on this technique are provided in Chapter 17.

Factors affecting airway resistance. Factors affecting the resistance to flow in the airways include the pattern of flow, the physical characteristics of the gas being breathed, and the size, shape, and caliber of the airways.

Two major types of airflow patterns characterize the movement of gases in the respiratory tract: laminar flow and turbulent flow.[15] A third pattern, transitional or tracheobronchial flow, represents a combination of the two primary types. The differences between these three flow patterns is illustrated in Fig. 8-11.

In laminar flow the gas moves in discrete cylindrical layers called laminae (layers) or streamlines. Because of frictional forces between the streamlines and the wall of the tube, movement of the outer layer (closest to the tube wall) is minimal. Toward the center of the tube, each layer impedes the next inner layer, but does so less and less. Thus, gas moving in a laminar pattern consists of concentric layers flowing parallel to the tube wall at linear flows that increase toward the center.[16]

Under conditions of laminar flow through a smooth, unbranched tube of fixed dimensions, the difference in pressure required to move a volume of gas through a tube per unit time (flow) is defined by Poiseuille's law:

$$\Delta P = \frac{n8l\dot{V}}{\pi r^4}$$

where ΔP is the driving pressure gradient in dynes per square centimeter, *n* is the viscosity of the gas, *l* is the tube length in centimeters, $\dot{V}$ is the gas flow in cubic centimeters per second, *r* is the tube radius in centimeters, and π and 8 are constants.[17]

If we are not interested in quantitative relationships but only in the general effects of changes in these parameters, the equation can be simplified by eliminating those factors that would not change significantly under the specified conditions. π and 8 are obvious constants. In a given subject, the tubing length, l (representing the airways) is also a constant at any given lung volume. Gas viscosity is also constant under normal physiologic conditions. Thus the above equation can be rewritten as a simple proportionality:

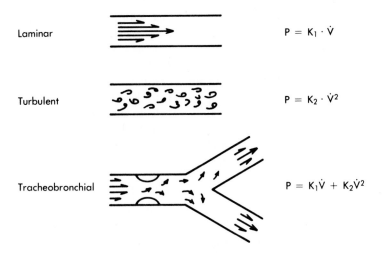

Fig. 8-11   The three patterns of flow: laminar, turbulent, and tracheobronchial. (From Moser KM and Spragg RG: Respiratory emergencies, ed 2, St Louis, 1982, The CV Mosby Co.)

$$\Delta P \cong \frac{\dot{V}}{r^4}$$

Or, rearranging to solve for $\dot{V}$:

$$\dot{V} \cong \Delta P r^4$$

In clinical pulmonary physiology, one of the most frequently encountered conditions is that involving narrowing of the airways through disease. The above proportionalities tell us that under conditions of laminar flow:

1. If the flow of gas is to remain constant, the delivery pressure must vary inversely with the fourth power of the airway's radius. Halving the tube radius will require a sixteen-fold increase in pressure to maintain a constant flow. Thus, to maintain stable ventilation in the presence of narrowing airways, we may need great increases in driving pressure.
2. If the delivery pressure of gas ventilating the lung remains constant, the flow of the gas will vary directly with the fourth power of the radius of the airway. Halving the tube radius will result in a sixteen-fold decrease in flow at a constant pressure. Therefore a small change in bronchial caliber can effect a tremendous change in the amount of gas flow through an airway.

Finally, with all other factors remaining constant, Poiseuille's law tells us that under conditions of laminar flow, the driving pressure is linearly proportional to the flow ($\dot{V}$) times a constant related to gas viscosity, tube length, and radius (K_1)[16]:

$$P = K_1 \times \dot{V}$$

Under certain conditions, the characteristics of gas flow through a tube undergo a significant change. The orderly pattern of concentric layers is no longer maintained. Molecular movement becomes chaotic, with the formation of irregular eddy currents. This type of pattern is called turbulent flow.[17]

The transition from a laminar to turbulent flow pattern depends on the interrelationship between several factors.[16] These factors, including gas density (d), gas viscosity (n), linear velocity (v), and tube radius (r), combine mathematically to determine Reynold's number (N_R):

$$N_R = \frac{v \times d \times 2r}{n}$$

Since the units used for each term cancel out, Reynold's number is dimensionless. Through a smooth-bore tube, laminar flow tends to degenerate into turbulent flow whenever Reynold's number exceeds 2000. If the wall of the tube is irregular, turbulent flow may occur at lower values of N_R.[12] In either case, the higher the linear velocity of the gas, the greater its density, the less its viscosity, and the greater the tube radius, the greater will be Reynold's number and the tendency toward turbulent flow.

Under conditions of turbulent flow, Poiseuille's law no longer applies. Instead, the difference in pressure required to move a volume of gas through a tube per unit of time (flow) is defined by the following equation[12]:

$$\Delta P = \frac{fl\dot{V}^2}{4\pi^2 r^5}$$

where ΔP is the driving pressure gradient, f is a friction factor that incorporates gas density, gas viscosity, and the roughness of the tube wall, l is the tube length, $\dot{V}$ is the gas flow, and r is the tube radius. In terms of the friction factor, as Reynold's number increases, density becomes more important and viscosity less so.[16]

The major difference between this formula and Poiseuille's law is the relationship between ΔP and $\dot{V}$. Whereas in Poiseuille's law, the driving pressure is linearly proportional to the flow, under conditions of turbulent flow, driving pressure is proportional to the square of the flow ($\dot{V}^2$). In equation form:

$$\Delta P \cong K_2 \times \dot{V}^2$$

where K_2 is a constant incorporating the friction factor (f), tube length, and radius.

Table 8-1 provides a comparison of driving pressures necessary with changing flows under laminar and turbulent conditions. As is evident, to double the flow under laminar conditions, one need only double the pressure. However, under conditions of turbulent flow, to double the flow, one must quadruple the driving pressure.

Transitional or tracheobronchial flow is a descriptive term given to the mixture of laminar and turbulent flows found in the normal respiratory tract. Combining the separate equations relating ΔP and $\dot{V}$ under laminar and turbulent conditions, we derive an approximation of the total driving pressure necessary to move gas throughout the respiratory tract, referred to as Rohrer's equation[16]:

$$\Delta P = (K_1 \times \dot{V}) + (K_2 \times \dot{V}^2)$$

Thus, for the lung as a whole, the driving pressure necessary to move gas throughout the respiratory tract represents the sum of the factors associated with laminar and turbulent flow. The magnitude of K_1 and K_2 expresses the relative contributions of these different flow patterns to overall airway resistance. To the extent that flow is mainly laminar, the driving pressure will vary linearly with the flow. On the other hand, when flow is mainly turbulent, the driving pressure will vary exponentially with the flow. All else being equal, laminar flow is most closely associ-

ated with gas viscosity, whereas turbulent flow relates best to gas density.

Distribution of airway resistance. Approximately 90% of the drop in pressure caused by frictional resistance to gas flow occurs in the nose, mouth, and large airways. Only about 10% of the total resistance to flow is attributable to airways less than 2 mm in diameter.[18] At first glance, this finding appears to contradict the fact that frictional resistance is inversely related to the radius of the conducting tube.

The reason for this apparent contradiction is revealed in Table 8-2, which provides values for the diameter, cumulative cross-sectional area, Reynold's number, and pressure differences (ΔP) associated with gas flow for selected portions of the upper and lower airways.[15] Consistent with our prior discussion of pulmonary anatomy (Chapter 6), branching of the tracheobronchial tree increases cross-sectional area throughout the system. Thus, as gas moves toward the alveoli, the combined "radius" of the conducting system increases dramatically. According to the laws of fluid dynamics, this increase in cross-sectional area causes a decrease in gas velocity that lowers Reynold's number, promotes a laminar flow pattern, and decreases the pressure drop caused by gas flow.

Reynold's number is highest in the mouth, trachea, and primary bronchi. Here, gas velocity is high and flow is turbulent. The resulting cumulative pressure drop of about 0.5 cm H_2O represents over 50% of the total pressure drop for the system as a whole. On the other hand, at the level of the terminal bronchioles, the total cross-sectional area has increased by over thirty-fold. Gas velocity is extremely low, and, as indicated by Reynold's number (3), flow is purely laminar. The difference in pressure, about 0.008 cm H_2O, represents less than 1% of the total pressure drop for the system as a whole.

Of course, the diameter of the airways are not constant, but change throughout the respiratory cycle. During inspiration, both the stretch of surrounding lung tissue and the widening transpulmonary pressure gradient increase the diameter of the airways. The greater the lung volume, the greater the influence of these factors on airway caliber. As depicted in Fig. 8-12, this increase in airway diameter at increasing lung volumes manifests itself in a proportionate decrease in airway resistance.[1]

Table 8-1 Comparison of Driving Pressures, Laminar vs Turbulent Flow

Flow ($\dot{V}$)	Driving pressure (ΔP)	
	Laminar	Turbulent
1	1	1
2	2	4
4	4	16
8	8	64
16	16	256

Nondimensional units demonstrating proportionate effect.

Table 8-2 Distribution of Airway Resistance (ΔP)

Order	Location	Diameter (mm)	Cum area (cm)	Reynold's number	ΔP cm H_2O	Cum ΔP cm H_2O
00	Mouth	20.0	3.0	2,986	0.170	0.170
0	Trachea	18.0	2.6	3,513	0.220	0.390
1	Primary bronchi	13.0	2.7	2,930	0.125	0.515
10	Bronchiole	1.63	20.6	47	0.016	1.036
16	Term bronchiole	0.50	92.7	3	0.008	1.089

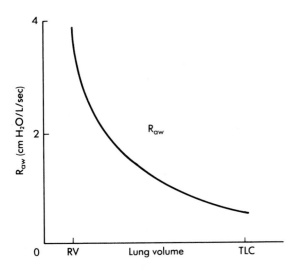

Fig. 8-12 Change in airways resistance (Raw) with change in lung volume. See text for discussion. (From Martin L: Pulmonary physiology in clinical practice: the essentials for patient care and evaluation, St Louis, 1987, The CV Mosby Co.)

On the other hand, as lung volume decreases toward residual volume, airway diameters decrease, and airway resistance rises dramatically. To fully understand the physiologic basis for this effect, and its importance in health and disease, we must take a closer look at the mechanics of exhalation.

Mechanics of exhalation

As previously discussed, airway caliber is determined by several factors. Foremost among these factors are the anatomic support provided to the airway and the pressure difference across its wall.

Anatomic support includes cartilage in the wall of the airway and the "traction" provided by surrounding elastic and connective tissue. As we already know, the larger airways depend mainly on cartilaginous support. Because smaller airways lack cartilage, they must depend on the structural support provided by the surrounding lung parenchyma.[19]

Airway caliber is also maintained by the difference in pressure that normally exists across the airway wall. Just as the transpulmonary pressure gradient is responsible for maintaining alveolar inflation, this pressure difference also helps stabilize the airways, particularly the small ones. As applied to the airways, the difference between the pressure outside their walls (the pleural pressure) and pressure inside the airway itself is called the *transmural pressure gradient*.

As we have learned, during normal, quiet breathing pleural pressure is usually negative, and airway pressure varies minimally around zero. Thus the transmural pressure gradient during normal, quiet breathing is negative, ranging between -5 cm H_2O and -10 cm H_2O. This neg-

ative transmural pressure gradient helps maintain the caliber of the small airways.

However, during forced exhalation, active contraction of the expiratory muscles may cause the pleural pressure to rise above atmospheric pressure, thereby reversing the transmural pressure gradient and eliminating the support it otherwise provides. Should this positive transmural pressure gradient exceed the supporting force provided by the surrounding lung parenchyma, the small airways may actually collapse.

Fig. 8-13 demonstrates this phenomenon as applied to the normal lung. In this example, forceful contraction of the expiratory muscles has caused the transthoracic pressure to rise, thereby increasing pleural pressure from its normal negative value to $+20$ cm H_2O. Alveolar pressure during forced exhalation represents the sum of the pleural pressure ($+20$ cm H_2O in this example) and that due to the elastic forces tending to cause alveolar contraction ($+10$ cm H_2O)[2]:

$$P_{alv} = P_{pl} + P_{recoil}$$
$$P_{alv} = 20 \text{ cm } H_2O + 10 \text{ cm } H_2O$$
$$P_{alv} = 30 \text{ cm } H_2O$$

This initial upstream pressure drops as gas flows from the alveoli toward the airway opening. Moving downstream toward the airway opening, the transmural pressure continually drops. At some point along the airway the pressure inside its wall equals the pressure outside in the pleural "space." This point is referred to as the *equal pressure point*, or EPP. Downstream, beyond this point, the pleural pressure exceeds the pressure inside the airway. The resulting negative transmural pressure gradient encourages airway compression and can lead to actual collapse.[6]

This airway compression increases expiratory airway resistance, thereby limiting flow. In fact, once the EPP is reached, greater expiratory effort will only further increase pleural pressure and restrict flow.[20] This "check-valve" mechanism is responsible for the characteristic leveling of flows at lower lung volumes that is observed in forced exhalation tests of pulmonary function (see Chapter 17).

In healthy subjects the EPP occurs only at lung volumes well below the resting expiratory level. This is because the additional anatomic support provided by the surrounding lung parenchyma tends to oppose the collapsing force created by the negative transmural pressure gradient.

However, in conditions like pulmonary emphysema, the elastic tissue normally responsible for supporting the small airways is destroyed. This destruction of elastic tissue has two major effects: (1) it increases the lung compliance, thereby decreasing its elastic recoil; and (2) it abolishes the major anatomic factor responsible for small airway support.[19]

As shown in Fig. 8-14, these factors have a significant effect on exhalation mechanics. Assuming the patient with emphysema is capable of developing a force expiratory ef-

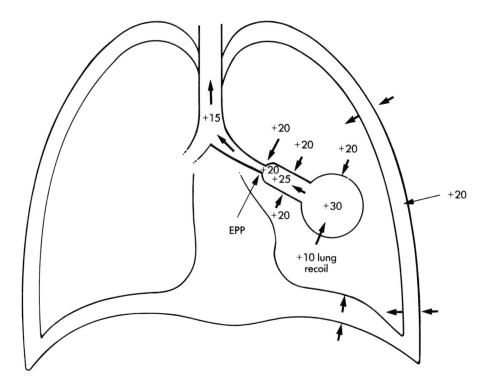

Fig. 8-13   Generation of equal pressure point (EPP) in normal lungs: pleural pressure (Ppl) 20 cm H_2O. This figure shows generation of the EPP when Ppl is 20 cm H_2O during forced exhalation. Alveolar pressure is the sum of Ppl (20 cm H_2O) plus lung elastic recoil pressure (10 cm H_2O), or 30 cm H_2O. Airway pressure falls continually from the alveolus to the mouth. At the EPP, pressure within the airway equals Ppl. Further toward the mouth, airway pressure falls below Ppl, resulting in a narrowed airway and limitation of airflow.   (From Martin L: Pulmonary physiology in clinical practice: the essentials for patient care and evaluation, St Louis, 1987, The CV Mosby Co.)

fort comparable to that developed in the normal individual, pleural pressure also rises to +20 cm H_2O. However, because of the decreased elastic recoil of the lung tissue (P_{recoil} = +5 cm H_2O), the generated alveolar pressure is only +25 cm H_2O. Moreover, because of the loss of elastic tissue, the small airways are more prone to collapse. In combination, these factors cause the EPP to "move" further upstream (toward the alveoli) than in the healthy lung. Airway collapse, therefore, occurs earlier and at higher volumes than in the normal subject. The result is premature trapping of air in the lung.

This condition of air trapping is a common complication of chronic bronchopulmonary disease, often posing a management problem for the respiratory care practitioner. A major consequence of chronic air trapping, because of the loss of elastic tissue, is a gradual elevation of the resting end-expiratory lung volume. As shown in Fig. 8-15, this produces an increase in both the functional residual capacity and the residual volume. Over time, there is a progressive increase in the size of the thorax, especially its anteroposterior diameter. The resulting physical abnormality is called a "barrel chest."

WORK OF BREATHING

Even during normal quiet breathing, work must be done by the respiratory muscles.[21] Normally this work involves the energy expenditure needed to overcome both the elastic and frictional forces opposing inflation. During normal quiet breathing the work accomplished during expiration is recovered from the potential energy that is "stored" in the expanded lung-thorax. However, forced exhalation requires that additional work be performed by the expiratory muscles. How much work is involved in forced expiration depends on the mechanical properties of the lungs and thorax, as previously described.

We can assess the work of breathing in two different but complementary ways.[16] The assessment of mechanical work involves measurement of the physical parameters of force and distance. Assessment of metabolic work involves measurement of the oxygen cost of breathing.

Mechanical work of breathing

In traditional physical terms, work done on an object is defined as the product of the force exerted on the object

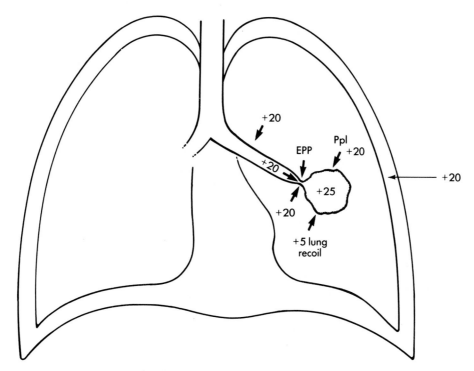

Fig. 8-14 EPP in emphysematous lungs. Despite maximal expiratory effort from total lung capacity, Ppl is 20 cm H_2O, but lung elastic recoil pressure is only 5 cm H_2O (compare with Fig. 8-13). As a result, airway driving pressure in the emphysematous lungs is only 25 cm H_2O. Airway driving pressure dissipates further down the airway and equals the Ppl (EPP) at a point earlier than it is reached in healthy lungs. As a result, the airways narrow or collapse at a larger lung volume than is normal. In patients with emphysema, airway collapse is contributed to by the weakened bronchial walls. (From Martin L: Pulmonary physiology in clinical practice: the essentials for patient care and evaluation, St Louis, 1987, The CV Mosby Co.)

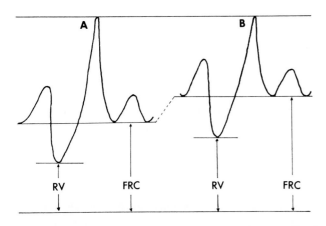

Fig. 8-15 Sketch **A** shows the resting level before, and **B** after, the effect of long-standing airway resistance and/or loss of lung elasticity, as the expansile thoracic springs dominate the pulmonary. Both functional residual capacity and residual volume enlarge. As disease progresses, loss of pulmonary flexibility decreases the expiratory reserve volume, further enlarging the residual volume, and continuing distention may depress the diaphragm to expand the total lung capacity.

times the distance it is moved, measured either in dyne·centimeters (CGS) or joules (SI):

$$\text{Work} = \text{Force} \times \text{distance}$$

Since pressure equals force per unit area (distance^2), and volume is the cube of length (distance^3), the product of pressure *(P)* and volume *(V)* has the same dimension as work:

$$P \times V = \text{Force/area} \times \text{volume}$$
$$P \times V = \text{Force/distance}^2 \times \text{distance}^3$$

or

$$P \times V = \text{Force/distance}^2 \times (\text{distance}^2 \times \text{distance})$$

Cancelling out the distance^2 in both numerator and denominator yields:

$$P \times V = \text{Force} \times \text{distance}$$

Therefore, the mechanical work of breathing can be calculated as the product of the change in pressure across the respiratory system times the resulting change in volume[22]:

$$\text{Work of breathing} = \Delta P \times \Delta V$$

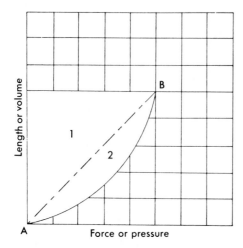

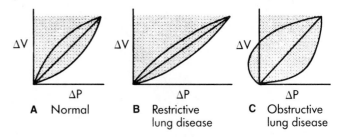

Fig. 8-17   Analysis of the work of breathing (shaded areas) for **A,** a healthy subject; **B,** a patient with restrictive ventilatory impairment; and **C,** a patient with chronic diffuse obstructive bronchopulmonary disease. (From Slonim NB and Hamilton LH: Respiratory physiology, ed 5, St Louis, 1987, The CV Mosby Co.)

Fig. 8-16   Point *A* is the resting level, and *B* is end-inspiration. *Dashed A-B* represents the pressure-volume relationship of pure elastic resistance, and *curved A-B* the "drag" added by nonelastic friction. At *B,* where airflow momentarily ceases, nonelastic resistance is inactive because it is dependent on movement. The curved line thus disappears, leaving only the elastic resistance of stretch. Areas *1* and *2* represent the work of overcoming elastic nonelastic resistance, respectively.

Since the respiratory muscles comprise part of the resistance offered by the chest wall, the total mechanical work of breathing cannot be easily measured during spontaneous breathing. However, total mechanical work can be readily determined during artificial ventilation, provided that the respiratory muscles are completely at rest. For this determination, the change in lung volume is related to the pressure difference between the airway opening and the body surface.[21]

Because we are dealing with the change in one variable (pressure) as related to the change in another (volume), determination of the mechanical work of breathing involves integral calculus. In simple terms, however, integration of the pressure × volume relationship yields an area on the volume-pressure curve of the lung.

Fig. 8-16 portrays a simple volume-pressure relationship for a single inspiration. Change in pressure is plotted on the x-axis, and change in volume is plotted on the y-axis. Thus the product of pressure × volume represents an area on the graph. The greater the area, the greater the amount of work.

Point *A* represents the resting end-expiratory level, with no air flow. Point *B* is equivalent to the pressure and volume occurring at end-inspiration. If we were to slowly inflate the lungs, stopping at several points along the way to plot the volume and pressure changes, we would obtain the straight dashed line *A-B*. Because conditions during these measurements are static, the straight line connecting these points represents the change in volume for a given change in pressure due solely to the elastic properties of the lungs. Thus the slope of straight line *A-B* is the compliance of the lungs. The work done to overcome these

purely elastic forces opposing inflation is represented by the triangular area *l*.

On the other hand, should we reinflate the lungs and measure their changes in pressure and volume during dynamic conditions of gas flow, the straight line relationship no longer pertains. Instead, a curved (solid) line is obtained between points *A* and *B*. This curve represents the additional "drag" imposed on inflation by frictional opposition to tissue and gas movement, consisting mainly of airway resistance. At points of zero flow *(A and B)*, frictional resistance is nonexistent, and the curve rejoins the static compliance line. The work done to overcome opposition caused by these frictional forces is represented by the loop labeled as area *2*.

The total mechanical work of breathing for this single breath is the sum of the work necessary to overcome both the elastic and frictional forces opposing inflation. Graphically, this is represented as the sum of areas *1* and *2*. In health, about two thirds of the total work of breathing is attributable to elastic forces opposing ventilation, with the remaining third caused by frictional resistance to gas and tissue movement.

In diseased states, the work of breathing can dramatically increase. Fig. 8-17 graphically compares the mechanical work of breathing exhibited by a normal subject *(A)* to that observed in a patient with decreased lung compliance or restrictive disease *(B)*, and a patient with increased airway resistance, or obstructive disease *(C)*. Here, both inspiratory and expiratory work are portrayed, with the shaded area of each graph corresponding to the total work done for a complete breath of equal volume.

The area of the volume-pressure curves in both diseased states is greater than that observed with the normal subject, indicating an increase in the mechanical work of breathing. However, close inspection reveals that the reasons for this increase in the mechanical work are different. In the patient with restrictive lung disease, the area of the volume-pressure curve is greater because the slope of the static component (compliance) is less than normal. On the other hand, the area of the volume-pressure curve in the

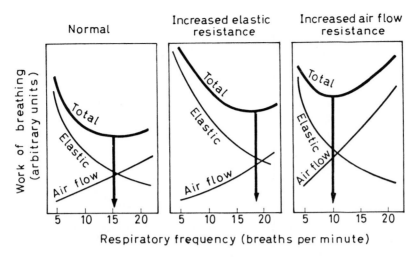

Fig. 8-18 Work done against airflow and elastic resistance together equal total work. Under normal circumstances, the total work of breathing is at a minimum at about 15 breaths per minute (left). For the same minute volume, but with increased elastic resistance (low compliance), minimum work is performed at higher frequencies (middle). However, with increased air flow resistance (right), minimum work occurs at lower rates of breathing. (From Nunn JF: Applied respiratory physiology, ed 2, London, 1977, Butterworth & Co.)

patient with obstructive lung disease is greater because the loop associated with frictional resistance is markedly widened (the leftward "bulge" of the loop indicates positive pleural pressure during expiration).

Even in normal subjects, the mechanical work of breathing is dependent on the pattern of ventilation. Whereas large tidal volumes tend to increase the elastic component of work, high frequencies tend to increase frictional work. In transition among breathing patterns, such as occurs between quiet breathing and exercise, normal individuals "automatically" adjust tidal volume and breathing frequency to minimize the work of breathing.

As depicted in Fig. 8-18, similar adjustments occur in diseased states.[13] Individuals with disorders characterized by an increased elastic work of breathing, such as pulmonary fibrosis, tend to assume a rapid and shallow breathing pattern. For these patients, such a pattern results in the minimum mechanical work necessary to effectively ventilate the lungs. On the other hand, patients with obstructive disorders tend to assume the pattern best able to reduce the frictional work of breathing. In this pattern, breathing tends to be slow and deep.

Exactly how these adjustments in breathing patterns are made is a question subject to considerable debate. However, current knowledge suggests that the gamma-efferent system of the respiratory muscles is primarily responsible (see Chapter 10). Regardless of the underlying mechanism, the body's ability to minimize respiratory work by varying breathing patterns is another good example of efficient homeostasis.

Metabolic work of breathing

To perform their work, the respiratory muscles consume oxygen. Thus the oxygen consumption of the respiratory

muscles reflects their energy requirements and provides an indirect measure of the work of breathing.[23]

The oxygen cost of breathing is assessed by determining the total oxygen consumption of the body at rest and at increased levels of ventilation produced either voluntarily or by carbon dioxide breathing.[21] Provided there are no other factors acting to increase oxygen consumption, the added O_2 uptake is attributed to the metabolism of the respiratory muscles.

The oxygen cost of breathing in normal individuals is approximately 0.5 to 1.0 ml/L of increased ventilation, an amount representing less than 5% of total body oxygen consumption.[21] At high levels of ventilation, however, the oxygen cost of breathing becomes progressively greater.

Of particular importance to the respiratory care practitioner is the fact that in certain diseased states the oxygen cost of breathing increases dramatically with increased levels of ventilation. Fig. 8-19 plots the oxygen consumption of the respiratory muscles (ml/min at STPD) at various levels of ventilation for a normal subject and for a patient with emphysema, a severe obstructive impairment. As ventilation increases, the oxygen consumption of the emphysematous patient's respiratory muscles increases at a much faster rate than that of the normal subject. In fact, this abnormally high oxygen cost of breathing represents a primary limiting factor to exercise in such patients.

THE DISTRIBUTION OF VENTILATION

The distribution of ventilation throughout the normal lung is not uniform. Reasons for this unevenness in the distribution of ventilation are many, involving both regional and local factors.[24] In health, the factors causing uneven ventilation help explain why the lung falls short of

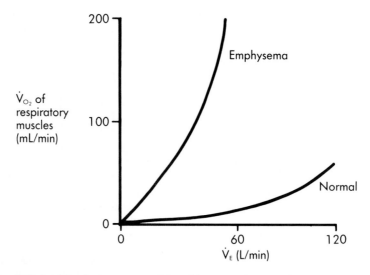

Fig. 8-19 Relationship of oxygen cost of breathing to expiratory minute volume for a healthy subject and for a patient with bronchitis-emphysema syndrome. (From Slonim NB and Hamilton LH: Respiratory physiology, ed 5, St Louis, 1987, The CV Mosby Co. After Campbell EJM, Westlake EK, and Cherniack RM: J Appl Physiol 11:303, 1957.)

being a perfect organ for gas exchange (see Chapter 9). In disease, normal variations in the distribution of ventilation can dramatically worsen and cause significant, even life-threatening, deficiencies in gas exchange. In fact, as described in detail in Chapter 15, the maldistribution of ventilation in diseased states represents the primary cause of impaired oxygen and carbon dioxide exchange.

Regional factors

Two major factors affect the regional distribution of gas in the normal lung: (1) relative differences in thoracic expansion, and (2) regional transpulmonary pressure gradients.[25] In combination, these factors cause proportionately more ventilation to go to the base and periphery of the lung during inspiration than to its apices and more central zones.

Differences in thoracic expansion. Differences in the configuration of the thoracic bony structures and the action of the respiratory muscles cause proportionately more expansion at the lung base than at its apex. In fact, when adjusted for the amount of lung tissue, expansion of the lower part of the chest is about 50% greater than that of the upper chest.[2] Moreover, the action of the diaphragm is such that the lower lobes and segments of the lung are preferentially inflated.

Transpulmonary pressure gradients. Although we have previously described the transpulmonary pressure gradient as if it were equal in all portions of the thorax, it actually varies substantially, both from outside to inside, and from top to bottom.

At any given level of alveolar inflation, the transpulmonary pressure gradient is directly related to the pleural pressure. Since the pleural pressure represents the pressure

on the outer surface (periphery) of the lung, its effect lessens as one moves inward toward more centrally located alveoli. Thus, changes in the transpulmonary pressure gradient are greatest for peripheral alveoli and least for those located in the central zones.[2] Therefore, peripheral alveoli tend to expand proportionately more than their more central counterparts.

Of greater significance in affecting the regional distribution of ventilation are top to bottom differences in pleural pressure, especially in the upright lung.[8] Because of the weight of the upright lung and the effect of gravity, pleural pressure increases by about 0.25 cm H_2O for each centimeter distance from the lung apex to its base. Whereas pleural pressure at the apex is about −10 cm H_2O, pleural pressure at the base is only about −2.5 cm H_2O.[7] Because of these differences in pleural pressures, the transpulmonary pressure gradient at the top of the upright lung is greater than that at the bottom. Alveoli at the apex are therefore maintained at a higher resting volume than those at the base.

Although at a higher resting volume than those at the base, alveoli at the apex expand less during inspiration. Reinspection of the pressure-volume curve of the lung helps explain this phenomenon. As shown in Fig. 8-20, alveoli at the lung apex "sit" on the upper portion of the pressure-volume curve. Because the curve here is relatively flat, a given change in pressure results in only a small change in volume.

On the other hand, alveoli at the lung base are positioned on the middle portion of the pressure-volume curve. Because the curve here is relatively steep, a given change in pressure results in a much larger change in volume.

Therefore, for a given transpulmonary pressure gradi-

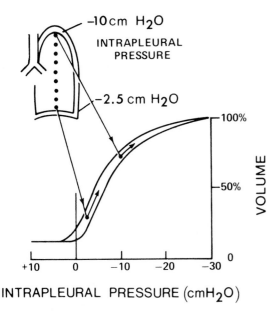

-10cm H₂O
INTRAPLEURAL PRESSURE
-2.5 cm H₂O

100%

50%

0

VOLUME

+10   0   -10   -20   -30

INTRAPLEURAL PRESSURE (cmH₂O)

Fig. 8-20 Causes of regional differences in ventilation down the lung. Due to the weight of the lung and the influence of gravity, the intrapleural pressure at the apex is more negative than at the base. Thus alveoli at the apex are maintained at a higher *resting* inflation volume than those at the base. However, alveoli at the apex reside on the higher portion of the pressure-volume curve, whereas those at the base are positioned on the lower, *steeper* portion. Thus, for an equal change in intrapleural pressure, alveoli at the base expand more on inspiration than those at the apex. (From West JB: Respiratory physiology: the essentials, ed 3, Baltimore, 1985, Williams & Wilkins Co.)

ent, these alveoli will expand more than those at the apex. In fact, the base of the upright lung receives about four times as much ventilation as does the apex.[7]

Although of lesser magnitude, these gravity-dependent differences are also observed in recumbent subjects. When lying on the back, a person's ventilation is still greatest in the "bottom" or dependent zones of the lung, in this case the posterior regions. Likewise, lying on the side causes more ventilation to go to the dependent zones, in this case mainly the lower lung.

Local factors

In addition to these regional factors, alveolar filling and emptying is also affected by local factors. Of particular importance in this regard are differences in the mechanical properties of the individual respiratory units and their accompanying airways. Although these local factors contribute to uneven ventilation in health, their primary influence on distribution of gases occurs in diseased states.

In concept, a simplified respiratory unit consists of an elastic element, the alveolus, and a resistive element, the airway. For a given transpulmonary pressure gradient, the change in alveolar volume that will occur and the time required to affect this change will depend on both the compliance and resistance of the unit as a whole.[8]

Looking at compliance alone, the greater the distensibility of the unit, the greater the volume change for a given transpulmonary pressure gradient. However, units with high compliance have less elastic recoil than normal and will tend to fill and empty more slowly than normal units. On the other hand, units with low compliance (high elastic recoil) fill less and fill and empty faster than normal.

Resistance in the airway leading to the alveolus will also affect emptying and filling. As shown in Fig. 8-21, the amount of a given driving pressure that actually reaches the distal portion of a lung unit depends on the caliber of its airway. Fig. 8-21, *A*, portrays a normal, unobstructed airway. The pressure drop between the beginning of the airway (Pa) and the terminal alveolus (PA) is minimal. Since little pressure is lost in transit through the airway, most of the original driving pressure is available for alveolar inflation.

In Fig. 8-21, *B,* the airway is obstructed between points *b1* and *b2,* creating high resistance to gas flow. Consequently, a substantial drop in pressure ($P_{b1} - P_{b2}$) occurs across the obstruction. Now less of the original driving pressure is available for alveolar inflation, resulting in less volume change. Moreover, the unit in Fig. 8-21, *B,* will fill and empty slower than the normal unit in Fig. 8-21, *A.*

Time constant. In reality, the elastic and flow resistive properties of the lung units cannot be treated in isolation. Together, compliance and resistance determine local rates of alveolar filling and emptying. The relationship between the compliance and resistance of a lung unit can be quantified in a mathematical expression called the *time constant.* The time constant is simply the product of the unit's compliance and resistance:

$$\text{Time constant} = C \times R$$

Substituting the appropriate units for both compliance and resistance into the above formula, we see that the product of these two variables is indeed a time, expressed in seconds:

$$\text{Time constant} = \text{liters/cm H}_2\text{O} \times \text{cm H}_2\text{O/liter/second}$$
$$= \text{liters/cm H}_2\text{O} \times \text{cm H}_2\text{O/liter/second}$$
$$= \text{seconds}$$

According to this formula, a lung unit will have a long time constant when its resistance is high, when its compliance is high, or both. Lung units with long time constants will take more time to fill and empty than units with normal compliance and resistance.

On the other hand, a lung unit with a short time constant would have either low resistance, low compliance, or both. These units will take less time to fill and empty than units with normal compliance and resistance.

Fig. 8-22 demonstrates the effect of time constants on the local distribution of ventilation in the lung. If the time available for inflation is constant, units with long time

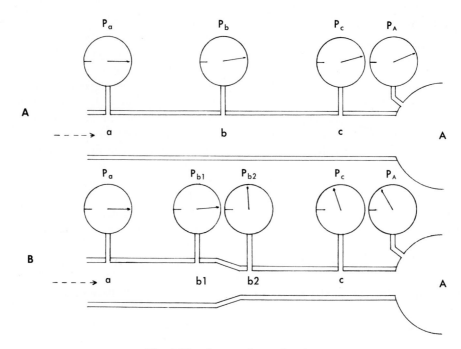

Fig. 8-21 See text for explanation.

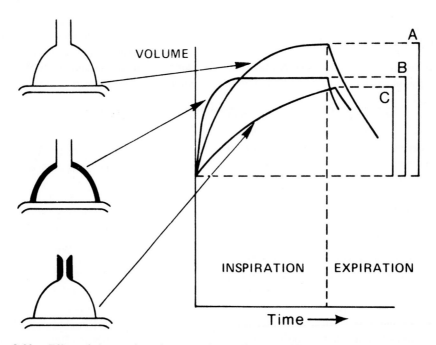

Fig. 8-22 Effect of changes in resistance and compliance on filling and emptying of lung units inflated with equal pressures. Lung unit A has normal resistance and compliance, and fills and empties at a normal rate (normal time constant). Lung unit B has normal resistance but low compliance, fills and empties faster than normal (low time constant), but at a lower volume. Lung unit C has normal compliance but high resistance. It fills and empties slower than normal (high time constant), but also at a lower volume. (From West JB: Respiratory physiology: the essentials, ed 3, Baltimore, 1985, Williams & Wilkins Co.)

constants fill less and empty slower than normal units. Units with short time constants also fill less than normal (because of the low compliance), but quickly fill and empty. In either case, the amount of ventilation going to the abnormal unit is less than that received by the unit with normal compliance and resistance.

Frequency dependence of compliance. Although local in origin, variations in time constant can have a substantial effect on ventilation throughout the lung as a whole. This effect is most evident in diseases characterized by chronic small airway obstruction, such as occurs in emphysema. In such cases, the time constants of many lung units are increased above normal. These lengthened time constants are mainly caused by increased resistance to flow in the small airways, although the loss of normal tissue elastic recoil also contributes to slowed filling and emptying.

Should the rate of breathing increase under these conditions, a unit with a long time constant will fill less and fill and empty slower than one with normal compliance and resistance. Should the high rate of breathing be maintained, more and more of the inspired gas will go to fewer and fewer lung units. With more of the inspired volume going to less lung units, a greater transpulmonary pressure gradient will be required to maintain an equivalent volume exchange. Thus the compliance of the lung will appear to decrease as breathing frequency increases.

This phenomenon, called *frequency dependence of compliance,* is used clinically as a sensitive test of small airways disease.[2] Because assessment of the frequency dependence of compliance involves measuring the change in volume for a given change in transpulmonary pressure during breathing, the compliance value obtained is not a truly static measure. Instead, the term dynamic compliance is used to indicate the effect of resistance on transpulmonary pressure gradients in the dynamic state.

Fig. 8-23 compares the dynamic compliance of a normal subject and one with small airways disease at increasing frequencies of breathing. Whereas the dynamic compliance of the normal subject remains stable as breathing frequency increases, that of the individual with small airways disease decreases progressively.

Obviously, the decrease in dynamic compliance that occurs in patients with small airways disease at higher frequencies of breathing has substantial clinical importance. As compliance drops, the work of breathing increases and with it the oxygen consumption of the respiratory muscles. Moreover, the distribution of ventilation worsens, further impairing oxygen and carbon dioxide exchange. In combination, these factors severely limit the ability of individuals with small airways disease to tolerate increased ventilatory demands, such as those occurring during exercise. More details on the practical aspects of these limitations and their importance in cardiopulmonary rehabilitation are provided in Chapter 34.

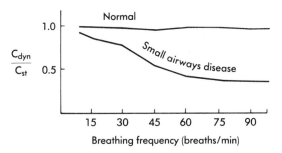

Fig. 8-23 Dynamic compliance. Normally, dynamic compliance is approximately the same as static compliance when the respiratory rate increases. In the presence of small airways disease, dynamic compliance falls relative to static compliance. See text for discussion. (From Martin L: Pulmonary physiology in clinical practice: the essentials for patient care and evaluation, St Louis, 1987, The CV Mosby Co.)

EFFICIENCY AND EFFECTIVENESS OF VENTILATION

Ventilation serves primarily as a mechanism for excretion of the gaseous by-product of metabolism, carbon dioxide. Ideally, this process should be conducted in both an efficient and effective manner. By efficient, we mean that the process should involve as little waste as possible. By effective, we mean that the process should adequately meet body needs.

Efficiency of ventilation

Even in health, the process of ventilation is not efficient. Ventilation is inefficient because substantial amounts of inspired gas are "wasted" on each breath. Wasted ventilation is ventilation that does not participate in gas exchange.

Ventilation is wasted because the lungs are essentially a dead end, as opposed to a continuous exchange circuit. In a continuous exchange circuit, such as that occurring in the circulatory system, fluid flows in and out through separate pathways. Under such conditions, all of the fluid can participate in the exchange and none is wasted.

In a dead-end exchange circuit, on the other hand, fluid must move in and out through the same pathway. Therefore, some of the fluid volume must occupy space in the pathway leading to the exchange area. Because this fluid volume will not have an opportunity to participate in exchange, it is considered wasted.

Minute ventilation. To understand how much ventilation is wasted, we must first determine the total ventilation. By convention, total ventilation is assessed over a standard time period of 1 min. The total amount of gas moving into or out of the lungs during this period is thus called the *minute ventilation.* Traditionally, expired volume is measured, and minute ventilation is symbolized as $\dot{V}_E$. Minute ventilation therefore is calculated as the product of the rate or frequency of breathing (f) times the expired tidal volume:

$$\dot{V}_E = f \times V_T$$

Substituting normal average values for a 70 kg subject, we calculate a normal minute ventilation of 6000 ml or 6.0 L:

$$\dot{V}_E = f \times V_T$$
$$\dot{V}_E = 12 \times 500 \text{ ml}$$
$$= 6000 \text{ ml/min}$$

Obviously, the minute ventilation varies according to the size of the individual and the metabolic rate, ranging from about 5.0 to 10.0 L per minute in the resting state.

Dead space ventilation. Because the lung is a dead end, as opposed to a continuous exchange circuit, not all of the minute ventilation participates in gas exchange. Some of this minute volume must occupy space in the conducting zones of the lung. Since the conducting zones of the lung do not participate in gas exchange, the volume occupying this space will be wasted. Clinically, wasted ventilation is referred to as *dead space.*

Anatomic dead space. The volume constituting the conducting zone of the lungs, including the upper airway, is called the anatomic dead space, abbreviated as V_{Danat}. V_{Danat} averages about 1 ml per pound of normal body weight. Thus, for an individual weighing 150 lb, V_{Danat} is about 150 ml.

Anatomic dead space does not contribute to gas exchange because it is rebreathed. During normal expiration, the first 150 ml of exhaled gas come from the anatomic dead space, and the remaining 350 ml from the alveoli. At the end of exhalation, the airways contain 150 ml of gas that has already undergone gas exchange in the alveoli. With the next inhalation this 150 ml volume will be rebreathed. Thus only about 350 ml of "fresh" or unrebreathed gas reaches the alveoli per breath.

Anatomic dead space is assessed using the single-breath nitrogen test, as described by Fowler.[26] As shown in Fig. 8-24, the nitrogen concentration of expired air is analyzed after a subject breathes 100% oxygen. During the first portion of expiration (coming solely from the conducting zones of the lung), 100% oxygen is exhaled and the nitrogen concentration remains at zero. As anatomic dead space gas begins mixing with gas coming from the alveoli, the nitrogen concentration rises abruptly. Eventually, the nitrogen concentration reaches a plateau, stabilizing at a level equivalent to that coming solely from the alveoli. The anatomic dead space is derived by estimating the middle point of the nitrogen curve.

Alveolar ventilation. To distinguish it from rebreathed gas or dead space volume, the amount of fresh gas reaching the alveoli per breath is called the *alveolar ventilation,* symbolized as V_A. V_A may be calculated by subtracting the anatomic dead space (V_{Danat}) from the tidal volume (V_T):

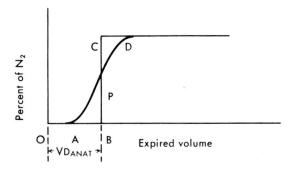

Fig. 8-24 Anatomic deadspace determination. The rise in concentration of nitrogen during a single expiration, after a breath of 100% O_2, is illustrated. Only the initial portion of the breath is included. As the subject expires, the N_2 concentration rises slowly at first as pure deadspace gas is exhaled; then as bronchial air is expired, the N_2 concentration rises abruptly. Since different parts of the lungs empty at different rates, the change from pure deadspace air to alveolar gas appears as an S-shaped curve. By constructing a square wave front *(BC)* so that the areas *ABP* and *DCP* are equal, the anatomic deadspace can be estimated as being equal to the volume expired up to point *B.* (From Ruppel G: Manual of pulmonary function testing, ed 4, St Louis, 1986, The CV Mosby Co.)

$$V_A = V_T - V_{Danat}$$

or, substituting average normal values:

$$V_A = 500 \text{ ml} - 150 \text{ ml}$$
$$= 350 \text{ ml}$$

Rather than calculating V_A on a breath-by-breath basis, we usually determine the amount of fresh gas reaching the alveoli per minute. This alveolar minute ventilation, abbreviated as $\dot{V}_A$, is simply the product of the frequency of breathing (f) times the alveolar ventilation per breath (V_A):

$$\dot{V}_A = f \times V_A$$

Since $V_A = V_T - V_{Danat}$, the above formula may be rewritten as:

$$\dot{V}_A = f \times (V_T - V_{Danat})$$

Substituting average normal values for V_T and V_{Dant}, we calculate a normal alveolar minute ventilation of about 4200 ml or 4.2 L:

$$\dot{V}_A = f \times (V_T - V_{Danat})$$
$$\dot{V}_A = 12 \times (500 \text{ ml} - 150 \text{ ml})$$
$$\dot{V}_A = 12 \times 350 \text{ ml}$$
$$\dot{V}_A = 4200 \text{ ml/min}$$

Alternatively, the amount of anatomic dead space ventilation *per minute* in normal subjects may be calculated as the difference between the total minute ventilation and the alveolar ventilation per minute:

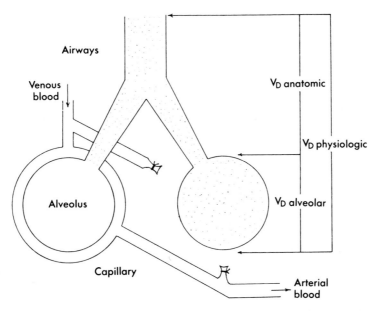

Fig. 8-25 The three types of dead space are shown in this sketch, which schematically represents two alveoli, their supporting airways, and capillaries. One alveolus is normally perfused and ventilated; but the capillary to the other is shown as if it were tied off and removed, so that the alveolus is freely ventilated but not perfused. The relationships of the dead spaces are indicated, as defined in the text.

$$\dot{V}_{Danat} = \dot{V}_E - \dot{V}_A$$

$$\dot{V}_{Danat} = 6000 \text{ ml} - 4200 \text{ ml}$$

$$= 1800 \text{ ml/min}$$

Thus nearly a third (1800 of 6000 ml) of the total ventilation per minute in normal subjects is wasted as rebreathed anatomic dead space.

Alveolar dead space. The above calculations assume that all the fresh gas reaching the alveoli participates in gas exchange. In health, this assumption is generally true. However, in certain disease states, some alveoli may receive adequate ventilation, but still not participate in gas exchange. These alveoli are ventilated but not perfused by the pulmonary circulation. Without perfusion by the pulmonary circulation, gas exchange cannot occur. Thus the volume of gas ventilating unperfused alveoli also is wasted ventilation or dead space.

To distinguish this abnormal wasted ventilation from the normal anatomic dead space, the volume of gas ventilating unperfused alveoli is called *alveolar dead space,* abbreviated as V_{Dalv}. The existence of significant amounts of alveolar dead space always indicates the presence of a pathologic abnormality, usually of the pulmonary circulation. A common clinical example of an abnormality of the pulmonary circulation that would increase V_{Dalv} is a pulmonary embolism. By blocking a portion of the pulmonary circulation, a pulmonary embolism can obstruct perfusion to otherwise normally ventilated alveoli, thereby creating alveolar dead space. Of course, this abnormal alveolar dead space occurs in addition to the pre-existing normal anatomic dead space, thereby further decreasing the efficiency of ventilation.

Physiologic dead space. The sum of anatomic and alveolar dead space is called physiologic dead space, abbreviated as V_{Dphy}:

$$V_{Dphy} = V_{Danat} + V_{Dalv}$$

Fig. 8-25 schematically portrays the relationship between the three types of dead space ventilation. As indicated, the total amount of wasted ventilation, or physiologic dead space, equals the sum of that normally attributed to the conducting airways (anatomic dead space) and the abnormal component resulting from alveoli that are ventilated but not perfused by the pulmonary circulation (alveolar dead space).

Since physiologic dead space includes both the normal and abnormal components of wasted ventilation, it is the preferred clinical measure of ventilation efficiency. For this reason, clinical assessment of alveolar ventilation employs this combined measure of wasted ventilation, as in the following modified formula:

$$\dot{V}_A = f \times (V_T - V_{Dphy})$$

or

$$\dot{V}_A = \dot{V}_E - \dot{V}_{Dphy}$$

Physiologic dead space is measured clinically using a modified form of the Bohr equation:

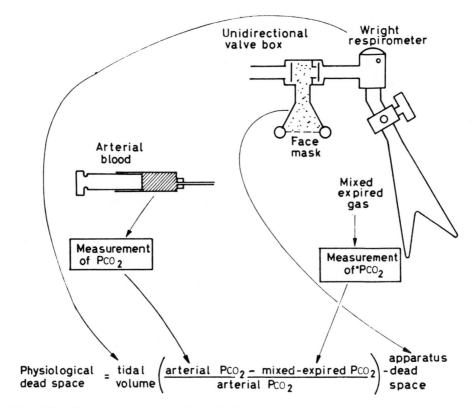

$$\text{Physiological} \atop \text{dead space} = \text{tidal} \atop \text{volume} \left(\frac{\text{arterial } P_{CO_2} - \text{mixed-expired } P_{CO_2}}{\text{arterial } P_{CO_2}} \right) \text{apparatus} \atop \text{-dead space}$$

Fig. 8-26   Clinical measurement of physiologic dead space. Arterial blood and mixed-expired air are collected simultaneously over 2-3 minutes in a gas-impermeable bag, while tidal volume is measured with a respirometer. Values for P_{CO_2} are then substituted into the Bohr equation, with a correction made for the rebreathed volume or mechanical dead space of the apparatus (stippled area). (From Nunn JF: Applied respiratory physiology, ed 2, London, 1977, Butterworth & Co.)

$$V_{Dphy} = \left[V_T \times \left(\frac{Pa_{CO_2} - P\bar{E}_{CO_2}}{Pa_{CO_2}} \right) \right] - V_{Dmec}$$

where V_{Dphy} is the physiologic dead space, V_T is the average tidal volume, Pa_{CO_2} is the partial pressure of CO_2 in the arterial blood, and $P\bar{E}_{CO_2}$ is the average partial pressure of CO_2 in the mixed expired air. V_{Dmec}, or the mechanical dead space, represents a correction factor for that portion of the patient's expired air that is rebreathed through the connecting apparatus.

The procedure for deriving V_{Dphy} in the laboratory or at the bedside is shown in Fig. 8-26. A sample of the patient's exhaled air is collected and measured over 2 to 3 min using a nonrebreathing valve, respirometer, and leak-free gas collection bag. The volume of the apparatus's mechanical dead space should be previously obtained by water displacement measurement. The larger the volume of mixed expired air collected, the greater the accuracy of the calculation.

During the period of expired gas collection, an arterial blood sample is drawn. The values for Pa_{CO_2} and $P\bar{E}_{CO_2}$ are then obtained via standard blood gas analysis and entered into the modified Bohr equation. As an example, if the arterial P_{CO_2} is reported to be 40 mm Hg, the mixed

expired P_{CO_2} is 20 mm Hg, the average tidal volume is 500 ml, and the mechanical dead space is 100 ml, then:

$$
\begin{aligned}
V_{Dphy} &= V_T \times \left[\left(\frac{Pa_{CO_2} - P\bar{E}_{CO_2}}{Pa_{CO_2}} \right) \right] - V_{Dmec} \\
&= \left[500 \times \left(\frac{40 - 20}{40} \right) \right] - 100 \\
&= [500 \times 0.50] - 100 \\
&= 250 - 100 \\
&= 150 \text{ ml}
\end{aligned}
$$

Dead space–to–tidal volume ratio. For clinical purposes, physiologic dead space is usually expressed as a ratio to the tidal volume. This ratio, abbreviated as V_D/V_T, provides a useful numeric index of the total amount of wasted ventilation (anatomic and alveolar dead space) per breath. As such, the V_D/V_T ratio represents the primary clinical measure of the efficiency of ventilation.

Using the data derived in the prior example, the V_D/V_T ratio is calculated as follows:

$$V_{Dphy}/V_T = 150/500$$
$$V_{Dphy}/V_T = 0.30$$

According to this calculation, the physiologic dead space for this patient is approximately one third of the tidal volume. This ratio varies among individuals with different volumes, having a normal range of about 0.2 to 0.4.

Clinical significance. Table 8-3 demonstrates the effect of changes in various parameters on alveolar ventilation. Even in normal subjects, alveolar ventilation depends on the relationship between the frequency of breathing and tidal volume. High frequencies and low tidal volumes result in a high proportion of wasted ventilation per minute. On the other hand, the most efficient breathing pattern, that which wastes the least proportion of ventilation per minute, is slow and deep breathing.

In disease states, an increase in V_{Dphy} will cause a decrease in alveolar ventilation, unless compensation occurs. Since an increased frequency of breathing, of and by itself, only worsens the problem, effective compensation for an increase in V_{Dphy} requires that the tidal volume be increased. Increased tidal volumes increase the elastic work of breathing and, with it, the oxygen consumption of the respiratory muscles. Since these increased demands cannot always be met, not all patients with an increase in V_{Dphy} can effectively compensate for the additional wasted ventilation. In such cases, alveolar ventilation will no longer be adequate to meet body needs.

Effectiveness of ventilation

Ventilation is effective when the body's need for removal of carbon dioxide is adequately met. Under resting metabolic conditions, the body produces about 200 ml of CO_2 per minute. This production of carbon dioxide must be matched by a sufficient level of alveolar ventilation per minute to ensure effective excretion.

The relative balance between carbon dioxide production and alveolar ventilation determines the level of this gaseous product of metabolism in the lungs and in the blood. Specifically, the partial pressure of CO_2 in the alveoli and blood is directly proportional to its production ($\dot{V}_{CO_2}$) and inversely proportional to its rate of excretion via alveolar ventilation ($\dot{V}_A$):

$$P_{CO_2} \cong \frac{\dot{V}_{CO_2}}{\dot{V}_A}$$

Normally, the alveolar and arterial partial pressures of carbon dioxide are in close equilibrium at approximately 40 mm Hg. Should the level of alveolar ventilation fall, the rate of carbon dioxide production will exceed its rate of excretion, and the P_{CO_2} will rise above its normal value of 40 mm Hg. Ventilation that is insufficient to meet metabolic needs is termed *hypoventilation*. Hypoventilation is always indicated by the presence of an elevated Pa_{CO_2}.

On the other hand, should the level of alveolar ventilation rise, the rate of carbon dioxide production will fall short of its rate of excretion, and the P_{CO_2} will fall below its normal value of 40 mm Hg. Ventilation in excess of metabolic needs is termed *hyperventilation*. Hyperventilation is always indicated by the presence of a lower than normal Pa_{CO_2}.

Hyperventilation must not be confused with the increase in ventilation that normally occurs in response to increased metabolic rates, such as would be observed during exercise. Under such circumstances, ventilation rises in proportion to the increase in carbon dioxide production, and the P_{CO_2} remains in the normal range. The normal increase in ventilation that occurs with increased metabolic rates is termed *hyperpnea*.

The effectiveness of ventilation is, therefore, determined by assessment of the partial pressure of carbon dioxide, specifically that measured in the arterial blood. Ventilation is effective when the Pa_{CO_2} is maintained within the normal limits of 35 to 45 mm Hg.

Ineffective ventilation occurs whenever carbon dioxide production and alveolar ventilation are out of balance. Hypoventilation is ineffective because carbon dioxide excretion is inadequate to meet metabolic needs. Hyperventilation is ineffective because wasteful amounts of energy (work) are being expended needlessly.

Unfortunately, there is no direct and consistent correlation between measures of ventilatory volumes and the effectiveness of ventilation. The presence of either hypoventilation or hyperventilation must therefore be determined by arterial blood gas analysis.

Table 8-3 Changes in Alveolar Ventilation (ml) Associated with Changes in Rate, Volume, and Physiologic Dead Space

	Rate of breathing	Tidal volume	Minute ventilation	Physiologic dead space	Alveolar ventilation
Normal	12	500	6000	150	4200
High rate, low volume	24	250	6000	150	2400
Low rate, high volume	6	1000	6000	150	5100
Increased dead space	12	500	6000	300	2400
Compensation for increased dead space	12	650	7800	300	4200

SUMMARY

Ventilation is the mechanical movement of air into and out of the lungs. This process is accomplished via the action of the respiratory muscles on the thorax. This action creates the pressure gradients necessary to overcome the elastic and frictional forces opposing the expansion of the lungs and thorax, and the movement of gas and tissues during active breathing.

In overcoming the elastic and frictional forces opposing inflation, work is performed by the respiratory muscles. During normal quiet breathing, the work accomplished during expiration is recovered from the potential energy that is "stored" in the expanded lung-thorax. However, forced exhalation requires that additional work be performed by the expiratory muscles. How much work is involved in breathing depends on the mechanical properties of the lungs and thorax.

These mechanical properties also affect the distribution of ventilation. In combination, regional and local factors make the lung a less than perfect organ for gas exchange. In disease, normal variations in the distribution of ventilation can dramatically worsen and cause significant deficiencies in gas exchange.

As a mechanism for excretion of carbon dioxide, the process of ventilation ideally should be both efficient and effective. Because of its design, even the normal lung wastes a portion of ventilation on each breath. Changes in the pattern of breathing also affect the efficiency of ventilation. Pathophysiologic abnormalities can dramatically increase the amount of wasted ventilation, making it difficult for the lung to effectively excrete its carbon dioxide load.

Ultimately, ventilation is considered effective when the body's need for removal of carbon dioxide is adequately met. This requires that the production of carbon dioxide be matched by a sufficient level of alveolar ventilation per minute to ensure effective excretion. The desired end result is maintenance of a normal arterial P_{CO_2} with maximum efficiency and minimum work.

REFERENCES

1. Fishman AP: Assessment of pulmonary function, New York, 1980, McGraw-Hill Book Co.
2. Martin L: Pulmonary physiology in clinical practice: the essentials for patient care and evaluation, St Louis, 1987, The CV Mosby Co.
3. Report of the ACCP-ATS Joint Committee on Pulmonary Nomenclature, Chest 67:583, 1975.
4. Tisi GM: Pulmonary physiology in clinical medicine, ed 2, Baltimore, 1984, Williams & Wilkins Co.
5. Peters RM: The mechanical basis of respiration, Boston, 1969, Little, Brown & Co.
6. Green JF: Mechanical concepts in cardiovascular and pulmonary physiology, Philadelphia, 1977, Lea & Febiger.
7. Green JF: Fundamental cardiovascular and pulmonary physiology, ed 2, Philadelphia, 1987, Lea & Febiger.
8. West JB: Respiratory physiology: the essentials, ed 3, Baltimore, 1985, Williams & Wilkins Co.
9. Murray JF: The normal lung, ed 2, Philadelphia, 1986, WB Saunders Co.
10. Von Neergaard K: Neue auffassungen uber einen grundbegriff der atemmechanik. Die retraktionkraft der lunge, abhangig von der oberflachenspannung in der alveolen, Z Ges Exp Med 66:373, 1929.
11. Clements JA et al: Pulmonary surface tension and alveolar stability, J Appl Physiol 16:444, 1972.
12. Jacquez JA: Respiratory physiology, New York, 1979, McGraw-Hill Book Co.
13. Cherniack RM, and Cherniack L: Respiration in health and disease, ed 3, Philadelphia, 1983, WB Saunders Co.
14. Foster RE et al: The lung: physiologic basis of pulmonary function tests, ed 3, Chicago, 1986, Year Book Medical Publishers.
15. Olson DE, Dart GA, and Filley GF: Pressure drop and fluid flow regime of air inspired into the human lungs, J Appl Physiol 28:482-484, 1970.
16. Slonim NB and Hamilton LH: Respiratory physiology, ed 5, St Louis, 1985, The CV Mosby Co.
17. Whitaker S: Introduction to fluid mechanics, Englewood Cliffs, NJ, 1968, Prentice-Hall.
18. Ferris BG Jr, Mead J, and Opie LH: Partitioning of respiratory flow resistance in man, J Appl Physiol 19:653-658, 1964.
19. Nunn JF: Applied respiratory physiology, ed 2, London, 1977, Butterworth & Co.
20. Robinson DR, Chaudhary BA, and Speir WS: Expiratory flow limitation in large and small airways, Arch Intern Med 144:1457, 1984.
21. Altose MD: Pulmonary mechanics. In Fishman AP, (editor): Assessment of pulmonary function, New York, 1980, McGraw-Hill Book Co.
22. Otis AB: The work of breathing, Physiol Rev 34:449-458, 1954.
23. Cournand A et al: The oxygen cost of breathing, Trans Assoc Am Phys 67:162-173, 1954.
24. Macklem PT: Relation between lung mechanics and ventilation distribution, Physiologist 16:580-588, 1973.
25. Milic-Emili J et al: Regional distribution of inspired gas in the lung, J Appl Physiol 21:749-759, 1966.
26. Fowler WS: Lung function studies. II. The respiratory dead space, Am J Physiol 154:405-416, 1948.

9

Gas Exchange and Transport

G. Woodward Gross
Craig L. Scanlan

Ventilation, or the mechanical movement of gas into and out of the lungs, is only one component of human respiration. The process of respiration demands that respired gases be distributed throughout the lungs, exchanged with the pulmonary capillary blood, and transported to and from the tissues in as efficient a manner as possible.

Normally, these respiratory processes of gas exchange and transport are accomplished in a well-integrated manner under a wide variety of circumstances. In disease states, however, one or more of these critical processes may become impaired, causing physiologic imbalances that can compromise function or even threaten survival. At such times, respiratory care intervention may be the only way to maintain or restore a level of function consistent with life.

OBJECTIVES

For these reasons, it is essential that respiratory care practitioners have in-depth knowledge of both the normal processes of gas exchange and transport and the mechanisms by which various pathophysiologic abnormalities affect these components of respiration. To that end, this chapter will provide a rigorous review of these physiologic processes, with an emphasis on normal relationships. Specifically, after completion of this chapter, the reader should be able to:

1. Delineate the normal gradients in oxygen and carbon dioxide partial pressures between the atmosphere and tissues;
2. Explain, using mathematical formulas, the determinants of alveolar oxygen and carbon dioxide partial pressures;
3. Apply pertinent physical laws in the determination of factors affecting diffusion at the alveolar-capillary membrane;
4. Describe the normal relationship between ventilation and perfusion in the healthy lung and its effect on local gas tensions in various lung zones;

5. Differentiate between the mechanisms by which oxygen and carbon dioxide are transported in the blood and the factors affecting their carriage to and from the tissues.

KEY TERMS

Most terms used in this chapter are defined in context. The following terms are introduced without explicit definition, but may be found in the text glossary:

absorption	hydrostatic
acidosis	hyperbaric oxygenation
alkalosis	hyperpyrexia
amino acid	hypothermia
anemia	hypoxemia
buffer	nitrite
congenital	placenta
conjugated protein	polypeptide
cyanotic heart disease	porphyrin
electrolytic	septic shock
enzyme	spectrophotometry
equilibrate	thrombus
erythrocyte	transfusion

DIFFUSION

Whole body diffusion gradients

Although enhanced by various mechanisms, the actual movement of respired gases between lungs and the body tissues depends mainly on the simple physical process of gaseous diffusion. For this process to provide an adequate supply of oxygen and removal of carbon dioxide, partial pressure gradients of sufficient magnitude and proper direction must exist throughout the body.

These normal diffusion gradients for both oxygen and carbon dioxide are shown schematically in Fig. 9-1. For oxygen, there is a stepwise downward "cascade" of partial

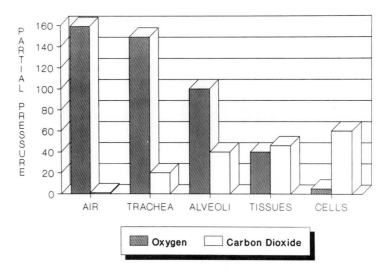

Fig. 9-1   Diffusion "cascades" for oxygen and carbon dioxide.

pressures from the normal atmospheric P_{IO_2} of 159 mm Hg to an average low point of 40 mm Hg or less at the level of the systemic capillaries. The intracellular P_{O_2}, estimated to be 5 mm Hg or less, provides the final gradient necessary for movement of oxygen into the cell.[1]

Likewise, a gradient of partial pressures exists for carbon dioxide. In this case, however, the direction of the gradient is reversed, from an estimated high of 60 mm Hg or more in the cells, to a low of less than 1 mm Hg in room air. This reverse cascade governs the movement of carbon dioxide from the tissues to the lungs and, with the aid of ventilation, out to the atmosphere.

Determinants of alveolar gas tensions

Effective exchange of oxygen and carbon dioxide in the lungs depends on the maintenance of diffusion gradients for these gases between the alveoli and pulmonary capillaries. Pulmonary capillary gas tensions depend mainly on the rate of cellular metabolism in relation to the state of tissue perfusion, and therefore is beyond the direct control of the clinician. Alveolar oxygen and carbon dioxide tensions, however, can be directly affected by clinical intervention. For this reason, respiratory care practitioners must have a sound understanding of the factors determining gaseous partial pressures in both the normal and abnormal exchange units of the lung.

Alveolar carbon dioxide tensions. The alveolar partial pressure of carbon dioxide, or P_{ACO_2}, is directly proportional to the body's production of carbon dioxide ($\dot{V}_{CO_2}$) and inversely proportional to the level of alveolar ventilation ($\dot{V}_A$).[2] Using a constant of 0.863 to convert $\dot{V}_{CO_2}$ from STPD to BTPS, these relationships can be expressed in the following mathematical formula:

$$P_{ACO_2} = \frac{\dot{V}_{CO_2} \times 0.863}{\dot{V}_A}$$

Given a normal $\dot{V}_{CO_2}$ of 200 ml/min and a normal alveolar ventilation of 4.2 L/min, application of the above formula yields a P_{ACO_2} of approximately 40 mm Hg:

$$P_{ACO_2} = \frac{200 \times 0.863}{4.2}$$
$$\cong 40 \text{ mm Hg}$$

Elevation of the P_{ACO_2} above this level will occur if (1) the body's carbon dioxide production increases, (2) alveolar ventilation decreases, or (3) both conditions pertain.[3] Likewise, a decrease in P_{ACO_2} below this normal level will occur if carbon dioxide production decreases or alveolar ventilation increases. Normally, however, complex respiratory control mechanisms maintain the P_{ACO_2} within a range of 35 to 45 mm Hg under a wide variety of conditions (see Chapter 10).

Alveolar oxygen tensions. Unlike carbon dioxide, oxygen constitutes a substantial portion of the inspired air. The alveolar partial pressure of oxygen, or P_{AO_2}, therefore is determined mainly by its partial pressure in the inspired gas. Applying Dalton's law (Chapter 4), the partial pressure of inspired oxygen must equal its fractional concentration (F_{IO_2}) times the total barometric pressure, or P_B:

$$P_{IO_2} = F_{IO_2} \times P_B$$

At sea level, (P_B = 760 mm Hg), the partial pressure of inspired oxygen is calculated as:

$$P_{IO_2} = 0.2095 \times 760 \text{ mm Hg}$$
$$= 159 \text{ mm Hg}$$

Correcting for water vapor pressure. Once entering the respiratory tract, oxygen molecules are effectively "displaced" by water vapor during the humidification process that occurs in the nose and upper airways. The resulting partial pressure of oxygen in the trachea is lowered by an amount equal to the water vapor pressure of saturated gas at body temperature (see Fig. 9-1). Given that the water vapor pressure, or P_{H_2O}, is 47 mm Hg at a normal body temperature of 37°C, the corrected partial pressure of inspired oxygen may be calculated according to the following formula:

$$P_{O_2} \text{ (tracheal)} = F_{IO_2} \times (P_B - P_{H_2O})$$

or

$$P_{O_2} \text{ (tracheal)} = F_{IO_2} \times (P_B - 47 \text{ mm Hg})$$

Substituting normal values at sea level into the equation, we calculate a tracheal P_{O_2} of approximately 149 mm Hg:

$$P_{O_2} \text{ (tracheal)} = 0.2095 \times (760 \text{ mm Hg} - 47 \text{ mm Hg})$$
$$= 149 \text{ mm Hg}$$

Accounting for carbon dioxide. As oxygen moves into the respiratory zones of the lung, it is further diluted or displaced by carbon dioxide. However, rather than simply subtract the P_{ACO_2}, as we did for water vapor pressure, a correction must be made for the relative difference between the amount of carbon dioxide that diffuses into the alveoli per minute ($\dot{V}_{CO_2}$) and the amount of oxygen that diffuses out of the alveoli per minute ($\dot{V}_{O_2}$).[4] This difference, expressed as the proportion $\dot{V}_{CO_2}/\dot{V}_{O_2}$, is called the respiratory exchange ratio or R.* Although it varies through the lung, R averages 0.8, indicating slightly greater O_2 uptake than CO_2 excretion.

Moreover, for any given respiratory exchange ratio, the partial pressure of CO_2 in alveolar gas is linearly related to the alveolar partial pressure of oxygen. Thus the P_{ACO_2} must also be corrected for the amount of oxygen in the inspired air, or F_{IO_2}.

Correcting the P_{ACO_2} for both the respiratory exchange ratio and the fractional concentration of oxygen in the inspired air is accomplished as follows:

$$\text{Corrected } P_{ACO_2} = \frac{P_{ACO_2}}{R} \times [1 + F_{IO_2}(R-1)]$$

Alveolar air equation. Applying this corrected P_{ACO_2} to the calculation of the partial pressure of oxygen in the alveoli, we derive the classic form of the alveolar air equation[3]:

$$P_{AO_2} = F_{IO_2}(P_B - P_{H_2O}) - \frac{P_{ACO_2}}{R}[1 + F_{IO_2}(R-1)]$$

In clinical practice it is common to drop the F_{IO_2} correction for alveolar carbon dioxide. Moreover, since the alveolar P_{CO_2} cannot easily be measured directly, and since the arterial P_{CO_2} closely approximates the alveolar level of this

gas, we commonly substitute the P_{aCO_2} for the P_{ACO_2}, thus deriving a clinical estimation form of the alveolar air equation:

$$P_{AO_2} = F_{IO_2}(P_B - P_{H_2O}) - \frac{P_{aCO_2}}{R}$$

As an example, if the $F_{IO_2} = 0.2095$, the $P_B = 760$ mm Hg, the $P_{H_2O} = 47$ mm Hg, the $P_{aCO_2} = 40$ mm Hg, and the $R = 0.8$, we can estimate the normal alveolar partial pressure of oxygen as follows:

$$P_{AO_2} = 0.2095(760 \text{ mm Hg} - 47 \text{ mm Hg}) - \frac{40 \text{ mm Hg}}{0.8}$$
$$= 149 \text{ mm Hg} - 50 \text{ mm Hg}$$
$$\cong 100 \text{ mm Hg}$$

In clinical practice, when the F_{IO_2} is greater than 0.60, the correction for R can be dropped, yielding the following simplified form of the alveolar air equation[3]:

$$P_{AO_2} = F_{IO_2}(P_B - P_{H_2O}) - P_{aCO_2}$$

Changes in alveolar gas partial tensions. Other than carbon dioxide, oxygen, and water vapor, alveoli normally contain nitrogen. As an inert gas, nitrogen takes no part in gas exchange, simply occupying space and exerting a stable partial pressure equivalent to that remaining after subtracting the other gas tensions:

$$P_{AN_2} = P_B - (P_{AO_2} + P_{ACO_2} + P_{H_2O})$$
$$P_{AN_2} = 760 \text{ mm Hg} - (100 \text{ mm Hg} + 40 \text{ mm Hg} + 47 \text{ mm Hg})$$
$$P_{AN_2} = 760 \text{ mm Hg} - (187 \text{ mm Hg})$$
$$P_{AN_2} = 573 \text{ mm Hg}$$

With the alveolar water vapor tension constant at 47 mm Hg, and the P_{AN_2} constant at 573 mm Hg, the only partial pressures that change in the normally ventilated and perfused alveolus are oxygen and carbon dioxide. Based on the alveolar air equation, and assuming a constant F_{IO_2} of 0.21, the P_{AO_2} should vary inversely with the P_{ACO_2}.

Since the P_{ACO_2} is itself inversely related to the level of alveolar ventilation, we would expect increases in $\dot{V}_A$ to simultaneously decrease P_{ACO_2} and increase P_{AO_2}. Decreases in $\dot{V}_A$ should have the opposite effect. As indicated in Fig. 9-2, this is precisely what occurs. With a constant carbon dioxide production, a fall in $\dot{V}_A$ causes a proportionate rise in P_{ACO_2}; this rise in P_{ACO_2} causes a proportionate fall in P_{AO_2}. Likewise, an increase in $\dot{V}_A$ causes a drop in P_{ACO_2} and a resultant rise in P_{AO_2}.[5]

The magnitude of this latter change is governed by the limited ability of the lungs to lower the P_{ACO_2}. In combination, regulatory control mechanisms and the elevated workload associated with increased alveolar ventilation prevent decreases in P_{ACO_2} much below 15 to 20 mm Hg.[3] When breathing room air, the highest P_{AO_2} one could ex-

---

*Not to be confused with the respiratory quotient (RQ), or whole body ratio of CO_2 production to O_2 consumption, the respiratory exchange ratio varies throughout the lung. For the lung as a whole, R is normally equal to 0.8.

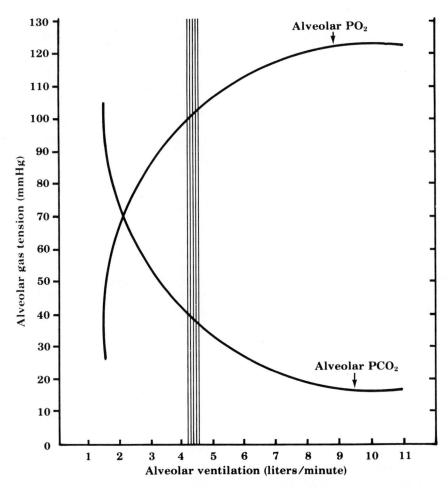

Fig. 9-2   The effect of alveolar ventilation on alveolar gases. (From Pilbeam SP: Mechanical ventilation: physiological and clinical applications, Denver, 1986, Multi-Media Publishing, Inc.)

pect to observe at sea level would be in the range of 120 to 130 mm Hg.

Because the total combined partial pressure of oxygen and carbon dioxide when breathing room air is approximately 140 mm Hg, one can estimate the effect of a change in P_{ACO_2} on P_{AO_2} using the following rule of thumb:

$$P_{AO_2} \cong 140 \text{ mm Hg} - P_{ACO_2}$$

Of course, this rule of thumb is based on the assumption that the respiratory exchange ratio remains stable at a normal value of 0.8. In reality, even in the normal lung, the respiratory exchange ratio varies substantially. Variations from the ideal respiratory exchange ratio are the result of imbalances in the amount of ventilation and perfusion occurring throughout the normal lung.[6] However, before discussing the important relationship between pulmonary ventilation and perfusion, we must first analyze the mechanism by which respiratory gases are exchanged between the alveoli and the blood and the blood and the tissues.

Mechanism of diffusion

Not long ago respiratory physiologists thought that gas exchange in the lung was an active process of secretion and absorption. Today, we know that the movement of respiratory gases throughout the respiratory and cardiovascular system depends on the relatively simple physical phenomenon of gaseous diffusion.

Barriers to diffusion. As described in Chapter 4, diffusion is the physical process whereby gas molecules move from an area of relatively high partial pressure to an area of low partial pressure. Because all motion requires some driving force, diffusion depends on a pressure gradient. The two gases with which we are concerned, oxygen and carbon dioxide, not only must diffuse from one area to another, but also must move through formidable barriers. The barrier to gaseous diffusion in the lung is the alveolar-capillary membrane. At the cellular level, gases must transverse a similar barrier between the systemic capillary and the tissue cell wall. Thus, for gases to pass throughout the system, pressure gradients must be sufficient to overcome these barriers to diffusion. Of primary concern to the

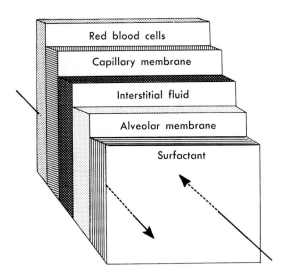

Fig. 9-3   The five barriers through which O_2 and CO_2 pass at the alveolocapillary membrane. (From McLaughlin AJ Jr: Essentials of physiology for advanced respiratory therapy, St Louis, 1977, The CV Mosby Co.)

respiratory care practitioner is the nature of diffusion at the site of external respiration, that is, the alveolar-capillary membrane.

Fig. 9-3 portrays a schematic representation of the alveolar-capillary membrane. For CO_2 or O_2 to move between alveolus and plasma in the pulmonary capillary, four "layers" must be transversed: the pulmonary surfactant layer, the alveolar epithelial membrane, the interstitial fluid space, and the capillary endothelial membrane.[7] Moreover, for these gases to pass into and out of the red blood cell, they also must transverse the erythrocyte cell membrane.

Fick's law of diffusion. The bulk movement of gases ($\dot{V}$) through biologic membranes is described according to the relationships specified in Fick's law of diffusion[8]:

$$\dot{V}_{gas} \cong \frac{A \times D}{T} (P_1 - P_2)$$

where *A* is equal to the cross-sectional area available for diffusion, *D* is the diffusion coefficient of the gas, *T* is the thickness or distance across the membrane, and $P_1 - P_2$ represents the difference in partial pressures of the gas, or partial pressure gradient, across the membrane.

According to this formula, the volume of a gas diffusing across a biologic membrane per unit of time will be greatest when the cross-sectional area, gas diffusion constant, and partial pressure gradient are all large, and the distance across the membrane is small. Conversely, a small cross-sectional area, low gas diffusion constant, small partial pressure gradient, or large diffusing distance can, alone or in combination, impede gaseous diffusion.

Given that the cross-sectional area and distance across the alveolar-capillary membrane is relatively constant in

the normal lung, we will focus our primary attention on the gaseous diffusion gradients that exist in the respiratory zone, and the relative difference in the ease with which oxygen and carbon dioxide diffuse across this biologic membrane.

Pulmonary diffusion gradients. For gas exchange to occur between the alveolus and pulmonary capillary, a difference in partial pressures ($P_1 - P_2$) must exist. Fig. 9-4 schematically portrays the magnitude and direction of these gradients for both oxygen and carbon dioxide.

As previously described, the partial pressures of oxygen and carbon dioxide in the ideal alveolus are determined mainly by the inspired oxygen concentration (FIO_2) and level of alveolar ventilation relative to carbon dioxide production. Although at any given moment these pressures will vary according to the ventilatory cycle, samples of alveolar air taken from a subject breathing room air at sea level will yield an average PO_2 of 100 mm Hg and an average PCO_2 of 40 mm Hg.

Mixed venous blood returning to the lungs has a lower partial pressure of oxygen (40 mm Hg) and a higher partial pressure of carbon dioxide (46 mm Hg) than alveolar gas. Therefore, two pressure gradients are established: one between alveolar and venous oxygen tensions (100 mm Hg − 40 mm Hg), and a smaller one between venous and alveolar carbon dioxide (46 mm Hg − 40 mm Hg).

Oxygen, therefore, diffuses from the alveolus into the pulmonary blood. As blood flows past the alveolus, it takes up oxygen, leaving the capillary with a PO_2 in close equilibrium with the alveolar oxygen tension of around 100 mm Hg. Simultaneously, carbon dioxide diffuses in the opposite direction until the capillary blood PCO_2 equilibrates with the alveolar PCO_2. This "arterialized" blood thus leaves the capillary with a PCO_2 of about 40 mm Hg.

Diffusion coefficients. In addition to the partial pressure gradient, the volume of a gas diffusing across a biologic membrane per unit of time is directly proportional to its diffusion coefficient. The diffusion coefficient represents a standardized measure of the milliliters per minute of a gas that will diffuse a distance of 1 μm over a square centimeter area with a pressure gradient of 760 mm Hg (1 atm).[9]

Since gas movement through the alveolar-capillary membrane is essentially diffusion through a liquid barrier, the diffusion coefficient must take into account both the density of the gas and its solubility in the liquid. Graham's law states that the diffusion coefficient of a gas in the gas phase is inversely proportional to the square root of its density (or gram molecular weight [gmw]).

$$D \cong \frac{1}{\sqrt{gmw}}$$

The solubility coefficient represents a standardized measure of the volume of a gas that can dissolve in 1 ml of a given liquid at standard pressure (760 mm Hg) and speci-

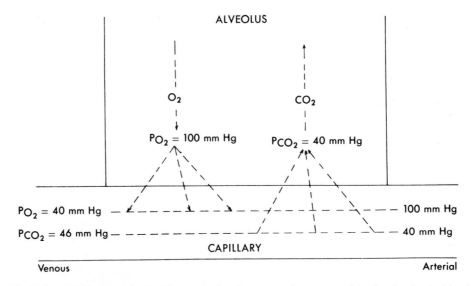

Fig. 9-4   Ventilation maintains the mean alveolar gas tensions as noted in the sketch. As blood enters the venous end of the pulmonary capillary, it loses its carbon dioxide and takes up oxygen, until these two gases are in equilibrium with the mean alveolar tensions, and it leaves the capillary as arterial blood.

fied temperature. The diffusion coefficient of a gas through a liquid is directly proportional to its solubility coefficient.

Therefore, the diffusion coefficient applicable to gas movement across the alveolar-capillary membrane must be directly proportional to the solubility coefficient of the gas and inversely proportional to the square root of its gram molecular weight:

$$D \cong \frac{\text{Sol. Coeff.}}{\sqrt{\text{gmw}}}$$

Given that the solubility coefficient of oxygen in plasma at 37°C is 0.023 ml/760 mm Hg, and for carbon dioxide is 0.510 ml/760 mm Hg, we may compare the relative ease with which each diffuses across the alveolar-capillary membrane:

$$D_{oxygen} \cong \frac{0.023}{\sqrt{32}} \qquad D_{carbon\ dioxide} \cong \frac{0.510}{\sqrt{44}}$$
$$\cong 0.004 \qquad\qquad \cong 0.077$$

$$\frac{D_{carbon\ dioxide}}{D_{oxygen}} \cong \frac{0.077}{0.004} \cong \frac{19}{1}$$

Therefore, because of its higher solubility in plasma, carbon dioxide has a diffusion coefficient about 20 times greater than that of oxygen. In the normal lung, this difference explains why a much smaller pressure gradient (6 mm Hg) is required to move CO_2 across the alveolar-capillary membrane than that required to move comparable amounts of oxygen (60 mm Hg). Moreover, this difference in diffusibility explains why disorders that impair the lung's diffusion capacity have little effect on carbon dioxide movement across the alveolar-capillary membrane.[10] That such disorders can and do impede the movement of

oxygen from alveolus into the pulmonary capillary circulation is caused entirely by oxygen's lower diffusion coefficient.

Time limitations to diffusion. For blood to leave the pulmonary capillary adequately oxygenated, it must spend sufficient time in contact with the alveolus to allow complete equilibration. Because of its higher diffusion coefficient, carbon dioxide movement across the alveolar-capillary membrane is seldom affected by time limitations. However, the time available for oxygen diffusion from the alveolus into the pulmonary circulation can be critical. Should insufficient time be available for equilibration of oxygen partial pressures, blood leaving the respiratory zone may not be fully oxygenated.

The time available for diffusion in the lung is a function of the rate of blood flow through the pulmonary circulation. As shown in Fig. 9-5, blood normally spends about 0.75 sec traversing the pulmonary capillary.[5] This time is more than sufficient to ensure complete gaseous equilibration of oxygen across the alveolar-capillary membrane.[11]

Should blood flow increase, as during heavy exercise, time spent in the pulmonary capillary can decrease by as much as two thirds, down to about 0.25 sec.[11] Even this short time frame is adequate to ensure that gaseous equilibration takes place, as long as no other factors are present to impede diffusion.

However, when disorders that impede diffusion are associated with conditions that increase cardiac output, rapid blood flow through the pulmonary circulation can further impair the ability of the lung to provide adequate oxygenation.[5] Fever and septic shock are good examples of clinical conditions that can limit the time available for diffusion by increasing the rate of blood flow through the lung.

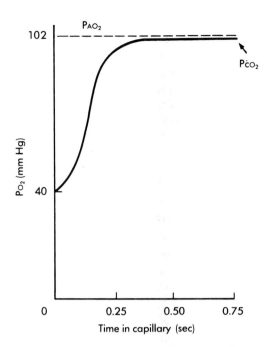

Fig. 9-5 Alveolar-capillary P_{O_2} gradient. Normal transit time for a red blood cell in the pulmonary capillary is approximately 0.75 sec. Blood P_{O_2} reaches near equilibrium with alveolar P_{O_2} (P_{AO_2}) well before the end of capillary transit time. (From Martin L: Pulmonary physiology in clinical practice: the essentials for patient care and evaluation, St Louis, 1987, The CV Mosby Co.)

Measurement of diffusion capacity. In cardiopulmonary physiology, knowledge of the diffusing capacity of the lung is sometimes helpful in evaluating pathologic conditions. The diffusing capacity of the lung (D_L) is defined as the number of milliliters of a specific gas that diffuses across the alveolar-capillary membrane into the bloodstream each minute, for each millimeter of mercury (mm Hg) difference in the pressure gradient.

Although oxygen itself can be used to measure the diffusion capacity of the lung, it is more common to employ low concentrations (0.25% to 0.40%) of carbon monoxide. Carbon monoxide is preferred over oxygen as the test gas because its higher affinity for hemoglobin keeps its capillary partial pressure extremely low, thereby minimizing the effect of variations in blood flow on the measurement.[4]

The average normal value for the diffusing capacity of the lung at rest (D_{LCO}), as measured by a single-breath carbon monoxide test, is about 27 ml/min/mm Hg.[5] Since oxygen has a diffusion coefficient about 1.23 times greater than that of carbon monoxide at body temperature, one may convert the value obtained with carbon monoxide to that applicable for oxygen by multiplying D_{LCO} by this factor. Details on the theory underlying the measurement of diffusing capacity, and the clinical implications of abnormal test results, are provided in Chapter 17.

Systemic diffusion gradients. The discussion of gradients so far has centered about the alveolar-capillary membrane. However, for a complete picture of diffusion, we must include the equally important gradients at the systemic or tissue level.

Partial pressure gradients at the level of the systemic capillaries can be visualized as the reverse of those in the lung. As the metabolism of the cell depletes its store of oxygen, the intracellular P_{O_2} drops below that of the blood entering the arterial end of the capillary. Oxygen thus diffuses from the systemic capillary blood (P_{O_2} = 100 mm Hg) to the tissues ($P_{O_2} < 40$ mm Hg). Simultaneously, carbon dioxide diffuses from the tissues ($P_{CO_2} > 46$ mm Hg) into the capillary blood (P_{CO_2} = 40 mm Hg).

Once equilibration is achieved, blood leaves the systemic capillaries as venous blood, with gas tensions roughly in equilibrium with those at the tissue level, that is, a P_{O_2} of about 40 mm Hg, and a P_{CO_2} of about 46 mm Hg. Just as "arterialized" blood reflects the events occurring in the respiratory zone of the lung, this venous blood reflects the metabolic state of the tissues, as related to their blood flow. For this reason, assessment of the events occurring at the tissue level, especially tissue oxygenation, require measurement of venous blood parameters. The collection and use of venous blood in the assessment of tissue oxygenation is discussed further in Chapter 31.

VARIATIONS FROM IDEAL GAS EXCHANGE

Up to this point, we have focused almost exclusively on the balance between gas partial pressures in a "perfect" alveolus, that is, one with ideal ventilation and blood flow. In reality, the normal lung is an imperfect organ of gas exchange. This is evident clinically in the measurement of arterial partial pressures of oxygen in normal subjects.

Theoretically, if all the blood leaving the lung were to pass through "ideal" gas exchange units with a P_{AO_2} of 100 mm Hg, the partial pressure of oxygen in the arterialized blood should be equal to that in the alveoli, 100 mm Hg. In reality, the P_{aO_2} of normal subjects at sea level is approximately 5 to 10 mm Hg less than the calculated P_{AO_2}.

This normal difference between alveolar and arterial oxygen partial pressures is called the *alveolar-arterial oxygen tension gradient*, abbreviated as $P_{(A-a)O_2}$. Two factors account for this normal difference: (1) the existence of anatomic shunts in the circulation, and (2) regional differences in ventilation and blood flow occurring in the lung.[4]

Anatomic shunts

An anatomic shunt represents a direct connection between the right (venous) and left (arterial) circulations. A right-to-left anatomic shunt occurs when a portion of the venous blood flow totally bypasses the pulmonary capillary circulation, thereby never contacting the areas of gas exchange. This venous blood enters the arterial circulation without picking up oxygen or removing excess carbon dioxide, which results in "diluting" the oxygen content and raising the partial pressure of carbon dioxide in the arterial blood in proportion to the amount of shunted flow. Two such anatomic shunts exist in the normal human circulation: the bronchial venous drainage and the thebesian venous drainage.

As discussed in Chapter 6, as much as two thirds of the return flow of the bronchial circulation (venous blood) empties into the pulmonary veins (arterialized blood). Although the relative amount of flow through this anatomic shunt is small, it results in a measurable decrease in oxygen content in the blood returning to the left atrium through the pulmonary venous circulation.

The thebesian drainage consists of small veins draining a portion of the coronary circulation and emptying into both atria of the heart. Those that communicate with the left atrium mix venous blood with arterial, thereby lowering the oxygen content of the arterial blood.

In combination, these normal anatomic shunts account for some 70% to 80% of the difference between the observed and expected levels of arterial oxygenation in normal subjects. The remainder of this difference is attributable to normal inequalities in ventilation and perfusion that occur throughout the lung.

Regional inequalities in ventilation and perfusion

The normal respiratory exchange ratio of 0.8 assumes that ventilation and perfusion in the pulmonary exchange units are in stable balance, with about one unit of alveolar ventilation ($\dot{V}_A$) being provided for each unit of pulmonary capillary blood flow ($\dot{Q}_c$). However, if $\dot{Q}_c$ is kept constant, and $\dot{V}_A$ increases, we would expect the alveolar P_{CO_2} to fall, and the alveolar P_{O_2} to rise. On the other hand, with $\dot{Q}_c$ constant, if $\dot{V}_A$ were to decrease, the alveolar P_{CO_2} should rise, and the alveolar P_{O_2} should fall.[6]

Changing the rate of blood flow will also disrupt the ideal balance in alveolar gas partial pressures. If $\dot{V}_A$ is kept constant, but $\dot{Q}_c$ increases, carbon dioxide will be delivered to the alveolus faster than it can be removed, and oxygen will be taken up faster than it can be restored. This will result in an increase in alveolar P_{CO_2}, and a fall in alveolar P_{O_2}. Should pulmonary capillary blood flow fall (decreased $\dot{Q}_c$), alveolar gas tensions would change in the opposite direction.

The ventilation-perfusion ratio ($\dot{V}_A/\dot{Q}_c$). Changes in $\dot{V}_A$ and $\dot{Q}_c$ are expressed as a ratio, $\dot{V}_A/\dot{Q}_c$, called the ventilation-perfusion ratio. An ideal ratio of 1.0 indicates that ventilation and perfusion in the pulmonary exchange units are equal. A high $\dot{V}_A/\dot{Q}_c$ indicates that ventilation is greater than normal, perfusion is less than normal, or both. Regardless of cause, a high $\dot{V}_A/\dot{Q}_c$ will result in higher than normal alveolar P_{O_2} and lower than normal alveolar P_{CO_2}.[13]

On the other hand, a low $\dot{V}_A/\dot{Q}_c$ indicates that ventilation is less than normal, perfusion is greater than normal, or both. Regardless of cause, a low $\dot{V}_A/\dot{Q}_c$ will result in lower than normal alveolar P_{O_2} and higher than normal alveolar P_{CO_2}.

Effect of alterations in the $\dot{V}_A/\dot{Q}_c$ ratio. Obviously, these changes in local ventilation and perfusion will affect the exchange rate for both carbon dioxide and oxygen, thereby altering R. Fig. 9-6 graphically portrays the effect of alterations in $\dot{V}_A/\dot{Q}_c$ on the respiratory exchange ratio (R), plotting all possible values of alveolar P_{O_2} and P_{CO_2}.[6]

Note that when ventilation and perfusion are in perfect equilibrium ($\dot{V}_A/\dot{Q}_c = 1.0$), the respiratory exchange ratio equals 0.8. At this point, the alveolar P_{O_2} and P_{CO_2} approximate the ideal values of 100 and 40 mm Hg, respectively.

As the $\dot{V}_A/\dot{Q}_c$ rises above 1.0 (following the curve to the right), the ratio of carbon dioxide excretion to oxygen uptake (R) also increases, resulting in a rise in alveolar P_{O_2} and a fall in alveolar P_{CO_2}. At the extreme right of the graph, perfusion is zero, and the $\dot{V}_A/\dot{Q}_c$ is infinitely large. At this point, there is ventilation with no accompanying perfusion, and the constituency of alveolar gas equals that of inspired air ($P_{O_2} = 150$ mm Hg; $P_{CO_2} = 0$ mm Hg). Exchange units with an infinite $\dot{V}_A/\dot{Q}_c$ ratio represent alveolar deadspace, as defined in Chapter 8. In the normal lung, alveolar deadspace is essentially nonexistent.

As the $\dot{V}_A/\dot{Q}_c$ drops below 1.0 (following the curve to the left), the ratio of carbon dioxide excretion to oxygen uptake (R) decreases, resulting in a drop in alveolar P_{O_2} and an increase in alveolar P_{CO_2}. At the extreme left of the graph, ventilation is zero, resulting in a $\dot{V}_A/\dot{Q}_c$ ratio of 0. At this point, there is perfusion with no accompanying ventilation, and the constituency of alveolar gas approximates that of mixed venous blood ($P_{O_2} = 40$ mm Hg; $P_{CO_2} = 46$ mm Hg). Exchange units with a $\dot{V}_A/\dot{Q}_c$ ratio of 0 provide no gas exchange whatsoever. Therefore blood passing through these units remains venous in character. When mixed with the arterial circulation, such blood has the same effect as that coming from right-to-left anatomic shunts. To distinguish their effect from that caused by anatomic shunts, exchange units with a $\dot{V}_A/\dot{Q}_c$ ratio of 0 are referred to as *alveolar shunts*. Whereas small anatomic shunts are considered normal, alveolar shunts always indicate a pathologic alteration in function.

Although alveolar deadspace and shunts do not exist in the normal lung, ($\dot{V}_A/\dot{Q}_c$ is never zero or infinity), ventilation-perfusion ratios do vary substantially from the ideal. Reasons for this variation and its effect on gas exchange are the focus of the following discussion.

Causes of regional differences in $\dot{V}_A/\dot{Q}_c$. Regional variations in $\dot{V}_A/\dot{Q}_c$ in the normal lung are due mainly to the effect of gravity, and, therefore, are most evident in the upright posture. Although gravity affects the distribution of both blood flow and ventilation in the lung, the effect on perfusion is greater than that on ventilation.

Perfusion. Because the pulmonary circulation is a low pressure system, the amount of blood flow in the upright lung varies considerably from top to bottom. As delineated in Chapter 6, hydrostatic pressures in the pulmonary circu-

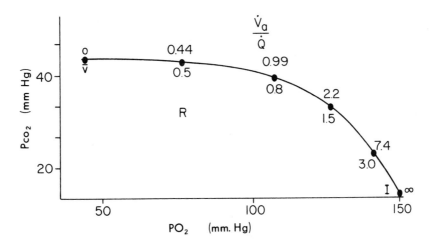

Fig. 9-6   A curve may be drawn that joins the points (representing the values of P_{O_2} and P_{CO_2}) that are determined by given values for the respiratory exchange ratio (R), the ventilation/perfusion ratio ($\dot{V}_A/\dot{Q}$), the composition of mixed venous blood ($\bar{v}$), and inspired air (I). (From Cherniack RM and Cherniack L: Respiration in health and disease, ed 3, Philadelphia, 1983, WB Saunders Co.)

lation decrease about 1 cm H_2O for every centimeter distance from the lung base to its apex.[8] Toward the apex of the lung, perfusion is minimal (low $\dot{Q}_C$). Moving down the lung, perfusion increases linearly in proportion to the hydrostatic pressure, such that the lung base receives nearly 20 times as much blood flow as the apex.[8]

Ventilation. Regional differences in ventilation in the lung also occur, but are less drastic than those observed for perfusion. Like perfusion, ventilation also increases from lung apex to base. The reason for these regional differences in ventilation, as discussed in Chapter 8, is the effect of gravity on intrapleural pressures.

Pleural pressures decrease by about 0.25 cm H_2O for each centimeter distance from the lung base to its apex, such that apical pleural pressures (about -10 cm H_2O) are about 7.5 cm H_2O less than pleural pressures at the lung base.[8] Because of these differences in pleural pressures, the transpulmonary pressure gradient at the top of the upright lung is greater than that at the bottom. Alveoli at the apex are, therefore, maintained at a higher resting volume than those at the base. However, because of their relative position on the steeper portion of the pressure-volume curve (see Chapter 8), alveoli at the base of the lung will expand more than alveoli at the apex during inspiration. The result is that about four times as much ventilation goes to the base of the upright lung than to the apex.

Fig. 9-7 summarizes the relationship between ventilation and perfusion in the normal upright lung. As is evident, both blood flow and ventilation decrease from bottom to top, but blood flow decreases proportionately more than does ventilation.[6] At the bottom of the lung, blood flow is greater than ventilation, resulting in a low $\dot{V}_A/\dot{Q}_C$. Moving up the lung, blood flow decreases more than ventilation, such that toward the middle, the two are approxi-

mately equal ($\dot{V}_A/\dot{Q}_C = 1.0$). Progressing toward the apex, ventilation begins to exceed blood flow, resulting in an increasing $\dot{V}_A/\dot{Q}_C$ ratio.

Of course, these regional differences in ventilation and perfusion alter the respiratory exchange ratio, thereby affecting the partial pressures of oxygen and carbon dioxide in the alveoli.[6] At the apex of the upright lung (where the $\dot{V}_A/\dot{Q}_C$ ratio is approximately 3.3), R is about 2.0, the alveolar P_{O_2} averages 132 mm Hg, and the alveolar P_{CO_2} is maintained at about 28 mm Hg. On the other hand, at the lung bases (where the $\dot{V}_A/\dot{Q}_C$ ratio is approximately 0.6), R is about 0.66, the alveolar P_{O_2} averages 89 mm Hg, and the alveolar P_{CO_2} is maintained at about 42 mm Hg.

Obviously, these deviations from the ideal balance of ventilation and perfusion help explain why gas exchange within the lung is not perfect. Were all blood to pass through ideal exchange units, arterial partial pressures of oxygen and carbon dioxide would be equivalent to those in a perfectly ventilated and perfused alveolus. However, the majority of blood flows through exchange units at the base of the lung. Here blood flow exceeds ventilation (low $\dot{V}_A/\dot{Q}_C$), and P_{O_2} levels are lower and P_{CO_2} levels higher than those in a perfect exchange unit. When this relatively large volume of blood combines with the smaller volume coming from the apex, the result is a mixture with less oxygen and more carbon dioxide than that provided by an ideal gas exchange unit.[4]

In reality, ventilation-perfusion inequalities always have a greater effect on the exchange of oxygen than on the transfer of carbon dioxide.[3] To understand this complex phenomenon (discussed in detail in Chapter 15), we must first analyze the differences in how these two respiratory gases are transported in the blood.

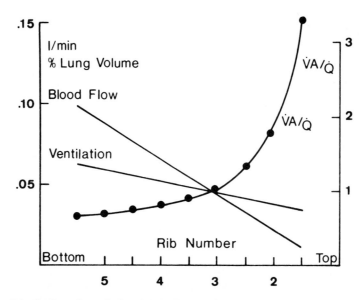

Fig. 9-7 Distribution of ventilation, blood flow, and ventilation-perfusion ratio up the normal upright lung. Straight lines have been drawn through the ventilation and blood flow data. Because blood flow falls more rapidly than ventilation with distance up the lung, the ventilation-perfusion ratio rises, slowly at first, then rapidly. (From West JB: Ventilation/bloodflow and gas exchange, Oxford, 1970, Blackwell Scientific Publishers.)

OXYGEN TRANSPORTATION

Oxygen is carried in the blood in two different states.[14] A small portion of oxygen is carried in the dissolved state in simple physical solution with the plasma and erythrocyte intracellular fluid. The vast majority of oxygen is carried in reversible chemical combination with hemoglobin within the erythrocyte.

Physically dissolved oxygen

As oxygen molecules diffuse into the blood from the alveoli, they immediately dissolve in the plasma and erythrocyte intracellular fluid. According to Henry's law, the amount of oxygen that dissolves in the plasma is directly proportional to its solubility coefficient and inversely proportional to the temperature. Assuming a constant body temperature of 37°C, 0.023 ml of oxygen will dissolve in each milliliter of plasma at a P_{O_2} of 760 mm Hg.[15]

In clinical practice, it is customary to measure and record dissolved blood gases in milliliters of gas per deciliter (100 ml) of plasma, or ml/dL (the older terms volumes% or vol% are equivalent to ml/dL). Since 0.023 ml O_2/ml plasma is equal to 2.3 ml O_2/100 ml plasma, 2.3 ml/dL of oxygen are carried in physical solution at a pressure of 760 mm Hg P_{O_2}. Dividing 2.3 by 760 derives a constant equivalent to the milliliters per deciliter of oxygen physically dissolved for each mm Hg P_{O_2}:

$$\text{ml/dL } O_2/\text{mm Hg } P_{O_2} = 2.3/760 = 0.003$$

The amount of oxygen that dissolves in plasma at any P_{O_2} can be calculated by simply multiplying this factor times the partial pressure of oxygen in the blood:

$$\text{Dissolved oxygen (ml/dL)} = P_{O_2} \times 0.003$$

Fig. 9-8 portrays this equation in graphic form. The relationship between the partial pressure of oxygen and the amount that dissolves in the plasma is direct and linear. For example, in normal arterial blood with its Pa_{O_2} of about 100 mm Hg, the dissolved oxygen equals approximately 0.3 ml/dL, or 0.3 ml of oxygen for each 100 ml of plasma. However, if a subject breathes pure oxygen, the arterial P_{O_2} could reach 673 mm Hg. In such a case, the amount of dissolved oxygen would proportionately increase to about 2.0 ml/dL. In a hyperbaric chamber breathing pure oxygen at 3 atm of pressure (2280 mm Hg), a subject may carry as much as 6.5 ml/dL dissolved oxygen in the plasma, enough alone to supply most tissue needs!

However, this partial pressure of oxygen is neither normally available nor physiologically tolerable to the lung. Instead of relying solely on dissolved oxygen for transport, the body has developed a unique and efficient chemical means for carrying this essential gas.

Chemically combined oxygen

The nature of hemoglobin. Most of the oxygen carried in the body is chemically combined with hemoglobin (Hb) in the erythrocytes. Hemoglobin is a conjugated protein consisting of four linked polypeptide chains (the globin portion), each of which is combined with a porphyrin complex called heme. The four polypeptide chains of the hemoglobin molecule are coiled together into a ball-like structure, the shape of which is critically important in determining its binding with oxygen.[1]

As shown in Fig. 9-9, each heme complex contains a

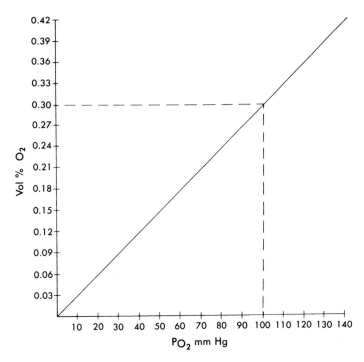

Fig. 9-8   The relationship between the number of milliliters of oxygen dissolved in blood and its consequent partial pressure is linear. Each 0.003 ml of oxygen dissolved in 100 ml of blood (vol% of O_2) exerts a pressure of 1 mm Hg. The *dashed line* emphasizes the fact that arterial blood, with an average P_{O_2} of 100 mm Hg, has 0.3 ml of oxygen dissolved in each 100 ml.

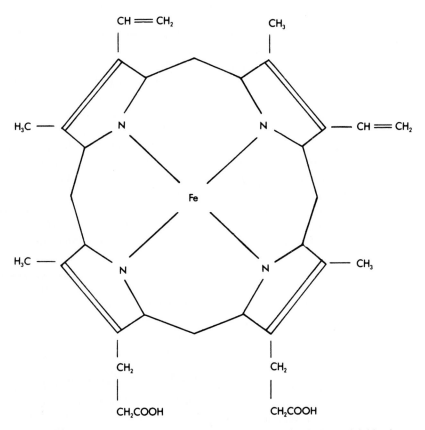

Fig. 9-9   Structure of heme. (From Lane EE and Walker JF: Clinical arterial blood gas analysis, St Louis, 1987, The CV Mosby Co.)

centrally located ferrous iron ion (Fe^{++}) that, in the reduced or deoxygenated state, has four unpaired electrons.[16] In this configuration, reduced hemoglobin (Hb^-) is a relatively weak acid. As such, Hb^- serves as an important blood buffer for hydrogen ions, a factor critically important in CO_2 transport (addressed subsequently).

It is at the ferrous iron ion site that oxygen molecules bind, one for each protein chain. On the addition of oxygen, all electrons become paired, and the hemoglobin is converted from its reduced state (Hb^-) to its oxygenated state (Hbo_2, or oxyhemoglobin).

Oxygen carrying capacity of hemoglobin. With the knowledge that each molecule of hemoglobin can combine with four molecules of oxygen, we can calculate the maximum amount of oxygen that can be carried by each gram of hemoglobin. With a molecular weight of approximately 66,700, 1 mol of hemoglobin weighs 66,700 g. This weight of hemoglobin ideally can combine with 4 mol of oxygen. Since 1 mol of oxygen at STPD is equivalent to 22.4 L or 22,400 ml (Avagadro's law), 66,700 g of hemoglobin can chemically combine with $4 \times 22,400$ ml oxygen. To calculate the amount of oxygen carried by each gram of hemoglobin, simply divide the volume equivalent of 4 mol of oxygen by the gram molecular weight of hemoglobin:

$$\frac{4 \times 22,400 \text{ ml/mol}}{66,700 \text{ g/mol}} = 1.34 \text{ ml/g*}$$

Therefore, each gram of hemoglobin is capable of carrying about 1.34 ml of oxygen. Given an average hemoglobin content in whole blood of 15 g/100 ml (15 g/dL), we may calculate the oxygen carrying capacity of the blood resulting from chemical combination with hemoglobin:

$$1.34 \text{ ml/g} \times 15 \text{ g/100 ml} = 20.1 \text{ ml/100 ml}$$
$$= 20.1 \text{ ml/dL}$$

Clearly, as compared with the blood's limited ability to carry oxygen in simple physical solution (0.3 ml/dL), the addition of hemoglobin increases the capacity for oxygen transport by nearly seventy-fold! Whether this remarkable capacity of hemoglobin to carry oxygen is actually achieved, however, depends on its saturation.

Hemoglobin saturation. The degree of saturation of the hemoglobin molecule with oxygen, Sao_2, represents a simple ratio of the amount of oxygen actually combined with hemoglobin (its content), compared with the amount of oxygen hemoglobin is capable of carrying (its capacity).[16] Hemoglobin saturation is always expressed as a percentage

of this ratio of content/capacity, and calculated according to the following formula:

$$Sao_2 = \frac{[Hbo_2]}{[Hb^-] + [Hbo_2]} \times 100$$

where $[Hbo_2]$ equals the amount of oxygenated hemoglobin (the content), and the term $[Hb^-] + [Hbo_2]$ equals the total hemoglobin available to carry oxygen, both reduced and oxygenated (the capacity).

For example, if there were a total of 15 g/dL Hb in the blood ($Hb^- + Hbo_2$), of which 7.5 g were oxyhemoglobin (Hbo_2), the Sao_2 would be calculated as:

$$Sao_2 = \frac{7.5}{15} \times 100$$
$$= 50\%$$

In this example, the hemoglobin is said to be "50% saturated," meaning that only half the available hemoglobin is actually carrying oxygen, with the remainder existing in the reduced or unoxygenated state. In actual clinical practice, we directly measure both Sao_2 and total hemoglobin content ($[Hb^-] + [Hbo_2]$) and thereby derive the $[Hbo_2]$.

The oxyhemoglobin dissociation curve. The degree of hemoglobin saturation with oxygen is determined by its affinity for this gas at various partial pressures of oxygen. The relationship between the saturation of hemoglobin with oxygen and Po_2 is described by the oxyhemoglobin dissociation curve.[14]

Unlike dissolved O_2, the amount of oxygen combined with hemoglobin is not linearly related to Po_2, but is described by an S-shaped curve (Fig. 9-10). The relatively flat upper part of the curve describes the normal operating range for arterial blood. Because the slope is minimal in this area, minor fluctuations in arterial oxygen tension, resulting from disease or environmental abnormalities, have little affect on hemoglobin saturation, indicating a strong affinity of hemoglobin for oxygen. For instance, with a normal arterial Po_2 of 100 mm Hg, hemoglobin is approximately 97% saturated with oxygen. Were some abnormality to reduce the Pao_2 to 65 mm Hg, the hemoglobin would still be about 90% saturated with oxygen.

However, below a Po_2 of 60 mm Hg, the curve steepens dramatically. In the normal operating range of the tissues, a given drop in oxygen partial pressure produces a precipitous drop in hemoglobin saturation, indicating a lessening affinity for oxygen. This relative decrease in the affinity of hemoglobin for oxygen represents a normal physiologic mechanism that assures release of large amounts of oxygen in the systemic capillaries in response to relatively small decreases in tissue Po_2.

Total oxygen contents of the blood

The total amount of oxygen carried in a given volume of blood, or total oxygen content, must equal the sum of that in physical solution and that chemically combined with he-

---

*Some controversy exists concerning the amount of oxygen that can combine with hemoglobin. Some investigators believe that the theoretic maximum is 1.39 ml/g hemoglobin, although in vivo this capacity has not been obtained. Although some texts use 1.36 ml/g, the value of 1.34 is still widely accepted and, therefore, retained for this section.

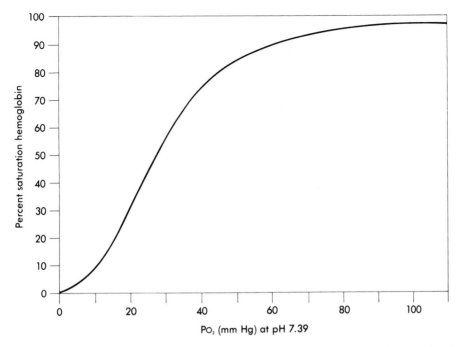

Fig. 9-10   The oxygen dissociation curve plots the relation between hemoglobin saturation (y-axis) and plasma Po_2 (x-axis). (From Lane EE and Walker JF: Clinical arterial blood gas analysis, St Louis, 1987, The CV Mosby Co.)

moglobin. Total oxygen content is abbreviated as Cxo_2, with the "x" referencing the type of blood being measured. Typically, "x" will be replaced with either an "a," indicating arterial blood, or a "v," indicating venous blood (see Chapter 3).

To calculate total oxygen content, we must know three values: the partial pressure of oxygen in the blood (Po_2), the total hemoglobin content (Hb in g/dL), and the hemoglobin saturation (Sao_2). Given these values, we proceed in three steps. First, we calculate the dissolved oxygen. Second, we calculate the oxygen chemically combined with hemoglobin. Third, we add the amount of oxygen dissolved to that chemically combined, thereby deriving the total (dissolved + chemically combined).

For example, let us assume that we obtain a sample of normal arterial blood with a Po_2 of 100 mm Hg, which contains 15 g/dL of Hb that is 97% saturated with oxygen. As a first step, we calculate the amount of dissolved oxygen by multiplying the Pao_2 times 0.003:

$$Dissolved\ O_2 = Po_2 \times 0.003$$
$$Dissolved\ O_2 = 100 \times 0.003$$
$$= 0.30\ ml/dL$$

To calculate the amount of oxygen chemically combined with hemoglobin, we multiply the hemoglobin content (15 g/dL) times its carrying capacity (1.34 ml/g) times the saturation of hemoglobin with oxygen (derived from the oxyhemoglobin dissociation curve):

$$Chemically\ combined\ O_2 = Hb\ (g/dL) \times 1.34\ ml/g \times Sao_2$$
$$Chemically\ combined\ O_2 = 15\ g/dL \times 1.34\ ml/g \times 97\%$$
$$= 19.50\ ml/dL$$

Adding the amount of oxygen dissolved to that oxygen chemically combined with hemoglobin yields the total arterial oxygen contents, or Cao_2:

$$Cao_2 = Dissolved\ O_2 + chemically\ combined\ O_2$$
$$= 0.30\ ml/dL + 19.50\ ml/dL$$
$$= 19.80\ ml/dL$$

Of course, we may also apply this approach to calculate the total oxygen content of blood returning from the tissues after unloading its oxygen. By comparing the difference in oxygen content between the point of oxygen loading (the lungs) and the point of oxygen unloading (the tissues), we can gain important insight into the overall mechanism of oxygen transportation.

Normal loading and unloading of oxygen (arterial-venous differences)

Fig. 9-11 employs the oxyhemoglobin dissociation curve to depict the events of oxygen loading at the lungs and unloading at the tissues, relative to changes in hemoglobin saturation and oxygen content of arterial and venous blood. Point Ⓐ represents normal values for arterial blood, with point Ⓥ indicating normal venous parameters.

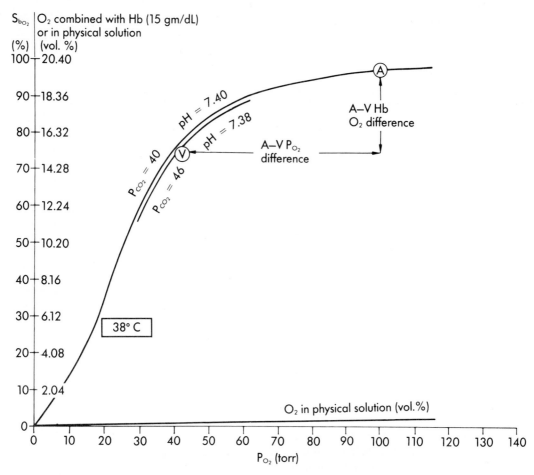

Fig. 9-11   The oxyhemoglobin dissociation curve, showing the basic relationship of blood O_2 transport. Its shape has great physiologic importance. The full curve above applies to the arterial blood of healthy man at rest, whereas the small section to its right applies to venous blood. Point *A* represents normal values for arterial blood, and point *V,* for venous blood. Changes in CO_2 pressure, pH, or temperature displace the oxyhemoglobin dissociation curve to the right or left. A physiologic shift from the venous to the arterial curve takes place as blood flows through the pulmonary capillaries, losing CO_2 and increasing in pH. The reverse shift occurs as blood flows through the systemic capillaries. Note that this effect, termed the Bohr shift, facilitates O_2 uptake in the lungs and O_2 dumping in the tissues. Note also the relatively small amount of O_2 carried by the blood in physical solution in the physiologic range of O_2 pressure.   (From Slonim NB and Hamilton LH, ed 5, St Louis, 1987, The CV Mosby Co.)

Blood leaving the lungs (point Ⓐ) is equilibrated with the alveolar P_{O_2} of about 100 mm Hg. At this P_{O_2}, the hemoglobin is approximately 97% saturated with oxygen. When arterial blood perfuses body tissues and equilibrates with the oxygen-poor cells, its P_{O_2} drops to the venous level of about 40 mm Hg, with a concurrent drop in saturation to approximately 73% (point Ⓥ). This portion of the curve, between a P_{O_2} of 100 mm Hg and 40 mm Hg, represents the difference in partial pressures between the points of oxygen loading and unloading, abbreviated $P(a-v)_{O_2}$.

To assess the actual change in oxygen content of the blood between the points of oxygen loading and unload-

ing, we must know the amount of hemoglobin in the blood. Using a normal hemoglobin content of 15 g/dL, and knowing the saturation of hemoglobin with oxygen at each possible P_{O_2}, we can calculate total oxygen contents at any P_{O_2} in the manner previously described. The y-axis of Fig. 9-11 provides this information for us, in P_{O_2} increments of 10 mm Hg. Table 9-1 summarizes the difference between the oxygen content of these normal arterial and venous points.

As indicated in Table 9-1, the difference between the arterial and venous oxygen contents is normally about 5 ml/dL. This *arterial-venous oxygen contents difference*, abbreviated $C(a-v)_{O_2}$, represents the amount of oxygen given up to the tissues by every 100 ml of blood on each pass through the systemic capillaries. Obviously, this value reflects the mean of the body as a whole, with different organ systems extracting more or less oxygen according to need.

Fick equation. Since the $C(a-v)o_2$ indicates oxygen extraction in proportion to blood flow, knowledge of this value, in combination with total body oxygen consumption, may be used to calculate cardiac output. The Fick equation relates these factors as follows:

$$\dot{Q}_T = \frac{\dot{V}o_2}{C(a-v)o_2 \times 10}$$

where $\dot{Q}_T$ equals cardiac output in L/min, $\dot{V}o_2$ equals total body oxygen consumption in ml/min, and $C(a-v)o_2$ equals the arterial-venous oxygen contents difference in ml/dL, with a factor of 10 used to convert ml/dL to ml/L. Given a normal $\dot{V}o_2$ of 250 ml/min and a normal $C(a-v)o_2$ of 5 ml/dL, we may calculate a normal cardiac output as:

$$\dot{Q}_T = \frac{250 \text{ ml/min}}{5 \text{ ml/dL} \times 10}$$

$$\dot{Q}_T = \frac{250 \text{ ml/min}}{50 \text{ ml/L}}$$

$$\dot{Q}_T = 5.0 \text{ L/min}$$

Significance of the $C(a-v)o_2$. According to this formula, if the oxygen consumption remains constant, a decrease in cardiac output will manifest itself by an increase in the $C(a-v)o_2$. Conversely, should cardiac output rise and oxygen consumption remain constant, the $C(a-v)o_2$ will fall proportionately. Although the Fick method of calculating cardiac output has generally been replaced by other techniques, the principle relating $C(a-v)o_2$ to perfusion regularly is applied in the monitoring of tissue oxygenation at the bedside. More details on these methods are provided in Chapter 31.

Factors affecting oxygen loading and unloading

In addition to the shape of the oxyhemoglobin curve, the loading and unloading of oxygen is affected by several important factors. Among those most important in clinical practice are: (1) the hydrogen ion concentration of the blood (pH), (2) the body temperature, and (3) the concentration of certain organic phosphates in the erythrocyte. Also affecting the loading and unloading of oxygen are

variations in the chemical structure of hemoglobin (some normal and others pathologic) and chemical combinations of hemoglobin with substances other than oxygen, in particular, carbon monoxide.

Hydrogen ion concentration of the blood (pH). The mechanism and clinical significance of blood pH changes are discussed in detail in Chapter 10. At this point, all we need to understand is that the affinity of hemoglobin for oxygen is significantly affected by changes in blood pH.

Bohr effect. The effect of variations in blood pH on the affinity of hemoglobin for oxygen is called the Bohr effect. As shown in Fig. 9-12, the Bohr effect manifests itself in changes in the relative position of the oxyhemoglobin dissociation curve. A decrease in pH shifts the curve to the right, and an increase in pH shifts it to the left.[17] This alteration in position of the curve is attributed to changes in the strength of the loose chemical bonds between the amino acids forming the hemoglobin chains. These changes alter the shape of the molecule as a whole, thereby increasing or decreasing the accessibility of the heme complex for oxygen binding.

As blood pH drops and the curve shifts to the right, the hemoglobin saturation for a given Po_2 falls, indicating that the affinity of hemoglobin for oxygen has decreased. Conversely, as blood pH rises and the curve shifts to the left, the hemoglobin saturation for a given Po_2 rises, indicating that the affinity of hemoglobin for oxygen has increased.

Physiologic significance. Even within the narrow range in which blood alternates between its arterial and venous states, the Bohr effect has physiologic importance. As illustrated in Fig. 9-13, blood pH varies about 0.03 unit between the normal venous and arterial points. As blood becomes venous, its carbon dioxide content rises, resulting in a decrease in pH from about 7.40 to 7.37. As a result, the oxyhemoglobin curve shifts slightly to the right, lowering the affinity of hemoglobin for oxygen. With this lowered affinity for oxygen, hemoglobin more readily gives up its oxygen, thus facilitating its unloading at the tissues.

Conversely, when venous blood returns to the lungs, the pH increases to the arterial point of 7.40. This rise in pH shifts the oxyhemoglobin curve to the left, thereby increasing the affinity of hemoglobin for oxygen and enhancing its uptake from the alveoli. The Bohr effect thus facilitates pulmonary uptake and tissue delivery of oxygen.[14]

Effect of wide fluctuations in pH. According to the Bohr effect, even when there is no change in Po_2, variation in blood pH can substantially modify the oxygen carrying capacity of the blood. Fig. 9-13 illustrates the effect that wide fluctuations in pH can have on the blood's oxygen carrying capacity. As an example, with a Pao_2 of 50 mm Hg, there is approximately a 15% difference in hemoglobin saturation between the pH values of 7.20 and 7.60.

Because the blood is able to maintain a higher oxygen saturation in a state of alkalosis than in acidosis, one might

Table 9-1 Oxygen Content of Arterial and Venous Blood

	Arterial O_2 (ml/dL)	Venous O_2 (ml/dL)
Combined O_2 ($1.34 \times 15 \times$ Sat)	19.5	14.7
Dissolved O_2 ($Po_2 \times 0.003$)	0.3	0.1
Total O_2 content	19.8	14.8

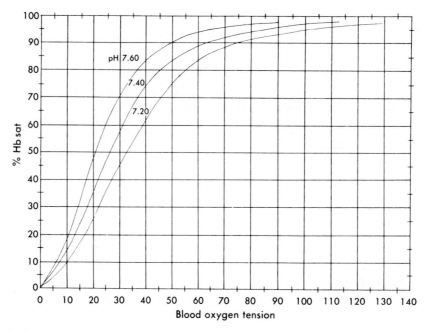

Fig. 9-12   Oxygen dissociation curve of blood at 37°C, showing variations at three pH levels. For a given oxygen tension, the higher the blood pH, the more the hemoglobin holds onto its oxygen, maintaining a higher saturation.

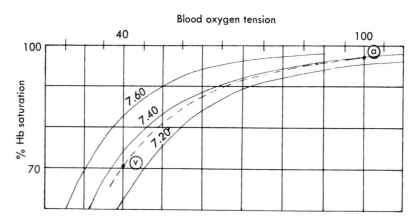

Fig. 9-13   Bohr effect. The *dashed line* indicates the physiologic shift in oxygen dissociation curve as changing blood carbon dioxide content alters blood pH between arterial, ⓐ, and venous, ⓥ, points.

presume that alkalosis is a desirable state. Comparison of the performance of both the pH 7.60 and pH 7.20 dissociation curves (see Fig. 9-13) demonstrates that this premise is false.

Assuming a hemoglobin concentration of 15 g/dL and complete oxygen equilibration at arterial and venous Po_2 levels of 100 mm Hg and 40 mm Hg, respectively, we read oxygen saturations of 98% for arterial blood and 84% for venous blood on the pH = 7.60 curve. Likewise, we read corresponding saturations of 94% and 62% on the pH = 7.20 curve. We can now compare the $C(a-v)o_2$ between the arterial and venous points for each abnormal pH value, and compare them with the normal $C(a-v)o_2$, as outlined in Table 9-2.

Although there is less than 1 ml/dL difference between the two abnormal pH blood samples at the arterial point, after tissue perfusion the $C(a-v)o_2$ of the blood with the low pH is more than double that of the blood with a pH of

Table 9-2   Arterial-Venous Oxygen Difference at Three pH Levels

| | Total O_2 (ml/dL) | | a−v (ml/dL) O_2 |
	Arterial	Venous	
pH 7.60	20.0	17.0	3.0
pH 7.40	19.8	14.8	5.0
pH 7.20	19.2	12.6	6.6

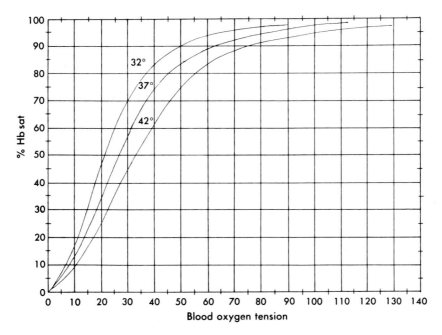

Fig. 9-14   Oxygen dissociation curve of blood at a pH of 7.40, showing variations at three temperatures. For a given oxygen tension, the lower the temperature, the more the hemoglobin holds onto its oxygen, maintaining a higher saturation.

7.60. This indicates that hemoglobin in blood with a lower than normal hydrogen ion concentration (high pH) holds its oxygen more strongly, making it less available to tissues than that normally provided.

This does not mean that a low blood pH is beneficial. Indeed, hemoglobin in blood with a low pH more readily releases oxygen to the tissues. However, the damaging effects of an increase in hydrogen ion concentration that are marked by a low pH more than outweigh any benefits gained in the ease of tissue oxygen extraction. Physiologically, maintenance of normal levels of arterial oxygen saturation, in conjunction with a pH in the normal range, assures both adequate loading and unloading of oxygen from hemoglobin.

Body temperature. In addition to variations in pH (and associated changes in Pco_2), alterations in body temperature influence the position of the oxyhemoglobin dissociation curve. As shown in Fig. 9-14, a drop in body temperature shifts the curve to the left, resulting in a higher hemoglobin saturation for a given Po_2, and thereby a greater affinity of hemoglobin for oxygen. Conversely, as body temperature rises, the curve shifts to the right, indicating a decrease in the affinity of hemoglobin for oxygen.

Like the Bohr effect, variations in the affinity of hemoglobin for oxygen caused by temperature changes enhance normal oxygen uptake and delivery.[14] At the tissue level, variations in temperature are directly related to metabolic rate, such that areas of high metabolic activity have higher temperatures. In areas such as exercising muscle, higher temperatures decrease the affinity of hemoglobin for oxygen, thereby enhancing its release to the tissues. In clinical practice, this same phenomenon occurs body wide under conditions of hyperpyrexia. Conversely, in hypothermia, the oxygen demands of the tissues are greatly reduced, and hemoglobin need not give up as much of its oxygen.

Because temperature influences hemoglobin saturation, and because patients' temperatures may vary substantially over time, it is customary to measure oxygen tension at a standard temperature of 37°C, correcting both tension and saturation to the patient's actual temperature by the use of tabulated factors or nomograms.

Organic phosphates. In the area of general metabolism, organic phosphates play vital roles in many cellular biochemical reactions and are essential to the transfer of energy on which cellular function depends. Within the past few years, attention has been directed to the involvement of phosphates in respiration. The two most significant organic phosphates in this regard are 2,3-diphosphoglycerate (2,3-DPG) and adenosine triphosphate (ATP). In the interest of brevity and because of its relatively greater importance, we describe 2,3-DPG as the prototype.[18,19]

At 0.85 mol/mol Hb, 2,3-DPG is the most abundant phosphate in the erythrocyte.[16] 2,3-DPG is synthesized via the metabolic pathways of glucose metabolism and can form a loose chemical bond with subunits of the globin chains of the unsaturated hemoglobin molecule. In combining with hemoglobin, 2,3-DPG stabilizes the molecule in its unsaturated configuration, thereby reducing its affinity for oxygen.[20] Indeed, without the existence of 2,3-DPG, the affinity of hemoglobin for oxygen would be so great that normal oxygen unloading would be impossible. The ability of 2,3-DPG to decrease the affinity of hemoglobin for oxygen is in direct proportion to its concentration within the erythrocyte.

Therefore, increased concentrations of 2,3-DPG shift the oxyhemoglobin dissociation curve to the right, promoting oxygen unloading at the tissues. Conversely, a shortage of this important organic phosphate within the erythrocyte will shift the curve to the left, increasing the affinity of hemoglobin for oxygen, and impairing its capacity to unload oxygen.

Changes in the intracellular level of 2,3-DPG occur during the events of normal gas exchange in the erythrocyte, and in response to certain chronic conditions. These factors, and their clinical significance, are outlined below.

Changes in pH. Intracellular 2,3-DPG concentrations vary directly with changes in pH, about 5% for each 0.01 unit pH change. Although an increase in pH immediately shifts the oxyhemoglobin curve to the left (the Bohr effect), the primary pH change increases intracellular 2,3-DPG, causing a slower compensatory shift back toward the original position. Conversely, a drop in pH will immediately shift the oxyhemoglobin curve to the right, but because of decreasing intracellular levels of 2,3-DPG, the curve will tend to move back toward its normal position. Several hours are required for these compensatory changes in 2,3-DPG levels.[20]

Chronic hypoxemia. Unlike the secondary change that occurs in 2,3 DPG levels with alterations in pH, chronic hypoxemia causes a primary and sustained elevation in intracellular 2,3-DPG concentrations.[21] This change maintains a right shift of the oxyhemoglobin curve, increasing the availability of oxygen to the tissues. This adaptive response is seen in normal individuals living at high altitudes and among those with pathologic conditions characterized by long-standing arterial hypoxemia, such as cyanotic congenital heart disease, chronic cardiovascular insufficiency, and chronic obstructive lung disease.

Anemia. Intracellular 2,3-DPG levels increase about 0.23% for each gram per deciliter drop in hemoglobin.[22] Like the response to chronic hypoxemia, this change represents an adaptation that may compensate for up to half the oxygen deficit caused by the loss of erythrocytes. Unlike the response to chronic hypoxemia, the increased 2,3-DPG levels observed with anemia can occur within minutes.[20] Moreover, this rapid response may account for the common observation that hypoxic symptoms are not always present in patients with severe anemia.

Banked blood. Banked blood exhibits a substantial decrease in 2,3-DPG levels over time, such that after 1 week of storage, the concentration of this organic phosphate is about one third normal.[20] This change shifts the oxyhemoglobin curve to the left, thereby decreasing the availability of oxygen to the tissues. Large transfusions of banked blood more than a few days old may therefore severely compromise oxygen delivery, even in the presence of a normal Po_2.

Abnormal hemoglobins. Also affecting the loading and unloading of oxygen are the presence of abnormal variants in the structure of the hemoglobin molecule. Normal adult hemoglobin is abbreviated HbA. Abnormal hemoglobins are given different letter designations, often according to the geographic locale where they were first identified. Thus HbR is the abbreviation for hemoglobin Rainier, and HbK the shorthand for hemoglobin Kansas. Each of the abnormal forms vary according to the composition of the amino acids in the polypeptide chains of the globin portion of the molecule. Over 120 abnormal hemoglobins have been identified, and even in normal individuals, anywhere from 15% to 40% of the circulating hemoglobin may have a structure different from normal HbA.[16,23]

Abnormal molecular structures. Variations in the composition of the amino acids in the polypeptide chains of the molecular structure alter its shape, either increasing or decreasing the accessibility of the heme portion to oxygen. Changes in the accessibility of the heme complex result in greater or lesser affinity for oxygen, and are manifested by a shift in the oxyhemoglobin curve. HbC (Chesapeake), HbR (Rainier), and HbY (Yakima) exhibit varying degrees of increased affinity for oxygen, with the latter causing a clinically significant shift to the left. HbK, on the other hand, has a lesser affinity for oxygen than HbA, causing a dramatic shift of the oxyhemoglobin curve to the right.[24]

Despite significant differences in the oxygen affinity exhibited by the abnormal hemoglobins, individuals with substantial percentages of these variants have near normal arterial-venous oxygen contents differences $(C(a-v)o_2)$, indicating adequate O_2 delivery to the tissues. Compensation probably occurs through changes in cardiac output and/or erythrocyte production.

Sickle cell anemia also represents a condition caused by an abnormal hemoglobin variant. Genetically determined, sickle cell anemia results from substitution of a single amino acid on two of the four chains of the globin moiety, producing HbS. HbS has less affinity for oxygen than HbA. More important from a clinical standpoint, however, is the fact that deoxygenated HbS is less soluble than either oxygenated HbS or HbA. In its deoxygenated form, HbS can actually crystallize within the erythrocyte, causing the characteristic deformation in the shape of the cell. This increases the fragility of the erythrocyte, and raises the possibility of thrombus formation.[4]

Oxidized hemoglobin (methemoglobin). Normally, the iron ion of the heme complex exists in the ferrous state (Fe^{++}). If oxidized, the ferrous iron loses an electron, changing to the ferric state (Fe^{+++}). This abnormal form of hemoglobin, called methemoglobin (metHb), cannot bind with oxygen and is therefore useless in oxygen transport.

Oxidation of hemoglobin to methemoglobin produces a condition called methemoglobinemia, comparable in effect to other forms of anemia. The most common cause of methemoglobinemia is nitrite poisoning. However, a large number of oxidizing agents, including aniline, paraaminosalicylic acid, and phenylhydrazine, can have a similar effect.[16] Congenital methemoglobinemias, though rare, also exist. These may be associated with a specific enzyme deficiency, either acquired or inherited.

In large quantities, methemoglobin gives the blood a characteristic brownish color. This produces a slate-gray skin coloration that may be confused with cyanosis.[1] The actual presence of methemoglobin can only be confirmed by absorption spectrophotometry. Treatment of methemoglobinemias caused by poisoning from oxidants involves removing the offending chemical and restoring the hemoglobin back to its ferrous state with a reducing agent such as methylene blue or ascorbic acid.

Fetal hemoglobin. During fetal life and for up to 1 year after birth, the blood has a high proportion of a hemoglobin variant called fetal hemoglobin (HbF). HbF exhibits a greater affinity for oxygen than adult hemoglobin, as manifested by a left shift of the oxyhemoglobin curve.[25] Given the characteristically low Po_2 available at the placenta, this left shift facilitates the loading of oxygen at the site of maternal-fetal gas exchange. Because of the relatively low pH of the fetal environment, unloading of oxygen at the cellular level is not greatly affected. After birth, however, this enhanced affinity for oxygen is less advantageous, and the fetal hemoglobin gradually is replaced over the first year of life with HbA. However, the production of HbF in adults can be stimulated by anemia.[20]

Carboxyhemoglobin. The affinity of hemoglobin for carbon monoxide (CO) is about 200 to 300 times greater than that for oxygen. Thus, even extremely low concentrations of this product of incomplete combustion will quickly displace oxygen from the hemoglobin molecule, forming HbCO, or carboxyhemoglobin. A carbon dioxide partial pressure of as low as 0.12 mm Hg can result in as much as 50% saturation of hemoglobin with carbon monoxide.[20] Because carboxyhemoglobin is useless for oxygen transport, each gram of hemoglobin that is saturated with carbon monoxide is equivalent to the absolute loss of a comparable amount of this pigment, as occurs in other types of anemia. For example, 50% saturation of hemoglobin with carbon monoxide has the same effect as an anemia with a hemoglobin content of 7.5 ml/dL. Moreover, the combination of carbon monoxide with hemoglobin shifts the oxyhemoglobin to the left, further interfering with oxygen delivery to the tissues. The treatment for carbon monoxide poisoning involves administration of as high a partial pressure of oxygen as possible, sometimes requiring the use of a hyperbaric chamber.[26]

Measurement of hemoglobin affinity for oxygen

Variations in the affinity of hemoglobin and its abnormal variants can be quantified using a measurement called the P_{50}. The P_{50} is defined as the partial pressure of oxygen at which the hemoglobin is 50% saturated, standardized to a pH of 7.40. A normal P_{50} is approximately 26.6 mm Hg. Conditions resulting in a decrease in hemoglobin affinity for oxygen (a shift of the oxyhemoglobin curve to the right) result in an increase in the P_{50} above normal. Conditions associated with an increase in hemoglobin affinity for oxygen (a shift of the oxyhemoglobin curve to the left) result in a decrease in the P_{50} below normal. For example, given a normal hemoglobin content of 15 g/dL, a 4 mm Hg increase in P_{50} would result in about 1 to 2 ml/dL more oxygen being unloaded at the tissues than when the P_{50} is normal.[27] Fig. 9-15 graphically demonstrates the application of the P_{50} measurement, summarizing how the major factors previously discussed affect the affinity of hemoglobin for oxygen.

CARBON DIOXIDE TRANSPORTATION

Fig. 9-16 portrays the physical and chemical events of gas exchange at the level of the systemic capillaries. At the level of the pulmonary capillaries, all events occur in the opposite direction. Although the primary focus here is carbon dioxide transport, Fig. 9-16 also includes the basic elements of oxygen exchange, previously discussed. Oxygen exchange is included here not only for completeness; the exchange and transport of these two gases are closely related.

Transport mechanisms

From 50 to 60 ml/dL of carbon dioxide are carried in the blood in three forms: (1) dissolved in physical solution, (2) chemically combined with protein, and (3) ionized as bicarbonate.[14]

Dissolved carbon dioxide. As with oxygen, CO_2 produced by the tissue cells dissolves in the plasma and intracellular fluid of the erythrocytes. Unlike oxygen, however, CO_2, which exists in physical solution in the blood, plays an important role in transport, accounting for about 10% of the total released at the lungs. This is because of the higher solubility coefficient of CO_2 in the plasma and the resultant greater proportion of this gas transported in physical solution.

Most of the carbon dioxide that goes into physical solution does not remain in that state. Instead, it chemically combines with other constituents of the blood, including protein and water.

Chemically combined with protein. Molecular carbon dioxide has the capacity to chemically combine with free amino groups (NH_2) of protein molecules (Prot), forming a carbamino compound:

$$Prot\text{-}NH_2 + CO_2 \rightleftharpoons Prot\text{-}NHCOO^- + H^+$$

About 1% of the carbon dioxide that leaves the tissue cells combines with plasma proteins to form these carbam-

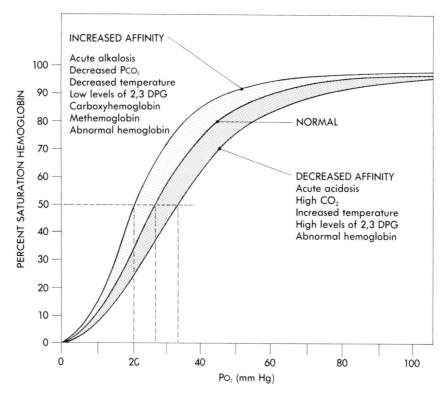

Fig. 9-15   Conditions associated with altered affinity of hemoglobin for O_2. P_{50} is the Pa_{O_2} at which hemoglobin is 50% saturated, normally 26.6 mm Hg. A lower than normal P_{50} represents increased affinity of hemoglobin for O_2; a high P_{50} is seen with decreased affinity. Note that variation from the normal is associated with decreased (low P_{50}) or increased (high P_{50}) availability of O_2 to tissues *(dotted lines)*. The shaded area shows the entire oxyhemoglobin dissociation curve under the same circumstances. (From Lane EE and Walker JF: Clinical arterial blood gas analysis, St Louis, 1987, The CV Mosby Co.)

ino compounds.[10] This fraction of carbon dioxide is relatively insignificant.

A larger fraction (about 20%) of the carbon dioxide combines with erythrocyte hemoglobin to form a carbamino compound called carbamino-Hb.[14] The resulting H^+ ions (see the above equation) are buffered by the reduced hemoglobin (Hb^-) made available by the concurrent release of oxygen to the tissues. The availability of additional sites for H^+ buffering has the effect of increasing the affinity of hemoglobin for CO_2. Moreover, because reduced hemoglobin is a weaker acid than oxyhemoglobin, pH changes associated with the release of the H^+ ions during the formation of carbamino-Hb are minimized. Although the carbamino-Hb constitutes only about 20% of the total carbon dioxide transported, it accounts for nearly 30% of that released at the lungs.

Ionized as bicarbonate. Of the CO_2 that dissolves in plasma, a small portion (about 5%) chemically combines with water in a process called hydrolysis. Hydrolysis of CO_2 initially forms carbonic acid, which quickly ionizes into hydrogen and bicarbonate ions[5]:

$$CO_2 + H_2O \rightleftharpoons H_2CO_3 \rightleftharpoons HCO_3^- + H^+$$

The resulting H^+ ions are buffered by the plasma proteins in much the same way as hemoglobin buffers H^+ within the red blood cell. However, the rate of this hydrolysis reaction in the plasma is extremely slow, and the amount of hydrogen and bicarbonate ions formed by this mechanism is minuscule.

The major portion of the transported carbon dioxide (about two thirds, or 63%) undergoes hydrolysis inside the erythrocyte, a reaction greatly enhanced by an enzyme catalyst called carbonic anhydrase (CA). The resulting H^+ ions are buffered by the imidazole group ($R-NHCOO^-$) of the reduced hemoglobin molecule. Again, the concurrent conversion of oxyhemoglobin to reduced hemoglobin facilitates the buffering of the H^+ ions, thereby enhancing the loading of CO_2 as carbamino-Hb.

As the hydrolysis of CO_2 continues, HCO_3^- ions begin to accumulate in the erythrocyte. To maintain a concentration equilibrium across the erythrocyte cell membrane, some of these anions diffuse outward into the plasma. Because the red blood cell is not freely permeable to cations, electrolytic equilibrium must be maintained via an inward migration of anions. This is accomplished by the shift of chloride ions (Cl^-) from the plasma into the erythrocyte, a

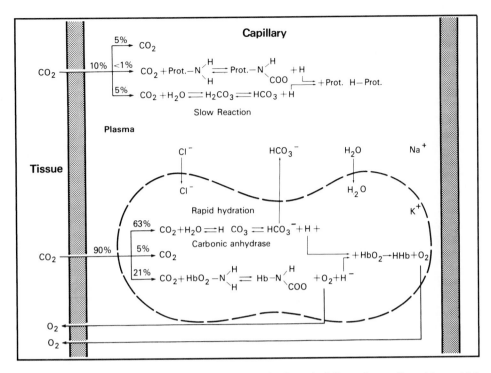

Fig. 9-16 Summary diagram of the various fates of CO_2 as it diffuses from cells and interstitial space into the peripheral capillaries prior to its transport toward the venous circulation. (From Martin DE and Youtsey JW: Respiratory anatomy and physiology, St Louis, 1988, The CV Mosby Co.)

process called the *chloride shift*, or the Hamburger phenomenon.

Carbon dioxide dissociation curve

Just as there is a relationship between blood Po_2 and oxygen saturation of hemoglobin, there is also a relationship between blood Pco_2 and content of carbon dioxide. This relationship is graphically portrayed via the carbon dioxide dissociation curve, shown in Fig. 9-17.

The first point to note is the influence that oxygen saturation has on the relationship between blood Pco_2 and content of carbon dioxide. We already know that carbon dioxide levels, through their influence on pH, modify the oxygen dissociation curve (Bohr effect). As shown in Fig. 9-17, *A*, it also is apparent that hemoglobin saturation with oxygen affects the position of the carbon dioxide dissociation curve. The influence of hemoglobin saturation with oxygen on CO_2 dissociation is called the *Haldane effect*. As previously explained, this phenomenon is attributable to changes in the affinity of hemoglobin for CO_2 that occur as a result of its buffering of H^+ ions.

Fig. 9-17, *A*, shows the curves of carbon dioxide dissociation for three levels of blood oxygen saturation, two of which are physiologic values, and the third an extreme value provided for contrast. These might be called "laboratory curves," since they are experimentally determined by subjecting samples of *whole blood* to various oxygen saturations and measuring the carbon dioxide content of each at different carbon dioxide tension exposures.

The purpose of the curves is to show how carbon dioxide dissociates from the blood as its partial pressure changes. The graphs indicate how this relationship depends on oxygen saturation. Fig. 9-17, *B*, shows selected segments of the curves to include the physiologic range of Pco_2, from the arterial point (ⓐ) with a Pco_2 of 40 mm Hg, Sao_2 of 97.5%, and carbon dioxide content of 48 ml/dL; to the venous point (ⓥ), with a Pco_2 of 46 mm Hg, Svo_2 of 70%, and carbon dioxide content of 53 ml/dL. Since oxygen saturation changes from arterial to venous blood, the true physiologic carbon dioxide dissociation curve must lie somewhere between the two "laboratory curves" for arterial and venous saturation. Such a curve is shown as the dashed line in Fig. 9-17, *B*.

At point ⓐ, the high Sao_2 decreases the capacity of the blood to hold CO_2, thus encouraging the unloading of this gas at the lungs. At point ⓥ, the lower Svo_2 increases the capacity of blood to hold CO_2, thus encouraging its uptake from the tissues.

Table 9-3 compares and contrasts the total carbon dioxide content of both arterial and venous blood plasma according to its major components. Here, "combined CO_2" is equivalent to carbamine compounds plus bicarbonate, while "dissolved CO_2" is that portion in simple physical solution in the plasma and erythrocyte water. Note that the

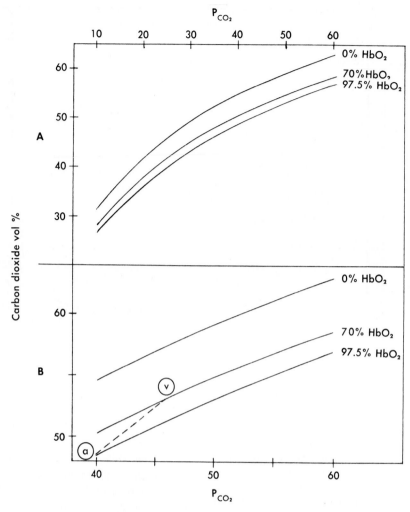

Fig. 9-17 Haldane effect and carbon dioxide dissociation curves. **A,** The relationship between carbon dioxide content and tension at three levels of hemoglobin saturation. **B,** Close-up of the curves between P_{CO_2} of 40 mm Hg and 60 mm Hg (see text for details). (Modified from Comroe JH Jr et al: The lung, ed 2, Chicago, 1962, Year Book Medical Publishers.)

Table 9-3 Carbon Dioxide Content of Arterial and Venous Blood Plasma

	Arterial		Venous	
	ml/dL	[mM/L]	ml/dL	[mM/L]
Combined CO_2	55.60	24.0	59.00	27.1
Dissolved CO_2	2.78	1.2	3.13	1.4
Total CO_2	58.38	25.2	62.13	28.5
P_{CO_2}	40 mm Hg		46 mm Hg	

amounts of CO_2 are expressed in both gaseous volume equivalents (ml/dL) and as millimoles per liter (mM/L). This latter measure of the chemical combining power of CO_2 in physiologic solutions is critical in understanding the role of this gas in acid-base balance.

Relationship of CO_2 to acid-base balance

Of critical importance in the maintenance of acid-base homeostasis is the relationship between the carbon dioxide that is carried as bicarbonate (a salt) and that which exists as carbonic acid (a weak acid). Together, this salt and its weak acid form the primary buffer system of the body, ensuring that fluctuations in H^+ concentrations have a minimal affect on changes in pH.

Because H_2CO_3 concentrations cannot be measured directly, we estimate the concentration of this weak acid. Since the amount of carbon dioxide that is hydrolyzed in the plasma to carbonic acid is directly proportional to the amount in physical solution, we may use the concentration of dissolved CO_2 to derive an estimate of the H_2CO_3.

As indicated in Table 9-3, the ratio of combined CO_2 (24 mEq/L) to that physically dissolved in the arterial blood (1.2 mEq/L) is maintained at a remarkably constant ratio of 20:1. Maintenance of this ratio ensures that the pH of the blood will stay within normal limits. Likewise, deviation from this ratio will result in abnormal shifts in pH. These important concepts will be pursued in depth in the next chapter.

SUMMARY

The exchange of oxygen and carbon dioxide between the atmosphere and the tissue cells depends mainly on the physical process of gaseous diffusion. Although anatomic shunts and regional differences in ventilation and perfusion make the lung a less than perfect organ of gas exchange, normal partial pressure gradients at the alveolar-capillary membrane are sufficient to ensure rapid movement of oxygen and carbon dioxide between the alveoli and pulmonary circulation.

The loading of these respired gases at the lung, and their unloading at the tissues, is further enhanced by specialized blood gas transport mechanisms. These mechanisms mutually facilitate each other, so that the process of oxygen uptake and delivery assists in the excretion and removal of carbon dioxide. Moreover, carbon dioxide transport plays a critical role in the regulation of acid-base homeostasis.

Normally, these processes are well integrated and maintained in a constant state of balance. However, abnormalities in structure or function can alter this balance and potentially disrupt the normal exchange and transport of respired gases between the atmosphere and the tissue cells.

Under such conditions, restoration of normal gas exchange and transport is a primary goal of respiratory care.

REFERENCES

1. Nunn JF: Applied respiratory physiology, ed 2, Kent, England, 1977, Butterworth & Co.
2. Tisi GM: Pulmonary physiology in clinical medicine, ed 2, Baltimore, 1984, Williams & Wilkins Co.
3. Martin L: Pulmonary physiology in clinical practice: the essentials for patient care and evaluation, St Louis, 1987, The CV Mosby Co.
4. West JB: Respiratory physiology—the essentials, ed 3, Baltimore, 1985, Williams & Wilkins Co.
5. Foster RE et al: The lung: physiologic basis of pulmonary function tests, ed 3, Chicago, 1986, Year Book Medical Publishers.
6. West JB: Ventilation-perfusion relationships, Am Rev Respir Dis 116:919, 1977.
7. Divertie MB and Brown AL Jr: The fine structure of the normal alveolocapillary membrane, JAMA 187:938, 1964.
8. Green JF: Fundamental cardiovascular and pulmonary physiology, ed 2, Philadelphia, 1987, Lea & Febiger.
9. Weast RC, editor: Handbook of chemistry and physics, ed 69, Cleveland, 1988, Chemical Rubber Co. Pub.
10. Comroe JH: Physiology of respiration, ed 2, Chicago, 1974, Year Book Medical Publishers.
11. Roughton FJW: The average time spent by the blood in the human lung capillary, and its relation to the rates of carbon monoxide uptake and elimination in man, Am J Physiol 143:621, 1945.
12. Harris EA et al: The normal alveolar-arterial oxygen tension gradient in man, Clin Sci Mol Med 46:89, 1974.
13. Murray JF: The normal lung, ed 2, Philadelphia, 1986, WB Saunders Co.
14. Roughton FW: Transport of oxygen and carbon dioxide. In Handbook of physiology, Sect 3, Respiration, vol 1, Washington, DC, 1964, American Physiological Association.
15. Peters JP and Van Slyke DD: Quantitative clinical chemistry, vol 2, Baltimore, 1931, Williams & Wilkins Co.
16. Lane EE and Walker JF: Clinical arterial blood gas analysis, St Louis, 1987, The CV Mosby Co.
17. Astrup P: Red-cell pH and oxygen affinity of hemoglobin, N Engl J Med 283:202, 1970.
18. Benesch R and Benesch RE: Intracellular organic phosphates as regulators of oxygen release by hemoglobin, Nature 221:618, 1969.
19. Klocke RA: Oxygen transport and 2,3-diphosphoglycerate (DPG), Chest 62 Suppl:79s, 1972.
20. Slonim NB and Hamilton LH: Respiratory physiology, ed 5, St Louis, 1985, The CV Mosby Co.
21. Oski FA et al: Red-cell 2,3-diphosphoglycerate levels in subjects with chronic hypoxemia, N Engl J Med 280:1165, 1969.
22. Torrance J et al: Intraerythrocyte adaptation to anemia, N Engl J Med 283:165, 1970.
23. Nagel RL and Bookchin RM: Human hemoglobin mutants with abnormal oxygen binding, Sem Hematol 11:385, 1974.
24. Parer JT: Oxygen transport in human subjects with hemoglobin variants having altered oxygen affinity, Respir Physiol 9:43, 1970.
25. Gregory IC: The oxygen and carbon dioxide capacities of fetal and adult hemoglobin, J Physiol (Lond) 236:625, 1974.
26. Norkool DM and Kirkpatrick JN: Treatment of acute carbon monoxide poisoning with hyperbaric oxygen: a review of 115 cases, Ann Emerg Med 14:1168, 1985.
27. Miller MF: Laboratory evaluation of pulmonary function, Philadelphia, 1987, JB Lippincott Co.

10

Acid-Base Balance and the Regulation of Respiration

Craig L. Scanlan

A central component of body homeostasis is the maintenance of a narrow range of pH. Although this range differs among various tissues and organ systems, deviations in the hydrogen ion concentration of 25% or more (a pH above 7.5 or below 7.3) can alter intracellular enzyme activity and increase the irritability of nerve and muscle tissue, especially that of the heart.[1] Survival is unlikely when the pH of body fluids drops below 7.0 or exceeds 7.8.

Normal metabolic processes of the body produce in excess of 24,000 mM of acid per day.[2] Therefore, mechanisms must exist to (1) prevent this acid load from causing wide fluctuations in pH, and (2) remove or excrete these by-products of metabolism. Several buffer systems assist in preventing wide fluctuations in pH in the body fluids. Excretion of body acids is accomplished by both the kidneys and lungs.

The respiratory system plays a vital role in both components of acid-base homeostasis. Indeed, the primary mechanisms involved in the regulation of breathing balance acid excretion to acid production through minute to minute changes in ventilation. Disorders of the respiratory system, including alterations in neural control mechanisms, can disrupt this delicate balance, thereby altering normal acid-base homeostasis.

For this reason, respiratory care practitioners must be capable of assessing patients' acid-base balance and the influence of the respiratory system on pH homeostasis. This critical ability requires in-depth knowledge of normal and abnormal acid-base chemistry and its relationship to the neural control of breathing.

OBJECTIVES

After completion of this chapter, the reader should be able to:

1. Compare and contrast the role of the body buffer systems, lungs, and kidneys in normal acid-base homeostasis;

2. Apply the concept of ionization constant to the calculation of the pH of the bicarbonate buffer system (the Henderson-Hasselbalch equation);

3. Employ the parameters of the Henderson-Hasselbalch equation to differentiate among the four primary (uncompensated) and four secondary (compensated) states of acid-base imbalance;

4. Compare the four primary states of acid-base imbalance according to underlying causes, and mechanisms of compensation and correction;

5. Interrelate the various physiologic processes responsible for regulating ventilation;

6. Describe the responses of the neural and chemical control mechanisms under abnormal conditions, including selected acid-base disorders.

KEY TERMS

Most terms used in this chapter are defined in context. The following terms are introduced without explicit definition, but may be found in the text glossary:

afferent
cerebrospinal
corticosteroid
diencephalon
efferent
glomerulus
Guillain-Barré syndrome
isopleth
ketoacidosis
mesencephalon
nephron
nomogram
paresthesia
peritubular

pickwickian syndrome
reabsorption
rostral
salicylate
semipermeable
tetany
titratable
transect
vagotomy
ventrolateral

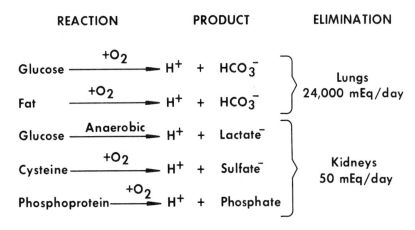

Fig. 10-1 Condensed chemical reactions show the products of several important metabolic pathways and the routes by which H^+ is eliminated. (From Murray JF: The normal lung, ed 2, Philadelphia, 1986, WB Saunders Co.)

ACID-BASE CHEMISTRY

Maintaining normal acid-base balance is one of the body's more important functions, and one in which respiration plays a major role. The body's goal in acid-base homeostasis is to maintain a balance between acid production and acid excretion while preventing large changes in the pH of its internal environment.

Normal aerobic metabolism of carbohydrates and fats results in the production of carbon dioxide (CO_2). In solution, CO_2 forms the weak carbonic acid, which dissociates into H^+ and HCO_3^- (Fig. 10-1). Since this acid exists in equilibrium with gaseous carbon dioxide, it is called a *volatile acid,* that is, an acid that can be excreted in its gaseous form. Some 24,000 mM of CO_2 are eliminated from the body daily via normal ventilation.[2]

Nonvolatile or *fixed acids* are also produced continuously, primarily from the catabolism of proteins (see Fig. 10-1). Examples of fixed acids regularly produced by the body include sulfuric acid (H_2SO_4) and phosphoric acid (H_2PO_4). Other acids, such as lactic acid, can be produced by the incomplete oxidative metabolism of carbohydrates and fats. Compared to the daily production of CO_2, the amount of fixed acid produced by the body is small, averaging approximately 1 mEq of acid/kg of body weight, or about 50 to 70 mM per day.[2] The kidney is responsible for removal of the body's fixed acid load.

If mechanisms that buffer and excrete both volatile and fixed acids were not present, normal acid production would continually increase the hydrogen ion concentration of body fluids and eventually cause cell death. The following discussions address the mechanisms applied to buffer and excrete the acid by-products of metabolism.

Body buffer systems

A buffer system represents a physiologic mechanism designed to counteract the effects of adding acid (or alkali) to body fluids, thereby limiting large changes in hydrogen ion concentration and preventing wide swings in pH.[3] Chemically, a buffer system consists of a weak acid and its alkaline salt or base.

Blood contains two primary buffer systems: the bicarbonate system and the nonbicarbonate system. The bicarbonate buffer system consists of the weak acid, carbonic acid (H_2CO_3), and its base, sodium bicarbonate ($NaHCO_3$). The nonbicarbonate buffer system consists mainly of phosphates and proteins, including hemoglobin.[4]

The total quantity of all blood buffers capable of binding hydrogen ions is called the *total buffer base,* abbreviated as BB. Normal buffer base (NBB) ranges from 48 to 52 mEq/L.[5]

The approximate contribution of the various blood buffers to the normal buffer base is summarized in Table 10-1. The bicarbonate buffer system, both within and outside the erythrocyte, is the most important of all blood buffer mechanisms.

Table 10-1 Approximate Contribution of Blood Buffers to Total Buffering Capacity

Buffer category	Percent buffering in whole blood
BICARBONATE	
Plasma bicarbonate	35
Erythrocyte bicarbonate	18
Total bicarbonate	53
NONBICARBONATE	
Hemoglobin	35
Plasma proteins	7
Organic phosphate	3
Inorganic phosphate	2
Total nonbicarbonate	47

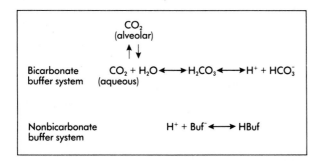

Fig. 10-2   Bicarbonate and nonbicarbonate buffer system. The two systems are in equilibrium with each other. (From Martin L: Pulmonary physiology in clinical practice: the essentials for patient care and evaluation, St Louis, 1987, The CV Mosby Co.)

The chemical actions of the two primary buffer systems are shown in simplified equations in Fig. 10-2. For simplicity, the conjugate component of the nonbicarbonate buffer system is represented as "Buf," with HBuf being the weak acid and Buf$^-$ being the base of the buffer pair.

Although Fig. 10-2 portrays these two systems separately, in reality they exist in equilibrium with each other. For this reason, measuring the components of either the bicarbonate or nonbicarbonate buffer system will provide an accurate overall picture of acid-base relationships in the blood.[1]

Normally, the bicarbonate buffer system is used as the focus for acid-base analysis. Not only is it the major contributor to the blood's buffering capacity, it is the easiest component to measure. Moreover, as shown in Fig. 10-2, the bicarbonate buffer system is an open buffer system, meaning that its acid component (carbonic acid) is volatile and readily excreted through the lungs in large quantities. In its gaseous form (CO_2), the volatile acid of the bicarbonate buffer system is highly diffusible across cell membranes. As a result, the chemical actions of this buffer system occur quickly within the body's cells.[1] For these reasons, our focus on blood buffers will emphasize the bicarbonate buffer system, addressing the role of the nonbicarbonate system as necessary.

Buffer action. If a strong acid is added to a buffer pair, the chemical reaction will yield a weak acid and neutral salt. Conversely, if a strong base is added to a buffer pair, the result will be a weak alkaline salt and water.

Thus, if hydrogen chloride is added to the carbonic acid/sodium bicarbonate buffer system, this strong acid will react with the bicarbonate of the buffer:

$$HCl + \frac{H_2CO_3}{NaHCO_3} \rightarrow H_2CO_3 + NaCl$$

This converts the strong acidity of hydrogen chloride to the relatively weak acidity of carbonic acid, thereby preventing a large drop in pH.

Similarly, if sodium hydroxide is added to this buffer system, it will react with the acid component of the pair:

$$NaOH + \frac{H_2CO_3}{NaHCO_3} \rightarrow NaHCO_3 + HOH$$

The strong alkalinity of sodium hydroxide is thus "buffered" into the relatively weak alkalinity of sodium bicarbonate. Eventually the buffer will be used up, but in the meantime the [H$^+$] of the reaction, and thus the pH, will change gradually rather than abruptly.

Calculating the [H$^+$] of a buffer solution. In a true buffer pair, the weak acid is slightly ionized, whereas its accompanying base is almost completely ionized.[6] The resulting [H$^+$] of the solution is proportionate to the ratio between the molar concentration of the free acid and the acid "bound" by base as the salt. The [H$^+$] of any buffer pair can be calculated if the concentration of the components and the ionization constant of the acid are known.

For example, the chemical dissociation of carbonic acid in solution occurs as follows:

$$H_2CO_3 \rightleftharpoons H^+ + HCO_3^- \text{ (very slight ionization)}$$

As described in Chapter 5, the ionization constant for this electrolytic dissociation is calculated as the product of the ionized components divided by the un-ionized component[6]:

$$K_{ac} = \frac{[H^+][HCO_3^-]}{[H_2CO_3]}$$

Rearranging the equation to solve for [H$^+$] yields the following:

$$[H^+] = K_{ac}\frac{[H_2CO_3]}{[HCO_3^-]}$$

In a buffer pair, most of the acid remains un-ionized (the characteristic of a weak acid). Therefore the concentration of un-ionized acid in the numerator of the preceding ratio essentially is the same as the known acid concentration that was used to prepare the buffer.

On the other hand, the base component of the buffer pair (sodium bicarbonate) is almost completely ionized (characteristic of a strong base):

$$NaHCO_3 \rightleftharpoons Na^+ + HCO_3^- \text{ (complete ionization)}$$

Therefore, the concentration of the bicarbonate ion in the denominator of the above equation is essentially the same as the total molar concentration of the base used in the buffer.

Thus, the above ionization equation for a weak acid can be rewritten to express the ionization of the buffer system as a whole. This is done by substituting the molar concentration of the buffer salt in place of the bicarbonate ion:

$$H^+ \text{ (m/L)} = K_{ac} \times \left[\frac{H_2CO_3 \text{ (m/L)}}{NaHCO_3 \text{ (m/L)}} \right]$$

According to this equation, the molar concentrations of hydrogen ions present in the bicarbonate buffer system are equal to the product of the ionization constant of the weak acid times the ratio of the concentrations of the weak acid and base components of the buffer pair.[3-6] As applied to buffer systems in general, we may write a generic equation for calculating their hydrogen ion concentrations:

$$H^+ = K_{ac} \times \frac{acid}{base}$$

pH and the Henderson-Hasselbalch equation. As compared with other electrolytes in the blood, hydrogen ions are present in minute quantities. Table 10-2 compares the plasma ion concentrations of the major cations found in the plasma.[1] The concentration of hydrogen ions is several hundred thousand times less than the other major electrolytes. Despite their comparatively low concentration, hydrogen ions exert profound effects on body chemistry.

Although the hydrogen ion concentration can be and is often measured in molar equivalents (normally 40 billionths of a mole or 40 nM), it is more commonplace to apply a negative logarithmic function to quantify the concentration of this critical cation. This measure, termed pH, is the negative log of the hydrogen ion concentration used as a positive number.[6] To relate pH to the generic buffer ionization equation previously derived, we simply multiply both sides of the equation by the log to the base 10, as in the following steps:

$$H^+ = K_{ac} \times \frac{acid}{base}$$

$$\log H^+ = \log \left[K_{ac} \times \frac{acid}{base} \right]$$

Since the $\log(a \times b) = \log a + \log b$:

$$\log H^+ = \log K_{ac} + \log \left[\frac{acid}{base} \right]$$

Multiplying both sides of the equation by -1 yields:

$$-\log H^+ = -\log K_{ac} - \log \left[\frac{acid}{base} \right]$$

Substituting the term "p" for the "$-\log$" of H^+ and K we derive:

$$pH = pK_{ac} - \log \left[\frac{acid}{base} \right] \quad or \quad pH = pK + \log \left[\frac{base}{acid} \right]$$

Table 10-2   Plasma Ion Concentrations

Ion*	nmol/L	mEq/L
H^+	40	4×10^{-5}
K^+	4,000,000	4
Ca^{++}	2,500,000	5
Mg^{++}	1,000,000	2
Na^+	140,000,000	140

*K^+, Potassium ion; Ca^{++}, calcium ion; Mg^{++}, magnesium ion; Na^+, sodium ion.
From Martin L: Pulmonary physiology in clinical practice: the essentials for patient care and evaluation, St Louis, 1987, The CV Mosby Co.

Note the use of the term pK. Similarly to pH, pK is defined as the negative log of the equilibrium constant of the acid component of the buffer system, used as a positive number.

Substituting sodium bicarbonate for the base and carbonic acid for the weak acid, we derive a basic equation for calculating the pH of the blood bicarbonate buffer system, better known as the Henderson-Hasselbalch equation:

$$pH = pK + \log \left[\frac{NaHCO_3}{H_2CO_3} \right]$$

Under normal physiologic conditions, the carbonic acid ionization constant (K) has a value of 7.85×10^{-7}, which is converted by calculation into a pK of 6.11. Therefore (rounding 6.11 to 6.1):

$$pH = 6.1 + \log \left[\frac{NaHCO_3}{H_2CO_3} \right]$$

Also, the importance of the numerator of the equation lies in the bicarbonate ion, since it represents the buffer base component. Thus:

$$pH = 6.1 + \log \left[\frac{HCO_3^-}{H_2CO_3} \right]$$

Moreover, laboratory techniques make it easier to determine the amount of dissolved carbon dioxide in the blood than the actual carbonic acid content. Because the dissolved carbon dioxide is directly proportional to the blood carbonic acid, the concentration of dissolved carbon dioxide can be substituted in the equation for carbonic acid[5]:

$$pH = 6.1 + \log \left[\frac{[HCO_3^-]}{[dissolved\ CO_2]} \right]$$

The dissolved carbon dioxide content (mM/L) in the denominator of the equation can be derived directly from the measured partial pressure of carbon dioxide in the blood. This is accomplished by multiplying the P_{CO_2} by a conversion factor of 0.03. Derivation of this factor is provided in the box below.

DERIVATION OF THE CONVERSION FACTOR FOR DISSOLVED CARBON DIOXIDE

1 mol CO_2	= 22,300 ml at 760 mm Hg pressure
1 mM CO_2	= 22.3 ml
Sol coeff of CO_2 at 760 mm Hg	= 0.51 ml CO_2/ml plasma
Thus ml CO_2/ml plasma at any P_{CO_2}	= $P_{CO_2} \times 0.51/760$
Thus ml CO_2/L plasma	= $P_{CO_2} \times 0.51 \times 1000/760$
Thus mM CO_2/L plasma	= $P_{CO_2} \times 0.51 \times 1000/760 \times 22.3$
	= $P_{CO_2} \times 0.03014$

Finally, as applied in clinical practice for determination of blood pH, the Henderson-Hasselbalch equation takes the following form:

$$pH = 6.1 + \log \left[\frac{[HCO_3^-]}{[PCO_2 \times 0.03]} \right]$$

Measurement and computation. In evaluating these relationships, we can measure in the laboratory certain blood values, which we then apply to the equation for whatever information is desired. Of the three variables in the Henderson-Hasselbalch equation, any one can be calculated if the other two are known.

In actual cardiopulmonary practice, modern blood-gas analyzers allow concurrent measurement of the pH, PCO_2, and PO_2 on the same blood sample.[7] Assuming that an arterial blood sample has a normal pH of 7.40 and a normal $PaCO_2$ of 40 mm Hg, the Henderson-Hasselbalch equation would allow derivation of the blood bicarbonate value as follows:

$$pH = 6.1 + \log \frac{[HCO_3^-]}{[PCO_2 \times 0.03]}$$

$$7.40 = 6.1 + \log \frac{[HCO_3^-]}{[40 \times 0.03]}$$

$$7.40 = 6.1 + \log \frac{[HCO_3^-]}{[1.2 \; mM/L]}$$

Rearranging to solve for HCO_3 yields the normal value for bicarbonate in the arterial blood (expressed in mEq/L):

$$[HCO_3^-] = 1.2 \times [antilog (7.40 - 6.1)]$$
$$= 1.2 \times [antilog (1.3)]$$
$$= 1.2 \times 20$$
$$= 24 \; mEq/L$$

Just as the HCO_3^- can be derived if we know the pH and PCO_2, so too can we calculate the pH or PCO_2 if the other values are known. The various forms of the Henderson-Hasselbalch equation necessary to derive any one unknown value are provided in the box below.

FORMS OF HENDERSON-HASSELBACH EQUATION USED TO COMPUTE AN UNKNOWN VALUE

To calculate the pH if the PCO_2 and HCO_3^- are known:

$$pH = 6.1 + \log \frac{[HCO_3^-]}{(PCO_2 \times 0.03)}$$

To calculate the PCO_2 if the pH and HCO_3^- are known:

$$PCO_2 = \frac{[HCO_3^-]}{[(0.03 \times antilog(pH - 6.1)]}$$

To calculate the HCO_3^- if the pH and PCO_2 are known:

$$[HCO_3^-] = (0.03 \times PCO_2) \times antilog(pH - 6.1)$$

Although a respiratory care practitioner equipped with an appropriate hand calculator and log tables can quickly derive unknowns from this equation, in clinical practice such manipulations generally are unnecessary. Modern blood-gas analyzers automate these computations, quickly deriving the HCO_3 value from the measured pH and PCO_2.

Computations involving the Henderson-Hasselbalch equation may also be accomplished using a variety of acid-base alignment nomograms.[5] The nomogram shown in Fig. 10-3 is useful for this purpose and can also aid the user in understanding the relationships among the variables involved in acid-base homeostasis.[1] The nomogram plots PCO_2 on the X-axis. pH and $[H^+]$ in nM/L are plotted on the Y-axis. HCO_3^- isopleths fan out from the lower left. By plotting the two known values and drawing intersecting lines, the third unknown easily can be derived.

Acid excretion

The body's buffer systems represent the first line of defense against the accumulation of hydrogen ions. However, if it were not for mechanisms to continually excrete the acid by-products of metabolism, body buffers would be quickly exhausted, and the pH of body fluids would rapidly drop to lethal levels.

Acid excretion is shared in a complementary fashion by the lungs and kidneys. The lungs can excrete only volatile acid (CO_2), but are capable of quickly removing vast quantities of this by-product of metabolism. The kidneys, on the other hand, function to remove fixed acids, but do so only at a relatively slow pace.[8] In health, the acid excretion mechanisms of these two organ systems remain in delicate balance. In disease, compromise or failure of one system can be partially offset by a compensatory response of the other. Failure of both systems obviously will result in rapid acid accumulation and, without correction, death of the organism.

The lungs. The lungs are responsible for the excretion of the volatile acid H_2CO_3. Because CO_2 is the end product of normal oxidative metabolism, the amount of H_2CO_3 formed is over 500 times that of all other acids combined.[2] In addition to this pathway, H_2CO_3 also is produced by the reaction of fixed acids with the bicarbonate buffer system. H_2CO_3 generated via both pathways is eliminated as CO_2 through the lungs. Some 24,000 mM of CO_2 are removed from the body daily via normal ventilation.

In reality, excretion of CO_2 does not, by itself, remove hydrogen ions.[2] Rather, the chemical reaction that releases this gas binds active hydrogen ions into harmless molecular combinations with water:

$$H^+ + HCO_3^- \leftrightharpoons H_2CO_3 \leftrightharpoons H_2O + CO_2$$

As described in Chapter 9, CO_2 excretion is directly proportional to the level of alveolar ventilation. Normally, the level of CO_2 in both the lungs and blood is maintained in a narrow range by sensitive and rapidly responding neural control mechanisms. These neural control mechanisms

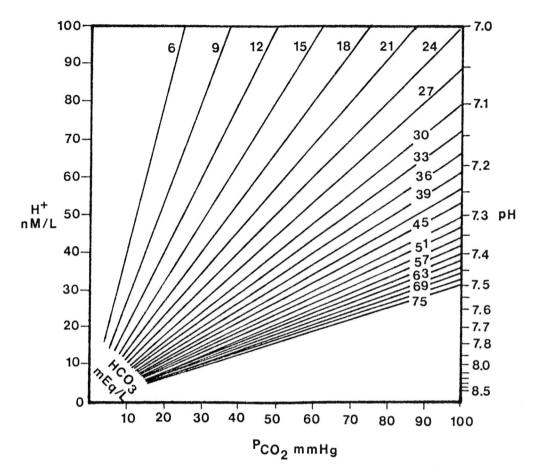

Fig. 10-3   Graphic solution of the Henderson-Hasselbalch equation. (From Martin L: Pulmonary physiology in clinical practice: the essentials for patient care and evaluation, St Louis, 1987, The CV Mosby Co.)

maintain near constant levels of CO_2 by carefully monitoring changes in hydrogen ion concentration, thereby constantly altering CO_2 excretion to match its production. More detail on these regulatory mechanisms is provided in the last section of this chapter.

The kidneys. Nonvolatile or fixed acids are not in equilibrium with an excretable gas. Therefore, such acids must be removed in solution by the kidneys. The process by which the kidneys perform this critical task is called *acidification of the urine*.[8]

Acidification of the urine involves two interrelated functions: reabsorption and generation of HCO_3^-, and actual elimination of fixed acids. Because these mechanisms occur in separate portions of the nephron, they are often considered separate functions. However, from the standpoint of overall body acid-base homeostasis, the retention of base (reabsorption of HCO_3^-) has the same effect as the excretion of acid.

Reabsorption of HCO_3^-. Because bicarbonate is freely filtered by the glomerulus, this important buffer would be quickly depleted unless it were actively reabsorbed. At a normal serum bicarbonate concentration of 24 mEq/L and normal glomerular filtration rates of 180 L/day, some 3600

to 4800 mEq of bicarbonate are reclaimed from the blood daily. Eighty to ninety percent of the bicarbonate reabsorption occurs in the proximal tubules, with the remainder of the filtration taking place in the distal tubules.[9]

Bicarbonate and chloride ions are selectively reabsorbed from the glomerular filtrate with sodium cations via active transport mechanisms. However, as compared to chloride, HCO_3^- is a poorly diffusible anion. Therefore, its transport is facilitated by conversion into the highly diffusible molecular CO_2.[8,9]

Fig. 10-4 portrays the mechanism by which the kidneys transport bicarbonate from the tubular lumen, through the tubular cells, and back to the peritubular capillaries. Hydrogen (H^+) ions cross the luminal membrane of tubular cells and react with the filtered bicarbonate (HCO_3^-) in the urine to form carbonic acid (H_2CO_3). The H_2CO_3 in the urine of the tubules breaks down into CO_2 and H_2O, and the CO_2 diffuses into the tubular cell. Within the tubular cells, CO_2 rapidly combines with water and dissociates into HCO_3^- and H^+, a reaction catalyzed by the enzyme carbonic anhydrase, found in high concentrations in the proximal tubular cells. While the H^+ produced in this reaction passes back into the tubule, it is exchanged for so-

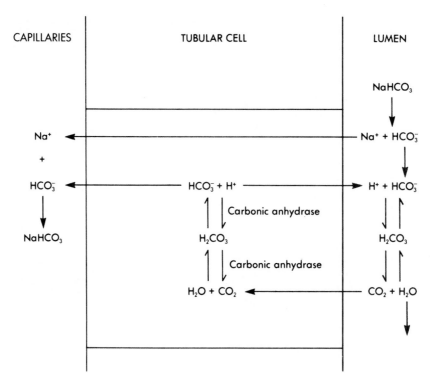

Fig. 10-4   Mechanism of bicarbonate reabsorption. (Modified from Lane EE and Walker JF: Clinical arterial blood gas analysis, St Louis, 1987, The CV Mosby Co.)

dium (Na^+), freeing up an HCO_3^- ion. At the same time, the bicarbonate generated within the tubular cells moves into peritubular capillaries, accompanied by the sodium cation. Therefore, for each H^+ secreted, one bicarbonate ion is returned to the blood. Interestingly, the bicarbonate ion that returns to the peritubular capillary is not the same one that entered the tubular lumen.

The rate of reabsorption of HCO_3^- in the proximal tubules is inversely proportional to the reabsorption of Cl^- ions.[2,8] If HCO_3^- is to be conserved, the kidneys will selectively reabsorb this buffer, at the expense of Cl^- reclamation. On the other hand, if the maintenance of acid-base homeostasis demands increased excretion of HCO_3^-, Cl^- will be preferentially retained.

Any remaining bicarbonate is reabsorbed in the distal tubule by a mechanism similar to that occurring in the proximal tubule. Although this process reclaims large amounts of bicarbonate, thus preserving the buffer capacity of the blood, only a small amount of hydrogen ions are excreted. Therefore, other mechanisms must exist to enhance H^+ removal.

Elimination of fixed acid. Two processes exist to enhance H^+ removal: the acidification of hydrogen phosphate (HPO_4^{--}), and the production of ammonium (NH_4^+) via the deamidization of protein.

The acidification of (HPO_4^{--}) occurs when H^+ ions combine with the phosphate buffers of the nonbicarbonate buffer system. As shown in Fig. 10-5, one of the two

Na^+ ions of the dissociated sodium hydrogen phosphate (Na_2HPO_4) is reabsorbed with HCO_3^- in exchange for an H^+ ion. The H^+ ion combines with HPO_4^{--} to form sodium dihydrogen phosphate (NaH_2PO_4), excreted in the urine as titratable acid. As with the process of bicarbonate reabsorption, for each H^+ secreted and exchanged with sodium, one bicarbonate ion is returned to the blood.

The acidification of HPO_4^{--} accounts for about one third to one half of the kidney's excretion of the body's fixed acid load.[8,9] However, the amount of acid excreted by this mechanism is limited by the amount of buffers present in the glomerular filtrate.

Most fixed acid is excreted by the kidneys in the form of ammonium ions (NH_4^+). The excretion of H^+ ions as ammonium ions enables the kidney to rid the body of large amounts of excess acid without lowering the urinary pH below 4.5.

As shown in Fig. 10-6, renal tubular cells produce ammonia (NH_3) by the deamidization of protein amino acids, especially glutamine. Ammonia freely diffuses across the cell membrane into the tubular lumen, where it readily combines with hydrogen ions to form ammonium ions. Because ammonium ions are not readily diffusible across the tubular cell membranes, they are excreted with the urine. Again, for each H^+ excreted by this mechanism, one Na^+ ion is exchanged, accompanied by a bicarbonate anion.

Normally, between one half and two thirds of the

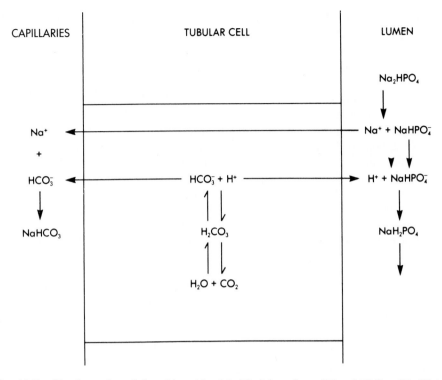

Fig. 10-5   The formation of titratable acid. (Modified from Lane EE and Walker JF: Clinical arterial blood gas analysis, St Louis, 1987, The CV Mosby Co.)

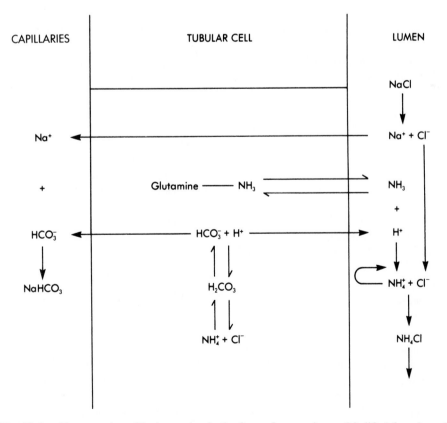

Fig. 10-6   The excretion of hydrogen ion in the form of ammonium. (Modified from Lane EE and Walker JF: Clinical arterial blood gas analysis, St Louis, 1987, The CV Mosby Co.)

body's production of nonvolatile acid is excreted as ammonium ions. Because this mechanism does not depend on the buffers being present in the glomerular filtrate, the kidneys can greatly increase the production of ammonia when the body needs to excrete excess acid. However, because ammonia production in the tubular cells is enzyme dependent, 2 to 5 days are required before this mechanism can reach its maximum capacity.

In combination, the reabsorption of HCO_3^- and the elimination of fixed acids by the kidneys serve two critical roles. First, both processes conserve sodium. Of more importance in the regulation of acid-base balance, however, is the fact that HCO_3^- is reabsorbed in proportion to the amount of H^+ that is excreted. In this manner, the bicarbonate buffer that is depleted in the first-line defense against hydrogen ions is fully restored, and homeostasis is maintained.[2]

ACID-BASE IMBALANCES

In health, the combined activity of the body buffer systems, the lungs, and the kidneys assures that acid-base homeostasis is maintained under a wide variety of conditions. However, should any of these three components fail, this balance can be disrupted.

Normal acid-base balance

Normally, the renal mechanisms of fixed acid buffering and excretion maintain an arterial blood bicarbonate concentration of 24 mEq/L, while the lungs excrete carbon dioxide to maintain a constant blood level equivalent to a $Paco_2$ of 40 mm Hg.[3-6] Based on these normal values, we may compute a normal pH of 7.40:

$$pH = 6.1 + \log \frac{[HCO_3^-]}{(Pco_2 \times 0.03)]}$$

$$pH = 6.1 + \log \left[\frac{24}{1.2}\right]$$

$$pH = 6.1 + \log [20]$$

$$pH = 7.4$$

Since pK is constant at 6.1, it is important to note that pH is determined by the ratio of the concentrations of buffer to weak acid, not their absolute values. Therefore, as long as the ratio of HCO_3^- buffer to weak acid (H_2CO_3) is 20:1, the pH will be normal.

Abnormal pH values

In health, the body maintains the arterial blood pH within a narrow normal range of 7.35 to 7.45. However, variations from this normal range can and do occur. When the blood pH is higher than normal (above 7.45), a state of *alkalemia* exists. When the blood pH is lower than normal (below 7.35), a state of *acidemia* exists.[10] Unfortunately,

knowledge of the pH alone provides little useful information regarding the process underlying an abnormal value. Indeed, as will be demonstrated, an abnormal acid-base state can exist with a normal pH.

Primary acid-base abnormalities

To analyze the processes underlying acid-base imbalances, we need to return to the Henderson-Hasselbalch equation. Beyond providing the basis for computing the parameters of acid-base balance, the Henderson-Hasselbalch equation can assist in understanding the interrelationships that occur between the various components of acid-base balance, particularly those underlying abnormal acid-base states.

As we know, the HCO_3^- component of the Henderson-Hasselbalch equation relates primarily to renal buffering and excretion of the body's fixed acid load. Likewise, the H_2CO_3 component of the equation relates primarily to the excretion of the volatile acid load by the lungs. Based on this understanding, we can rewrite the equation to reflect in concept these critical components of acid-base balance:

$$pH \propto \frac{\text{Fixed acid buffering (HCO}_3^-\text{) by kidneys}}{\text{Volatile acid regulation (CO}_2\text{) by lungs}}$$

According to this conceptual formula, the pH will rise if either the buffer capacity increases (kidneys) or the volatile acid (CO_2) decreases (lungs). On the other hand, if either the buffer capacity decreases or CO_2 increases, the pH will fall.

Thus alkalemia (a high pH) can be caused by either an increase in buffer base (as indicated by an increase in HCO_3^-) or a decrease in CO_2. Likewise, acidemia (a low pH) can be caused by either a decrease in buffer base (as indicated by a decrease in HCO_3^-) or an increase in CO_2. Because two primary causes can be associated with an abnormally high pH, and two primary causes can be associated with an abnormally low pH, there exists four primary abnormal acid-base processes (Table 10-3).

Table 10-3   Primary Acid-Base Disturbances

pH change	Primary abnormality	Designation
Alkalemia (increased pH)	Decreased Pco_2 Increased HCO_3	Respiratory alkalosis Metabolic (nonrespiratory) alkalosis
Acidemia (decreased pH)	Increased Pco_2 Decreased HCO_3	Respiratory acidosis Metabolic (nonrespiratory) acidosis

Respiratory processes. Since changes in CO_2 are primarily a function of the lung, imbalances resulting solely from this component are considered respiratory in origin. Respiratory processes resulting in acidemia are termed respiratory acidosis. Respiratory acidosis occurs whenever the denominator of the equation (CO_2) rises ($\rightarrow$ = normal or no change, $\uparrow$ = increased, $\downarrow$ = decreased):

$$\downarrow pH \propto \rightarrow HCO_3^- / \uparrow Paco_2 \text{ (respiratory acidosis)}$$

Respiratory processes resulting in alkalemia are termed respiratory alkalosis. Respiratory alkalosis occurs whenever the denominator of the equation (CO_2) falls:

$$\uparrow pH \propto \rightarrow HCO_3^- / \downarrow Paco_2 \text{ (respiratory alkalosis)}$$

Metabolic processes. On the other hand, changes in HCO_3^- are primarily caused by variations in buffer capacity, or fixed acid load, that is metabolic or nonrespiratory in origin. Metabolic processes resulting in acidemia are termed metabolic acidosis. Metabolic acidosis occurs whenever the numerator of the equation (HCO_3^-) falls:

$$\downarrow pH \propto \downarrow HCO_3^- / \rightarrow Paco_2 \text{ (metabolic acidosis)}$$

Metabolic processes resulting in alkalemia are termed metabolic alkalosis. Metabolic alkalosis occurs whenever the numerator of the equation (HCO_3^-) rises.

$$\uparrow pH \propto \uparrow HCO_3^- / \rightarrow Paco_2 \text{ (metabolic alkalosis)}$$

Restoring a normal pH

The goal of acid-base homeostasis is maintenance of a normal pH. There are two means by which an abnormal pH may be restored: compensation and correction.

Compensation. Since the pH is proportionate to the ratio of fixed acid buffering capacity (controlled by the kidneys) to volatile acid excretion (controlled by the lungs), a primary failure of one organ system can be compensated for by the other. In compensation, the system not primarily affected assumes responsibility for returning the pH to normal.[11] Compensation represents a normal response of the body to a failure in one component of the acid-base regulatory mechanism.

As an example, should the $Paco_2$ rise to 60 mm Hg because of hypoventilation (respiratory acidosis), the pH would fall to approximately 7.23:

$$pH = 6.1 + \log \left[\frac{24}{(60 \times 0.03)} \right]$$

$$pH = 6.1 + \log [13]$$

$$pH = 7.23$$

By increasing the amount of HCO_3^- buffer in the numerator of the equation to 36 mEq/L (via increased renal reabsorption of bicarbonate), the original normal ratio of buffer to acid (20:1) is restored and the pH is returned to 7.40:

$$pH = 6.1 + \log \left[\frac{36}{(60 \times 0.03)} \right]$$

$$pH = 6.1 + \log \left[\frac{36}{1.8} \right]$$

$$pH = 6.1 + \log [20]$$

$$pH = 7.40$$

Likewise, if a metabolic or nonrespiratory process alters HCO_3^- concentrations above or below normal, the lungs will respond by increasing or decreasing their excretion of CO_2 in an attempt to restore the normal ratio of base to acid, and thereby return the pH toward normal.

Table 10-4 summarizes the four primary acid-base disorders and the compensatory responses that normally characterize the body's efforts to restore pH values back toward normal.[1] Large arrows indicate the direction of the changes caused by the primary disturbance; small arrows indicate the nature of the compensatory response.

Obviously, compensatory responses require that the unaffected system be functioning normally. Otherwise, compensation will either not occur or, if it occurs, will be less than effective. Moreover, the speed with which compensation occurs varies substantially according to the organ system responsible. More details on these compensatory processes, including their clinical applications, are provided in the following sections.

Correction. In compensation for an acid-base abnormality, the system not primarily affected assumes responsibility for returning the pH to normal. On the other hand, correction of an acid-base abnormality aims to restore the pH toward normal by treatment of the aberrant component. For example, correction of the acute respiratory acidosis in the above example would require that the $Paco_2$ be lowered back to its normal value of 40 mm Hg. This could be accomplished by increasing alveolar ventilation to match CO_2 production, thereby restoring the pH back toward its normal value of 7.40.

In general, actions designed to correct acid-base abnor-

Table 10-4   Primary Event and Compensatory Response for Acid-Base Disorders

Acid-base disorder	Primary event		Compensatory response	
Metabolic acidosis	$\downarrow pH \simeq$	$\dfrac{\downarrow HCO_3^-}{Paco_2}$	$\downarrow pH \simeq$	$\dfrac{\downarrow HCO_3^-}{\downarrow Paco_2}$
Metabolic alkalosis	$\uparrow pH \simeq$	$\dfrac{\uparrow HCO_3^-}{Paco_2}$	$\uparrow pH \simeq$	$\dfrac{\uparrow HCO_3^-}{\uparrow Paco_2}$
Respiratory acidosis	$\downarrow pH \simeq$	$\dfrac{HCO_3^-}{\uparrow Paco_2}$	$\downarrow pH \simeq$	$\dfrac{\uparrow HCO_3^-}{\uparrow Paco_2}$
Respiratory alkalosis	$\uparrow pH \simeq$	$\dfrac{HCO_3^-}{\downarrow Paco_2}$	$\uparrow pH \simeq$	$\dfrac{\downarrow HCO_3^-}{\downarrow Paco_2}$

From Martin L: Pulmonary physiology in clinical practice: the essentials for patient care and evaluation, St Louis, 1987, The CV Mosby Co.

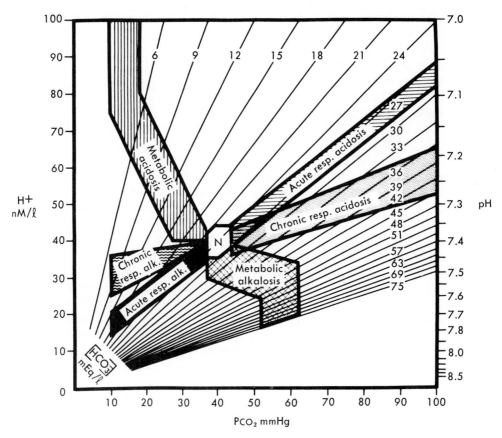

Fig. 10-7   Acid-base map. (See text for description.) (Reprinted from Goldberg M et al: JAMA 223:1973. Copyright 1973, American Medical Association.)

malities must focus on removing the underlying cause of the disturbance. Moreover, correction of compensated acid-base abnormalities must be done slowly and with extreme care. Otherwise, correction potentially can cause rapid and potentially harmful fluctuations in pH.

CLINICAL ACID-BASE STATES

The effective management of acid-base imbalances requires accurate identification of the patient's underlying acid-base status. Although respiratory care practitioners primarily are involved in implementing treatment plans designed to correct respiratory acid-base abnormalities, the metabolic component cannot be overlooked. Indeed, certain metabolic acid-base abnormalities (both primary and compensatory) result from disorders of the cardiopulmonary system. For this reason, the skilled respiratory care clinician must be able to distinguish among the clinical manifestations and potential underlying causes of all common acid-base disturbances.

Graphic interpretation

Given the complexity of clinical acid-base chemistry, it is sometimes helpful to visualize various acid-base states

with a graphic "map." Fig. 10-7 illustrates such a map. The map portrays various acid-base states as overlays on the nomogram previously used to graphically solve the Henderson-Hasselbalch equation. The areas of acid-base abnormalities surrounding a central normal axis are plotted as 95% confidence bands, based on the clinical and statistical analysis of a large number of patients. Intersects outside the mapped areas indicate mixed acid-base problems.

Although no substitute for either sound knowledge of acid-base chemistry or clinical acumen, maps such as these are particularly useful as learning aids. For this reason, we will frequently refer to Fig. 10-7 as we further explore the major categories of acid-base imbalances.

Systematic clinical assessment

In analyzing an acid-base problem, it is helpful to approach the data using a series of systematic steps.[12,13] This approach helps avoid the tendency to jump to conclusions and ensures that all relevant information is applied to solve the problem at hand. We will apply the following approach in the interpretation of selected examples of acid-base imbalances:

Step 1—categorize the pH. If pH is within normal range, either a normal acid-base status, a completely compensated acid-base disorder, or a mixed acid-base disorder is present. A normal acid-base status is obvious by a normal Pa_{CO_2} (35 to 45 mm Hg) and plasma bicarbonate (22 to 26 mm Hg). If plasma bicarbonate and Pa_{CO_2} are both abnormal with a normal pH, either a fully compensated or mixed acid-base disorder is present.

If pH is below 7.35, acidemia is present and an acidosis is most likely the primary problem. If pH is greater than 7.45, alkalemia is present and an alkalosis is most likely the primary disturbance.

Step 2—determine the respiratory involvement. Inspect the Pa_{CO_2}. If the Pa_{CO_2} is normal and the pH is not, the abnormal process is of nonrespiratory origin (skip to step 3). If the Pa_{CO_2} is elevated (greater than 45 mm Hg) and there is an acidemia present, the primary disturbance is most likely respiratory acidosis. If the Pa_{CO_2} is low (less than 45 mm Hg) and there is an alkalemia present, the primary disturbance is most likely respiratory alkalosis. Other alterations in Pa_{CO_2} are most likely compensatory for a metabolic disturbance.

Step 3—determine the metabolic involvement. Inspect the plasma HCO_3^-. If the HCO_3^- is normal and the pH is not, the abnormal process is of respiratory origin (see step 2). If the HCO_3^- is elevated (greater than 26 mEq/L) and there is an alkalemia present, the primary disturbance is most likely metabolic alkalosis. If the HCO_3^- is low (less than 26 mEq/L) and there is an acidemia present, the primary disturbance is most likely metabolic acidosis. Other alterations in HCO_3^- are most likely compensatory for a respiratory disturbance.

Step 4—assess for compensation. Once the acid-base disorder is identified as respiratory or metabolic, look for the degree of compensation occurring. Respiratory acidosis is compensated for by elevation of plasma HCO_3^-; a respiratory alkalosis is compensated for by a decrease in plasma HCO_3^-. Metabolic acidosis is compensated for by a decrease in Pa_{CO_2}; metabolic alkalosis is compensated for by an elevation of Pa_{CO_2}.

If the pH is on the acid side of 7.40 (7.35 to 7.39), the acid-base component that would lend itself to acidosis (either increased Pa_{CO_2} or decreased plasma HCO_3^-) is the primary imbalance. If the pH is on the alkaline side of 7.40 (7.41 to 7.45), the acid-base component that would lend itself to alkalosis (either decreased Pa_{CO_2} or increased plasma HCO_3^-) is the primary disturbance.

Respiratory acidosis

Respiratory acidosis is a primary physiologic process that causes an increase in the arterial P_{CO_2} or hypercapnia.[1,13] When not complicated by other acid-base problems, respiratory acidosis lowers the pH of the blood. An acute rise in P_{CO_2} of 20 mm Hg will lower the pH by about 0.10 unit.

Causes. Hypercapnia may result from either simple hypoventilation or an altered $\dot{V}_A/\dot{Q}_C$ ratio, particularly an in-

---

COMMON CAUSES OF RESPIRATORY ACIDOSIS

WITH NORMAL LUNGS

CNS depression
  Anesthesia
  Sedative drugs
  Narcotic analgesics
Neuromuscular disease
  Poliomyelitis
  Myasthenia gravis
  Guillain-Barré syndrome
Trauma
  Spinal cord
  Brain
  Chest wall
Severe restrictive disorders
  Obesity (Pickwickian syndrome)
  Kyphoscoliosis

WITH ABNORMAL LUNGS

Chronic obstructive pulmonary disease
Acute airway obstruction (late phases)

---

crease in physiologic dead space. In either case, alveolar ventilation is inadequate to meet the metabolic demands for CO_2 excretion, and the Pa_{CO_2} rises.

Respiratory acidosis resulting from simple hypoventilation is associated mainly with nonrespiratory disorders in which depression of the central nervous system or impaired respiratory muscle action affect an otherwise normal lung. Respiratory acidosis due to $\dot{V}_A/\dot{Q}_C$ abnormalities is associated mainly with chronic obstructive pulmonary disease. The common causes of respiratory acidosis in both the normal and abnormal lung are summarized in the boxed material.[7,9,12]

As indicated on the acid-base map (see Fig. 10-7), if the process causing the disturbance is acute in onset, the patient with respiratory acidosis will exhibit an elevated arterial P_{CO_2}, decreased arterial pH, and a normal or slightly elevated serum HCO_3^-. A clinical example of acute respiratory acidosis, including analysis, is provided as Case Study 1.

Compensation. Compensation for respiratory acidosis begins as soon as the carbon dioxide starts to accumulate. The normally functioning kidney attempts to increase reabsorption of bicarbonate to keep pace with the rising levels of dissolved carbon dioxide.[2]

The kidney uses two mechanisms to regulate the essential electrolyte levels.[14,15] First, it preferentially reclaims the bicarbonate anion at the expense of chloride, thereby increasing the Cl^- concentration of the urine and decreas-

ACID-BASE CASE STUDY 1
Acute (uncompensated) respiratory acidosis

The patient is a 35-year-old Hispanic woman admitted to the emergency room with a diagnosis of heroin drug overdose. Her breathing is shallow and slow. Arterial blood gas analysis reveals the following:

pH:	7.30
$Paco_2$:	55 mm Hg
HCO_3^-:	27 mEq/L

- **STEP 1** *Categorize the pH*

  The pH is below normal, indicating the presence of an acidemia.

- **STEP 2** *Determine the respiratory involvement*

  The Pco_2 is elevated above normal, indicating hypoventilation as a contributing factor for the acidemia (possible respiratory acidosis).

- **STEP 3** *Determine the metabolic involvement*

  The HCO_3^- is slightly elevated above normal; however, this is within the expected range for acute respiratory acidosis (1 mEq for each 10 to 15 mm Hg increase in Pco_2).

- **STEP 4** *Assess for compensation*

  As explained under step 3, the HCO_3^- is within the expected range for acute respiratory acidosis, therefore there is no evidence of metabolic compensation.

- **CONCLUSION**   *Acute (uncompensated) respiratory acidosis.*

ACID-BASE CASE STUDY 2
Chronic (compensated) respiratory acidosis

The patient is a 73-year-old white man being treated on an outpatient basis for pulmonary emphysema, diagnosed some 7 years ago. His breathing is labored at rest, with marked use of accessory muscles. Arterial blood gas analysis reveals the following:

pH:	7.33
$Paco_2$:	64 mm Hg
HCO_3^-:	34 mEq/L

- **STEP 1** *Categorize the pH*

  The pH is slightly below normal, indicating the presence of a mild acidemia.

- **STEP 2** *Determine the respiratory involvement*

  The Pco_2 is above normal, indicating hypoventilation as a contributing factor in the acidemia (possible respiratory acidosis).

- **STEP 3** *Determine the metabolic involvement*

  The HCO_3^- is substantially elevated above normal. Because there is a mild acidemia present, a primary metabolic alkalosis is ruled out. Compensation for the respiratory acidosis is a possibility.

- **STEP 4** *Assess for compensation*

  The HCO_3^- is about 8 to 10 mEq above normal; this is consistent with a compensatory response by the kidneys (about 4 mEq/L for each 10 mm Hg rise in Pco_2).

- **CONCLUSION**   *Chronic (compensated) respiratory acidosis.*

---

ing its level in the plasma. Second, the kidney increases the exchange of sodium for H^+ via the acidification processes previously described.

If the onset of respiratory acidosis is acute, renal compensation may not be able to keep up with the rising carbon dioxide on a minute-by-minute basis, and the compensatory bicarbonate reabsorption and urine acidification may not reach its maximum efficiency for 3 or 4 days. However, the clinician will usually start to see evidence of a response within 24 hours.

On the other hand, if the respiratory acidosis develops slowly, as is often seen in the course of chronic pulmonary disease, the compensatory process may adjust proportionately to the acidosis. In such instances, pH levels may be kept stable at or near the low end of the normal range. This is often referred to as "chronic" respiratory acidosis (Case Study 2). In such cases the underlying process is still present; renal compensation simply masks the effect by preventing a serious drop in pH. Examination of arterial blood still reveals an elevated Pco_2, the hallmark of respiratory acidosis. However, as demonstrated in the example (see Case Study 2), the HCO_3^- is elevated above normal.[16] Moreover, serum Cl^- would be decreased, and the pH of the urine would be below normal.

The absolute upper limit of the kidney's ability to compensate for respiratory acidosis is unknown. One study concluded that renal compensation was rarely complete for a $Paco_2$ greater than 70 mm Hg.[14] Other clinical case reports have demonstrated compensation for, and good tolerance of, arterial Pco_2 levels as high as 90 mm Hg.[15]

Differentiating between acute and chronic respiratory acidosis is complicated by the fact that plasma HCO_3^- concentrations are not governed solely by the kidneys. As indicated earlier, increased levels of dissolved CO_2 increase H_2CO_3 concentrations. According to the principles of mass action, the resulting dissociation of carbonic acid into its ionic components is enhanced, thereby increasing the levels of HCO_3:

$$CO_2 + H_2O \rightleftharpoons H_2CO_3 \rightleftharpoons H^+ + HCO_3^-$$

Careful inspection of the acute respiratory acidosis region in Fig. 10-7 demonstrates this effect. As the Pco_2 rises above normal, a small but measurable increase in HCO_3^- immediately occurs.[2,5] This increase in HCO_3^- is not the result of renal compensation. Rather, it is solely attributable to the "push" of the above dissociation reaction to the right.

As a rule of thumb, acute respiratory acidosis can be expected to raise the HCO_3^- by about 1 mEq/L for each 10 to 15 mm Hg increase in P_{CO_2}. On the other hand, if renal compensation is occurring, as in chronic respiratory acidosis, the plasma HCO_3^- can be expected to increase by about 4 mEq/L for each 10 mm Hg rise in P_{CO_2} (see Fig. 10-7).[12]

To clarify these relationships, some laboratories report an additional value called the *standard bicarbonate*. The standard bicarbonate is defined as the plasma concentration of HCO_3^- in mEq/L that would exist if the P_{CO_2} were normal (40 mm Hg). In concept, this measure eliminates the effect of dissolved CO_2 on HCO_3^- levels, thereby facilitating assessment of the metabolic component of acid-base balance. However, as a calculated rather than measured value, the derivation of standard bicarbonate has substantial theoretical shortcomings.[2] For this reason, its use generally has been abandoned for other metabolic indices, specifically the measurement called *base excess*.

Base excess (BE) is defined as the difference between the normal buffer base (NBB) and the actual buffer base (BB) in a whole blood sample, expressed in mEq/L[17]:

$$BE = NBB - BB$$

A normal BE is +/−2 mEq/L. A positive BE (greater than +2 mEq/L) indicates a gain of base or loss of acid from nonrespiratory causes. A negative BE or base deficit exists when the difference between the normal buffer base (NBB) and the actual buffer base (BB) is less than −2 mEq/L. A base deficit indicates a shortage of base or excess of acid from nonrespiratory causes.[5,17]

Because BE quantifies only the metabolic contribution in an acid-base disturbance, it helps fine-tune the analysis when compensation or mixed disorders occur. Base excess is derived by graphic solution of a nomogram developed by Siggaard-Andersen.[5] Derivation of BE requires prior measurement of the blood pH, Pa_{CO_2}, and hemoglobin concentration.

In acute or uncompensated respiratory acidosis, BE would always fall within the normal range. On the other hand, when renal compensation is occurring in response to a chronic respiratory acidosis, BE would be elevated above the normal range because of the increased levels of plasma HCO_3^-.

Correction. As previously described, correction of an acid-base abnormality aims to restore the pH toward normal by treatment of the aberrant component. In acute or uncompensated respiratory acidosis, this may be accomplished by increasing alveolar ventilation and thereby lowering the Pa_{CO_2}. In chronic or compensated respiratory acidosis, the pH already has been adjusted toward normal by renal retention of HCO_3^-. In this case, a rapid increase in alveolar ventilation will quickly raise the pH above normal, further complicating the acid-base imbalance.[7]

Respiratory alkalosis

Respiratory alkalosis is a primary physiologic process that causes a decrease in the arterial P_{CO_2} or hypocapnia.[1] When not complicated by other acid-base problems, respiratory alkalosis raises the pH of the blood. An acute drop in P_{CO_2} of 10 mm Hg will raise the pH by about 0.10 unit.

Causes. As with respiratory acidosis, the processes underlying respiratory alkalosis may occur in patients with normal lungs or those with pulmonary disease.[2] In either case, alveolar ventilation is excessive in relation to metabolic demands for CO_2 excretion, the cardinal definition of hyperventilation. As indicated in the boxed material, respiratory alkalosis occurring in patients with normal lungs generally is attributable to disorders causing stimulation of the central nervous system. On the other hand, respiratory alkalosis occurring in patients with cardiopulmonary disorders is most likely caused by one of two factors: arterial hypoxemia or direct stimulation of certain parasympathetic receptors located in the lung parenchyma. Both mechanisms will be described later in this chapter.

A third cause of respiratory alkalosis in patients receiving respiratory care is iatrogenically induced hyperventilation. An iatrogenic condition represents a problem or complication resulting from treatment. Iatrogenically induced hyperventilation is most commonly associated with the application of mechanical ventilators. Overzealous artificial ventilation can quickly result in acute respiratory alkalosis. A transient respiratory alkalosis may also occur when drawing an arterial blood gas, resulting from patient anxiety or pain. Such results can easily be misinterpreted un-

---

COMMON CAUSES OF RESPIRATORY ALKALOSIS

WITH NORMAL LUNGS
Anxiety
Fever
Stimulant drugs
CNS lesions
Pain
Sepsis
Hypobarism (high altitude)

WITH ABNORMAL LUNGS
Hypoxemia-causing conditions
    Acute asthma
    Pneumonia
Stimulation of vagal lung receptors
    Pulmonary edema
    Pulmonary vascular disease

EITHER
Iatrogenic hyperventilation

ACID-BASE CASE STUDY 3
Acute respiratory alkalosis

A distraught 77-year-old man enters the hospital and is found to have ingested large doses of aspirin (acetylsalicylic acid) in a suicide attempt. The patient exhibits rapid and deep breathing, has slurred speech, and complains about tingling in the extremities. Arterial blood gas analysis reveals the following:

$$
\begin{array}{ll}
\text{pH:} & 7.57 \\
\text{Paco}_2\text{:} & 23 \text{ mm Hg} \\
\text{HCO}_3^-\text{:} & 21 \text{ mEq/L}
\end{array}
$$

- **STEP 1** *Categorize the pH*

    The pH is substantially above normal, indicating the presence of an alkalemia.

- **STEP 2** *Determine the respiratory involvement*

    The P_{CO_2} is well below normal, indicating hyperventilation as a contributing factor in the alkalemia (possible respiratory alkalosis).

- **STEP 3** *Determine the metabolic involvement*

    The HCO_3^- is slightly lower than normal; because there is an alkalemia present, a primary metabolic acidosis is ruled out. Compensation for the respiratory alkalosis is a possibility.

- **STEP 4** *Assess for compensation*

    The drop in HCO_3^- is within the expected range for acute respiratory alkalosis (1 mEq for each 5 mm Hg decline in P_{CO_2}). Therefore no compensation has taken place.

- **CONCLUSION** *Acute respiratory alkalosis.*

ACID-BASE CASE STUDY 4
Compensated (chronic) respiratory alkalosis

A 27-year-old man is admitted to the hospital with a persistent case of bacterial pneumonia that has not responded to 6 days of ambulatory care with antimicrobials. He exhibits a mild cyanosis and labored breathing. Arterial blood gas analysis (breathing room air) reveals the following:

$$
\begin{array}{ll}
\text{pH:} & 7.46 \\
\text{Paco}_2\text{:} & 26 \text{ mm Hg} \\
\text{HCO}_3^-\text{:} & 18 \text{ mEq/L} \\
\text{Pao}_2\text{:} & 53 \text{ mm Hg}
\end{array}
$$

- **STEP 1** *Categorize the pH*

    The pH is slightly above normal, indicating the presence of a mild alkalemia.

- **STEP 2** *Determine the respiratory involvement*

    The P_{CO_2} is well below normal, indicating hyperventilation as a contributing factor in the alkalemia (possible respiratory alkalosis).

- **STEP 3** *Determine the metabolic involvement*

    The HCO_3^- is substantially lower than normal; because there is an alkalemia present, a primary metabolic acidosis is ruled out. Compensation for the respiratory alkalosis is a possibility.

- **STEP 4** *Assess for compensation*

    The HCO_3^- is about 8 mEq below normal; this is consistent with a compensatory response by the kidneys (about 5 mEq/L for each 10 mm Hg drop in P_{CO_2}).

- **CONCLUSION** *Compensated (chronic) respiratory alkalosis.*

less the clinician responsible for obtaining the sample notifies those responsible for the analysis of the patient's acid-base status.

Clinical manifestations. An early indicator of acute respiratory alkalosis is paresthesia. Later, neural reflexes become hyperactive, and true tetanic contractions can occur. Because a rapid decrease in P_{CO_2} produces marked contraction of cerebral arterioles, respiratory alkalosis can also impair cerebral circulation.[18] Depending on its severity, this reduction in blood flow to the brain can cause symptoms ranging from speech difficulty to muscular paralysis. Hypocapnia also predisposes the patient to serious disturbance in myocardial conductivity, resulting in potentially life-threatening cardiac arrhythmias.[1] Case Study 3 provides a clinical example of acute respiratory alkalosis, including the acid-base analysis.

Compensation. Compensation for respiratory alkalosis is accomplished by an increased renal excretion of bicarbonate, retention of chloride, and a reduction in both the formation of ammonia and excretion of titratable HPO_4^{--}. This lowers the blood bicarbonate level, bringing the acid-base ratio back toward 20:1 and reducing the pH back toward normal (Case Study 4).

As with respiratory acidosis, the expected change in plasma HCO_3^- with respiratory alkalosis depends on the magnitude and the longevity of the problem. Whereas in acute respiratory alkalosis the HCO_3^- can be expected to drop by about 1 mEq/L for each 5 mm Hg decline in P_{CO_2}, patients with chronic or compensated respiratory alkalosis tend to exhibit a 5 mEq/L decrease in HCO_3^- for every 10 mm Hg decrement in P_{CO_2}.[12]

Correction. As with respiratory acidosis, correction of respiratory alkalosis aims to restore the pH back toward normal. Normally this is accomplished indirectly by elimination or treatment of the stimulus causing increased alveolar ventilation. In general, only iatrogenically induced respiratory alkalosis is directly managed by decreasing alveolar ventilation.

Metabolic (nonrespiratory) acidosis

Metabolic, or nonrespiratory, acidosis is a primary physiologic process that causes a decrease in the plasma bicarbonate, a condition called hypobasemia.[1,10] When not complicated by other acid-base imbalances, metabolic acidosis lowers the pH of the blood.

COMMON CAUSES OF METABOLIC
(NONRESPIRATORY) ACIDOSIS

LOSS OF BASE (NORMAL ANION GAP)
Direct loss of bicarbonate

Diarrhea
Pancreatic fistula
Carbonic anhydrase inhibition

Chloride retention

Renal tubular acidosis
Chloride administration
    NH_4Cl
    Parenteral nutrition (arginine/lysine)

GAIN OF ACID (INCREASED ANION GAP)
Metabolically produced

Diabetic ketoacidosis
Alcoholic ketoacidosis
Lactic acidosis
Renal insufficiency (phosphate, sulphate retention)
Starvation

Drug or chemical induced

Salicylate intoxication
Carbenicillin therapy
Methanol (formic acid)
Ethylene glycol (oxalic acid)
Paraaldehyde (acetic acid)

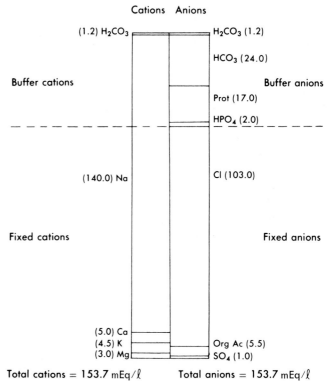

Fig. 10-8   Balance between fixed and buffer electrolytes of plasma.

Causes. Metabolic, or nonrespiratory, acidosis is associated with either a gain in fixed (nonvolatile) acids or an excessive loss of buffer base.[2] The boxed material delineates the common clinical disorders associated with each of these two major categories of metabolic acidosis. Regardless of the underlying cause, the hallmark of metabolic acidosis is a reduction in the buffering capacity of the blood, as manifested by a low HCO_3^- and a large negative base excess (BE).

Although the end result of all types of metabolic acidosis is the same (a decreased HCO_3^- or negative BE), the effective clinical management of this acid-base disorder demands that the underlying cause be clearly established. In most cases a careful history and related clinical assessment will allow the clinician to distinguish between metabolic acidosis resulting from a gain in fixed acids and that caused by an excessive loss of base. However, in some situations, this difference is not so clear.

Differentiating between the various types of metabolic acidosis often requires further analysis of the plasma electrolytes. In metabolic disorders, acid-base balance depends, in part, on the balance between the plasma cations and anions.[11] The former consist of sodium, calcium, potassium, and magnesium; the latter, bicarbonate, protein,

(serum protein and hemoglobin), phosphate, chloride, sulfate, and organic acids. As shown in Fig. 10-8, the sum of the anions must equal the sum of the cations.

In clinical practice, the only electrolytes commonly measured are Na^+, K^+, Cl^-, and HCO_3^-. The relative balance between cations and anions is therefore determined by calculating the difference between the total of the two primary anions (Cl^- and HCO_3^-) and the two primary cations (Na^+ and K^+). This computation is called the anion gap[1]:

$$Anion\ gap = (Na^+ + K^+) - (Cl^- + HCO_3^-)$$

Usually, K^+ is ignored in the computation. Therefore the normal anion gap range is about 8 to 16 mEq/L.[1] An anion gap greater than 16 mEq/L is usually caused by metabolic acidosis, specifically those types of metabolic acidosis associated with a gain in unmeasured organic acids (see boxed material). Such unmeasured organic acids include lactic acid, ketones (beta-hydroxybutyric acid and acetoacetic acid), salicylic acid, formic acid, and oxalic acid. Lactic acid and ketones are metabolically produced, whereas salicylic acid, formic acid, and oxalic acid represent ingested anions. Metabolic acidosis caused by renal insufficiency also causes an increased anion gap because of the retention of phosphate and sulphate anions.

On the other hand, not all types of metabolic acidosis elevate the anion gap. Specifically, conditions in which the acidosis is caused by either a loss of HCO_3^- or gain of Cl^-

ACID-BASE CASE STUDY 5
Compensated metabolic acidosis

A 38-year-old man has suffered for weeks from severe diarrhea without medical attention. Arterial blood gas analysis reveals the following:

pH:	7.33
Pa_{CO_2}:	26 mm Hg
HCO_3^-:	13 mEq/L
BE:	−11 mEq/L

- STEP 1   *Categorize the pH*

  The pH is slightly below normal, indicating the presence of an acidemia.

- STEP 2   *Determine the respiratory involvement*

  The P_{CO_2} is below normal, indicating hyperventilation. However, because there is an acidemia present, the presence of a primary respiratory alkalosis is ruled out. The low P_{CO_2} may be a compensatory response to a primary metabolic problem (possible metabolic acidosis).

- STEP 3   *Determine the metabolic involvement*

  The HCO_3^- is substantially lower than normal; given the low pH, this low HCO_3^- signals a possible metabolic acidosis. This is confirmed by the large base deficit (−11 mEq/L).

- STEP 4   *Assess for compensation*

  The hyperventilation previously described must represent a compensatory response to the primary metabolic acidosis.

- CONCLUSION   *Compensated metabolic acidosis.*

(as opposed to a gain of acid) generally will not increase the anion gap (see boxed material). In these situations, bicarbonate loss and chloride retention offset each other, keeping the anion gap within normal limits.

Because of the characteristic elevation of serum chloride, nonrespiratory acidosis with a normal anion gap is called *hyperchloremic metabolic acidosis.* Hyperchloremic metabolic acidosis may be caused by any condition in which HCO_3^- is lost or Cl^- is gained. Among the most common causes of bicarbonate loss are diarrhea, pancreatic fistula, and renal tubular acidosis. Chloride ingestion may also cause hyperchloremic metabolic acidosis. Ammonium chloride (NH_4Cl) ingestion is a primary cause of hyperchloremic metabolic acidosis, as are amino acid–chloride formulas used in parenteral nutrition (hyperalimentation).

Compensation. Compensation for metabolic acidosis occurs via an increase in the excretion of volatile acid (CO_2) by the lungs. In this manner, the ratio of bicarbonate to H_2CO_3 is raised toward a normal of 20:1, restoring the pH toward its normal range. Case Study 5 provides an example of compensated metabolic acidosis.

COMMON CAUSES OF METABOLIC (NONRESPIRATORY) ALKALOSIS

INCREASE IN BASE

Administration/ingestion of HCO_3
Hypochloremia
    Diuretic therapy
    Contraction of blood volume

LOSS OF FIXED ACID

Severe vomiting
Nasogastric suction
Hypokalemia
    Potassium deficiency
    Corticosteroids

Because the response of the normal respiratory system to metabolic acidosis is rapid, uncompensated metabolic acidosis is rare.[12] Therefore one expects the P_{CO_2} of a patient with metabolic acidosis to be below normal. Indeed, if a metabolic acidosis is confirmed and the P_{CO_2} is normal or high, a ventilatory disorder must coexist.

Correction. As with the other acid-base abnormalities, correction of metabolic acidosis aims to restore the pH to normal. Normally this is accomplished by treatment of the underlying process causing the gain of acid or loss of base. However, because respiratory compensation normally accompanies metabolic acidosis, the pH may already be adjusted toward normal. Corrective action in these situations must not be accomplished too quickly. Otherwise the pH may swing rapidly above normal, further complicating the acid-base imbalance.

Metabolic (nonrespiratory) alkalosis

Metabolic or nonrespiratory alkalosis is a primary physiologic process that causes an increase in the plasma bicarbonate, a condition called hyperbasemia.[1,10] When not complicated by other acid-base imbalances, metabolic alkalosis raises the pH of the blood.

Causes. Metabolic or nonrespiratory alkalosis is associated with either a loss of fixed (nonvolatile) acids or an excessive gain of buffer base.[19] The boxed material lists the common clinical disorders associated with each of these two major categories of metabolic alkalosis. Regardless of underlying cause, the hallmark of metabolic alkalosis is an increase in the buffering capacity of the blood, as manifested by an elevated HCO_3^- and a positive base excess (BE).

Metabolic alkalosis caused by ingestion or administration of excessive HCO_3^- is a relatively rare occurrence. This is because the normal kidneys can rapidly excrete excessive loads of HCO_3^-. More commonly, metabolic alkalosis is caused by either gastric loss of fixed acid, as with

ACID-BASE CASE STUDY 6
Metabolic alkalosis

An 83-year-old woman with heart disease has been taking a powerful diuretic to remove excess edema fluid from her legs and help keep her free of pulmonary edema. Her blood gases and serum electrolytes reveal the following:

pH:	7.58
$Paco_2$:	48 mm Hg
HCO_3^-:	44 mEq/L
BE:	+19 mEq/L
Serum K^+:	2.5 mEq/L
Serum Cl^-:	95 mEq/L

- **STEP 1** *Categorize the pH*

    The pH is substantially above normal, indicating the presence of an alkalemia.

- **STEP 2** *Determine the respiratory involvement*

    The Pco_2 is slightly above normal, indicating a mild hypoventilation. However, because there is an alkalemia present, the existence of a primary respiratory acidosis is ruled out. The elevated Pco_2 may be a compensatory response to a primary metabolic problem (possible metabolic alkalosis).

- **STEP 3** *Determine the metabolic involvement*

    The HCO_3^- is substantially higher than normal; given the high pH, this elevated HCO_3^- signals a metabolic alkalosis. This is confirmed by the large base excess (+19 mEq/L). Further, the low serum K^+ and Cl^- indicate a hypokalemic/hypochloremic metabolic alkalosis.

- **STEP 4** *Assess for compensation*

    Although there is a slight elevation in the Pco_2, compensation for the metabolic alkalosis is minimal. This lack of compensation is consistent with the presence of hypokalemic metabolic alkalosis.

- **CONCLUSION** *Uncompensated metabolic alkalosis.*

---

severe vomiting or nasogastric suctioning, or by augmented renal excretion of H^+, K^+, or Cl^- (Case Study 6).

Augmented renal excretion of H^+, K^+, or Cl^- can be caused by administration of certain diuretic agents or corticosteroids or can occur in conjunction with clinical entities such as Cushing's syndrome or aldosteronism.[8] Both types of metabolic alkalosis are associated with disruptions in normal electrolytic exchange in the kidney.

Normally the kidney reabsorbs about 80% of the filtered sodium with Cl^- or bicarbonate anions. The remainder of the sodium is exchanged for cations, specifically H^+ and K^+. In the presence of reduced serum chloride (hypochloremia), HCO_3^- is preferentially reabsorbed over chloride, and more sodium must be exchanged for H^+ and K^+. In combination, these factors increase serum HCO_3^- and enhance acid excretion, thereby causing metabolic alkalosis.

In the presence of reduced serum potassium (hypokalemia), more sodium must be exchanged for H^+, also enhancing acid excretion and causing metabolic alkalosis. Interestingly, hypokalemia can be both a cause and effect of metabolic alkalosis.[19] Low potassium levels, such as occur with a potassium deficiency, cause alkalosis via the mechanism just described. However, in the presence of a metabolic alkalosis caused by excessive base, the kidneys attempt to retain H^+. In such situations, K^+ will be preferentially excreted, causing hypokalemia.

Compensation. The expected compensatory response to metabolic alkalosis is CO_2 retention via hypoventilation.[20] However, this response generally is not observed, especially in hypokalemic metabolic alkalosis.

The failure to compensate for hypokalemic metabolic alkalosis may be explained, in part, by the cation exchange that occurs across cellular membranes in this condition.[2] As serum K^+ decreases, K^+ ions diffuse out of the cells in exchange for H^+ ions. This increase in intracellular hydrogen ion concentration, especially in the respiratory chemoreceptive centers, offsets the influence of the extracellular alkalosis, thereby maintaining a normal stimulus to breathe.

If carbon dioxide retention occurs in response to metabolic alkalosis, its magnitude eventually is blunted by the decrease in Pao_2 that occurs with hypoventilation.

Correction. Correction of metabolic alkalosis aims to restore normal fluid volume and electrolyte concentrations, especially potassium and chloride levels. This may be accomplished by administration of chloride containing compounds. If hypokalemia is a primary factor, KCl is the preferred corrective agent. Metabolic alkalosis caused by excessive corticosteroids is often resistant to chloride therapy because of the kidney's inability to retain this electrolyte.

Mixed acid-base states

It is obvious that combinations of disorders may occur in the same patient.[21,22] Mixed acid-base disorders are most common among critically ill patients. Considering the high intensity of involvement of respiratory care practitioners with the critically ill, these complex acid-base problems will be encountered frequently.

Any of the two primary respiratory states may coexist with any of the two primary metabolic states, and patients with simultaneous respiratory and metabolic disease often present complicated pictures. Moreover, an imbalance in one direction can theoretically be offset by an imbalance in the other, with a resulting normal pH. Differentiation between these many possibilities demands that laboratory data be integrated with information relevant to the full clinical status of the patient. Only by integrating these perspectives can the respiratory care practitioner understand and appropriately participate in the management of such combined acid-base disorders.

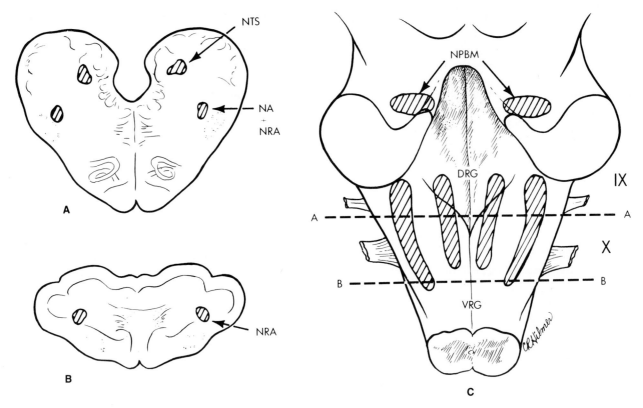

Fig. 10-9   Diagram of central respiratory centers in the midbrain. **A,** Transverse section of the medulla oblongata slightly rostral to the obex at the level indicated by the dashed line *AA* in **C. B,** Transverse section of the medulla slightly caudal to the obex at the level indicated by the dashed line *BB* in **C. C,** Dorsal view of the medulla and pons, showing the location of central respiratory neuron groups: *NTS,* nucleus solitarius; *NA,* nucleus ambiguus; *NRA,* nucleus retroambigualis; *NPBM,* nucleus parabrachialis medialis; *DRG,* dorsal respiratory group; *VRG,* ventral respiratory group; *IX,* ninth cranial (glossopharyngeal) nerve; and *X,* tenth cranial (vagus) nerve. (From Slonim NB and Hamilton LH: Respiratory physiology, ed 5, St Louis, 1987, The CV Mosby Co.)

REGULATION OF RESPIRATION

For the lungs to effectively exchange respired gases and participate in acid-base homeostasis, a control or regulatory mechanism must exist. Exactly how these diverse and sometimes conflicting roles are integrated is an ongoing subject of inquiry.

Contemporary studies of the regulation of respiration have made it clear that the control mechanisms underlying this process are exceedingly complex.[23,24] Even today, our knowledge in this area is incomplete and often speculative. Our focus will be to apply what is currently known in this area to the clinical practice of respiratory care.

Rhythmicity of breathing

Among the best known facts regarding the regulation of breathing is that the rhythmic cycle of inspiration and expiration is primarily mediated via the central nervous system.[25] Moreover, we know that this cycle originates in the brainstem, mainly from neurons located in the medulla.[26,27]

Medullary respiratory "centers."   By use of microelectrodes, clusters of neurons having activity patterns linked with inspiration and expiration have been identified (Fig. 10-9).[28,29] A dorsal respiratory group of neurons is located on either side of the medulla, in the nucleus of the tractus solitarius (NTS). These dorsal neurons appear to be the primary source of inspiratory activity, probably through direct efferent innervation of the phrenic nerves. Moreover, the dorsal respiratory group appears to receive afferent impulses through the IX and X cranial nerves. These nerves are responsible for transmitting sensory impulses from the lungs, airways, and peripheral chemoreceptors to the brainstem.

A ventral respiratory group of neurons is located in the ventrolateral portion of the medulla, in the region of the nucleus ambiguus (NA) and nucleus retroambigualis (NRA). The more rostral neurons of the ventral respiratory group have mainly inspiratory activity, while those more caudal are primarily expiratory in function. Unlike the dorsal neurons, the ventral respiratory group receives no afferent input.

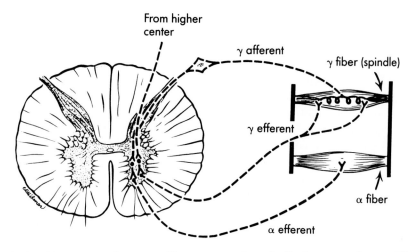

Fig. 10-10   The extravagal gamma-efferent system is a feedback system that modifies the breathing pattern. (From Slonim NB and Hamilton LH: Respiratory physiology, ed 5, St Louis, 1987, The CV Mosby Co.)

Until recently, it was thought that these dorsal and ventral groups served, respectively, as inspiratory and expiratory "centers." Moreover, it was believed that the cyclical pattern of inspiration and expiration was simply a result of self-excitation and mutual inhibition between these groups. Recent evidence suggests that this explanation may be an oversimplification.[30-33] We simply do not know how this area generates the rhythmicity.

Pons. If the brainstem is transected above the medulla, spontaneous respiration continues, although in a more irregular pattern. This finding has led to the conclusion that the pons is not involved in the genesis of rhythmic breathing, but may only serve to modify the activity of the lower medullary centers. Indeed, recent evidence suggests that the neurons of the pons, unlike their medullary counterparts, have no periodic activity.[34]

As shown in Fig. 10-9, two localized collections of neurons in the pons have been shown to influence the medullary respiratory centers: the apneustic center (located at the level of the area vestibularis) and the pneumotaxic center (located in the region of the nucleus parabrachealis medialis [NPBM]). Until recently, the apneustic center was thought to enhance the activity of the inspiratory neurons in the medulla, being inhibited by either pneumotaxic stimulation or vagal afferent input via the pulmonary stretch receptors (the Hering-Breuer reflex).

Recent research suggests that the apneustic center may instead serve as the "off switch" by which normal inspiration is terminated.[35] In this explanation, the "off switch" is activated by either pneumotaxic stimulation or vagal afferent input. This theory helps explain the inspiratory spasms (apneustic breathing) that occur with suppression of the pneumotaxic center or blockage of vagal afferent input to the brainstem. However, the exact details on how the pontine and medullary centers interact or modify the basic cyclical rhythm are still being sought.[30-33]

Gamma-efferent feedback system. Impulses generated by the brainstem respiratory centers are delivered over efferent pathways to the respiratory muscles, causing their contraction. How much these muscles contract, however, is determined by a separate regulatory mechanism common to all skeletal muscle. This system is called the gamma-efferent feedback system.

The gamma-efferent feedback system represents a reflex arc that automatically adjusts muscle contractions to accommodate varying loads. As shown in Fig. 10-10, impulses arising from the brainstem centers travel over efferent nerves to both the alpha and gamma fibers. As both fibers contract, stretch receptors in the spindle of the gamma fibers send impulses back to the spinal cord over gamma-afferent pathways, in proportion to the change in spindle tension. In turn, the reflex impulses arising from the stretch receptors are transmitted to the alpha fibers over alpha-efferent pathways.

As long as muscle contraction is unopposed, both the alpha and gamma fibers will shorten to the same degree, and increases in spindle tension will be minimal. However, if the shortening of the muscle fibers meets resistance, the tension in the stretch receptors of the spindle will increase. An increase in the tension on the spindle fiber stimulates the ventral horn motorneurons of the cord and, via the gamma-efferent portion of the arc, causes further contraction of the main muscle (alpha) fibers.

An increase in tension on the respiratory muscle spindle fibers will occur whenever the transpulmonary pressure gradient is increased, as with an increase in airway resistance or a decrease in lung or thoracic compliance (see Chapter 8). These conditions impose an increased load on the respiratory muscles, to which the gamma-efferent system responds by increasing its strength of contraction. In this manner, muscle contractions are automatically adjusted to accommodate the varying loads associated with changes in the mechanical properties of the lungs and thorax.

Sustained increases in gamma-afferent activity occur when the effort required to contract the muscle exceeds the actual shortening, as would be the case with a decrease in compliance. Current theory suggests that such conditions affect the brainstem centers by causing early cessation of inspiration.[34] This theory explains, in part, the increased frequency of breathing associated with conditions that lower lung or thoracic compliance.

Influence of higher centers. Stimulation of selected neurons in the mesencephalon (midbrain) and diencephalon (hypothalamus and thalamus) can augment tidal volume, respiratory rate, or both.[2] These responses may simply represent a general increase in the "arousal" reaction of the reticular activating system.

Modification of the basic respiratory rhythm more commonly occurs via the cerebral cortex.[34] Good examples of the modifying influence of the cerebral cortex are the variations in a breathing pattern that occur with breath-holding, voluntary hyperventilation, isometric muscular efforts, singing, crying, and swallowing. However, the ability of the cerebral cortex to override the basic cyclical pattern established by the medullary centers is limited. This limitation is caused by the strong influence of other factors on the regulation of breathing, particularly the chemical constituency of the blood and cerebrospinal fluid.

Chemical regulation of respiration

It has long been known that the normal rhythmic pattern of breathing is modified by a variety of chemical stimuli, particularly hypercapnea, acidemia, and hypoxia. Research conducted over the past 75 years has demonstrated that the major factor responsible for changes in ventilation is neural input to the medullary centers through specialized structures called *chemoreceptors*.[36-38] A chemoreceptor is a group of nerve cells that senses and responds to changes in the chemical composition of its fluid environment.

There are two sets of chemoreceptors: the central or medullary chemoreceptors and the peripheral chemoreceptors. The central chemoreceptors lie on the ventrolateral surfaces of the medulla in proximity to the exit of cranial nerves IX and X. The peripheral chemoreceptors are located in the bifurcations of both carotid arteries and the arch of the aorta. Afferent neurons from the carotid bodies ascend as part of the carotid nerve to join the glossopharyngeal nerve. The afferent nerve fibers from the aortic bodies enter the vagal nerve pathways usually along with the recurrent laryngeal nerves.

Both the central and peripheral chemoreceptors send impulses to the medullary center, and while there are similarities in their functions, there are also significant differences. These differences are most pronounced in their relative response to CO_2 and O_2.

Response to carbon dioxide. Carbon dioxide exerts the primary chemical influence on breathing. High inspired

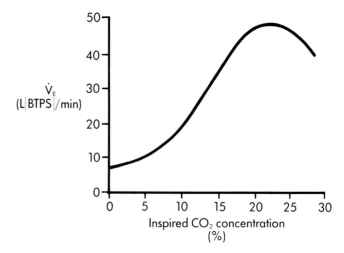

Fig. 10-11   Ventilatory response to CO_2 concentration in inspired gas.   (From Slonim NB and Hamilton LH: Respiratory physiology, ed 5, St Louis, 1987, The CV Mosby Co.)

partial pressure of carbon dioxide has a direct stimulating effect on ventilation (Fig. 10-11). Ventilation increases gradually as inspired CO_2 concentrations rise to 8% to 10%. Concentrations in the 10% to 20% range cause a proportionately greater increase in ventilation. However, at concentrations in the 20% range, CO_2 exerts a depressant effect on both ventilation and the central nervous system as a whole, not unlike an anesthetic gas.

Early experiments demonstrated that this effect resulted, in part, from changes in the chemical environment of the brainstem. Perfusion of the ventricles of the brain with fluid containing a high Pco_2 or low pH stimulated breathing. On the other hand, perfusion with fluid containing a low Pco_2 or high pH depressed respiration. These findings pointed to the existence of a central chemoreceptive area.

Central chemoreceptors. The central chemoreceptors have primary responsibility for sensing and responding to changes in blood levels of CO_2. However, these specialized cells are not in direct contact with the blood. Instead, they are exposed to the circulating cerebrospinal fluid (CSF), which is separated from the blood by a semipermeable membrane referred to as the blood-brain barrier.

The blood-brain barrier is relatively impermeable to hydrogen and bicarbonate ions, but is freely permeable to molecular carbon dioxide. Elevations in blood CO_2 therefore cause rapid diffusion of this gas into the CSF, where it dissociates into H^+ and HCO_3^-, lowering the CSF pH. Current knowledge suggests that it is the low pH of the CSF, and not the high CO_2, that causes stimulation of the central chemoreceptors. Thus, increased levels of CO_2 in the blood increase ventilation indirectly by altering the pH of the CSF, and thereby stimulating the central chemoreceptors. The central chemoreceptors, in turn, signal the medullary centers to increase ventilation.

Exactly how these various inputs are integrated remains unknown. However, the effectiveness of this central mechanism for chemical control is so extraordinary that the Pa_{CO_2} normally does not vary more than about 3 mm Hg over the course of a day.

Peripheral chemoreceptors. Early research demonstrated that when blood high in CO_2 or low in O_2 perfused the left ventricle and first part of the aorta, stimulation of breathing occurred. However, such stimulation was observed only when the vagus nerves were intact. Later investigations showed a similar effect with the carotid arteries. These findings pointed to the existence of peripheral chemoreceptors.

As compared with the central chemoreceptors, the carotid and aortic bodies are not very sensitive to CO_2 changes.[37] In general, the Pa_{CO_2} must rise 20 to 30 mm Hg above normal before a significant increase in ventilation occurs. For this reason it is estimated that less than a third of the response to hypercapnea in normal subjects is a result of the activity of the peripheral chemoreceptors.

The peripheral chemoreceptors are also responsive to changes in H^+. This response occurs even in the presence of normal or low partial pressures of CO_2, as might be observed in metabolic acidosis. However, the response to changes in blood pH is less sensitive than that to CO_2. The pH must change by 0.05 to 0.1 units before a ventilatory response is observed.

Although the peripheral chemoreceptors are stimulated by hypercapnea and acidemia, their primary role appears to be in response to hypoxia.

Response to oxygen lack. Whereas the body's response to hypercapnea occurs with small increases in P_{CO_2}, the response to hypoxia requires a substantially greater deviation from normal before ventilation is increased. Ventilation is not stimulated significantly until inspired concentrations fall to 12% or less, equivalent to an arterial Po_2 between 50 and 60 mm Hg. In normal individuals living at sea level, the hypoxic stimulus to breathing is not considered part of the regular mechanism controlling respiration.[34]

Moreover, in contrast to hypercapnea, which acts both centrally and peripherally, hypoxia appears to stimulate breathing solely through the peripheral chemoreceptors. In fact, if the peripheral chemoreceptors are removed, arterial hypoxemia actually suppresses ventilation, presumably by depression of the medullary centers.

The peripheral chemoreceptors respond to decreased partial pressures of oxygen, rather than an actual decrease in the oxygen content of the blood. This sensitivity to Pa_{O_2} is explained, in part, by the extraordinarily high blood flow they receive in comparison with their metabolic rates.[37] Because the arterial-venous oxygen content difference $(C(a-v)O_2)$ of the peripheral chemoreceptors is extremely small, most of their oxygen needs are met by the small amount of dissolved O_2 in the plasma. Therefore, a decrease of sufficient magnitude in either the Po_2 or blood flow will stimulate the peripheral chemoreceptors, causing

an increase in afferent input to the medullary centers and a proportionate increase in ventilation.

The sensitivity of the peripheral chemoreceptors to Pa_{O_2}, as opposed to Ca_{O_2}, explains why conditions in which the arterial oxygen content is low but the oxygen partial pressure is normal do not stimulate breathing. Such conditions include anemia and carbon monoxide poisoning.

Interactions. The occurrence of hypercapnea and hypoxemia together result in an additive effect on ventilation.[34] As shown in Fig. 10-12, in the presence of hypoxemia, the ventilatory response to hypercapnea occurs earlier and is greater than when the Po_2 is normal. Likewise, in the presence of hypercapnea, the ventilatory response to hypoxemia is augmented. In clinical practice, these interactions help explain the differential effect of and response to hypercapnea and hypoxemia in patients with respiratory insufficiency and failure.

Reflex control of respiration

In addition to input provided by the chemoreceptors, the respiratory centers of the brainstem constantly receive and process other sensory information. This information arises from a variety of mechanical sensors called proprioceptors. Impulses from these proprioceptors travel over afferent pathways of the vagus nerve to the medullary respiratory centers, where they are integrated with other input to vary the breathing pattern.

Proprioceptive mechanisms thus provide the third major regulatory influence on respiration, termed *reflex control*.[39,40] The major reflex control mechanisms include: the Hering-Breuer inflation reflex, Head's paradoxic reflex, the deflation reflex, airway irritant reflexes, a vascular congestive reflex, and the baroreceptor reflex to changes in systemic perfusion pressures.

Inflation reflex (Hering-Breuer reflex). The Hering-Breuer inflation reflex originates in specialized stretch receptors located primarily in the bronchi and bronchioles. These stretch receptors progressively discharge nerve impulses during inflation of the lung. Because such impulses continue as long as intratracheal pressure remains high, the stretch receptors responsible for the Hering-Breuer reflex are called "slowly adapting" receptors. These impulses travel through the vagus nerve to the apneustic center.

Traditionally the inflation reflex was thought to modulate the depth of inspiration by inhibiting apneustic center activity. However, recent experimentation in animals indicates that these receptors mainly influence the duration of the expiratory pause occurring between breaths, rather than the depth of inspiration. Moreover, it now appears that the inflation reflex is weak or absent during normal quiet breathing in healthy adults. The only evidence of a strong inflation reflex in humans is among newborn infants.[2]

Head's paradoxic reflex. When the afferent pathways for the Hering-Breuer reflex are blocked by cooling the va-

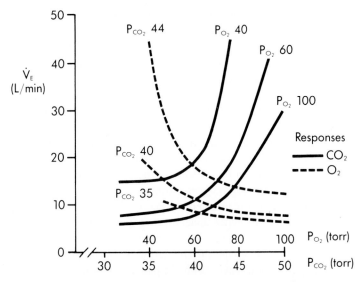

Fig. 10-12   Set of curves illustrating the ventilatory response to hypercapnia and hypoxia. The curves were constructed from published data. The solid lines represent the ventilatory response to P_{CO_2} at constant P_{O_2}. The broken lines represent the response to P_{O_2} at constant P_{CO_2}. (From Slonim NB and Hamilton LH: Respiratory physiology, ed 5, St Louis, 1987, The CV Mosby Co.)

gus nerve, inflation of the lung causes an additional inspiratory effort. This response, called Head's paradoxic reflex, is also initiated through sensory stimulation of pulmonary stretch receptors. However, as compared with those responsible for the Hering-Breuer reflex, the stretch receptors involved in Head's reflex are stimulated mainly by rapid volume changes. Hence these receptors are referred to as "rapidly adapting."

Head's reflex may be the basis for the occasional deep breath or sigh that punctuates normal breathing, thereby preventing alveolar collapse or microatelectasis. It may also be responsible for maintaining high tidal volumes during exercise and the successive gasping exhibited by newborn infants as they progressively inflate their lungs at birth.[34]

Deflation reflex. Injury to the lung or chest wall that causes deflation results in an increased force and frequency of inspiratory effort. This response, which is distinct from the Hering-Breuer reflex, is referred to as the deflation reflex. Like Head's reflex, the deflation reflex is initiated through sensory stimulation of rapidly adapting stretch receptors located primarily in the bronchi and bronchioles. The deflation reflex may help explain the hyperpnea that is frequently observed with chest compression and pneumothorax. Because the deflation reflex is observed mainly in response to injury, it is sometimes referred to as a nociceptive reflex.[2]

Irritation reflexes. Irritant receptors are located in the subepithelial tissues of the larger airways, mainly in the posterior wall of the trachea, and at the bifurcations of the larger bronchi. Not active during normal breathing, these receptors respond to a variety of mechanical, chemical, and physiologic stimuli, including physical manipulation or irritation, inhalation of noxious gases, histamine-induced bronchoconstriction, asphyxia, and microembolization of the pulmonary arteries. Stimulation of the irritant receptors can result in bronchoconstriction, hyperpnea, reflex closure of the glottis, and cough. These responses are readily observed at the bedside during procedures such as tracheobronchial intubation or bronchoscopy and can be mitigated by the application of local anesthetics.

Reflex response to pulmonary capillary congestion. Pulmonary embolism, pulmonary edema, and congestive heart failure all can evoke a rapid, shallow, breathing pattern. That such a pattern is abolished by vagotomy demonstrates its reflex origin.

The source of this reflex response is thought to be the juxtopulmonary capillary receptors, called "J" receptors. These receptors originally were considered part of the deflation reflex. Recent research indicates that the prime role of the J receptors is in response to increases in pulmonary capillary pressures.[2] Besides causing rapid, shallow, breathing, stimulation of the J receptors can result in bradycardia, hypotension, and expiratory narrowing of the glottis. J receptor stimulation also may contribute to the sensation of dyspnea accompanying pulmonary vascular congestion.[2]

Baroreceptor reflexes. It has long been observed that a decrease in arterial blood pressure results in hyperventilation, and an increase in arterial blood pressure causes hypoventilation.[34] This reflex is mediated primarily by the aortic and carotid baroreceptors (described in Chapter 7).

The hyperventilation that occurs with decreased perfusion pressures slightly increases arterial oxygen content, thereby providing a small increment in oxygen delivery. Of perhaps more importance is the potential increase in venous return that would result from such a breathing pattern. However, these effects are minimal, and the actual role of the baroreceptor reflex in the regulation of respiration remains unknown.

Integrated responses

Fig. 10-13 provides an integrated perspective on the interaction among the three major mechanisms involved in the regulation of respiration. The basic rhythmicity of the breathing pattern is established by the medullary and pontine centers. The response of the respiratory muscles to varying mechanical loads is adjusted via the gamma-efferent feedback system. Modification to the basic breathing pattern occurs via input from local and peripheral chemoreceptors in the aortic and carotid bodies, and from proprioceptors located in the lung parenchyma. In addition, input from higher brain centers provides voluntary control when necessary. In combination, these control

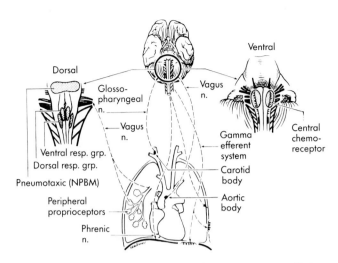

Fig. 10-13   The system that regulates pulmonary ventilation and generates the breathing pattern. (From Slonim NB and Hamilton LH: Respiratory physiology, ed 5, St Louis, 1987, The CV Mosby Co.)

mechanisms normally assure that ventilation is efficient, that gas exchange is adequate, and that acid-base homeostasis is maintained.

When faced with abnormal circumstances, these control mechanisms must adjust their activity to maintain as near a normal level of body function as possible. As with any deviation from normal, such adjustments represent a compromise. Good examples of adjustments made by the regulatory mechanisms are those that occur in chronic hypoxemia, chronic hypercapnea, and metabolic acidosis.

Chronic hypoxemia. An initial reduction in arterial Po_2 is immediately detected by the peripheral chemoreceptors, causing an immediate increase in ventilation. The resulting hyperventilation lowers blood CO_2 levels, causing diffusion of this gas out of the cerebrospinal fluid. As CO_2 leaves the CSF, brain pH rises, causing a suppression of ventilation. This secondary action slightly offsets the initial hypoxic stimulus, resulting in a lower level of hyperventilation than would otherwise occur.

Beyond the acute phase, continued low arterial Po_2 levels provoke a series of compensatory responses designed to improve oxygen delivery and restore a normal pH.

Within a few hours, active transport of HCO_3^- out of the CSF begins, causing a lowering of its pH to normal. As the pH of the CSF is restored to normal, the early secondary suppression to ventilation is removed, and a new balance (with greater hyperventilation) is established.

In essence, chronic hypoxemia causes the medullary chemoreceptors to be "reset" to maintain a lower than normal Pco_2. Under such circumstances, should the hypoxic stimulus be removed, hyperventilation will continue, although at a lesser magnitude. As the Pco_2 rises over time, CSF HCO_3^- will rise, and ventilation will eventually be restored to normal.

Chronic hypercapnea. An acute increase in arterial Pco_2 causes an immediate increase in ventilation via stimulation of both the peripheral and central chemoreceptors. Should the hypercapnea persist, the kidneys begin to preferentially retain bicarbonate and excrete chloride and fixed acids. At the same time, the rise in Pco_2 and resultant drop in pH in the CSF causes active inward migration of HCO_3^- across the blood-brain barrier.

The rise in CSF HCO_3^- brings its pH back toward normal. However, as the pH is adjusted toward normal, the central chemoreceptive drive to increase ventilation becomes blunted. Moreover, the responsiveness to additional increases in CO_2 is suppressed. In combination, these factors allow the Pco_2 to rise further, creating a potentially vicious cycle.

However, as long as one is breathing room air, the rise in $Paco_2$ causes a reciprocal fall in the Pao_2. When this fall in Pao_2 is of sufficient magnitude (below 60 to 70 mm Hg), the peripheral chemoreceptors are again stimulated, this time by the arterial hypoxemia. Therefore, despite the loss of central sensitivity to CO_2, ventilation is maintained via a hypoxic stimulus.

With the main drive to breathe being arterial hypoxemia, elimination of this stimulus can result in depression of ventilation, increased hypercapnea, and even death. The potential for this oxygen-induced hypoventilation underlies the use of controlled low-flow oxygen therapy in patients with chronic hypercapnea, as described in Chapter 25.

Chronic (compensated) metabolic acidosis. A rise in fixed acid in the blood lowers its pH, quickly causing stimulation of the peripheral chemoreceptors and hyperventilation. The lowered blood Pco_2 causes a similar decrease in the CSF Pco_2, thereby raising its pH. This CSF alkalosis causes a secondary central inhibition to ventilation that partially blunts the initial peripheral stimulation.

As with chronic hypoxia, if the hyperventilation persists, active transport of HCO_3^- out of the CSF begins, causing a lowering of its pH to normal. As the pH of the CSF is restored to normal, the early secondary suppression to ventilation is removed, and a new balance (with greater hyperventilation) is established. Moreover, the central chemoreceptors are "reset" to this lower level of CO_2, and become more sensitive to increases in the CSF level of this gas.

If the metabolic acidosis is rapidly corrected, hyperventilation will persist, and the patient will swing from a compensated metabolic acidosis to an acute respiratory alkalosis. Events such as these explain the persistent hyperventilation observed with rapid correction of compensated metabolic acidosis, as in the treatment of renal tubular acidosis by dialysis or diabetic ketoacidosis by insulin.[2]

SUMMARY

Metabolic processes of the body produce in excess of 24,000 mM of acid per day. Normal acid-base homeostasis involves minimizing pH changes resulting from this acid load and removing or excreting these by-products of metabolism. Buffer systems serve as the first line of defense in preventing wide fluctuations in pH in the body fluids. Excretion of body acids is accomplished by both the kidneys and lungs.

Imbalances in acid-base homeostasis can arise from alterations in respiratory or metabolic function, from ingestion of chemicals or drugs, or as a result of treatment. Compensatory mechanisms of the body minimize the effect of these imbalances via adjustments of the system not affected. Correction of acid-base imbalances requires that the system primarily affected be restored to normal function.

In this regard, the respiratory system plays a vital role. In addition to regulating gas exchange, the mechanisms controlling respiration are intimately involved in acid-base balance. For these reasons, understanding the role of the respiratory system in acid-base balance is a critical prerequisite to the provision of comprehensive and quality respiratory care.

REFERENCES

1. Martin L: Pulmonary physiology in clinical practice: the essentials for patient care and evaluation, St Louis, 1987, The CV Mosby Co.
2. Murray JF: The normal lung, ed 2, Philadelphia, 1986, WB Saunders Co.
3. Winters RW, Knud E, and Dell RB: Acid-base physiology in medicine, Copenhagen, 1967, The London Co.
4. Filley G: Acid-base and blood gas regulation, Philadelphia, 1971, Lea & Febiger.
5. Siggaard-Andersen O: The acid-base status of the blood, ed 4, Baltimore, 1974, Williams & Wilkins Co.
6. Jones NL: Blood gases and acid-base physiology, New York, 1980, Brian C. Decker.
7. Shapiro BA, Harrison RA, and Walton JR: Clinical application of blood gases, ed 3, Chicago, 1982, Year Book Medical Publishers.
8. Narins RG: Acid-base metabolism. In Gonick HC, editor: Current nephrology, vol 1, Boston, 1977, Houghton Mifflin Co.
9. Lane EE and Walker JF: Clinical arterial blood gas analysis, St Louis, 1987, The CV Mosby Co.
10. ACCP-ATS Joint Committee on Pulmonary Nomenclature: Pulmonary terms and symbols, Chest 67:583, 1975.
11. Rose BD: Clinical physiology of acid-base and electrolyte disorders, New York, 1977, McGraw-Hill Book Co.
12. Wilkins RL: Interpretation of blood gases. In Wilkins RL, Sheldon RL, and Krider SJ: Clinical assessment in respiratory care, St Louis, 1985, The CV Mosby Co.
13. Flenley DC: Blood-gas and acid-base interpretation, Basics of RD 10:1, September 1981.
14. Refsum HE: Acid-base disturbances in chronic pulmonary disease, Ann NY Acad Sci 133:142, 1966.
15. Petty TL and Neff TA: Renal function in respiratory failure, JAMA 217:82, 1971.
16. Robin ED: Abnormalities of acid-base regulation in chronic pulmonary disease, with special reference to hypercapnia and extracellular alkalosis, N Engl J Med 268:917, 1963.
17. Collier CR, Hackney JD, and Mohler JD: Use of extracellular base excess in diagnosis of acid-base disorders: a conceptual approach, Chest 61:65, 1972.
18. Nunn JF: Applied respiratory physiology, ed 2, Kent, England, 1977, Butterworth & Co.
19. Selden DW and Rector FC Jr: The generation and maintenance of metabolic alkalosis, Kidney Int i:306, 1972.
20. Goldring RM: Respiratory adjustments to chronic metabolic alkalosis in man, J Clin Invest 47:188, 1968.
21. McCurdy DK: Mixed metabolic and respiratory acid-base disturbances: diagnosis and treatment, Chest 62:355, 1972.
22. Narins RG and Emmett M: Simple and mixed acid-base disorders: a practical approach, Medicine 59:161, 1980.
23. Mitchell RA and Berger AJ: Neural regulation of respiration, Am Rev Respir Dis 111:206, 1975.
24. Berger AJ, Mitchell RA, and Severinghaus JW: Regulation of respiration, N Engl J Med 297:92-97, 138-143, 194-201, 1977.
25. Euler CV: Brain stem mechanisms for the generation and control of breathing pattern. In Fishman AF et al, editors: Handbook of physiology, Sect 3, The respiratory system, vol 2, Control of breathing, Bethesda, 1986, American Physiological Society.
26. Bradley GW: Control of breathing pattern. In Widdicombe JG, editor: International review of physiology, vol 14, Baltimore, 1974, University Park Press.
27. Cohen MI: Central determinants of respiratory rhythm, Ann Rev Physiol 43:91-104, 1981.
28. Kalia MP: Anatomical organization of central respiratory neurons, Ann Rev Physiol 43:105-120, 1981.
29. Long SE and Duffin J: The medullary respiratory neurons: a review, Can J Physiol Pharmacol 62:161-182, 1984.
30. Feldman JL: Interactions between brainstem respiratory neurons, Fed Proc 40:2384-2388, 1981.
31. Wang SC and Ngai SH: Respiration coordinating mechanisms of the brain stem: a few controversial points, Ann NY Acad Sci 109:550, 1963.
32. Merrill EG: Where are the real respiratory neurons? Fed Proc 40:2389-2394, 1974.
33. Richter DW, Ballantyne D, and Remmers JH: How is the respiratory rhythm generated? A model, News Physiol Sci 1:109-112, 1986.
34. Slonim NB and Hamilton LH: Respiratory physiology, ed 5, St Louis, 1985, The CV Mosby Co.
35. Cohen MI and Feldman JL: Models of respiratory phase-switching, Fed Proc 36:2367-2374, 1977.
36. Sorenson SC: The chemical control of ventilation, Acta Physiol Scand (Suppl) 361:1-72, 1971
37. Torrance RW: Arterial chemoreceptors. In Widdicombe JG, editor: International review of physiology, vol 2, Baltimore, 1974, University Park Press.
38. Fitzgerald RS and Lahiri S: Reflex response to chemoreceptor activity. In Fishman AF et al, editors: Handbook of physiology, Sect 3, The respiratory system, vol 2, Control of breathing, Bethesda, 1986, American Physiological Society.
39. Coleridge HM and Coleridge JCG: Reflexes evoked from the tracheobronchial tree and lungs. In Fishman AF et al, editors: Handbook of physiology, Sect 3, The respiratory system, vol 2, Control of breathing, Bethesda, 1986, American Physiological Society.
40. Widdicombe JG: Reflex control of breathing. In Widdicombe, JG, editor: International review of physiology, vol 2, Baltimore, 1974, University Park Press.

Essentials for Patient Care

SECTION

Essentials for Patient Care

11

Health Communication

Robin A. Harvan

The dynamic nature of health care delivery has magnified the challenges involved in relationships among health professionals and patients. The current health care system is characterized by changing priorities, settings, services, technologies, and funding patterns. More than ever, health professionals such as respiratory care practitioners are being held accountable to provide both technically competent and personalized, humane care.[1] Thus technical knowledge and skills alone are no longer viewed as a sufficient basis for practice.

Moreover, the provision of quality health care is becoming increasingly dependent on complex and demanding interactions among a vast array of health professionals. Implicit in this renewed emphasis on a team approach to health care delivery is the need for open, ongoing, and effective communication among health care providers. In fact, in this new environment the effectiveness with which health professionals fulfill their helping roles will be measured mainly by their skills in human communication.[2]

OBJECTIVES

This chapter will thus focus on skills of communication and human interaction within the context of the modern health care delivery system. Rather than prescribing strict formulations of what to say and how to behave, we will take a more descriptive approach to health communication as a complex and dynamic process. Specifically, after completion of this chapter, the reader will be able to:

1. Differentiate between the concepts of communication in general and health communication in particular;

2. Define the importance of communication as related to both patient care and professional performance and job satisfaction;

3. Distinguish by example among the various levels of health communication;

4. Apply various communication models to derive a common set of principles governing communication in the health care setting;

5. Differentiate among the determinants of effective verbal and nonverbal communication, as related to the practitioner's role as both speaker and listener;

6. Outline the key considerations necessary for effective communication to occur in professional-patient, professional-professional, professional-family, and patient-family relationships.

KEY TERMS

Most terms used in this chapter are defined in context. The following terms are introduced without explicit definition but may be found in the text glossary:

acronym	hierarchical
animosity	interdisciplinary
auditory	interpersonal
autonomy	intrapersonal
disposition	jargon
empathetic	multidimensional
encode	pantomime
esthetic	transaction
feedback	treatment regimen

THE NATURE OF COMMUNICATION IN HEALTH CARE

Almost everyone agrees that communication plays an important role in the delivery of health care. Nonetheless, the importance of communication in both patient and professional interaction is generally underestimated. This viewpoint is based, in part, on an overly simplistic notion of the nature of the communication process. For respiratory care practitioners to develop good health communication skills, they must first understand both the nature of the communication process in general and its importance and complexity as applied to health care.

Definitions of communication

Many definitions of the term communication have been given. Rather than attempt to provide a single definition,

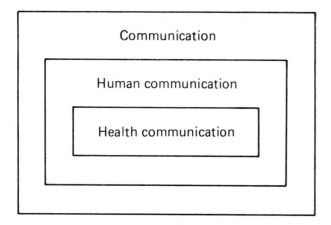

Fig. 11-1 Relationship between three kinds of communication. (From Northouse PG and Northouse LL: Health communication: a handbook for health professionals, Englewood Cliffs, NJ, 1985 Prentice-Hall.)

we will examine the concept by distinguishing between different kinds of communication. Proceeding from general to specific, we will focus on the relationship between communication, human communication, and health communication (Fig. 11-1).

In general, communication is a term used to refer to any dynamic process whereby meaning is shared. As illustrated in Fig. 11-1, human communication is a subset of communication in general, to be distinguished from other types of communication that do not involve human beings, such as communication among lower animals. Human communication thus refines the definition of communication to include its human dimensions.

Human communication therefore represents any dynamic process whereby information, meanings, and rules are shared among individuals. Given this human dimension, a multitude of human qualities are involved in this sharing process of exchange. For example, these uniquely human qualities include personal feelings, attitudes, dispositions, values, and motivations.

Health communication is, then, a subset of human communication. Health communication is concerned with promotion of health or prevention of illness within our society and with making the health care system run to the satisfaction of both patients and practitioners. Health communication is the "cement" that binds, coordinates, and integrates human efforts to treat and prevent human suffering caused by illness and disease.[3] The focus of health communication, therefore, is on specific health-related interactions, including the factors that influence these interactions.

Importance of health communication

Clearly, communication is a fundamental part of our social existence. Likewise, communication plays a vital role in health care. Health care, after all, is a human enterprise, with social relationships at its core. Health communication consists of both the health-related interactions that occur as

a component of these social relationships and the various factors that influence these interactions.[3]

Because of the diversity of the relationships and the health-related interactions, communication has a tremendous effect on health care delivery. Communication influences the evaluation and treatment of patients, including their compliance with treatment regimens, their satisfaction with services, and even their emotional well-being. Communication also affects the morale and performance of health professionals.[1,4]

Respiratory care personnel treat, manage, control, and perform diagnostic evaluations in the care of patients with deficiencies and abnormalities of the cardiopulmonary system. With care of patients as the primary aim of the profession, effective communication skills in managing professional-patient interactions are essential.

The interactions that occur as a component of these relationships can influence the professional's ability to identify the patient's health problems, evaluate the patient's progress, and make recommendations for respiratory care. The outcomes of treatment may also be affected by communication. Through effective communication, the respiratory care practitioner can help patients cope with hospitalization and obtain maximum benefit from respiratory care procedures, thereby helping to improve both patients' emotional well-being and the outcomes of therapy.

With regard to the influence of communication on morale and performance, most respiratory care practitioners function within complex health care organizations. Within this context, communication among health care professionals, including both informal interactions and communication along formal organizational lines of authority, exerts a profound influence on one's job satisfaction, performance, and productivity.

It is therefore essential that respiratory care practitioners explore and reflect on the nature and extent of communication required in their chosen profession. In doing so, they will quickly discover that communication skills will determine, in large measure, both the quality of respiratory care services and the satisfaction realized in the provision of such services.

Complexity of communication in health care

Communication is so much a part of our personal lives that it can easily be taken for granted. If communication is viewed simply as an act of sending a message to be received by someone else, without consideration of its complexities, the process is likely to fail. Even in the best case, communication failure can result in misunderstandings between the parties involved. In the worst case, communication failure can cause personal animosity and mistrust. In clinical practice, communication failure may result in unexpected, unsatisfactory, or even adverse outcomes for the patient.

It is therefore critically important that respiratory care practitioners understand the complexity of communication

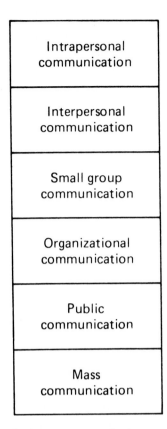

Fig. 11-2 Basic human communication contexts. (From Ruffner M and Burgoon M: Interpersonal communication, New York, 1981, Holt, Rinehart & Winston.)

and recognize the many factors that can contribute to communication problems. Only by doing so can the practitioner identify the unique strengths and weaknesses that characterize his or her own communication skills. In turn, only through the identification of one's own strengths and weaknesses can improvements be made.

Levels of health communication

As illustrated in Fig. 11-2, health communication can occur at many different levels.[2] These levels include mass communication, public communication, organizational communication, small-group communication, interpersonal communication, and intrapersonal communication.

A good example of the relationship among these various levels of health communication is the recent effort of the US Public Health Service to reduce risk factors and increase public awareness of the hazards of smoking (see Chapter 33 for details). At the level of mass communication, these efforts have included national mass media campaigns (via television, radio, and newspaper channels) designed to inform the public of the hazards of smoking. At the level of public communication, governmental and private-sector activity (such as that conducted by the American Lung Association) has used presentations, speeches, and public addresses to communicate the need to rid society of smoking. Organizational communication activities

have focused on establishment of smoke-free areas or the banning of smoking altogether. Small-group communication efforts have provided peer support for persons who seriously intend to quit smoking, while interpersonal health communication interactions, such as one-on-one teaching efforts between a respiratory care practitioner and a smoking patient, provide opportunities for learning, reinforcement, and follow-up. Last and most important is the level of intrapersonal communication. It is "self-talk" about health issues, such as the need to refrain from or quit smoking, that will ultimately determine one's health-directed behavior.

MODELS OF COMMUNICATION

Models are used to help explain both the nature of communication and the variables that affect the process. Each of the following selected models highlights particular components of the communication process. Admittedly, each model has limitations in representing the full complexity of human communication. When taken together, however, these models can help the respiratory care practitioner establish a personal framework by which one's skills in communication can be examined and enhanced.

General communication models

The Shannon-Weaver model. One of the earliest general models of communication was developed in 1949 by Shannon and Weaver.[5] As illustrated in Fig. 11-3, this model is of a one-way or linear nature, portraying communication in a manner not unlike the process of radio, television, or telephone transmission.

The Shannon-Weaver model represents communication as a pathway by which a message is "sent" from a source to its destination. In this model, a source selects the information and "encodes" it as a message. Encoding involves the translation of the information into selected verbal and nonverbal symbols, such as words, numbers, or gestures.

Once the message is encoded, it is "transmitted" by a signal through a "channel" to a receiver. For example, transmission over a channel may involve audible sounds or visual images. The receiver then "decodes" the message, which is sent to a particular destination.

Whereas electronic coding and decoding is a relatively consistent and predictable process, this element of human communication is much more complex. All too often we assume that the meaning of a message is the same to both sender and receiver. In fact, cultural and ethnic group differences, as well as individual variations in education and experience, can have a dramatic effect on the process of communication.

The General Motors Corporation learned this lesson well when it attempted to market its Chevrolet Nova automobile to the Spanish-speaking countries of Central and South America. Whereas "Nova" communicated a stellar image to English-speaking Americans, the rough transla-

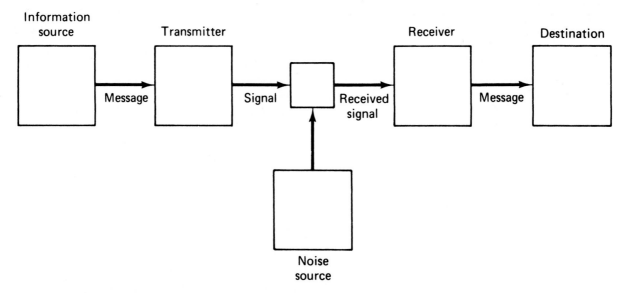

Fig. 11-3 Shannon-Weaver communication model. (From Shannon CE and Weaver W: The mathematical theory of communication, Champaign, Ill, University of Illinois Press, Copyright 1949 by The University of Illinois Press.)

tion of the name (that is, "no va") was taken by those of Spanish origin to mean "does not go." Needless to say, the car did not readily sell under that name!

The Shannon-Weaver model also introduced the concept of "noise" as applied to human communication. Just as noise interferes with the transmission of electronic signals, so, too, can noise disturb the transmission or reception of human communication.

In the context of human communication, noise represents sensory, physical, psychologic, or emotional distractions. A simple example of sensory noise in health communication would be an actual environmental distraction, such as activities occurring in the next bed. Physical noise might include a patient's pain or depressed level of consciousness.

More complex and harder to discern are the psychologic or emotional components of noise. A good example of these types of noise might be the severe anxiety of the patient during an acute attack of asthma or the withdrawal that characterizes some terminally ill patients.

Of course, the psychologic and emotional components of noise are not necessarily limited to the patient. A respiratory care practitioner still angry over an earlier encounter with a physician could bring this "noise" to the bedside of the next patient visited. Likewise, a practitioner with strong negative feelings against homosexuals might allow this element of noise to influence communication with a victim of AIDS.

The SMCR model. Similar in concept to the Shannon-Weaver model is the SMCR model of communication.[6] SMCR is an acronym for four key components of communication highlighted by the model: the source, the message, the channel, and the receiver (Fig. 11-4).

This model extends our understanding of the communication process by identifying a variety of contributing factors associated with each of its four major components. First, the model emphasizes the importance of the communication skills of both sender and receiver. On the basis of this concept, it becomes clear that effective communication is a two-way process and that receiving skills, such as listening, are as important a part of the process as are sending skills, such as speaking.

According to this model, however, communication skill is only one of many human factors affecting the process. Additional human factors involved in a communication interaction include the attitudes, knowledge, and social and cultural backgrounds of both the sender and the receiver. To the extent that these related factors are common to both sender and receiver, the likelihood of effective communication is enhanced. On the other hand, differences in the attitudes, knowledge, or social or cultural backgrounds of the sender and the receiver can contribute to difficulties in communication between the parties in the process.

The fact that differences in attitudes and values can serve as a barrier to effective communication has already been highlighted. With regard to the effect that knowledge differences have on communication, the health professional–patient relationship, by definition, is characterized by a large gap in technical knowledge. Clearly, any attempt to communicate with a patient at the same level of knowledge as might be used in a professional-peer interaction is inappropriate and likely to fail. Finally, anyone who has visited a different country, even one in which English is the primary language, can attest to the importance of social and cultural differences in communication.

The SMCR model also highlights the fact that a commu-

Source	Message	Channel	Receiver
Communication skills	Elements	Seeing	Communication skills
Attitudes	Structure	Hearing	Attitudes
Knowledge	Content	Touching	Knowledge
Social system	Treatment	Smelling	Social system
Culture	Code	Tasting	Culture

Fig. 11-4   SMCR model. (From Berlo DK: The process of communication: an introduction to theory and practice, New York, 1960, Holt, Rinehart & Winston.)

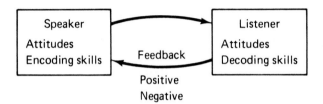

Fig. 11-5   A simple model of the speech communication process. (From Miller GR: An introduction to speech communication, ed 2, Indianapolis, 1972, The Bobbs-Merrill Co.)

nicated message consists of more than just content; specifically, it demonstrates that the elements, structure, treatment, and coding of the message can also affect how it is received and interpreted. Finally, the SMCR model demonstrates that the channel of communication may involve more than just sight and hearing and that other sensory input may accompany or substitute for visual or auditory communication. One need only think how touch, for example, can be used to communicate compassion, empathy, love, anxiety, and fear—all without words.

The speech communication model. More recently, the key role of feedback in the communication process was highlighted in a model proposed by Miller (Fig. 11-5).[7] In this model, the speaker encodes a message, which is influenced by his or her attitudes. The message is then sent and decoded by the listener, who is also influenced by his or her attitudes. The listener (receiver) then sends positive or negative feedback to the sender who, in turn, responds to this new information. This process demonstrates the dynamic nature of communication and the importance of feedback in social transactions.

As an example of the importance of feedback in communication, let us consider the simple situation of a class lecture. If the content or presentation is considered boring to the listeners, the lecturer will normally receive feedback through such physical cues as the inattentiveness or restlessness of the audience. Of course, the good lecturer will recognize these cues and alter the content or style of presentation accordingly. A more pertinent clinical example

might be the anger or hostility expressed by a patient during an interview in which she reveals her prior bad experiences with a respiratory care practitioner. Clearly, this feedback can and should be used to alter the message provided by the sender; specifically, it should be used in an attempt to regain the patient's confidence and trust.

Health communication models

To help explain human communication that occurs in the special context of health care, several authors have developed models specific to this setting. The two models selected for discussion here are the King interaction model and the Northouse health communication model.

The King interaction model. The King model was designed specifically to represent the interactive communication process between a professional nurse and a patient.[8] As shown in Fig. 11-6, a professional-patient transaction involves collaborative assessment and definition of health-related goals. Together, the professional and the patient make judgments and take communicative action (verbal or nonverbal) on the basis of their personal perceptions. These personal perceptions, in turn, lead to reactions and reciprocal interactions. Along with the feedback mechanism, the transactions are a result of this reciprocal relationship.

Clearly, in emphasizing the importance of mutual goal setting as a component of health communication, this model recognizes that communication in the health care setting represents a means to an end, that is, a collaboratively agreed upon set of expectations that satisfies both the professional and the patient. Implicit in this model is the importance of the health professional and the patient sharing their expectations and attempting to resolve differences in a mutually satisfactory way. Underlying this model is the principle of patient autonomy and patient rights, as discussed further in Chapter 12.

The Northouse model. The Northouse health communication model (Fig. 11-7) combines many of the key elements described by others while placing the process within the overall context of health care.[2] This broader view of

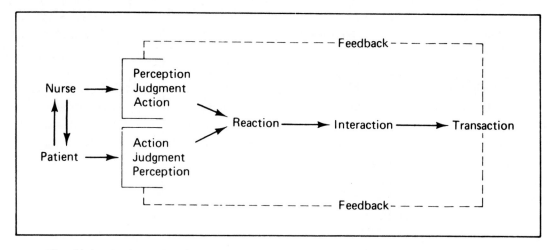

Fig. 11-6   An interaction model. An approach to the nurse-client communication process. (From King IM: Toward a theory of nursing: general concepts of human behavior, New York, 1971, John Wiley & Sons, Inc.)

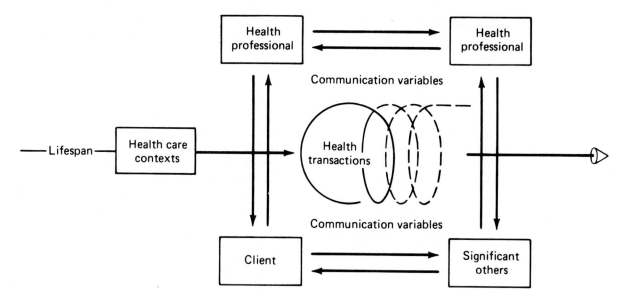

Fig. 11-7   Health communication model. (From Northouse PG and Northouse LL: Health communication: a handbook for health professionals, Englewood Cliffs, NJ, 1985, Prentice-Hall.)

communication incorporates a developmental approach that focuses on the interactions that occur within various kinds of health-directed relationships. Specifically, the model identifies four primary types of health communication interaction: peer (professional-professional) relationships, professional-patient (client) relationships, professional-family relationships, and patient-family relationships.

These primary elements of the model include the context for communication, the participants, and the actual communication transactions. As with the SMCR model, several key variables are identified as influential and contributing factors to the process. Considered together, these elements illustrate that health communication is a transactional, multidimensional process by which persons (health professionals, clients, and significant others) interact with

each other on health-related issues in a mutual effort to maintain or improve the client's health.

Implications of health communication models

In light of the concepts developed in these various communication models, it is clear that several common principles underlie the process of human communication in general and health communication in particular.[1,2,9] First, we must recognize that communication is a dynamic, ongoing, and constantly changing process. This concept forces us to recognize that communication is not a static event but that it constantly changes because of a number of diverse variables that affect the interaction.

Second, we must recognize that human communication is a form of symbolic interaction. In communication, we use symbols to express meaning. These symbols may be verbal (words) or nonverbal (facial expressions or gestures). For effective communication to occur, such symbols must have the same meaning to both sender and receiver. To the extent that the meaning differs between sender and receiver, effective communication is unlikely.

Even when the meaning of our symbols is shared among the participants in a communication interaction, certain sensory, physical, psychological, or emotional distractions may disturb the transmission of a message. Although it is impossible to entirely eliminate this "noise," the skillful communicator will attempt to minimize the influence of these distractions, thereby increasing the likelihood that the message will be received as intended.

Third, we must acknowledge that human communication is transactional in nature. Contrary to the concepts expressed in the early models of communication, it has become increasingly apparent that communication is a two-way process in which participants are mutually influenced by the interaction.

Fourth, we must acknowledge that the context within which human communication occurs affects its outcomes. This implies that the environment, physical surroundings, and settings can and do have an effect on the communication process.

Finally, we must recognize that human communication has multiple purposes. Because there may be various reasons for communicating, the motivations and intentions that underlie our messages may differ according to the purpose of the interaction and its circumstances.

DETERMINANTS OF EFFECTIVE COMMUNICATION

Having explored the general nature of the communication process, we will now focus on the determinants of effective communication. First, we will look at the health professional as speaker; this will be followed by an analysis of the critical and often overlooked role of the health professional as listener. These viewpoints will emphasize the important dimensions of verbal communication, including listening skills. Then we will explore the importance of the nonverbal dimensions of the communication process.

The health professional as speaker

As a health professional, the respiratory care practitioner frequently must communicate verbally to achieve one of several purposes, including one or more of the following:

- *To establish rapport with another individual,* such as a colleague, a patient, or a member of the patient's family;
- *To obtain information,* such as during a patient interview;
- *To relay pertinent information,* as when informing a physician of a patient's progress;

- *To give instructions,* as when teaching a patient how to perform a lung function test; and
- *To persuade others to action,* as when one attempts to convince a patient to quit smoking.

To effectively achieve these goals, the respiratory care practitioner must consider four basic dimensions of verbal communication: (1) the actual presentation of the material, including the vocabulary used, the clarity of the message, and the way the material is organized; (2) the tone and volume of one's voice; (3) one's attitude as speaker or presenter; and (4) one's credibility as speaker or presenter.[1,10]

With regard to presentation of the material, the practitioner must use the appropriate vocabulary. The mastery of appropriate vocabulary means knowing when and how to use professional jargon.[10] In professional-patient or professional-family interactions, it may be necessary to translate technical jargon into terms the lay person can understand.

The clarity of the message will also determine how and how well it is received. The old admonition to "think before you speak" has its merits. The meaning of the message should initially be clear to the practitioner if it is to be communicated with clarity to others. This may also be applicable to the overall organization of the material. Beginning, progressing through, and ending a communication are important skills to master for effective interactions.

The tone and volume of the speaker's voice constitute another determinant of successful verbal communication. Moods, emotions, and other variables can be interpreted from the speaker's voice as the channel of communication. Therefore the health professional needs to be sensitive to the hidden messages that may be sent by tone and volume as well as by the spoken word.[10] The attitude of the speaker can also influence the message of the spoken word. Attitudes can be communicated through the verbal communication of the message as well as through the nonverbal dimension of communication.

Finally, there is the consideration of the credibility of the speaker. To be perceived as credible, health professionals must take care to see that they are competent, of high character, and able to display good will appropriately.[1]

The health professional as listener

By recognizing that human communication is a two-way process, we must also acknowledge that our listening abilities are as important as our verbal skills. A great deal of time in our professional work day is spent listening to others. It is therefore essential that respiratory care practitioners develop and apply effective listening skills.

Types of listening. As with the initiation or presentation of a communication message, there are different types of listening. Smith[11] has developed a hierarchical categorization of various types of listening, ranging from the most complex (listed first) to the least complex (listed last):

- *Analytical*—listening for specific kinds of information and arranging them into categories;

- *Directed*—listening to answer specific questions;
- *Attentive*—listening for general information to understand the total picture;
- *Exploratory*—listening because of one's own interest in the subject that is being discussed;
- *Appreciative*—listening for esthetic pleasure, such as listening to music;
- *Courteous*—listening because one feels obligated to listen;
- *Passive*—listening as in overhearing something, not being attentive to the matter being discussed.

Generally, in their role as health professionals, respiratory care practitioners will be involved in the more complex levels of listening. For example, analytic listening serves as the basis for most patient interviews, as detailed in Chapter 13. Directed listening would be appropriate when the practitioner gives the patient an opportunity to ask questions about a specific procedure or treatment regimen. Attentive listening would be helpful in ascertaining patients' feelings about their hospitalization or their level of anxiety regarding their illness. Effective listening thus requires the respiratory care practitioner to recognize the appropriate type of listening required in a given situation.

Of course these more complex types of listening are generally goal directed, with some specific purpose in mind. There are other times when the respiratory care practitioner should serve simply as a courteous listener. Taking the time to listen to a patient's story of personal experiences or a description of his hometown confirms the patient's self-worth and humanness in what is all too often an unfriendly and cold environment. In fact, courteous listening can often be as important a therapeutic tool as any technical intervention.

The listening process. Listening may also be viewed as a process consisting of several key components. As shown in Fig. 11-8, this process includes four key stages: hearing, attention, understanding, and remembering.[12] As with communication models in general, a message is sent from a source (sender) to the listener (receiver).

Hearing represents the simple physical process of receiving sound waves. Obviously, impaired hearing, which is common in elderly patients, can negatively affect the listening process. A patient's hearing impairment must be recognized and compensated for by the health professional.

Attention is the second stage of the listening process. Attention is an active mental process that involves discrimination among the many audible signals that may be present and the sorting out of those that are important and relevant to the communication process from those that are simple distractions. Given the nature of the hospital environment, with its various machine sounds, public address announcements, and the seemingly constant background talk of others in the surroundings, proper attention can be difficult to achieve for both the patient and the health professional.

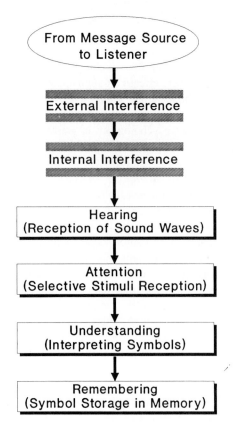

Fig. 11-8   Barker's four-stage listening model. (Redrawn from Barker LL: Communication, ed 2, Englewood Cliffs, NJ, 1981, Prentice-Hall.)

The stage of *understanding* as a component of listening is equivalent to the "decoding" process previously described in our analysis of communication models. Both verbal and nonverbal symbols must be given meaning by the listener. Ideally, what the listener understands should have the same meaning as what the sender intended, but this is not always the case. Of course, since understanding is an internal process, it is impossible to confirm without feedback between sender and listener.

The last stage of listening is *remembering* or "storing" the symbols, however understood, in one's memory. This component of the process is particularly important in the analytic, directed, and attentive types of listening, as information must be remembered to be used.

Clearly, disruption of any one or more of the key elements included in this model can have a negative effect on the final reception of a communicated message. Many of the following guidelines for effective listening focus on one or more of these elements of the listening process and how best to remove or minimize factors that impinge on the proper reception of a message.

Guidelines for effective listening. Since effective listening is a two-way street, the respiratory care practitioner should always have two goals in mind when communicating with others. First, using the methods and suggestions that follow, the practitioner must constantly try to improve his or her own listening skills. Second, the practitioner must learn to ascertain whether and how accurately the party or parties involved have properly received and processed the message sent.[10]

Several simple suggestions may be considered for improving one's own listening skills. First, the practitioner should learn to stop talking—to practice silent listening and to avoid interrupting the speaker during an interaction. Studies have consistently shown that, with the exception of patient interviews, health professionals consistently dominate communication interactions with patients.[13]

Second, the practitioner must learn to concentrate. Concentration involves focusing one's attention on the speaker and the message and avoiding or minimizing distractions and interferences in the environment.

Third, the practitioner must learn to be tolerant—to maintain composure, to control emotions, and to avoid premature judgments. Among the most pervasive problems in listening are allowing emotions such as anger or anxiety to distort our understanding and drawing conclusions before a speaker completes his or her thoughts or arguments. One helpful way to control emotions during difficult communication interactions is to purposefully delay one's response. In this respect, the old practice of counting to ten is truly a helpful approach. Likewise, jumping to conclusions can be avoided by purposefully reserving judgment, extending one's silence, or trying to take the other person's point of view, no matter how offensive or absurd it may initially seem. Limiting one's judgment to content, rather than to style or delivery, may also help avoid these common problems.

In regard to confirming others' reception of communicated messages, the practitioner must learn to listen empathetically.[1] Empathetic listening involves five key components: attending, paraphrasing, requesting clarification, perception checking, and reflecting feelings.

Attending involves the use of gestures and posture that communicate one's attentiveness, as well as being on the lookout for similar nonverbal cues coming from the other party. Attending also involves confirming remarks, such as "I see what you mean."

Paraphrasing, or repeating the other's response in one's own words, is a useful technique to confirm that understanding has taken place between the parties involved in the interaction. Overuse of paraphrasing, however, can become irritating to some persons.

Requesting clarification begins with an admission of misunderstanding on the part of the listener, with the intent being to better understand the message through restatement or the use of alternative examples or illustrations. As with paraphrasing, overuse of this technique can hamper effective communication, especially if used in a condescending or patronizing manner. Requests for clarification should thus be used only when truly necessary and should always be nonjudgmental in nature.

Perception checking involves confirming or refuting the more subtle components of a communication interaction, such as messages that are implied but not stated. For example, the practitioner might "sense" that a patient is unsure of the need for a treatment. In this case, the practitioner might check this perception by saying: "You don't seem to be sure that you need this treatment. Is that correct?" Of course, by verifying or refuting this perception, both the professional and the patient will come to better understand each other.

Finally, *reflecting feelings* involves the use of statements as "verbal mirrors" to better ascertain the emotions of the other party. Nonjudgmental statements, such as "You seem to be anxious about (this situation)," provide the opportunity for the other person to express and reflect on his or her emotions and can help confirm or deny their true feelings.

In summary, by combining silence, concentration, and tolerance with empathetic feedback, the respiratory care practitioner can expect to enhance his or her listening skills, thereby increasing the likelihood of effective communication with both peers and patients.

Nonverbal communication in health care

To understand the full complexity of health interactions among professionals, patients, and family members, one needs to be aware of the contributions made by the nonverbal dimension of the communication process.[2] In fact, one should not be surprised to learn that nonverbal communication has consistently been found to be a more powerful means of transmitting messages than verbal communication.[14]

Nonverbal communication includes such elements as body movement, facial expression, eye behavior, voice tone, space, touch, and physical characteristics. These elements may be used either to substitute for verbal communication or to enhance, reinforce, or contradict verbally communicated messages.[10] Pantomime and demonstration are good examples of how nonverbal communication can substitute for verbal communication. On the other hand, when we use nonverbal communication to enhance, reinforce, or contradict verbal messages, we are participating in *metacommunication*.

Pantomime and demonstration substitute for the spoken word through an enactment of the message. Demonstration is useful in patient instruction when a particular activity is to be repeated by the patient. Pantomime is especially useful for interactions with a person who has a perceptual or hearing impairment. If the health professional is proficient only with the English language, pantomime may also be useful with non-English-speaking persons.

Metacommunication does not completely substitute for verbal communication. Rather, metacommunication involves actions and behaviors that accompany our words and consequently modify their meaning. Facial expressions, eye behavior, body positions, posture, hand gestures, physical appearance, and touch can all modify the meaning of our words.[10] For example, it has been said that "the eyes are the mirrors of the soul." So, too, may be the overall facial expressions of the individual. A smile, a frown, a gaze, or a stare can modify an intended message. Sitting or standing, leaning forward, or keeping one's distance also affects the communication process. One's physical appearance, body movements, and gestures can influence the process and outcomes of an interaction. In addition, touch can take a variety of forms and convey a diversity of meanings.

Generally, the verbal and nonverbal components of a communication should enhance and reinforce each other. For example, the practitioner who combines a verbal message in a compassionate tone ("You're going to be all right now") with the confirming touch of the hand is sending a much stronger message to the anxious patient than that provided by either component alone. On the other hand, consider the same verbal message delivered by a practitioner in a brusque manner while purposely avoiding eye contact with the patient. Which message would the patient be inclined to believe?

Obviously, contradictory verbal and nonverbal information can frequently lead to misunderstandings and misinterpretations. For this reason alone, the respiratory care practitioner must be sensitive to the nonverbal dimension of communication and be attentive to the nonverbal cues and behaviors that accompany verbal interactions with patients and colleagues.

COMMUNICATION IN HEALTH CARE RELATIONSHIPS

We have previously identified four major types of interaction that exist in the health care setting: the professional-patient relationship, the professional-professional relationship, the professional-family relationship, and the patient-family relationships.[2] These relationships and selected factors that represent potential barriers to effective communication are illustrated in Fig. 11-9.

Professional-patient relationships

The nature of each professional-patient relationship is influenced by the personal and professional characteristics that both patient and professional bring to the relationship.[2,10] Characteristics such as needs, perceptions, attitudes, motivations, and values represent variables in communication that play a crucial role in health-related interactions. For the health professional, intrapersonal communication is essential to knowing one's self. Personal recognition and reflection thus constitute the first step toward effective interaction with others.

In the professional-patient relationship, understanding the patient's role and the nature of that role must be considered. The fact that a patient is in need of respiratory care, for example, typifies feelings of loss that may be associated with the patient's self-image, independence, and privacy.[10] Patients also must deal with hospitalization, the financial strain of health care costs, or the often frightening technologic aspects of diagnostic and therapeutic procedures.

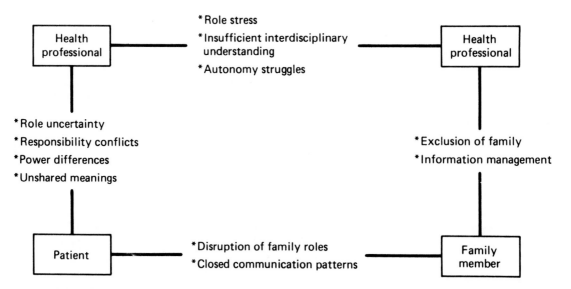

Fig. 11-9 Potential barriers to effective communication among participants in health care settings. (Redrawn from Northouse PG and Northouse LL: Health communication: a handbook for health professionals, Englewood Cliffs, NJ, 1985, Prentice-Hall.)

Professional-professional relationships

With today's complex and dynamic system of health care, the delivery of quality health care services often depends on cooperation and collaboration among many types of health professionals. It is important, therefore, that respiratory care practitioners understand the various roles and responsibilities of all members of the health care team with whom they interact. Insufficient interdisciplinary understanding can cause professionals to make too little use of one another's unique areas of expertise or to become embroiled in "turf" negotiations.[2] With the provision of quality patient care the primary aim of all health professions, health professionals must be able to relate the roles and functions of health team members in various health care settings to individual and societal health-related needs.

Professional-family relationships

Blind focus solely on the patient can cause one to underestimate the importance of family members in improving and maintaining the patient's health status. Although first demonstrated in the area of neonatal care,[15] the importance of family involvement in the provision of health care cannot be overstated.

For family members to maintain their supportive role in health care, they need to have effective communication with health professionals.[2] Therefore, attention should be given to this supportive role and the appropriateness of family member inclusion in the health communication process.

Patient-family relationships

Equally important is the recognition of relationships between the patient and his or her family members. Each affects and influences the other. This recognition may help the respiratory care practitioner attain a better understanding of the patient. In addition, communication with family members in a way that facilitates their supportive communication with one another may enhance the patient-family relationship and also relationships with other members of the health care team.[2]

SUMMARY

Human communication represents a dynamic process whereby information, meanings, and rules are shared between individuals. Health communication is a subset of human communication concerned with promotion of health or prevention of illness within our society and with making the health care system run to the satisfaction of both patients and practitioners.

Despite the fact that the effectiveness with which health professionals fulfill their helping roles is determined largely by their skills in communication, its importance in both patient and professional interaction is generally underestimated. Communication influences the evaluation and treatment of patients, including their compliance with treatment regimens, their satisfaction with services, and even their emotional well-being. Communication also affects the morale and performance of health professionals.

Several common principles underlie the process of communication. Communication is a dynamic process of symbolic interaction influenced by a host of sensory, physical, psychologic, emotional, and environmental factors. Further, communication represents a two-way interaction in which participants are mutually influenced by the exchange. Finally, communication can and does serve multiple purposes.

Whether it be in professional-patient, professional-professional, professional-family, or patient-family relationships, the respiratory care practitioner must constantly assume the dual roles of both effective speaker and attentive listener. In doing so, one will quickly discover that these skills provide the foundation for both the provision of quality respiratory care services and the mutual satisfaction to be derived from these helping relationships.

REFERENCES

1. Klinzing D and Klinzing D: Communication for allied health professionals, Dubuque, Iowa, 1985, William C Brown.
2. Northouse PG and Northouse LL: Health communication, Englewood Cliffs, NJ, 1985, Prentice-Hall, Inc.
3. Pettegrew LS et al, editors: Explorations in provider and patient interaction, Louisville, Ky, 1982, Humana, Inc.
4. DiMatteo MP: A social-psychological analysis of physician-patient rapport: toward a science of the art of medicine, J Soc Issues 35:17-31, 1979.
5. Shannon C and Weaver W: The mathematical theory of communication, Champaign, Ill, 1949, University of Illinois Press.
6. Berlo DK: The process of communication: an introduction to theory and practice, New York, 1960, Holt, Reinhart & Winston.
7. Miller GR: An introduction to speech communication, ed 2, Indianapolis, 1972, Bobbs-Merrill Co, Inc.
8. King IM: Toward a theory of nursing: general concepts of human behavior, New York, 1971, John Wiley & Sons, Inc.
9. Ruffner M and Burgoon M: Interpersonal communication, New York, 1981, Holt, Reinhart & Winston.
10. Purtilo R: Health professional/patient interaction, ed 3, Philadelphia, 1984, WB Saunders Co.
11. Smith E: Improving listening effectiveness, Tex Med 71:98-100, 1975.
12. Barker LL: Communication, ed 2, Englewood Cliffs, NJ, 1981, Prentice-Hall, Inc.
13. Bain DJL: Doctor-patient communication in general practice, Med Ed 10:125-131, 1976.
14. Argyle M, Alkema F, and Gilmour R: The communication of friendly and hostile attitudes by verbal and non-verbal signals, Eur J Soc Psych 1:385-402, 1971.
15. Sameroff AJ: Psychologic needs of the parent in infant development. In Avery GB, editor: Neonatology: pathophysiology and management of the newborn, ed 3, Philadelphia, 1987, JB Lippincott Co.

12

Ethical and Legal Implications of the Practice

Raymond S. Edge

Conventional knowledge and technical standards of good practice are generally adequate to ensure that respiratory care practitioners fulfill their roles competently and that the needs and expectations of the patients they serve are met. However, there can arise special circumstances in which prevailing technical standards provide an insufficient basis for our choices and actions. Often these special circumstances involve ethical issues or the law.

Ethics and law provide social sanctions and functions that help society maintain order and continuity. Professional ethics guide respiratory care practitioners, in their dealings with others, toward actions that are designed to bring about a particular result. In respiratory care, the ideal result would be restoration of health to the patient. Law, unlike ethics, sets not an ideal but, rather, a minimum standard for social behavior. The force behind law is some enforceable punishment, while for ethics it is expulsion from the society of respiratory care practitioners.

OBJECTIVES

Clinical practice is an arena in which knowledge of both legal and ethical principles is needed. It is the intent of this chapter to develop the knowledge base necessary to apply these perspectives to practice. Specifically, after completion of this chapter, the reader should be able to:

1. Define the basic goal of the respiratory care professional code of ethics;

2. Relate the respiratory care code of ethics to the six basic principles of biomedical ethics;

3. Describe the two basic biomedical ethics viewpoints and show how they relate to the dichotomy so often found in ethical decision making;

4. Delineate the basic information that needs to be gathered before a reasoned ethical decision is made;

5. Define the differences between civil and criminal law and relate them to current practice;

6. Describe the nature and elements of a malpractice suit and relate the various torts to current practice;

7. Relate the current practice of respiratory care to professional liability;

8. Describe the nature of unlawful and unethical practice as it relates to the diversification of the respiratory care into home care and durable medical equipment supplies;

9. Relate the process of licensure to increased legal responsibility and liability;

10. Explain how the emerging physician-patient relationship, centered on patient autonomy and responsibility, is shaping the ethical and legal aspects of practice.

KEY TERMS

Most terms used in this chapter are defined in context. However, because of its unique content, a separate glossary of legal terms appears at the end of the chapter.

ETHICAL DILEMMAS OF PRACTICE

The growth of respiratory care as a profession has been closely associated with a rather remarkable series of advances in medical technology and treatment protocols, coupled with rising expectations of an ever-growing and sophisticated patient population. These changes in the health care environment not only have helped create this new specialty but also have changed the landscape of medicine, creating a new world of previously unfaced ethical and legal dilemmas. In this new world of practice, much of the geography still lies uncharted and is yet to be mapped by ethicists and lawyers.

The approaches used to address ethical issues in health care practice range from the specific to the general. Specific guidance in resolving ethical dilemmas is usually provided by a professional *code of ethics*. A more general approach is to apply the concepts and principles of *ethical theory* to decisions involving moral issues. We will explore each of these approaches in terms of its usefulness in making sound ethical choices.

Codes of ethics

The code of ethics for the profession of respiratory care (see box opposite) represents a set of general principles and rules developed to bring about a desired or ideal result: the restoration of patient health. Codes for different specialties or professions might well differ from that governing respiratory care, as they may seek a different goal.

Ethical codes, then, depend on a specialized group's decision concerning what is needed to achieve an ideal good, rather than on general morality or personal value systems. Personal ethics or morals grow out of the individual's particular world view and are shaped by the experiences of one's cultural past. Personal ethics or morals are the social screen by which individuals decide what ought to be, based on social convention and community expectations. These systems of evaluation provide individuals with general rules of conduct that determine which actions, such as lying and stealing, are inherently wrong.[1]

In a complex world, values help set priorities and give life meaning and structure. While it would be desirable and less stressful if the respiratory care practitioner's professional code always matched his or her personal value system, this is unlikely. Unfortunately, in clinical practice there are many instances in which personal values may conflict with what is found to be medically and legally acceptable or ethical. In a pluralistic society, it would be a remarkable code of ethics that managed to fit each respiratory care practitioner's personal value system all the time.

Another limitation of professional codes of ethics, such as that applicable to respiratory care, is their narrow focus. Unfortunately, codes of ethics often represent overly simplistic or proscriptive ideas of how to deal with patent misbehavior or flagrant abuses of authority over which few would disagree.

The really difficult moral decisions stem from situations in which two or more right choices are incompatible, in which the choices represent different priorities, or in which there are limited resources to achieve the desired priorities. As the American Hospital Association notes, reduction of these issues to simple formulations is no easy task. The number and complexity of ethical dilemmas have grown dramatically because of the increasing sophistication of medical science and technology, concerns about practical limits on financial resources for health care, changes in society, and growing emphasis on the autonomy of the individual.[2]

AARC CODE OF ETHICS

The principles set forth in this document define the basic ethical and moral standards to which each member of the American Association for Respiratory Care should conform.

1. The respiratory care practitioner shall practice medically acceptable methods of treatment and shall not endeavor to extend his practice beyond his competence and the authority vested in him by the physician.
2. The respiratory care practitioner shall continually strive to increase and improve his knowledge and skill and render to each patient the full measure of his ability. All services shall be provided with respect for the dignity of the patient, unrestricted by considerations of social or economic status, personal attributes, or the nature of health problems.
3. The respiratory care practitioner shall be responsible for the competent and efficient performance of his assigned duties and shall expose incompetence and illegal or unethical conduct of members of the profession.
4. The respiratory care practitioner shall hold in strict confidence all privileged information concerning the patient and refer all inquiries to the physician in charge of the patient's medical care.
5. The respiratory care practitioner shall not accept gratuities for preferential consideration of the patient. He shall not solicit patients for personal gain and shall guard against conflicts of interest.
6. The respiratory care practitioner shall uphold the dignity and honor of the profession and abide by its ethical principles. He should be familiar with existing state and federal laws governing the practice of respiratory therapy and comply with those laws.
7. The respiratory care practitioner shall cooperate with other health care professionals and participate in activities to promote community and national efforts to meet the health needs of the public.

Resolution of these more complex problems requires a more general approach than that provided by a code of ethics. This more general perspective is provided by the broad principles of ethical theory.

Principles of ethical theory

Health specialties, such as respiratory care, have as the basis of their codes of ethics a common core of broad ethical principles. Any consideration of ethical principles eventually must address the meaning of such terms as right, good, and obligatory. Obviously, in the absence of some benchmark of what constitutes morally justifiable behavior, it is possible to argue in favor of almost any position.

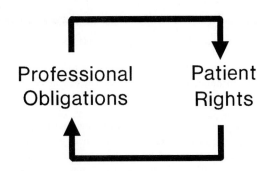

Fig. 12-1   Reciprocal relationship between professional obligations and patient rights.

Contemporary ethical principles underlying modern bioethics have evolved from many sources, including the conceptions of natural law espoused by Aristotle and Aquinas, Judeo-Christian formulations of morality, Kant's analysis of universal duties, and the values orientations that characterize modern political systems, especially those embodied in our democratic form of government. Although some controversy exists, most ethicists agree that autonomy, veracity, nonmaleficence, beneficence, confidentiality, and justice represent the primary guiding principles in moral decision making.

As applied to professional practice, each of these ethical principles consists of two components: a professional duty and a patient right (Fig. 12-1). For example, the principle of autonomy obliges health professionals to uphold others' freedom of will and freedom of action. The principle of beneficence obliges us to further the interests of others, either by promoting their good or by actively preventing their harm. The principle of justice obliges us to ensure that others receive what they rightfully deserve or legitimately claim.

Embodied in each duty is a reciprocal patient right, such as the right to autonomous choice, the right not to be harmed, and the right to fair and equitable treatment. From these general principles of rights and obligations, one can generate more specific rules, such as those included in a code of ethics.

Autonomy.   The principle of autonomy acknowledges patients' personal liberty and their right to decide on their own course and to follow through a plan freely agreed on by themselves.

It is from this principle that rules concerning informed consent are derived, for to decide freely a person must have adequate information to comprehend the available options. A corollary to rules of informed consent, derived from experiences with the holocaust of World War II, is that individuals must not only be given the information but also be "situated as to exercise free power of choice, without the intervention of any element of force, fraud, deceit, duress, over-reaching or other ulterior form of constraint or coercion" (The Nuremberg Code, Rule 1).

Autonomy, then, has two basic requirements: (1) *freedom to decide,* which depends on information and comprehension, and (2) *freedom to act without coercion,* which depends on respect for personal autonomy granted by health professionals and the families involved.

Thus, under the principle of autonomy, the respiratory care practitioner's use of deceit or coercion to get a patient to reverse his or her decision to refuse a treatment would be considered unethical, as would threatening a patient who did not wish to sign a consent form.

Unfortunately, the principle of autonomy is one that is often recognized and appreciated more in the abstract than in practice. There is a tendency among health workers to assume that, by virtue of their training or experience, they know what is best for the patient. This view, called *paternalism,* has long been a mainstay of health care practice, as evident in the following excerpts from the 1848 Medical Code of Ethics[3]:

Obligations of patients to their physicians

The obedience of a patient to the prescriptions of his physician should be prompt and implicit. He should never permit his own crude opinion as to their fitness to influence his attention to them.

Duties of physicians to their patients

A physician should not be forward to make gloomy prognostications, because they savor of empiricism, by magnifying the importance of his services in the treatment or cure of disease. But he should not fail, on proper occasions, to give to the friends of the patients timely notice of danger when it really occurs; and even to the patient himself if absolutely necessary.

In the past, medical care was based mainly on good bedside manner and often on poor science. Patients were made well as much by faith in the caring and authority of the caregiver as by the notions and nostrums prescribed. Today medicine has given up much of its home-based art for the benefits of modern science. The rising expectations of the population, as well as the heavy involvement of government and third-party payers, has created a new consumerism. Inherent in this new consumerism is the expectation that the lay person is to be given greater responsibility and authority in decision making with respect to personal health care.

Robert Veatch of the Kennedy Institute of Ethics believes that the old ethic of patient benefit is now outmoded and should be replaced by an ethic of patient responsibility.[4,5] Many authorities think that the growing conflict between patient autonomy and the paternalism of health care providers is the central crisis in medical relationships today.[6]

To aid patients and health care professionals with regard to the expectation of greater patient autonomy and shared decision making, the American Hospital Association has published *The Patients' Bill of Rights* (see box on p. 267). This document, although lacking the force of law, pro-

AMERICAN HOSPITAL ASSOCIATION PATIENT'S BILL OF RIGHTS

1. The patient has the right to considerate and respectful care.
2. The patient has the right to obtain from his physician complete current information concerning his diagnosis, treatment, and prognosis in terms the patient can be reasonably expected to understand. When it is not medically advisable to give such information to the patient, the information should be made available to an appropriate person in his behalf. He has the right to know, by name, the physician responsible for coordinating his care.
3. The patient has the right to receive from his physician information necessary to give informed consent prior to the start of any procedure and/or treatment. Except in emergencies, such information for informed consent should include but not necessarily be limited to the specific procedure and/or treatment, the medically significant risks involved, and the probable duration of incapacitation. Where medically significant alternatives for care or treatment exist, or when the patient requests information concerning medical alternatives, the patient has the right to such information. The patient also has the right to know the name of the person responsible for the procedures and/or treatment.
4. The patient has the right to refuse treatment to the extent permitted by law and to be informed of the medical consequences of his action.
5. The patient has the right to every consideration of his privacy concerning his own medical care program. Case discussion, consultation, examination, and treatment are confidential and should be conducted discreetly. Those not directly involved in his care must have the permission of the patient to be present.
6. The patient has the right to expect that all communications and records pertaining to his care should be treated as confidential.

7. The patient has the right to expect that within its capacity a hospital must make reasonable response to the request of a patient for services. The hospital must provide evaluation, service, and/or referral as indicated by the urgency of the case. When medically permissible, a patient may be transferred to another facility only after he has received complete information and explanation concerning the needs for and alternatives to such a transfer. The institution to which the patient is to be transferred must first have accepted the patient for transfer.
8. The patient has the right to obtain information as to any relationship of his hospital to other health care and educational institutions insofar as his care is concerned. The patient has the right to obtain information as to the existence of any professional relationships among individuals, by name, who are treating him.
9. The patient has the right to be advised if the hospital proposes to engage in or perform human experimentation affecting his care or treatment. The patient has the right to refuse to participate in such research projects.
10. The patient has the right to expect reasonable continuity of care. He has the right to know in advance what appointment times and physicians are available and where. The patient has the right to expect that the hospital will provide a mechanism whereby he is informed by his physician or a delegate of the physician of the patient's continuing health care requirements following discharge.
11. The patient has the right to examine and receive an explanation of his bill regardless of source of payment.
12. The patient has the right to know what hospital rules and regulations apply to his conduct as a patient.

Reprinted with permission of the American Hospital Association, Copyright 1972.

vides excellent insight into the emerging patient-provider relationship. A careful reading of this document provides the respiratory care practitioner with a helpful guide in addressing issues in this vital and changing arena.

Many states have adopted specific legislation giving the patient "the fundamental right to control the decisions relating to their own medical care, including the decision to have life-sustaining procedures withheld or withdrawn in circumstances where such persons are diagnosed as having a terminally and irreversible condition."[7]

Veracity. The principle of veracity is often linked to autonomy, especially in the area of informed consent. In general, veracity binds both the health giver and the patient to tell the truth. The nature of the health process is such that both parties involved are best served in an envi-

ronment of trust and mutual sharing of all necessary information.

The problems associated with the principle revolve around such issues as "benevolent deception" for the patient's own good, where the decision is made to withhold the truth so that the patient can be prepared, or in cases in which patients state that they do not want the truth if it is bad news.

When the physician decides to withhold the truth from a conscious, alert, well-oriented adult, the decision affects the interactions between all the health care providers and the patient and has a chilling effect on the rapport necessary for good care. In a recent poll by the Louis Harris group, 94% of the Americans surveyed indicated that they wanted to know everything about their cases, even the dismal facts.[8] Outside of pediatrics, and in rare cases where there is evidence that the truth would lead to a disaster such as suicide, giving the patient the truth, in as palatable a manner as possible, is probably the best policy.[1,9,10]

Nonmaleficence. In the Hippocratic oath taken as they enter practice, physicians swear to "never use treatment to injure or wrong the sick." This generally accepted principle of nonmaleficence obligates the health care practitioner to never harm the patient and, further, to actively prevent harm where possible.

In a simpler time this was an easier principle to uphold in practice, but now many of the procedures performed and pharmaceuticals used have undesirable secondary effects. For example, we might ask whether it is ethical to give high doses of steroids to asthmatic patients, knowing the many harmful consequences of these drugs.

Some ethicists suggest that the solution to these dilemmas of the double effect lie in the first intent.[10,11] In these cases the harmful effect is viewed as an indirect or unintended result. Four conditions are required for an action that helps but may harm the patient to be considered ethical: (1) the action itself must be good, (2) the individual must intend only the good effect, (3) the adverse effects cannot be a means to a good end, and (4) there must be a proportionately grave reason for permitting the adverse effect, that is, there must be a favorable balance between the good and adverse effects.[1]

Beneficence. In its simplest meaning, the principle of beneficence requires that the health practitioner go beyond doing no harm and actively contribute to the health and well-being of the patients served. Within this dictum lie many quality-of-life issues, for medicine today possesses the technology to keep some persons alive well beyond any rational good to themselves. This presents real dilemmas for those who are confronted with the ability to prolong life but not the ability to restore any human qualities. In these cases some interpret the principle of beneficence to mean that they must do everything possible to promote life, regardless of how useful that life might be to the patient. Other health care professionals in the same situation might see the principle as being better served by doing nothing and allowing death to occur without heroic measures.

In most of these cases, patients are not in a position to decide for themselves and the matter is left to the family, the health care team, ethics committees, or, at times, the legal system. Decision makers are aided in the selection of an authentic choice if the patient has made his or her wishes known or has filed a "living will" or durable power of attorney (see box above). In the past, living wills have been ignored by health practitioners, and their legal weight has been challenged in court. In recent years, however, state legislatures have begun to support these documents. Beginning with the 1976 California law, more than 30 other states have now adopted similar legislation.[8,12]

EXAMPLE OF A LIVING WILL

To My Family, My Physician, My Lawyer
And All Others Whom It May Concern

Death is as much a reality as birth, growth, maturity, and old age—it is the one certainty of life. If the time comes when I can no longer take part in decisions for my own future, let this statement stand as my expression of my wishes and directions, while I am still of sound mind.

If at such a time the situation should arise in which there is no reasonable expectation of my recovery from extreme physical or mental disability, I direct that I be allowed to die and not be kept alive by medications, artificial means, or "heroic measures." I do, however, ask that medication be mercifully administered to me to alleviate suffering even though this may shorten my remaining life.

This statement is made after careful consideration of and is in accordance with my strong convictions and beliefs. I want the wishes and directions here expressed carried out to the extent permitted by law. Insofar as they are not legally enforceable, I hope that those to whom this Will is addressed will regard themselves as morally bound by these provisions.

The professions have also been active in addressing the complex issues involved in life support technologies. For example, the AMA Council on Ethical and Judicial Affairs has recently provided physicians with a set of broad guidelines related to the withholding or withdrawing of life-prolonging medical treatments (see box on p. 269).

Confidentiality. The principle of confidentiality is founded in the Hippocratic oath and was reiterated by the World Health Association in 1948. It obliges the health practitioner to "respect the secrets which are confided . . . even after the patient has died." Like many of the other fundamental principles of biomedical ethics, the principle is often balanced against other principles, such as beneficence.

A classic confidentiality case that occurred in California involved a young man who had voluntarily visited an outpatient psychiatric unit for evaluation. During his time with the psychologist, he related that he was planning to kill a particular young woman. The psychologist had security officers hold the fellow, but during this period he appeared normal and demanded to be released. Given the voluntary nature of the visit and the fact that the man appeared normal, he was released.

The decision of the health professional not to restrain the patient or to warn the young woman was based on the principle of patient confidentiality. The tragedy of this case is that the patient did kill the young woman as indicated.

When the parents of the murdered woman learned that the psychologist and security officers were aware of the

AMERICAN MEDICAL ASSOCIATION

STATEMENT ON WITHHOLDING OR WITHDRAWING LIFE-PROLONGING MEDICAL TREATMENT

The social commitment of the physician is to sustain life and relieve suffering. Where the performance of one duty conflicts with the other, the preferences of the patient should prevail. If the patient is incompetent to act in his own behalf and did not previously indicate his preferences, the family or other surrogate decisionmaker, in concert with the physician, must act in the best interest of the patient.

For humane reasons, with informed consent, a physician may do what is medically necessary to alleviate severe pain, or cease or omit treatment to permit a terminally ill patient to die when death is imminent. However, the physician should not intentionally cause death. In deciding whether the administration of potentially life-prolonging medical treatment is in the best interest of the patient who is incompetent to act in his own behalf, the surrogate decisionmaker and physician should consider several factors, including: the possibility for extending life under humane and comfortable conditions; the patient's values about life and the way it should be lived; and the patient's attitudes toward sickness, suffering, medical procedures, and death.

Even if death is not imminent but a patient is beyond doubt permanently unconscious, and there are adequate safeguards to confirm the accuracy of the diagnosis, it is not unethical to discontinue all means of life-prolonging medical treatment.

Life-prolonging medical treatment includes medication and artificially or technologically supplied respiration, nutrition or hydration. In treating a terminally ill or permanently unconscious patient, the dignity of the patient should be maintained at all times. (I,III,IV,V)

Section 2.20 of *Current Opinions of the Council on Ethical and Judicial Affairs of the American Medical Association*, 1989. Reprinted with permission.

threat to their daughter's life and had made no effort to warn her of the potential for harm, they sued. The court ruled for the parents, stating that the obligation of confidentiality toward the patient was of a lesser nature than the obligation to the innocent party.[10] The main ethical controversy around confidentiality concerns the assessment of whether more harm is done by occasionally breaching confidentiality or by always respecting it, regardless of the consequences.

Confidentiality in health care provider–patient relationships is not considered an absolute obligation in most professional codes of ethics. The American Medical Association Code of Ethics, Section 9, provides the following guidelines: "A physician may not reveal the confidences entrusted to him in the course of medical attendance or the deficiencies he may observe in the character of patients, unless he is required to do so by law or unless it becomes necessary in order to protect the welfare of the individual or of the community."

Unfortunately, confidentiality often is breached not as a rational decision, such as when a choice is made between competing principles or when the legal process demands that information be revealed. Rather, confidentiality is breached more often by a careless "slip of the tongue." Such social trading in gossip regarding patients is unprofessional, unethical, and (in certain cases) illegal.

Confidential information, once highly protected, is now easy to obtain through unauthorized access to computerized data. Clinical data are available for close scrutiny by the clerical staff, laboratory personnel, and other health care providers. The widespread use of these data systems represents a real threat to patient confidentiality.

Potential violations of the patient's right to privacy in patient populations such as those with acquired immune deficiency syndrome (AIDS) pose a special threat, as disclosure may result in economic, psychologic, or bodily harm to the patient. The respiratory care practitioners would do well to adhere to the dictum found in the Hippocratic oath: "What I may see or hear in the course of the treatment or even outside of treatment of the patient in regard to the life of men, which on no account one must spread abroad, I will keep to myself, holding such things to be shameful to be spoken about."

Justice. The principle of justice requires that like cases should be treated alike and that those that are different should be treated differently. Under this principle, we find such issues as the fair distribution of care.

In an environment of rising expectation regarding health care, issues of justice are coming to the forefront as policy makers wrestle with questions of how much care can be provided and on what basis. Current population trends indicate that in the year 2000 the number of persons over 75 years of age will have increased by 30% from the 1980s.[13] The nation is rapidly approaching a period in history when those contributing to the financial resources of our health care system will be smaller in number than those who rely on its resources. Such nations as Great Britain have long found it necessary to set up criteria for rationing certain kinds of care. Under England's health care system, for example, the government will not pay for kidney dialysis for patients over the age of 55 years.[8]

As health care reimbursement policies in the US change, our society is beginning to question the level of care that citizens can claim or legitimately expect. Distributive justice deals with the proper apportionment of benefits and burdens in a society, as represented by taxes and subsidies. Questions of justice seem rather straightforward and possible when seen as abstract policies, guidelines, or legislation designed to allocate scarce resources. It is more difficult to address questions related to care of individual

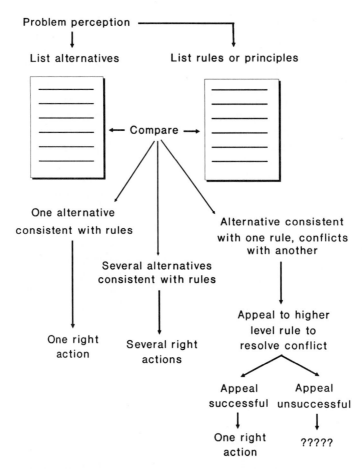

Fig. 12-2 The formalist approach to ethical decision making. (Redrawn from Brody H: Ethical decisions in medicine, ed 2, Boston, 1981, Little, Brown & Co.)

patients, such as "Can we deny needed care to individuals on the basis of their inability to pay?"

A second form of justice seen in the practice of medicine is retributive justice, which calls for recovery of damages incurred as a result of the action of others. Damage awards in civil cases of medical malpractice or negligence are examples of retributive justice. Industries that have been found to pollute or produce harmful agents, such as asbestos, have been sued for damages as a form of retribution. Pulmonary function technologists have long been part of the process that determines the amount of loss suffered and the degree of impairment caused by industrial agents that cause lung damage.

Ethical viewpoints and decision making

In decisions pertaining to ethical issues, a dichotomy is often found. One group of practitioners may attempt to adhere to a strict interpretation of ethical principles such as those just described, whereas others seek to decide the issue solely on a case-by-case basis, considering only the potential good (or bad) results of the decision.

These different approaches represent the two dominant ethical viewpoints that have come to shape modern ethical

reasoning.[14-17] The former approach, which attempts to consistently apply a set of rules and principles, is called *formalist* reasoning. The latter approach, in which the consequences of the act serve as the basis for decision making, is called *consequentialist* reasoning.

Formalism. Formalist thought asserts that certain features of an act itself determine its moral justifiability. Within this framework, standards of right and wrong are formulated in terms of ethical principles or rules that function apart from the consequences of a particular action. An act is considered morally justifiable if—and only if—it upholds the rules or principles that apply.

The major objection to formalist reasoning lies in its potential for inconsistency. Critics of formalist reasoning insist that no principle or rule can be framed that does not admit exceptions. Moreover, claim these critics, no principles or rules can be framed that do not admit conflicts.

The previous scenario regarding confidentiality of psychiatric information is a good example of the problems inherent in the formalist perspective. Basically, this case involved a conflict between the principle of confidentiality and the principle of justice, that is, the right of society to be protected from persons with harmful intent. The court

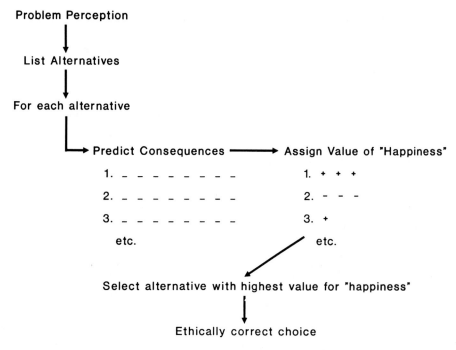

Fig. 12-3   The consequentialist approach to ethical decision making. (Redrawn from Brody H: Ethical decisions in medicine, ed 2, Boston, 1981, Little, Brown & Co.)

decision highlighted the fact that principles must admit exceptions, particularly that the principle of confidentiality does not always apply.

Conflicts among competing principles can be resolved only when they are given a "weight" or relative priority. In this way, various alternatives are compared with a set of prioritized rules. As shown in Fig. 12-2, if one or more alternatives are consistent with all applicable rules or principles, the decision is easy.[18] On the other hand, if there is a conflict among rules, the decision maker must appeal to the higher-level rule to resolve the conflict. As indicated in the figure, this approach may not always be successful (indicated by the ?????? following "appeal is unsuccessful").

Consequentialism. From the consequentialist perspective, the basic criteria by which we judge rightness or wrongness of an act is the relative amount of good (over evil) that a particular action brings about. The most common application of consequentialism judges acts according to the principle of utility. In its simplest form, the principle of utility aims to promote the greatest general good for the greatest number.

As shown in Fig. 12-3, the consequentialist approach requires the practitioner to identify all alternative actions and, for each, assign a value of "happiness" or the relative amount of good over evil brought into being.[18] According to this framework, the ethically correct choice is simply that which would result in the greatest general good or happiness among those involved in the situation.

Critics of this approach claim that it suffers from two fundamental flaws: first, the "calculus" involved in pro-

jecting and weighing the amount of good over evil that might result from alternative actions is not always possible; second, reliance on the principle of utility to the exclusion of all else can result in actions that are incompatible with ordinary judgments regarding the rights and obligations inherent in human interactions.

A classic example of the inconsistency of consequentialist reasoning with ordinary judgments can be seen in the true World War II case of the battle for North Africa. In this scenario, there were two groups of soldiers, but only enough antibiotics for one. One group required the medication to treat syphilis contracted in the local brothels; the other group needed antibiotics to manage wounds acquired in battle. Thus the dilemma arose as to who should receive the antibiotics.

From the formalist perspective, the decision as to who should receive the antibiotics would be based on some concept of justice, such as giving priority to the sickest or to those most in need. However, the actual decision made in this case was a consequentialist one, based not on the desire to justly distribute the drug but, rather, on the need to obtain a quick victory, with as few casualties as possible. Thus, in this scenario, the scarce medication was given to those who were "wounded" in the brothels rather than in battle, as they could be restored quickly and returned to the front lines to aid the war effort.[9]

Mixed approaches. Mixed approaches to moral reasoning attempt to capitalize on the strengths inherent in these two major lines of ethical thought. One approach, called rule utilitarianism, represents a variation of consequentialist reasoning. Under this framework, the question is not which act or practice has the greatest utility but which rule or principle would promote the greatest good if it were generally accepted.

For example, the rule utilitarian would consider truth telling a necessary ethical principle, not so much because of its intrinsic moral "rightness" but because its application would promote the greatest good in professional-patient relationships. Specifically, if this rule were not followed consistently, it would be impossible for the patient and the health professional to establish a trusting relationship.

The rule utilitarian approach is probably the most appealing and useful to health professionals. Its appeal is derived in part from its ability to address both the human rights and obligations and the consequences inherent in our actions. Moreover, rule utilitarianism seems best able to accommodate the modern realities of human experience that so often impinge on the day-to-day practice of health care delivery.

Comprehensive decision-making models

To aid in the process of decision making in bioethics, several comprehensive, or mixed-approach, models have been developed. Fig. 12-4 shows one example of a comprehensive ethical decision-making model that incorporates the best components of formalism and consequentialism.[18] In this approach, the ethical problem is framed in terms of the conditions and of who is affected. Initially, an action is chosen on the basis of a prospective determination of its consequences. However, the potential consequences of this preliminary decision are then compared to the human values underlying the problem. The "short test" of this comparison of consequences to human values is a simple restatement of the Golden Rule: "Would I be satisfied to have this action taken on me?" The preliminary decision is considered ethically justifiable if—and only if—it passes this test of human values.

A simpler but nonetheless comprehensive model has been proposed by Francoeur.[10] Under this framework, ethical decision making involves eight key steps: (1) identification of the problem or issue, (2) identification of the individuals involved, (3) identification of the ethical principle(s) that apply, (4) identification of who should make the decision, (5) identification of the role of the practitioner, (6) consideration of the alternatives, including their possible long- and short-term consequences, (7) making the decision (including the decision not to act), and (8) following the decision to observe its consequences.

Decision-making models notwithstanding, respiratory care practitioners are often at a double disadvantage in the arena of biomedical ethics, as they are faced not only with living with their own decisions but also with supporting the decisions of their physician colleagues. Unless excellent communication is maintained, misunderstandings can occur. Such misunderstandings may be contributing fac-

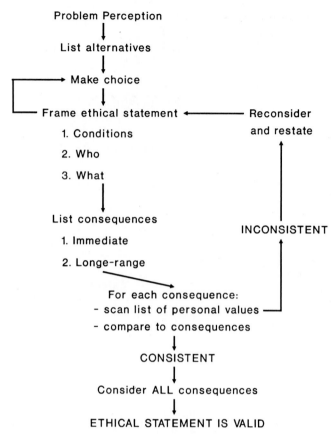

Fig. 12-4 A comprehensive ethical decision-making model. (Redrawn from Brody H: Ethical decisions in medicine, ed 2, Boston, 1981, Little, Brown & Co.)

tors in the high job stress, burnout, and early attrition that have characterized respiratory care.

The addition of classes in biomedical ethics, coupled with decision-making and communication skills, is needed to prepare graduates for the often confusing and frustrating practice found in today's clinics. The specialty requires practitioners who can go beyond simple assertions of their beliefs of rightness or wrongness and provide justifications that are both right and reasoned.

LEGAL ISSUES AFFECTING RESPIRATORY CARE

Unfortunately, there are times when the decisions cannot be made within the confines of the medical community and the patients served. These problems often find their way to the courts for arbitration. The problem of professional liability for physicians is immense, and it is estimated that one of four physicians in this country will be sued this year. In Florida one third of the obstetricians have stopped delivering babies because of the potential liability risk. In a recent poll, 38% of the responding surgeons said they were restricting their practices and 27%

said that they might retire early as a consequence of the current liability situation.[19] In *Megatrends,* John Naisbitt noted that the average malpractice jury verdict award was $1 million, triple the average in 1980.[20] Adjusted for inflation, this would be equivalent to about $2 million today. Clearly, the costs, losses, frustration, and distraction brought about by the current level of legal intervention into medical practice is a national crisis.

Systems of law

In our legal system, the law is divided into two broad classes: criminal and civil. Criminal law deals with acts or offenses against the welfare or safety of the public. Offenses against criminal law are punishable by fines, imprisonment, or both. In these cases the accuser is the state and the person prosecuted is the defendant. Three gradations of criminal acts are recognized by the law: (1) offenses, such as disorderly conduct or traffic violations; (2) misdemeanors, such as small thefts, perjury, conspiracies, and assaults without the use of weapons; and (3) felonies, which include major robberies, assault with a dangerous weapon, rape, arson, and murder.[21] A respiratory care practitioner would usually not be involved in a problem involving criminal law, except as mentioned below under criminal malpractice.

Civil laws protect individuals from others who might take unfair and unlawful advantage of them. A person who believes that his or her rights have been interfered with can seek redress from the courts. In these cases, the person bringing the complaint is known as the plaintiff and the person accused of the wrong is the defendant. Civil courts decide between the two parties with regard to the degree of wrong and the level of restitution required.[21] The category of civil law best related to the practice of medicine and respiratory care is tort law.

Tort law. A claim of private or civil wrong or injury, other than breach of contract, for which the court will provide a remedy in the form of damages, is known as a tort. The word tort refers to any legal wrong committed on a person or property independent of contract. Causes for the complaints may range from assault and battery to invasion of privacy. However, the most common torts brought against health care professionals fall into the categories of malpractice or negligence.[21-24]

Malpractice. Malpractice is defined as professional misconduct, unreasonable lack of skills or fidelity in professional or judicial duties, evil practice, or unethical conduct. There are three classifications of malpractice: (1) criminal malpractice, including such crimes as assault and battery or euthanasia, which are handled separately in criminal courts; (2) civil malpractice, such as negligence or a practice that falls below a reasonable standard, which is handled in civil courts; and (3) ethical malpractice, which includes violations of professional ethics and may result in censure or disciplinary actions by licensure boards.[21,22]

Negligence. The tort of negligence is concerned with the compensation of a person for loss or damages arising from the unreasonable behavior of another. The normal standard for the claim is the imposed duty not to cause risk or harm to others, the standard being that which a reasonable and prudent person should have foreseen and avoided. With health care providers, a higher standard than that of the average man is recognized, as health professionals are considered to owe a special duty to patients and to act with special skill and attention.[25-27]

In negligence cases, breach of duty often involves the matter of foreseeability. Cases in which the patient falls, is burned, is given the wrong medication, or is harmed by defects in an apparatus often revolve around the duty to anticipate the harm.[25,28,29] Duty can be defined as an obligation to do a thing, a human action exactly conformable to the law that requires us to obey.[21]

For the tort of negligence to be a valid claim, it must have three elements[21,23,24]:

1. The health care provider must owe a legal duty to the patient, such duty being established by a patient-provider relationship.
2. The established duty was breached by provision of a standard of care that falls below that owed to the patient. The usual standard of care owed is that recognized nationally or the general standard as determined by the training of the individual practitioner.
3. The breach of duty caused actual harm or injury to the individual. The injured party must file the lawsuit within the time frame established by the statute of limitations. The claim must be supported by a preponderance of evidence to prevail.

Res ipsa loquitur. The legal principle, *res ipsa loquitur,* meaning "the thing speaks for itself," is sometimes invoked to show that the harm would not ordinarily have happened if those in control had used appropriate care.[21] *Res ipsa loquitur* is a principle that allows negligence to be established by inference. Three basic elements are necessary to justify invocation of this principle[21,22,30]:

1. The harm was such that it would not normally occur without someone's negligence.
2. The action responsible for the injury was under the control of the defendant.
3. The injury did not result from any contributing negligence or voluntarily assumed risk on the part of the injured party.

The classic example of "the thing speaks for itself" would be a nasopharyngeal airway that becomes displaced and lodged inside a patient's nose. Limitations to the use of *res ipsa loquitur* have been developed to protect the practitioner from suits arising from cases in which the practice was adequate but the results were unsuccessful.

Strict liability. Strict liability is a theory in tort law that can be used to impose liability without fault in situations where injury occurred under conditions of reasonable care.[21,26] The most common cases of strict liability are those involving the use of dangerous products or techniques. Courts have imposed the application of this principle on the manufacturers and distributors of some products used in medical treatments, as well as on the hospitals for their administrative and mechanical services, but have generally refused to extend this doctrine to professional services.

Intentional torts. An intentional tort is a wrong perpetrated by one who intends to do that which is forbidden by law. This is in contrast with negligence, in which the professional fails to exercise an adequate degree of care in doing what is otherwise permissible. The acts must be intentionally done to produce the harm or done with the belief that the result was substantially certain to follow. These torts are more serious than the tort of negligence, in that the defendant intended to commit the wrong.[23] As a result, punitive as well as actual damages may be awarded. Examples of intentional torts are those that involve defamation of character, invasion of privacy, deceit, infliction of mental distress, and assault and battery.[21]

Within the hospital, the unwarranted discussion of the patient's condition, diagnosis, or treatment for purposes other than the necessary exchange of information between health care providers is always deemed suspect in regard to defamation of character.

Under the general title of defamation of character are the torts of libel and slander. *Slander* is the oral defamation of a person by speaking unprivileged or false words by which his or her reputation is damaged. *Libel* is printed defamation by written words, cartoons, and such representations as to cause the individual to be avoided or held in contempt.[21] Libel or slander does not exist unless it is seen or heard by a third person. If the practitioner directs his or her remarks only to the person involved, it is not slanderous. If, on the other hand, the remark is made in the presence of a third party, it might constitute slander.

Caution with regard to unauthorized disclosure of information about a patient is especially critical in cases involving a disease such as AIDS, which often carries a high degree of medical and social stigma. The patient has a legal right to expect that all information regarding his or her disease will be held in strict confidence.

The states of California and Wisconsin now have civil liability and criminal penalties for the release of confidential HIV test results where the breach of confidence results in economic, psychologic, or bodily harm to the patient.

An *assault* is an intentional act that places another person in fear of immediate bodily harm. Threatening to injure someone is considered an act of assault. *Battery*, on the other hand, represents unprivileged, nonconsensual physical contact with another person. In the classic act of assault and battery, one person threatens and actually injures another.

While battery is an unusual charge against clinicians, because of the nature of their work, it is one that creates special problems. The major element of battery is physical contact without consent. When a practitioner performs a procedure without the patient's informed consent, this contact may be considered battery.[31] In most instances, there is an *implied consent* created when the patient solicits care from the physician, which allows for ordinary procedures to be performed without written consent. In all cases of unusual, difficult, or dangerous procedures, such as surgery, the courts require written consent. For this reason, to avoid the possibility of being accused of battery, practitioners should always explain all procedures involving physical contact to the patient before their initiation.

The defenses that can be applied to intentional torts lie generally in two areas. The first is that there was a lack of intent to create the harm, as only clinicians who engage in intentional conduct are liable. If, in the performance of the care, the practitioner fainted and, in doing so, caused the injury, he or she would not be liable under intentional tort theories, as the action was not voluntary. The second acceptable defense is that the patient gave consent to the procedure. If the patient consented to the action, knowing the risks involved, the practitioner would not be liable.[32] Thus consent by the patient for both nonroutine and routine procedures should be obtained before care is rendered.

Breach of contract. Breach of contract is a much rarer malpractice claim than negligence. This claim is based on the theory that when a health professional renders care, there is established a professional-patient relationship that gives rise to a contract, either implicit or explicit by law.[21,23] Essentially, the contract binds the health professional to regard the patient's welfare as the foremost concern, to act only in his behalf, to protect his life, preserve his health, relieve suffering, and protect his privacy. When, as a result of the services rendered under this contract, the patient is injured, the patient may claim that the failure to competently perform the service is a breach of the contract.

Like all other professionals, respiratory care practitioners are responsible for their actions.[33] When these actions result in the injury of another, the injured party may turn to the courts for redress. If the practitioner, while acting for the physician, injures the patient through some negligent act, the patient may sue both the practitioner and the physician.

Civil suits

Civil suits can be brought for many reasons, such as to challenge a law or to enjoin an activity. However, as in the case of malpractice suits, most seek monetary damages. The following scenario is an example of a situation that might involve the respiratory care practitioner in such a case. In this scenario, the physician means to order 0.5 ml of a bronchodilator for his 3-year-old asthmatic patient, but instead inadvertently writes a prescription for 5 ml of the drug. As a result of the overdose given by the respiratory care practitioner, the child dies.

A clearly articulated legal principle in negligence is that the duty owed to the patient is commensurate with the patient's needs. In short, the more vulnerable the patient, the greater the caregiver's duty to protect.[25,27] Under this principle, when the order is not clear or seems inappropriate, clinicians have an obligation to clarify rather than risk harm.

Suit could be brought against the physician for negligence in ordering the overdose, against the nurses and the respiratory care practitioner for failing to recognize that the dose was inappropriate for the child, and possibly against the pharmacist for failing to gain adequate information as to the nature of the patient so that an appropriate dose could be calculated. The plaintiff would base the secondary charges against the nurses and the allied health practitioners on the theory that liability would be incurred by those who missed an opportunity to correct the first wrongdoer's mistake.[29]

Steps in a civil suit. The basic steps of such a civil suit are as follows[21,22,34]:

1. A petition or complaint is filed in the appropriate court for that jurisdiction. The complaint is a statement of the material facts upon which the plea for judicial relief is based.

2. A summons is served on the accused by the officer of the court, and the defendants must file their answers with the court, responding to each allegation within a specified period of time.

3. Normally at this time the persons who have received the summons or complaint naming them as defendants contact their insurer. The insurer assigns an attorney to defend the suit; the assigned counsel represents the insured rather than the insurer. In many multiple-defendant cases, each defendant would have a separate attorney.

4. After the complaints have been filed with the courts and the defendants notified, there are pretrial activities by both parties to elicit all the facts in a situation. These activities are known as the discovery phase. This preliminary fact-finding stage is used by the attorneys to narrow the legal issues and expand the liability and defense theories. During the discovery phase each party may submit a series of written questions (interrogatories) that must be answered under oath. An example of this might be the plaintiff's question as to which physicians supervised the practitioner or the defendants' request for a list of all physicians who treated the plaintiff during the last 5 years.

5. A deposition is taken. This is an oral testimony, transcribed as it is given in the presence of all attorneys involved in the suit. The deposition establishes a record of the events in the case and allows the attorneys to judge the effectiveness of the individuals as witnesses. The defendant should cooperate and be completely candid with his attorney with regard to the deposition. A cardinal rule for the process is that the person tell the truth, without embellishment, speculation, or volunteered information. In that the deposition is in regard to material that is more familiar to the clinician than to the lawyers involved, the practitioner can approach the questioning with a certain degree of confidence. Before signing the document, the deponent is allowed to read a copy of the transcription and to make corrections. A person named as a defendant should prepare for the deposition by reviewing all records of the incident and by discussing the issues with the lawyer. Often a review of other depositions given is helpful, in that it familiarizes the person with the process.

Court appearance. Court appearance is very important, and the clinician who is called to testify must appear honest, competent, and sincere. During cross-examination the plaintiff's attorneys can be very aggressive and abusive or gentle and soft spoken. Either way, the practitioner should understand that the attorney is working for his client. All the material given in deposition applies equally to the courtroom. Above all else, the practitioner should tell the truth. If the initial facts contained in the formal deposition are correct, one need not fear cross-examination in court. Under civil law, the court will then decide the merits of the case, determine who committed the wrong, and determine the level of restitution to be made.

Medical supervision

Respiratory care practitioners are required by their scope of practice to work under competent medical supervision. This requirement creates not only a professional relationship but a legal one as well. If the practitioners are employed by the physician, the physician is liable for their actions. The legal framework for this liability is found in the principle of *respondeat superior,* which translates to mean "let the master answer."[21,22,35]

Under this legal doctrine, the physician assumes responsibility for wrongful actions on the part of the practitioner, as long as such dereliction occurred in the course of the employer-employee relationship. For this liability to be incurred, two conditions must be met: (1) the act must be within the scope of employment and (2) the injury caused must be from an act of negligence.

If the practitioner acted outside his or her scope of practice as outlined by either licensure laws or institutional regulations, the court would need to decide whether the physician would still be liable. If, for instance, the practitioner, while in the patient's room to deliver an aerosol treatment, went beyond the normal scope of practice and adjusted cervical traction, thereby causing injury, it is doubtful that the physician could be held fully responsible. However, under the principle of *respondeat superior,* the hospital, as a corporate entity, could be held responsible for the actions of its employees.[32,35]

Historically, respiratory care practitioners have not been named individually as defendants in malpractice cases, since the law has generally not yet recognized their role as specialized health care providers. Either the hospital or the physician is usually named as the defendant for the acts of the practitioner. The practitioner in these cases has been viewed simply as an employee, merely carrying out the orders of a superior. However, with the increased application of state licensure regulations governing the practice of respiratory care, this relative protection from liability is rapidly changing.

Scope of practice

One measurement of professionalism in an occupation is the extent to which the group is willing to direct its own development and regulate the activities of others within the specialty. This self-direction is done primarily through state licensure boards, which attempt to ensure that the professional exhibits a minimum level of competence.

Licensure laws and regulations. Within the new legislation for licensure is always a clause indicating scope of practice. The scope-of-practice statutes give the general guidelines and parameters for the clinician's practice (see box). Deviation from the statutory mandates could be a source of legal problems as the specialty seeks to add new duties. Practitioners must inform themselves of the limitations to the scope of care and seek amendments to the licensure regulations as they expand their practices. Ideally, the original language of a licensure law should be broad enough to account for changes in practice without requiring continual amendment.

Implications for the practitioner. The Jolene Tuma case gives some indication of the problems associated with going beyond the legal scope of practice.[15] In this case Ms. Tuma, a nurse, counseled a patient on alternate forms of cancer therapy, such as Laetrile and nutritional therapies. The state board of licensure sought to remove her license for unprofessional conduct on the grounds that this form of counseling went well beyond the scope of practice as indicated in her practice act. Ms. Tuma retained her license on the basis that the nurse practice act did not identify unprofessional conduct clearly enough. She was, however, enjoined from continuing with any further acts of this nature.

Providing emergency care without physician direction. One unique area that allows practice without the direction of a competent physician is that of rendering emergency medical care to injured persons. The "Good Samaritan" laws protect citizens from civil or criminal liability for any acts of omission that occur during attempts to give emergency aid. Most states have legislated Good Samaritan statutes to encourage professionals to give needed emergency medical assistance. It is necessary for this aid to be given in good faith and free from possible charges of gross negligence or willful misconduct. However, it is unlikely that the practitioner would be protected for giving aid, such as performing a tracheostomy, that clearly went beyond the expected skills of that individual or beyond

---

BASIC ELEMENTS OF A PRACTICE ACT

Some practice acts will emphasize one area over another, but the majority of the acts will address the following elements:

1. Scope of professional practice
2. Requirements and qualifications for licensure
3. Exemptions
4. Grounds for administrative action
5. Creation of an examination board and processes
6. Penalties and sanctions for unauthorized practice

---

that which could be defined as first aid. Good Samaritan laws in general apply only to roadside accidents and emergency situations outside the hospital.[22]

INTERACTION OF ETHICS AND THE LAW

A good example of the interaction of ethics and the law in respiratory care results from the diversification of the field into home care and durable medical equipment supply. This diversification has led to new relationships between these elements of the health care system and has created the real potential for both unethical and unlawful activity.

For example, if the practitioner accepts some remuneration, such as a finder's fee or a percentage of the total lease costs, for referring patients to a particular home care company or equipment service, he or she should be prepared to face charges of unethical and perhaps illegal practice.

Statute 42 of the US Code 139nn deals directly with the legal component of this problem. According to this code, anyone who knowingly or willfully solicits, receives, offers, or pays directly or indirectly any remuneration in return for Medicare business is guilty of a criminal offense. Violation of this statute carries the potential for a prison sentence, a $25,000 fine, or both.[36] If the practitioner is aware that others are engaged in these practices, he should report these activities to the US Department of Health and Human Services or the Judicial Committee of the AARC.

To aid the clinician in maintaining an ethical stance on these new issues, the AARC has established a position statement with regard to ethical performance of respiratory home care (see box on p. 277).

SUMMARY

If ethical reasoning is to be of any value to those who must apply its concepts, it must account for the reality of human experience and take its rightful place among the many considerations that compete for our attention. These

---

AARC STATEMENT IN REGARD TO THE ETHICAL PERFORMANCE OF RESPIRATORY HOME CARE

The Code of Ethics of the AARC applies to all respiratory care practices regardless of the environment in which care may be delivered. In general, the following definition of conflict of interest is provided:

Under no circumstances should any respiratory care practitioner engage in any activity which compromises the motive for the provision of any therapy procedures, the advice or counsel given patients and/or families, or in any manner profit from referral arrangements with home care providers.

Specifically, conflict of interest shall be defined as: any act of a respiratory care practitioner during or outside the practitioner's principal employment for which the practitioner receives any form of consideration for:

  a. The referral of patients to specific home care providers.

  b. The solicitation of others for specific home care provider referrals.

  c. Recommendations for ordering of specific therapy procedures and/or equipment.

  d. Recommendations for the continuation of unwarranted procedures and/or equipment.

  e. The association of any practitioner with any home care provider, when profit or revenue generation influences the selection, evaluation, or continuation of any home care procedure and/or equipment.

  f. Individuals who are either employed by or receive remuneration from both health care institutions which may refer patients and by durable medical suppliers who offer respiratory home care must openly disclose this relationship to both parties.

  g. Institutionally based respiratory care practitioners who have significant ownership interest in a durable medical equipment company which provides respiratory home care must openly disclose this relationship to the employing institutions, Medicare Part B carriers, and all others who may be involved in the referral process. The practitioner must remove himself from the process of patient referrals to that provider.

Awareness of activities that may be viewed as being a conflict of interest and in violation of the Code of Ethics of the AARC shall be documented and sent to the Judicial Committee of the AARC.

---

considerations include (1) factual premises and beliefs, such as the definition of death, (2) legal concepts, such as tort laws, and (3) externally imposed mandates or expectations, such as hospital accreditation standards.

In many instances, such considerations uphold our underlying moral convictions and strengthen support for a given decision or action. The real challenge to the respira-

tory care practitioner arises when moral principles dictate one course of action and factual knowledge, legal concepts, or external expectations dictate another.

Respiratory care is an occupation that aspires to professional status. Long ago, Socrates demanded that professionals acknowledge the social context of their activities and that they recognize their obligations toward the segment of society that they profess to serve. As our analysis of ethical reasoning and the law has made clear, only by identifying, justifying, and prioritizing basic principles of human values can the respiratory care practitioner resolve the difficult questions of professional behavior in consistent ways. To the extent that clearly articulated principles guide our choices and actions, all involved will be well served.

Glossary of legal terms

actual damages Compensation for actual injuries or losses, such as medical expenses, lost wages, etc.

affidavit A written statement of facts given voluntarily under oath.

allegation A written statement by a party to a suit concerning what the party expects to prove.

assault Any conduct that creates a reasonable apprehension of being touched in an injurious manner. No actual touching is required to prove assault.

battery An unconsented actual touching that causes injury.

breach of contract Failure, without legal excuse, to carry out the terms of a legal agreement.

breach of duty Failure to complete an assignment that is legal and agreed upon.

bribery, commercial The advantage that one competitor secures over fellow competitors by secret and corrupt dealing with employees or agents or prospective purchasers.

brief A written statement prepared by an attorney arguing a case in court. A brief contains a summary of the facts of the case, the pertinent acts to include those who had the right of control over the negligent actions.

burden of proof The requirement of proving facts in dispute on an issue raised between the parties in a case.

citation Any legal reference, usually cites the law book, volume number, and the section or page number.

civil action Action brought to enforce, redress, or protect private rights. This includes all types of actions other than criminal proceedings.

civil law The body of law every particular nation, commonwealth, or city has established peculiarly for itself. These laws are concerned with civil or private rights and remedies.

claim To demand as one's own or as one's right; to assert; to urge; to insist.

coercion Compulsion; constraint; compelling by force or arms or threat. The force may be actual, direct, implied, or legal.

compensation Payment of damages. Giving an equivalent or substitute of equal value for a loss sustained.

complainant One who applies to the courts for legal redress by filing a complaint. One who instigates prosecution or who prefers accusation against a suspected person.

complaint The first document filed in court by the plaintiff to begin a suit.

concurrent tortfeasors Those whose independent, negligent acts combined at one point in time to cause injury to a third party.

consumer An individual who purchases, uses, maintains, and disposes of products and services.

contract, express An actual agreement between parties whose terms are stated orally or written at the time the agreement is made.

contract, implied A contract not created or evidenced by the explicit agreement of the parties but inferred by the law, as a matter of reason and justice from their acts or conducts, making it a reasonable assumption that a contract existed between them by tacit understanding.

defendant The person denying the party against whom relief or recovery is sought in an action or suit. Also, the accused in a criminal case.

deposition The testimony of a witness taken on interrogatories. The deposition can be either oral or written.

deponent One who testifies to the truth of certain facts. One whose deposition is given.

due process of law Law in its regular course of administration through courts of justice.

duty A human action that is exactly conformable to the laws that require us to obey them. It is a legal or moral obligation.

false imprisonment The unlawful arrest or detention of a person without warrant, by an illegal warrant, or by an illegally executed warrant.

informed consent A general principle of law which states that a physician has a duty to disclose what a reasonably prudent physician in the medical community in the exercise of reasonable care would disclose to his patient as to whatever grave risks of injury might be incurred from a proposed course of treatment. The patient exercising ordinary care for his own welfare and faced with a choice of undergoing the proposed treatment may therefore intelligently exercise his judgment by reasonably balancing the probable risks against the probable benefits.

intent The design, resolve, or determination with which a person acts. It refers only to the state of mind with which the act is done or omitted.

interrogatories A set or series of written questions drawn up for the purpose of being addressed to a party, witness, or other person having information of interest in the case.

negligence The failure to do something that a reasonable person guided by ordinary considerations would do. Also, the doing of something that a reasonable and prudent person would not do.

negligence, contributory The act of doing something or failing to do something that results in the want of ordinary care on the part of the complaining party. This act or omission occurs concurrently with the defendant's negligence and is the proximate cause of injury. Cause in the plaintiff's harm.

patient-physician privilege The right of a patient to refuse to divulge or have divulged by his physician, the communications made between him and his physician.

petition A formal written request addressed to some governmental authority. It is usually a formal written application to a court requesting judicial action on a certain matter.

plaintiff A person who brings an action. A person who seeks remedial relief for an injury to his rights.

pleading The formal allegations by the parties of their respective claims and defenses.

power of attorney An instrument authorizing another to act as one's agent or attorney.

reasonable man doctrine The standard that one must observe to avoid liability for negligence is the standard of the reasonable man. This standard includes the foreseeability of harm to an individual.

redress Satisfaction or equitable relief for an injury sustained.

res ipsa loquitur "The thing speaks for itself." Rule of evidence whereby negligence of alleged wrongdoer may be inferred from the mere fact that the accident happened.

respondeat superior "Let the master answer." This maxim means that the master is liable in certain cases for the wrongful acts of his servant. The doctrine is inapplicable where injury occurs while the servant is acting outside the legitimate scope of authority.

statute An act of the legislature declaring, commanding, or prohibiting something.

statute of limitations A statute declaring that no suit shall be maintained nor any criminal charge be made unless brought about within a specified period of time after the right accrued.

tort A legal wrong committed on a person or property independent of contract.

tortfeasor A wrongdoer. The person who commits or is guilty of a tort.

REFERENCES

1. Fowler MD and Ariff JL: Ethics at the bedside, Philadelphia, 1987, JB Lippincott Co.
2. American Hospital Association: Values in conflict: resolving ethical issues in hospital care, Chicago, 1985, The Association.
3. Katz J: The silent world of doctor and patient, New York, 1986, The Free Press.
4. Veatch RM: A theory of medical ethics, New York, 1981, Basic Books.
5. Veatch RM: Models for ethical medicine in a revolutionary age, Hastings Center Report 2:1-2, June 1973.
6. Beauchamp TL and McCullough LB: Medical ethics, Englewood Cliffs, NJ, 1984, Prentice-Hall.
7. Cook SE and Anderson CC: The current medical malpractice crisis, Schumpert Med Q pp. 106-111, Nov. 1987.
8. Scully TC and Scully C: Playing God, New York, 1987, Simon & Schuster.
9. Bok S: Lying: moral choice in public and private life, New York, 1978, Vintage Books, Inc.
10. Francoeur RT: Biomedical ethics, a guide to decision making, New York, 1983, A Wiley Medical Publications.
11. Ramsey P and McCormick R, editors: Doing evil to achieve good, Chicago, 1978, Loyola University Press.
12. Dennis C: The power of attorney book, Berkeley, 1985, Nolo Press.
13. Evans RE: Health care technology and the inevitability of resource allocation and rationing decisions, JAMA 249:2208-2219, 1983.
14. Beauchamp TL and Childress JF: Principles of biomedical ethics, ed 3, New York, 1989, Oxford University Press.
15. Purtillo RB and Cassel CK: Ethical dimensions in the health professions, Philadelphia, 1981, WB Saunders Co.
16. Frankena WK: Ethics, ed 2, Englewood Cliffs, NJ, 1973, Prentice-Hall.
17. Ross WD: The right and the good, Oxford, England, 1930, Clarendon Press.
18. Brody H: Ethical decisions in medicine, ed 2, Boston, 1981, Little, Brown & Co.
19. Todd JS: The problem of professional liability, Schumpert Med Q, pp. 112-118, Nov. 1987.
20. Naisbett J: Megatrends: ten directions for transforming our lives, ed 6, New York, 1983, Warner Books.
21. Black HC: Black's law dictionary, St Paul, Minn, 1983, West Publishing Co.
22. Hemelt MD and Mackert ME: Dynamics of law in nursing and health care, Reston, Va, 1982, Reston Pub Co.
23. Fiesta J: The law and liability, New York, 1983, Wiley Medical.
24. Murchison I, Nichols TS, and Hanson R: Legal accountability in the nursing process, St Louis, 1982, The CV Mosby Co.
25. Cushing M: Who transcribed that order, Am J Nurs 86:1107-1108, Oct. 1986.
26. Gaare R: Introduction to the legal system of bioethics, Biolaw, Frederick, Md, 1988, University Publications of America.
27. Wooten v US, 574. Supp. 200 (1982); affirmed 722 f.2d 743 (1983) (duty owed patient is commensurate with the patient's needs).
28. Burks v Christ Hospital, 19 Ohio St 2d, 249 NE2d 829 (failure to follow procedures results in liability for patient's fall).
29. Norton v Argonaut Insurance Co, 144 So2d 249 (La Ct App 1962) (nurse held liable for overdose after failure to clarify confusing medication order).
30. Ybarra v Spangard, 25 Cal 2nd 486, 154 p 2d 687 (1944) Supreme Court of Ca (injury held under principle of res ipsa loquitur).
31. Burton v Leftwich, 123 So 2d 766 (La Ct App 1960) (damages recovered after assault by practitioner).

32. Hogue E: Nursing and legal liability, New York, 1985, National Health Pub.
33. Morrison v MacNamara, 407 A 2d 555 (DC 1979) (nonphysician found liable for improper performance of laboratory test).
34. Cushing M: How a civil suit starts, Am J Nurs 85:655-656, June 1985.
35. Bernardi v Community Hospital Association, 166 Colo 280, 443 P 2d 708 (1968) Supreme Court of Colorado (hospital held responsible under principle of respondiat superior).
36. Larson K: DME referrals: what's legal and what's not, AARTimes 10(8):28-31, 1986.

BIBLIOGRAPHY

Blendon RJ: Health policy choices for the 1990s, Issues Science Technol 2:65, 1986.

Eisendrath SJ and Jonson AR: The living will, help or hindrance? JAMA 249:2054-2058, 1983.

Epstein D: Medicare fraud, abuse, and respiratory therapy, AARTimes 9(10):21-26, Oct 1985.

Krekeler K: Critical care nursing and moral development, Crit Care Nurs Q 10:1-10, September 1987.

Leikin SL: An ethical issue in pediatric cancer care: nondisclosure of a fatal prognosis, Pediatr Ann 10:37-41, 44-45, 1981.

Starr P: The social transformation of American medicine, New York, 1982, Basic Books.

The President's Commission for the Study of Ethical Problems in Medicine and Biomedical and Behavioral Research: Washington, DC, 1983, US Government Printing Office (10 reports).

13

General Patient Care

Frances W. Quinless

Respiratory care practitioners share general responsibilities for providing safe and effective patient care with other members of the health care team. General patient care responsibilities shared among all health professionals include basic patient observation and assessment, the provision of physical and psychologic support, the implementation of various safety measures, and the careful and accurate documentation of care. The purpose of this chapter is to provide a foundation of knowledge necessary to effectively discharge these general aspects of patient care.

OBJECTIVES

This chapter provides an overview of the general patient care responsibilities regularly assumed by the respiratory care practitioner. Specifically, after completion of this chapter, the reader will be able to:

1. Recognize the value of astute observation as a tool for the assessment of patients with respiratory dysfunction;
2. Describe the specific guidelines for critically observing patients with respiratory dysfunction;
3. Recognize the importance of the interview process as a means of collecting initial and ongoing patient data;
4. Appreciate the factors that enhance or hinder interpersonal communication;
5. Understand the interrelationships of observation and interviewing in the patient assessment process;
6. Describe general physical support measures for the care of patients with respiratory dysfunction;
7. Appreciate the importance of psychologic support measures for the care of patients experiencing acute, chronic, or terminal respiratory illness;
8. Delineate the basic safety considerations involved in

patient care, including patient movement, patient ambulation, and electrical and fire safety;
9. Describe the need for and methods of documenting patient care for the medical record.

KEY TERMS

Most terms used in this chapter are defined in context. The following terms are introduced without explicit definition, but may be found in the text glossary:

ampere	hyperreflexia
Babinski reflex	hypnotic
bruit	hypothalamus
cephalocaudal	incoherent
depersonalize	intravascular
diaphoresis	microampere
disequilibrium	mottling
dorsalis pedis	nonflammable
dyspnea	opiate
egocentrism	popliteal
embolus	stasis
hemithorax	tibial
hemoptysis	turgor

GENERAL PATIENT ASSESSMENT

As a key member of the health care team, the respiratory care practitioner must be proficient in the basic techniques used to assess a patient's status. The three primary assessment skills are observation and inspection, interviewing, and the measurement of vital signs.

Observation and inspection

Observation and inspection are among the first steps in the classic model of physical examination, as described in detail in Chapter 16. Besides providing essential information about the patient, these initial assessment steps are useful in determining the acuity of the problem at hand and the possible need for immediate intervention by the health care team.

Section on vital signs excerpted from Wilkins, RL: Techniques of physical examination. In Wilkins RL, Sheldon RL, and Krider SJ: Clinical assessment in respiratory care, St Louis, 1985, The CV Mosby Co.

Patient observation follows an established set of guidelines and involves both direct inspection and scrutiny of the patient's interaction with the environment. These guidelines provide an organizing structure for data collection that, with practice, will allow the practitioner to assess a patient's respiratory status in a quick and efficient manner.

Assessment of the environment. Because the patient and the environment interact continuously, good observational assessment must take into account key environmental factors. For example, a very dry, hot room may aggravate or intensify respiratory symptoms in a patient with chronic obstructive pulmonary disease. Likewise, an asthmatic child may experience an acute asthmatic attack during periods of environmental stress.

In the hospital, the environment should be assessed for comfort, cleanliness, provision of proper equipment, and safety considerations (discussed later in this chapter). The practitioner should observe how the patient "fits" the environment. Representative questions to be addressed in assessing the hospital environment include the following: Is the patient relaxed in appearance? Does the patient appear comfortable? Are the patient's material needs within easy reach? Is the temperature and humidity of the room appropriate? Is the lighting adequate? Is the patient's bed positioned to allow window viewing?

Patient observation and inspection. Once environmental factors are considered, the practitioner should systematically proceed through a series of observations. At a minimum, observational assessment should include: (1) the patient's overall appearance, (2) the patient's mental status, and (3) specific signs associated with respiratory dysfunction.

In conducting these observations, the practitioner must try to take a holistic, or system-wide, perspective. For example, acute respiratory insufficiency can affect other organ systems, such as the central nervous system or the cardiovascular system. As observation proceeds, findings indicating pulmonary dysfunction should be grouped and prioritized for significant patterns from which decisions can be made.

Overall appearance of the patient. The first few seconds of an encounter with a patient will usually help reveal both the acuity and severity of the problem at hand. These "initial impressions" should determine the course of subsequent assessment. If, for example, the patient's general appearance indicates an acute and potentially life-threatening problem, therapeutic intervention must be instituted at once, with more thorough assessment postponed until the patient is stabilized. On the other hand, if the initial impressions indicate that the patient is stable and not in immediate danger, a complete assessment can be conducted.

Basic indicators useful in assessing the overall appearance of the patient include facial expression, degree of

alertness, level of anxiety or distress, positioning, and personal hygiene. Facial expressions can help reveal the presence of pain or anxiety. Simple observation of the patient's alertness and level of anxiety or distress help determine both the severity of the problem at hand and the degree of patient cooperation one can realistically expect. Observation of the position assumed by the patient may also be useful in assessing the severity of the problem and the patient's response to it. Finally, observational assessment of personal hygiene indicators can help reveal information useful in determining both the duration and impact of the problem at hand.

Observation of mental status. After observing the overall appearance of the patient, the practitioner should quickly assess the patient's mental status. The importance of this component of observation is based on the fact that a patient's mental status influences, and is influenced by, his or her respiratory status. For example, severe anxiety may worsen an asthmatic patient's sensation of breathlessness and create further respiratory embarrassment via stimulation of both sympathetic nervous system and hormonal responses. Similarly, low arterial oxygen content, or hypoxemia, may impair central nervous system function, thereby causing confusion, stupor, or even unconsciousness.

By simply being with a patient, certain observable characteristics can be noted. The first important characteristic is the patient's orientation to time, place, and person (self and significant others). If this simple assessment indicates that the patient is alert and oriented to his or her environment, the practitioner should continue to assess the nature of interactions between both the patient and other health professionals and the patient and his or her significant others. Such clinical observations will assist the practitioner in responding effectively and appropriately to the patient, to the patient's significant others, and to other health team members.

If the patient is not alert and does not appear oriented to time, place, or person, the practitioner should try to objectively determine and describe the patient's level of consciousness. Although in-depth neurologic assessment is beyond the scope of this text, a practitioner can objectively describe a patient's level of consciousness using a relatively simple rating scale. The boxed material on p. 282 outlines such a scale, using the terms confused, delirious, lethargic, obtunded, stuporous, and comatose. As indicated, each of these clinical terms is associated with certain observable patient behaviors or responses to external stimuli.

Inspection for respiratory system signs. After assessing the patient's mental status, the practitioner should carefully inspect the patient for signs of respiratory system dysfunction. Such inspection must occur in a well-structured, organized, and logical pattern. Recalling that symmetry is a basic trait of the human body, the practitioner should observe the respiratory system in a comparative

LEVELS OF CONSCIOUSNESS

CONFUSED

- Exhibits slight decrease of consciousness
- Is slow in mental responses
- Has decreased or dulled perception
- Is incoherent in thought

DELIRIOUS

- Confused
- Easily agitated
- Irritable
- Exhibits hallucinations

LETHARGIC

- Sleepy
- Arouses easily
- Responds appropriately when aroused

OBTUNDED

- Awakens only with difficulty
- Responds appropriately when aroused

STUPOROUS

- Does not completely awaken
- Has decreased mental and physical activity
- Exhibits response to pain and deep tendon reflexes
- Is slow to respond to verbal stimuli

COMATOSE

- Is unconscious
- Does not respond to stimuli
- Does not exhibit voluntary movement
- Exhibits possible signs of upper motor neuron dysfunction (Babinski reflex present and hyperreflexia)
- Loss of reflexes with deep or prolonged coma

COMMON NORMAL RESPIRATORY SIGNS DETERMINED BY INSPECTION

- Thoracic symmetry during breathing
- Shoulders at same level with convex shape from neck to lateral borders
- Ribs are higher posteriorly than laterally
- Each anterior hemithorax projects further forward than the sternum
- Costal angle approximately 90 degrees—increases with inspiration
- Anteroposterior thorax diameter is less than the transverse diameter
- Spine straight
- Abdomen and thorax rise/protrude synchronously during inspiration
- Inspiration shorter than expiration (normal ratio of 1:2 to 1:3)
- Accessory muscles of respiration *not* used during quiet breathing
- Respiratory rate between 10 and 20 respirations per minute (adults)

racic activity (intercostal retraction, intercostal bulging, chest protrusions, etc); (6) the use of accessory muscles of respiration during quiet breathing; and (7) the expectoration of sputum. The box above summarizes the major normal respiratory signs that can be determined by simple observation in adult patients. The box on p. 283 includes common deviations noted from observation.

In summary, astute and systematic observation represents a critical component of general patient assessment. Through the proper application of observation skills, the practitioner can gather information essential in tailoring a respiratory care plan to the patient's individual needs. However, whenever possible, respiratory care planning also requires direct collection of data from the patient. This is accomplished via the patient interview.

Patient interviewing

Interviewing supplements inspection and observation by providing the patient's own perspective on the problem at hand. Although interviewing is the most common method for gathering objective historical data, its most important role is in revealing a patient's *subjective* impressions about his or her illness, ie, its symptoms. For this reason, the interview is often the most crucial aspect of general patient assessment. The interview process also serves as the foundation on which the subsequent interpersonal relationship between patient and practitioner develops.

As with observation, good interviewing is a learned skill. Once learned and properly applied, the results of patient interviewing contribute to rational clinical decision

manner, carefully noting deviations occurring from side to side. Moreover, to prevent gaps in data collection, the practitioner should apply a cephalocaudal or "head-to-tail" approach to inspection. Last, the practitioner should try to observe the patient's respiratory status throughout changes in posture, changes in rate and depth of breathing, and during speech. Ideally, these observations should occur with the thorax unclothed.

A systematic framework for observation of the patient must compare what is observed with what would be expected in normal individuals. Key elements in this systematic approach include observation of the following: (1) the rate and depth of respirations (including the relative time spent in inspiration and expiration); (2) the basic pattern of breathing (abdominal versus thoracic); (3) the relative anteroposterior dimensions of the thorax; (4) the symmetry and magnitude of thoracic motion (unilateral, decreased, or increased motion); (5) the presence of abnormal tho-

---

COMMON RESPIRATORY DEVIATIONS NOTED VIA OBSERVATIONS

ABNORMAL BREATHING

Tachypnea
Bradypnea
Periodic apnea
Hyperpnea
Pleuritic breathing
Cheyne-Stokes breathing
Excessive sighing
Markedly prolonged expiratory time

ASYMMETRY OF MOTION OF THORACIC STRUCTURE

Unilateral breathing
Thoracic cage deformities or bulging
Increased anteroposterior diameter

PRESENCE OF PRONOUNCED VENOUS PATTERN ON THORAX

---

making. As an added benefit, the development of effective interviewing skills can assist the practitioner in realizing greater self-awareness and personal growth.

Once interviewing skills become second nature, the practitioner will be able to assist patients in establishing a trusting relationship and openly confiding their problems and personal concerns. This interpersonal communication process may also help patients learn more about themselves. Finally, an appropriately conducted interview may serve both therapeutic and educational goals, thereby assisting the patient and practitioner in working together toward a common end. Communication focused on common health-related goals is termed therapeutic communication.

Therapeutic communication. As indicated in Chapter 11, effective communication occurs when two individuals agree on the message that has occurred between them. Whereas general social communication need not have a specific goal, therapeutic communication is planned and organized with a specific goal in mind.

Therapeutic communication is most effective when (1) the communication is initiated by the health professional; (2) the patient's specific health problem or health care is the focus of the communication; (3) the goal of the communication is to obtain information that will be useful in the resolution of a health problem or for the general improvement of health status; and (4) the decision to terminate communication is made by the patient.

In therapeutic communication, the health professional is responsible for implementing and focusing the communication toward a specific goal. However, this responsibility must be at least partially shared by the patient. For the patient, sharing in this process means being open and honest.

Practitioners must therefore establish a climate that encourages mutual trust and respect.

Therapeutic communication occurs within a complex context. As shown in Fig. 13-1, this context includes sensory and emotional factors; environmental factors; verbal and nonverbal components of the communication process; and the values, beliefs, feelings, habits, and preoccupations of both the professional and the patient.

Therapeutic communication between practitioner and patient is most effective when the practitioner is well prepared. Knowing as much as possible about a patient *prior to interviewing* helps the practitioner focus the interview process. Moreover, having this prior knowledge can increase the patient's confidence in the practitioner's skills and decrease the time required for the interview.

Conducting an interview. Given the diversity of goals served by the interview process, the strict specification of procedural steps is inappropriate. Instead, this section focuses on elements common to good interviewing. Specifically, we look first at key preparatory steps (including establishment of an appropriate climate) and then provide general operating guidelines useful in structuring a successful patient interview.

Preparation. Prior to initiating a patient interview, the practitioner should determine its necessity. If it is possible to obtain the information through other sources, a full interview may not be necessary. In fact, recognizing when not to interview is as important a skill as interviewing itself.

Preparation for the interview should also take into account the nature and severity of a patient's illness. As previously indicated, these factors can significantly affect the interviewing process. Sensitivity to these factors will enhance a practitioner's interviewing skills.

Illness may be accompanied by severe anxiety, fear, depression, anger, and other emotional responses. Pain affects the perception of sound, the interpretation of auditory stimuli, and the response to these stimuli. Medications, especially opiates, sedatives, and hypnotics, will obviously affect mental status and the patient's response to questions. An individual suddenly transformed into a "patient" may experience denial of the illness, which may also affect interview responses. Where necessary, validation of a patient's responses should be provided through family members or other health professionals.

In regard to a patient's illness, data previously collected by observation should determine both the style and focus of the interview. In some cases, the acuity and severity of a patient's illness (as determined by rapid observation and inspection) may simply make it impossible to interview a patient at a given time. For example, a patient with severe dyspnea, tachypnea, and diaphoresis is not a good candidate for interview. These signs and symptoms speak for themselves and demand immediate intervention.

In general, when a team of practitioners is simulta-

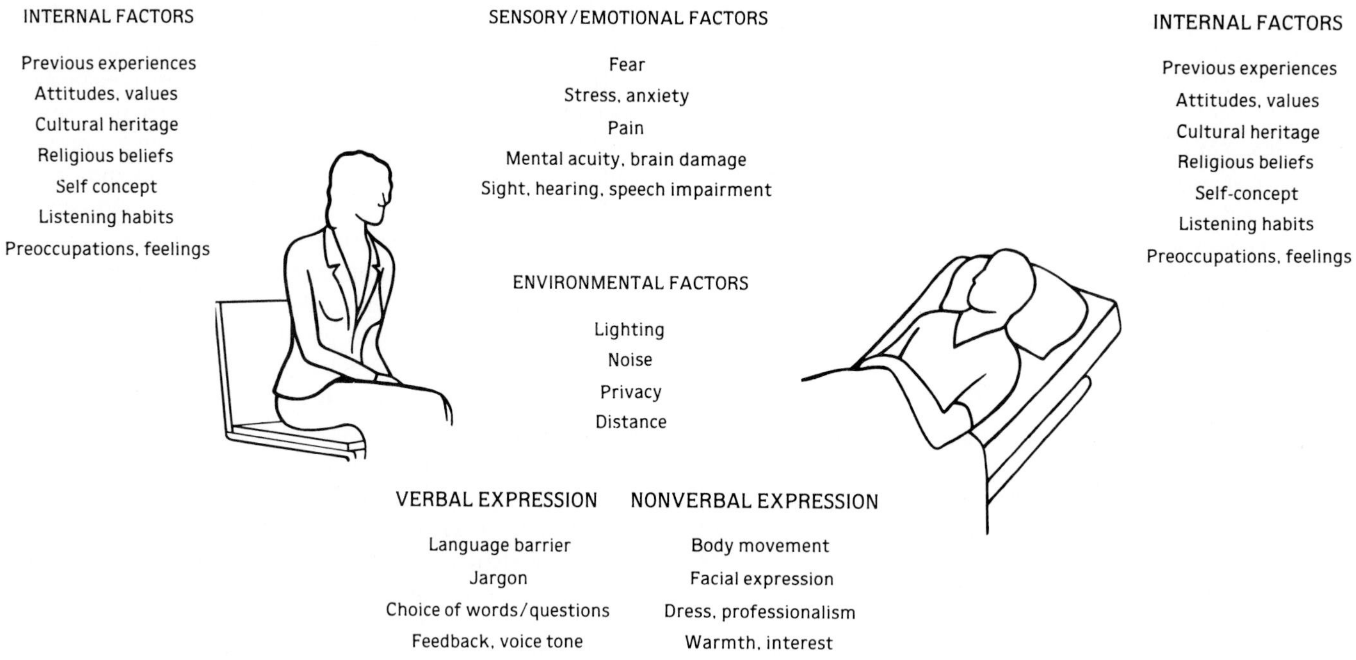

INTERNAL FACTORS

Previous experiences
Attitudes, values
Cultural heritage
Religious beliefs
Self concept
Listening habits
Preoccupations, feelings

SENSORY/EMOTIONAL FACTORS

Fear
Stress, anxiety
Pain
Mental acuity, brain damage
Sight, hearing, speech impairment

INTERNAL FACTORS

Previous experiences
Attitudes, values
Cultural heritage
Religious beliefs
Self-concept
Listening habits
Preoccupations, feelings

ENVIRONMENTAL FACTORS

Lighting
Noise
Privacy
Distance

VERBAL EXPRESSION

Language barrier
Jargon
Choice of words/questions
Feedback, voice tone

NONVERBAL EXPRESSION

Body movement
Facial expression
Dress, professionalism
Warmth, interest

Fig. 13-1   Factors influencing communication. (From Wilkins RL, Sheldon RL, and Krider SJ: Clinical assessment in respiratory care, St Louis, 1985, The CV Mosby Co.)

neously caring for a patient (as during certain emergencies), the interview process ideally should be delegated to a single member of the team. Besides being an unnecessary burden for patients, having to express the same information over and over again to several professionals can decrease patient confidence in the total team effort.

Once the practitioner decides to conduct an interview, he or she should first review the patient's medical record. The medical record will assist the practitioner in determining the present complaint, the past medical and surgical history, and pertinent family and social information. Obtaining this information will assist the practitioner in structuring the interview around a general goal and specific objectives. Moreover, when the patient has already been interviewed, but additional information is still needed, prior review of the medical record will help decrease redundant questions.

The practitioner should also assure (as much as possible) that the physical environment is conducive to interviewing. At a minimum, the room used should be quiet and comfortable. Efforts must also be made to maintain patient privacy. During those times when these conditions cannot be met, the practitioner should at least make the patient aware of his or her concerns for privacy and comfort. Such empathetic concern will help establish mutual trust between patient and practitioner.

Once the decision is made to conduct an interview, practitioners should introduce themselves by name, professional role, and purpose for being with the patient. One should always use the patient's full name and title, such as

"Ms. Johnson." Depersonalizing terms such as "Grandma" must be avoided. The practitioner should also determine if the timing for the interview is appropriate, thereby immediately involving the patient in the decision-making process.

Finally, preparation for the interview should take into account the relative physical positions taken by patient and practitioner. To avoid uncomfortable or intimate contact, the distance between the patient and the practitioner should be at least a few feet. In addition, positions that indicate power or authority over the patient should be avoided. Ideally, both the patient and practitioner should be on eye level to indicate mutual respect. Moreover, the practitioner should avoid standing over a patient or leaning casually against a bed or wall.

Establishing a climate. Good preparation for a patient interview helps establish a climate conducive to effective patient-practitioner interaction. In establishing the climate, the practitioner should avoid reading a checklist type of interview with paper, pen, and clipboard in hand. This hurried approach may give the message that time is being needlessly wasted on the patient. A calm and unhurried demeanor should be used in the interview process. Also, the practitioner should try to reduce the interview to the most salient questions. In this manner, one can avoid rushing through the process in an interrogatory manner.

Additional factors that can help establish a good climate include the following: (1) the credibility established by the professional via his or her general demeanor, dress, and perceived competency (as related to patient expectations);

(2) the acceptance by the practitioner of the patient's humanity (despite one's personal opinions regarding certain behaviors); (3) the practitioner's display of professional objectivity without personal defensiveness, bias, or an overly judgmental attitude; and (4) the practitioner's display of a caring, empathetic (versus sympathetic) attitude.

Factors that may have a negative influence on the interview process include: (1) a practitioner's attitude of control, power, or superiority over the patient; (2) the failure of the practitioner to attend to the patient's physical or emotional responses or cues during the process, especially by display of hurried conduct; (3) the practitioner's display of a judgmental or biased attitude; (4) the practitioner's demand for patient compliance to his or her own schedule or rules, eg, with suppression of patient digressions; and (5) the practitioner's treatment of the patient as a member of a specific group, culture, or ethnic orientation, rather than as an individual.

In addition to these negative factors, there are recognized verbal and nonverbal communication behaviors that hinder the interviewing process (see Fig. 13-1). Body language is the single most influential of these negative behaviors. Gestures, facial expressions, and postures that suggest impatience or lack of commitment immediately alert both the patient and his or her significant others to a professional's noncaring demeanor. Verbal communications that discourage patient openness include biased responses, false reassurance, expressions that discourage negative emotions or feelings, leading or closed statements or questions, and inappropriate changing of topics.

Finally, practitioners should be aware that they often evade topics that create personal discomfort or stress during an interview. This may erect a barrier in the relationship. Since interviewing is a growth process for both the interviewer and the patient, the practitioner will gradually become aware of personally uncomfortable topics. This self-awareness may become a springboard for improving interviewing skills.

General guidelines. Given good initial preparation and the establishment of an appropriate climate, the practitioner should then structure the interview according to the following general guidelines:

1. Determine the subjective information needed to plan specific respiratory care interventions;
2. Prepare an interview schedule with specific questions needed to obtain the information required;
3. Prepare a general opening question for the interview schedule; the information obtained may guide or focus the remainder of the interview;
4. Guide the patient carefully in the questioning process, maintaining focus while allowing digression;
5. Guide the patient through the interview using the following interpersonal communication techniques:
   Facilitation—techniques that assist or encourage the patient to respond. Examples include nonverbal behavior such as maintaining eye contact, leaning toward the patient, nodding the head; and verbal communication such as "please go on," "go on," or "explain that to me again."
   Clarification—techniques that seek clearer information from the patient. Examples include questions such as "I don't understand what you have just said. Please explain that to me again" and statements or questions that help the practitioner understand a patient's response that may have been initially vague or unclear.
   Reflection—restating what the patient has said. For example, the practitioner might respond to a patient's complaint of orthopnea with the following questions: "So your shortness of breath goes away when you sit up? Do other positions help ease your breathing?" Reflection often leads to more detail on the part of the patient. It may also "buy" the interviewer time to develop or alter strategy.
   Empathy—verbal or nonverbal communication that informs the patient the practitioner understands the feelings or emotions being expressed. Examples of verbal expressions indicating an empathetic response include statements such as "Yes, I understand your concern," or "I can see why you are so upset." Empathetic responses like these help secure a therapeutic relationship. Such responses do not necessarily imply that the practitioner agrees with the patient's emotions; they simply communicate that the expression of such feelings is acceptable.
   Interpretation—verbal expressions that help the practitioner draw inferences from the patient's verbal and nonverbal responses. For example, "You seem to be anxious about (this situation)" provides the opportunity for the patient to express his or her emotions, and can help the practitioner validate the patient's true feelings.

6. When exploring the patient's symptoms, use probing questions to elaborate on the onset, characteristics, and course of each subjective complaint. The box on p. 286 outlines the approach taken to the analysis of a symptom. As previously discussed, a patient's subjective evaluation of a symptom is related to individual factors such as pain tolerance and perception. Thus, one should evaluate the intensity or severity of a symptom in terms of its observable interference with the patient's ability to function.

In summary, the planning and delivery of individualized respiratory care requires both a knowledge of the patient's complaints and concerns and a climate of mutual understanding and respect. An appropriately planned and conducted patient interview can serve both purposes, thereby contributing to more effective and more humane respiratory care.

ANALYSIS OF A SYMPTOM

ONSET OF SYMPTOM
- Date
- Time
- Onset, ie, gradual or sudden?
- Precipitating events (eg, injury, exertion)
- Predisposing factors (eg, age, infection, pregnancy, environment, drugs, or other therapeutic agents or treatments)

CHARACTERISTICS OF SYMPTOM
- Quality
- Consistency
- Duration
- Quantity
- Location
- Radiation
- Intensity
- Aggravating factors
- Relieving factors
- Associated symptoms

COURSE OF SYMPTOM
- Timing (eg, acute, chronic, recurrent acute, daily, periodic)
- Therapy (prescribed or nonprescribed)—effective or otherwise?

Vital signs

Assessment of vital signs represents the most frequent clinical measurement made by health professionals. The vital signs provide important diagnostic information and may reveal the first clue of adverse reactions to treatment. The four basic vital signs are body temperature, pulse rate, respiratory rate, and blood pressure.

Body temperature. The normal body temperature for most individuals is approximately 98.6°F (37°C) with a range from 97°F to 99.5°F and with daily variations of 1° to 2°F. The body temperature usually is lowest in the early morning and highest in the late afternoon. Metabolic functions occur optimally when the body temperature is within the normal range.

Maintenance of the body temperature in the normal range is done by the balancing of heat production with heat loss. If the body were not able to discharge the heat generated by metabolism, temperature would rise approximately 2°F per hour. The hypothalamus plays an important role in regulating heat loss and can initiate peripheral vasodilation and sweating in an effort to dissipate body heat. The respiratory system also helps in the removal of excess heat through ventilation. When the inspired gas is cooler than the body temperature, the airways warm the gas to body temperature. Exhalation aids in the dissipation of ex-

cess body heat. When the inspired gas is heated to near body temperature, as with heated aerosols, generators, or humidifiers, this mechanism is not functional.

An elevation of body temperature above normal can result from disease or from normal activities such as exercise. Temperature elevation associated with disease is called *fever,* and the patient is said to be *febrile.* Fever often occurs as a result of viral or bacterial organisms invading the body and producing an infection.

A fever increases the metabolic rate of the body, producing an increase in both oxygen consumption and carbon dioxide production. For every 1°C elevation of body temperature, oxygen consumption and carbon dioxide production increase approximately 10%. The demand for an increase in the supply of oxygen and removal of carbon dioxide must be met by an increase in both circulation and ventilation. Examination of the febrile patient often reveals an increase in heart and breathing rates. For the patient with significant cardiac or pulmonary disease, this increased demand may overtax the cardiopulmonary systems.

When the body temperature is below normal, *hypothermia* exists. Hypothermia is not common but can occur in individuals with severe head injuries that damage the hypothalamus and in individuals suffering from prolonged exposure to cold. When the body temperature is below normal, the hypothalamus initiates shivering in an effort to generate energy and vasoconstriction to conserve body heat.

Because hypothermia reduces oxygen consumption and carbon dioxide production by the body tissues, the patient with hypothermia may exhibit slow, shallow breathing and a reduced pulse rate. Mechanical ventilators in the control mode may need significant adjustments in the depth and rate of delivered tidal volumes as the body temperature of the patient varies above and below normal.

The body temperature is most often measured at one of the three sites; the mouth, axilla, or rectum. Rectal temperatures most accurately reflect actual body-core temperature. Oral temperature measurement is the most acceptable for the awake, adult patient, but this method should not be used with infants, comatose patients, or orally intubated patients. After the patient has ingested hot or cold liquid or has been smoking, a 10- to 15-minute waiting period is required before an accurate oral temperature can be obtained. The axillary temperatures of infants and small children who do not tolerate rectal thermometers may be taken safely.

The oral temperature is not affected significantly by simple oxygen administration via nasal cannula or mask. For this reason, it is not necessary to remove the oxygen or take rectal temperatures of patients receiving simple oxygen therapy.

However, the oral temperature may not be a valid measure of body temperature in patients breathing heated or cooled aerosol via face masks. There is a tendency for oral temperatures to be increased slightly with the application of heated aerosol and decreased slightly with cool aerosol inhalation. In these cases, when absolute accuracy is essential, the rectal route should be employed.

Pulse rate. The peripheral pulse should be evaluated for rate, rhythm, and strength. The normal pulse rate for adults is 60 to 100 beats per minute and is regular in rhythm. A pulse rate exceeding 100 beats per minute is termed *tachycardia.* Common causes of tachycardia include exercise, fear, anxiety, low blood pressure, anemia, fever, reduced arterial blood oxygen levels, and certain medications. A pulse rate below 60 beats per minute is termed *bradycardia.* This is less common, but can occur as a side effect of medications and with certain cardiac arrhythmias.

The amount of oxygen delivered to the tissues depends on the ability of the heart to pump oxygenated blood. The amount of blood pumped through the circulatory system (cardiac output) is a function of heart rate and stroke volume. When the oxygen content of the arterial blood falls below normal, usually from lung disease, the heart tries to compensate by increasing the cardiac output to maintain an adequate oxygen delivery to the tissues. Increases in cardiac output are accomplished, in part, by an increase in heart rate. For this reason the heart is an important dimension to monitor in patients with lung disease.

The most common site for evaluation of the pulse is a radial artery. The examiner's second and third finger pads are used in assessment of the radial pulse (Fig. 13-2). Ideally, the pulse rate should be counted for 1 min. The following characteristics of the pulse should be noted and documented: (1) rate—is it normal, high, or low; (2) rhythm—is it regular, consistently irregular, or irregularly irregular; (3) amplitude—are there any changes in the amplitude of the pulse in relation to respiration; are there changes in amplitude from one beat to another; and (4) presence of thrills (palpable turbulence in flow) or bruits (auscultatory turbulence in flow). If the patient's wrist is held too far above the level of his heart, the pulse may be difficult to obtain.

Other common sites available for assessment of the pulse include the carotid, brachial, femoral, temporal, popliteal, posterior tibial, and dorsalis pedis (Fig. 13-3). When the blood pressure is abnormally low, the more centrally located pulses, such as the carotid and femoral pulses, are identified more easily than the peripheral pulse. If the carotid site is used to obtain a pulse, great care must be taken to avoid the carotid sinus area. Mechanical stimulation of the carotid sinus can evoke a strong parasympathetic response and cause bradycardia or even asystole.

Spontaneous ventilation may influence the strength of the pulse. When the patient's pulse strength decreases with spontaneous inhalation, it is referred to as *pulsus paradoxus. Pulsus alterans* is an alternating succession of

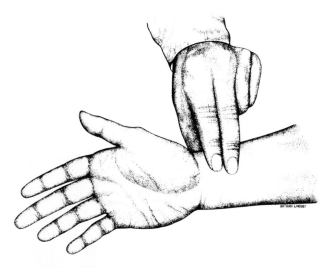

Fig. 13-2 Technique for assessment of radial pulse. (From Wilkins RL, Sheldon RL, and Krider SJ: Clinical assessment in respiratory care, St Louis, 1985, The CV Mosby Co.)

strong and weak pulses and usually is not related to respiratory disease.

Respiratory rate. The normal resting adult rate of breathing is 12 to 20 breaths per minute. *Tachypnea* is the term used to describe respiratory rates above normal. Rapid respiratory rates may be associated with exercise, fever, arterial hypoxemia, metabolic acidosis, anxiety, and pain. A slow respiratory rate, referred to as *bradypnea,* is uncommon but may occur in patients with head injuries or hypothermia, as a side effect of certain medications such as narcotics, and in patients with drug overdoses. Along with the rate, the pattern of breathing should be assessed.

The respiratory rate is counted by watching the abdomen or chest wall move in and out with breathing. With practice, even the subtle breathing movements of the normal individual at rest can be identified easily. In some patients the examiner may need to place a hand on the patient's abdomen to confirm the breathing rate.

Ideally, the patient should be unaware that the respiratory rate is being counted. One successful method to accomplish this is to count the respiratory rate immediately after evaluating the pulse, while maintaining the fingers on the radial artery.

Blood pressure. The arterial blood pressure is the force exerted against the wall of the arteries as the blood moves through the arterial vessels. Arterial *systolic* blood pressure is the peak force exerted during contraction of the left ventricle. *Diastolic* pressure is the force occurring when the heart is relaxed. *Pulse pressure* is the difference between systolic and diastolic pressures. The normal pulse pressure is 35 to 40 mm Hg. When the pulse pressure is less than 30 mm Hg, the peripheral pulse is difficult to detect.

The arterial blood pressure is determined by the force of

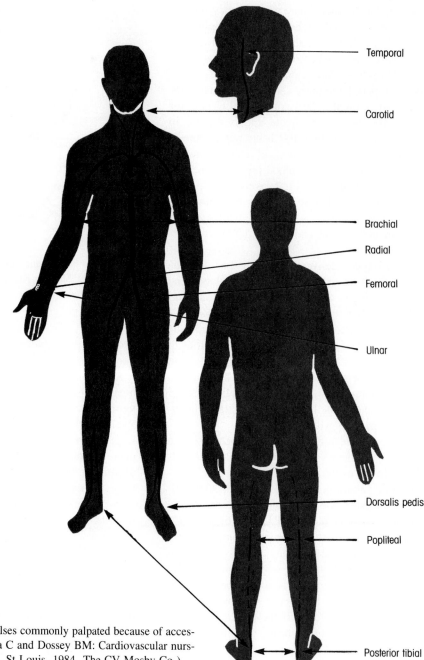

Temporal

Carotid

Brachial

Radial

Femoral

Ulnar

Dorsalis pedis

Popliteal

Posterior tibial

Fig. 13-3   Arterial pulses commonly palpated because of accessibility. (From Guzzetta C and Dossey BM: Cardiovascular nursing: bodymind tapestry, St Louis, 1984, The CV Mosby Co.)

left ventricular contraction, the peripheral vascular resistance, and the blood volume (see Chapter 7). Normal systolic pressures range from 95 to 140 mm Hg, with an average of 120 mm Hg. Normal diastolic pressures range from 60 to 90 mm Hg, with an average of 80 mm Hg. The blood pressure is recorded with systolic listed over diastolic; for example, 120/80 mm Hg.

A blood pressure persistently above 140/90 mm Hg is termed *hypertension*. Hypertension may result from an increase in the force of ventricular contraction or an elevation of peripheral vascular resistance. Severe hypertension can cause central nervous system abnormalities (such as

headaches, blurred vision, and confusion), uremia, congestive heart failure, or cerebral hemorrhage leading to stroke.

Hypotension is defined as a blood pressure less than 95/60 mm Hg. It may occur as the result of peripheral vasodilation, left ventricular failure, or low blood volume. With hypotension, perfusion of vital body organs may be significantly reduced. Without adequate circulation, oxygen delivery to the tissues can be impaired, and tissue hypoxia may occur. For this reason prolonged hypotension must be guarded against.

Changes in posture may produce abrupt changes in the

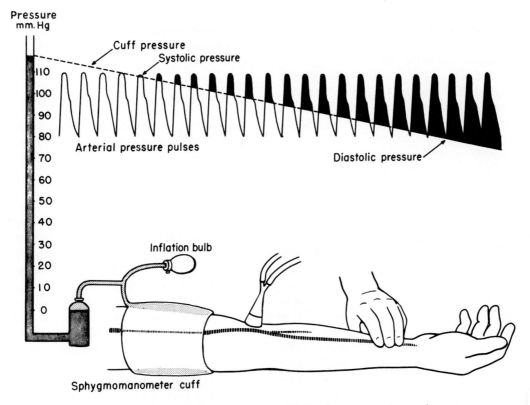

Pressure
mm. Hg

Cuff pressure
Systolic pressure

Arterial pressure pulses

Diastolic pressure

Inflation bulb

Sphygmomanometer cuff

Fig. 13-4   Auscultatory method for measuring arterial blood pressure, using a sphygmomanometer and a stethoscope. (From Rushmer RR: Structure and function of the cardiovascular system, ed 2, Philadelphia, 1976, WB Saunders Co.)

arterial blood pressure in the hypovolemic patient. When healthy individuals move from the supine to the sitting position, their blood pressure changes very little. However, when hypovolemia is present, the blood pressure may decrease significantly when the patient assumes an elevated position. This condition, referred to as *postural hypotension,* can be confirmed by measuring the blood pressure in both the supine and sitting positions. Rapid drops in arterial blood pressure caused by postural hypotension can cause a reduction in cerebral blood flow and lead to syncope, or fainting. Postural hypotension is generally treated either with fluid administration or vasoactive drugs. Untreated or nonresponsive, postural hypotension must always be taken into account when moving or ambulating a patient.

The most common technique for measuring arterial blood pressure is the auscultatory method, which uses a blood pressure cuff (sphygmomanometer) and a stethoscope (Fig. 13-4). When the cuff is applied to the upper arm and pressurized to exceed systolic blood pressure, the brachial blood flow is stopped. As the pressure in the cuff is released slowly to a point just below systolic pressure, blood flow intermittently passes the obstruction. Partial obstruction of the arterial blood flow creates a turbulent flow, producing vibrations called *Korotkoff sounds.* Korotkoff sounds can be heard over the brachial artery distal to the obstruction with the aid of a stethoscope.

To measure the blood pressure, a deflated cuff is

wrapped snugly around the upper arm with the lower edge of the cuff 1 inch above the antecubital fossa. The brachial pulse is palpated, and the cuff is inflated to a pressure 30 mm Hg higher than the point at which the pulse was obliterated. The bell of the stethoscope is placed over the site of the brachial artery. Then the cuff is deflated at a rate of 2 to 3 mm Hg per second while observing the manometer.

The systolic blood pressure is recorded from the point at which the initial Korotkoff sounds are heard. The point at which the sounds become muffled is recorded as the diastolic pressure. This muffling sound is the final change in the Korotkoff sounds just before they disappear. At this point the cuff pressure is equal to the diastolic pressure, and no turbulent sounds are created. The examiner must be careful to perform the procedure rapidly, since the pressurized cuff is impairing circulation to the forearm and hand. Since cuff pressures are only estimates of pressure based on blood flowing through an artery, anything that alters flow in the artery may result in erroneous blood pressure measurements.

Common mistakes that can result in erroneous high-cuff pressure measurements include the following:

1. Too narrow a cuff. (Cuff and bladder width should be at least the diameter of the arm.)
2. Cuff applied too tightly.
3. Cuff applied too loosely. (When the loose bladder is inflated, the edges rise so the portion pressing on the artery has a tourniquet effect.)

4. Excessive pressure placed in the cuff during measurement.
5. Inflation pressure held in the cuff.
6. Incomplete deflation of cuff between measurements.

A low pressure reading may be obtained if the cuff is too wide; however, this produces errors in the range of 3 to 5 mm Hg rather than the 40 mm Hg error often obtained when using too narrow a cuff.

Erroneous diastolic pressure measurement may occur when pressure is maintained on the artery so that laminar flow is not reestablished. Since turbulent flow can be heard, muffling and/or disappearance of sound may not occur. Causes include applying the cuff too tightly and pressing the stethoscope too tightly over the artery. When both muffling and disappearance of the sound occur, both pressures are recorded (120/80/60). Static electricity, ventilators, extraneous room sounds, and presence of an *auscultatory gap* may also cause erroneous cuff measurements. An auscultatory gap is a 20 to 40 mm Hg drop with no sound between the first systolic sound and the continuous pulse sound. Inflating the cuff until the palpated radial pulse can no longer be felt prevents missing the "opening snap." When an auscultatory gap is heard, both the opening snap pressure and the pressure where continuous pulses were heard should be recorded (160/140/80).

The systolic blood pressure usually decreases slightly with normal inhalation. This decrease in systolic blood pressure is more significant during a forced maximal inhalation. When the systolic pressure drops more than 6 to 8 mm Hg during inhalation at rest, a definite abnormality exists; this is termed *paradoxical pulse*. The mechanism responsible for this fluctuation in blood pressure centers around the negative intrathoracic pressure created by the respiratory muscles during inhalation. The negative intrathoracic pressure facilitates venous return to the right ventricle and discourages arterial blood flow out of the left ventricle. Additionally, the increased venous return to the right ventricle increases the right ventricular filling pressure, which causes the interventricular septum to distend toward the left ventricle. This results in reduced left ventricular filling, reduced stroke volume, and decreased systolic blood pressure simultaneous with inhalation.

The fluctuation in systolic blood pressure with ventilation can be identified most accurately with a sphygmomanometer; however, if the pulse can be felt to wane with inspiration in several accessible arteries, paradoxical pulse is present. To confirm and quantify the presence of paradoxical pulse, a blood pressure cuff must be used. The cuff is inflated until no sounds are heard with the stethoscope bell over the brachial artery, and then it is gradually deflated until sounds are heard on exhalation only. The cuff pressure then is reduced slowly until sounds are heard throughout the respiratory cycle. The difference between these two pressure readings indicates the degree of paradoxical pulse. A reading in excess of 6 to 8 mm Hg is significant.

The presence of paradoxical pulse may occur with acute airway obstruction such as asthma or constrictive pericarditis.

PATIENT SUPPORT TECHNIQUES

Patient support techniques complement focused care by ensuring that patients' basic needs are met. Effective support techniques must attend to both the physical and psychologic needs of the patients.

Physical support

General physical support techniques for patients experiencing respiratory dysfunction include positioning, medications, activity, hydration, and clearance of secretions.

Positioning. For patients experiencing respiratory dysfunction, the high Fowler's position, with support from a firm mattress or chair and pillows, is the one of choice. Patients will assume this position automatically if conscious. Providing an over-bed stand with pillows will help them acquire needed relaxation and sleep. More detail on patient positioning is provided in the following section on safety considerations.

Medications. All medications taken by the patient must be carefully reviewed for mechanisms of action and potential adverse reactions. The medication regimen is best delineated through a team approach including the respiratory care practitioner, physician, pharmacist, nurse, and patient. The patient should be informed of the actions and possible reactions to drugs administered. Education is critical for compliance.

Activity. Acute or chronic respiratory dysfunction often taxes a patient's total energy requirements. For the patient, all other activities become inconsequential in comparison with breathing. Thus, in the short term, a patient may develop venous stasis with resultant thrombi and pulmonary emboli due to relative inactivity. In the long term, the patient may develop muscular atrophy, venous stasis, and embolization due to inactivity. Patients must be educated to maintain mobility, even while in bed. Appropriate activities (usually conducted under the auspices of the physical therapy staff) include isometric exercises, flexion and contraction of the knee and ankle, and foot rotation. General mobility (as tolerated) must be encouraged, especially for postoperative patients. Patients with chronic disease should be enrolled in a pulmonary rehabilitation program. Among the activities included in such programs are physical conditioning exercises, which help prevent muscle atrophy due to disuse (see Chapter 34). Details on patient activity, including ambulation techniques, are presented in the section on safety considerations.

Hydration. Adequate hydration plays an essential role in maintaining the normal volume and viscosity of respiratory tract secretions. General body dehydration can result in viscous, tenacious secretions. Moreover, systemic dehydration can result in a decrease in circulating blood volume, which can lead to tachycardia and an increase in cardiac work load.

In the hospital, the adequacy of a patient's systemic hydration is monitored by ongoing assessment of several related parameters. These parameters include the vital signs (particularly blood pressure and pulse), urine output, weight changes, skin turgor, mental status, presence of edema, and lung sounds.

In many elderly individuals, especially those with chronic illnesses, the mechanisms responsible for maintaining fluid balance do not function normally. Particularly common in such patients is a weak thirst response. For this reason, these patients must be taught to maintain an adequate fluid intake by recognizing other signs of dehydration, such as concentrated urine and rapid weight loss. Moreover, to help maintain a normal volume and viscosity of respiratory tract secretions, patients with chronic obstructive pulmonary disease must be shown how to adequately humidify their home environment. In general, this is most safely accomplished via evaporative humidification equipment (as opposed to devices that create particulate aerosols). More detail on humidification approaches is provided in Chapter 23.

Removal of pulmonary secretions. Secretions in the pulmonary tract must be kept loose and mobile. If loose, these secretions can be mobilized via various techniques for expectoration or suction. Chest percussion, vibration, and postural drainage enable secretions to be "forced" into the main respiratory passages for easy removal. Patients should be taught abdominal diaphragmatic breathing and coughing exercises to increase inspiratory capacity and stimulate expectoration. These techniques are especially valuable in postoperative patients at risk for the complications of hypoventilation (ie, atelectasis and pneumonia). Postural drainage is a technique that helps mobilize secretions from small airways into larger airways for expectoration or suctioning. Techniques designed to help mobilize secretions are described in detail in Chapter 27.

Psychologic support

The nature of psychologic support given patients depends, in part, on the stage of their illness. In this context, we may differentiate between three general approaches: (1) psychologic support for the patient with an acute, life-threatening illness, (2) psychologic support for the patient with a chronic disorder, and (3) psychologic support for the terminally ill.

Acute conditions. Patients experiencing acute respiratory insufficiency should be cared for according to the general principles of crisis management. A crisis is a time-limited event that leads to disequilibrium. Patients with acute respiratory insufficiency experience an abrupt disequilibrium in meeting their most basic physiologic need, that is, oxygen and carbon dioxide exchange.

Acute conditions generally require physician leadership and a team effort. The practitioner must recognize his or her specific functions in crisis situations and not cause undue duplication of effort. A disorganized, leaderless team is inefficient and may worsen the patient's anxiety. Likewise, an anxious team transfers this anxiety to the patient.

For the respiratory care practitioner, several principles are helpful in dealing with such crises. The first and most important consideration is to initiate all respiratory care interventions in a competent, efficient, and confident manner. Patients experiencing acute respiratory insufficiency need immediate help for survival. During this phase, the practitioner should avoid any actions that might cause additional patient stress, such as demanding additional patient information.

The second principle in crisis management is to ensure that all interventions are explained to the patient during the process. In these situations, decision making is primarily in the hands of the health team. Patients should not be expected to make serious, life-sustaining decisions when experiencing severe respiratory insufficiency. To a great extent, the health team assumes control of, and responsibility for, the patient's survival.

After resolution of the immediate crisis, the patient must be carefully followed. Such follow-up helps determine the most appropriate post-crisis management. During the post-crisis phase, the importance of the patient's subjective responses must not be overlooked. Although patient emotions may have relatively little effect during a life-threatening crisis, these responses can dramatically affect the patient's post-crisis course. For this reason, both objective and subjective data should be obtained to plan the post-crisis management approach. The following specific points bear emphasis:

1. Patients should be fully informed of the specifics of the respiratory crisis. They need to know the cause of the problem, the evolution of it, and the nature of subsequent interventions. Patients need to "decode" the stimuli they experience during their crisis. This will help them better understand their situation in both cognitive and emotional terms.

2. Physical assessment should be conducted regularly to both assess the patient's progress and to monitor the development of potential complications.

3. Assessment should include determination of patients' coping mechanisms and their emotional response to the crisis. Although a crisis typically causes disequilibrium, it can also lead to personal growth. Health team members should foster patients' self-awareness using the techniques of facilitation, clarification, reflection, interpretation, and empathy previously discussed. Patients should be encouraged to talk about the crisis, with the health care professional serving as an active listener. Patients exhibiting unhealthy responses should be referred to other health professionals as required.

For example, denial of a crisis may help the patient survive the immediate episode; however, continued denial may negatively affect patient involvement in post-crisis care, and thus prolong recovery.

4. In cooperation with patients and other health care team members, the practitioner should develop individual post-crisis respiratory care plans. Where appropriate, these plans should include educational as well as therapeutic objectives. Consideration must be given to including each patient's family in this planning process.

Chronic conditions. Patients with chronic respiratory disease face a set of circumstances substantially different from those with acute illnesses. By definition, a chronic disease produces signs and symptoms for variable lengths of time, is associated with a long course, and results in only partial recovery. Chronic respiratory disease may additionally result in some combination of physical, emotional, interpersonal, financial, and social losses.

A major factor involved in the competent care of such individuals is the practitioner's orientation toward chronic disease. All too often, patients with chronic illnesses are "labeled" according to their disability, rather than treated as individuals with unique needs and responses. Ideally, the practitioner should first recognize the patient as a person, and only then as a patient with a specific illness. Respect of the patient's dignity and wishes is critical to effective long-term care.

This individualized approach to chronic disease and disability can be fostered by (1) viewing the patient as an individual, not an illness or a set of symptoms; (2) giving the patient control over his or her life, including participating in the selection of interventions; (3) educating the patient on disease management in the context of his or her home and work environment; and (4) recognizing the patient's priorities as the major determinant of respiratory interventions.

These principles will help the practitioner develop a trusting, therapeutic relationship with the patient. Ultimately, this therapeutic relationship will assist the practitioner in evaluating the patient's self-esteem and aid in the identification of the patient's goals, both short- and long-term.

Finally, patients with chronic illnesses (and their families) must be able to make sound decisions regarding the use of community resources, financial assistance programs, home health agencies, and medical equipment providers. Such choices require accurate and comprehensive information, usually provided by selected members of the health care team. As a critical member of that team, the respiratory care practitioner can play a vital role in the subsequent provision of long-term care. Key components of this care, including patient education, pulmonary rehabilitation, and home care, are discussed in more detail in Chapters 33 to 35.

Terminal illnesses. Research on the dying process indicates that the terminally ill tend to move through a series of common stages, which include denial, anger, depression, bargaining, and acceptance.

Although commonalities in the process have been identified, dying is still a uniquely individual event. For this reason, there are no hard and fast "rules" for providing psychologic support to the terminally ill. Instead, the practitioner responsible for the care of a terminally ill patient should simply strive to (1) help the patient cope with the illness, (2) provide comfort and relief from pain, (3) maintain the patient's dignity and self-worth, and (4) help the patient reach the acceptance stage of the process.

To care for the terminally ill patient, practitioners must first be aware of their own attitudes and feelings about death. Dying patients require humanistic care; however, a practitioner's fear of death may hinder truly open and humane care for the very people who require it most. There are, however, certain aspects of caring that can help patients reach the critical phase of acceptance.

Practitioners must feel comfortable with death and be aware of their own philosophy of life and death. Such awareness on the part of the practitioner can help the patient recognize his or her own beliefs and values regarding death. In addition, practitioners must accept death as the inevitable outcome of caring for the terminally ill. Efforts to prevent death under such circumstances are futile; victory cannot be attained despite current technology. Once this conclusion is reached and agreed to by the health care team, the respiratory care practitioner can relax and fully attend to the patient's individual needs and desires.

Perhaps the most difficult perspective in working with the terminally ill is patience. Unfortunately, our acute care orientation often makes it difficult to be patient with the dying patient. Patience with the dying process is essential if patients are to die in the manner they deem most comfortable. In addition to patience, letting patients die in a self-defined manner, ie, one not defined by the practitioner, requires true sincerity and empathy.

Another important component of psychologic support for the terminally ill is trust. A patient's death will be more comfortable when a trusting relationship has been established with the practitioner. The practitioner should make a commitment to care for the patient throughout the dying process. Beyond providing for the patient's physical needs, caring involves the courage to remain with the patient throughout this process, and to experience the event on a human, as opposed to simply clinical, level. Caring also involves hope, ie, hope that life has been meaningful and that the trusting relationship established between patient and practitioner is of true value.

Unfortunately, the pain and suffering associated with death is often treated with narcotics, sedatives, and tranquilizers, rather than with an open giving of the health care team to the patient. Pain should be treated without fear of addicting the patient; however, drugs need not be given in amounts that cause confusion and lethargy. Providing an appropriate mix of pain relief and caring, members of the health care team may decrease the discomfort associated with a terminal disease process.

Finally, isolating the terminally ill is a problem found in many hospitals. This isolation not only causes loneliness for the patient, but also shields the practitioner from the discomfort associated with dealing with death. Both social and emotional loneliness may develop in patients through hospital rituals that isolate the dying. To provide effective and meaningful care for the terminally ill, practitioners must avoid this tendency toward isolation and directly involve themselves in both the trepidation and reverence that surrounds this most human of all experiences.

SAFETY CONSIDERATIONS

Patient safety must always be a paramount consideration in the delivery of respiratory care. Although the respiratory care practitioner does not usually have full control of the patient environment, efforts must be made to minimize safety hazards and patient risks whenever possible. The key areas of potential risk common to most patients receiving respiratory care are (1) patient movement and ambulation, (2) electrical hazards, and (3) fire hazards.

Patient movement and ambulation

Basic body mechanics. Posture is defined as the relationship of the body parts to each other both in resting and activity states. Good body posture is necessary for psychologic, physiologic, and safety reasons. Improper body posture may affect appearance and place inappropriate stress on certain bones, muscles, and organs. Good body mechanics represent postures to be assumed by patients and practitioners in various activities that minimize the likelihood of injury.

Fig. 13-5 illustrates the correct and incorrect body mechanics for lifting heavy objects. Fig. 13-6 applies this concept to lifting and moving a patient.

Moving the patient in bed. Conscious people assume positions in bed that are most comfortable for them. For example, patients with acute or chronic respiratory dysfunction often assume a high Fowler's position, with arms flexed and thorax leaning forward. This position assists them in attaining maximal inspiration with a minimum of effort. In other cases, however, patients may be required to assume certain positions for therapeutic reasons. Good examples of situations requiring special positioning include neurosurgical patients and patients with hip replacement.

Fig. 13-7 demonstrates the correct technique for lateral movement of a bed-bound patient. Fig. 13-8 illustrates the ideal method for moving a conscious patient toward the head of a bed. Fig. 13-9 shows the proper technique for assisting a patient to the bedside position for dangling or transfer to a chair.

Ambulation. Ambulation is necessary for normal body functioning. Bed rest, even with appropriate passive and/or active range-of-joint movement exercises, produces a myriad of adverse effects on physiology. Progressive am-

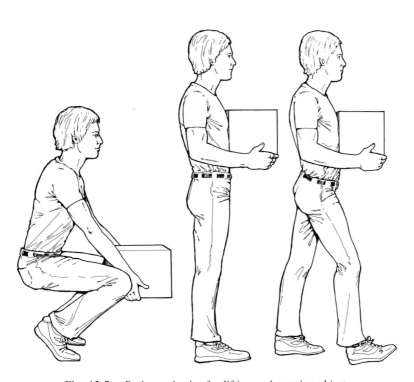

Fig. 13-5   Body mechanics for lifting and carrying objects.

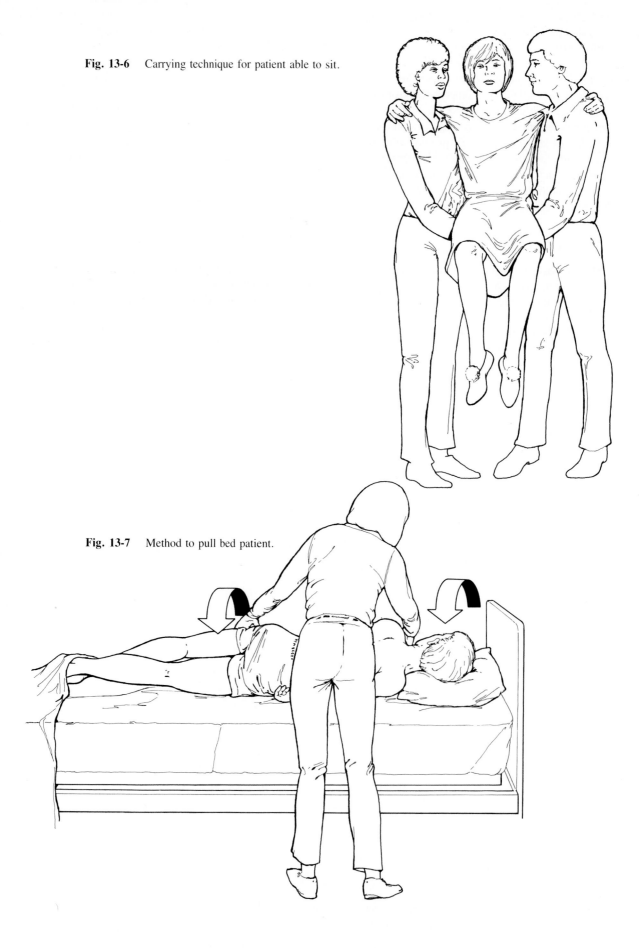

Fig. 13-6   Carrying technique for patient able to sit.

Fig. 13-7   Method to pull bed patient.

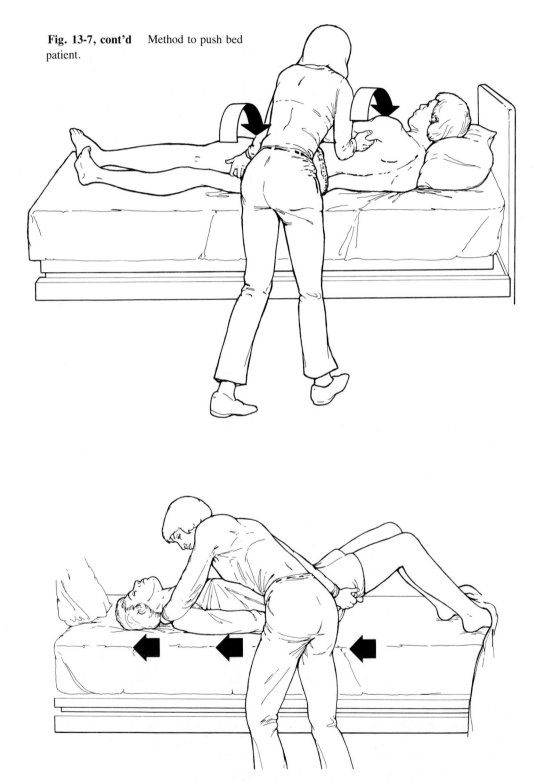

Fig. 13-7, cont'd Method to push bed patient.

Fig. 13-8 Method to move patient up in bed with patient's assistance.

Fig. 13-9   Method to assist in patient dangling at side of bed.

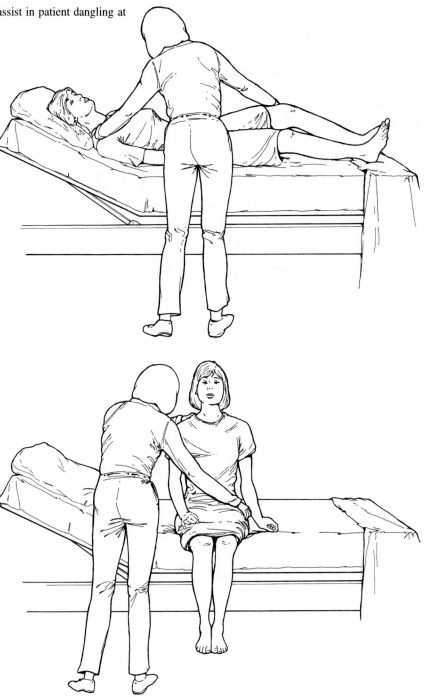

bulation for a hospitalized patient is approached in an orderly and safe fashion by all health team members.

Ambulation is initiated if the patient is physiologically stable and free from severe pain. Thus the patient must be assessed prior to ambulation. The most critical factors necessary for ambulation are stable vital signs and absence of severe pain. Safe patient movement includes the following steps: (1) placing the bed in a low position and locking its wheels; (2) placing all equipment close to the patient to prevent dislodgment during ambulation (eg, intravenous equipment, nasogastric tube, surgical drainage tubes); (3) moving the patient toward the proximal side of bed; (4) assisting the patient to sit in bed (ie, arm under proximal shoulder and one under distal axilla); (5) placing one hand under the patient's distal knee and gradually rotating the patient so that legs are dangling off bed; (6) letting the patient remain in this dangling position until dizziness or light-headedness abate (encouraging the patient to look forward rather than look at the floor may help); (7) assisting the patient to a standing position; (8) encouraging the patient to breathe easily and unhurriedly during this initial change to a standing posture; (9) walking with the patient using no, minimal, or moderate support (ie, moderate support requires the assistance of two practitioners, one on either side of the patient); and (10) limiting walking to approximately 5 to 10 min for the first exercise.

The patient must be monitored during walking. The practitioner should note the patient's level of consciousness, color, breathing, strength or weakness, and complaints throughout the activity. The practitioner should ensure that emergency seats are available if the patient becomes uncomfortable. Patients must be encouraged to progressively ambulate until no assistance is required.

Electrical safety

With the proliferation of electrical equipment in hospitals, the potential for electrical accidents has multiplied. These problems have been compounded by the fact that invasive devices, such as internal catheters and pacemaker wires, make patients more susceptible to the dangers of electric shock. Because respiratory care often involves operation of electrical devices in the presence of electrically susceptible patients, practitioners must understand the fundamentals of electrical safety.

Physiologic effects of electrical current. Current is the primary factor determining the effect of a shock. Voltage and resistance are important only because they determine how much current will flow.

The harmful effects of electrical current depend on (1) the amount of current flowing through the body, (2) the duration with which this current is applied, and (3) the path the current takes through the body.

For example, as long as a person is insulated by normal clothing and shoes and is in a dry environment, a 120 volt (V) shock may be hardly felt. However, if the same person were standing without shoes on a wet floor, the same voltage could prove fatal. This difference in effect is due to differences in the resistance to current and the amount of current that actually flows through the body. In the first case, resistance is high. Therefore, current flow through the body is low. In the second situation, resistance is low, and the current flow is dangerously high.

A shock hazard can exist only if the electrical "circuit" through the body is complete. Even when voltage is applied to an internal conductor, a current will not flow unless there is a second conductor to complete the circuit. Therefore, two electrical connections to the body are required for a person to receive a shock. In electrical devices, these connections typically consist of a "hot" wire and a "neutral" wire. The neutral wire completes the circuit by taking the electrical current to a "ground." A ground is simply a low resistance pathway to a point of zero voltage, such as the earth (thus the term "ground").

Once such a pathway is established, the direction the electrical current takes through the body will determine the extent of the shock hazard. Normally, the skin offers great resistance to the flow of electrical current. However, this resistance is strongly affected by moisture. Depending on the amount of moisture present, electrical resistance across the intact body can vary from over 1 million ohms (for very dry skin) to less than 1000 ohms (for wet skin).

If the high resistance normally offered by dry skin is bypassed, as in patients with pacemaker wires or saline-filled intravascular catheters, current can readily flow into the body, causing damage to its vital organs. Even urinary catheters and catheters used to drain fluid from the body may represent a conducting path. The heart is particularly sensitive to electric shock. Experiments with dogs have demonstrated that ventricular fibrillation can occur when currents as low as 20 microamperes (μA) (one 20 millionth of an ampere) are applied directly to the heart. Although potentially lethal, a current this low is not normally perceptible.

Therefore, according to the pathway current takes through the body and the magnitude of that current, we may differentiate between two different types of shock hazards: *macroshock* and *microshock*. A macroshock hazard exists when a relatively high current (usually greater than 1 milliampere [mA] or 1/1000 ampere [A]) is applied externally to the skin. A microshock hazard, on the other hand, exists when a small, usually imperceptible current (usually less than 1 mA) is allowed to bypass the skin and follow a direct, low-resistance pathway into the body. Patients susceptible to microshock hazards are termed *electrically sensitive* or *electrically susceptible*. Table 13-1 summarizes the differential effect of these two types of electrical shock hazards.

Preventing shock hazards. Most shock hazards are caused by inappropriate or inadequate grounding. These can be eliminated or minimized by attending to a few basic rules regarding patient and equipment grounding.

General precautions. General precautions, applicable to all patient situations, include (1) never grounding the patient and (2) always ensuring that all patient-related equipment is properly grounded.

1. **Do not ground the patient.** The primary purpose of electrical safety measures is to ensure that the patient does not become part of an electrical circuit. If a patient is grounded, he or she can become part of an electrical circuit. In such cases, patient contact with any source of electrical voltage will cause current to flow through the body. Eliminating the electrical path to ground from the patient will eliminate the possibility of current flow. Therefore, ensuring that the patient is isolated from an electrical ground is the first and foremost method of minimizing electrical shock hazards.

Unfortunately, isolating the patient from a ground connection is not always easy. For example, older ECG equipment typically used the right leg lead as a patient ground. Since many patients on continuous ECG monitors have other electrical apparatuses in contact with the body, this is an obvious hazard. Modern ECG monitors overcome this problem via the use of isolation transformers, which isolate the patient from ground.

In addition to ECG equipment, other patient devices, such as indwelling catheters, may close an electrical circuit by providing a conducting pathway to ground. For this reason, all devices connected to a patient should be checked to ensure that the patient is isolated from electrical ground.

2. **Ground electrical equipment near the patient.** All electrical equipment, such as lights, electric bed motors, and monitoring or therapeutic instruments used in patient care, should be connected to grounded outlets with three-wire cords. In these cases, the third (ground) wire prevents the dangerous buildup of voltage that can occur on the metal frames of some electrically powered equipment.

Modern electrical devices used in hospitals are designed so that their frames are grounded, but their connections to the patient are not. In this manner, all electrical devices within the reach of the patient are grounded, but the patient remains isolated from ground. Unfortunately, since the ground wire is simply a protection device and not part of the main circuit, equipment will continue to operate normally even if the ground wire is broken. Therefore, all electrical equipment, particularly those devices used with electrically

susceptible patients, must be checked for appropriate grounding on a regular basis.

For equipment in use, a faulty ground may be revealed by a tingling sensation that occurs when the metal parts of a piece of equipment are touched. The presence of such tingling indicates improper grounding and the possibility of a serious current leakage. In these cases the practitioner must ensure that the faulty equipment is immediately taken out of service.

Precautions for electrically sensitive patients. Additional precautions should be followed by the practitioner when the patient is considered electrically susceptible because of the presence of indwelling catheters or pacemaker wires.

1. **Avoid contact with transcutaneous conductors.** The practitioner should avoid contacting a bare pacemaker wire or the conducting part of a catheter while simultaneously touching any metal object with the other hand. This precaution is necessary to prevent closing the electrical circuit between the patient and a ground. This hazard can be minimized by covering exposed pacemaker wires with a nonconducting material, such as plastic or rubber.

2. **Connect all electrical equipment to a common ground.** If two pieces of electrical equipment have different grounds, a malfunction in one could produce a voltage difference between the two instruments, and thus a flow of current. For this reason the practitioner should make sure that all electrical devices being used with a microshock-sensitive patient are connected to wall outlets having a common low-resistance ground. In most modern hospitals, patient areas have a special

Table 13-1 Effects of Electric Shock

Amperes	Milliamperes (mA)	Microamperes (μA)	Effects
APPLIED TO SKIN (MACROSHOCK)			
6 or more	6000 or more	more than 6,000,000	Sustained myocardial contraction followed by normal rhythm; temporary respiratory paralysis; burns, if small area of contact
0.1 to 2-3	100 to 3000	100,000	Ventricular fibrillation; respiratory center intact
0.050	50	50,000	Pain, fainting, exhaustion,* mechanical injury; heart and respiratory function intact
0.016	16	16,000	"Let go" current, muscle contraction
0.001	1	1000	Threshold of perception; tingling
APPLIED TO MYOCARDIUM (MICROSHOCK)			
		100	Ventricular fibrillation

Physiologic effects of AC shocks applied for one second to the trunk or directly to the myocardium. Duration of exposure and current pathway are major determinants of human response to electrical shock.

electrical panel to which all electrical equipment should be connected. These panels usually provide the optimum in safe grounding for equipment and should be used exclusively for connecting equipment to a power source.

Modern electrical equipment has made possible great advances in health care, and the use of sophisticated electronic devices will undoubtedly increase. The benefits of such devices can be maintained without shock hazards if proper attention is paid to the grounding of equipment and the electrical isolation of the patient from hazardous current paths. The respiratory care practitioner can contribute to this effort by maintaining a close watch on the ground wires of equipment, noting frayed wires or other obvious electrical hazards, and scrupulously following the key precautions just described.

Fire hazards

To start any fire, three conditions must be met: (1) flammable material must be present, (1) oxygen must be present, and (3) the flammable material must be heated to or above its ignition temperature. To the extent that all three conditions are present, the likelihood of a fire is high. On the other hand, removal of one or more of these conditions can prevent a fire from occurring or extinguish a fire once it has started.

Because of the widespread use of oxygen concentrations above those normally found in the ambient atmosphere, the potential for fire is a particularly important consideration in respiratory care. Although oxygen is nonflammable, it greatly accelerates the rate of combustion. The relationship between the burning intensity of a combustible substance and the amount of ambient oxygen is direct but not simple. Burning speed increases with an increase in the concentration of oxygen or with an increase in total pressure of a constant gas concentration. Therefore, both oxygen concentration and partial pressure influence the rate of burning.

The safe application of oxygen demands that flammable materials and potential ignition sources be removed from the vicinity of use. Flammable materials include cotton, wool, polyester fabrics, and bedclothing; paper materials; plastics; and certain lotions or salves, such as petroleum jelly. The most common potential ignition sources are smoking materials, sparks from electrical equipment, or static electrical discharges.

To minimize the fire hazards associated with oxygen use the practitioner should ensure, wherever possible, that flammable materials are not used in its presence. This is particularly important whenever oxygen enclosures, such as tents or croupettes, are used.

In terms of sources of ignition, the practitioner must ensure that smoking is not allowed in rooms where oxygen is in use. Great care must be taken to avoid electrical equipment capable of generating high-energy sparks, such as

exposed switches. Moreover, all appliances that transmit house current should be kept out of oxygen enclosures.

A frequent source of worry is the presence of static electrical sparks generated by the friction of movements of the patient in bed or by uniforms of personnel rubbing against bed clothing. For any spark to ignite flammable material, the spark must be able to generate enough heat energy to start the process.

Studies with oxygen concentrations varying from 21% to 100% show that static electrical sparks applied to such fabrics as vinyl plastic canopies, tissue paper, nylon, wool, cotton, muslin, and dacron-cotton can cause ignition. However, ignition generally occurs only at elevated oxygen concentrations and only with a barrage of sparks at a frequency of 60 per minute. Under no circumstances did a single spark produce a fire.

Such studies suggest that, even in the presence of high oxygen concentrations, the overall hazard from static sparks with the materials in common use is very low. In general, solitary static sparks do not have sufficient heat energy to raise common materials to their flash points. The minimal risk that may be present can be further reduced by maintaining the relative humidity in oxygen enclosures at 60% or greater.

DOCUMENTATION

Legally, documentation of the care given to a patient means that care was rendered; lack of documentation means that care was not given. Hospital accrediting agencies critically evaluate the medical records of patients. Medical records include progress notes, flow sheets, and checklists. Again, if the practitioner does not document care given (ie, patient assessment data, interventions, and evaluation of care rendered), the practitioner and the hospital may be accused of patient neglect. Adequate documentation of care is only valuable in reference to standards and criteria of care. Respiratory care departments, like all departments in health care facilities, must generate their standards of patient care. For each standard, criteria must be delineated against which the adequacy of patient care can be measured. Documentation must reflect these standards.

Documentation should be succinct. Only the single most appropriate word or phrase should be written on medical records. The language must be that universally accepted for the health sciences. For example, abbreviations can only be those of the hospital's accepted abbreviation list. Brevity and use of appropriate language drastically reduce the practitioner's documentation time. The practitioner must document only what is, not one's interpretation or judgment. Assessments of data must be clearly within one's professional domain. When a practitioner is unable to interpret data obtained, it is valuable to state so in the

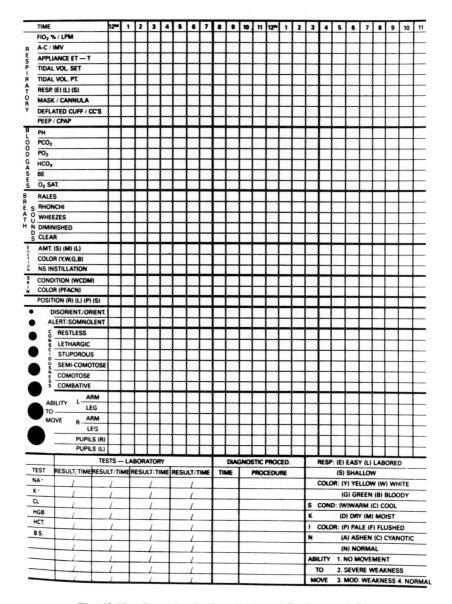

Fig. 13-10   Example of a flow sheet used for documentation.

record and contact another professional for advice or referral.

The problem-oriented medical record (POMR) method of charting is a clear and logical format used by health care professionals to document care. This structured approach calls for information to be written relative to each specific problem identified for the patient. Information relative to each problem is written in the SOAP format as shown in the box on p. 301.

If used correctly by all professionals involved in the care of the patient, the evaluation of a plan is included in the subsequent notations. Flow sheets are designed to succinctly report data and to decrease time in documentation. Fig. 13-10 provides an example of a flow sheet used for documentation. When used properly in conjunction with problem-oriented notes or narrative notes, the flow sheet provides a wealth of valuable data quickly.

An alternate method of documenting is the paragraph or narrative note format. This method employs a separate section in the medical record for notes made by specific groups of professionals. For example, sections will include physicians' notes, nurses' notes, or any notes from members of the health care team. This format is more free flowing than the POMR style. Professionals are charged with documenting succinctly information that would also be contained in the POMR style; however, the information is not labeled according to specific problems. With this format, the burden of logical thinking is on the practitioner. The format of documenting is secondary to the information contained within the notation. Thus clarity, brev-

EXAMPLE OF PROBLEM-ORIENTED RECORD ENTRY

PROBLEM 1: PNEUMONIA

2/12/89   *Subjective:* "My chest hurts when I take a deep breath."

Objective: Awake, alert, oriented to time, place, and person; sitting upright in bed with arms leaning over the bedside stand; pale and dry skin; respirations 26/min, thoracic in nature, shallow; pulse 98/min, regular and faint to palpation; BP 112/68, left arm, sitting position; bronchial breath sounds in lower posterior lung fields; occasionally expectorating thin, cloudy, yellow mucus.

Assessment: Pneumonia continues.

Plan: Therapeutic—assist with coughing and deep breathing at least q 2 hr; humidification treatments q 4 hr; percussion, clapping, and vibration q 4 hr; assist with ambulation as per physician orders and patient tolerance. Diagnostic—continue to monitor lung sounds prior to each treatment. Education—teach to cough and deep breathe; evaluate return demonstration.

ity, and accuracy are demanded in all formats of documentation.

SUMMARY

General patient care is a responsibility shared among all health professionals. The provision of safe, effective, and humane respiratory care demands that practitioners develop and apply these general patient care skills in consistent and considerate ways. Observation and interviewing skills represent a key component of the planning and evaluation process. Patient support techniques attend to the basic physical and psychologic needs of the individual with an acute, chronic, or terminal illness. Safety considerations protect patients from unnecessary risks and hazards. Finally, documentation assures that the care rendered is consistent with applicable professional standards and expectations and is available to all members of the health care team for continuing assessment and monitoring of patient progress.

BIBLIOGRAPHY

Benjamin A: The helping interview, ed 3, Boston, 1980, Houghton Mifflin Co.

Bruner J: Hazards of electrical apparatus, Anesthesiology 28:945-957, 1967.

Cair JB: Communicating and relating, Reading, Mass, 1979, Benjamin Cummings Pub. Co.

Carriere VK, Murdaugh C, and Janson-Bjerklie S: A framework for assessing pulmonary disease categories, Focus Crit Care 11(2):10-16, 1984.

Dalziel CF and Lee WR: Reevaluation of lethal electrical currents, IEEE Transactions on Industry and General Applications, vol IA-4, Sept/Oct 1968, p 467; vol IGA-4, 1968, p 676.

Dalziel CF: Electric shock hazards, IEEE Spectrum 9(2):41, 1972.

Dimond M and Jones SL: Chronic illness across the life span, Norwalk, Conn, 1983, Appleton-Century-Crofts.

Dudley D: Coping with chronic COPD: therapeutic options, Geriatrics 36:69-74, 1981.

Eggland ET: Teaching the ABCs of COPD, Nurs 87 17(1):60-64, 1987.

Enelow AJ and Swisher SN, editors: Interviewing and patient care, ed 3, Oxford, 1985, Oxford University Press.

Froelich RE: Clinical interviewing skills: a programmed manual for data gathering, evaluation, and patient management, St Louis, 1977, The CV Mosby Co.

Hames CC and Doyle HJ: Basic concepts of helping, New York, 1980, Appleton-Century-Crofts.

Hasler ME and Cohen JA: The effect of oxygen administration on oral temperature assessment, Nurs Res 31:265, 1982.

Kaufman JS and Woody JW: For patients with COPD: better living through teaching, Nurs 80 10(3):57-61, 1980.

Lambert VA and Lambert CE: Psychosocial care of the physically ill, Englewood Cliffs, NJ, 1985, Prentice-Hall, Inc.

Lim-Levy F: The effect of oxygen inhalation on oral temperature, Nurs Res 31:151, 1982.

McNett SC: Social support, threat, and coping responses and effectiveness in the functionally disabled, Nurs Res 36:98-103, 1987.

National Fire Protection Association: Safe use of electricity in hospitals, NFPA 76BM, Boston, 19??, The Association.

Nave CR and Nave BC: Physics for the health sciences, Philadelphia, 1985, WB Saunders.

Nerenz DR and Leventhal H: Self regulation in chronic illness. In Burish TG and Bradley LA, editors: Coping with chronic illness, New York, 1984, Academic Press.

Purtilo R: Health professional/patient interaction, ed 2, Philadelphia, 1978, WB Saunders.

Rebuck AS and Pengelly LD: Development of pulsus paradoxus in the presence of airway obstruction, N Engl J Med 288:66, 1973.

Reiser DE and Schmock CI, editors: Patient interviewing: the human dimension, Baltimore, 1980, Williams & Wilkins Co.

Scanlan CL: Electrical safety in respiratory therapy. Part I, Dallas, 1978, American Association for Respiratory Therapy.

Scanlan CL: Electrical safety in respiratory therapy. Part II, Dallas, 1978, American Association for Respiratory Therapy.

Segall A: The sick role concept: understanding illness behavior, J Health Social Behav 17:162-170, 1976.

Seidel HM et al: Mosby's guide to physical examination, St Louis, 1987, The CV Mosby Co.

Starmer CF, Whalen RE, and McIntosh HD: Hazards of electric shock in cardiology, Am J Cardiol 14:537-546, 1964.

Steeves RH and Kahn DL: Experiencing of meaning in suffering, Image 19:114-116, 1987.

Thompson LE: When caring is the only cure: managing the chronically ill patient, Nurs 87 17(1):58-59, 1987.

Ufema JK: How to talk to dying patients, Nurs 87 17(8):43-46, 1987.

Wood LA and Rambo BJ: Nursing skills for allied health services, ed 2, Philadelphia, 1977, WB Saunders.

Yonkman CA: Cool and heated aerosol and the measurement of oral temperature, Nurs Res 31:354, 1982.

Zerwekh JV: Comforting the dying dyspneic patient, Nurs 87 17(11):66-69, 1987.

14

Principles of Infection Control

Craig L. Scanlan
Halcyon St. Hill

Between 5% and 10% of all patients admitted to hospitals acquire an infection during their stay. It is estimated that these nosocomial infections directly increase health care costs by over a billion dollars per year. The indirect costs associated with hospital-acquired infections are even more staggering, amounting to some $5 to $10 billion per year in lost economic productivity.

Between 10% and 40% of all nosocomial infections are pulmonary in nature. Moreover, among all hospital-acquired infections, nosocomial pulmonary infections are those most frequently related to patient mortality. Historically, respiratory care–related equipment and procedures have been identified as a major cause of nosocomial infections. It is therefore essential that respiratory care practitioners be actively involved in efforts to reduce the incidence of hospital-acquired infections.

The incidence of hospital-acquired infections can be reduced only by strict adherence to infection control procedures, including techniques designed to (1) eliminate the sources of infectious agents, (2) create barriers to their transmission, and (3) monitor and evaluate the effectiveness of these control methods.

Effective application of infection control procedures is a major and ongoing responsibility of all respiratory care practitioners. Assumption of this important responsibility requires a general understanding of clinical microbiology and specific knowledge and skill in a variety of infection control procedures. This chapter provides foundation knowledge and skills necessary to fulfill this critical responsibility.

OBJECTIVES

On completion of this chapter the reader should be able to:

1. Apply the major categories of microorganisms to identify and describe those most pathogenic to humans;

2. Describe the three major elements necessary for the spread of infection in general and respiratory infections in particular;

3. Compare and contrast the various infection control methods used in respiratory care equipment processing;

4. Differentiate the various infection control techniques involved in the maintenance of in-use respiratory care equipment, the processing of reusable respiratory care equipment, and the use of fluids and medications;

5. Describe the appropriate use of general barrier methods of infection control;

6. Differentiate the special categories of patient isolation, including acceptable modification of these precautions;

7. Delineate the universal infection control precautions currently recommended by the Centers for Disease Control;

8. Describe the key components of a departmental bacteriologic surveillance program.

KEY TERMS

Most terms used in this chapter are defined in context. The following terms are introduced without explicit definition but may be found in the text glossary.

aerobic	dysphagia
anaerobic	empyema
cationic	endocarditis
CDC	endogenous
cellulitis	eukaryotic
conjunctivitis	extracorporeal
debilitated	facultative
debridement	faucial

gastroenteritis

glomerulonephritis

granulomatous

HIV

immunosuppressed

intrapartum

lymphoma

morphology

myositis

nonmotile

osteomyelitis

otitis media

pediculosis

phagocytosis

pleomorphic

procaryotic

RSV

septicemia

sporicidal

sporulation

tetany

thermophilic

transplacental

uremia

urethritis

virucidal

CLINICAL ASPECTS OF MICROBIOLOGY

Microbiology is the study of microorganisms, including bacteria, viruses, fungi, protozoa, and algae (Fig. 14-1). It is closely related to respiratory care practice in two fundamental ways. First, many disorders of the respiratory system are caused by microorganisms and treated, in part, by antimicrobial drugs. Second, as previously discussed, respiratory care–related equipment and procedures have been identified as a major cause of hospital-acquired infections. For these reasons, respiratory care practitioners must have a sound foundation of knowledge in both the general principles of microbiology and their clinical application.

This section focuses on the clinical aspects of microbiology, specifically those elements most directly related to infection control in the hospital. To this end, we assume that the reader is already familiar with the more general principles of microbiology.

Common infectious agents

All major categories of microorganisms, with the possible exception of the algae, are capable of invading a human host and causing disease. Using the standard classification scheme, we highlight the major infectious agents and describe their importance in both pulmonary medicine and hospital epidemiology.

Bacteria. Bacteria are the most common cause of nosocomial infections in the hospital setting. Bacteria are pro-

caryotic unicellular organisms that range in size from about 0.5 to 40 μm, and are found in three basic shapes: cocci (spherical forms), bacilli (rod-shaped forms), and spirochetes (helical or spiral forms). Identification of bacteria depends on both simple visual categorization by these shapes (morphologic analysis) and more detailed assessment of structural and metabolic characteristics.

Staining methods are one way to help further categorize bacteria. The gram stain takes advantage of differences in the chemical composition of the bacterial cell wall to broadly categorize bacteria into those that retain the initial basic stain after alcohol wash (gram-positive bacteria) and those that do not (gram-negative bacteria). The acid-fast stain (also called the Ziehl-Neelsen stain) is used specifically to help identify organisms in the genus *Mycobacterium*. *Mycobacterium*, such as the tuberculosis bacillus, are categorized as acid-fast organisms because they retain a carbolfuchsin stain even after an acid wash. More sophisticated staining and visualization techniques may be necessary to aid identification of some other bacteria.

Specialized metabolic tests, based on differences in the growth media used, in the metabolic need for oxygen, and in enzyme production, allow further categorization. In this manner, for example, *Staphylococcus aureus* could be identified as a gram-positive cocci that appears singly, paired, or in irregular clusters; produces the catalase and coagulase enzymes; and is capable of fermenting (anaerobically metabolizing) mannitol.

Whereas initial classification by staining can be accomplished immediately, metabolic tests require lengthy periods of culturing, often as long as 18 to 48 hours. In practical terms, these timelines mean that the treatment of an infectious disease must be initiated before final identification of the causative organism.

Table 14-1 summarizes the major bacteria that can be pathogenic to humans. The remainder of this section provides essential information on these infectious agents, grouped according to their major categories.

Gram-positive cocci. The most common respiratory bacterial pathogens in this category are *Staphylococcus aureus*, *Streptococcus pyogenes*, and *Streptococcus pneumoniae*, also known as *Diplococcus pneumoniae*.

Fig. 14-1 Branches of microbiology.

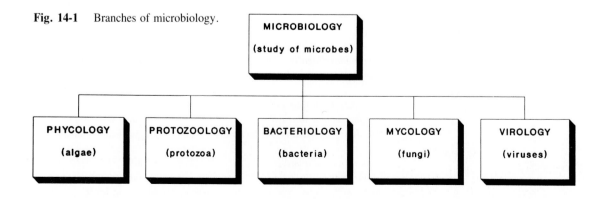

S aureus is an aerobic or facultative aerobic organism that is part of the normal flora of the skin and respiratory tracts. It is a common cause of skin disorders, but is also implicated in pneumonia and other organ or systemic infections, especially in the elderly, neonates, and those debilitated by other disease processes. It is easily killed via normal sterilization processes and is susceptible to most physical and chemical disinfectants. Outside the hospital, treatment of *S aureus* infection is usually with penicillin. *S aureus* strains causing in-hospital infections tend to be penicillin resistant. For this reason, nosocomial *Staphylococcus* infections usually are treated with penicillinase-resistant derivatives such as oxacillin and nafcillin.

Most streptococci are facultative anaerobes. Lansfield groups A, B, C, D, and G are the most common human pathogens. Group A beta-hemolytic streptococci, or *S pyogenes,* cause most human infections, including rheumatic fever, endocarditis, glomerulonephritis, septicemia, and scarlet fever. *S pneumoniae,* an alpha-hemolytic organism, is the primary cause of pneumococcal pneumonia, but is also responsible for acute infectious bronchitis, peritonitis, meningitis, and otitis media. Streptococci are readily killed in normal sterilization processes and are susceptible to most physical and chemical disinfectants. The primary drug used in the treatment of streptococcal infections is penicillin, with erythromycin and the cephalosporins employed as alternative antimicrobial agents.

Gram-negative cocci. The clinically important gram-negative cocci are *Neisseria gonorrhoeae* (the gonococcus) and *Neisseria meningitidis* (the meningococcus). Both are facultatively anaerobic to aerobic diplococci, growing best in an atmosphere of 3% to 10% carbon dioxide. *N gonorrhoeae* is the cause for the sexually transmitted gonorrhea infection. *N meningitidis* causes meningitis, but can also cause septicemia, especially in susceptible hosts. These gram-negative diplococci are readily killed in normal ster-

Table 14-1   Major Pathogenic Bacteria

Category	Organism	Disease
Gram-positive cocci	*Staphylococcus aureus*	Skin infections, pneumonia, enteritis
	Streptococcus pyogenes	Pharyngitis, rheumatic fever
	Streptococcus pneumoniae	Pneumonia, meningitis
Gram-negative cocci	*Neisseria gonorrhoeae*	Gonorrhea
	Neisseria meningitidis	Meningitis
Gram-negative coccobacilli	*Haemophilus influenzae*	Meningitis, pneumonia, epiglottitis
	Bordetella pertussis	Whooping cough
	Brucella	Brucellosis
Gram-positive spore-forming bacilli	*Bacillus anthracis*	Anthrax
	Bacillus cerus	Endocarditis
	Clostridium tetani	Tetanus
	Clostridium perfringens	Gas gangrene
	Clostridium botulinum	Botulism
Gram-positive non-spore-forming bacilli	*Corynebacterium diphtheriae*	Diphtheria
Gram-negative bacilli	*Escherichia coli*	Pneumonia, diarrhea, sepsis
	Klebsiella pneumoniae	Pneumonia, diarrhea, sepsis
	Serratia marcescens	Pneumonia, sepsis
	Shigella dysenteriae	Diarrhea, dysentery
	Salmonella typhi	Diarrhea, sepsis
	Proteus vulgaris	Pneumonia, sepsis
	Pseudomonas aeruginosa	Pneumonia, sepsis
	Bacteroides fragalis	Endocarditis, pneumonia
	Legionella pneumophilia	Legionellosis
Acid-fast bacilli	*Mycobacterium tuberculosis*	Tuberculosis (classic)
	Mycobacterium kansasii	Atypical tuberculosis
	Mycobacterium avium-intracellulare	Atypical tuberculosis
Spirochetes	*Treponema pallidum*	Syphilis
	Leptospirae	Conjunctivitis
	Borrelia	Recurrent fever

ilization processes and are susceptible to most physical and chemical disinfectants. Treatment of *N gonorrhoeae* infections is usually with penicillin G or ampicillin. *N meningitidis* can also be managed with penicillin, usually in combination with chloramphenicol.

Gram-negative coccobacilli. Morphologically, some bacteria fall between the cocci and bacilli in shape. These are called coccobacilli. The coccobacilli most often implicated as human pathogens are gram-negative, facultative, nonmotile organisms capable of capsule formation. Because the capsule protects these organisms against the action of certain key body defense mechanisms, such as phagocytosis, the encapsulated forms are more virulent than the noncapsulated forms.

Haemophilus influenzae is the most important gram-negative coccobacilli responsible for respiratory infections. In its encapsulated form, *H influenzae* is the primary cause of bacterial meningitis in small children. *H influenzae* is also a cause of pneumonia, bronchitis, epiglottitis, and otitis media in children.

The noncapsulated form of *H influenzae* is commonly found as part of the normal flora of the upper respiratory tract. For this reason, most adult infections with *H influenzae* occur in hosts with compromised defense mechanisms. *H influenzae* is readily killed through normal sterilization processes and is susceptible to most physical and chemical disinfectants. Existing *H influenzae* infections are treated with ampicillin, chloramphenicol, or the cephalosporins.

Other gram-negative coccobacilli of clinical importance are *Bordetella pertussis* and the *Brucella* species. *B pertussis* causes whooping cough, a highly communicable disease that, if not treated, can be fatal, especially in infants. Currently, the best treatment is prevention by immunization, although this approach is not without hazard. Once infected with *B pertussis,* patients are usually treated with erythromycin, tetracycline, and chloramphenicol.

Brucella species are primarily pathogenic to animals and only secondarily to humans. Cattle, pigs, sheep, and goats are carriers of this species. In humans, infection with *Brucella* organisms is called brucellosis, or undulant fever. Tetracycline and streptomycin are the antibiotics of choice.

Gram-positive bacilli. Gram-positive bacilli are further divided into two major categories: those that form spores and those that do not.

Gram-positive spore-forming bacilli. Bacterial sporulation is a protective mechanism that increases the resistance of the organism to adverse environmental conditions. The protoplasm within a bacterial spore can stay alive for many years. For example, most vegetative bacteria (non-spore-forming bacilli) cannot endure temperatures beyond 150°F. On the other hand, some spore-forming bacilli can withstand live steam at 212°F for or more. Spore-forming bacteria also are highly resistant to certain chemical disinfectants that easily kill vegetative bacteria.

Two clinically significant genera of bacilli are capable of spore formation: the genus *Bacillus* and the genus *Clostridium. Bacillus* organisms are mainly aerobic, although some are facultative. *Bacillus anthracis* is the most virulent, causing anthrax in both animals and humans. Invasion of the blood or respiratory system with this organism can have fatal consequences. The pulmonary infection is characterized by severe edema and hemorrhaging. Septicemia may also occur. Penicillin or erythromycin are the antibiotics of choice for anthrax infections. *Bacillus cerus* is the more common but less virulent pathogen in this genus. This organism has been associated with endocarditis, pulmonary and wound infections, and food poisoning. As with anthrax, treatment is with penicillin or erythromycin.

Clostridium organisms are obligate anaerobes. The three most common organisms in this genus that are pathogenic to humans are *Clostridium tetani* (the cause of tetanus), *Clostridium perfringens* (one of the causes of gas gangrene), and *Clostridium botulinum* (the cause of botulism).

C tetani is found mainly in the soil, but may exist in the human intestinal tract. The organism gains entry to the body through piercing wounds or abrasions. Toxins produced by the organism cause tetany of certain skeletal muscle groups. Without treatment, tetanus can result in death from respiratory failure. Treatment involves prompt administration of the tetanus antitoxin, with concurrent use of anticonvulsants and sedatives (see Chapter 19). Mechanical ventilation may be necessary to support some victims.

C perfringens also enters the body through deep wounds, causing either an anaerobic cellulitis (not severe) or anaerobic myositis (true gas gangrene). Toxemia and death may result from the later type of infection. Gas gangrene is treated by wound debridement in conjunction with administration of tetracycline and penicillin. Oxygen under pressure (hyperbaric oxygen) may also be useful in limiting further tissue involvement.

C botulinum causes botulism, a noninfectious disease caused by ingestion of the potent toxin produced by this organism. The toxin affects the cranial nerves, causing double vision, dizziness, dysphagia, and respiratory embarrassment, potentially leading to respiratory failure. As with tetanus, botulism is treated with an antitoxin (see Chapter 19). Since introduction of this antitoxin, mortality rates for botulism have dropped from near 60% to as low as 12%. Prevention, however, remains the first line of defense, involving careful food preparation and preservation.

In their spore phase, spore-forming bacilli are the most difficult microorganisms to kill. Steam autoclaving or ethylene oxide sterilization provides the only absolute assurance that these resistant forms of life are destroyed. The difference between true sterilization and disinfection is defined in terms of sporicidal action. Although some chemical solutions can kill spore-forming bacilli, exposure times are often too lengthy to be practical.

Gram-positive non-spore-forming bacilli. Corynebacterium diphtheriae is the most important organism in this category. Facultative, nonmotile, and pleomorphic (many-shaped), *C diphtheriae* is the causative agent for diphtheria, both the cutaneous form and the more familiar respiratory (or faucial) disease. Invasion of the mucous membranes of the upper respiratory tract produces the typical gray-white pseudomembranous coating that leads to life-threatening upper airway obstruction. Typical treatment of the acute disease includes establishment of an emergency endotracheal airway and diphtheria antitoxin, followed by a regimen of erythromycin or the cephalosporins.

C diphtheriae is readily killed through normal sterilization processes and is susceptible to most physical and chemical disinfectants. Widespread immunization against diphtheria in the US has greatly decreased the incidence of this disease.

Gram-negative enteric bacilli. Gram-negative enteric bacilli, also called coliform bacteria, are found in the digestive tract of all animals, including humans. Most are facultative anaerobes belonging to the family Enterobacteriaceae. Some produce toxins generically called bacteriocins. Among the most important of the enteric bacteria are *Escherichia coli, Klebsiella pneumoniae, Serratia marcescens, Shigella dysenteriae,* and members of the *Proteus* and *Salmonellae* genera. Members of the family Pseudomonadaceae will also be described here. Although not true enterics, the Pseudomonadaceae are often isolated in screening procedures for coliforms and lead to infections similar to those caused by the Enterobacteriaceae.

E coli is part of the normal flora of the intestinal tract, and normally is not pathogenic. *E coli* is a common cause of urinary tract infections and can result in pneumonia, neonatal meningitis, and septicemia in debilitated or immunosuppressed patients. *E coli* can also cause a dysentery-like intestinal infection.

K pneumoniae is an opportunistic organism that frequently colonizes the upper respiratory tract of hospitalized patients. Lower respiratory tract invasion, commonly secondary to a pre-existing pneumonia of other origin, can cause a severe secondary pneumonia with tissue necrosis. *K pneumoniae* can also cause septicemia in exposed children. It is resistant to many antibiotics, but the cephalosporins and chloramphenicol have been used with variable success.

S marcescens can often be cultured from "aseptic" solutions used to fill humidifiers and nebulizers and is also commonly isolated from the hands of hospital personnel. Also opportunistic in nature, it commonly causes a primary infection in patients with indwelling catheters and a secondary infection among those being treated for gram-positive pneumonias. Gentamicin is the antimicrobial of choice.

S dysenteriae and members of the *Salmonella* genera all cause intestinal infection via the ingestion of contaminated food or water. *Salmonella typhi* causes dysentery, gastroenteritis, and typhoid fever, a systemic disease. Infection with *S dysenteriae* also causes gastroenteritis and may result in septicemia. Systemic salmonellosis is treated mainly with chloramphenicol, while *Shigella* infections respond best to ampicillin.

Proteus infections, on the other hand, are normally spread by direct contact, causing secondary intestinal, urinary, and respiratory tract infections. *Proteus* infections respond best to ampicillin, cephalothin, or the aminoglycosides.

Gram-negative enteric bacilli are readily killed through normal sterilization processes and are susceptible to most physical and chemical disinfectants. However, the enterics are highly resistant to lesser forms of infection control, such as bacteriostatic detergents. Some species even thrive in certain soap and detergent solutions!

Of all the members of the family Pseudomonadaceae, *Pseudomonas aeruginosa* is the most significant. *P aeruginosa* is a motile, aerobic bacillus commonly found in soil and water. In the hospital, it can be cultured from sinks, soap trays, drinking water, food, and respiratory care equipment. It is estimated that 10% or more of hospital-acquired infections are caused by this opportunistic organism, which is particularly virulent among burn patients and those receiving immunosuppressive drugs. *P aeruginosa* is highly resistant to many antibiotics, with carbenicillin, gentamicin, and the cephalosporins among the few effective antimicrobial agents.

Gram-negative anaerobic bacilli. Gram-negative anaerobic bacilli are the most numerous group of microorganisms in the human intestinal tract and the oral cavity. *Bacteroides* organisms are the most common gram-negative, obligate anaerobe rods involved in hospital-acquired infections. *Bacteroides* organisms can cause a wide variety of localized infections, including endocarditis, osteomyelitis, pneumonia, empyema, and urinary tract infections. Systemic *Bacteroides* infections can occur following perforation of abdominal viscera or after septic abortion. Because this species is particularly slow-growing, *Bacteroides* infections are often not recognized. Antimicrobial treatment of *Bacteroides* infections includes clindamycin for *Bacteroides fragilis,* and erythromycin and chloramphenicol for other species. Gram-negative anaerobic bacilli such as *Bacteroides* are readily killed through normal sterilization processes and are susceptible to most physical and chemical disinfectants.

Legionella pneumophilia. *L pneumophilia* is an aerobic bacillus that stains poorly and appears to be gram-negative. It is treated separately here because it does not grow on common culture media and is difficult to identify. It appears to colonize in water and has been found in air-conditioning units, shower heads, and respiratory care equipment. The infection does not appear to be communicable between patients and is probably acquired by direct inhalation of aerosols carrying the organism. *L pneumophilia* causes a high fever, chills, myalgia, nausea, and diarrhea, and can progress to a life-threatening pneumonia (see Chapter 19). Treatment is usually with erythromycin, although tetracycline and rifampin may be used. *L pneumophilia* is readily killed via normal sterilization processes and is susceptible to most physical and chemical disinfectants.

Acid-fast bacilli (Mycobacteria). Acid-fast bacilli, such as *Mycobacterium tuberculosis*, are non-spore-forming, nonmotile, small aerobic organisms found throughout the environment. In addition to *M tuberculosis*, other acid-fast bacilli pathogenic to humans include *Mycobacterium kansasii*, *Mycobacterium avium-intracellulare*, and *Mycobacterium leprae*.

M tuberculosis causes the chronic granulomatous infection most often localized to the lung. Pulmonary tuberculosis is classically transmitted by aerosol droplets and droplet nuclei produced by coughing. Although much less common, *M kansasii* and *M avium-intracellulare* produce similar infections, but are usually spread through contaminated water. As such, they have caused nosocomial infections among patients undergoing invasive procedures like renal dialysis and extracorporeal circulation.

Both *M tuberculosis* and *M kansasii* are treated with a combination of agents, including isoniazid, rifampin, pyrazinamide, and ethambutol. A vaccine (bacille Calmette-Guérin, or BCG) can immunize individuals against *M tuberculosis* (see Chapter 19). Formerly a rare form of mycobacterial infection, *M avium-intracellulare* is now appearing with some frequency among AIDS patients and is highly resistant to most antimicrobials. All mycobacteria can be killed by normal sterilization processes. However, with the exception of the spore-formers, mycobacteria are significantly more resistant to chemical disinfection than most other bacteria.

Spirochetes. Spirochetes pathogenic to humans belong mainly to the family Spirochaetaceae. These include members of the genera *Treponema*, *Borrelia*, and *Leptospira*. *Treponema pallidum* causes the sexually transmitted disease syphilis, which is treated successfully with penicillin. Members of the genus *Borrelia* are transmitted by insect vectors and can cause an infectious process characterized by recurrent fever. *Borrelia* infections are treated with erythromycin or tetracycline.

Leptospira species can cause infection of the central nervous system, kidneys, liver, or lungs. Direct contact with infected rats or contaminated water is the most common source of infection. Penicillin, tetracycline, and streptomycin are the antibiotics of choice.

Viruses. Viruses are the smallest identified organisms. For example, the polio virus is less than 0.03 μm in diameter. Viruses are obligate intracellular parasites, consisting solely of a core of nucleic acid surrounded by a lipoprotein coat. Viruses replicate by invading host cells through the cell membrane. Depending on the virus involved, these infections can be transmitted by essentially all common routes.

Although some antiviral drugs exist, immunization is currently the most important approach in controlling viral infections. All pathologic viral agents are killed via normal sterilization processes; most are susceptible to common physical and chemical disinfection processes.

Viruses may be classified according to either their structure or nucleic acid composition. In terms of nucleic acid composition, there are two basic categories: DNA viruses and RNA viruses (Table 14-2).

The major pathogenic DNA viruses are smallpox (variola), herpes simplex, hepatitis, varicella-zoster, the Epstein-Barr virus, and the adenoviruses. Herpes simplex causes a variety of human infections, including genital and neonatal herpes. Hepatitis infections are of two major types: A and B. Type A, or infectious hepatitis, is normally transmitted via contaminated food, water, milk (the vehicle route), or by contact with contaminated blood. Type B, or serum hepatitis, is transmitted mainly through contact with contaminated blood or body fluids. Of the two, hepatitis B causes the most severe infections, with mortality rates of 10% or more. Varicella-zoster virus is the cause of chickenpox and shingles. Epstein-Barr virus is the major causative agent in infectious mononucleosis. The adenoviruses, of which there are over 30 immunologic types, are a common source of both childhood infections and endemic respiratory tract infections in adults.

The most common disease-producing RNA viruses are the rhinoviruses, responsible for over a third of all upper respiratory tract infections. More virulent RNA viruses include those causing influenza; the respiratory syncytial, parainfluenza, and coxsackie viral infections; measles; mumps; rubella (German measles); poliomyelitis; rabies; encephalitis; yellow fever; and the human immunodeficiency virus (HIV) responsible for the acquired immune deficiency syndrome (AIDS).

Influenza viruses are of three major types: A, B, and C. Type B is the most common cause of yearly influenza epidemics, for which immunization is the only prevention. Influenza epidemics are a major source of concern in hospital infection control because of the effect of the infection on debilitated patient groups, especially those with pre-existing chronic lung disease. The parainfluenza virus, related to the mumps virus, is a common cause of croup (laryngotracheal bronchitis) in infants. Respiratory syncytial virus (RSV) is the predominant cause of bronchiolitis in children less than 1 year old.

The human immunodeficiency virus (HIV) responsible for AIDS alters the body's immune response by directly attacking the T lymphocytes (including the T helper cells) of the immune system (see Chapter 19). Current epidemiologic and laboratory knowledge indicates that the transmission of AIDS is limited to one of three routes: (1) sexual contact, (2) parenteral exposure via contaminated intravenous needles, and (3) transplacental and/or intrapartum perinatal exposure. Transfusion with contaminated blood is also a risk factor. However, recent implementation of mandatory serologic testing of donated blood for HIV antibodies has dramatically reduced the risk of this route as a source of transmission.

Given the high probability of exposure of certain hospital personnel to blood and body fluids, both the hepatitis B and, more recently, the HIV viruses have become the focus of hospital infection control efforts. Infection of hospital personnel with the hepatitis B virus occurs at a rate some ten times greater than in the general population, mainly through contact with contaminated blood, blood products, or other body fluids. In most cases, overt carelessness or neglect of standard infection control protocols has been identified as the reason for acquisition of the hepatitis B infection. Nonetheless, given the fact that exposure to hepatitis B is not entirely preventable, it is recommended that all health care personnel at high risk be immunized against this viral agent.

Regarding the HIV virus, data gathered recently by the Centers for Disease Control (CDC) indicates (1) that AIDS is no more prevalent among health care personnel than in the general population and (2) that 95% of the health care

personnel who have contracted AIDS probably did so through high-risk behaviors (such as drug abuse or extensive homosexual contact) not associated with their jobs. As with hepatitis B, the incidence of AIDS among health care workers not exhibiting high-risk behaviors has been attributed mainly to carelessness or neglect of infection control procedures. Unfortunately, at the time of this writing, no human vaccine exists for the HIV virus.

Clearly, transmission of these blood and body fluid-borne viral agents in the hospital is preventable, but only with rigorous and careful adherence to specified infection control protocols. More details on the methods for preventing transmission of infections via the blood and body fluid route in general, and those applicable to AIDS in particular, are provided later in this chapter.

Rickettsiae and chlamydiae. Like viruses, rickettsiae and chlamydiae are both obligate intracellular parasites, meaning they require a living host for replication. However, unlike viruses, both exhibit a cellular organization more like bacteria. Both are extremely small organisms, generally less than a μm in size. Transmission of rickettsiae is mainly via the vector (insect) route, whereas chlamydiae may be transmitted via the airborne route (psittacosis) or via direct contact, particularly genital.

Table 14-2 Viruses that Cause Disease in Humans

Virus	Acid	Transmission route	Diseases
Influenza	RNA	Respiratory tract	Tracheobronchitis, pneumonia, susceptibility to bacterial pneumonia
Parinfluenza	RNA	Respiratory tract	Upper respiratory disease, croup, pneumonia
Respiratory Syncytial	RNA	Respiratory tract	Bronchitis Bronchiolitis, pneumonia
Measles	RNA	Respiratory tract	Rash, systemic illness, pneumonia, encephalomyelitis
Mumps	RNA	Respiratory tract	Parotitis, orchitis, pancreatitis, encephalitis
Adeno	DNA	Respiratory tract, conjunctivae	Tracheobronchitis, pharyngitis, conjunctivitis
Rhino	RNA	Respiratory tract	Mild upper respiratory tract, "colds"
Coxsackie	RNA	? Respiratory tract ? Gut	Systemic, meningitis, tracheobronchitis, myocarditis
Hepatitis	DNA	Gut	Hepatitis, systemic disease
Rabies	RNA	Bites, or saliva on cut	Fatal CNS damage
Polio	RNA	Gut, CNS	Systemic damage
Herpes simplex	DNA	Oral, genital, eye	Blisters, latent infection, keratoconjunctivitis
Varicella	DNA	Respiratory tract	Vesicles (all ectodermal tissues), skin, mouth, respiratory tract
Rubella	RNA	Respiratory tract	Systemic mild illness, rash, congenital anomalies in embryo
Cytomegalovirus	DNA	Not known	Usually latent disseminated disease in newborn and "crippled host"
HIV	RNA	Blood, body fluids	AIDS

The common rickettsial diseases affecting humans, including their etiologic agents and vectors, are summarized in Table 14-3. Ninety percent of all rickettsial infections in the US are Rocky Mountain spotted fever, caused by *Rickettsia rickettsii*. Antimicrobial treatment includes a regimen of tetracycline and chloramphenicol.

Chlamydial diseases are less common in the US than those caused by rickettsiae. However, *Chlamydia trachomatis*, the infectious agent in trachoma, is the most common cause of blindness in the world. *C trachomatis* can also result in a nongonococcal urethritis and newborn conjunctivitis (by contact with the mother's genital tract). *Chlamydia psittaci* causes psittacosis (ornithosis), a highly infectious pneumonia transmitted by contact with parrots, parakeets, pigeons, and other birds. Chlamydial infections are normally treated with tetracycline.

Organisms belonging to the genera rickettsiae and chlamydiae are readily killed through normal sterilization processes and are susceptible to most physical and chemical disinfectants.

Mycoplasmas. Mycoplasmas were first identified as causative agents in a severe pneumonia affecting cattle. They were originally thought to be viruses because of their extremely small size and resultant ability to pass through bacterial filters. However, like bacteria, mycoplasmas grow on artificial media.

Mycoplasmas, formerly known as pleuropneumonia-like organisms or PPLO, have no rigid cell wall, are pleomorphic, and do not retain the gram stain. *Mycoplasma pneumoniae* is the primary pathogen in this genus, causing primary atypical pneumonia. The infection is spread mainly by contact with respiratory tract secretions and treated by tetracycline or erythromycin. Identification of the organism is difficult, usually requiring comparative serologic studies. Mycoplasmas are readily killed through normal sterilization processes and are susceptible to most physical and chemical disinfectants.

Fungi. The fungi include both molds and yeasts. Fungi are ubiquitous organisms, having a preference for warm, moist environments such as found in the hospital. As compared with bacteria, fungi are much larger and possess a more complex and highly organized structure (eukaryotic cell structure). They may reproduce either sexually by fusion or asexually by spore formation.

Fungal infections, called mycoses, are of two general types: (1) those that occur in otherwise healthy individuals and (2) those associated with decreased host resistance (opportunistic infections). Primary fungal infections occurring in otherwise healthy people include those caused by *Coccidioides immitis, Histoplasma capsulatum, Blastomyces dermatitidis,* and *Cryptococcus neoformans*. Common opportunistic fungal infections include those caused by *Candida albicans, Aspergillus fumigatus,* and *Nocardia asteroides*. Opportunistic fungal infections are a major problem in most hospital settings because of the large number of debilitated and immunosuppressed patients.

Fungi are readily killed through normal gas or autoclave sterilization processes and are susceptible to most physical and chemical disinfectants. Table 14-4 summarizes the common infectious fungal disorders.

Protozoa. Protozoal infections are prevalent in many tropical areas of the world and may also be found under conditions of crowding and poor sanitation. Amebiasis, malaria, and trypanosomiasis are examples of these protozoal infections. Because of their unique distribution, their importance in US hospital infection control is minimal.

Recently, however, a protozoal-type organism called *Pneumocystis carinii* has gained substantial attention as an opportunistic infection in patients with an abnormal or altered immunologic status, particularly those suffering from the acquired immune deficiency syndrome (AIDS).

Pneumocystis carinii is most probably a protozoan with both intracellular and intercellular life stages. Infection with *P carinii* causes an acute interstitial pneumonia with fatality rates in excess of 50%. Treatment is with co-trimoxazole or pentamidine isethionate. Pneumocystis appears to be killed via normal sterilization processes. However, because of difficulty in isolating this organism, its susceptibility to common physical and chemical disinfectants has not undergone evaluation.

Table 14-3   Rickettsial Diseases of Humans

Group	Principal diseases	Etiologic agent	Reservoir in nature	Usual occurrence
Typhus	Epidemic typhus	*Rickettsia prowazekii*	Man, lice	Worldwide winter and spring
	Murine typhus	*Rickettsia mooseri*	Rats and rat fleas	Worldwide where rats abound
Spotted fever	Rocky Mountain spotted fever	*Rickettsia rickettsii*	Ticks	North and South America
	Rickettsial pox	*Rickettsia akari*	Mite	New York City, Boston
Q fever	Q fever	*Rickettsia burnetii (Coxiella burnetii)*	Ticks; infected cattle and sheep	Probably worldwide
Trench fever	Trench fever	*Rickettsia quintana*	Body lice, humans	Europe, Africa, North America

SPREAD OF INFECTION

Three elements must be present for an infection to spread: a source of infecting organisms, a susceptible host, and a mode of organism transmission.

Source

The primary sources of infectious agents in the hospital are people (patients, personnel, or visitors) and inanimate objects that have become contaminated, such as equipment and medications. People may have an acute disease, may be in the incubation period of the disease, or may simply be colonized by an infectious agent, with no apparent symptoms. People may also serve as their own source of infectious agents via endogenous flora. This latter mechanism is called *autogenous* infection.

Microorganisms differ in their relative pathogenicity or virulence. Highly virulent organisms need only be present in small numbers to cause an infectious response. On the other hand, microorganisms that are relatively avirulent must be present in extremely large numbers to cause infection in an immunocompromised host.

Most cases of nosocomial pneumonia are caused by bacteria. Aerobic gram-negative bacilli and aerobic gram-pos-itive cocci each account for approximately 40% of all reported cases of nosocomial pneumonia.

Host

The mere presence and growth of microorganisms in a host, without tissue invasion, damage, or toxin response, is called *colonization*. Whether a colonized patient actually develops an infection depends on the relative virulence of the organism and the host's resistance to the infectious agent present.

Patients' resistance to infectious agents varies greatly. Some individuals may be immune or able to resist colonization by a pathogenic organism. Others exposed to the same infecting organism may become asymptomatic carriers. Still others may develop clinical disease. Persons with diabetes mellitus, lymphoma, leukemia, neoplasia, or uremia and those treated with certain antimicrobials, corticosteroids, irradiation, or immunosuppressive agents may be particularly susceptible to infection. Age, chronic debilitating disease, shock, coma, traumatic injury, or surgical procedures also increase the susceptibility of patients to infection.

The high incidence of gram-negative bacterial pneumo-

Table 14-4   Major Fungal Infections

Organism	Disease	Comments
Coccidioides immitis	Coccidioidomycosis	Also called San Joaquin fever because of prevalence in southwest US; initial illness like influenza; some patients progress to severe systemic infection; transmission via airborne dusts
Cryptococcus neoformans	Cryptococcosis	Also known as torulosis; acquired via contact with bird excreta; causes solitary pulmonary nodule in most cases; may progress to fatal meningoencephalitis in some
Histoplasma capsulatum	Histoplasmosis	Acquired via contact with soil containing fecal matter from birds and bats; prevalent in Mississippi valley area; mimics tuberculosis
Blastomyces dermatitidis	Blastomycosis	Acquired via contact with soil contaminated with animal feces; frequently disseminates to skin, bones, GI tract, kidneys, and brain
Candida albicans	Candidiasis	Occurs almost exclusively in immunosuppressed patients; similar in presentation to tuberculosis; may disseminate to brain and meninges
Aspergillus fumigatus	Aspergillosis	Occurs in three forms: (1) allergic, (2) invasive (common in immunosuppressed patients or those with hematologic malignancies), and (3) "fungus ball" or aspergilloma colonization in pulmonary cavitary lesions; invasive form is the most serious

nias in the hospital is believed to be the result of factors that promote colonization of the pharynx with these organisms. Colonization dramatically increases in patients with severe underlying illness and predisposes such patients to gram-negative pneumonias.

In terms of nosocomial pneumonias in general, three fourths of cases occur in patients who have had surgical operations, especially those involving the chest or abdomen. In such patients, impairment of normal swallowing and respiratory clearance mechanisms allows bacteria to enter and remain in the lower respiratory tract. Instrumentation of the respiratory tract, anesthesia, surgical pain, and use of narcotics and sedatives all increase the susceptibility of the host.

The risk of pneumonia is not the same for all surgical patients. Patients at highest risk include the elderly, the severely obese, those with chronic obstructive pulmonary disease or a history of smoking, and those with an artificial airway in place for prolonged periods of time.

Patients with an artificial airway (endotracheal or tracheostomy tube) are at high risk for acquiring a nosocomial pneumonia for several reasons. Typically, patients requiring prolonged intubation or a tracheostomy already have one or more factors predisposing to infection, such as severe chronic obstructive lung disease. Another risk factor may be increased upper airway colonization with aerobic gram-negative bacteria. Moreover, since the artificial airway bypasses the normal protective mechanisms of the upper airway, bacteria are afforded greater access to the lower respiratory tract. Finally, manipulation of these tracheal tubes increases the likelihood of cross-contamination, particularly during suctioning procedures.

Pneumonia resulting from certain pathogens occurs primarily in immunocompromised hosts. Immunosuppression may be pharmacologically induced, as in patients who have received a renal transplant, or may result from an underlying disease process, such as AIDS. Regardless of underlying cause, immunocompromised hosts are particularly likely to develop opportunistic pneumonias caused by (1) viruses (such as cytomegalovirus), (2) parasites (such as *P carinii*), or (3) fungi (such as *C albicans*).

Transmission

Transmission of microorganisms occurs via four major routes: contact, vehicle, airborne, and vectorborne. Some microorganisms may be transmitted by more than one route. For example, the HIV virus can spread either by direct contact (sexual intercourse) or by indirect contact with a contaminated inanimate object (needles). Examples of the common routes for transmission of selected microorganisms are provided in Table 14-5.

Contact transmission. Contact transmission is the most important and most frequent route for transmission of nosocomial infections. Methods of contact transmission include (1) direct contact, (2) indirect contact, and (3) droplet contact.

Direct contact involves direct physical transfer between a susceptible host and an infected or colonized person. Sexually transmitted diseases such as gonorrhea and syphilis are transmitted by direct contact. In the hospital setting, direct contact transmission can occur when a colonized or infected practitioner turns a patient, changes a tracheostomy dressing, or performs other procedures requiring direct contact. This is the common mode of transmission for many nosocomial *Staphylococcus* and enteric bacterial infections. Direct contact can also occur between patients.

Indirect contact involves contact of a susceptible host with a contaminated intermediate object. Inanimate objects that can harbor infectious agents are called *fomites*. Common fomites include clothing, dressings, instruments, or equipment. For example, indirect patient contact with a contaminated nebulizer is a common mode for transmission of *P aeruginosa* in the hospital. Contaminated needles can serve as a vehicle for indirect contact transmission of both hepatitis B and HIV infections.

Droplet contact transmission occurs when an infectious agent enters the conjunctivae, nose, or mouth of a susceptible host via contact with an infected person or carrier who is coughing or sneezing. This is considered "contact" transmission rather than airborne, since droplets usually travel no more than 3 ft. Measles and streptococcal pneumonia are examples of infections transmitted via the droplet contact route.

Vehicle transmission. Vehicle transmission occurs when a susceptible host is exposed to an infectious agent transmitted through contaminated food or water. Salmonellosis and hepatitis A are examples of food vehicle-

Table 14-5   Routes of Infectious Disease Transmission

Mode	Type	Examples
Contact	Direct	Hepatitis A, venereal disease, HIV, *Staphylococcus* organisms, enteric bacteria
	Indirect	*Pseudomonas* organisms, enteric bacteria, hepatitis B, HIV
	Droplet	Measles, *Streptococcus* organisms
Vehicle	Waterborne	Shigellosis, cholera
	Foodborne	Salmonellosis, hepatitis A
Airborne	Aerosols	Legionellosis
	Droplet nuclei	Tuberculosis, diphtheria
	Dust	Histoplasmosis
Vectorborne	Ticks and mites	Rickettsial diseases
	Mosquito	Malaria
	Flea	Bubonic plague

transmitted infection. Shigellosis and cholera are examples of waterborne infections.

Airborne transmission. Airborne transmission occurs when an infectious agent is disseminated in the air, either by aerosol droplets, droplet nuclei, or dust particles. Aerosol droplets are small, water-based particles ranging in size from 50 to 100 μm. Aerosol droplets may be mechanically produced by aerosol generators or created by coughing and sneezing. Droplet nuclei are the residue of evaporated water droplets. Because of their smaller size (0.5 to 12 μm), droplet nuclei can remain suspended in the air for extremely long periods of time. Dust or dirt particles, usually greater than 50 μm in size, act as minute fomites.

Organisms carried in this manner can be widely dispersed by air currents before being inhaled by or deposited on a susceptible host. Legionellosis (legionnaires' disease) is probably transmitted via actual aerosol droplets. Tuberculosis is a classic example of an infection transmitted via droplet nuclei. Most fungal infections are transmitted via the airborne route on dust particles.

Vectorborne transmission. Vectorborne transmission occurs when an animal, especially an insect, is responsible for transferring an infectious agent from one host to another. Vectorborne transmissions such as malaria (mosquito vector) are of major concern in tropical countries. Although vectorborne transmissions are also responsible for many types of infections in the US (including Lyme disease), they are of little significance in hospital-acquired infections.

Spread of infection into the lungs

Spread of infectious agents into the lungs occurs by one or more of three major routes: (1) aspiration of oropharyngeal secretions; (2) inhalation of aerosol droplets, droplet nuclei, or dust particles containing infectious agents; and (3) blood-borne spread from a distant site of infection.

Of these routes, aspiration is believed to cause most cases of bacterial pneumonia, both nosocomial and community-acquired. The likelihood of aspiration is greatest in persons with abnormal swallowing mechanisms. Such patients usually have one or more of the following risk factors: (1) a decreased level of consciousness, (2) dysphagia from neurologic or esophageal disorders, or (3) a nasogastric tube. Patients who have undergone instrumentation of the respiratory or gastrointestinal tracts are also at high risk for aspiration.

INFECTION CONTROL METHODS

Infection control aims to break the chain of events causing the spread of infectious agents. This may be accomplished by (1) eliminating the source of infecting organisms, (2) decreasing the susceptibility of hosts, or (3) interrupting the route(s) of organism transmission.

Decreasing the susceptibility of hosts is the most difficult and least feasible approach to infection control. Hos-

pital efforts to achieve this end focus mainly on selective immunization programs for employees. Depending on the relative risks involved, hospital personnel are often required to undergo immunization for tuberculosis (BCG vaccine), diphtheria, tetanus, influenza, and hepatitis.

With the exception of the BCG vaccination, these approaches do not address the potential for spread of bacterial infections. Moreover, such immunization programs provide no assurances that patients and visitors are comparably protected. For this reason, we will focus on the two alternative approaches to infection control, that is, eliminating the source and interrupting the route(s) of transmission.

Eliminating the source of infectious agents

It is impossible to totally eliminate the source of all infectious microorganisms. This is the reason for a multifaceted approach to infection control. Nonetheless, standard infection control procedures must begin with efforts to remove or minimize the number of offending organisms present in the patient environment.

Infection control procedures designed to eliminate the source of infectious agents fall into two major categories: general sanitation measures and specialized equipment processing.

In the presence of a filthy environment, efforts to implement all other infection control procedures will be useless. General sanitation measures attend to the overall cleanliness of the environment. The goal of general sanitation is to reduce the number of microorganisms in the environment to a level deemed safe by public health standards.

Particularly important in the hospital setting are sanitary laundry management, food preparation, and housekeeping. Environmental control of the air (via specialized ventilation systems) and water complement these efforts.

The goal of specialized equipment processing is to render equipment linked to infection transmission free of microbial contamination or to reduce contamination to such a low level that the risk of infection is minimal.

Specialized equipment processing involves decontamination, sterilization, and disinfection of inanimate objects or vehicles that can harbor and transmit infectious agents. *Decontamination* is the process whereby contaminants are removed from objects, usually by simple physical means, such as washing. *Sterilization* is a process that renders objects free from all living organisms. True sterilization kills both the vegetative and spore forms of all bacteria, fungi, yeast, and viruses. *Disinfection* is a process that destroys the vegetative form of pathogenic organisms. Unlike sterilization, disinfection may not kill spore-forming bacteria.

Decontamination. The first step in specialized equipment processing is decontamination. Decontamination procedures are designed to remove infectious materials, particularly organic residues, from equipment that has been used. Where possible, this is accomplished by complete disassembly and a manual or automated wash in appropriate disinfectant detergents. Objects that cannot be immersed, such as certain electrical equipment, should at least be surface disinfected with a 70% alcohol solution or the equivalent. Where possible, these items should undergo subsequent ethylene oxide sterilization.

Careful rinsing of washed equipment is necessary to ensure that any soap or detergent residues are removed. Such residues can be irritating to human tissue and mucous membranes, and may decrease the effectiveness of subsequent sterilization or disinfection procedures. Moreover, when reassembly of decontaminated equipment must be done prior to subsequent processing, care must be taken not to cause recontamination. Aseptic reassembly should be preceded by a vigorous hand scrub and ideally conducted in a filtered hood designed for this purpose. Decontaminated equipment should never be allowed to sit on open counters for prolonged periods of time.

Although careful decontamination will remove most infectious material from processed equipment, it cannot totally eliminate the risk of infection. For this reason, most equipment must undergo either sterilization or disinfection.

Sterilization. Sterilization may be accomplished by either physical or chemical means. Both methods appear to kill microorganisms via denaturation, coagulation, or inactivation of essential proteins. Table 14-6 compares and contrasts the major methods of sterilization.

Physical methods of sterilization. The most common physical method used to sterilize respiratory care equipment is heat. Other less common physical methods of sterilization include ionizing radiation and ultrasonic vibrations.

Heat. For most objects, heat is the most practical and efficient method of sterilization. However, both the temperature and the length of exposure necessary for sterilization vary considerably for individual categories of organisms. In general, the higher the temperature, the shorter the time necessary for true sterilization.

Heat sterilization would be simple without bacterial spores. The bacterial spore is probably the most resistant form of life known; some will survive the temperature of boiling water for several hours. There is no standard pattern of heat resistance for spores, since their resistance varies not only from species to species, but also within the same species under different conditions of age or growth. For this reason, all heat sterilization methods must be sufficient enough to kill the most resistant bacterial spore forms.

Common methods of heat sterilization include incineration, boiling, autoclaving (moist heat under pressure), and dry heat.

Incineration, or burning, is used as a method of sterilization only when the object has no further use or is so contaminated with virulent organisms as to prohibit its reuse. Although incineration is the surest method of sterilization, its use is limited.

Boiling water at sea level (100°C) readily destroys vegetative forms of pathogenic organisms. However, some bacterial spores can withstand boiling for long periods; thus, one cannot be certain of complete sterilization by using boiling water. Moreover, since water boils at lower temperatures at high altitudes, sterilization using boiling water may be ineffective, particularly with thermophilic organisms.

Moist heat, or steam under pressure, is the most efficient sterilization agent. Steam under pressure, using an autoclave, quickly coagulates cell proteins. The time necessary to achieve sterilization depends on both the temperature and pressure. As the pressure increases, temperature increases and time decreases. For example, at 15 psi, the temperature of steam is 121°C, and 15 min is required for full sterilization. On the other hand, if the pressure is

Table 14-6   Comparison of Sterilization Methods

Method	Applicable equipment	Advantages	Disadvantages
Incineration	Disposables; grossly contaminated articles	Surest method; simple	Limited use; may result in air pollution
Boiling	Metals; heat-resistant plastics	Inexpensive; simple	Time-consuming; altitude dependent; may damage some equipment
Autoclave	Metal instruments; linens	Inexpensive; fast; nontoxic; prewrapping of items	May damage heat-or moisture-sensitive equipment
Dry heat	Laboratory glassware; metal instruments	Inexpensive; simple; nontoxic	Damages heat-sensitive equipment
Ionizing radiation	Foods; some medical supplies	Fast; effective; prewrapping of items	Expensive; toxic by-products may be produced
Ethylene oxide	Heat-sensitive items	Effective; prewrapping of items	Time-consuming; expensive; toxic residues must be removed by aeration

raised to 20 psi, the temperature increases to 126°C, and the sterilization time decreases to 10 min. A pressure of 15 psi at 121°C is the combination most commonly employed for sterilization.

For autoclaving to be effective, the chamber atmosphere must be free of air and contain only steam. Most autoclaves are equipped with controls that automatically evacuate the air before the steam pressure is allowed to rise to 15 psi. Moreover, items placed in the autoclave must be properly packed to ensure exposure. Unfortunately, many of the materials used in the manufacture of respiratory equipment will not withstand the high temperatures and pressures of the autoclave. For this reason, application of steam heat for respiratory care equipment processing is limited.

Dry heat sterilization is accomplished in an oven like that used in a home. Dry heat sterilization requires considerably higher temperatures for complete effectiveness than does steam sterilization. As with steam sterilization, there is no definite standard, but a temperature of 160° to 180°C applied over 2 hours is the most common approach. Dry heat is ideal for most glass and metal objects. However, as with the steam autoclave, most common materials used in respiratory care cannot undergo dry heat sterilization.

Ionizing radiation. Short-wavelength electromagnetic rays are an extremely effective sterilizing agent. Both x-rays and gamma rays can be used to this end, with gamma radiation the most common application. X-radiation is produced by electron generators similar to those used in diagnostic radiology. Gamma radiation is emitted from radioactive isotopes such as cobalt.

Ionizing radiation kills microorganisms either through destruction of the cellular nucleic acids or by ionization of intracellular water. Although many commercial products are sterilized in this manner, the required equipment and shielding costs are prohibitive for most hospitals. Moreover, in the dosage required to achieve sterilization, ionizing radiation can chemically alter some materials, creating toxic by-products.

Ultraviolet light is another ionizing source used in infection control. Ultraviolet light is effective in killing most bacteria, but it poorly penetrates most common materials. To be effective, ultraviolet light must have direct contact with the offending organisms. For this reason, ultraviolet light is not considered a true sterilizing agent. It may, however, be useful in reducing the microbial population of the air in operating rooms, nurseries, communicable-disease wards, and bacteriologic laboratories.

Ultrasound. In solution, ultrasonic vibrations at frequencies in the 100,000 to 400,000 MHz range are efficient in cleaning debris from soiled or contaminated equipment. At high amplitude and frequency, ultrasound vibrations also have been used in laboratory settings to disrupt microbial cell walls, thus causing sterilization. However, this process is lengthy, requiring 4 hours or more to achieve true sterilization. Moreover, removal of equipment from an ultrasonic bath without causing recontamination is difficult. For this reason, ultrasound should be considered mainly as an effective tool in equipment decontamination.

Chemical methods of sterilization. Chemical methods of sterilization include the use of ethylene oxide (ETO) gas and selected liquid solutions.

Ethylene oxide. Ethylene oxide is a potent sterilizing agent, whether used undiluted or in the diluted form (with Freon or carbon dioxide). Chemically, ethylene oxide acts on microorganisms by alkylation, or combination of the alkylene oxide with the sulphydryl, amino, carboxyl, or hydroxyl groups in the protein molecule. This action effectively kills all microorganisms.

Because ethylene oxide exists as a vapor at room temperature, it is readily diffusible and, therefore, effective under ambient conditions. The gas does not damage plastic or rubber materials. Moreover, because ethylene oxide readily penetrates packaging materials, articles to be sterilized can be packaged before being placed in the sterilizer. For these reasons, ethylene oxide gas is particularly useful as a sterilant for heat- and moisture-sensitive items that cannot be steam sterilized.

Proper use of ethylene oxide requires special attention to the preparation of materials, fulfillment of sterilization cycle parameters, and completion of aeration. Therefore, hospital personnel operating ethylene oxide equipment must be knowledgeable and skilled in all parameters of sterilization, including aeration procedures. Expert supervision should be provided to periodically observe and document appropriate disassembly, cleaning, packaging, sterilization, biologic control, and aeration procedures.

PREPARATION OF MATERIAL. Material to be sterilized with ethylene oxide should be surgically clean. Organic coatings such as blood or pus protect microorganisms and may prevent sterilization. All materials must be "towel dry." The ethylene oxide sterilization process depends on the presence of adequate, but not excessive, moisture. Materials must be free from water drops, which could interfere with sterilization. Particulate water droplets may also combine with ethylene oxide to form ethylene glycol (antifreeze), which can be irritating to tissues.

Prepared materials should be kept in an area where the relative humidity is 30% or more. Materials should never be force-dried before wrapping. Any caps, plugs, valves, or stylets should be removed from equipment to ensure gas penetration and contact. Hollow-bore needles and plastic or rubber tubing must be open at both ends and free from plugs. Syringes should be disassembled and packaged with the plungers outside the barrels.

WRAPPING MATERIALS. Materials used to wrap items for sterilization by ethylene oxide must be highly permeable to the gas. Suitable wrapping materials include double-thickness muslin or paper similar to that used in the steam autoclave. Several types of heat-sealed plastic and paper pouches and plastic films, such as 3 to 5 mil polyethylene, are specifically designed for ethylene oxide sterilization. Materials that are inadequately permeable to ethylene oxide and should not be used include aluminum foil, nylon film, Saran, Mylar, cellophane, polyamide, polyester, and polyvinylidene films.

LOADING THE STERILIZER. An ethylene oxide sterilizer should be loaded using the same principles that apply to an autoclave. Space must be provided between items to ensure gas circulation. Overloading may impede sterilization and must be avoided. The manufacturer's instructions concerning loading should always be followed.

STERILIZATION CYCLES. The manufacturer's instructions must be adhered to regarding all parameters of the sterilization cycle. Effective sterilization requires close attention to the time, temperature, gas concentration, and humidity requirements of the system used. Typical conditions for a sterilization cycle are 3 to 4 hours exposure to a gas concentration of 800 to 1000 mg/L at 50° to 56°C and 30% to 60% relative humidity. Higher relative humidity may increase the certainty of sterilization; some of the latest automatic sterilizers now appearing on the market control the humidity between 80% and 100%.

After completion of a sterilization cycle, the sterilizer door should be open for 5 minutes prior to unloading. Since ethylene oxide forms an explosive mixture with air, smoking must not be permitted in the area.

AERATION. Nonporous materials such as metal and glass absorb no ethylene oxide and may be used immediately following sterilization. However, ethylene oxide retained in porous materials following sterilization is toxic to human tissues and can cause severe chemical burns. For this reason, adequate aeration of gas-absorbent materials, such as plastic or rubber items, is essential. All items requiring aeration following sterilization must be identified at the time of packaging. After cycle completion, these items should be segregated from those composed exclusively of glass or metal and aerated long enough to ensure that any residual ethylene oxide is reduced to a safe level.

The actual aeration time required depends on several variables. These include the composition, form, and weight of the material sterilized; the type of ethylene oxide sterilization system; and the aeration temperature. The material requiring the longest aeration time is polyvinyl chloride, commonly known as PVC. Plastics such as polyethylene and polypropylene do not require as long a period of aeration. However, if the composition of an article is in doubt, it should be treated as if it were polyvinyl chloride. Also, any PVC materials previously sterilized by gamma radiation should never be sterilized by ethylene oxide, as considerable amounts of ethylene chlorohydrin will be formed.

Elimination of residual ethylene oxide from polyvinyl chloride takes about 7 days at room temperature. In an aeration cabinet at 50°C, residual ethylene oxide can gener-

ally be removed in about 12 hours; at 60°C only 8 hours are required. Of course, these are guidelines only. The manufacturer's instructions for a particular aerator must be consulted to determine required aeration times of common materials.

Chemical solutions. Several chemical solutions are available that can serve as sterilizing agents under appropriate conditions. However, in the clinical setting these agents are primarily applied as high-level disinfectants. For this reason, they will be discussed in the next section.

Disinfection. Disinfection destroys the vegetative form of pathogenic organisms. "High-level" disinfection aims to eliminate all vegetative bacteria, not just prevent the further growth of microorganisms.

As with sterilization processes, disinfection may be accomplished by either physical or chemical means. The most common physical disinfection technique used in respiratory care is pasteurization. Numerous chemical methods are available to disinfect respiratory care equipment.

Physical disinfection. Over the last decade, pasteurization has become an efficient and cost-effective method for disinfection of equipment used in respiratory care. Like boiling and steam under pressure, pasteurization uses moist heat to coagulate the cell protein of microorganisms. However, the temperatures used in this process are insufficient to kill bacterial spores.

The major spore-forming bacteria pathogenic to humans include *B anthracis*, *C tetani*, *C perfringens*, and *C botulinum*. Anthrax is a relatively rare organism, especially in the hospital setting. Although members of the genus *Clostridium* can produce lethal toxins (tetanus, botulism, and gas gangrene), these organisms are anaerobic and of little threat in the presence of free atmospheric oxygen. For this reason, the inability of the pasteurization process to kill bacterial spores is of minor practical concern.

The exposure time necessary to kill vegetative bacteria by pasteurization depends on temperature. The flash process, used mainly to disinfect liquids such as milk, consists of exposing the material to 72°C for a period of 15 seconds. More applicable to respiratory care equipment processing is the batch process. In the batch process, equipment is immersed in a water bath heated to 63°C for 30 minutes. Most respiratory care–related equipment can easily withstand these conditions without damage.

The major limitation of pasteurization is not the process itself, but the difficulty in preventing equipment recontamination following immersion. Special filtered dryers, used in conjunction with laminar-flow assembly hoods and scrupulous aseptic techniques, generally minimize the likelihood of recontamination.

Chemical disinfection. Chemical disinfection involves the application of chemical solutions to contaminated equipment or surfaces. Depending on their chemical makeup, these disinfectants may kill microorganisms by disruption of the cell membrane, coagulation or denaturation of cellular protein, alkylation of cellular enzymes, or oxidative reactions.

There are six major categories of chemical disinfectants used in clinical practice: the alcohols, the phenols and their derivatives, the halogens, the iodophors, the aldehydes, and the quaternary ammonium compounds. Each category of disinfectant has its own advantages and disadvantages. The selection of an appropriate agent, therefore, depends on the nature of the application at hand. Table 14-7 compares and contrasts the major chemical disinfection agents.

Alcohols. The bactericidal and fungicidal actions of the alcohols are apparently accomplished by protein denaturation. The bactericidal action of alcohols is directly related to their molecular weight. The two most common alcohols are isopropyl and ethyl alcohol, with isopropyl alcohol being slightly more effective as a disinfectant. Disinfection is most effective if the alcohol is in aqueous solution, with a 70% percent solution being the most widely used concentration.

When used in the appropriate concentrations, alcohols are effective in killing most vegetative bacteria, including *M tuberculosis*. However, alcohols generally are ineffective against bacterial endospores. Anthrax spores have been reported to have survived in alcohol for as long as 20 years.

Phenols. Lister first made use of phenol (carbolic acid) in the 1800s to reduce infections resulting from surgery. Phenol apparently causes injury to the cell membrane, but is also capable of inactivating enzymes and denaturing cellular proteins. Simple phenol in a 5% solution is rapidly effective against most vegetative forms of bacteria, including *M tuberculosis*. Phenols are also fungicidal. However, spores generally are not destroyed, and viruses are not particularly susceptible to phenolic action. Phenols tend to

stay active in the presence of organic matter and can remain active on surfaces long after application.

Attempts to reduce the toxicity of the phenolic compounds led to the synthesis of a number of derivative disinfectants. Two of the more common ones are hexylresorcinol and hexachlorophene. These phenolic derivatives were frequently incorporated into soap and detergent formulas to enhance the bacteriostatic activity of the surface-active agents. However, studies conducted on hexachlorophene in the early 1970s indicated that this agent could be absorbed through the skin and cause brain damage, particularly in infants. Consequently, since 1972 hexachlorophene is provided only by prescription.

Halogens. Of the halogens, chlorine and iodine are the only two used extensively as disinfectants. Chlorine, in either the gaseous state or chemical compound, is a potent and rapid-acting disinfectant. If not for its extreme toxicity, chlorine gas could be used as a sterilizing agent. Chlorine compounds are most effective in alkaline solutions; increased temperatures enhance their action. For disinfectant purposes, chlorine is commonly prepared as the hypochlorite (bleach) or chloramine solution. Unfortunately, the actions of chlorine preparations are significantly impaired by the presence of organic matter.

Iodine in alcohol solution (tincture of iodine) is one of the most popular wound and skin bactericidal agents. In weak solutions the activity of iodine is increased at an acid pH. In addition to its effectiveness against most vegetative bacteria, iodine has fungicidal, sporicidal, and virucidal action. High concentrations of iodine can cause tissue necrosis, and its staining properties limit its use with many materials.

Iodophors represent mixtures of iodine and surface-active organic compounds. Unlike tincture compounds, iodophors are water soluble, nonstaining, and less irritating

Table 14-7   Comparison of Chemical Disinfectant Agents

Agent	Example(s)	Bacteria	AFB	Spores	Fungi	Viruses*
Alcohols	Ethyl alcohol	+ +	+	− −	+ +	+(L)
	Isopropyl alcohol	+ +	+	− −	+ +	+(L)
Phenols	Amphyl	+ +	+	− −	+ +	+(L)
	Hexachlorophene	+	+	− −	+	+(L)
Halogens	Chlorine	+ +	+ +	+ +	+ +	+(L/H)
	Iodine	+ +	+ +	+	+ +	−
	Sodium hypochlorite	+ +	+	+	+ +	+(L)
Iodophors	Povidone	+ +	+	− −	+ +	+(L/H)
Aldehydes	Acid glutaraldehyde	+ +	+ +	+	+ +	+(L)
	Alkaline glutaraldehyde	+ +	+ +	+ +	+ +	+(L/H)
Quaternary ammoniums	Double quats	+	− −	− −	+	−
	Triple quats	+ +	+	− −	+ +	−

*Note: Activity depends on whether the virus is lipophilic (L) or hydrophilic (H).

to tissue. However, iodophors generally have less bactericidal activity than iodine tinctures.

Aldehydes. The two major aldehydes used for disinfection purposes are formaldehyde and glutaraldehyde. Aldehydes kill microorganisms via alkylation of cellular enzymes. Under appropriate conditions (described below), aldehydes are active against all living material. Under these circumstances, aldehydes may also be classified as sterilizing agents.

Formaldehyde is an excellent disinfectant when used as a gas. It is effective in closed areas as both a bactericide and fungicide. In an aqueous solution of approximately 37% formaldehyde, it is known as formalin. Formalin destroys vegetative bacteria and the spores of both bacteria and fungi; however, its poor penetration and irritating vapor limit its use mainly to specimen fixation.

Similar to formaldehyde, but without most of its undesirable properties, is glutaraldehyde. Glutaraldehydes kill microorganisms by denaturing cell protein. Two forms of glutaraldehyde are available for use as disinfectants and sterilizing agents: alkaline glutaraldehyde and acid glutaraldehyde.

Alkaline glutaraldehyde is a 2% glutaraldehyde solution buffered by $NaHCO_3$ to a pH between 7.5 and 8.5. Alkaline glutaraldehyde is bactericidal, tuberculocidal, fungicidal, and virucidal at room temperature in 10 minutes. Immersion in alkaline glutaraldehyde for 10 hours is required for full sterilization (sporicidal action).

Over time, alkaline glutaraldehyde gradually undergoes degradation and loses activity. Above a pH of 9, this process proceeds rapidly. In the pH range of 7.5 to 8.5, the degradation reaction is slowed down considerably so that full antimicrobial activity can be maintained for 4 weeks.

Acid glutaraldehyde acts most effectively in a pH range of 2.7 to 3.7. As with its alkaline counterpart, the acid preparation is bactericidal, tuberculocidal, fungicidal, and virucidal at room temperature. However, the acid preparation requires 20 minutes to achieve this high-level disinfection. Sterilization with acid glutaraldehyde can be accomplished in as little as 1 hour if the solution is heated to 60°C.

The major disadvantage of the glutaraldehydes is their irritating effect, particularly on the mucous membranes and eyes. Materials disinfected or sterilized in glutaraldehyde solutions must, therefore, be thoroughly rinsed and dried before use. Of course, these procedures increase the likelihood of recontamination.

Quaternary ammonium compounds. Quaternary ammonium compounds, or "quats," are cationic detergents containing ammonium ions. Quaternary ammonium compounds kill microorganisms mainly by disrupting their cell membrane. Inactivation of intracellular enzymes or the denaturation of proteins may also be involved in their disinfectant action.

When compared with most other chemical disinfectants, quaternary ammonium compounds are bland, nontoxic, and inexpensive. However, their bactericidal activity is selective. Quats are most active against gram-positive vegetative bacteria. Their disinfectant capabilities with gram-negative organisms, such as *P aeruginosa,* vary according to the formulation, concentration, and time of exposure. The sporicidal activity of quats is minimal, and the tuberculocidal and virucidal activity is questionable. Perhaps most important of all, the disinfectant activity of quaternary ammonium compounds tends to be neutralized by soaps and anionic detergents and reduced by contact with organic material and hard water.

Recently, manufacturers have increased the effectiveness of quaternary ammonium compounds by combining formulations. These formulations are called double or triple quats. Double or triple quat preparations provide low-level disinfection in 10 to 20 minutes and remain active for 1 to 4 weeks. Extreme care is required to thoroughly rinse soap and organic material from the equipment before processing, as the quats are neutralized by these materials. Dilution of these solutions with rinse water will alter the pH and reduce disinfectant activity. As with any liquid chemical disinfectant, processed equipment must be dried and reassembled carefully to prevent recontamination.

In general, these shortcomings restrict the use of quaternary ammonium compounds as disinfectants in the hospital setting. However, quats have become increasingly popular in the home care setting, replacing acetic acid as the most common home disinfectant. Generally, quats are more effective and less costly than acetic acid in achieving the low-level disinfection necessary to control most types of infection in the home setting. However, as indicated in Chapter 35, high-level disinfection in the home cannot be accomplished with quaternary ammonium compounds. For this reason, activated glutaraldehyde is recommended as the disinfectant of choice in the home care setting.

Interrupting routes of transmission

Complementing efforts to eliminate the source of infectious agents are activities designed to interrupt common routes of microorganism transmission. The two major infection control methods designed to interrupt organism transmission are equipment handling procedures and barrier/isolation techniques.

Equipment handling procedures.. Equipment handling procedures that help prevent transmission of microorganisms include maintenance of in-use respiratory care equipment, processing of reusable equipment, the use of disposables, and fluid and medication precautions.

Maintenance of in-use equipment. The in-use respiratory care equipment most likely to transmit infectious agents includes, in order of importance, large-reservoir jet nebulizers, ventilators and their associated circuitry, and oxygen therapy apparatuses.

The principal source for transmission of pathogenic microorganisms via respiratory care equipment are large-reservoir jet nebulizers. These reservoir nebulizers can become contaminated by the introduction of nonsterile fluids or air, by handling of the nebulizer cup, and by retrograde flow of contaminated delivery tubing condensate back into the reservoir. Once introduced, bacteria in the nebulizer reservoirs can multiply to sufficiently large numbers within 24 hours to cause infection if nebulized and inhaled.

To minimize the likelihood of reservoir nebulizers transmitting infectious agents, the following procedures should be scrupulously followed:

- Fluid reservoirs should be filled immediately before use. Fluid should not be added to replenish partially filled reservoirs. If fluid is to be added, the remaining old fluid should first be discarded.
- Tubing condensate should be discarded and not allowed to drain back into the reservoir.
- Large-volume jet nebulizers, medication nebulizers, and large-volume (cascade-type) continuous-use humidifiers and their reservoirs should be routinely changed and replaced with equipment that has been sterilized or has undergone high-level disinfection every 24 hours.
- Humidifiers or nebulizers that create droplets for purposes of room humidification should never be used.

In-use ventilator equipment and peripheral circuitry, especially their humidifiers and/or nebulizers, also are potential vehicle for the spread of infection. To decrease the likelihood of this respiratory care equipment transmitting infectious agents, the following procedures are recommended:

- Breathing circuits (including associated humidifiers and nebulizers) should be routinely changed and replaced with equipment that has been sterilized or has undergone high-level disinfection every 24 hours.
- When a ventilator is used to treat multiple patients, as with IPPB administration, the breathing circuit should be changed between patients and replaced with a sterilized or disinfected one.

Although posing considerably less threat, an oxygen therapy apparatus should also be treated as a potential vehicle for transmitting infectious agents. To minimize the possibility of this equipment transmitting infectious agents, the following procedures are recommended:

- Reusable small-volume oxygen humidifier reservoirs should be cleaned, rinsed, and dried daily before refilling.
- The tubing (including any nasal prongs) and any mask used to deliver oxygen from a wall outlet should be changed between patients.

Processing reusable equipment. Reusable equipment that is improperly processed represents another source for transmitting pathogenic microorganisms. General guidelines for decontamination, sterilization, and disinfection were previously discussed. Specific procedures to be followed in processing reusable, respiratory care equipment include the following:

- All respiratory care equipment to be sterilized or disinfected should be thoroughly cleaned to remove all blood, tissue, food, or other residue. It should be decontaminated before or during cleaning if it is marked "contaminated" and received from patients in certain types of isolation (see subsequent section).
- Respiratory care equipment that touches mucous membranes should be sterilized before use on other patients; if this is not feasible, it should receive high-level disinfection.
- Breathing circuits (including tubing and exhalation valves), medication nebulizers and their reservoirs, large-volume jet nebulizers and their reservoirs, and cascade humidifiers and their reservoirs should be sterilized or receive high-level disinfection.
- Since coupling chambers for ultrasonic nebulizers are difficult to disinfect adequately, these chambers should be gas-sterilized (ethylene oxide) or have at least 30 minutes of contact time with a high-level disinfectant.
- The internal machinery of ventilators and breathing machines need not be routinely sterilized or disinfected between patients.
- Bedside respirometers and other equipment used to monitor several patients in succession should not directly touch parts of the breathing circuit. Rather, extension pieces should be used between the equipment and breathing circuit and should be changed between patients. If no extension piece is used and such monitoring equipment is directly connected to contaminated equipment, the monitoring equipment should be sterilized or receive high-level disinfection before use on other patients.
- Once they have been used for one patient, manual resuscitation bags should be sterilized or receive high-level disinfection before use on other patients.

Disposable equipment. The use of disposable respiratory care equipment represents a major approach to preventing transmission of pathogenic microorganisms in the clinical setting. Depending on its use, disposable equipment may be provided presterilized or simply aseptically clean. In either case, inventory control is necessary to assure appropriate equipment usage and condition, usually according to the manufacturer's instructions. Under no conditions should disposable respiratory care equipment be reused.

Fluid and medication precautions. Fluids and medications represent a major source for the transmission of infectious agents. To minimize the possibility of fluids and medications serving as a vehicle for the spread of infection, the following procedures are recommended:

- Only sterile fluids should be used to fill nebulizers and humidifiers. These fluids should be dispensed aseptically. Contaminated equipment should not be allowed to enter or touch the fluid while it is being dispensed.

- After a large container (bottle) of fluid intended for use in a nebulizer or humidifier has been opened, unused fluid should be discarded within 24 hours.
- Either single-dose or multi-dose vials can be used for respiratory care. If multi-dose vials are used, they should be stored (refrigerated or at room temperature) according to directions on the label or package insert. Vials should be used no longer than the expiration date given on the label.

Barrier and isolation methods. Since a major route for the spread of nosocomial infections is by direct or indirect contact with infected persons, infection control measures that place "barriers" between the source and the susceptible host should help disrupt transmission of pathogenic microorganisms. General barrier-type precautions common in clinical practice include handwashing and the use of gloves, masks, and gowns. When used together with the physical separation of infected patients in specific disease categories, these general techniques are combined into isolation protocols.

Handwashing. Proper handwashing is the single most important means of preventing the spread of infection. In fact, if handwashing is done appropriately, glove and gown barrier precautions may have no additional benefit.

Respiratory care personnel should always wash their hands after contacting a patient, even when gloves are used. In addition, personnel should wash their hands after coming into contact with any body excretions (such as feces and urine) or wound, skin, or respiratory secretions. Hands should also be washed before performing invasive procedures, touching wounds, or touching patients who are at high risk for infection. Handwashing between all patient contacts is particularly critical in intensive care units and newborn nurseries.

When taking care of patients that are infected or colonized with virulent microorganisms, respiratory care practitioners should use antiseptics for handwashing, rather than simple soap and water. Antiseptics will inhibit or kill many microorganisms that may not be completely removed by normal handwashing. Moreover, good antiseptics have a residual effect that continues to suppress microbial growth well after handwashing. Such antiseptics should not be used as a substitute for adequate handwashing, however.

Gloves. In general, there are three major reasons for using gloves. First, gloves reduce the likelihood that health personnel will become infected by contacting infected patients. Second, gloves reduce the possibility of health personnel transmitting their own endogenous microbial flora to patients. Finally, gloves reduce the likelihood that health personnel will become colonized with microorganisms and carry them to other patients.

Under most conditions, the use of gloves to prevent colonization and transmission of microorganisms between patient contacts can be eliminated by proper attention to handwashing. However, since handwashing practices vary substantially both between and within hospitals, gloves represent a practical means of preventing transient hand colonization and spread of some infections. Moreover, recent concern over the spread of AIDS and other blood-borne pathogens suggests that barrier precautions, such as gloves, should be consistently used for all patients (details on the prevention of AIDS transmission follow).

For these reasons, gloves should be used by respiratory care practitioners whenever excretions, secretions, blood, or body fluids are likely to be contacted. The use of gloves is especially important wherever the risk of exposure to blood is increased and the infection status of the patient is unknown, such as in emergency care settings.

When gloves are indicated, disposable single-use gloves should be worn. Depending on their purpose, either sterile or aseptically clean gloves are chosen. Gloves should be changed after direct contact with a patient's excretions or secretions, even if in the middle of a treatment or procedure. Used gloves should be discarded into appropriate receptacles.

Masks. Masks help prevent the transmission of infectious agents via the airborne route. They protect the wearer from inhaling both large-particle aerosol droplets (transmitted by close contact) and the smaller droplet nuclei (true airborne transmission). The high-efficiency disposable masks are more effective than cotton gauze or paper tissue masks in preventing both aerosol particle and droplet nuclei spread.

If the infection is transmitted by large-particle aerosols, masks need only be used by those close to the patient. If the infection is spread over longer distances by air, masks should be used by all persons entering the room or area.

Masks also can prevent transmission of some infections that are spread by direct contact with mucous membranes. This is because masks discourage personnel from touching their eyes, nose, and mouth until after they have washed their hands and removed the mask.

All masks should fully cover both the nose and the mouth. Because masks become ineffective when moist, they should be discarded after single use. Masks should never be lowered around the neck and reused.

Gowns. Gowns protect clothing from contamination that might occur in patient care activities. Because such soiling occurs infrequently, gowns are not necessary for most patient care activities.

Gowns are indicated when clothes are likely to be soiled with infective secretions or excretions of a patient in isolation. Even when gross soiling is not anticipated, gowns are indicated for all persons entering the room of patients who have highly contagious disorders that can cause serious illness, such as varicella (chickenpox) or disseminated zoster.

As with gloves and masks, gowns should be worn only once and then discarded. In most circumstances, aseptically clean, freshly laundered, or disposable gowns are satisfactory. Sterile gowns may be necessary in some instances, as with extensive burns or wounds.

Isolation precautions. Isolation precautions are designed to prevent the spread of infectious agents among patients, personnel, and visitors.

There are two current approaches to selecting isolation precautions: disease-specific and categorical. The disease-specific method is based on detailed isolation specifications for each infectious disease, as provided by the Centers for Disease Control. The categorical method derives isolation categories by grouping diseases for which similar isolation precautions are indicated. Seven isolation categories are used: (1) strict isolation, (2) contact isolation, (3) respiratory isolation, (4) tuberculosis (AFB) isolation, (5) enteric precautions, (6) drainage/secretion precautions, and (7) blood/body-fluid precautions.

Strict isolation. Strict isolation is designed to prevent transmission of highly contagious or virulent infections that may be spread by both air and contact. Diseases requiring strict isolation include diphtheria, Lassa fever, pneumonic plague, smallpox, and varicella (chickenpox). The following box specifies the precautions to be taken in strict isolation.

Contact isolation. Contact isolation is designed to prevent transmission of highly contagious infections or colonizations that do not warrant strict isolation. Infections in this category include acute respiratory infections in infants and young children, including croup, colds, pharyngitis, bronchitis, viral pneumonias, influenza, and viral bronchiolitis; newborn gonococcal conjunctivitis; cutaneous diphtheria; disseminated herpes simplex; severe primary or neonatal impetigo; pediculosis; staphylococcal pneumonia; group A streptococcal pneumonia; rabies; rubella; scabies; and any major skin, wound, or burn infection that is draining and not covered. Also, contact isolation may be indicated when a patient is infected or colonized with bacteria proven resistant to multiple antibiotics.

All diseases or conditions requiring contact isolation are spread primarily by close or direct contact. Thus, masks, gowns, and gloves are recommended for anyone in close contact with patients having infections in this category. The box below specifies the precautions to be taken in contact isolation.

SPECIFICATIONS FOR CONTACT ISOLATION

1. Private room is indicated. In general, patients infected with the same organism may share a room. During outbreaks, infants and young children with the same respiratory clinical syndrome may share a room.
2. Masks are indicated for those who come close to the patient.
3. Gowns are indicated if soiling is likely.
4. Gloves are indicated for touching infective material.
5. Hands must be washed after touching the patient or potentially contaminated articles and before taking care of another patient.
6. Articles contaminated with infected material should be discarded or bagged and labeled before being sent for decontamination and reprocessing.

However, not all the precautions listed in the boxed material are necessary for all diseases. For example, masks and gloves are not generally necessary for the care of infants and young children with acute viral respiratory infections; gowns are not usually indicated for newborns with gonococcal conjunctivitis; and care of patients infected with resistant bacteria does not normally require masks unless a pneumonia is present. Because of these variations within the contact isolation category, some degree of "over-isolation" may occur.

Respiratory isolation. Respiratory isolation is designed to prevent transmission of infectious diseases via the droplet contact route. Direct and indirect contact transmission, although infrequent, can occur with some infections in this category.

Diseases requiring respiratory isolation include epiglottitis, meningitis, or childhood pneumonia due to *H influenzae,* measles, meningococcal pneumonia, mumps, and pertussis. The following box specifies the precautions to be taken in respiratory isolation.

Tuberculosis isolation (AFB). Tuberculosis, or AFB, isolation is designed for patients with pulmonary tuberculosis who have a positive sputum smear or a chest x-ray film that strongly suggests active disease. Laryngeal tuberculosis is also included in this category. The box below specifies the precautions to be taken in tuberculosis isolation.

SPECIFICATIONS FOR STRICT ISOLATION

1. Private room is indicated; door should be kept closed. In general, patients infected with the same organism may share a room.
2. Masks are indicated for all persons entering the room.
3. Gowns are indicated for all persons entering the room.
4. Gloves are indicated for all persons entering the room.
5. Hands must be washed after touching the patient or potentially contaminated articles and before taking care of another patient.
6. Articles contaminated with infective material should be discarded or bagged and labeled before being sent for decontamination and reprocessing.

SPECIFICATIONS FOR RESPIRATORY ISOLATION

1. Private room is indicated. In general, patients infected with the same organism may share a room.
2. Masks are indicated for those who come close to the patient.
3. Gowns are not indicated.
4. Gloves are not indicated.
5. Hands must be washed after touching the patient or potentially contaminated articles and before taking care of another patient.
6. Articles contaminated with infective material should be discarded or bagged and labeled before being sent for decontamination and reprocessing.

SPECIFICATIONS FOR TUBERCULOSIS (AFB) ISOLATION

1. Private room with special ventilation is indicated; door should be kept closed. In general, patients infected with the same organism may share a room.
2. Masks are indicated only if the patient is coughing and does not reliably cover mouth.
3. Gowns are indicated only if needed to prevent gross contamination of clothing.
4. Gloves are not indicated.
5. Hands must be washed after touching the patient or potentially contaminated articles and before taking care of another patient.
6. Articles are rarely involved in transmission of TB. However, articles should be thoroughly cleaned and disinfected or discarded.

In general, infants and young children with pulmonary tuberculosis do not require isolation precautions because they rarely cough, and, as compared with adults, their bronchial secretions contain few bacilli. To protect the patient's privacy, this category is visibly posted as AFB isolation.

Enteric precautions. Enteric precautions are designed to prevent infections that are transmitted by contact with feces. Diseases requiring enteric precautions include amebic dysentery; cholera; coxsackievirus disease; encephalitis; gastroenteritis caused by *E coli,* salmonellae, or shigellae organisms; type A viral hepatitis; poliomyelitis; viral meningitis; necrotizing enterocolitis; viral pericarditis or myocarditis; and any enteroviral infection or acute diarrhea suspected of being infectious.

Although most infections in this category cause gastrointestinal symptoms, some do not. For example, feces from patients infected with poliovirus and coxsackieviruses are infective, but these infections do not usually cause prominent gastrointestinal symptoms. The box below specifies the enteric precautions.

SPECIFICATIONS FOR ENTERIC PRECAUTIONS

1. Private room is indicated if patient hygiene is poor. A patient with poor hygiene does not wash hands after touching infective material, contaminates the environment with infective material, or shares contaminated articles with other patients. In general, patients infected with the same organism may share a room.
2. Masks are not indicated.
3. Gowns are indicated if soiling is likely.
4. Gloves are indicated if touching infective material.
5. Hands must be washed after touching the patient or potentially contaminated articles and before taking care of another patient.
6. Articles contaminated with infective material should be discarded or bagged and labeled before being sent for decontamination and reprocessing.

Drainage/secretion precautions. Drainage/secretion precautions are designed to prevent transmission of infections that occur by indirect contact with purulent material or drainage from an infected site. Infectious diseases included in this category result in the production of infective purulent material, drainage, or secretions. Examples include chlamydial infections, gas gangrene, conjunctivitis, minor infected decubiti ulcers, and minor or limited skin, wound, or burn infections. Infections caused by resistant microorganisms and major skin, wound, or burn infections require contact isolation. The following box specifies the precautions to be taken in drainage/secretion isolation.

SPECIFICATIONS FOR DRAINAGE/ SECRETION PRECAUTIONS

1. Private room is not indicated.
2. Masks are not indicated.
3. Gowns are indicated if soiling is likely.
4. Gloves are indicated for touching infective material.
5. Hands must be washed after touching the patient or potentially contaminated articles and before taking care of another patient.
6. Articles contaminated with infective material should be discarded or bagged and labeled before being sent for decontamination and reprocessing.

Blood/body-fluid precautions. Blood and body-fluid precautions are designed to prevent infections transmitted by direct or indirect contact with contaminated blood or body fluids. For some diseases included in this category, such as malaria, only blood is infective; for other diseases, such as hepatitis B and AIDS, both blood and body fluids may be infective.

Diseases requiring blood and body-fluid precautions include the acquired immunodeficiency syndrome (AIDS), hepatitis B, hepatitis (non-A, non-B), yellow fever, Colorado tick fever, leptospirosis, malaria, and primary or secondary syphilis with skin and mucous membrane lesions. The box below specifies the precautions to be taken in blood and body-fluid isolation.

Other considerations. Considerations related to the application of isolation procedures include the handling of contaminated articles and equipment, the use of needle and syringes, and the transportation and handling of laboratory specimens.

CONTAMINATED ARTICLES AND EQUIPMENT. Used articles that have been contaminated with infective material should be enclosed in an impervious bag before removal from the room of a patient on isolation precautions. Bagging is intended to prevent accidental exposure of both personnel and the environment to contaminated articles. A single bag is probably adequate if (1) the bag is strong and impervi-

ous and (2) bagging can be accomplished without contaminating the bag's outer surface. Otherwise, a double bagging procedure is necessary. Bags used for articles or waste materials that have been contaminated should be clearly labeled or color coded for this purpose.

Use of disposable articles reduces the possibility that equipment will serve as a source of transmission. However, disposable articles must be disposed of safely and adequately. Contaminated disposable equipment should be bagged, labeled, and disposed of in accord with both hospital and applicable local, state, or federal regulations.

Reusable patient-care equipment should be returned to the applicable processing area for decontamination and reprocessing. Contaminated equipment in bags should remain bagged until decontaminated or sterilized.

NEEDLES AND SYRINGES. All personnel should exercise extreme caution when handling used needles and syringes. To prevent accidental needle-stick injuries, used needles should not be recapped, but rather placed in a prominently labeled, puncture-resistant container that is designated solely for this purpose. Needles should never be bent or broken by hand, since this is a common cause of needle-stick injuries. If the patient's blood is infective, disposable syringes and needles are recommended. If reusable syringes are used, they should be treated as contaminated articles, using the precautions described above.

LABORATORY SPECIMENS. When gathering laboratory specimens (such as sputum), extreme care should be taken to prevent contamination of the external surface of the container. If the outside of the container is contaminated, it must be disinfected or placed in an impervious bag. To minimize the likelihood of leakage during transport, laboratory specimens should always be placed in a sturdy container with a secure lid. When a specimen comes from a patient on isolation precautions, the container normally should be placed in an impervious bag and appropriately labeled before removal from the room.

Modifications to standard isolation procedures. Isolation precautions may have to be modified for patients needing intensive care or emergency interventions. Whenever such changes are necessary, efforts must be made to ensure minimal risk to both patients and hospital personnel. As a general guideline, modification of any isolation protocol should never compromise adherence to the generic aseptic procedures, particularly conscientious handwashing with antiseptic solutions.

Intensive care. Patients requiring intensive care are usually among those at highest risk for acquiring serious nosocomial infections. There are several reasons for this increased risk. First, contact between patients and health personnel in an intensive care unit is more frequent than in other settings. Second, intensive care units typically cluster patients together in a confined area. Third, patients in the intensive care setting tend to have significantly less host resistance and consequently are more susceptible to

---

SPECIFICATIONS FOR BLOOD/ BODY-FLUID PRECAUTIONS

1. Private room is indicated if patient hygiene is poor. A patient with poor hygiene does not wash hands after touching infective material, contaminates the environment with infective material, or shares contaminated articles with other patients. In general, patients infected with the same organism may share a room.
2. Masks are not indicated.
3. Gowns are indicated for touching blood or body fluids.
4. Gloves are indicated for touching blood or body fluids.
5. Hands must be washed immediately if they are potentially contaminated with blood or body fluids and before taking care of another patient.
6. Articles contaminated with blood or body fluids should be discarded or bagged and labeled before being sent for decontamination and reprocessing.
7. Care should be taken to avoid needle-stick injuries. Used needles should not be recapped or bent; they should be placed in a prominently labeled, puncture-resistant container designated specifically for such disposal.
8. Blood spills should be cleaned up promptly with a solution of 5.25% sodium hypochlorite diluted 1:10 with water.

infection. Finally, patients in intensive care units are more likely to undergo multiple invasive procedures.

The isolation precaution that will be most modified in an intensive care setting is the use of a private room. Patients with serious, contagious infections should be placed in a private room, even if one is not available in the intensive care unit. When a private room or cubicle in the intensive care unit is not feasible, and if airborne transmission of infectious agents is not likely, it is acceptable to define an isolation area with physical barriers such as curtains or partitions, or by marking the area with floor tape. In addition, standard instructional cards should be posted to notify personnel and visitors regarding the applicable isolation precautions.

Newborns and infants. Isolation precautions for newborns and infants may have to be modified from those recommended for adults because of the general lack of private rooms for these patients.

Specifically, the grouping of infants together is permissible if (1) facilities and procedures provide assurances that appropriate handwashing is regularly performed by all personnel and (2) sufficient space (4 to 6 feet) is provided between patient care stations. Where used, enclosed incubators are satisfactory for limited isolation of infants, but should not be considered a primary means of infection control.

In addition to these precautions, grouping of patients with the same infection (cohorting) may be necessary. Cohorting is feasible only if the patients can be separated into a single large room with dedicated personnel.

Immunocompromised patients. Patients with conditions such as leukemia, cancer, or severe burns, or patients receiving therapies that suppress the immune system (body irradiation, steroid therapy, or immunosuppressive drugs) are highly susceptible to infection. In the past, these patients were assigned to a "protective isolation" category. Recent evidence indicates that this approach is no more useful in preventing infection than rigorous adherence to an appropriate handwashing protocol. This is because the most common source of infection in immunocompromised patients is their own (endogenous) flora.

Nonetheless, immunocompromised patients should be separated from patients with infectious diseases, preferably in a private room. Under these conditions, meticulous adherence to routine standards for asepsis are generally sufficient to minimize the risk of infection.

Burn patients. Most major burn wounds become infected within 48 to 72 hours after the initial incident. Therefore, care of patients with severe burns must involve concerted efforts to minimize wound colonization and prevent infection. Although isolation precautions and infection control methods for major burns vary, most burn centers enforce strict contact isolation procedures.

Special considerations with the HIV virus. As indicated earlier in this chapter, the HIV virus is causing ma-

jor concern in both the health care community and among members of the general population. Regarding its potential for transmission in the hospital setting, the National Centers for Disease Control have issued specific guidelines to minimize risk. These guidelines emphasize the application of universal blood and body-fluid precautions and provide special protocols for conducting invasive procedures.

Universal precautions. Since it is impossible to reliably identify all patients infected with the HIV virus or other blood-borne infectious agents, the CDC recommends that blood and body-fluid precautions be consistently used for all patients. Such an approach is particularly important in emergency care settings, where the risk of blood exposure is high and the infection status of the patient is usually unknown.

Specific CDC guidelines for universal precautions are provided in the box on p. 324. These guidelines reiterate and strengthen normal blood and body-fluid precautions. In fact, implementation of these universal blood and body-fluid precautions for all patients effectively eliminates that isolation category.

Precautions for invasive procedures. All health care personnel involved in invasive procedures must routinely use appropriate barrier precautions to prevent skin and mucous membrane contact with blood and other body fluids. Gloves and surgical masks are required for all invasive procedures. Protective eyewear and gowns or aprons are recommended for any procedure that could result in the generation of droplets or the splashing of blood or other body fluids. If hands or other skin surfaces become contaminated during an invasive procedure, the gloves should be removed and the affected area thoroughly washed.

As previously indicated, existing evidence indicates that the risk for hospital personnel becoming infected by the HIV virus through job-related activities is extremely small. Simple adherence to these CDC precautions further decreases this risk. Hospital personnel who are careful and meticulous in applying these standards should feel confident in delivering quality care to all their patients.

SURVEILLANCE

Surveillance is an ongoing process designed to ensure that infection control procedures are achieving their goal. Surveillance generally involves three interrelated components: (1) equipment-processing quality control, (2) routine sampling of in-use equipment, and (3) microbiologic identification. During major outbreaks of nosocomial infections, surveillance will also involve epidemiologic investigation.

The policies and procedures governing a hospital surveillance program are normally established by an infection control committee and administered by an infection control nurse or epidemiologist. Depending on institutional policy, surveillance may be a solely centralized function or may

CENTERS FOR DISEASE CONTROL (CDC) UNIVERSAL PRECAUTIONS

1. All health care workers should routinely use appropriate barrier precautions to prevent skin and mucous membrane exposure when contact with blood or other body fluids of any patient is anticipated. Gloves should be worn for touching blood and body fluids, mucous membranes, or nonintact skin of all patients, for handling items or surfaces soiled with blood or body fluids, and for performing venipuncture and other vascular access procedures. Gloves should be changed after contact with each patient. Masks and protective eyewear or face shields should be worn during procedures that are likely to generate droplets of blood or other body fluids to prevent exposure of mucous membranes of the mouth, nose, and eyes. Gowns or aprons should be worn during procedures that are likely to generate splashes of blood or other body fluids.

2. Hands and other skin surfaces should be washed immediately and thoroughly if contaminated with blood or other body fluids. Hands should be washed immediately after gloves are removed.

3. All health care workers should take precautions to prevent injuries caused by needles, scalpels, and other sharp instruments or devices during procedures; when cleaning used instruments; during disposal of used needles; and when handling sharp instruments after procedures. To prevent needle-stick injuries, needles should not be recapped, purposely bent or broken by hand, removed from disposable syringes, or otherwise manipulated by hand. After they are used, disposable syringes and needles, scalpel blades, and other sharp items should be placed in puncture-resistant containers for disposal; the puncture-resistant containers should be located as close as practical to the use area. Large-bore reusable needles should be placed in puncture-resistant containers for transport to the reprocessing area.

4. Although saliva has not been implicated in HIV transmission, to minimize the need for emergency mouth-to-mouth resuscitation, mouthpieces, resuscitation bags, or other ventilation devices should be available for use in areas in which the need for resuscitation is predictable.

5. Health care workers who have exudative lesions or weeping dermatitis should refrain from all direct patient care and from handling patient care equipment until the condition resolves.

6. Pregnant health care workers are not known to be at greater risk of contracting HIV infection than health care worker develops HIV infection during pregnancy, the infant is at risk of infection resulting from perinatal transmission. Because of this risk, pregnant health care workers should be especially familiar with and strictly adhere to precautions to minimize the risk of HIV transmission.

be decentralized to the various service departments. In the latter case, respiratory care practitioners will work directly with the infection control nurse or epidemiologist and the microbiology laboratory in implementing department-level surveillance procedures.

Equipment-processing quality control

Equipment-processing quality control involves monitoring and evaluating personnel adherence to procedures for equipment decontamination, sterilization, and disinfection. Supplementing this evaluation of the process must be assessment of the outcomes or results of equipment processing. Processing quality control must determine if the procedures used actually result in sterile or disinfected equipment. This is accomplished using both specially prepared processing indicators and culture sampling methods.

Processing indicators. As the name implies, processing indicators indicate whether a sterilization or disinfection process has done its job. There are two types of processing indicators: chemical and biologic.

Chemical indicators. Chemical indicators, usually impregnated on packaging tape, change color when exposed to specific conditions. Autoclave chemical indicators change color after exposure to a given temperature for a sufficient period of time. Likewise, chemical indicators used in ethylene oxide processing change color after exposure to a given concentration of the gas.

Chemical indicators provide visual evidence that a package has been through a sterilizing process. Since neither autoclave nor ethylene oxide processing changes the appearance of packs or packaging, indicator tape also helps distinguish between processed and unprocessed items.

However, while a chemical indicator gives visual, external evidence that a package has been through a sterilizer cycle, it cannot assure that either the process was truly effective or the items are truly sterile. To provide these assurances, biologic indicators are necessary.

Biologic indicators. Biologic indicators consist of strips of paper impregnated with an appropriate spore preparation. *Bacillus stearothermophilus* is the primary biologic indicator used for autoclave processes, while *Bacillus subtilis* is the organism of choice for ethylene oxide sterilization.

These spore strips are housed in a plastic capsule with a glass ampule that contains a selected growth medium, usually tryptic soy broth (Fig. 14-2). To prevent contamination with other organisms, but to ensure gas penetration, the capsule cap contains a bacterial filter.

The capsule is wrapped in the recommended packaging material and placed in the most inaccessible location in the sterilizer load (failure to observe this precaution can lead to a sterile biologic control in an unsterile load). After sterilization, the glass ampule in the capsule is crushed, exposing the spores to the growth medium. The capsule is then incubated according to the manufacturer's instruc-

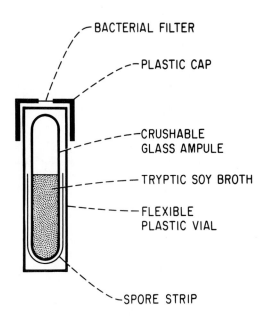

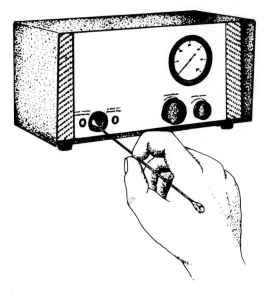

Fig. 14-2 Biologic sterilization indicator. The capsule contains a strip impregnated with bacterial spores, pH indicator, and culture medium in a crushable ampule. After removal from the sterilizer the ampule is crushed, releasing the culture medium onto the spore strip. A yellow color after incubation indicates incomplete sterilization. (Redrawn from Boyd and Hoerl: Basic medical microbiology, ed 3, Boston 1986, Little, Brown & Co.)

Fig. 14-3 Swab sampling. (From McLaughlin AJ: Manual of infection control in respiratory care, Boston, 1983, Little Brown.)

tions. Turbidity or color change in the growth medium after the specified incubation period indicates bacterial growth and failure of the sterilization process.

Unfortunately, the incubation period required to verify sterility of a given processing cycle can range from 1 to 3 days. This requires that the processed equipment be held from use until its sterility is assured. Obviously, this "down time" adds to the cost of care by demanding larger inventories of reusable equipment.

Nonetheless, the use of biologic indicators is an essential element in equipment-processing quality control. Biologic indicators should be used to verify all sterilization cycles. These indicators also are useful when experimenting with new packaging materials or modifications of processing procedures. Any deviation in procedure from that recommended by a sterilizer's manufacturer must be pretested with a biologic control.

Culture sampling. The use of processing indicators generally is limited to sterilization methods using heat, ionizing radiation, and gas. To monitor and evaluate the effectiveness of other procedures, especially pasteurization and chemical disinfection, bacteriologic samples are obtained and cultured from processed equipment. When performed correctly, culture sampling determines the level of residual bacteria remaining on this equipment, thereby providing information on the efficacy of the disinfection process.

Unfortunately, contamination during sampling proce-

dures is common, making equipment culture results difficult to interpret. Moreover, if adherence to disinfection protocols is carefully monitored, regular culture sampling is generally unnecessary. Therefore, in the absence of a nosocomial epidemic, regular culturing of processed equipment is not warranted.

Random sampling and culturing of stored items is used in assessing packaging adequacy and material shelf-life. Culturing also may be a useful tool when assessing a new disinfectant or disinfectant process. Finally, sampling of in-use equipment is a normal component of bacteriologic surveillance.

Sampling of in-use equipment

In addition to selected sampling of processed equipment, surveillance procedures usually involve random sampling and culturing of in-use equipment. The purpose of sampling and culturing in-use equipment is twofold: (1) it helps establish the frequency with which in-use items should be removed from use and reprocessed and (2) it can contribute to early identification of the source of nosocomial epidemics before they become widespread.

There are three common methods used to sample respiratory care-related equipment: (1) swab sampling, (2) liquid broths, and (3) aerosol impaction. Each method is designed to facilitate sample collection from particular equipment or equipment locations. Personnel responsible for departmental sampling of in-use equipment must be trained in these techniques.

Swab sampling. Swab sampling is used to obtain bacterial cultures from easily accessible surfaces of respiratory care equipment. As shown in Fig. 14-3, a specially prepared sterile swab is rubbed on the equipment surface at a single location. Each location sampled requires a new swab. Using aseptic techniques, the swab is placed either in a tube of sterile liquid broth or used to inoculate a plate of growth media. Information regarding the date, time, equipment source, and location from which the sample was taken must be provided. Samples are then transported to the microbiology laboratory for incubation and identification.

Liquid broths. Swab sampling cannot reach many parts of respiratory care equipment, especially inside of certain tubing delivery circuits. In these situations, sterile liquid broths are used to obtain a sample. Using aseptic techniques, the broth is poured into circuitry tubing and "swished" back and forth. Once exposed, the broth is poured into a sterile container for culturing. Labeling protocol is the same as with swab sampling.

Aerosol impaction. Given the fact that jet nebulizers are a major source for bacterial colonization and the spread of infection, it is often necessary to sample the actual particulate output of these devices. Sampling of liquid particle aerosols is accomplished by inertial impaction devices. These range in complexity from a simple funnel with attached culture plate to sophisticated, multichamber devices that segregate aerosol particles according to size. Regardless of the device used, asepsis must be maintained during equipment setup and sample collection. Labeling protocol is the same as with other sample collection methods.

Microbiologic identification

The hospital microbiology laboratory fulfills a central role in bacteriologic surveillance. Here, organisms are cultured, isolated, and identified according to a variety of specialized techniques and procedures.

Although the majority of its activities are provided as diagnostic services, the microbiology laboratory works closely with the infection control nurse or epidemiologist in support of the surveillance program. Regular diagnostic activities often reveal patterns of infection with certain microorganisms that can precede widespread outbreaks. When combined with ongoing surveillance activity, such information can prevent or minimize large-scale, in-hospital epidemics.

When the surveillance program is decentralized to the departmental level, respiratory care practitioners may work closely with the microbiology laboratory staff to develop, maintain, and evaluate the methods and procedures used to gather and interpret bacteriologic samples.

SUMMARY

Hospital-acquired infections represent a major problem in health care delivery, causing substantial morbidity and mortality and costing billions of dollars each year.

The incidence of hospital-acquired infections can be reduced only by strict adherence to infection control proce-

dures that include techniques designed to (1) eliminate the sources of infectious agents, (2) create barriers to their transmission, and (3) monitor and evaluate the effectiveness of these control methods. Effective application of infection control procedures is a major and ongoing responsibility of all respiratory care practitioners.

BIBLIOGRAPHY

American Association for Respiratory Therapy, Technical Standards and Safety Committee: Recommendations for respiratory therapy equipment: processing, handling and surveillance, Respir Care 22:928, 1977.

American College of Surgeons: Total care for burn patients: a guide to hospital resources, Bull Am Coll Surg 62:6-14, 1977.

American Hospital Association, Advisory Committee on Infections: Infection control in the hospital, ed 4, Chicago, 1979, The Association.

American Respiratory Care Foundation: Guidelines for disinfection of respiratory care equipment used in the home, Respir Care 33:801-808, 1988.

Association for the Advancement of Medical Instrumentation Z79 Subcommittee on Ethylene Oxide Sterilization: Ethylene oxide sterilization: a guide for hospital personnel, Respir Care 22(1):1977.

Baumgartner K: Bacterial control in inhalation therapy, Can J Inhal Ther 7:12, 1971.

Benarde MA and Hegh C: Ethylene oxide sterilization, Hospitals 44:62, 1970.

Centers for Disease Control: Recommendations for preventing transmission of infection with human T-lymphotropic virus type III/lymphadenopathy-associated virus in the workplace, MMWR 34:681-6, 691-5, 1985.

Centers for Disease Control: Acquired immunodeficiency syndrome (AIDS): precautions for health-care workers and allied professionals, MMWR 32:450-451, 1983.

Couperus JJ and Elder HA: Infectious disease aspect of respiratory therapy. In Burton GG and Hodgkin JE, editors: Respiratory care: a guide to clinical practice, ed 2, Philadelphia, 1984, JB Lippincott Co.

Darin J: Respiratory therapy equipment in the development of nosocomial respiratory tract infections, Curr Rev Respir Ther 4:83, 1985.

Deane RS, Mills EL, and Hamel AJ: Antibacterial action of copper in respiratory therapy apparatus, Chest 58:373, 1970.

Dixon RE et al: Aqueous quaternary ammonium antiseptics and disinfectants, JAMA 236:2415-2417, 1976.

Favero MS: Sterilization, disinfection, and antisepsis in the hospital. In Manual of clinical microbiology, ed 4, Washington, DC, 1985, American Society for Microbiology.

Garner JS and Favero MS: Guideline for handwashing and hospital environmental control, pub No 99-1117, Atlanta, 1985, Centers for Disease Control.

Garner JS and Simmons BP: Centers for Disease Control guideline for isolation precautions in hospitals, pub No 83-8314, Atlanta, 1983, Centers for Disease Control.

Gorman SP, Scott EM, and Russell AD: A review: antimicrobial activity, uses and mechanisms of action of glutaraldehyde, J Appl Bacteriol 48:161-190, 1980.

Howard BJ et al: Clinical and pathogenic microbiology, St Louis, 1987, The CV Mosby Co.

Johanson WG: Infectious complications of respiratory therapy, Respir Care 27:445, 1982.

McLaughlin AJ: Manual of infection control in respiratory care, Boston, 1983, Little, Brown & Co.

Nelson EJ: A new use for pasteurization: disinfection of inhalation therapy equipment, Respir Care 16:97, 1971.

Perkins JJ: Principles and methods of sterilization, ed 2, Springfield, Ill, 1983, Charles C Thomas, Publisher.

Reinarz JA et al: The potential role of inhalation therapy equipment in nosocomial pulmonary infection, J Clin Invest 44:831-839, 1965.

Rendell-Baker L and Roberts RB: Safe use of ethylene oxide sterilization in hospitals, Anesth Analg 49:919, 1970.

Rendell-Baker L and Roberts RB: The hazards of ethylene oxide, Anesthesiology 30:349, 1969.

Simmons BP: Guidelines for hospital environmental control, Infect Control 2:131-146, 1981.

Stonehill AA, Krop S, and Borick PM: Buffered glutaraldehyde: a new chemical sterilizing solution, Am J Hosp Pharm 20:458, 1963.

Williams WW: Guideline for infection control in hospital personnel, Infect Control 4(suppl):326-349, 1983.

Wright N: Methods and principles of sterilization, Hosp Management 109:65, 1970.

SECTION V

The Need for Respiratory Care

15

Patterns of Cardiopulmonary Dysfunction*

Craig L. Scanlan

Cardiopulmonary dysfunction exists when the lungs, heart, or vascular systems fail to fulfill their coordinated functions adequately and efficiently. In the most general terms, this means that there is impaired oxygen delivery to or carbon dioxide removal from the tissues or that the energy cost necessary to exchange these metabolites effectively is prohibitively excessive.

Based on this general definition, the majority of clinical disorders resulting in abnormal cardiopulmonary function may be grouped into one or more major patterns, including hypoxia, ventilation-perfusion ($\dot{V}/\dot{Q}$) imbalances, airway obstruction, pulmonary distention, and pulmonary restriction.

For the practitioner, a thorough understanding of these major patterns of pathophysiology provides the necessary foundation for the collaborative planning and implementation of quality respiratory care.

*Discussion on ventilation-perfusion imbalances adapted with permission from Martin L: Pulmonary physiology in clinical practice: the essentials for patient care and evaluation, St Louis, 1987, The CV Mosby Co.

OBJECTIVES

After completing this chapter, the reader will be able to:

1. Describe the primary abnormal physiologic processes underlying cardiopulmonary dysfunction;

2. Differentiate among the causes, physiologic effects, and clinical manifestations of hypoxia, both acute and chronic;

3. Explain how $\dot{V}/\dot{Q}$ imbalances affect the exchange of both oxygen and carbon dioxide between the lungs and pulmonary circulation;

4. Differentiate among the major causes, clinical manifestations, and treatment strategies employed in the following categories of cardiopulmonary dysfunction:
   Airway obstruction;
   Pulmonary distention;
   Pulmonary restriction.

KEY TERMS

Most terms used in this chapter are defined in context. The following terms are introduced without explicit definition but may be found in the text glossary:

aliquot	extravasate
anaphylaxis	fibrosis
atopic	hematopoiesis
bronchiectasis	hypothermia
buccal	ischemia
carboxyhemoglobinemia	methemoglobinemia
costrovertebral	myocardial infarction
cytochrome oxidase system	neurogenic
empyema	periosteum
endocarditis	sclera
epistaxis	somnolence
erythropoiesis	sulfhemoglobin

GENERAL CONCEPTS

Before analyzing the major clinical patterns of cardiopulmonary dysfunction, it is useful to assess the physiologic bases underlying all such deviations from normal function. In general, cardiopulmonary dysfunction exists when oxygen delivery to or carbon dioxide removal from the tissues is impaired or when the energy cost necessary to exchange these metabolites effectively is prohibitively excessive.

Impaired oxygen delivery

As discussed in Chapter 9, oxygen delivery to the tissues is a function of arterial oxygen content (CaO_2) multiplied by cardiac output ($\dot{Q}T$):

$$\text{Oxygen delivery} = CaO_2 \times \dot{Q}T$$

When oxygen delivery is inadequate to meet cellular needs, a condition of *hypoxia* exists. According to the above equation, hypoxia can occur if (1) the oxygen content of arterial blood is decreased, (2) cardiac output or perfusion is decreased, or (3) both conditions pertain.

A decrease in the oxygen content of the arterial blood is termed *hypoxemia*. Hypoxemia can result from a decreased Pa_{O_2}, a decrease in available hemoglobin, or hemoglobin saturation abnormalities. Alone or combined, these factors will lower the amount of oxygen available to the tissues. Thus, without a compensatory response by the cardiovascular system, a decrease in arterial oxygen content may result in tissue hypoxia.

A decrease in perfusion, even without hypoxemia, can also cause hypoxia. Decreased perfusion may be localized to a particular tissue region (ischemia) or generalized to the entire body (shock). Regardless of locale, the likelihood of tissue hypoxia is directly related to the severity of the flow disturbance, the length of the incident, and the metabolic rate of the affected tissues.

Impaired carbon dioxide removal

As presented in Chapter 10, impaired removal of carbon dioxide by the lung results in hypercapnia and respiratory acidosis. Of course, carbon dioxide levels are governed by the relationship between its production and excretion, as specified in the following formula:

$$Pa_{CO_2} = \frac{\dot{V}_{CO_2} \times 0.863}{\dot{V}_A}$$

Given this relationship, any disorder that lowers alveolar ventilation ($\dot{V}_A$) relative to metabolic need will impair carbon dioxide removal.

Clinically, a decrease in alveolar ventilation relative to metabolic need may occur when (1) the minute ventilation ($\dot{V}_E$) is inadequate, (2) the dead space ventilation per minute ($\dot{V}_{DS}$) is increased, or (3) an inadequate $\dot{V}_E$ and an increased $\dot{V}_{DS}$ coexist.[1] An inadequate $\dot{V}_E$ usually manifests itself as a simple reduction in tidal volumes and is usually associated with restrictive conditions, such as respiratory center depression, neuromuscular disorders, or impeded thoracic expansion (see the subsequent section on pulmonary restriction). An increase in $\dot{V}_{DS}$ may be caused by either rapid, shallow breathing (an increase in anatomic dead space per minute) or to the presence of areas of the lung with abnormally high $\dot{V}/\dot{Q}$ ratios (an increase in physiologic dead space per minute).

Regardless of underlying cause, a decrease in alveolar ventilation relative to metabolic need will always result in hypercapnia, or an elevated arterial P_{CO_2}. Since an elevated Pa_{CO_2} increases ventilatory drive in healthy subjects, the very existence of hypercapnia suggests the presence of other abnormalities of the respiratory apparatus. Specifically, the presence of hypercapnia indicates one of the following: (1) the patient is not responding normally to the elevated Pa_{CO_2}, (2) the patient is responding normally, but the signal is not getting through to the respiratory muscles, or (3), despite normal afferent and efferent response mechanisms, the lungs and chest bellows simply cannot provide adequate ventilation because of restrictive disease or muscular fatigue.[2]

Prohibitive energy costs

The lungs and the heart normally can meet the tissues' metabolic needs over a wide range of physiologic demands. During exercise, for example, it is not unusual for a healthy individual to maintain a fivefold increase in $\dot{V}_E$ and a tripling of cardiac output to meet the tissue needs for increased oxygen delivery and carbon dioxide removal.

However, even in healthy individuals, there is an upper limit to the amount of work that the respiratory and cardiovascular systems can perform. At a point determined, in part, by the individual's overall physical conditioning, lactic acidosis and muscle fatigue combine to limit continued exercise tolerance.

Of course, this upper limit of work tolerance is much lower for patients with respiratory or cardiovascular disease. In those with respiratory disease, the major factors limiting an increase in workload are an inadequate ventilatory reserve and dyspnea. Moreover, unlike healthy individuals, individuals with respiratory disease may exhibit an actual increase in P_{CO_2} at higher levels of energy expenditure, which can lead to respiratory failure.

On the other hand, in patients with cardiovascular disease, the major factor limiting an increase in work is the inability to increase cardiac output in response to increased metabolic needs. This may be caused by inadequate stroke volume, inadequate heart rate, or both, with inadequate stroke volume being the most common limiting factor. Regardless of underlying cause, these limitations lead to an early increase in lactic acid production (resulting from anaerobic metabolism) and hyperventilation. Sustained increases in workload may ultimately result in cardiac failure.

Thus, if the workload necessary to maintain normal oxygen delivery and carbon dioxide removal exceeds the ability of the lungs or heart to fulfill these functions, the body may have to accept an abnormal state of affairs to conserve energy. Thus, hypoventilation and hypercapnia may have to be "accepted" to avoid overt respiratory muscle fatigue, and a decreased cardiac output, with an increased $C(a-\bar{v})_{O_2}$, may have to be "accepted" in lieu of risking acute cardiac failure.

In summary, the three major physiologic disturbances underlying all forms of cardiopulmonary dysfunction are (1) impaired oxygen delivery, (2) impaired carbon dioxide removal, and (3) energy costs exceeding those which the respiratory and cardiovascular systems can maintain.

Associated with these major physiologic disturbances are a large number of discrete clinical disorders. In general, these numerous disorders may be grouped into one or more major pathophysiologic patterns, including hypoxia, ventilation-perfusion imbalances, airway obstruction, pulmonary distention, and pulmonary restriction.

HYPOXIA

Hypoxia exists when not enough oxygen is delivered to the tissues to meet their metabolic needs.[3,4] In this section we explore the major causes of hypoxia and its physiologic effects and clinical manifestations, followed by a brief discussion of treatment.

Causes

As previously discussed, hypoxia is usually caused by either a decrease in the oxygen content of arterial blood (hypoxemia) or a decrease in whole body cardiac output or local tissue perfusion. Both these conditions result in a decrease in delivery of oxygen to the tissues. A third major category of hypoxia, called histotoxic hypoxia or *dysoxia*, can occur in the presence of normal oxygen delivery to the tissues. Dysoxia represents an abnormal metabolic state in which the tissues are unable to use the oxygen made available to them.[5] The major causes of hypoxia and their primary indicators are summarized in Table 15-1.

Hypoxemia. A decrease in the oxygen content of the arterial blood, or hypoxemia, can result from a decreased Pa_{O_2}, a decrease in available hemoglobin, or hemoglobin saturation abnormalities. Alone or combined, these factors will lower the amount of oxygen carried to the tissues. Without a compensatory response by the cardiovascular system, a decrease in arterial oxygen content may result in tissue hypoxia.

Decreased Pa_{O_2}. A reduction in the partial pressure of oxygen in the arterial blood may result from a low ambient P_{O_2}, hypoventilation, impaired alveolar-capillary diffusion, right-to-left anatomic shunts, or $\dot{V}/\dot{Q}$ imbalance.

Low ambient P_{O_2}. Breathing a mixture of gases with a low concentration of oxygen at atmospheric pressure (760 mm Hg), or breathing air at pressures less than atmospheric, lowers the alveolar oxygen tension, thereby decreasing the Pa_{O_2}. A common example of this problem is encountered during travel to high altitudes, where the unaccustomed visitor often suffers the ill effects of hypoxia

Table 15-1   Causes of Hypoxia

Cause	Primary indicator	Mechanism	Example
HYPOXEMIA			
Low P_{IO_2}	Low P_{AO_2} Low Pa_{O_2}	Reduced P_B	Altitude
Hypoventilation	Low Pa_{O_2} High P_{CO_2}	Decreased $\dot{V}_A$	Drug overdose
Diffusion defect	Low Pa_{O_2} High $P_{(A-a)O_2}$ on air; resolves with O_2	Barrier at A-C membrane	Interstitial lung disease
Anatomic shunt	Low Pa_{O_2} High $P_{(A-a)O_2}$ on air; does not resolve with O_2	Blood flow between right and left sides of circulation	Congenital heart disease
$\dot{V}/\dot{Q}$ imbalance			
Low $\dot{V}/\dot{Q}$	Low Pa_{O_2} High $P_{(A-a)O_2}$ on air; resolves with O_2	Decreased $\dot{V}_A$ relative to perfusion	Chronic obstructive lung disease; aging
Physiologic shunt	Low Pa_{O_2} High $P_{(A-a)O_2}$ on air; does not resolve with O_2	Perfusion without ventilation	Atelectasis
HB deficiency			
Absolute	Low Hb content Reduced Ca_{O_2}	Loss of Hb	Hemorrhage
Relative	Abnormal Sa_{O_2} Reduced Ca_{O_2}	Abnormal Hb	Carboxyhemoglobin
REDUCED BLOOD FLOW	Increased $C(a-\bar{v})_{O_2}$ Decreased $C\bar{v}_{O_2}$	Decreased perfusion	Shock; ischemia
DYSOXIA	Normal Ca_{O_2} Increased $C\bar{v}_{O_2}$	Disruption of cellular enzymes	Cyanide poisoning; septic shock

A-C, alveolar-capillary; *Hb,* hemoglobin.

for several days. This condition is often referred to as acute mountain sickness.[6,7] The body's compensatory response to this form of chronic hypoxia is described later in this chapter.

Hypoventilation. Based on the alveolar air equation, and assuming a constant F_{IO_2}, the partial pressure of oxygen in the alveoli varies inversely with the P_{ACO_2} (see Chapter 9). Thus, a rise in the alveolar P_{CO_2}, or hypoventilation, is always accompanied by a proportionate fall in the alveolar P_{O_2}.

Impaired alveolar-capillary diffusion. Even in the presence of a normal alveolar P_{O_2}, pathologic changes in the alveolar-capillary membrane, such as may occur with fibrosis or interstitial edema, may limit diffusion of oxygen molecules into the pulmonary capillary blood, thereby lowering the P_{aO_2}. However, a pure diffusion limitation is a relatively uncommon cause of hypoxemia at rest. Limitations to diffusion, if present, generally manifest themselves only when the blood flow through the pulmonary circulation is increased, as during exercise (see Chapter 9).

Anatomic shunts. An anatomic shunt consists of a direct communication between the arterial and venous circulations. Small anatomic shunts, through the bronchial circulation and thebesian vessels, occur in healthy individuals. Abnormal anatomic shunts are the result of congenital defects, disease, or trauma. Congenital heart disease is the most common cause of anatomic shunting.

The two types of anatomic shunts are right to left and left to right. A right-to-left shunt exists when blood flows through the shunt from the venous to the arterial side of the circulation. Under these conditions, the low oxygen content of the venous blood will dilute the higher oxygen content of the arterial blood, lowering both the oxygen content and P_{O_2} in the resultant mixture.

A left-to-right shunt exists when blood flows through the shunt from the arterial to the venous side of the circulation and has little direct effect on the oxygen content of the arterial blood. However, to make up for the effective loss of arterial flow through the left-to-right shunt, the heart may have to increase the amount of blood it pumps per minute to satisfy tissue demands. For this reason, large left-to-right shunts can significantly increase the workload on the heart and may lead to cardiac failure.

Ventilation-perfusion imbalance. As described in Chapter 9, even in the normal lung the relationship between ventilation and perfusion is imperfect. In conjunction with the presence of small anatomic shunts, this normal $\dot{V}/\dot{Q}$ imbalance helps explain why the arterial P_{O_2} is always slightly less than the alveolar P_{O_2}.

In assessing reductions in P_{aO_2}, the clinician must also take into account the normal decrease in arterial oxygen tensions that occurs with aging. As shown in Fig. 15-1, when an individual breathes air at sea level, the "normal" $P_{(A-a)O_2}$ increases in a near-linear fashion with increasing age, resulting in a gradual decline in the P_{aO_2} over time.

One may estimate the expected P_{aO_2} in older adults using the following formula[8]:

$$\text{Expected } P_{aO_2} = 100.1 - (0.323 \times \text{age [yr]})$$

This progressive widening of the $P_{(A-a)O_2}$ over time is attributable to the normal loss of elastic recoil pressure in the aging lung and resultant changes in the distribution of ventilation to perfusion.

However, when blood perfuses areas of the lung where ventilation is abnormally reduced, or the amount of blood is abnormally excessive for the amount of ventilation present, the P_{aO_2} can become markedly reduced. The most obvious example of this type of $\dot{V}/\dot{Q}$ imbalance is the physiologic shunt. A physiologic shunt exists when a portion of the pulmonary blood perfuses unventilated alveoli ($\dot{V}/\dot{Q} = 0$). The result is similar to that previously described for a right-to-left anatomic shunt; that is, deoxygenated blood mixes with arterialized blood, lowering both the C_{aO_2} and the P_{aO_2}.

Of course, $\dot{V}/\dot{Q}$ ratios less extreme than this can and do occur. Indeed, low $\dot{V}/\dot{Q}$ ratios (less than 1 but greater than 0) are a more common cause of hypoxemia than are true physiologic shunts. Because of the clinical importance of this problem, its principles and consequences are discussed in some detail later in this chapter.

Hemoglobin deficiencies. A normal P_{aO_2} does not by itself guarantee adequate arterial oxygen content or delivery. For the arterial oxygen content to be adequate, there must also be sufficient quantities of normal hemoglobin in the circulating blood. Even with a normal P_{aO_2}, a deficiency in hemoglobin can result in hypoxia.

Hemoglobin deficiencies, or *anemias*, may be categorized as absolute or relative. An absolute hemoglobin deficiency occurs when the blood hemoglobin concentration is lower than normal. Relative hemoglobin deficiencies are caused by the displacement of oxygen from normal hemoglobin or the presence of abnormal hemoglobins.

Absolute hemoglobin deficiencies. A reduction in the blood hemoglobin concentration may be caused by a loss of circulating red blood cells, as occurs with hemorrhage, or by defective or inadequate erythropoiesis. Regardless of cause, a quantitative lack of circulating hemoglobin can seriously impair the blood's oxygen-carrying capacity, even with a normal supply (P_{aO_2}) and adequate diffusion.

Relative hemoglobin deficiencies. For adequate oxygenation, not only must there be enough hemoglobin, but it must be capable of normal oxygen transport. As described in Chapter 9, abnormal hemoglobin transport of oxygen may occur when normal hemoglobin is exposed to carbon monoxide (carboxyhemoglobinemia), when normal hemoglobin is oxidized to methemoglobin (methemoglobinemia), or when abnormal variants exist in the chemical structure of the hemoglobin.

With carboxyhemoglobinemia and methemoglobinemia, each gram of hemoglobin so affected is equivalent to the

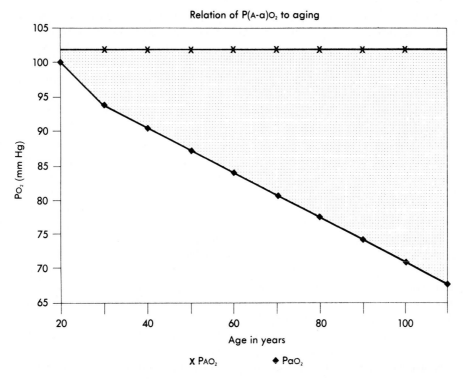

Fig. 15-1   The relationship of P(A-a)o$_2$ and aging. As Pao$_2$ naturally falls with age, P(A-a)o$_2$ increases at the rate of approximately 3 mm Hg each decade beyond 20 years. (From Lane EE and Walker JF: Clinical arterial blood gas analysis, St Louis, 1987, The CV Mosby Co.)

absolute loss of a gram of normal hemoglobin, as occurs in absolute anemia. Abnormal variants in the chemical structure of the hemoglobin have variable effects on oxygen transport, with those causing marked left shifts in the dissociation curve (thereby impeding oxygen unloading) having the greatest potential to cause hypoxia. HbC (Chesapeake), HbR (Rainier), and HbY (Yakima) all exhibit a greater affinity for oxygen than normal hemoglobin, with HbY having the greatest negative effect on oxygen unloading at the tissues.

Reduction in blood flow (shock or ischemia). Because oxygen delivery is a function of both arterial oxygen content and cardiac output, hypoxia can still occur in the presence of a normal Cao$_2$ if blood flow to the tissues is reduced. A reduction in blood flow to the tissues may be of two types—generalized circulatory failure (shock) or local reductions in perfusion (ischemia).

Generalized circulatory failure (shock). In the presence of generalized circulatory failure, such as may occur in cardiogenic, hypovolemic, neurogenic, septic, or anaphylactic shock, tissue oxygen deprivation is widespread. Although the body attempts to compensate for oxygen deprivation by directing blood flow to those organs most sensitive to hypoxia, this response is limited. Thus prolonged shock will ultimately result in irreversible damage to the central nervous system (CNS) and eventual cardiovascular collapse. The causes and clinical manifestations of shock

and the body's response to shock are discussed in Chapter 19.

Localized reductions in perfusion (ischemia). Even in the presence of adequate whole-body perfusion, local reductions in blood flow can cause hypoxia in delimited areas, resulting in anaerobic metabolism, metabolic acidosis, and eventual death of the affected tissue. Myocardial infarction and stroke (cerebrovascular accident) are good examples of conditions in which ischemia results in localized hypoxia and tissue death.

Dysoxia. Dysoxia is a form of hypoxia in which the cellular use of oxygen is abnormal. The best example of dysoxia is cyanide poisoning. Cyanide inactivates the intracellular cytochrome oxidase system, thereby preventing cellular use of oxygen. Septic shock may also disrupt cellular enzyme systems and hinder oxygen uptake by the tissues.

Physiologic effects

Mild hypoxia produces only minor physiologic changes. Hyperventilation is an early response to hypoxia in healthy subjects, and subtle changes in intellectual performance and visual acuity may be apparent. However, more severe hypoxia can result in the following[9]:

1. Pulmonary vasoconstriction resulting in pulmonary vascular hypertension;
2. An increased strain on the cardiovascular system caused by a compensatory increase in cardiac output;

3. Deleterious effects on myocardial function, especially in the presence of preexisting coronary artery disease;
4. Impaired renal function, with a tendency to retain sodium and water;
5. Altered CNS function, ranging from restlessness and disorientation to convulsions and permanent brain damage;
6. Anaerobic metabolism, lactic acid accumulation, and metabolic acidosis.

Clinical manifestations

Clinically, hypoxia may manifest itself in a number of ways, depending on its severity and duration (acute versus chronic). Table 15-2 compares and contrasts the major clinical findings associated with mild to moderate hypoxia with those typically observed in severe hypoxia. Two of these clinical manifestations, cyanosis and clubbing, warrant detailed discussion.

Cyanosis is one of the most commonly described clinical signs of severe hypoxia. It imparts a blue or blue-gray color to skin, mucous membranes, and nail beds and may be present in both acute and chronic hypoxia. This blue or blue-gray coloration is caused by the presence of abnormally high amounts of reduced or unsaturated hemoglobin in the blood.

Cyanosis may be categorized as either central or peripheral. Central cyanosis, observed best in the capillary beds of the lips or buccal membranes, is caused by a reduction in the hemoglobin saturation of arterial blood. Peripheral cyanosis, on the other hand, results from an excessive amount of reduced hemoglobin in the venous blood. An excessive amount of reduced hemoglobin in the venous blood occurs when oxygen extraction by the tissues is abnormally high, as occurs with poor perfusion or blood stasis.

Normally, capillary blood contains about 2.5 g/dL reduced hemoglobin (Hb^-).[10] For cyanosis to be detected, the capillaries generally must contain at least 5 g/dL Hb^-. Assuming a normal hemoglobin concentration of 15 g/dL and a normal arterial-venous oxygen content difference of 5 ml/dL, a mean capillary Hb^- content of 5 g/dL will occur when the arterial oxygen saturation, or Sao_2, drops below 80%. On a normal oxyhemoglobin dissociation curve, an Sao_2 of 80% corresponds to a Pao_2 of about 45 mm Hg. Thus, we would expect central cyanosis to be evident whenever the arterial Po_2 drops below this level.

However, since cyanosis depends on a specific concentration of unsaturated capillary hemoglobin, the relationship between its appearance and the presence of hypoxia is not always what one would expect. For example, when there is an absolute deficiency in the amount of circulating hemoglobin, as in anemia, there may not be enough unsaturated hemoglobin to produce central cyanosis until the arterial saturation drops well below 80%. Conversely, in polycythemia or erythrocytosis, the total concentration of circulating hemoglobin is increased. In this case, the amount of reduced hemoglobin may be sufficient to produce central cyanosis even though there is adequate oxygen delivery to the tissues. Moreover, if the cyanosis is peripheral, arterial oxygen content may be normal. In this case, the cyanosis is caused by poor capillary perfusion or blood stasis, not by reduced arterial oxygen content.

Last, evaluation of the presence and degree of cyanosis depends on the examiner's perception and is modified by factors such as the ambient lighting, the color of the skin, and the presence of abnormal blood pigments (e.g., methemoglobin or sulfhemoglobin). For these reasons, cyanosis must be considered an unreliable indicator of hypoxemia and hypoxia.[11]

Clubbing is one form of a more generalized process that affects bones and joints called hypertrophic osteoarthropathy.[12] Osteoarthropathy is a chronic inflammatory process that results in thickening of the periosteum, as evidenced on x-ray examination. Joints may also be swollen and inflamed. In a well-developed case there may be pain and disabling limitations to motion. Clubbing may occur early in the development of hypertrophic osteoarthropathy, or it may occur without long bone changes.

Clubbing is manifested by a bulbous swelling of the terminal phalanges of the fingers and toes. There is an increase in all diameters of the tips of the extremities, giving them a "drumstick" appearance. In contrast to the process found in long bones, pain is seldom a symptom of clubbing, even though the soft tissue swelling at the ends of the digits may be considerable.

Table 15-2 Clinical Manifestations of Hypoxia

	Mild to moderate	Severe
Respiratory findings	Tachypnea	Tachypnea
	Dyspnea	Dyspnea
	Paleness	Cyanosis
Cardiovascular findings	Tachycardia	Tachycardia, eventual bradycardia, arrhythmias
	Mild hypertension	
	Peripheral vasoconstriction	Hypertension and eventual hypotension
Neurologic findings	Restlessness	Somnolence
	Disorientation	Confusion
	Headaches	Blurred vision
	Lassitude	Tunnel vision
		Loss of coordination
		Impaired judgment
		Slow reaction time
		Manic-depressive activity
		Coma
Other		Clubbing

From Pilbeam SP: Mechanical ventilation, Denver, 1986, Multi-Media Publishing, Inc.

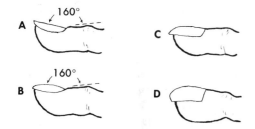

Fig. 15-2 Clubbing is characterized by marked curvature of the nail, a loss of the cuticular angle, an increase in the angle the surface of the nail makes with the terminal phalanx above the normal of 160 degrees, and a bulbous soft tissue swelling of the terminal phalanx. **A** and **B** show the contours of normal straight and curved nails; **C** and **D** represent increasing degrees of clubbing.

A characteristic feature of clubbing is the contour of the nail, which becomes rounded both longitudinally and transversely. Although such curvature may be seen in healthy individuals, the distortion of the nail in clubbing is marked by loss of the cuticular angle, that is, the angle between the junction of the skin and nail.

For purposes of illustration, Fig. 15-2 compares a normal flat nail, a normal curved nail, and early and late clubbing. Both normal nails exhibit a cuticular angle of less than 180 degrees. However, this normal angle is absent in fingers with clubbing. Associated with the loss of the cuticular angle in the early stages of clubbing is a "floating" nail base, or sponginess under the base of the nail, which allows it to be moved up and down with compression. Then, as the clubbing progresses from mild to severe, the degree of nail curvature gradually increases.

Despite the frequency with which clubbing is seen, its specific cause remains unknown. We do know that patients with this disorder demonstrate an increase in the width of the capillaries and an increased blood flow through the terminal portions of the affected digits.[13] In adults approximately 75% to 85% of all clubbing is associated with respiratory disease, such as lung tumors, bronchiectasis, or pulmonary fibrosis. Between 10% and 15% of patients with clubbing have an underlying cardiac disease, such as a congenital right-to-left shunt or chronic bacterial endocarditis. Patients with hepatic or gastrointestinal disorders make up an additional 10% of those with clubbing, with the remaining 5% associated with miscellaneous conditions. In children, clubbing is predominantly found with cystic fibrosis, bronchiectasis, empyema, and congenital heart disease.

Acute hypoxia. Acute hypoxia is caused by a rapid reduction of available oxygen, as from asphyxia, airway obstruction, blockage of alveoli by the fluid of edema or infectious exudate, abrupt cardiorespiratory failure, or acute hemorrhage. Regardless of cause, tachypnea and dyspnea are common, as is hyperventilation. However, in patients unable to increase their alveolar ventilation, tachypnea may result in hypoventilation, which will worsen an existing hypoxia.

Hypoxia produces a mental state like alcoholic intoxication.[14] Headache is a frequent complaint, and disorientation often occurs, although mental stimulation may be evident early on. However, as the hypoxia worsens, confusion and somnolence become apparent. Eventually, muscle coordination is lost, and judgment becomes impaired.[4] Finally, there is a loss of consciousness and coma.

As is evident from these signs, the most critical target organ of hypoxia is the CNS. With few exceptions, survival following acute hypoxia depends on its effect on the brain. One of the brain's early responses to hypoxia is vasodilation and an increased cerebral blood flow. However, because nerve tissue is so vulnerable to lack of oxygen, a few minutes of severe hypoxia may irreversibly damage brain cells. Comas of days' or weeks' duration are not uncommon, and the half-living vegetative existence of the not-quite-dead brain may be the most tragic consequence of hypoxia.

As previously described, other organs are also affected by hypoxia. Hypoxia strains the heart indirectly by causing tachycardia and pulmonary vasoconstriction. Hypoxia may also act directly on the myocardial fibers, causing a decrease in contractility, cardiac arrhythmias, or actual tissue death. Likewise, hypoxia interferes directly with the function of the renal tubular cells, compromising the kidney's ability to maintain normal electrolyte and water balance.

The depth of hypoxia the body can tolerate varies substantially. Obvious modifying variables include those related to the state of the circulation (especially the cerebral), the general body cellular health, the metabolic rate, and the rapidity and intensity with which therapy is instituted. Although some authorities suggest that an arterial Po_2 below 20 mm Hg is incompatible with life,[15] some patients have recovered from hypoxic incidents in which the arterial Po_2 was as low as 9 mm Hg. Moreover, some individuals have survived total asphyxia (as during cold water immersion) for more than 30 minutes. In these cases, survival has been attributed to the dramatic decrease in metabolic rate accompanying the whole-body hypothermia.

Chronic hypoxia. If hypoxia develops slowly, the body has time to make compensatory adjustments to minimize its effect. Diseases most likely to cause chronic hypoxia include parenchymal lung disorders (both destructive and fibrotic), chronic airway obstruction, congenital or acquired heart diseases, and chronic anemia.

Much of our knowledge regarding the body's response to chronic hypoxia has been learned by studying people born at or acclimatized to high altitudes. Many of these people live normal and active lives at partial pressures of oxygen in the same range as that found in patients at sea level who are suffering from hypoxia as a result of disease. Obviously, high-altitude dwellers must have physiologically adjusted to their "hypoxic" environment.

Although many of the details concerning pulmonary and cardiovascular adaptation to altitude are still under investigation, a few pertinent facts have been established. First, high-altitude dwellers tend to exhibit mild hyperventilation, which raises the alveolar Po_2, thereby partially offsetting the lower ambient Po_2. The resulting slight respiratory alkalosis is compensated for by increased renal excretion of HCO_3^-, yielding a normal blood and cerebrospinal fluid pH.

Supplementing this means of increasing the oxygen content of the arterial blood, high-altitude dwellers realize an increase in the amount of oxygen delivered to their tissues. This enhanced oxygen delivery caused by an increase in the amount of available hemoglobin and an increase in tissue vascularity. The increased amounts of hemoglobin available to the high-altitude dwellers occur through a larger red cell mass. This increased volume of circulating erythrocytes, called *secondary polycythemia*, is caused by an increased level of erythropoietin, a hormone that stimulates the bone marrow to produce red blood cells. The increase in vascularity is the result of an increase in the number of capillaries present in muscle, thereby decreasing the distance necessary for diffusion.

Last, whether born at or acclimatized to altitude, individuals who chronically breath low ambient partial pressures of oxygen tend to exhibit pulmonary arterial hypertension from hypoxic pulmonary vasoconstriction. Clinically, this pulmonary arterial hypertension manifests itself in changes in the electrocardiogram characteristic of right ventricular hypertrophy, such as right axis deviation.[16]

In a sense, the patient with chronic hypoxic resulting from a pulmonary or cardiovascular disorder is in a situation much like that of the high-altitude dweller, with the important difference being the presence of some underlying pathologic condition. For these patients, chronic hypoxia often results in persistent mental and physical fatigue. Mental responses may become sluggish and acuity diminished, and patients will frequently complain of an inability to perform even the simplest physical task without difficulty. As a rule, however, chronic hypoxia itself is not the primary cause of their disability; rather, it is the underlying disease responsible for the hypoxia that limits activity. For example, in patients with certain forms of chronic lung disease, it is the physical effort or work necessary to maintain adequate oxygen and carbon dioxide levels that is the real cause of disability, not the hypoxia itself.

As with high-altitude dwellers, a secondary polycythemia is common, although not always readily apparent. In some patients, this compensatory response to chronic hypoxia may be readily detected by examination of the blood hematocrit. Normally, the hematocrit does not exceed about 45%, but in secondary polycythemia it may rise above 55%. The hemoglobin content is similarly elevated from its usual upper limit of 15 g/dL to perhaps 20 g/dL, and measurement of the circulating erythrocytes will often show more than the normal concentration of about 5 million/mm^3.

However, these simple measures do not always reflect the hypoxic hematopoiesis responsible for polycythemia,[17] particularly in those patients in whom there is an associated increase in plasma volume. If great enough, this increase in plasma volume may result in normal values for those measurements that relate red blood cell numbers or hemoglobin content to blood volume. More definitive diagnostic tests, such as those measuring the circulating red blood cell mass, may be the only way to uncover an actual increase in erythrocytes.

However, enough patients show elevated hematocrits and hemoglobin contents to warrant a few remarks about the clinical significance of such findings. With a sufficient increase in the ratio of red blood cells to blood fluid, the viscosity of the blood rises, thereby increasing cardiac work and slowing blood flow. Sluggish blood flow, in turn, increases the likelihood of intravascular thromboses.[18] These detrimental effects probably become physiologically significant when the hematocrit reaches 55% to 60%, at which point any advantages gained by increasing the blood's oxygen-carrying capacity are nullified.[19]

As previously described, the patient with secondary polycythemia is usually cyanotic, despite an actual increase in the volume of oxygen carried by the blood. Patients often complain of headache, fullness in the head, nasal stuffiness, lethargy, difficulty in taking a deep breath, and epistaxis (nosebleed). The small vessels of the sclera (the white of the eye) may be grossly congested from an increased blood volume. Finally, the increased volume and viscosity of circulating blood can place an abnormally high work load on the heart, especially the less muscular right ventricle. In combination with the hypoxic pulmonary arterial hypertension, this increased cardiac work load can result in *cor pulmonale,* or right ventricular heart disease secondary to pulmonary disease.

Laboratory assessment

The laboratory assessment of hypoxia involves sampling, calculating, and measuring various blood parameters, including the Pao_2, the $P(A-a)o_2$, the Cao_2, and the $C\bar{v}o_2$ (oxygen content of the mixed venous blood). By combining these indicators, it is possible to identify the primary physiologic cause of the hypoxia (Table 15-3).

Except for hemoglobin deficiencies, all causes of reduced arterial oxygen content (hypoxemia) are associated with a reduced Pao_2. However, only hypoxemia caused by a diffusion defect, right-to-left shunting, and $\dot{V}/\dot{Q}$ imbalances manifests itself in an increased $P(A-a)o_2$ breathing room air. Administration of an increased Fio_2 will cause the $P(A-a)o_2$ to lessen in severity or resolve if the problem is a low $\dot{V}/\dot{Q}$ or a diffusion defect. However, the administration of a higher F_{IO_2} typically results in a widening of the $P_{(A-a)O_2}$ with right-to-left shunting, either anatomic or physiologic.

With hypoxemia in general, as long as the cardiovascular system can compensate for the reduction in arterial oxygen content by increasing cardiac output, the oxygen content of the mixed venous blood ($C\bar{v}_{O_2}$) can remain normal, and actual tissue hypoxia can be avoided. On the other hand, if the cardiovascular system cannot compensate, or if the hypoxemia is severe, the $C\bar{v}_{O_2}$ may drop, indicating the presence of tissue hypoxia.

In terms of hemoglobin deficiencies (without complicating problems), the Pa_{O_2} is often normal, as is the $P_{(A-a)O_2}$. Combined, these factors indicate a normal exchange of oxygen between the alveoli and pulmonary capillaries. However, the measured Ca_{O_2} will always be decreased because of the blood's decreased oxygen-carrying capacity.

As with hemoglobin deficiencies, when hypoxia is caused by reduced blood flow, the Pa_{O_2} and $P_{(A-a)O_2}$ may be normal. Moreover, the arterial oxygen content (Ca_{O_2}) may also be normal. The major laboratory abnormality signaling hypoxia caused by reduced blood flow is a reduction in the $C\bar{v}_{O_2}$, or oxygen content of the mixed venous blood.

Like hypoxia resulting from reduced blood flow, the Pa_{O_2}, $P_{(A-a)O_2}$, and Ca_{O_2} may all be normal in dysoxia. However, since this is a condition in which oxygen uptake by the tissues is abnormally low, the $C\bar{v}_{O_2}$ may be *higher* than normal because of failure of the cells to extract the oxygen delivered to them.

Another condition in which the $C\bar{v}_{O_2}$ may not be a use-ful indicator of the extent of tissue hypoxia is adult respiratory distress syndrome (ARDS). In these patients, the $C\bar{v}_{O_2}$ may not accurately reflect changes in cardiac output, oxygen delivery, or oxygen consumption of the tissues.[20]

Thus, with two major exceptions (dysoxia and ARDS), the "best" laboratory indicator of the presence or absence of hypoxia is the $C\bar{v}_{O_2}$. Unfortunately, the $C\bar{v}_{O_2}$ can only be obtained by invasive sampling of blood from the distal port of a pulmonary artery catheter. More details on the clinical assessment of oxygenation, as related to the management of patients in respiratory failure, are provided in Chapter 31.

Treatment

In patients with hypoxia, the primary therapeutic goal is to provide sufficient oxygen to the cells to preserve their normal function. Generally, this requires restoring satisfactory arterial oxygen content and ensuring adequate tissue perfusion while avoiding the hazards of high oxygen partial pressures (see Chapter 25). While hypoxia is being relieved, every effort must be made to correct the underlying pathologic condition(s) responsible for the inadequate availability of oxygen.

When hypoxemia is caused by a reduction in the alveolar P_{O_2}, a diffusion defect, or a moderately low $\dot{V}/\dot{Q}$, normal levels of arterial oxygenation can be achieved by simple oxygen therapy techniques, generally with an F_{IO_2} of less than 0.50. Details on the indications, methods of administration, and hazards of simple oxygen therapy are provided in Chapter 25.

When hypoxemia is caused by extremely low $\dot{V}/\dot{Q}$ ratios or physiologic shunting, even 100% oxygen may not be

Table 15-3   Assessment of Hypoxia

Cause	Pa_{O_2}	$P_{(A-a)O_2}$ Air	$P_{(A-a)O_2}$ O_2	Ca_{O_2}	$C\bar{v}_{O_2}$
HYPOXEMIA					
Low P_{IO_2}	− −	N	N	− −	N*
Hypoventilation	− −	N	N	− −	N*
Diffusion defect	− −	+ +	N	− −	N*
Anatomic shunt	− − −	+ + +	+ + + +	− −	N*
$\dot{V}/\dot{Q}$ imbalance					
Low $\dot{V}/\dot{Q}$	− −	+ +	+	− −	N*
Physiologic shunt	− − −	+ + +	+ + + +	− −	N*
Hb deficiency					
Absolute	N or − −	N	N	− −	− −
Relative	N or − −	N	N	− −	− −
REDUCED BLOOD FLOW	N	N	N	N	− −
DYSOXIA	N	N	N	N	+ +

*Venous oxygen content will remain normal only if cardiac output increases to compensate.
N, Normal; −, decreased; +, increased.

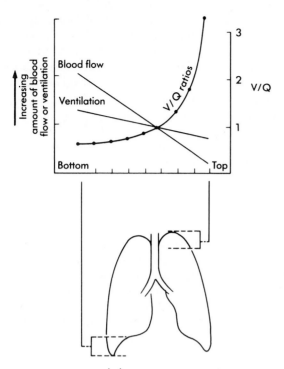

Fig. 15-3 Changes in V̇/Q̇ ratios in the upright lung. At the top of the lung, ventilation is greater than perfusion, resulting in high V̇/Q̇ ratios. From the top to the bottom of the lung, there is a progressive increase in both ventilation and perfusion. Since blood flow increases more than ventilation, the V̇/Q̇ ratios decrease and are lowest at the bottom of the lung. (From Martin L: Pulmonary physiology in clinical practice: the essentials for patient care and evaluation, St Louis, 1987, The CV Mosby Co.)

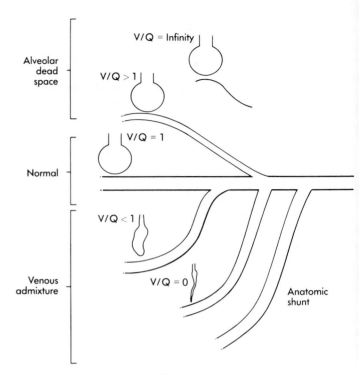

Fig. 15-4 The range of V̇/Q̇ ratios. See text for discussion. (From Martin, L: Pulmonary physiology in clinical practice: the essentials for patient care and evaluation, St Louis, 1987, The CV Mosby Co.)

sufficient to achieve a satisfactory arterial oxygen content. Instead, special methods of ventilatory support designed to open collapsed alveoli, such as CPAP or CMV with positive end-expiratory pressure (PEEP), may be necessary. These special methods of ventilatory support are described in detail in Chapters 29 and 30.

When secondary polycythemia complicates chronic hypoxia, phlebotomy may be useful. Withdrawal of venous blood, in increments of about 300 ml at intervals of 3 to 4 days, can lower the hematocrit and reduce blood viscosity. The clinical results are often rewarding, since patients feel better both physically and mentally and the progress of cor pulmonale is retarded.[19]

VENTILATION-PERFUSION IMBALANCES

As previously discussed, V̇/Q̇ imbalances are by far the most common physiologic cause for a reduced Pa_{O_2}. V̇/Q̇ imbalances are the primary mechanism causing hypoxemia in virtually all parenchymal lung diseases, such as asthma, atelectasis, bronchitis, emphysema, pneumonia, and pulmonary embolism. As we shall see, V̇/Q̇ imbalances also

are a common cause for impaired carbon dioxide removal in many clinical situations.

Definition

As used in clinical medicine, V̇/Q̇ imbalance refers to an abnormal deviation in the distribution of ventilation to perfusion among the lung's alveolar-capillary units. Normally, most lung units receive an amount of ventilation nearly equivalent to their blood flow, for example, 1 ml of air for each 1 ml of capillary blood flow. Such units are "balanced," with a V̇/Q̇ ratio of close to 1.0. When an alveolar-capillary unit has more ventilation than blood flow, the ratio for that unit is greater than 1.0; if more blood flow than ventilation is present, the ratio will be less than 1.0.

In reality, even the normal lung has some V̇/Q̇ mismatch (see Chapter 8). Because of the effects of gravity, some lung units are overventilated and some are overperfused. In the upright lung, both ventilation and perfusion are increased toward the bottom of the lung (Fig. 15-3). However, because perfusion increases more than ventilation, there is a change in V̇/Q̇ ratios from less than 1 at the bottom to more than 3 at the top of the lung. This slight mismatch in the normal lung explains, in part, why the arterial Po_2 is always slightly less than the alveolar Po_2.

Distribution of $\dot{V}/\dot{Q}$ ratios in disease

In disease states, the range of $\dot{V}/\dot{Q}$ imbalances becomes much greater than normal. Fig. 15-4 shows the possible range of $\dot{V}/\dot{Q}$ ratios. As shown in the top two units, to the extent that ventilation is greater than perfusion (a high $\dot{V}/\dot{Q}$), there is wasted ventilation or alveolar dead space. To the extent that ventilation is less than perfusion (low $\dot{V}/\dot{Q}$), the mixed venous blood passing through the pulmonary capillaries is exposed to less oxygen than normal and therefore leaves the alveolar region with a abnormally low oxygen content. When this poorly oxygenated blood mixes with blood that has been normally oxygenated, the result is a reduced arterial oxygen content and a reduced Pao_2.

In lung disease, deviations from the normal distribution of ventilation to perfusion usually result in both an excess wasted ventilation and poor oxygenation. Since a $\dot{V}/\dot{Q}$ imbalance makes the lung a less efficient organ for exchanging oxygen, the Pao_2 will be reduced. $\dot{V}/\dot{Q}$ imbalances also impair CO_2 exchange, although the effect on Pao_2 is usually more profound than on the partial pressure of arterial carbon dioxide. Reasons for this difference are discussed later in this section.

Shunts and venous admixture

"Shunt" is an overused word in pulmonary physiology and often means different things to different people. In its simplest definition, a shunt occurs whenever one thing bypasses another. In the lungs, the term shunt is commonly used when blood from the venous side of the circulation mixes with freshly oxygenated, or arterialized, blood. This right-to-left shunting lowers the oxygen content of the blood leaving the lungs, a condition called *venous admixture*.

Venous admixture can occur in three situations, only two of which are true shunts:

1. A right-to-left anatomic shunt occurs when blood bypasses the lungs through an anatomic channel, such as normally exists in the thebesian and bronchial circulations. Abnormal right-to-left anatomic shunts may occur in some forms of congenital heart disease and can develop in certain chronic lung diseases, such as bronchiectasis.
2. A right-to-left physiologic shunt occurs when a portion of the cardiac output perfuses unventilated alveoli. In this case, there is no abnormal connection between the venous and arterial circulations; rather, venous blood entering the lung follows its normal course but returns to the arterial circulation unchanged, that is, as poorly oxygenated venous blood. Physiologic shunting is often seen in conditions such as pulmonary edema, pneumonia, and atelectasis.
3. A low $\dot{V}/\dot{Q}$ ratio occurs when an area of the lung is poorly ventilated relative to its perfusion. In this case, the pulmonary blood is exposed to some alveolar air, but this is insufficient to achieve full oxygenation. Low $\dot{V}/\dot{Q}$ ratios account for most cases of hypoxemia seen clinically.

In terms of its effect on oxygenation, a right-to-left physiologic shunt is equivalent to a right-to-left anatomic shunt. In both cases, some unoxygenated blood bypasses the alveoli and mixes with oxygenated blood. Although both types of shunt cause a venous admixture, they differ in one important aspect from venous admixtures caused by low $\dot{V}/\dot{Q}$ ratios. Since shunted blood contacts no air, increasing the fraction of inspired oxygen (Fio_2) will not significantly improve oxygenation. In contrast, because blood in low $\dot{V}/\dot{Q}$ units is in contact with some air, oxygenation of blood perfusing these areas can be improved by increasing the Fio_2. Increasing the inspired oxygen concentration to 100% will completely oxygenate the blood that serves these units.

In the past, 100% oxygen was commonly administered to differentiate between hypoxemia caused by a low $\dot{V}/\dot{Q}$ and hypoxemia resulting from a right-to-left shunt. It is now known that breathing 100% oxygen can cause shunting by promoting the collapse of alveoli with low $\dot{V}/\dot{Q}$ ratios. This phenomenon, called absorption atelectasis, occurs because pure oxygen in poorly ventilated alveoli is quickly absorbed by the capillary blood, thereby lowering the total gas pressure responsible for maintaining the alveolus open. In the well-ventilated alveolus, oxygen uptake by the blood is balanced by its constant replenishment, thereby ensuring stability of the respiratory unit.

Effect of $\dot{V}/\dot{Q}$ imbalances on oxygenation and carbon dioxide removal

Oxygenation. It has been stated that $\dot{V}/\dot{Q}$ imbalances are the most common cause of hypoxemia. The mechanism of this type of hypoxemia can now be examined more closely. In Fig. 15-5, the arterial partial pressure of oxygen (Pao_2) is plotted against the arterial oxygen content; this is the oxygen dissociation curve for a hemoglobin content of 15 g/dL. The shape of the curve is the same as when Pao_2 is plotted against the percentage of oxygen saturation of hemoglobin. Note that the curve is nearly flat in the range of physiologic Pao_2 values (above 70 mm Hg) and falls steeply below 60 mm Hg. Points representing oxygen contents from three separate alveolar-capillary units are also shown. These units have $\dot{V}/\dot{Q}$ ratios of 0.1, 1.0, and 10.0. Note that the decrease in capillary oxygenation caused by the low $\dot{V}/\dot{Q}$ unit is not compensated for by the high $\dot{V}/\dot{Q}$ unit.

Units with low $\dot{V}/\dot{Q}$ ratios have low alveolar Po_2 values. Blood perfusing these units has a low end-capillary oxygen content. If there were a range of $\dot{V}/\dot{Q}$ units from 1.0 (normal) down to 0, the result could only be hypoxemia, since low oxygen contents would be mixing with normal oxygen contents. In fact, a $\dot{V}/\dot{Q}$ imbalance implies that at least some units are overventilated (high $\dot{V}/\dot{Q}$ ratios) while others are underventilated (low $\dot{V}/\dot{Q}$ ratios). However, if

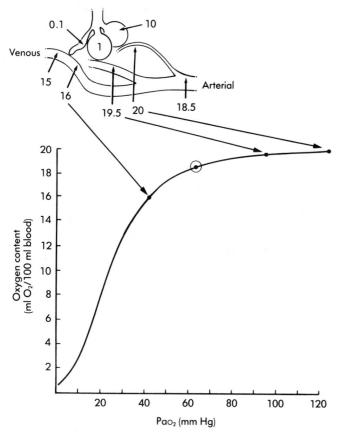

Fig. 15-5 Oxygen dissociation curve: Pa_{O_2} versus oxygen content. Oxygen content from alveolar-capillary units with $\dot{V}/\dot{Q}$ ratios of 0.1, 1, and 10 are, respectively, 16, 19.5, and 20.0 ml O_2/dL blood. Lines are drawn for each content to its point on the dissociation curve. The average oxygen content, 18.5 ml O_2/dL, is represented by a circle on the dissociation curve. Note that the arterial oxygen content after all the blood is mixed (18.5 ml O_2/dL) is lower than the oxygen content from the normal unit (19.5 ml O_2/dL) (From Martin L: Pulmonary physiology in clinical practice: the essentials for patient care and evaluation, St Louis, 1987, The CV Mosby Co.)

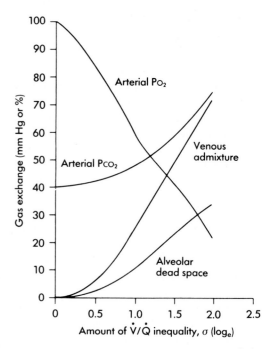

Fig. 15-6 Gas exchange effects from progressive $\dot{V}/\dot{Q}$ imbalance. $\dot{V}/\dot{Q}$ inequality and overall gas exchange in computer model of the lung. For this model, oxygen uptake and carbon dioxide output were kept constant. As the amount of $\dot{V}/\dot{Q}$ inequality increases (represented by a log scale on the abscissa), Pa_{O_2} decreases and Pa_{CO_2} increases; this occurs because $\dot{V}/\dot{Q}$ inequality causes increases in both venous admixture and alveolar dead space. (From Martin L: Pulmonary physiology in clinical practice: the essentials for patient care and evaluation, St Louis, 1987, The CV Mosby Co.)

blood from these areas with high $\dot{V}/\dot{Q}$ ratios is mixed with blood perfusing areas with low $\dot{V}/\dot{Q}$ ratios, the resulting P_{O_2} will always be lower than the average of the two.

This phenomenon occurs because the final Pa_{O_2} is determined not by an average of oxygen partial pressures coming from various lung units, but by an average of the oxygen contents. The oxygen dissociation curve shows that when aliquots of unequal oxygen content mix, the resulting P_{O_2} is not an average of the mixing P_{O_2} levels, but instead is an average of the mixing oxygen contents. Partial pressures of gases do not average out when equal aliquots of blood mix. It is the gas contents (i.e., oxygen and carbon dioxide) that mix and average out.

Since hemoglobin is almost fully saturated at a P_{O_2} of 100 mm Hg (see Fig. 15-5), an increase in oxygen partial

pressures above this level contributes little to increasing the blood's oxygen content. Thus, compared with those with normal $\dot{V}/\dot{Q}$ ratios (about 1.0), lung units with higher than normal $\dot{V}/\dot{Q}$ ratios cannot significantly raise the oxygen content of the blood. Although the final oxygen content still represents an average of that coming from all lung units, the resulting Pa_{O_2} is lower than would be predicted by averaging the P_{O_2} values from each pulmonary capillary.

The expected decrease in Pa_{O_2} and the increase in venous admixture resulting from progressive $\dot{V}/\dot{Q}$ imbalances are shown in Fig. 15-6. This figure represents a computer lung model in which cardiac output, minute ventilation, and oxygen uptake are kept constant and the effects of increasing $\dot{V}/\dot{Q}$ imbalance on gas exchange are analyzed. As can be seen, as the $\dot{V}/\dot{Q}$ imbalance worsens, the venous admixture increases. This increasing venous admixture is accompanied by a steady decline in the arterial P_{O_2}.

Carbon dioxide removal. As indicated in Fig. 15-6, $\dot{V}/\dot{Q}$ imbalances also impair carbon dioxide removal.[21] As the $\dot{V}/\dot{Q}$ imbalance worsens, the number of lung units ventilated but not perfused grows, resulting in a progres-

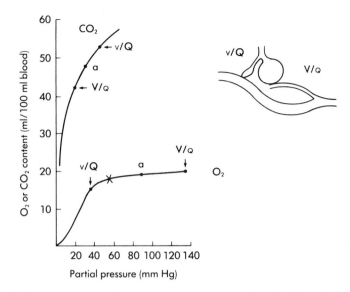

Fig. 15-7 $\dot{V}/\dot{Q}$ imbalance and the dissociation curves for carbon dioxide and oxygen. v/Q represents low $\dot{V}/\dot{Q}$ units, and V/Q represents high $\dot{V}/\dot{Q}$ units. See text for discussion. (From Martin L: Pulmonary physiology in clinical practice: the essentials for patient care and evaluation, St Louis, 1987, The CV Mosby Co.)

sive increase in physiologic dead space. In concept, this increase in physiologic dead space should result in a progressive rise in Pa_{CO_2} levels (as predicted by the model in Fig. 15-6). However, in clinical practice, the increase in Pa_{CO_2} levels that should occur with a $\dot{V}/\dot{Q}$ imbalance is not always apparent. Many patients who are hypoxemic resulting from a $\dot{V}/\dot{Q}$ imbalance have a low or normal Pa_{CO_2}.

This common clinical finding suggests that $\dot{V}/\dot{Q}$ imbalances tend to exert a greater effect on oxygenation than on carbon dioxide removal. Careful inspection of the oxygen and carbon dioxide dissociation curves supports this concept and helps explain why it is true. Fig. 15-7 shows the oxygen and carbon dioxide dissociation curves plotted on the same scale. The upper curve is for carbon dioxide; note that it is diagonal in the physiologic range. The lower curve is for oxygen; it is almost flat in the physiologic range. The x-axis plots the partial pressures of both oxygen and carbon dioxide; the y-axis plots their blood gas contents. Point *a* on each curve is the normal arterial point for both content and partial pressure.

To the right of the graph are two lung units, one having a low $\dot{V}/\dot{Q}$ ratio and one having a high $\dot{V}/\dot{Q}$ ratio. The content of oxygen and carbon dioxide in the blood from each type of unit is represented on the dissociation curves. The final carbon dioxide content is represented as point *a* on the carbon dioxide dissociation curve, arrived at by averaging the high and low $\dot{V}/\dot{Q}$ points on the carbon dioxide curve. Note that this is the same as the normal arterial point for carbon dioxide. The final oxygen content is point *x*, arrived at by averaging the high and low $\dot{V}/\dot{Q}$ points on the oxygen curve. Note that, compared with carbon diox-

ide, the point resulting from averaging the blood contents from the high and low $\dot{V}/\dot{Q}$ units for oxygen is substantially lower than its normal arterial point.

Thus the effect of low $\dot{V}/\dot{Q}$ units is to lower the P_{O_2} and raise the P_{CO_2}; the shape of the dissociation curves dictates that the respective contents will also change in the same direction. On the other hand, the effect of high $\dot{V}/\dot{Q}$ units is the opposite, that is, to raise the P_{O_2} and lower the P_{CO_2}. However, the shape of the dissociation curves dictates that this high $\dot{V}/\dot{Q}$ unit can reverse the high P_{CO_2} but not the low P_{O_2}. Thus any elevation of P_{CO_2} from low $\dot{V}/\dot{Q}$ units can be compensated for by a reduction in the P_{CO_2} in high $\dot{V}/\dot{Q}$ units. However, these high $\dot{V}/\dot{Q}$ units cannot compensate for the reduction of oxygen content, since the oxygen dissociation curve is nearly flat in the range of high P_{O_2} values.

However, for patients with $\dot{V}/\dot{Q}$ imbalances to compensate for the high P_{CO_2} levels in underventilated units, they must augment both their $\dot{V}_E$ and $\dot{V}_A$ (Fig. 15-8). Thus, patients who can increase their $\dot{V}_E$ in the face of a $\dot{V}/\dot{Q}$ imbalance will usually manifest hypoxemia along with either a normal or low Pa_{CO_2}.

Although the majority of patients with a $\dot{V}/\dot{Q}$ imbalance do not manifest hypercapnia, some do, particularly when the $\dot{V}/\dot{Q}$ imbalance is severe and chronic. This is because such patients are unable to sustain the necessary increase in $\dot{V}_E$. The most common example clinically is the patient with severe chronic obstructive pulmonary disease (COPD) whose $\dot{V}/\dot{Q}$ imbalance has resulted in a large amount of alveolar dead space. Such a patient must maintain an increased $\dot{V}_E$ to maintain a normal Pa_{CO_2}. However, if the energy costs required to maintain a high $\dot{V}_E$ are

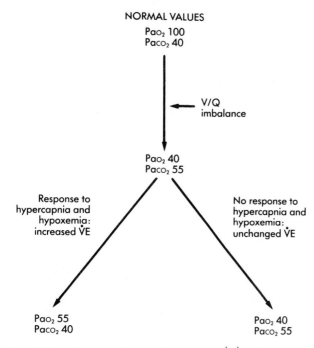

NORMAL VALUES
PaO_2 100
PaCO_2 40

V/Q
imbalance

PaO_2 40
PaCO_2 55

Response to
hypercapnia and
hypoxemia:
increased V̇E

No response to
hypercapnia and
hypoxemia:
unchanged V̇E

PaO_2 55
PaCO_2 40

PaO_2 40
PaCO_2 55

Fig. 15-8   Changes in PaO_2 and PaCO_2 from V̇/Q̇ imbalance. All values are mm Hg. See text for discussion. (From Martin L: Pulmonary physiology in clinical practice: the essentials for patient care and evaluation, St Louis, 1987, The CV Mosby Co.)

prohibitive, the patient will opt for less work and hence exhibit an elevated PaCO_2.

In such cases the basic cause of hypercapnia is an increase in physiologic dead space caused by a V̇/Q̇ imbalance. Thus, a V̇/Q̇ imbalance is not only the most common cause of hypoxemia, but, by the mechanism just explained, a primary factor in many cases of hypercapnia.

AIRWAY OBSTRUCTION

Obstruction of the airways is one of the most common causes of cardiopulmonary disability. Obstruction may be transient and reversible, or it may be permanent. We considered the effects of airway resistance on the mechanics of ventilation earlier and now concern ourselves with a description of the physiologic and pathologic changes brought about by obstruction.

Causes

The primary causes of airway obstruction are mucosal edema, bronchial spasm, increased secretions, and bronchiolar collapse (Fig. 15-9). Other causes of airway obstruction, such as inhaled foreign bodies or large tumors, are discussed in other chapters.

Mucosal edema. Edema represents an abnormal increase in the amount of interstitial fluid surrounding the body cells. Pathologic changes cause a shift of body water from the plasma to the intercellular spaces, with resulting

swelling of the affected area. Edema may be either localized or widespread. The most common example of edema of the respiratory tract is the nasal swelling and inflammation that accompanies the common cold (rhinitis). This same response can be visualized in the other portions of the respiratory tract. For example, edema resulting from a localized infection of the larynx and trachea in children, well known as "croup," can produce severe airway obstruction. Likewise, edema and airway narrowing caused by infection in the small bronchi and bronchioles of children results in a condition called bronchiolitis.

There are three major causes of edema of the respiratory tract:

1. Mechanical irritation or trauma to the respiratory mucosa, as from instrumentation, the presence of a foreign body, or the inhalation of caustic liquids or irritant fumes;
2. Infection in which the reaction represents the body's defense against the invading organisms;
3. Allergy to inhaled liquids or particulate matter, exemplified by the common allergic (atopic) bronchial asthma.

In acute edema, the respiratory mucosa becomes soft, spongy, and waterlogged. There is usually an accompanying arteriolar and capillary congestion, which adds to the swelling. If of short duration, acute edema may be easily reversible once its cause is removed. However, if the edema is long lasting or frequently recurring, as with chronic respiratory infections, it may become indurated, giving the tissue a permanent thickening and a firm, rather than soft, consistency. Such changes will markedly impair the normal mucociliary clearance mechanism.

Bronchial spasm. Spasm may be defined as involuntary and excessive muscle contraction. Common examples are found in extremity muscle cramps, spasm of neck muscles after injury, and intestinal cramps. Bronchial spasm represents the excessive and prolonged contraction of the involuntary smooth muscle fibers in the walls of the bronchi and bronchioles. Whether localized or widespread, bronchial spasm can seriously reduce airway lumens, thereby obstructing airflow.

In general, the causes of bronchial spasm are the same as those for edema, that is, mechanical irritation, infection, or allergy. As with edema, chronically recurring bronchial spasm can result in permanent histologic changes, in this case hypertrophy of the bronchial smooth muscle.

Increased secretions. By increased bronchial secretions we mean an actual increase in volume of secretions produced, an increase in their viscosity, or both. Although such reactions may follow exposure of the respiratory mucosa to many irritants, infection is the most frequent offender, and the common cold, with its abundance nasal secretions, is again a familiar example.

Bronchial secretions may be composed of many ingredi-

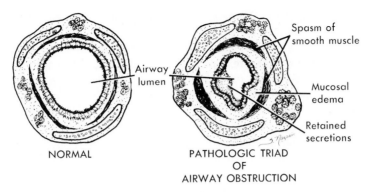

Fig. 15-9   Cross-sections of airways comparing normal with obstruction caused by pathologic triad. Note narrowed airway lumen (opening) in obstructed airway.

ents: mucus, secreted by the goblet cells and mucous glands of the bronchial mucosa; DNA and RNA (released from the nuclei and cytoplasm of disintegrating cells); and plasma fluid and proteins, including fibrinogen, escaping from pulmonary capillaries.[22]

Distinguishing between normal and abnormal secretions depends on the relative concentrations of their components. For clinical purposes, we can differentiate between two broad types of sputum—mucoid and purulent. Mucoid secretions generally represent a response by the airways to foreign matter invasion, infective or noninfective, in an attempt to remove the offending agent. One of the characteristics of a well-established chronic bronchitis is an actual increase in the number and size of mucous glands in the bronchial walls. The secretions produced will contain a high concentration of mucus in proportion to the other constituents.

Mucus contains mucoproteins, a combination of any of several proteins with substances known as mucopolysaccharides, and long-chain carbohydrate-containing compounds. These mucoproteins give respiratory tract secretions their characteristic viscosity. Thus, when stimulated to overproduce sputum by some irritative or pathologic process, the airways will contain larger amounts of fluid of a greater than normal viscosity. Viscosity of normal secretions can also be raised to abnormally high levels by simple dehydration. The importance of adequate systemic and airway hydration in maintaining normal function of the respiratory tract mucosa is considered in depth in Chapter 23.

Purulent secretions, on the other hand, are the result of invasion of the respiratory tract by pathogenic bacteria and the effect of such infection on the sputum. The natural inflammatory response to bacterial infection brings many leukocytes to the area, and they engage the invading organisms in destructive battle. The mucoid secretions, which are the first response, become grossly infiltrated with intact and fragmented bacteria, leukocytes, and tissue cells damaged by the process. Disruption of the cytoplasm and nuclei of the cells releases into the secretions a large amount of nucleoproteins, the DNA and RNA. It is principally the DNA protein that gives the secretions their purulent character and high viscosity. High concentrations of DNA also give purulent sputum its characteristic yellow to greenish discoloration. This is in distinct contrast to the colorless or frothy mucoid type.

If the bronchial inflammation is acute, the sputum may have streaks of dark red or brown from extravasated blood. Finally, depending on the offending bacteria or the presence of secondary or mixed infection, putrefactive organisms will often distinguish purulent sputum with a disagreeable odor.

As the volume and viscosity of respiratory tract secretions increase, the normal mucociliary clearance mechanism becomes less effective. Moreover, high-viscosity respiratory tract secretions cannot be as easily cleared by coughing. In combination, these factors can lead to retained secretions, mucus plugging, and atelectasis.

Bronchiolar collapse. Usually associated with chronic bronchopulmonary disease, bronchiolar collapse is a clinically important form of small airway obstruction that, in many patients, becomes the most critical factor in ventilatory disability. The conditions predisposing to bronchiolar collapse are most frequently found in the destructive lung diseases such as emphysema, bronchiectasis, and cystic fibrosis, with emphysema being by far the most important cause.

As discussed in Chapter 8, the caliber of the small airway is determined by two factors: (1) the structural support of the surrounding lung parenchyma and (2) the difference in pressure that normally exists across the airway wall, or transmural pressure gradient.

In conditions such as pulmonary emphysema, the elastic tissue normally responsible for radial support of the small airways is destroyed. This loss of elastic tissue has two major effects. First, it increases the compliance of the lung, thereby decreasing its elastic recoil. Second, it abolishes the major anatomic factor responsible for small airway support.[23]

During inhalation the negative intrapleural pressure dilates the small airways, as in the normal lung. During exhalation, however, the rising intrapleural pressure causes less of an increase in alveolar pressure (because of the loss of elastic recoil). Moreover, as intrapleural pressure rises, the bronchioles, lacking the normal support of the surrounding lung tissue, are readily compressed. When combined, these factors cause the equal pressure point (EPP) to "move" further upstream than in the healthy lung. Airway collapse therefore occurs earlier and at higher volumes than in the healthy subject. The result is premature trapping of air in the lung.

Patients in whom this condition is clinically significant are usually those who already have expiratory difficulty from their underlying disease and must exert exceptional effort during exhalation. Thus, the element of bronchiolar collapse can contribute to a steadily worsening disability.

In addition to its chronic influence on exhalation, bronchiolar collapse can produce an acute state referred to as *acute air trapping*. Frequently, without warning, a patient may suddenly be unable to complete a phase of exhalation already started. The chest is immobilized in a position of partial exhalation, and the patient is unable either to inhale or to empty the lungs further. The patient may struggle to move the chest and become severely cyanotic, especially in the face and neck.

Such an episode may be triggered by an unnoticed early expiratory effort of greater force than usual. As the sequence of events described previously comes into play after movement of part of the exhaled air, a number of bronchioles completely collapse, trapping the remainder of the tidal volume. Although frightening to the point of panic to patient and observers alike, these attacks are generally self-limiting. A series of lateral squeezes applied to both sides of the thorax will often supply sufficient spurts of air to overcome the collapse and empty the lungs. This technique is learned by many patients and especially by members of their families.

To prevent acute trapping and to accomplish the maximum exhalation with the minimum of effort, patients either learn spontaneously or are taught the technique of pursed-lip breathing. In this maneuver the patient slightly purses the lips while exhaling, deliberately prolonging exhalation and trying to maintain an even flow of air. This moderate obstruction at the mouth increases pressure in the upstream airways and moves the EPP further downstream toward the larger airways with cartilaginous support, thereby avoiding premature closure of the small airways.[1,24] Pursed-lip breathing may also increase the efficiency of ventilation by slowing the respiratory rate and increasing the tidal volume.[25]

Clinical manifestations

Obstruction greatly increases the work of breathing because of the elevated airflow resistance. Resistance to breathing may be more pronounced in one phase or the other of ventilation. For example, the laryngeal obstruc-

tion of childhood croup results in a marked increase in inspiratory resistance. This may necessitate a strong inspiratory effort, resulting in noticeable retraction of the sternum and epigastrium during inspiration. Moreover, the flow of air past the obstruction may produce a harsh sound known as a stridor.

Most often, however, obstruction is a major problem in chronic bronchopulmonary diseases, in which exhalation is impeded. In these cases, normal passive exhalation cannot overcome the high expiratory flow resistance, and exhalation often requires strenuous muscular effort. The tremendous work involved in moving air against obstruction uses so much physical energy that it constitutes one of the major factors in the disability of chronic pulmonary diseases. As described in Chapter 28, muscular fatigue may lead to hypercapnia, respiratory acidosis, and respiratory failure.

Whether inspiratory or expiratory, all obstructive disorders are characterized by impedance to the flow of air. In the pulmonary function laboratory, this flow impedance always manifests itself as a decrease in the rate of flow, as measured during the applicable phase of breathing (see Chapter 17). If the problem is mainly expiratory flow obstruction, expiration time is usually prolonged beyond that of inhalation, and often contraction of the upper abdomen is evident during the latter part of exhalation. If bronchospasm is extensive or mobile secretions are present, characteristic breath sounds can be heard during exhalation by auscultation or, at times, by the unaided ear. These breath sounds may include early inspiratory crackles, rhonchi, and wheezes. More detail on the physical signs and symptoms of obstructive lung disease is provided in Chapter 16.

Treatment

In general, the strategy for treating obstructive lung disorders depends on the underlying pathologic condition. For example, therapeutic intervention in reversible obstructive diseases such as asthma involves efforts to restore normal function by applying various drugs to reduce bronchial spasm and mucosal edema. On the other hand, when the disorder involves permanent damage to the lung parenchyma, such as occurs in chronic bronchitis and emphysema, therapy is mainly supportive and is directed at relieving symptoms and preventing complications. General considerations in the treatment of obstructive lung disorders are provided in Chapter 19. The various modes of respiratory care applicable to patients with obstructive lung disease are reviewed in detail in Section VI, "Basic Therapeutics."

PULMONARY DISTENTION

Pulmonary distention occurs when the resting lung volume is elevated above normal and results in an increased functional residual capacity and residual volume, a reduced inspiratory capacity, and a downward displacement of the diaphragm. If chronic, pulmonary distention causes a progressive increase in the size of the thorax, especially its anteroposterior diameter. The resulting physical abnormality is called a "barrel chest."

Causes

From a practical point of view, pulmonary distention usually refers to the hyperinflation characterizing pulmonary emphysema. Basically, emphysema is a destructive disease characterized by disruption of the alveolar walls. This destructive process converts the lung from an organ with a large number of relatively uniform and small air spaces into one with a smaller number of large air spaces. A consequence of this change in lung structure is a dramatic loss of elastic fibers and a marked unevenness in gas distribution throughout the lung.

Less well defined as a pathologic entity is the degenerative change that accompanies the aging process and that diminishes the tone of elastic tissue throughout the body. The loss of skin elasticity in older persons is a common observation, and apparently a similar phenomenon takes place in the lung. The increase in functional residual capacity (FRC) often seen with advancing age is sometimes referred to as "senile emphysema," although there is no concrete evidence that this constitutes a true disease state. However, this phenomenon is accompanied by a gradual and predictable decrease in the lung's ability to oxygenate the blood, as previously described.

Pulmonary distention may also occur in reversible airway obstruction, such as during an attack of acute bronchial asthma. In this condition, diffuse bronchial spasm is the outstanding feature, and during such an episode the FRC may be markedly increased. On subsidence and in the absence of complications, the resting thoracic level returns to normal.

Clinical manifestations

Regardless of underlying cause, the increased FRC, reduced inspiratory capacity, and downward displacement of the diaphragm that characterize pulmonary distention can have significant adverse effects on ventilation.

Increased functional residual capacity. An abnormal enlargement in the FRC simply prolongs the time necessary for the mixing of gases within the lung. However, since an enlarged FRC is usually accompanied by airway obstruction, large and variable-sized air spaces, or both, the distribution of inspired gas will be uneven. Uneven gas distribution results in an abnormal $\dot{V}/\dot{Q}$ relationship, as previously described.

An estimate of the evenness with which inspired air is distributed among the alveoli can be made in the pulmonary function laboratory (see Chapter 17). One technique involves the breathing of pure oxygen for several minutes, gradually washing out nitrogen remaining in the lung from previous air breathing. The exhaled air is monitored by an analyzer that measures the gradually decreasing concentration of nitrogen removed, and the time-concentration rela-

tionship is noted. In a lung disrupted by severe obstruction or variable-sized air spaces that empty in an irregular fashion, the time-concentration relationship will be markedly abnormal. Another technique uses the inhalation of a known concentration of inert helium; by measurement of the time it takes for the lung air to reach equilibrium with the inhaled gas, the distribution characteristic of the lung can be determined.

Reduced inspiratory capacity. The elevated end-expiratory resting level of the thorax and the low, flat diaphragm (described next) produce the inspiratory position of the thorax. Thus, at their resting level, the lungs are already in a position of partial inspiration. This encroachment on the inspiratory capacity limits the patient's ability to increase tidal volumes in response to exertional needs.

Low position of diaphragm. As the FRC rises, overdistention of the lung depresses and flattens the contour of the diaphragm. In this position, contraction of the diaphragm pulls the costal margin in and reduces the volume of the thorax during inhalation rather than enlarging it. With loss of effective use of the diaphragm, reduction in intrapleural pressure depends on contraction of the intercostals and the accessory ventilatory muscles. The pull of the accessory muscles causes an upward and outward displacement of the sternum and an increase in the sternal angle (the junction of the manubrium and body of the sternum, at the level of the second rib).

Negative intrapleural pressure, generated at a tremendous energy cost to the patient, also acts on the ineffective diaphragm, pulling it upward during inhalation, the so-called paradoxical ventilation. Thus, while the intercostals and accessories are working hard to enlarge the thorax, the rising diaphragm, sucked upward by their action, partially negates their efforts, and the net gain in thoracic volume is small in proportion to the physical effort expended. When inspiratory efforts are strenuous enough, not only is the diaphragm elevated during inhalation, but the abdominal wall is also retracted in a contrary manner.

Exhalation, lacking the effective use of the abdominals, is a slow process, depending on inadequate passive recoil and expiratory action of the intercostals. Moreover, during exhalation, rising intrapleural pressure drives down the diaphragm as the abdominal wall balloons outward. The clinical picture is one of a short, gasping inhalation, with extensive use of accessory muscles of ventilation and epigastric retraction, followed by a prolonged exhalation accompanied by varying degrees of epigastric protrusion.

Treatment

If the cause of pulmonary distention is chronic degenerative changes in the structure of the lung parenchyma, there is no effective treatment. In such cases, therapy is mainly supportive and includes rehabilitative activities designed to enhance more effective use of respiratory muscles (see Chapters 27 and 34). On the other hand, if the pulmonary distention is caused by a reversible obstructive disorder, such as occurs during an acute asthma attack, treatment is directed at the primary problem, that is, the airway obstruction.

PULMONARY RESTRICTION

Pulmonary restriction is a general term that encompasses a broad category of disorders with widely variable causes that share a common denominator, namely, a reduction in lung volume.

Causes

As listed in Table 15-4, there are six major categories of restrictive lung disease: skeletal-thoracic, neuromuscular, pleural, interstitial, alveolar, and abdominal.

Skeletal-thoracic causes. Some thoracic causes of restriction are the result of structural changes in the chest, while others are due to reduced flexibility. Kyphoscoliosis is a good example of a restrictive disorder caused by structural changes in the chest. Kyphoscoliosis is characterized by an abnormal curvature of the spine that, when it affects the dorsal segment, distorts the thoracic cage by compressing one side or the other. In general, it is produced by an imbalance between the bilateral skeletal muscle groups. Weakness of one muscle group allows unopposed traction by the other, with eventual tilting and rotation of the spine and chest cage.

Ankylosing spondylitis is a restrictive disorder in which the primary problem is reduced flexibility of the chest cage. In ankylosing spondylitis the vertebral bodies and the costovertebral joints become fused, causing a dramatic decrease in thoracic wall compliance.

Neuromuscular causes. Processes that interfere with the transfer of central neural output to the contracting muscles that expand the rib cage can also result in restrictive impairments. Included in this category are abnormalities of the spinal cord, peripheral nerves, neuromuscular junctions, and respiratory muscles. Some diseases in this category, such as poliomyelitis, can involve both the central respiratory control mechanism and the peripheral neuromuscular apparatus. Characterizing all these abnormalities is an inability to generate normal respiratory pressures, either automatically or intentionally.

Pleural disorders. Pleural disorders can result in restriction either through direct pathologic involvement of the pleural membranes themselves or as a result of space-occupying lesions. Pleurisy is an example of the former; pleural effusion, empyema, pneumothorax, and hemothorax are examples of the latter.

Interstitial disorders. Interstitial pulmonary disease processes predominantly involve chronic inflammatory or fibrotic changes. Chronic inflammatory processes, such as recurrent respiratory infections, often accompany chronic bronchopulmonary disease such as emphysema and follow such destructive disease processes as tuberculosis and bronchiectasis. Inhalation of inorganic dusts, such as oc-

curs in the industrial or occupationally related pneumoconioses, is the most common cause of fibrotic changes in the lung tissue.

Alveolar disorders. Alveolar restrictive processes involve changes in the area of the terminal respiratory unit, including the pulmonary capillary circulation. Pneumonia, an acute infectious process leading to alveolar consolidation, is a good example. Vascular congestion, such as occurs in cardiogenic pulmonary edema, can also result in restriction. In this case, increased fluid in the pulmonary interstitial spaces and in the alveoli causes a reduction in lung compliance.

Abdominal causes. Through immobilization of the diaphragm, abdominal conditions are a frequent cause of pulmonary restriction. Among the most common abdominal conditions restricting lung expansion are splinting, distention, and fluid accumulation.

Abdominal splinting, a rigid contraction of the musculature of the abdominal wall, is usually an unconscious reaction to pain from intra-abdominal disease or postoperative discomfort. Ventilation can be seriously impeded, and the combination of restriction and hypoventilation comprises a common respiratory complication of abdominal disease.

Abdominal distention results from excessive accumulation of gas or air in the stomach or intestinal tract. This may be so pronounced that the abdominal wall is pushed outward into a rounded dome under great tension.

An abnormal increase in abdominal fluid, referred to as *ascites,* is usually the result of liver disease, heart failure, or some pathologic condition causing widespread peritoneal irritation. Ascites interferes with diaphragmatic descent by the increased intra-abdominal pressure.

Table 15-4   Categories of Restrictive Pulmonary Disorders

Category	Examples
Skeletal-thoracic	Kyphoscoliosis
	Ankylosing spondylitis
CNS-neuromuscular	Cord transection
	Amyotrophic lateral sclerosis
	Guillain-Barré syndrome
	Myasthenia gravis
Pleural	Pleurisy
	Effusion-empyema
	Pneumothorax
	Hemothorax
Interstitial	Recurrent infections
	Pneumoconiosis
Alveolar	Pneumonia
	Pulmonary edema
Abdominal	Splinting
	Distention
	Ascites

Effect of restriction on ventilation

All restrictive disorders lower lung volumes. In particular, restriction reduces the vital capacity (VC); in severe instances the VC may not be much greater than the resting tidal volume. In this case, as with distention, there may be little or no inspiratory reserve volume to accommodate increased ventilatory demands.

In neuromuscular disorders the FRC is maintained near normal levels. However, because of inspiratory muscle weakness, total lung capacity decreases. On the other hand, expiratory muscle weakness causes an increase in the residual volume. As with restrictive disorders in general, both vital capacity and the maximum inspiratory pressure (negative inspiratory force) are diminished.

Only the interstitial and alveolar forms of restrictive disease actually result in a decrease in lung compliance. A decrease in lung compliance, in turn, can result in a maldistribution of ventilation and an increased work of breathing.

Treatment

The specific objectives in treating pulmonary restriction aim at removing the underlying cause. For example, the removal of pleural or abdominal fluid, or the repair of structural defects of the thorax, should alleviate the restriction to ventilation. Unfortunately, in many restrictive conditions, such as the pneumoconioses, there is no specific treatment available to correct the primary problem. In these cases, treatment is mainly supportive, with the goal to minimize symptoms and prevent further complications.

SUMMARY

When the lungs, heart, or vascular systems fail to fulfill their coordinated functions efficiently and adequately, a state of cardiopulmonary dysfunction is said to exist. One or more of three primary physiologic abnormalities underlies all cardiopulmonary dysfunction. Either oxygen delivery to or carbon dioxide removal from the tissues is impaired, or the energy cost necessary to exchange these metabolites effectively is prohibitively excessive.

If oxygen delivery to the tissues is inadequate to meet their metabolic needs, hypoxia is present. Hypoxia may result from either a decrease in the oxygen content of arterial blood (hypoxemia) or a decrease in tissue perfusion. A third major category of hypoxia, called histotoxic hypoxia or dysoxia, occurs when the cells cannot properly use the oxygen delivered to them.

Impaired carbon dioxide removal is always associated with a decrease in $\dot{V}_A$ relative to metabolic need, as clinically manifested by hypercapnia. Hypercapnia may be caused by an inadequate $\dot{V}_E$, increased $\dot{V}_{DS}$, or both.

Airway obstruction, pulmonary distention, and pulmonary restriction may affect both oxygen exchange and carbon dioxide removal, most commonly by altering the normal relationship between ventilation and perfusion in the lung. Moreover, each of these major patterns of cardiopulmonary dysfunction can result in an increase in the work of breathing, thereby making the energy cost necessary to exchange oxygen and carbon dioxide effectively prohibitively high.

An understanding of these major patterns of pathophysiology, including their causes, clinical manifestations, and general treatment approaches, provides the foundation for quality respiratory care.

REFERENCES

1. Martin L: Pulmonary physiology in clinical practice: the essentials for patient care and evaluation, St Louis, 1987, The CV Mosby Co.
2. West JB: Causes of carbon dioxide retention in lung disease, N Engl J Med 284:1232, 1971.
3. Editorial: Hypoxemia vs hypoxia, N Engl J Med 274:908, 1966.
4. Van Liere EJ and Stickney JC: Hypoxia, Chicago, 1963, University of Chicago Press.
5. Robins ED: Dysoxia: abnormal tissue oxygen utilization, Arch Intern Med 137:905, 1977.
6. Porter R and Knight J, editors: High altitude physiology: cardiac and respiratory aspects, London, 1971, Churchill Livingstone.
7. Sutton JR, Jones N, and Houston C, editors: Hypoxia: man at altitude, New York, 1982, Thieme-Stratton, Inc.
8. Sorbini CA et al: Arterial oxygen tension in relation to age in healthy subjects, Respiration 25:3, 1968.
9. Burrows B, Knudson RJ, and Kettrl LJ: Respiratory insufficiency, Chicago, 1975, Year Book Medical Publishers, Inc.
10. Cherniack RM, Cherniack L, and Naimark A: Respiration in health and disease, ed 2, Philadelphia, 1972, WB Saunders Co.
11. Hudson LD: Evaluation of the patient in acute respiratory failure, Respir Care 28:542-550, 1983.
12. Shulman LE: Hypertrophic osteoarthropathy, Bull Rheum Dis 7:135, 1957.
13. Field AS Jr and Gray FD Jr: The width of the nail fold capillary stream in clubbing, Dis Chest 41:631, 1962.
14. Barcroft J: Anoxemia, Lancet 2:485, 1920.
15. Campbell EJM: The management of acute respiratory failure in chronic bronchitis and emphysema, Am Rev Respir Dis 96:626, 1967.
16. Slonim NB and Hamilton LH: Respiratory physiology, ed 5, St Louis, 1985, The CV Mosby Co.
17. Shaw DB and Simpson T: Polycythemia in emphysema, Q J Med 30:135, 1961.
18. Comroe JH Jr: Physiology of respiration, ed 2, Chicago, 1974, Year Book Medical Publishers, Inc.
19. Filley GF: Pulmonary insufficiency and respiratory failure, Philadelphia, 1967, Lea & Febiger.
20. Mohsenifar Z et al: Relationship between O_2 delivery and O_2 consumption in the adult respiratory distress syndrome, Chest 83:267, 1983.
21. West JB: Ventilation/blood flow and gas exchange, ed 4, Oxford, 1980, Blackwell Scientific Publications, Ltd.
22. Tappan V and Zalar V: Pathophysiology of bronchial mucus, Ann NY Acad Sci 106:722, 1963.
23. Nunn JF: Applied respiratory physiology, ed 2, London, 1977, Butterworth Publishers.
24. Barach AL: In Petty TL, editor: Chronic obstructive pulmonary disease, New York, 1978, Marcel Dekker, Inc.
25. Mueller RE, Petty TL, and Filley GF: Ventilation and arterial blood gas changes induced by pursed lip breathing, J Appl Physiol 28:784, 1970.

16

Physical Assessment of the Patient

Robert L. Wilkins

The progression of respiratory care as a clinical science has placed increasing demands on practitioners to combine diagnostic skills within their repertoire of therapeutic modalities. The integration of assessment with treatment is a necessary outcome of the growing complexity of roles and functions assumed by respiratory care practitioners. No longer is it acceptable to initiate or alter therapeutic regimens without careful consideration of the underlying pathologic condition and its clinical manifestations. Decisions regarding the initiation, continuation, change, and discontinuation of therapy must be based on tangible clinical evidence. Although the prescribing physician has primary responsibility for making these determinations, the respiratory care practitioner is obliged to participate in the clinical decision-making process. To fulfill this role effectively, the practitioner must assume responsibility for the ongoing gathering and interpretation of relevant patient data.

Among the many sources of data on a patient's status, physical assessment provides foundation information on which most subsequent diagnostic testing depends. Moreover, when integrated with the planning and implementation of therapeutic regimens, physical assessment of the patient can serve as the basis for selecting appropriate interventions and monitoring patient progress toward predefined goals. Last, physical assessment findings help the practitioner better understand underlying pathophysiologic processes.

OBJECTIVES

The goal of this chapter is to provide the reader with the foundation knowledge necessary to conduct a physical assessment of the adult patient. Although assessment related to respiratory disorders will be emphasized, a broad view of other pertinent systems will be included. Specifically,

after completion of this chapter, the reader should be able to:

1. Outline the steps normally taken in a comprehensive physical assessment;

2. Interpret the findings obtained during initial observation;

3. Apply specific anatomic and general pathophysiologic knowledge in the systematic examination of the head, neck, thorax, lungs, precordium, abdomen, and extremities;

4. Relate the findings of physical assessment to general patterns of cardiopulmonary dysfunction.

KEY TERMS

Most terms used in this chapter are defined in context. The following terms are introduced without explicit definition but may be found in the text glossary:

anterolateral	laryngospasm
antecubital fossa	palmar
axillary	pneumothorax
bronchiolitis	posterolateral
cannula (oxygen)	sensorium
constrictive pericarditis	sphygmomanometer
epigastrium	subglottic
epiglottitis	supraglottic
hypervolemia/hypovolemia	ulnar
intubation (tracheal)	

Physical examination is the process of examining the patient for the physical signs of disease. It is an inexpensive way of obtaining immediate and pertinent information about the patient's health status. The four basic components of physical examination are inspection, palpation, percussion, and auscultation.

The patient initially is examined to help identify the correct diagnosis. Once a tentative diagnosis is determined, subsequent examinations are used to monitor the patient's

Adapted from Wilkins RL, Sheldon RL, and Krider SJ, editors: Clinical assessment in respiratory care, ed 2, St Louis, 1990, The CV Mosby Co.

hospital course and to evaluate the results of treatment. Each examination should be tailored according to the patient's history and the purpose of the examination. Through experience, the examiner learns which of the techniques described within this chapter should be employed in any situation. Each examination should be performed in a quiet, well-lighted room, and the examiner should avoid exposing the patient to any unnecessary discomfort.

The skills described within this chapter are not difficult to learn; however, proficiency is attained only with practice. The beginner first should practice the skills on healthy individuals to improve technique and, more important, to obtain an appreciation for normal variations. Abnormalities can be detected only by examiners who have developed an appreciation of normal body functions for comparison.

This chapter emphasizes the techniques of examination used in assessing the patient with respiratory disease. Because respiratory disease may alter indirectly other body systems, examination of the entire patient is important. The techniques used in examining the thorax and other body systems for the abnormalities often associated with respiratory disease are reviewed. The content of this chapter is presented in the typical order in which the physical examination is performed and recorded: initial impressions, assessment of the vital signs, and examination of the head, neck, thorax, abdomen, and extremities (see box opposite).

INITIAL ASSESSMENT

A review of the patient's history of present illness and past medical history before examination is helpful, especially if the examiner was not involved in acquiring the patient's medical history. This gives the examiner insight into the physical examination findings to be expected and suggests the techniques to emphasize. The history is generally followed by an initial assessment consisting of observational impressions and the measurement of vital signs.

Initial impressions

An initial impression is determined by observing the patient's level of consciousness and general state of health. This assessment identifies the acuteness of the patient's illness. If the patient demonstrates signs of acute, severe illness, the remainder of the physical examination may have to be limited to gathering only essential information. When the patient's condition is more stable, a thorough examination can be performed to identify all abnormalities.

Evaluation of the patient's level of consciousness is a simple but important task. Adequate cerebral oxygenation must be present for the patient to be conscious, alert, and

---

TYPICAL FORMAT FOR RECORDING THE PHYSICAL EXAMINATION

INITIAL IMPRESSION
Age, height, weight, and general appearance

VITAL SIGNS
Pulse rate, respiratory rate, temperature, and blood pressure

HEENT (HEAD, EARS, EYES, NOSE, AND THROAT)
Inspection findings

NECK
Inspection and palpation findings

THORAX
Lungs—inspection, palpation, percussion, and auscultation
Heart—inspection, palpation, and auscultation findings

ABDOMEN
Inspection, palpation, percussion, and auscultation findings

EXTREMITIES
Inspection and palpation findings

---

well oriented. The conscious patient also should be evaluated for orientation to time, place, and person. This is referred to as evaluating the patient's *sensorium*. The alert patient who is well oriented as to time, place, and person is said to be "oriented × 3," and sensorium is considered normal.

An abnormal sensorium and a loss of consciousness may occur when cerebral perfusion is inadequate or when poorly oxygenated blood is delivered to the brain. As cerebral oxygenation deteriorates, the patient initially is restless, confused, and disoriented. If tissue hypoxia worsens, the patient eventually may become comatose. An abnormal sensorium also may occur in chronic degenerative brain disorders, as a side effect of certain medications, and in drug overdose cases.

Obvious indicators of the patient's general state of health usually are recorded as part of the initial impression. Statements regarding the patient's height, weight, apparent versus actual age, and obvious degree of illness may be included.

Vital signs

The assessment of vital signs, that is, body temperature, pulse rate, respiratory rate, and blood pressure, was covered in detail in Chapter 13. Typically, vital signs are measured as a component of the initial patient assessment.

These measures provide important diagnostic information and may reveal the first clue of adverse reactions to treatment.

EXAMINATION OF THE HEAD AND NECK

Head

An examination of the head first should identify the patient's facial expression. This may help determine if the patient is in acute distress or suffering from physical pain. The facial expression also can help to evaluate alertness, mood, general character, and mental capacity. Abnormalities identified during inspection of the face produced by respiratory disease include nasal flaring, cyanosis, and pursed-lip breathing. Nasal flaring is identified by observing the external nares flare outward during inhalation. This occurs especially in neonates with respiratory distress and indicates an increase in the work of breathing.

When respiratory disease results in reduced oxygenation of the arterial blood, cyanosis may be detected, especially around the lips and oral mucosa. Cyanosis may be difficult to detect, especially in a poorly lighted room. Although the presence of cyanosis suggests that tissue oxygenation is less than optimal, further investigation is indicated. The absence of cyanosis, however, does not indicate that tissue oxygenation is adequate, because a sufficient hemoglobin concentration must exist before cyanosis can be identified (see Chapter 15).

Patients with chronic obstructive lung disease may use pursed-lip breathing during exhalation. This technique often is taught to patients and even may be used by patients who have not had instruction on its benefits. Some patients naturally begin to pucker their lips during exhalation to provide a slight resistance to the exhaled breath. This resistance theoretically provides a slight back pressure in the small airways during exhalation and prevents their premature collapse.

Neck

Inspection and palpation of the neck are of value in determining the tracheal position and in estimating the jugular venous pressure (JVP). Normally, the trachea is located centrally in the neck when the patient is facing forward. The midline of the neck can be identified by palpating the suprasternal notch at the base of the anterior neck. The midline of the trachea should be directly below the center of the suprasternal notch.

The trachea may be shifted from midline with unilateral upper lobe collapse, pneumothorax, pleural effusion, or lung tumors. The trachea shifts toward the collapsed lung but away from the pneumothorax, pleural effusion, or lung tumor. Abnormalities in the lower lung fields may not shift the trachea unless the defect is severe.

The JVP is estimated by examining the level of the column of blood in the jugular veins. JVP reflects the volume

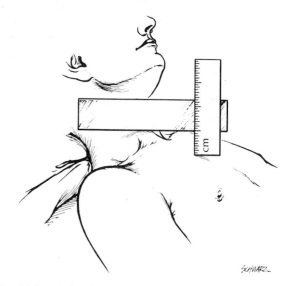

Fig. 16-1   Estimation of jugular venous pressure. (From Malasanos L et al: Health assessment, ed 4, St Louis, 1990, The CV Mosby Co.)

and pressure of the venous blood in the right side of the heart. Both the internal and external jugular veins can be assessed, although the internal jugular is most reliable. Individuals with obese necks may not have visible neck veins, even with distention.

In the supine position the neck veins of a healthy individual are full. When the head of the bed is elevated gradually to a 45-degree angle from horizontal, the level of the column of blood descends to a point no more than a few millimeters above the clavicle with normal venous pressure. With elevated venous pressure, the neck veins may be distended as high as the angle of the jaw, even when the patient is sitting upright. The degree of venous distention can be estimated by measuring the distance the veins are distended above the sternal angle. The sternal angle has been chosen universally, since its distance above the right atrium remains relatively constant (about 5 cm) in all positions. With the head of the bed elevated to a 45-degree angle, venous distention greater than 3 to 4 cm above the sternal angle is abnormal (Fig. 16-1).

Exact quantification of the jugular pressure in terms of centimeters above the sternal angle is difficult and probably exceeds the accuracy needed for most observers. A simple grading scale of normal, increased, and markedly increased is acceptable.

The level of jugular venous distention may vary with breathing. During inhalation the level of the column of blood may descend toward the thorax and return to the previous position with exhalation. For this reason, JVP should always be estimated at the end of exhalation.

The most common cause of jugular venous distention is right ventricular failure, which may occur secondary to left ventricular failure or chronic hypoxemia. Hypoxemia

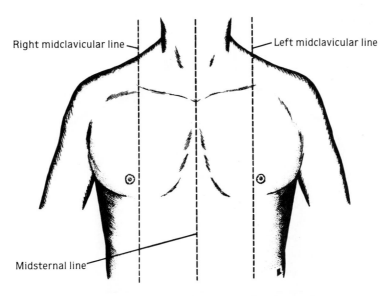

Fig. 16-2   Imaginary lines on anterior chest wall.

causes pulmonary vasoconstriction and increases the resistance of blood flow through the pulmonary vasculature, increasing the work load on the right ventricle. Persistent lung disease with hypoxemia may result in right ventricular failure and jugular venous distention. Jugular venous distention also may occur with hypervolemia and when the venous return to the right atrium is obstructed by mediastinal tumors.

EXAMINATION OF THE THORAX AND LUNGS

Lung topography

To perform an accurate physical assessment of the respiratory system, the examiner must understand how the lungs are situated within the chest. Topographic (surface) landmarks of the chest are helpful in identifying the location of underlying structures and in describing the location of abnormalities.

Imaginary lines. On the anterior chest the midsternal line divides the chest into two equal halves. The left and right midclavicular lines parallel the midsternal line and are drawn through the midpoints of the left and right clavicles, respectively (Fig. 16-2).

The midaxillary line divides the lateral chest into two equal halves. The anterior axillary line parallels the midaxillary line and is situated along the anterolateral chest. The posterior axillary line is also parallel to the midaxillary line and is located in the posterolateral chest (Fig. 16-3).

Three imaginary vertical lines are described on the posterior chest. The midspinal line divides the posterior chest into two equal halves. The left and right midscapular lines parallel the midspinal line and pass through the inferior angles of the scapulae in the relaxed upright individual (Fig. 16-4).

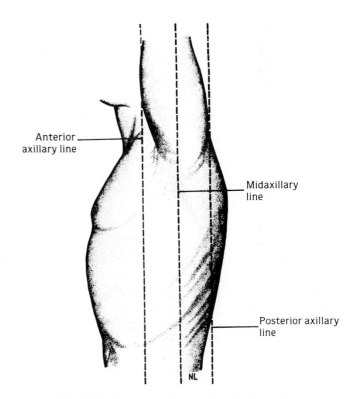

Fig. 16-3   Imaginary lines on lateral chest wall.

Thoracic cage landmarks. On the anterior chest the suprasternal notch is located at the top of the manubrium and can be located by palpating the depression at the base of the neck. Directly below this notch is the sternal angle, which also is referred to as the angle of Louis. Identification of the sternal angle can be achieved by palpating down from the suprasternal notch until the ridge between

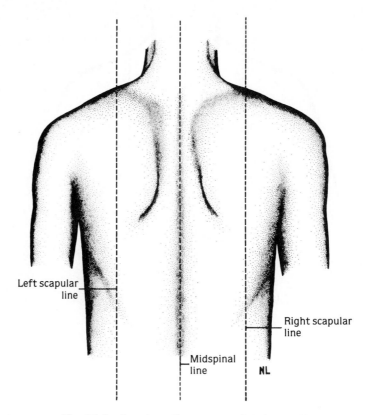

Fig. 16-4   Imaginary lines on posterior chest wall.

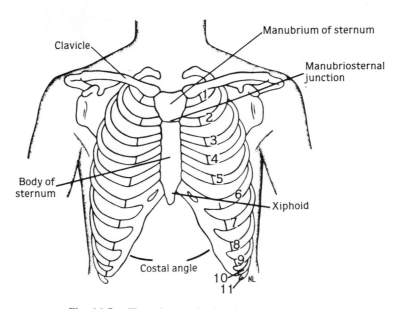

Fig. 16-5   Thoracic cage landmarks on anterior chest.

the body of the sternum and the manubrium is identified. This important landmark is visible in most individuals. The second rib articulates with the top of the corpus sterni at this point (Fig. 16-5). Rib identification on the anterior chest now can be accomplished with this as a reference point. It is recommended that ribs be counted to the side of the sternum, since individual costal cartilages that attach

the ribs to the sternum are not identified as easily near the sternum.

On the posterior chest, the spinous processes of the vertebrae are useful landmarks (Fig. 16-6). The spinous process of the seventh cervical vertebra (C-7) usually can be identified by having the patient extend the head and neck forward and slightly down. At the base of the neck the

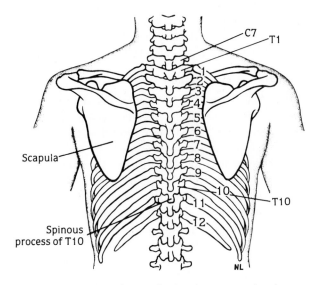

Fig. 16-6 Thoracic cage landmarks on posterior chest.

most prominent spinous process that can be visualized and palpated is C-7. The spinous process just below C-7 belongs to the first thoracic vertebra (T-1). The scapular borders also can be useful landmarks on the posterior chest. With the patient's arm raised above the head, the inferior border of the scapula approximately overlies the oblique fissure that separates the upper from the lower lobes on the posterior chest.

Lung fissures. Between the lobes of the lungs are the interlobar fissures. Both lungs have an oblique fissure that begins on the anterior chest at approximately the sixth rib at the midclavicular line. This fissure extends laterally and upward until it crosses the fifth rib on the lateral chest in the midaxillary line and continues on the posterior chest to approximately T-3 (Figs. 16-7 and 16-8).

The right lung also has a horizontal fissure that separates the right upper lobe from the right middle lobe. The horizontal fissure extends from the fourth rib at the sternal border around to the fifth rib at the midaxillary line. The left lung rarely has a horizontal fissure.

Fig. 16-7 Topographic position of lung fissures on anterior chest.

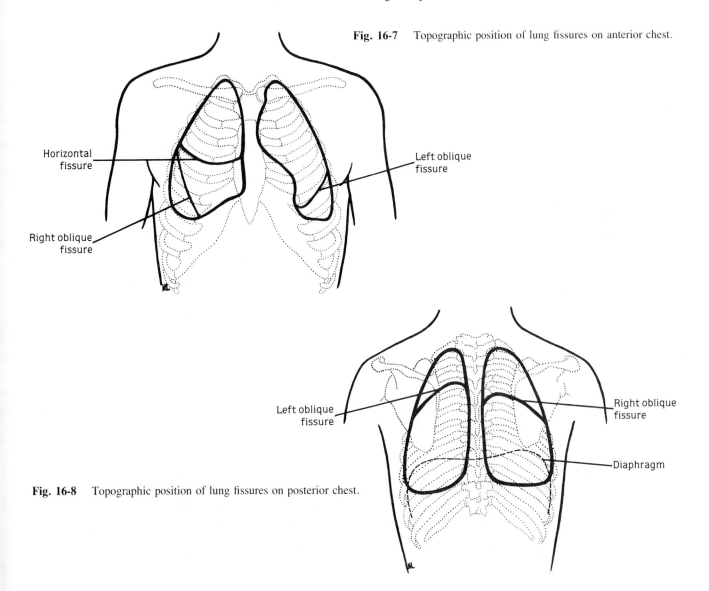

Fig. 16-8 Topographic position of lung fissures on posterior chest.

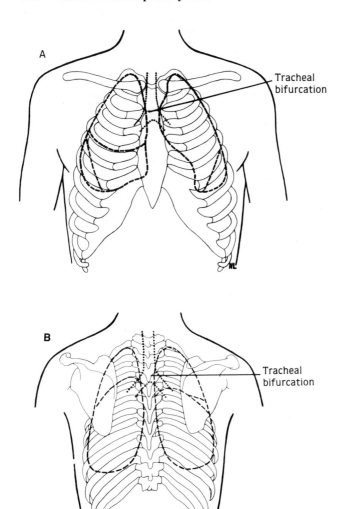

A

Tracheal bifurcation

B

Tracheal bifurcation

Fig. 16-9   Topographic position of tracheal bifurcation and lung borders on anterior chest, **A,** and posterior chest, **B.**

Tracheal bifurcation. The carina is located approximately beneath the angle of Louis on the anterior chest and at about T-4 on the posterior chest (Fig. 16-9).

Diaphragm. The diaphragm is a dome-shaped muscle that lies between the thoracic and abdominal cavities and moves up and down during normal ventilation. At the end of a tidal expiration the right dome of the diaphragm normally is located at the level of T-9 posteriorly and the fifth rib anteriorly. On the left side, the diaphragm normally comes to rest at end expiration at T-10 posteriorly and the sixth rib anteriorly. The right hemidiaphragm is usually a little higher anatomically than the left hemidiaphragm because of the placement of the liver.

Lung borders. Superiorly on the anterior chest the lungs extend 1 to 2 cm above the medial third of the clavicles. At end expiration, the inferior borders on the anterior chest extend to approximately the sixth rib at the midclavicular line and to the eighth rib on the lateral chest wall. On the posterior chest the superior border extends to T-1 and varies inferiorly with ventilation between approximately T-9 and T-12 (see Fig. 16-9).

Techniques of examination

Inspection. Visual examination of the chest is of value in assessing the thoracic configuration and the pattern and effort of breathing. For adequate inspection the room must be well lighted and the patient should be sitting upright. When the patient is too ill to sit up, the examiner must carefully roll the patient to one side in an effort to examine the posterior chest. Male patients should be stripped to the waist. Female patients should be given some type of drape to prevent embarrassing exposure of the breasts.

Thoracic configuration. The normal adult thorax has an anteroposterior diameter less than the transverse diameter. The anteroposterior diameter normally increases gradually with age and prematurely increases in patients with certain types of chronic obstructive lung disease. This abnormal increase in anteroposterior diameter is called *barrel chest.* When the anteroposterior diameter increases, the slope of the ribs lose their normal 45-degree angle in relation to the spine and become more horizontal (Fig. 16-10).

Other abnormalities of the thoracic configuration include the following:

Pectus carinatum	Sternal protrusion anteriorly
Pectus excavatum	Depression of part or all of the sternum, which can produce a restrictive lung defect
Kyphosis	Spinal deformity in which the spine has an abnormal anteroposterior curvature
Scoliosis	Spinal deformity in which the spine has a lateral curvature
Kyphoscoliosis	Combination of kyphosis and scoliosis; may produce a severe restrictive lung defect as a result of poor lung expansion

Breathing pattern and effort. At rest, the normal adult has a consistent rate and rhythm of ventilation. Breathing effort is minimal on inhalation and passive on exhalation. Men typically breathe with their diaphragm, causing the stomach to move slightly outward during inhalation. Women tend to use a combination of intercostal muscles and the diaphragm, producing more chest wall movement than men. Table 16-1 describes the abnormal patterns of breathing.

Any respiratory abnormalities that increase the work of breathing may cause the accessory muscles of ventilation to become active, even at rest. This is common in acute and chronic diffuse airway obstruction, acute upper airway

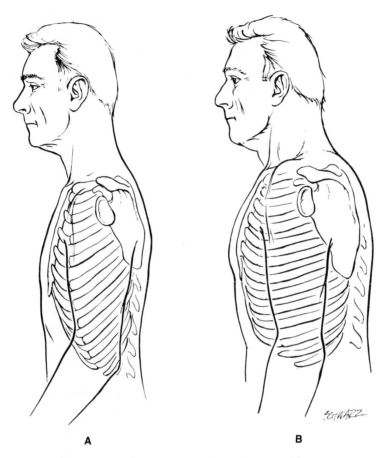

Fig. 16-10   A, Patient with normal thoracic configuration. **B,** Patient with increased anteroposterior diameter. Note contrasts in angle of slope of ribs and development of accessory muscles. (From Malasanos L et al: Health assessment, ed 4, St Louis, 1990, The CV Mosby Co.)

Table 16-1   Abnormal Breathing Patterns

Pattern	Characteristics	Causes
Apnea	No breathing	Cardiac arrest
Biot's	Irregular breathing with long periods of apnea	Increased intracranial pressure
Cheyne-Stokes	Irregular type of breathing; breaths increase and decrease in depth and rate with periods of apnea	Diseases of central nervous system Congestive heart failure
Kussmaul's	Deep and fast	Metabolic acidosis
Apneustic	Prolonged inhalation	Brain damage
Paradoxic	Portion or all of chest wall moves in with inhalation and out with exhalation	Chest trauma, diaphragm paralysis
Asthmatic	Prolonged exhalation	Obstruction to airflow out of lungs

obstruction, and disorders that reduce lung compliance.

The diaphragm may be nonfunctional in patients with spinal injuries or neuromuscular disease and have severely limited function in patients with chronic obstructive lung disease. When this occurs, the accessory muscles of ventilation may also become active.

In patients with emphysema, the lungs lose their elastic recoil and become hyperinflated. This results in the diaphragm's being pushed down into a less functional position. The accessory muscles then must assist ventilation by raising the anterior chest in an effort to increase thoracic volume. When the accessory muscles are producing a "clavicular lift" of more than 5 mm in this situation, lung function tests have demonstrated consistently the presence of severe obstructive lung disease.[1]

Palpation. Palpation is the art of touching the chest wall in an effort to evaluate underlying lung structure and function. Palpation is performed to (1) evaluate vocal fremitus, (2) estimate thoracic expansion, and (3) assess the skin and subcutaneous tissues of the chest.

Vocal fremitus. The term vocal fremitus refers to the vibrations created by the vocal cords during phonation. These vibrations transmit down the tracheobronchial tree and through the alveoli to the chest wall. When these vibrations are felt on the chest wall, it is called *tactile fremitus.*

During the assessment of tactile fremitus, the patient is directed to repeat the words "ninety-nine" while the examiner systematically palpates the thorax. The examiner can use the palmar aspect of the fingers or the ulnar aspect of the hand as illustrated in Fig. 16-11. If one hand is used, it should be moved from one side of the chest to the corresponding area on the other side. The anterior, lateral, and posterior chest wall should be evaluated.

The vibrations of tactile fremitus may be increased, decreased, or absent. Increased fremitus results from the transmission of the vibration through a more solid medium. The normal lung structure is a combination of solid and air-filled tissue. Any condition that tends to increase the density of the lung, such as the consolidation occurring with pneumonia, results in an increased intensity of fremitus. If the area of consolidation is not in connection with a patent bronchus, fremitus will not be increased but will be absent or decreased.

A reduced tactile fremitus often is present in patients who are obese or overly muscular. Also, when the pleural space lining the lung becomes filled with air (pneumothorax) or fluid (pleural effusion), the vocal fremitus is reduced significantly or is absent.

In patients with emphysema the lungs become hyperinflated with a significant reduction in the density of lung tissue. In this situation the vibrations transmit poorly through the lung tissue, resulting in a bilateral reduction in tactile fremitus. The bilateral reduction in tactile fremitus is more difficult to detect than the unilateral increase in fremitus

associated with lobar consolidation. The causes of abnormal tactile fremitus are summarized as follows:

Increased
  Pneumonia
  Lung tumor or mass
  Atelectasis
Decreased
  Unilateral
    Bronchial obstruction with mucus plug or foreign object
    Pneumothorax
    Pleural effusion
  Diffuse
    Chronic obstructive lung disease
    Muscular or obese chest wall

The passage of air through airway(s) containing thick secretions may produce palpable vibrations referred to as *rhonchial fremitus.* Rhonchial fremitus often is identified during inhalation and exhalation and may clear if the patient produces an effective cough. It frequently is associated with a coarse, low-pitched sound that is audible without a stethoscope.

Thoracic expansion. The normal chest wall expands symmetrically during deep inhalation. This expansion can be evaluated on the anterior and posterior chest. Anteriorly, the examiner's hands are placed over the anterolateral chest with the thumbs extended along the costal margin toward the xiphoid process. On the posterior chest the hands are positioned over the posterolateral chest with the thumbs meeting at approximately the eighth thoracic vertebra (Fig. 16-12). The patient is instructed to exhale slowly and completely while the examiner's hands are positioned as described. When the patient has exhaled maximally, the examiner gently secures the tips of the fingers against the sides of the chest and extends the thumbs toward the midline until the tip of each thumb meets at the midline. The patient then is instructed to take a full, deep breath. The examiner should make note of the distance each thumb moves from the midline. Normally, each thumb moves an equal distance of approximately 3 to 5 cm.

Diseases that affect expansion of both lungs cause a bilateral reduction in chest expansion. This is seen commonly with neuromuscular diseases and chronic obstructive pulmonary disease. A unilateral (one-sided) reduction in chest expansion occurs with respiratory diseases that reduce the expansion of one lung or a major part of one lung. This may occur with lobar consolidation, atelectasis, pleural effusion, and pneumothorax.

Skin and subcutaneous tissues. The chest wall can be palpated to determine the skin's general temperature and condition. When air leaks from the lung into subcutaneous tissues, fine beads of air produce a crackling sound and sensation when palpated. This condition is referred to as *subcutaneous emphysema,* and the sensation produced on palpation is called *crepitus.*

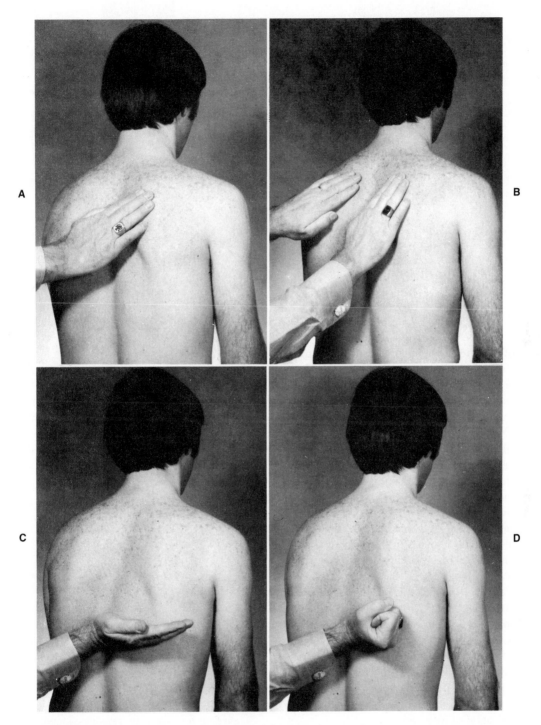

Fig. 16-11   Palpation for assessment of vocal fremitus. **A,** Use of palmar surface of fingertips. **B,** Simultaneous application of fingertips of both hands. **C,** Use of ulnar aspect of hand. **D,** Use of ulnar aspect of closed fist. (From Prior JA, Silberstein JS, and Stang JM: Physical diagnosis: the history and examination of the patient, ed 6, St Louis, 1982, The CV Mosby Co.)

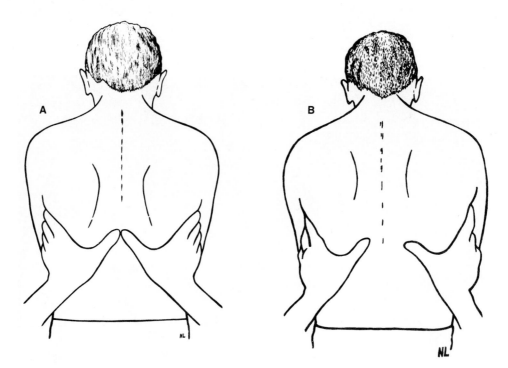

Fig. 16-12   Estimation of thoracic expansion. **A,** Exhalation. **B,** Maximal inhalation.

Percussion of the chest. Percussion is the art of tapping on a surface in an effort to evaluate the underlying structure. Percussion of the chest wall produces a sound and a palpable vibration useful in evaluating the underlying lung tissue. The vibration created by percussion penetrates the lung 5 to 7 cm below the chest wall.

The technique most often used in percussion of the chest wall is termed mediate or indirect percussion. The examiner places the middle finger of the left hand (if the examiner is right-handed) firmly against the chest wall parallel to the ribs with the palm and other fingers held off the chest. The tip of the middle finger on the right hand or the lateral aspect of the right thumb strikes the finger against the chest near the base of the terminal phalanx with a quick, sharp blow. Movement of the hand striking the chest should be generated at the wrist and not the elbow or shoulder (Fig. 16-13).

The percussion note is clearest if the examiner remembers to keep the finger on the chest firmly against the chest wall and to strike this finger and immediately withdraw. The two fingers should be in contact only for an instant. As one gains experience in percussion of the chest, the feel of the vibration created becomes as important as the sound in the evaluation of lung structures.

Percussion over lung fields. Percussion of the lung fields should be done systematically, consecutively testing comparable areas on both sides of the chest. Percussion over the bony structures and breasts of the female is not of value and should be avoided. Asking patients to raise their arms above their shoulders will help move the scapulae laterally and minimize their interference with percussion on the posterior chest wall.

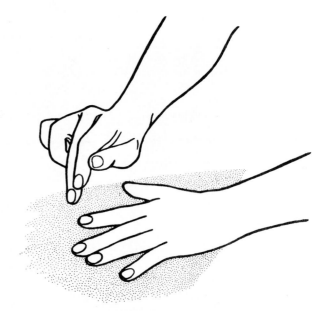

Fig. 16-13   Technique for indirect chest percussion.

The sounds generated during percussion of the chest are evaluated for intensity (loudness) and pitch. Percussion over normal lung fields produces a sound moderately low in pitch that can be heard easily. This sound is best described as normal resonance. When the percussion note is louder and lower in pitch than normal, the resonance is said to be increased. Percussion may produce a sound with characteristics just the opposite of resonance, referred to as dull or flat. This sound is high pitched, brief, and not loud.

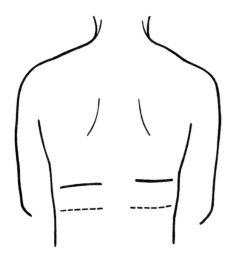

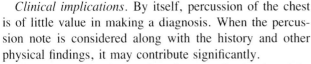

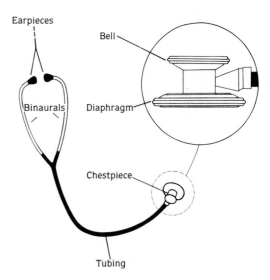

Fig. 16-14   Assessment of diaphragmatic excursion by percussion. Horizontal lines indicate position of diaphragm at maximal inhalation and exhalation.

Fig. 16-15   Acoustic stethoscope.

Clinical implications. By itself, percussion of the chest is of little value in making a diagnosis. When the percussion note is considered along with the history and other physical findings, it may contribute significantly.

Any abnormality that tends to increase the density of the lung tissue, such as the consolidation of pneumonia, lung tumors, or alveolar collapse (atelectasis), results in a loss of resonance and a dull percussion note over the affected area. Percussion over pleural spaces filled with fluid, such as blood or water, also results in a dull or flat percussion note.

An increase in resonance is detected in patients with hyperinflated lungs. Hyperinflation can occur as a result of acute bronchial obstruction (asthma) or chronic obstructive disease such as emphysema. The percussion note also can increase in resonance when the pleural space contains large amounts of air (pneumothorax).

Limitations. Unilateral abnormalities are easier to detect than bilateral abnormalities because the normal side provides an immediate comparison. The dullness heard from percussion over consolidation is a distinct sound that is easier to detect than the subtle increase in resonance associated with hyperinflation or pneumothorax.

Percussion of the chest has limitations that are often clinically important. Abnormalities that are small or more than 5 cm below the surface are not likely to be detected during percussion of the chest.

Diaphragmatic excursion. The range of diaphragm movement may be estimated by percussion and is done best on the posterior chest wall (Fig. 16-14). To estimate diaphragm movement, the patient first is instructed to take a deep, full inspiration and hold it. The examiner then determines the lowest margin of resonance by percussing over the lower lung field and moving downward in small increments until a definite change in the percussion note is detected. The patient then is instructed to exhale maxi-

mally, holding this position while the percussion procedure is repeated. The examiner should work rapidly to prevent the patient from becoming short of breath. The normal diaphragm excursion during a deep breath is about 5 to 7 cm. The range of diaphragm movement is less than normal in patients with certain neuromuscular diseases or severe pulmonary hyperinflation.

The exact range of movement and position of the diaphragm is difficult to determine by percussion.[2] This is because the diaphragm is a dome-shaped muscle with the center of the dome 15 cm beneath the surface of the posterior chest. Percussion only can approximate the position and degree of movement.

Auscultation of the lungs. Auscultation is the process of listening for sounds produced in the body. Auscultation over the thorax is performed to identify normal or abnormal lung sounds. A stethoscope is used during auscultation to promote better transmission of sounds to the examiner. Whenever auscultation is performed, the room must be as quiet as possible.

Stethoscope. The stethoscope possesses four basic parts: a bell, a diaphragm, tubing, and earpieces (Fig. 16-15). The bell detects a broad spectrum of sounds and is of particular value when listening to low-pitched sounds, such as those produced by the heart. It also is valuable in auscultation of the lungs in certain situations, as in the emaciated patient where rib protrusion restricts placement of the diaphragm flat against the chest. The bell piece should be pressed lightly against the chest when attempting to auscultate low-frequency sounds. If the bell is pressed too firmly against the chest wall, the skin will be stretched under the bell and may act as a diaphragm, filtering out certain low-frequency sounds.

The diaphragm piece is used most often in auscultation of the lungs, since most lung sounds are of relatively high frequency. It also is useful in listening to high-frequency heart sounds. The diaphragm piece should be pressed firmly against the chest so that external sounds are not heard.

The ideal tubing should be thick enough to exclude external noises and approximately 25 to 35 cm (11 to 16 inches) long. Longer tubing may compromise sound transmission, and shorter tubing is often inconvenient in reaching the patient's chest.

The stethoscope should be examined regularly for cracks in the diaphragm, wax or dirt in the ear pieces, and other defects that may interfere with the transmission of sound. It should be wiped off with alcohol on a regular basis to prevent a buildup of microorganisms.

Technique. When possible, the patient should be sitting upright in a relaxed position. The patient should be instructed to breathe a little deeper than normal with the mouth open. Inhalation should be active and exhalation passive. The bell or diaphragm must be placed directly against the chest wall, since clothing may alter lung sounds or produce distorted sounds. The tubing should not rub against any objects, since this may produce extraneous sounds. Auscultation of the lungs should be systematic, including all lobes on the anterior, lateral, and posterior chest. It is recommended that the examiner begin at the base, compare side with side, and work toward the lung apexes. The examiner should begin at the lung bases because certain abnormal lung sounds (described later) that primarily occur in the dependent lung zones may be altered by several deep breaths. At least one full ventilatory cycle should be evaluated at each stethoscope position. The common errors of auscultation that should be avoided are summarized in the box on p. 363.

Four characteristics of breath sounds should be specifically listened for by the examiner. First, the pitch (vibration frequency) should be identified. Second, the amplitude or intensity (loudness) is noted. Third, the distinctive characteristics are listened for and noted. Fourth, the dura-

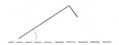

Fig. 16-16 Diagrammatic representation of normal breath sound. Upstroke represents inhalation, and downstroke represents exhalation; length of upstroke represents duration; thickness of stroke represents intensity; angle between upstroke and horizontal line represents pitch.

tion of inspiratory sound is compared with expiration. The acoustic characteristics of breath sounds can be illustrated in breath sound diagrams (Fig. 16-16). The characteristics of the normal breath sounds are described in Table 16-2. Examiners first must be familiar with the characteristics of normal breath sounds before they can expect to identify the subtle changes that may signify respiratory disease.

Terminology. In healthy individuals the sounds heard over the trachea have a loud, tubular quality. These are referred to as *bronchial* or *tracheal* breath sounds. Bronchial breath sounds are high-pitched sounds with an expiratory component equal to or slightly longer than the inspiratory component.

A slight variation to bronchial breath sounds is heard around the upper half of the sternum on the anterior chest and between the scapulae on the posterior chest. These sounds are not as loud as bronchial breath sounds, are slightly lower in pitch, and have equal inspiratory and expiratory components. They are referred to as *bronchovesicular* breath sounds.

When the examiner auscultates over the lung parenchyma of a healthy individual, soft, muffled sounds are heard. These sounds, referred to as *vesicular* or *normal* breath sounds, are lower in pitch and intensity (loudness) than bronchial breath sounds. Vesicular sounds are most difficult to hear and are heard primarily during inhalation

Table 16-2 Characteristics of Normal Breath Sounds

Breath sound	Pitch	Intensity	Location	Diagram of sound
Vesicular or normal breath sounds	Low	Soft	Peripheral lung areas	
Bronchovesicular	Moderate	Moderate	Around upper part of sternum, between scapulae	
Bronchial	High	Loud	Over trachea	

COMMON ERRORS OF AUSCULTATION

ERRORS	CORRECT TECHNIQUE
Listening to breath sounds through the patient's gown	Placing bell or diaphragm directly against the chest wall
Allowing tubing to rub against bed rails or patient's gown	Keeping tubing free from contact with any objects during auscultation
Attempting to auscultate in a noisy room	Turning television or radio off
Interpreting chest hair sounds as adventitious lung sounds	Wetting chest hair before auscultation if thick
Auscultating only the "convenient" areas	Asking alert patient to sit up; rolling comatose patient onto side to auscultate posterior lobes

---

with only a minimal exhalation component (see Table 16-2).

Respiratory disease may alter the intensity of normal breath sounds heard over the lung fields. A slight variation in intensity is difficult to detect even for experienced clinicians. Breath sounds are described as *diminished* when the intensity decreases and *absent* in extreme cases. Breath sounds are described as *harsh* when the intensity increases. When harsh breath sounds have an expiratory component equal to the inspiratory component, they are described as *bronchial* breath sounds.

Abnormal sounds or vibrations produced by the movement of air in the lungs are termed *adventitious sounds*. Most adventitious lung sounds can be classified as either continuous or discontinuous sounds. Continuous lung sounds are defined as having a duration longer than 25 msec. (This definition is derived from recording and spectral analysis of lung sounds. Examiners are not expected to time the lung sounds.) Discontinuous lung sounds are characteristically intermittent, crackling, or bubbling sounds of short duration, usually less than 20 msec.[3]

The terminology used to describe abnormal lung sounds has had a confusing history. As a result, there has been a lack of standardization among clinicians.[4] Fortunately, the American Thoracic Society and the American College of Chest Physicians formed a committee to address the issue of pulmonary nomenclature. Their work first was published in 1975 and suggested that the term *rales* be used to describe discontinuous types of abnormal lung sounds and that the term *rhonchi* be used to describe continuous types of sounds.[5]

The committee published updated reports in 1977 and 1981 that advocated the term *crackles* for describing discontinuous types of lung sounds instead of the more popular term rales.[6,7] Rales has been used in the past as the term for both continuous and discontinuous types of abnormal lung sounds. However, the committee decided that the term crackles may be better suited for describing discontinuous types of lung sounds. Although the use of the term rales has declined since the committee's recommendations, it remains a popular term among many clinicians.[8] The up-

dates also suggested that high-pitched continuous types of abnormal lung sounds be described as *wheezes* and that rhonchi be used specifically for low-pitched continuous sounds. For the remainder of this text, to be consistent with these recommendations, the term crackles is used to indicate discontinuous lung sounds; wheezes is used for high-pitched continuous lung sounds; and rhonchi is used for low-pitched continuous lung sounds.

Another continuous sound heard primarily over the larynx and trachea during inhalation, when upper airway obstruction is present, is known as *stridor*. This is a loud, low-pitched sound that frequently may be heard without a stethoscope.

The reader should be aware that since there is a lack of standardization of lung sound terminology among clinicians, authors of other publications may use different terms to describe abnormal lung sounds. Table 16-3 provides a list of alternative terms that may be used by others.

When abnormal lung sounds are identified, their location and specific characteristics should be noted. Abnormal lung sounds may be high or low pitched, loud or faint, scanty or profuse, and inspiratory or expiratory (or both). The timing during the respiratory cycle should be noted also, for example, late inspiratory. The examiner must pay close attention to these characteristics for abnormal lung sounds because they help determine the lungs' functional

Table 16-3 Recommended* Terminology for Lung Sounds Versus Alternative Terminology

Recommended term	Classification	Alternative terms
Crackles	Discontinuous	Rales Crepitations
Wheezes	High-pitched, continuous	Sibilant rales Musical rales Sibilant rhonchi
Rhonchi	Low-pitched, continuous	Sonorous rales Low-pitched wheeze

*According to the Ad Hoc Pulmonary Nomenclature Committee of ATS/ACCP.

status. This is further discussed in the following paragraphs.

Mechanisms and significance of lung sounds. The exact mechanisms responsible for the production of normal and abnormal lung sounds are not fully known. However, there is enough agreement among investigators to allow a general description. This knowledge should give examiners a better understanding of the lung sounds frequently heard through a stethoscope.

Normal breath sounds. Lung sounds heard over the chest of the healthy individual are generated primarily by turbulent flow in the larger airways.[9,10] Turbulent flow creates audible vibrations in the airways, producing sounds that are transmitted through the lung and the chest wall. As the sound travels to the lung periphery and the chest wall, it is altered by the filtering properties of normal lung tissue. Normal lung tissue is known to act as a low-pass filter, which means it preferentially passes low-frequency sounds. This filtering effect can be demonstrated easily by listening over the periphery of the lung while a subject speaks. The muffled voice sounds are difficult to understand because of the lung's filtering properties.

This filtering phenomenon accounts for the characteristic differences between bronchial breath sounds heard directly over larger airways and vesicular sounds heard over the periphery of the lung. Normal vesicular lung sounds essentially are filtered bronchial breath sounds.

Abnormal breath sounds. Bronchial breath sounds also can be classified as abnormal lung sounds when heard over peripheral lung regions. Bronchial breath sounds may replace the normal vesicular sound when the lung tissue increases in density as occurs in atelectasis and pneumonia. When the normal air-filled lung tissue becomes consolidated, the filtering effect is lost, and similar sounds are heard over large upper airways and the consolidated lung.[11]

Diminished breath sounds. Diminished breath sounds occur when the sound intensity at the site of generation (larger airways) is reduced or when the transmission properties of the lung or chest wall are reduced. The intensity of sound created by turbulent flow through the bronchi is reduced with shallow or slow breathing patterns. Obstructed airways and hyperinflated lung tissue inhibit normal transmission of sounds through the lungs. Air or fluid in the pleural space and obesity reduce the transmission of breath sounds through the chest wall.

In patients with chronic airflow obstruction, the intensity of vesicular breath sounds often is reduced markedly throughout all lung fields. This is primarily the result of poor sound transmission through hyperinflated lung tissue as occurs with emphysema. Shallow breathing patterns also contribute to reduced breath sound intensity in patients with chronic obstructive lung disease. Studies have been done correlating the intensity of vesicular lung sounds with pulmonary function tests, and these studies have provided some useful conclusions. A definite, diffuse reduction in breath sound intensity is strong evidence that obstructive pulmonary disease is present and that a significant reduction in expiratory flow rates exists. Normal breath sound intensity heard throughout the lung fields nearly excludes the possibility that significant chronic obstructive abnormalities are present. Mild reductions in breath sound intensity are less predictive.[12-14]

Wheezes and rhonchi. Wheezes and some rhonchi are generated by the vibration of the wall of a narrowed or compressed airway as air passes through at high velocity.[9,11] The diameter of an airway may be reduced by bronchospasm, mucosal edema, or foreign objects. The pitch of the wheeze is independent of the length of the airway but is related directly to the degree of narrowing. The greater the narrowing, the higher the pitch. Low-pitched continuous sounds (rhonchi) often are associated with the presence of excessive secretions in the airways. A sputum flap vibrating in the airstream may produce rhonchi that clear after the patient coughs.

The significance of expiratory wheezing during unforced breathing has been studied, and several useful conclusions have been reached. Patients with chronic airflow obstruction who do not wheeze are not likely to have significant improvements of expiratory flow rates (measured by spirometry) after bronchodilators. Patients with chronic airflow obstruction who wheeze are more likely to have significant improvement in their expiratory flow rate after bronchodilators. When unforced expiratory wheezing is intense, spirometry consistently demonstrates moderate to severe airway obstruction. Less intense wheezing is associated with a wide range of obstructive defects.[15] Wheezing heard during a forceful expiratory maneuver is identified commonly in individuals with obstructed and unobstructed airways and is of no predictive value.

Crackles. Crackles often are produced by the movement of excessive secretions or fluid in the airways as air passes through. In this situation crackles are usually coarse and are heard during inspiration and expiration. They often clear if the patient coughs and may be associated with rhonchial fremitus.

Crackles also occur in patients without excess secretions when collapsed airways pop open during inspiration.[9,16-19] The crackling sound in this situation is caused by the explosive-type equalization of pressure between the collapsed airways and the patent airways above. Airway closure may occur in peripheral bronchioles or in more proximal bronchi. The source of the crackles in this situation may be suggested by certain characteristics described in the following paragraphs.

Larger, more proximal bronchi may close during expiration when there is an abnormal increase in bronchial compliance or if the retractive pressures around the bronchi are low. In this situation crackles usually occur early in the inspiratory phase and are referred to as early inspiratory crackles (Fig. 16-17). Early inspiratory crackles are usually scanty but may be loud or faint. They often are trans-

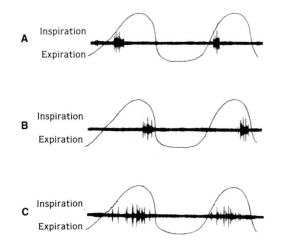

Fig. 16-17 Timing of inspiratory crackles. **A,** Early inspiratory crackles. **B,** Late inspiratory crackles. **C,** Paninspiratory crackles.

mitted to the mouth and are not silenced by a cough or change in position. They most often occur in patients with chronic obstructive lung diseases such as chronic bronchitis, emphysema, and asthma and may indicate that a more severe airway obstruction is present.[17]

Peripheral alveoli and airways may close during exhalation when the surrounding intrathoracic pressure increases. Crackles produced by the sudden opening of peripheral airways usually occur late in the inspiratory phase and are referred to as late inspiratory crackles. They are more common in the dependent regions of the lungs where transmural pressure gradients during exhalation predispose the peripheral airways to collapse. They often are identified in several consecutive respiratory cycles, producing a recurrent rhythm. They may clear with changes in posture or if the patient performs several deep inspiratory maneuvers. Coughing or maximal exhalation by the patient may cause late inspiratory crackles to reappear. Patients with

respiratory disorders that reduce lung volume (restrictive disorders)—such as atelectasis, pneumonia, pulmonary edema, and fibrosis—are most likely to have the late inspiratory type of crackles (Table 16-4).[17]

The presence of inspiratory crackles generally is considered an abnormal physical finding but may occur in healthy individuals in certain situations.[20,21] Fine inspiratory crackles can be identified in healthy subjects during inhalation from low lung volumes (after maximal exhalation). In addition, an end-expiratory cough may result in the identification of late inspiratory crackles that were not present after a normal expiratory effort. Since crackles can be elicited from normal subjects during inspiration from low lung volumes, they are not necessarily abnormal lung sounds. Perhaps fine, late inspiratory crackles should be considered abnormal only when they occur during inhalation from a resting lung volume.

Pleural friction rub. A pleural friction rub is a creaking or grating type of sound that occurs when the pleural surfaces become inflamed and the roughened edges rub together during breathing, such as occurs with pleurisy. It may be heard only during inhalation but often is identified during both phases of breathing. Pleural friction rubs often sound similar to coarse crackles but are not affected by coughing. The intensity of pleural rubs may increase with deep breathing.

Voice sounds. If inspection, palpation, percussion, or auscultation of the patient's chest suggests any respiratory abnormality, vocal resonance is assessed. Vocal resonance is produced by the same mechanism as vocal fremitus described earlier. The vibrations created by the vocal cords during phonation travel down the tracheobronchial tree and through the peripheral lung units to the chest wall. The patient is instructed to repeat the words "one, two, three," or "ninety-nine" while the examiner listens over the chest wall with a stethoscope, comparing the sides. The normal, air-filled lung tissue filters the voice sounds, significantly

Table 16-4 Application of Adventitious Lung Sounds

Lung sounds	Possible mechanism	Characteristics	Causes
Wheezes	Rapid airflow through obstructed airways caused by bronchospasm, mucosal edema	High-pitched; most often occur during exhalation	Asthma, congestive heart failure, bronchitis
Stridor	Rapid airflow through obstructed airway caused by inflammation	High-pitched; often occurs during inhalation	Croup, epiglottitis, postextubation
Crackles			
Inspiratory and expiratory	Excess airway secretions moving with airflow	Coarse and often clear with cough	Bronchitis, respiratory infections
Early inspiratory	Sudden opening of proximal bronchi	Scanty, transmitted to mouth; not affected by cough	Bronchitis, emphysema, asthma
Late inspiratory	Sudden opening of peripheral airways	Diffuse, fine; occur initially in the dependent regions	Atelectasis, pneumonia, pulmonary edema, fibrosis

reducing intensity and clarity. Pathologic abnormalities in lung tissue alter the transmission of voice sounds, resulting in either increased or decreased vocal resonance.

An increase in intensity and clarity of vocal resonance resulting from enhanced transmission of vocal vibrations is referred to as *bronchophony*. Bronchophony indicates an increase in lung tissue density, as can occur in the consolidation phase of pneumonia. Bronchophony is easier to detect when unilateral and often is associated with bronchial breath sounds, dull percussion note, and increased vocal fremitus.

Vocal resonance is reduced in similar lung abnormalities that result in reduced breath sounds and decreased tactile fremitus. Hyperinflation of lung parenchyma, pneumothorax, bronchial obstruction, and pleural effusion all reduce the transmission of vocal vibrations through the lung or chest wall, producing decreased vocal resonance.

When the spoken voice increases in intensity and its character takes on a nasal or bleating quality, it is referred to as *egophony*. Egophony may be identified over areas of the chest where bronchophony is present. The exact reason for this change in voice-sound character is unknown. It is identified most easily by having the patient say "e-e-e." If egophony is present, the "e-e-e" will be heard over the peripheral chest wall with the stethoscope as an "a-a-a." Egophony usually is identified only over an area of compressed lung above a pleural effusion.

Whispering pectoriloquy may be a helpful physical finding, especially in patients with small or patchy areas of lung consolidation. The patient is instructed to whisper the words "one, two, three" while the examiner listens over the lung periphery with a stethoscope, comparing the sides. Whispering creates high-frequency vibrations that are filtered out selectively by normal lung tissue and normally heard as muffled, low-pitched sounds. However, when consolidation is present, the lung loses its selective transmission quality, and the characteristic high-pitched sounds are transmitted to the chest wall with clarity.

Auscultatory percussion of the chest. A technique that combines auscultation and percussion is known as auscultatory percussion. The procedure is simple to perform and only requires a stethoscope. The examiner percusses on the patient's manubrium with the index finger and one hand while auscultating over the posterior lung fields, comparing both sides.

The advantage of auscultatory percussion over conventional percussion is the increased sensitivity to lung abnormalities.[22] Guarino demonstrated this advantage in his study of 30 patients with unilateral lung disease. Of the 30 patients studied, 28 had abnormal chest x-ray films with normal or equivocal findings during conventional percussion. In the majority of cases, the auscultatory percussion technique readily detected the abnormalities. Before this method can be accepted widely, however, confirmation by other studies is needed.

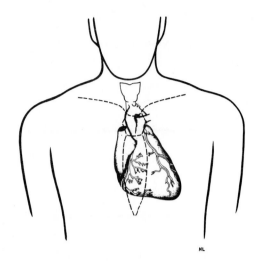

Fig. 16-18   Topographic position of heart.

EXAMINATION OF THE PRECORDIUM

As mentioned previously, chronic diseases of the lungs may frequently be associated with abnormalities in other body systems. Recognition of these abnormalities is helpful in identifying respiratory disease and in quantifying its severity. Because of the close working relationship between the heart and lungs, the heart is especially at risk for developing problems secondary to lung disease. The techniques for physical examination of the chest wall overlying the heart, or *precordium,* include inspection, palpation, and auscultation. Percussion is of little or no value in the examination and is omitted. For the sake of convenience most clinicians examine the precordium simultaneously with the lungs.

Review of heart topography

The heart lies between the lungs within the mediastinum and is situated so that the right ventricle is more anterior than the left ventricle. The upper portion of the heart consists of both atria and is referred to commonly as the base of the heart. The base lies directly beneath the upper-middle portion of the body of the sternum. The lower portion of the heart, which consists of the ventricles, is referred to as the apex. The apex points downward and to the left, extending to a point near the midclavicular line, and usually lies directly beneath the lower left portion of the corpus sterni and near the costal cartilage of the fifth rib (Fig. 16-18).

Inspection and palpation

The purpose of inspecting and palpating the precordium is to identify any normal or abnormal pulsations. Pulsations on the precordium are affected by the thickness of the chest wall and the quality of the tissue through which the vibrations must travel. The normal apical impulse is produced by the thrust of the contracting left ventricle and

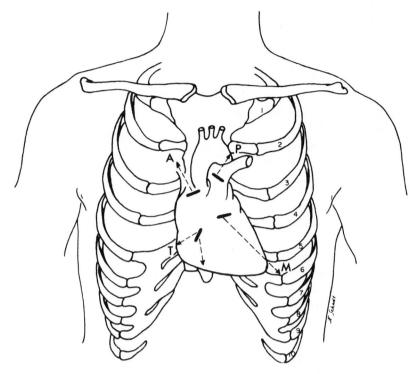

Fig. 16-19 Anatomic and auscultatory valve area. Location of anatomic valve sites is represented by solid bars. Arrows designate transmission of valve sounds to their respective auscultatory valve areas. *M,* Mitral valve; *T,* tricuspid valve; *A,* aortic valve; *P,* pulmonic valve. (From Prior JA, Silberstein JS, and Stang JM: Physical diagnosis: the history and examination of the patient, ed 6, St Louis, 1982, The CV Mosby Co.)

usually is identified near the midclavicular line in the fifth intercostal space. This systolic thrust, referred to as the *point of maximal impulse,* or PMI, may be felt and visualized in many healthy individuals.

Right ventricular hypertrophy, a common manifestation of chronic lung disease, often produces a systolic thrust that is felt and possibly visualized near the lower left sternal border. The palmar aspect of the examiner's right hand is placed over the lower left sternal border for identification. Right ventricular hypertrophy may be the result of chronic hypoxemia, pulmonary valve disease, or pulmonary hypertension.

In patients with chronic pulmonary hyperinflation (emphysema), identification of the apical impulse is more difficult. The increase in anteroposterior diameter and the alteration in lung tissue contribute to poor transmission of the vibrations of systole to the surface of the chest. Therefore in patients with pulmonary emphysema the intensity of the PMI may be reduced or not identifiable.

The PMI may shift to the left or right with shifts in the mediastinum. Pneumothorax or lobar collapse often shifts the mediastinum, resulting in a shift of the PMI toward the lobar collapse but usually away from the pneumothorax. Patients with emphysema and low, flat diaphragms may have the PMI located in the epigastric area.

The second left intercostal space near the sternal border is referred to as the *pulmonic* area and is palpated in an effort to identify accentuated pulmonary valve closure. Strong vibrations may be felt in this area with pulmonary hypertension or valvular abnormalities (Fig. 16-19).

Auscultation of heart sounds

Normal heart sounds primarily are created by closure of the heart valves. The first heart sound (S_1) is produced by the sudden closure of the mitral and tricuspid valves (atrioventricular) during contraction of the ventricles. When systole ends, the ventricles relax and the semilunar valves (pulmonic and aortic) close, creating the second heart sound (S_2). Because the left side of the heart has a significantly higher pressure created during systole, closure of the mitral valve is louder and contributes more than the closure of the tricuspid valve to S_1 in the healthy individual. For the same reason, closure of the aortic valve usually is more significant in producing S_2. Whenever the atrioventricular or semilunar valves do not close simultaneously, a split heart sound is heard. A slight splitting of S_2 is normal and often occurs as the result of normal spontaneous ventilation. The normal splitting of S_2 is increased during inhalation because of the decrease in intrathoracic pressure, which improves venous return to the right side of the heart and further delays pulmonic valve closure.

A third heart sound (S_3) may be identified during diastole. S_3 is thought to be produced by rapid ventricular filling immediately after systole. The rapid distention of the ventricles causes the walls of the ventricles to vibrate and produce a sound of low intensity and pitch. It is best heard over the apex. It is normal in healthy children and is referred to as physiologic S_3 in this situation. In other situations, however, an S_3 is abnormal. For example, in an older patient with a history of heart disease, an S_3 is a definite abnormality and may signify myocardial infarction.

A fourth heart sound (S_4) is produced by mechanisms similar to S_3. It may occur in healthy individuals or be considered a sign of heart disease.

Auscultation of the heart sounds may identify alterations in the loudness of either S_1 or S_2. A reduction in the intensity of heart sounds may be the result of cardiac or extracardiac abnormalities. Extracardiac factors include alteration in the tissue between the heart and the surface of the chest. Pulmonary hyperinflation, pleural effusion, pneumothorax, and obesity make identification of both S_1 and S_2 difficult. S_1 and S_2 intensity also may be reduced when the force of ventricular contraction is poor, as in heart failure, or when valvular abnormalities exist.

Pulmonary hypertension produces an increased intensity of S_2 as a result of more forceful closure of the pulmonic valve; this is referred to as an increased P_2. A lack of S_2 splitting with inhalation also may be the result of pulmonary hypertension. An increased P_2 is identified best over the pulmonic area of the chest.

Cardiac murmurs are identified whenever the heart valves are incompetent or stenotic. Murmurs usually are classified as either systolic or diastolic. Systolic murmurs are produced by an incompetent atrioventricular valve or a stenotic semilunar valve. An incompetent atrioventricular valve allows a back flow of blood into the atrium, usually producing a high-pitched "whooshing" noise simultaneously with S_1. A stenotic semilunar valve produces a similar sound created by an obstruction of blood flow out of the ventricle during systole.

Diastolic murmurs are created by an incompetent semilunar valve or a stenotic atrioventricular valve. An incompetent semilunar valve allows a back flow of blood into the ventricle simultaneously with or immediately after S_2. A stenotic atrioventricular valve obstructs blood flow from the atrium into the ventricles during diastole and creates a turbulent murmur.

A murmur also may be created by rapid blood flow across normal valves. In summary, murmurs are created by (1) a back flow of blood through an incompetent valve, (2) a forward flow through a stenotic valve, and (3) a rapid flow through a normal valve.

Auscultation of heart sounds usually is done at the same time the lung sounds are identified. The bell and diaphragm pieces of the stethoscope are used. The heart sounds may be easier to identify by requesting that the patient lean forward or lay on the left side, since this anatomically moves the heart closer to the chest wall. When the peripheral pulses are difficult to identify, auscultation over the precordium may provide an easier method of identifying the heart rate.

EXAMINATION OF THE ABDOMEN

An in-depth discussion of examining the abdomen is beyond the scope of this book; however, a review of the abnormalities associated with respiratory diseases is presented.

The abdomen should be inspected and palpated for evidence of distention and tenderness. Abdominal distention and pain may cause impairment of the diaphragm and contribute to respiratory insufficiency or failure. It may inhibit the patient from coughing and deep breathing, both of which are important in preventing respiratory complications in the postoperative patient.

Palpation and percussion are used on the right upper quadrant of the abdomen in an effort to estimate the size of the liver (Fig. 16-20). Among its many causes, an enlarged liver may be observed in patients with chronic right heart failure occurring secondary to chronic respiratory

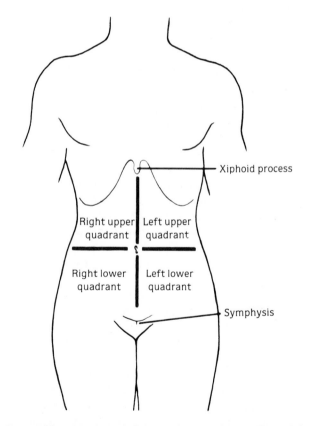

Fig. 16-20 Division of abdomen into quadrants. (From Prior JA, Silberstein JS, and Stang JM: Physical diagnosis: the history and examination of the patient, ed 6, St Louis, 1982, The CV Mosby Co.)

disease. In such cases, the venous blood flow returning to the right ventricle is reduced and major veins and organs may become engorged. The hepatic vein that empties into the inferior vena cava may become engorged in this situation, and the liver enlarges. This is referred to as *hepatomegaly*.

To identify hepatomegaly, the superior and inferior borders of the liver are identified by percussion. Normally, the liver spans about 10 cm at the midclavicular line. If the liver extends more than 10 cm, it is considered enlarged.

EXAMINATION OF THE EXTREMITIES

Respiratory disease may result in numerous abnormalities identified during inspection of the extremities. These abnormalities include digital clubbing, cyanosis, and pedal edema. Each is discussed briefly.

Clubbing

Clubbing of the digits is a significant manifestation of cardiopulmonary disease (see Chap. 15). The mechanism responsible for clubbing is not known, but it often is associated with a chronic decrease in oxygen supply to the body tissues in general. It is identified most commonly in patients with bronchogenic carcinoma, chronic obstructive lung disease, and chronic cardiovascular disease.

Clubbing is characterized by a painless enlargement of the terminal phalanges of the fingers and toes that requires years to develop. As the process of clubbing advances, the angle of the fingernail to the nail base advances past 200 degrees, and the base of the nail feels spongy. The profile view of the digits allows easier recognition of clubbing (Fig. 16-21).

Cyanosis

Examination of the digits should identify either the presence or absence of cyanosis in any patient suspected of having respiratory disease. The transparency of the fingernails and skin covering the digits allows cyanosis to be detected readily in this area. Cyanosis occurs whenever 5.0 mg/dL of reduced hemoglobin exists; thus the intensity of cyanosis increases with the amount of hemoglobin in the blood. Patients with a high hemoglobin concentration (polycythemia) develop cyanosis at a lesser degree of tissue hypoxia, whereas patients with low hemoglobin concentrations (anemia) have severe hypoxia before cyanosis occurs. The presence of cyanosis may indicate that the lungs are not oxygenating the blood optimally, but tissue hypoxia may not be severe, especially if polycythemia is present. Additionally, not all hypoxic states produce cyanosis (see Chapter 15). Peripheral cyanosis may also be a sign of inadequate perfusion.

Pedal edema

Patients with chronic respiratory disease may have pedal edema as a manifestation of their chronic disease. Since

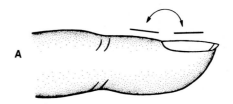
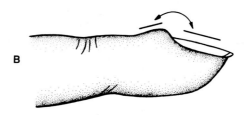
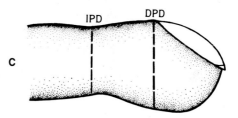

Fig. 16-21   A, Normal digit configuration. **B,** Mild digital clubbing with increased hyponychial angle. **C,** Severe digital clubbing; depth of finger at base of nail *(DPD)* is greater than depth of interpharyngeal joint *(IPD)* with clubbing.

hypoxemia produces pulmonary vasoconstriction, the right ventricle must work harder than normal whenever significant hypoxemia exists. This chronic work load on the right ventricle may result in right ventricular hypertrophy and poor venous blood flow to the heart. When the venous return to the right side of the heart is reduced, the peripheral blood vessels engorge, resulting in an accumulation of fluid in the subcutaneous tissues of the ankles, referred to as *pedal edema*. The ankles most often are affected, since they naturally are maintained in a gravity-dependent position throughout the day. The edematous tissues pit (indent) when pressed firmly with the fingertips. Pitting edema should be evaluated for the level of occurrence above the ankle in an effort to quantify the degree of right ventricular failure. For example, pitting edema occurring at a level well above the knee is more significant than pitting edema around the ankles only.

Capillary refill

Assessment of capillary refill is performed by pressing firmly for a brief period on the fingernail and identifying the speed at which the blood flow returns. When cardiac output is reduced and digital perfusion is poor, capillary refill is slow, taking several seconds to appear. In healthy individuals with good cardiac output and digital perfusion, capillary refill normally should take less than 3 seconds.

Peripheral skin temperature

When the heart does not circulate the blood at a sufficient rate, compensatory vasoconstriction occurs in the extremities to shunt blood toward the vital organs. The reduction in peripheral perfusion results in a loss of warmth in the extremities. Palpation of the patient's feet and hands may provide general information about perfusion. Cool extremities usually indicate inadequate perfusion.

Actual extremity temperature can be measured and compared with room temperature. The extremity should be at least 2°C warmer than room temperature (unless room temperature is equal to or greater than body temperature). When there is less than a 2°C difference, perfusion is reduced; an 0.5°C difference indicates that the patient has serious perfusion problems.

PHYSICAL SIGNS OF RESPIRATORY DISEASE

The techniques of physical examination provide an inexpensive and rapid method to identify important clinical abnormalities of the cardiopulmonary system. The initial evaluation of the patient with acute disease, requiring rapid assessment and treatment, should identify the adequacy of tissue oxygenation and pulmonary function with regard to ventilation and oxygenation.

Tissue oxygen availability is a function of cardiac output and the content of oxygen in the arterial blood. The most accurate assessment of arterial oxygenation is done through analysis of an arterial blood gas sample; however, in certain situations in which time is of the essence or when blood gases are not available, clinical signs and symptoms must be relied on. Clinical signs of acute hypoxemia include tachycardia, hypertension, tachypnea, cyanosis, restlessness, and confusion. Clinical signs of reduced cardiac output and poor tissue perfusion include hypotension, cool extremities with weak or absent pulse, poor capillary refill, semiconsciousness or coma, peripheral cyanosis, reduced urinary output, and tachycardia.

Chronic hypoxemia also may result in right ventricular hypertrophy and failure. This condition, referred to as cor pulmonale, is clinically evidenced by pedal edema, loud pulmonic valve closure, jugular venous distention, hepatomegaly, and a systolic heave at the lower left sternal border.

By itself, the physical examination usually cannot confirm a specific diagnosis, but it can suggest certain pathologic abnormalities of the lungs. When the physical findings are considered along with the history and the other diagnostic procedures discussed in this section, a more specific diagnosis can be supported. Table 16-5 summarizes the characteristic abnormal physical findings and possible causes of common pulmonary disorders. Rather than focusing on specific respiratory diseases, the following discussion emphasizes patterns of abnormalities.

Table 16-5 Physical Signs of Abnormal Pulmonary Pathology

Abnormality	Initial impression	Inspection	Palpation	Percussion	Auscultation	Possible causes
Acute airways obstruction	Appears acutely ill	Use of accessory muscles	Reduced expansion	Increased resonance	Expiratory wheezing	Asthma, bronchitis
Chronic airways obstruction	Appears chronically ill	Increased antero-posterior diameter, use of accessory muscles	Reduced expansion	Increased resonance	Diffuse reduction in breath sounds; early inspiratory crackles	Chronic bronchitis, emphysema
Consolidation	May appear acutely ill	Inspiratory lag	Increased fremitus	Dull note	Bronchial breath sounds; crackles	Pneumonia, tumor
Pneumothorax	May appear acutely ill	Unilateral expansion	Decreased fremitus	Increased resonance	Absent breath sounds	Rib fracture, open wound
Pleural effusion	May appear acutely ill	Unilateral expansion	Absent fremitus	Dull note	Absent breath sounds	Congestive heart failure
Local bronchial obstruction	Appears acutely ill	Unilateral expansion	Absent fremitus	Dull note	Absent breath sounds	Mucous plug
Diffuse interstitial fibrosis	Often normal	Rapid shallow breathing	Often normal; increased fremitus	Slight decrease in resonance	Late inspiratory crackles	Chronic exposure to inorganic dust
Acute upper airway obstruction	Appears acutely ill	Labored breathing	Often normal	Often normal	Inspiratory or expiratory stridor or both	Epiglottitis, croup, foreign body aspiration

Acute airways obstruction

Respiratory distress is usually apparent because of the observation of tachypnea, tachycardia, intercostal retraction in inspiration, and use of the accessory muscles. Paradoxical pulse may be present and usually indicates severe airway obstruction. Expiratory wheezes and rhonchi may be present but may diminish as bronchial obstruction improves or worsens. The lungs are hyperinflated diffusely, resulting in bilateral reduction in tactile and vocal fremitus, reduced vesicular-type breath sounds, and a mild to moderate increase in resonance with percussion. As bronchial obstruction resolves, the physical findings return to normal. Asthma, acute exacerbations of bronchitis, bronchiolitis, or foreign body aspiration may produce this clinical picture.

Chronic airways obstruction (Fig. 16-22)

At rest the patient may not appear in respiratory distress. The respiratory rate may be normal, but prolongation of the expiratory phase with pursed-lip breathing often is noted. An increase in the anteroposterior diameter of the chest, referred to as a barrel chest, is often noted. Large supraclavicular fossae may be present. The intercostal spaces retract with inspiration, and accessory muscles are used in an effort to lift the anterior chest wall during inspiration, resulting in a "clavicular lift" during inhalation. Breath sounds often are reduced markedly bilaterally and become absent in more severe cases. Adventitious lung sounds that may be identified include early inspiratory crackles, rhonchi, and wheezes. Tactile and vocal fremitus are reduced, and resonance with percussion is increased. The diaphragm is low, flat, and relatively immobile. Bilateral chest expansion is reduced significantly with quiet and deep breathing. In contrast to acute bronchial obstruction, the abnormalities do not resolve. Emphysema and chronic bronchitis may produce this type of clinical picture.

Consolidation (Fig. 16-23)

Consolidation of the lung parenchyma occurs when the alveoli fill with fluid and exudate as a result of a bacterial or viral pneumonia or when a parenchymal tumor develops. The patient usually appears acutely ill and febrile and breathes more rapidly than normal.

Examination of the chest may identify increased tactile and vocal fremitus, bronchial breath sounds, and a dull percussion note over the area(s) of consolidation. Bronchophony, egophony, and whispering pectoriloquy may be present. Inspiratory crackles may be identified, especially later in the progression of pneumonia as the consolidation resolves. Expansion of the affected side may be reduced.

Pneumothorax (Fig. 16-24)

Air in the pleural space may result in significant abnormalities, depending on the extent of the pneumothorax and underlying lung dysfunction. A small pneumothorax may go unnoticed; however, when lung compression is signifi-

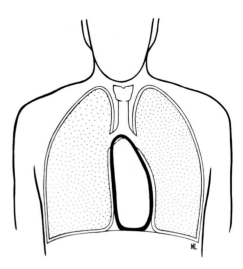
Fig. 16-22   Chronic pulmonary hyperinflation with low, flat diaphragm and small, narrow heart.

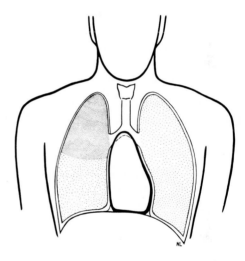
Fig. 16-23   Right upper lobe consolidation.

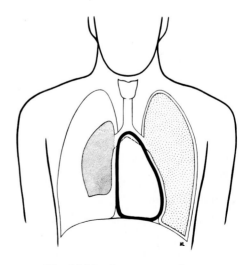
Fig. 16-24   Large pneumothorax.

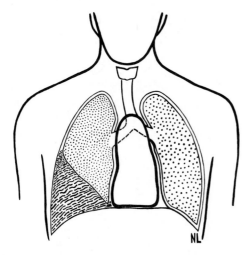

Fig. 16-25   Large pleural effusion.

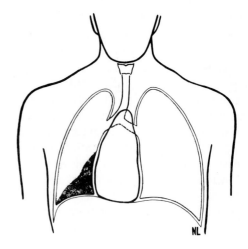

Fig. 16-26   Atelectasis of right lower lobe.

cant, the patient appears acutely short of breath. Over the pneumothorax, chest expansion is reduced, the percussion note is increased in resonance, breath sounds are absent, and tactile fremitus is absent. The trachea and mediastinal contents shift away from the affected side with tension in the pleural space as may occur in positive pressure breathing. If the pneumothorax is severe enough to disrupt cardiac function, blood pressure will decrease.

Pleural effusion (Fig. 16-25)

The patient with fluid in the pleural space may not appear ill, depending on the cause and size of the effusion. The trachea may be shifted toward the opposite side with larger pleural effusions. The percussion note is dull or flat, tactile fremitus is absent, and breath sounds are reduced or absent over the effusion. Near the upper limit of the effusion, bronchial breath sounds may be heard; this is caused by compression of the underlying lung.

Acute local bronchial obstruction with atelectasis (Fig. 16-26)

A sudden complete obstruction of a major bronchus may occur as the result of a mucus plug, bronchogenic carcinoma, or an aspirated foreign body. Distal to the obstructed bronchus, lung parenchyma collapses, resulting in a sudden loss of volume on the affected side. Consequently, the trachea and mediastinal contents shift toward the affected side. The shift may increase during inspiration and decrease with expiration. Over the affected area, chest expansion is reduced, percussion note is dull or flat, tactile fremitus is reduced or absent, and breath sounds are reduced or absent.

Diffuse interstitial fibrosis

The patient is usually in no acute distress at rest but has significant dyspnea on exertion. The respiratory pattern usually is rapid and shallow. Fine, late inspiratory crackles

are a common finding with auscultation; they are not influenced by body position or coughing. The percussion note is reduced slightly throughout all lung fields. In more severe chronic cases the signs of cor pulmonale may be evident.

Acute upper airway obstruction

The patient with an acute upper airway obstruction appears in acute distress with labored and often noisy breathing. The accessory muscles commonly are used during inhalation. With supraglottic obstruction, inspiratory time may be prolonged; subglottic obstruction usually prolongs expiratory time. Inspiratory stridor may be heard without a stethoscope. Breath sounds often are clear, but the sounds of upper airway obstruction may be transmitted to the peripheral chest, making it difficult to identify vesicular or other adventitious breath sounds. The lungs usually are normal to percussion and palpation. Since the patient is at risk, he or she should not be left alone, and assessment must be quick and accurate to allow proper treatment. Epiglottitis, foreign body aspiration, laryngospasm, or croup may produce these types of findings.

SUMMARY

Physical assessment of patients with disorders of the respiratory system provides important information that, combined with other clinical diagnostic and monitoring procedures, helps confirm the presence of certain pathophysiologic processes and provides a basis for selecting and altering therapeutic regimens.

By applying the methods of inspection, palpation, percussion, and auscultation, the respiratory care practitioner can differentiate among major patterns of cardiopulmonary dysfunction, recognize changes in patient status, and determine a patient's response to therapeutic intervention. Effective application of these skills thus enhances the practitioner's ability to individualize patient care, thereby increasing the likelihood of achieving the outcomes desired.

REFERENCES

1. Anderson CL, Chankar PS, and Scott JH: Physiological significance of sternomastoid muscle contraction in chronic obstructive pulmonary disease, Respir Care 25:937, 1980.
2. Williams TJ, Ahmand D, and Morgan WK: A clinical and roentgenographic correlation of diaphragmatic movement, Arch Intern Med 141:878, 1981.
3. Murphy RLH, Holford E, and Knowler W: Visual lung sound characterization by time-expanded waveform analysis, N Engl J Med 296:968, 1977.
4. Andrews JL and Badger TL: Lung sounds through the ages, JAMA 241:2625, 1979.
5. Report of the ACCP-ATS Joint Committee on Pulmonary Nomenclature, Chest 67:583, 1975.
6. Report of the ATS-ACCP Ad Hoc Subcommittee on Pulmonary Nomenclature, ATS News 3:5, 1977.
7. Report of the ATS-ACCP Ad Hoc Subcommittee on Pulmonary Nomenclature, ATS News 2:8, 1981.
8. Wilkins RL, Dexter JR, and Smith JR: Survey of adventitious lung sound terminology in case reports, Chest 85:523, 1984.
9. Forgacs P: The functional basis of pulmonary sounds, Chest 73:399, 1978.
10. Murphy RLH and Holford SK: Lung sounds, Basics RD 8: March 1980.
11. Donnerberg RL et al: Sounds transfer function of the congested canine lung, Br J Dis Chest 74:23, 1980.
12. Bohadana AB, Peslin R, and Uffholtz H: Breath sounds in the clinical assessment of airflow obstruction, Thorax 33:345, 1978.
13. Pardee NE et al: Combinations of four physical signs as indicators of ventilator abnormality in obstructive pulmonary syndromes, Chest 77:354, 1980.
14. Pardee NE, Martin CJ, and Morgan EH: A test of the practical value of estimating breath sound intensity, Chest 70:341, 1976.
15. Marini JJ et al: The significance of wheezing in chronic airflow obstruction, Am Rev Respir Dis 120:1069, 1979.
16. Forgacs P: Crackles and wheezes, Lancet 2:203, 1967.
17. Nath AR and Capel LH: Inspiratory crackles, early and late, Thorax 29:223, 1974.
18. Nath AR and Capel LH: Inspiratory crackles and mechanical events of breathing, Thorax 29:695, 1974.
19. Forgacs P: Lung sounds, Br J Dis Chest 63:1, 1969.
20. Thacker RE and Kraman SS: The prevalence of auscultatory crackles in subjects without lung disease, Chest 81:672, 1982.
21. Workum P et al: The prevalence and character of crackles (rales) in young women without significant lung disease, Am Rev Respir Dis 126:921, 1982.
22. Guarino JR: Auscultatory percussion of the chest, Lancet 2:1332, 1980.

BIBLIOGRAPHY

Bates B: Physical examination, ed 2, Philadelphia, 1983, JB Lippincott Co.

Cherniack RM, Cherniack L, and Naimark A: Respiration in health and disease, ed 3, Philadelphia, 1983, WB Saunders Co.

Forgacs P: Lung sounds, London, 1978, Bailliere Tindall.

Judge RD and Zuidema GD: Methods of clinical examination, ed 4, Boston, 1982, Little, Brown & Co.

Malasanos L et al: Health assessment, ed 3, St Louis, 1990, The CV Mosby Co.

Prior JA and Silberstein JS: Physical diagnosis: the history and examination of the patient, ed 6, St Louis, 1982, The CV Mosby Co.

Wilkins RL, Hodgkin JE, and Lopez B: Lung sounds: a practical guide, St Louis, 1988, The CV Mosby Co.

17

Basic Pulmonary Function Measurements

John W. Youtsey

The primary functions of the lung are oxygenation of mixed venous blood entering the pulmonary capillaries from the pulmonary arteries and removal of excess carbon dioxide before the blood returns to the heart via the pulmonary veins. The ability of the lungs to perform these functions depends on the integrity of the airways, the function of the diaphragm and thoracic muscles, the status of the cardiovascular system, and the condition of the lung tissues themselves.

Pulmonary function testing can provide valuable information concerning these important clinical variables, thereby assisting in the diagnosis and assessment of pulmonary disorders. A variety of tests are now available to help in the diagnosis and evaluation of respiratory disease. For the respiratory care practitioner, a working knowledge of these tests and the ability to interpret their findings is an essential prerequisite in the planning and implementation of effective patient care.

OBJECTIVES

This chapter provides an introduction to the key concepts and procedures underlying the clinical application of pulmonary function testing in respiratory care. After completion of this chapter, the reader should be able to:

1. Describe the general goals and identify specific uses for pulmonary function testing as a component of respiratory care;

2. Differentiate by definition among the various conventional tests of lung volumes, capacities, and flows;

3. Describe the clinical test methods commonly employed in the measurement of lung volumes, capacities, and flows;

4. Differentiate the clinical test methods used to obtain supplementary information regarding pulmonary function;

5. Apply pulmonary function data to distinguish among the major patterns of pulmonary disease.

KEY TERMS

Most terms used in this chapter are defined in context. The following terms are introduced without explicit definition but may be found in the text glossary:

consolidation	parenchyma
distensibility	plethysmography
effort-dependent	pneumotachometer
effort-independent	rehabilitation
elastance	reliability
equilibration	spirometer
fibrosis	tangent
kymograph	transducer
neoplasm	validity
nomogram	

GENERAL PRINCIPLES IN PULMONARY FUNCTION TESTING

A complete evaluation of pulmonary function requires multiple lung function studies. Such studies will measure lung volumes and capacities, flows, diffusion capacities, and the distribution of ventilation. With the use of a combination of these tests, a complete and quantitative picture of lung function can be developed.

Purposes of pulmonary function testing

A clinical approach to pulmonary function testing should emphasize the gathering of both diagnostic and therapeutic information. Too often pulmonary function tests are used merely to verify a suspected diagnosis. However, pulmonary function testing has both diagnostic and therapeutic roles.

General considerations or questions that should be addressed in the diagnostic and therapeutic aspects of pulmonary function testing and evaluation are delineated in Table 17-1. Specific purposes of assessing pulmonary function include the following:

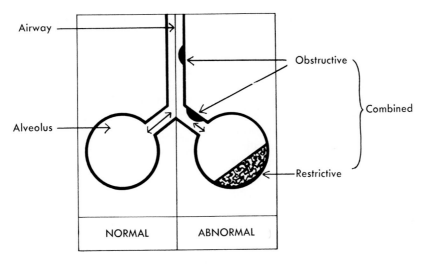

Fig. 17-1 Diagram of the physiologic aspects of pulmonary (lung) disease.

1. *To screen for pulmonary disease.* Screening programs can detect functional or mechanical lung change caused by disease in the general population and in individual workers or other high-risk groups.
2. *To evaluate surgical risk.* Preoperative evaluation can identify those patients who may have an increased risk of pulmonary complications after surgery.
3. *To assess disease progression.* Evaluation not only can help make or verify the initial diagnosis; it can also be used as an evaluation of disease progression or the reversibility of the disease.
4. *To assist in the determination of pulmonary disability.* Evaluation can also be used to determine the degree of disability caused by occupational lung diseases, such as anthracosilicosis (black lung disease). Such findings may be used to validate claims for financial compensation.
5. *To modify the therapeutic approach to patient care.* Evaluation may also be helpful in the selection or modification of a specific therapeutic approach to patient care, such as the response to certain drugs or the assessment of a rehabilitation exercise protocol.

Table 17-1 Basic Questions for Clinical Pulmonary Function Testing

Diagnostic	Therapeutic
Is lung disease present?	Is the disease reversible?
What type of lung disease?	To what degree is the disease reversible?
What degree of lung disease?	Is rehabilitation feasible?
Single or multiple diseases present?	Can rehabilitation be objectively evaluated?
Can multiple diseases be separated?	Can rehabilitation be subjectively evaluated?

Physiologic considerations

Pulmonary function testing provides the basis for classifying pulmonary diseases into three major physiologic categories: obstructive lung diseases, restrictive lung diseases, and combined lung diseases. Fig. 17-1 summarizes these physiologic considerations in pulmonary function testing.

Obstructive lung disease is characterized by decreased flows, especially on forced expiration. The primary factor in obstructive airway disease is an increase in airway resistance. This may be caused by bronchospasm, increased pulmonary secretions, and/or a breakdown of the structural support system of small airways (bronchioles). As a result, airflow is decreased. Pulmonary function parameters that signify obstructive disease processes include (1) increased airway resistance; (2) decreased forced expiratory flows; and (3) air trapping.

Restrictive lung disease is characterized by decreased lung volumes. The primary factor in restrictive lung disease is a decrease in compliance (distensibility). This can be a result of changes in the lung tissues (parenchyma), the chest wall, or both. This decrease in lung compliance is usually the result of lung inflammation, fibrotic lung disease, neoplasms, or thoracic wall abnormalities, such as kyphoscoliosis.

Neuromuscular diseases can also result in decreased lung volumes, mainly by affecting the function of the respiratory muscles. In these circumstances lung and thoracic compliance may be normal, but the patient is simply unable to generate sufficient pressure differences to take a full, deep breath.

Combined lung disease involves a decrease in both flows and volumes. For this reason, it is necessary to look at the relationships between both parameters, as measured and predicted.

Testing overview

Although arbitrary, pulmonary function testing can be divided into two categories: conventional and supplementary. The conventional or clinical spirometry division consists of the measurement of lung volumes and capacities and expiratory flows. Most hospitals are technically capable of providing these testing measurements. Furthermore, methods of clinical spirometry have been used for many years and are easily performed. For the majority of patient care situations, the conventional pulmonary function tests provide the essential clinically useful information.

Supplementary pulmonary function tests consist of the measurement of pulmonary compliance, diffusion, lung scans, closing volumes, flow volume curves and loops, and plethysmography. These tests are normally used in specific clinical situations, in pulmonary research, or where conventional testing has not adequately clarified the patient's status.

CONVENTIONAL PULMONARY FUNCTION TESTS

Conventional pulmonary function tests can be divided into two further categories: those measuring lung volumes and capacities and those measuring flow. Specific tests under each category provide the information necessary to differentiate the major categories of pulmonary disease.

Lung volume and capacity tests

The lung can be subdivided into separate volumes of gas. These volumes can be added together in various combinations called lung capacities. A lung capacity consists of two or more lung volumes. There are four lung volumes and four lung capacities (Fig. 17-2).

The majority of lung volumes are recorded and measured by means of simple spirometry; however, the residual volume and therefore the total lung capacity and the functional residual capacity cannot be measured directly during simple spirometry.

Definitions. Lung volumes and capacities recorded and measured through simple spirometry include the following:

tidal volume (V_T) the volume of air that is inhaled or exhaled from the lungs during quiet breathing.
inspiratory reserve volume (IRV) the maximum volume of air that can be inhaled following a normal quiet inspiration.
inspiratory capacity (IC) the maximum amount of gas that can be inhaled following a normal quiet exhalation. The inspiratory capacity is the sum of the tidal volume and the inspiratory reserve volume (IC = V_T + IRV).
expiratory reserve volume (ERV) the amount of gas that can be exhaled from the lung following a normal quiet exhalation.
vital capacity (VC) the maximum amount of gas that can be exhaled following a maximum inhalation of gas (or the maximum amount of gas that can be inhaled following a maximum exhalation). The vital capacity equals the sum of the inspiratory reserve volume, the tidal volume, and the expiratory reserve volume (VC = ERV + V_T + IRV).

Lung volumes and capacities that cannot be measured directly with the use of simple spirometry include the following:

residual volume (RV) the volume of gas remaining in the lungs after a complete exhalation.
functional residual capacity (FRC) the amount of gas left in the lungs following a normal quiet exhalation (also known as resting expiratory level). The functional residual capacity equals the sum of the residual volume and the expiratory reserve volume (FRC = RV + ERV).
total lung capacity (TLC) the maximum volume of gas in the lungs at the end of a maximum inhalation. The total lung capacity equals the sum of the vital capacity and the residual volume (TLC = VC + RV).

Clinical test procedures. Clinical test procedures vary according to the volume or capacity being measured. Some measurements can be accurately conducted at the bedside whereas others require specialized equipment found only in a pulmonary function laboratory.

Tidal volume. The V_T is easily measured directly from a simple spirogram (see Fig. 17-2). The patient is asked to breathe normally into a spirometer or other appropriate instrument that has either a kymograph or a similar recording device attached. For the purpose of test validity and standardization, the patient should be in a sitting position and a nose clip should be used. The patient breathes through a tight-fitting mouthpiece until a normal rhythm is established. It generally takes the patient 2 to 3 minutes to adjust to the nose clip and mouthpiece. Since the tidal volume will vary normally from breath to breath, an average V_T is a more reliable measurement. The total volume of air ($\dot{V}$) moved during either inhalation or exhalation for a period of time (usually 1 minute) should be measured. This total volume is then divided by the ventilatory rate (f). The following formula can be used to calculate the V_T:

$$V_T = \frac{\dot{V}}{f}$$

where f is the ventilatory rate or frequency and $\dot{V}$ is the volume of air inhaled or exhaled in a given time period (usually 1 minute).

The normal V_T is approximately 500 ml for the average healthy adult, with a range of about 100 ml. There is a great deal of variation in the normal population, and measurements beyond the normal range (400 to 600 ml) are not necessarily indicative of a disease process. Normal V_T values are often observed in both restrictive and obstructive lung diseases. Therefore the V_T alone is not a valid indicator of lung disease.

Inspiratory capacity. The IC is also measured directly from a spirogram. The patient is asked to breathe in maximally at the end of a normal exhalation. Fig. 17-2 demonstrates that the IC is composed of two lung volumes: the V_T and the IRV. The following formula demonstrates this relationship between lung volumes and capacities:

$$IC = V_T + IRV$$

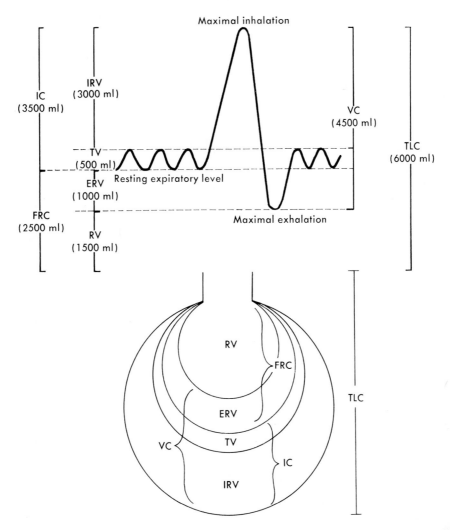

Fig. 17-2 Lung volumes and capacities. Representation of a normal spirogram and the divisions of lung volumes and capacities. Numbers shown are for comparison for an average sized, young adult.

The normal IC is approximately 3000 to 4000 ml, again with a significant variation in the normal population. The IC will represent around 75% to 80% of the VC and around 55% to 60% of the TLC. Like the V_T measurements, normal values can be observed in both obstructive and restrictive lung diseases. However, IC generally will be reduced in both restrictive and obstructive lung diseases. Increases usually mean that the patient was not truly at the resting expiratory level when the test was performed.

Inspiratory reserve volume. IRV, a component of the IC, is usually not measured during spirometry. Like both the V_T and the IC, it can be normal in both restrictive and obstructive diseases. It is not a significant clinical measure of lung mechanics.

Expiratory reserve volume. ERV is measured directly from the spirogram. The patient is asked to breathe normally for a few breaths and then exhale maximally. ERV is that volume of air exhaled between the resting expiratory level and the maximum exhalation level on the spirogram.

The normal ERV is approximately 1000 ml and represents around 20% to 25% of the VC. It can be either normal or reduced in obstructive and restrictive lung diseases.

Vital capacity. The VC is measured from the spirogram by the patient inhaling as deeply as possible and then exhaling fully, taking all the time necessary to exhale completely. A similar test, called the forced vital capacity (FVC), requires completion of the same maneuver; however, the patient must exhale as forcibly and quickly as possible.

The normal range for VC is 4000 to 5000 ml and represents approximately 80% of the TLC. Normal values can vary significantly, depending on age, sex, and test position. Weight is not a factor in predicting normal values. Because of this, various nomograms are available for pre-

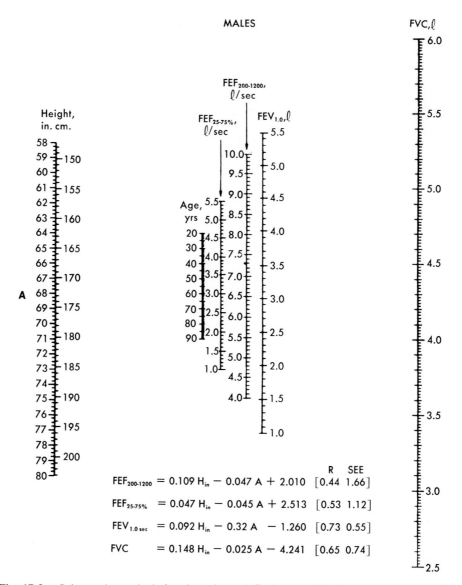

MALES

FEF$_{200-1200,}$ ℓ/sec

FEF$_{25-75\%,}$ ℓ/sec

FEV$_{1.0,}$ ℓ

FVC, ℓ

Height, in. cm.

Age, yrs

A

FEF$_{200-1200}$ = 0.109 H$_{in}$ − 0.047 A + 2.010   R   SEE   [0.44   1.66]

FEF$_{25-75\%}$ = 0.047 H$_{in}$ − 0.045 A + 2.513   [0.53   1.12]

FEV$_{1.0\,sec}$ = 0.092 H$_{in}$ − 0.32 A   − 1.260   [0.73   0.55]

FVC   = 0.148 H$_{in}$ − 0.025 A − 4.241   [0.65   0.74]

Fig. 17-3   Spirometric standards for, **A,** males and, **B,** females (BTPS). (From Morris JF, Koski WA, and Johnson LC: Am Rev Resp Dis 103(1):57, 1971.)

dicting normal values. Fig. 17-3 represents typical nomograms for predicting spirometric values for men and women.

A decrease in VC occurs in restrictive lung diseases. In early to moderate obstructive lung diseases, the VC may be normal or reduced. In severe obstructive lung diseases, the VC is generally reduced. A reduction can occur in two ways: (1) a reduction in TLC, which is observed in restrictive lung diseases, and/or (2) an increase in RV, which is observed in some types of obstructive lung disease.

An FVC will generally be significantly less than a normal VC in patients with obstructive lung disease. This is primarily a result of airway collapse during the forced expiration and the resultant air trapping (see Chapter 8). To be significant, the difference between the VC and the FVC should be greater than 10%.

Residual volume and functional residual capacity. Measurements of RV and FRC are important pulmonary function tests. Both are usually elevated in obstructive lung diseases. The normal RV is approximately 1500 ml and represents about 25% of the TLC.

RV, FRC, and TLC cannot be measured directly with simple spirometry. In fact, one must know the RV to measure the TLC and the FRC. Most indirect pulmonary function tests actually measure the FRC. By using the formula RV = FRC − ERV, the RV can be calculated. The three most commonly used methods for measurement of RV are (1) helium dilution, (2) nitrogen washout, and (3) body plethysmography.

Helium dilution test. The helium dilution test is also called the closed-circuit method. The principle is based on the dilution of helium in a closed-spirometer system. A

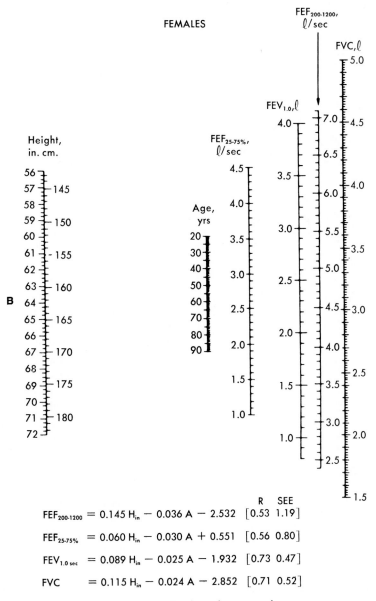

FEF$_{200-1200}$ = 0.145 H$_{in}$ − 0.036 A − 2.532 [0.53 1.19]

FEF$_{25-75\%}$ = 0.060 H$_{in}$ − 0.030 A + 0.551 [0.56 0.80]

FEV$_{1.0 sec}$ = 0.089 H$_{in}$ − 0.025 A − 1.932 [0.73 0.47]

FVC   = 0.115 H$_{in}$ − 0.024 A − 2.852 [0.71 0.52]

Fig. 17-3, cont'd   For legend see opposite page.

known volume and concentration of helium (He) is introduced into the spirometer system. Following a normal exhalation, the patient is connected to the system. While the patient is connected, carbon dioxide is eliminated through a carbon dioxide absorbent and oxygen is added at a rate equal to the oxygen consumption. The patient rebreathes the gas in the system until an equilibrium is reached. This usually takes less than 7 minutes; however, in patients with severe obstructive lung disease it can take up to 30 minutes for equilibrium of the helium between the patient and the spirometer system to occur (Fig. 17-4).

Two major calculations are necessary before the residual volume itself is calculated:

1. The volume in the spirometer system must be known:

$$V = \frac{He\ added\ (ml)}{\%\ He\ (first\ reading)}$$

2. The functional residual capacity must be calculated:

$$FRC = \frac{(He_1 - He_2)}{He_2} \times V \times BTPS\ correction\ factor$$

where FRC is the functional residual capacity; V is the volume in the spirometer system; He$_1$ is the initial concentration of helium before the patient is connected to the system; He$_2$ is the final equilibrated concentration of helium; and the BTPS correction factor is the constant used to convert volume to body temperature and pressure saturated. Once the FRC is known, the RV is calculated by subtracting the ERV from the FRC:

$$RV = FRC - ERV$$

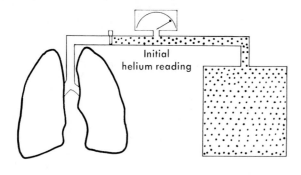

Initial
helium reading

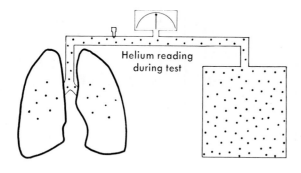

Helium reading
during test

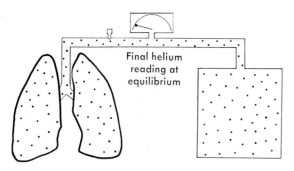

Final helium
reading at
equilibrium

Fig. 17-4   Indirect spirometric method for measuring the functional residual capacity and the residual volume. Helium dilution method.

The end expiratory level or FRC is a more reliable point from which to measure as compared to the RV, since starting the test at RV requires maximal expiratory effort by the patient.

Nitrogen washout test. Also called the open-circuit method, this test is based on the principle that the patient inhales pure oxygen from the spirometer system and washes the nitrogen from the lungs. It is assumed that the nitrogen concentration in the lungs is in equilibrium with the atmosphere (approximately 79%). The patient's exhaled gas is monitored and its volume and nitrogen percentages are measured. The patient breathes 100% oxygen for approximately 7 minutes, until complete washout occurs (Fig. 17-5). The test must be performed in a completely closed system since the leakage of room air would alter the measured nitrogen percentage. As in the helium

dilution test, the patient is connected to the system at the end expiratory level. In this manner, an accurate FRC can be reliably assessed.

The following formula is used to determine the FRC by the nitrogen washout method:

$$V_1N_1 = V_2N_2$$

or

$$V_1 = \frac{V_2N_2}{N_1}$$

where V_1 is FRC, the volume of gas in the lungs at end expiratory level; N_1 is nitrogen percentage in the lungs at the beginning of the test; V_2 is expired volume; and N_2 is nitrogen percentage in the spirometer at the end of the test. As before, the RV is determined by subtracting the ERV from the FRC.

Body plethysmography. The plethysmograph consists of a sealed chamber in which the patient sits (Fig. 17-6). Pressure transducers (electronic manometers) measure pressure both at the airway and in the chamber. An electronically controlled shutter allows the airway to be occluded periodically; thus airway pressure changes are measured under conditions of no airflow. According to Boyle's law ($k = V \times P$), volume changes in the thorax create volume changes in the chamber, which in turn are reflected by pressure changes in the chamber.

During the test, the patient is placed in the chamber, connected to the mouthpiece, and asked to breathe normally through the mouthpiece. At end inspiration and end expiration there is no airflow, and the alveolar pressure is equal to the airway pressure at that time. At a specific time (end expiration, for example) the shutter is occluded, and the various volume and pressure values are measured. As applied to the body plethysmography, Boyle's law ($k = V \times P$) can be rewritten as follows:

$$PV = (P + \Delta P)(V + \Delta V)$$

where P is the pressure in the lungs at end expiration (atmospheric); ΔP is the change in pressure produced by the respiratory efforts (as sensed by the airway pressure transducer); V is the volume of gas in the lungs at end expiration or FRC; and ΔV is the change in gas volume in the lungs produced by the respiratory efforts (as sensed by the box pressure transducer). By solving for V (the FRC), the equation can be rearranged as follows:

$$V \text{ (FRC)} = \frac{\Delta V}{\Delta P} (P + \Delta P)$$

Since ΔP is negligible as compared to P (atmospheric pressure), the equation can be rewritten to yield the following clinical simplification:

$$V \text{ (FRC)} = P \text{ (atmospheric pressure)} \times \frac{\Delta V}{\Delta P}$$

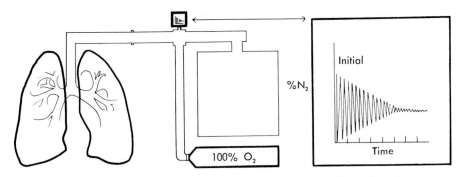

Fig. 17-5   Indirect spirometric method for measuring the functional residual capacity and residual volume. Nitrogen washout method.

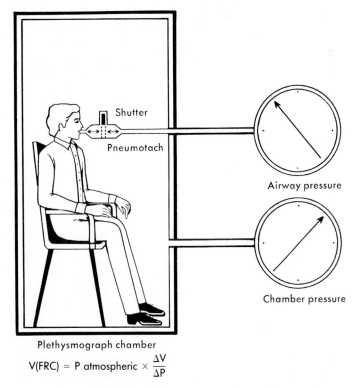

Plethysmograph chamber

$$V(FRC) = P \text{ atmospheric} \times \frac{\Delta V}{\Delta P}$$

Fig. 17-6   Body plethysmography method for measuring lung volumes. ΔV is the change in gas volume in the lungs, as sensed by the chamber pressure manometer. ΔP is the change in pressure produced by the respiratory efforts of breathing against the shutter, as sensed by the airway pressure manometer.

Because the body plethysmography method of FRC determination actually measures the total amount of gas in the thorax, the values obtained may be substantially larger than those that result from either helium dilution or nitrogen washout techniques. Such a difference would occur whenever there is gas in the thorax that is not in communication with the airways, as might be the case in pneumothorax and pneumomediastinum.

Total lung capacity.   TLC is the sum of the VC and the RV. Each can be measured as described previously. TLC is the only truly diagnostic single parameter in spirometry. It is always elevated in obstructive lung diseases and reduced in chronic restrictive lung diseases. Certain acute disorders, such as pulmonary edema, atelectasis, and consolidation, will also cause a reduction in TLC.

Interpretation of lung volumes and capacities.   When one is interpreting lung volumes and capacities, as well as all pulmonary function testing results, several factors should be considered:

1. Patient history. A patient history should include age,

sex, height, weight, weight gains or losses, and vital signs. A family history of pulmonary or cardiac diseases should be ascertained. The patient should be questioned concerning allergies, current medications, recent illnesses, and general information about the home and work environment.

2. Patient cooperation. All test procedures should be explained thoroughly before actual testing begins. It should be determined whether the patient is capable, either physically or mentally, of full cooperation. This is important in determination of the validity of certain test results.

3. Predicted values. Test results are usually reported in relation to normal predicted values. These values are based on the patient's age, sex, and height. Test results, however, should always be evaluated against the total patient picture.

In addition, the various lung volumes and capacities should be looked at collectively. Table 17-2 summarizes lung volume and capacity changes that occur in obstructive and restrictive lung diseases.

Tests of expiratory airflow volumes

The simple spirogram along with predicted average or normal values, can provide clues to detect respiratory disorders (restrictive, obstructive, or combined). With the exception of the TLC, which is diagnostic of disease, the other values alone do not provide sufficient information.

Tests that measure airflow volumes provide important information relating to the actual function of the lungs, the degree of impairment, and often the general location (large airways, small airways, etc) of the primary problem. To gather this additional information, tests that measure the actual pulmonary mechanisms are needed. Timed forced expiratory volume measurements (FEV_t) provide a great deal of information. Such tests measure the ability of the patient to maximally exhale and in the shortest period of time. FEV_t tests are recorded with spirometry equipment. In recent years the use of electronic instruments and computers has simplified the calculation of the various FEV_t tests.

Definitions. Conventional measures of airflow volumes include the following:

forced vital capacity (FVC) the maximum volume of gas the patient can exhale as forcefully and as quickly as possible. It will be less than the normal slow VC when airway collapse and air trapping are present. The FVC is usually measured in liters.

forced expiratory volume, half second ($FEV_{0.5}$) the maximum volume of gas a patient can exhale during the first half second during an FVC maneuver.

forced expiratory volume, 1 second (FEV_1) the maximum volume of gas a patient can exhale during the first second during an FVC maneuver.

forced expiratory volume, 3 seconds (FEV_3) the maximum volume of gas a patient can exhale during the first 3 seconds during an FVC maneuver.

forced expiratory volume percent (FEV%) the percentage of the *measured* FVC that a given FEV_t represents.

The following additional measures are not actually FEVs, but are included under this section because of their relationship to the other tests of expiratory airflow:

forced expiratory flow, 200-1200 ($FEF_{200-1200}$) a measure of the average expiratory flow during the early phase of exhalation. Specifically, it is a measure of the flow for 1 L of expired gas immediately following the first 200 ml of expired gas. Originally this test was called the maximum expiratory flow (MEFR). The test is recorded in liters per minute (L/min) or liters per second (L/s).

forced expiratory flow, 25%-75% (FEF_{25-75}) a measure of the average expiratory flow during the middle 50% phase of exhalation. The first quarter and the last quarter of the exhalation are ignored. The flow of the middle 50% is thus measured. The test is recorded in liters per minute or liters per second.

maximum voluntary ventilation (MVV) the maximum volume of gas a patient can move during 1 minute. Previously it was called the maximum breathing capacity (MBC). The results are expressed in liters per minute. The test is usually run for 10, 12, or 15 seconds and a value is calculated in liters per minute.

peak expiratory flow (PEF) the maximum flow at which a patient can exhale during a forced expiration. The test results are recorded in liters per second or liters per minute.

Clinical test procedures. Expiratory airflow volumes are generally measured and analyzed either manually or by computerized methods. Regardless of approach, those responsible for testing must be well versed in the principles underlying each analysis and the procedures for obtaining valid results.

Forced vital capacity. The FVC is easily measured with simple spirometry as well as electronic devices. The pa-

Table 17-2   Lung Volumes and Capacities in Pulmonary Disease

Test	Obstructive disease	Restrictive disease
Tidal volume (V_T)	Normal or elevated	Normal or reduced
Inspiratory capacity (IC)	Normal or reduced	Normal or reduced
Expiratory reserve volume (ERV)	Normal or reduced	Normal or reduced
Vital capacity (VC)	Normal or reduced	Reduced
Residual volume (RV)	Increased	Normal or reduced
Functional residual capacity (FRC)	Increased	Normal or reduced
Total lung capacity (TLC)	Increased	Reduced

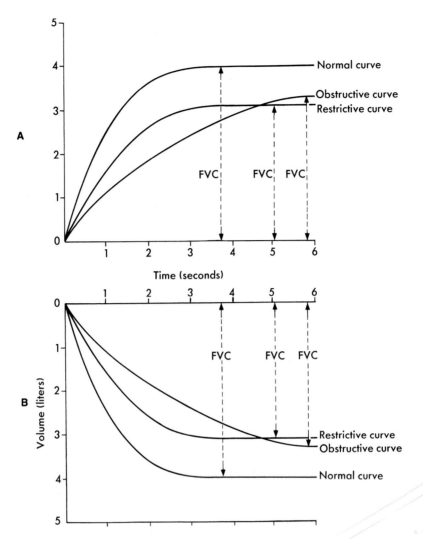

Fig. 17-7   Forced vital capacity curves comparing normal, obstructive ...d restrictive disorders. **A** shows curves as they appear on commonly available spirometer⁻ ...an tracings beginning at the bottom left corner. **B** shows same curves as they appear on so⁻ ..spirometers that begin tracings at upper left corner.

tient is asked to exhale as forcibly and as quickly as pos⁻ ble into the spirometer or pneumotachometer. The ; atient should breathe in maximally and exhale as qui⁻.ly as possible. It is necessary to coach the patien⁻ ⁻ achieve his or her maximum exhalation pos⁻⁻.⁻. The significance of this test has already b⁻⁻. uiscussed. Fig. 17-7 demonstrates FVCs from common spirometer tracings for the normal, obstructive, and restrictive states. The FVCs in both the obstructed and restricted curves are shown reduced below normal. The primary difference between the curve in the patient with restrictive disease as compared with the patient with obstructive disease is the slope of the curve.

Forced expiratory volume timed. The FEV during a specified time interval (0.5, 1, or 3 seconds) determines the maximum volume of gas that can be exhaled during the forced capacity maneuver in those time intervals. The patient is asked to perform an FVC maneuver as previ-

ously described. The spirometer drum moves at a preset speed. With the horizontal axis as the time interval, the exhaled volume can be measured directly from the spirometer for a specific time period (Fig. 17-8). The volume must be corrected to BTPS. The predicted values for the FEV_1 can be calculated directly from nomograms, as provided in Fig. 17-3.

It is more clinically valuable to look at the FEV_t as it is related to the patient's FVC. Therefore

$$FEV\% = \frac{FEV_t}{FVC} \times 100$$

Normal values for the FEV% are listed in Table 17-3. Patients with obstructive pulmonary disease will show a reduction in the FEV_t% whereas patients with restrictive disorders will generally show normal FEV_t% as compared

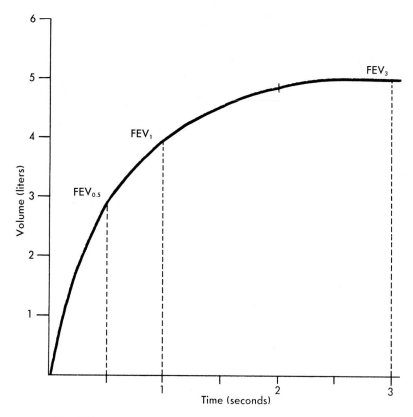

Fig. 17-8   Forced expiratory volumes for 0.5, 1, and 3 seconds.

with their measured FVC. If compared with normal prediction values, however, the FEV_t, expressed as a volume, will be reduced.

Forced expiratory flows, 200-1200 and 25%-75%. The $FEF_{200-1200}$ and FEF_{25-75} represent average flows that occur during specific intervals on the FVC curve. These flows were originally described as maximum expiratory flows; therefore the $FEF_{200-1200}$ was called the maximum expiratory flow (MEFR) and the FEF_{25-75} was called maximum midexpiratory flow (MMEF).

Both measurements can be made on a simple spirogram where a timed FVC is recorded. For the $FEF_{200-1200}$ test, the time interval is marked between the 200 ml point and the 1200 ml point. A straight line is drawn between these points, and the line is extended to intersect two 1-second

Table 17-3   Normal Clinical Ranges for Forced Expiratory Volumes Timed (FEV_t) as a Percentage of the FVC (FEV%)

Test (FEV%)	Normal clinical range*
$FEV_{0.5}$	50-70%
FEV_1	70-83%
FEV_2	84-93%
FEV_3	94-97%

*Decreases with age.

time lines (Fig. 17-9). The volume of air measured between the two time lines can be read from the spirogram and is recorded as a flow in liters per second. The volume measured must be corrected to BTPS.

The FEF_{25-75} is a measure of the flow during the middle portion of the FVC or the time necessary to exhale the middle 50%. The only limitation is that the first 25% and the last 25% of the FVC are ignored. A straight line is drawn between the points that represent 25% and 75%. Again, the line is extended through two 1-second lines, and the volume is measured and corrected to BTPS (Fig. 17-10).

Both the FEF_{25-75} and the $FEF_{200-1200}$ measure the average flow rate in a specific time period. The difference between the two depends on where, during the FVC curve, the measurement is made. The normal $FEF_{200-1200}$ is usually greater than 5 L/s (300 L/min). Since the test is done at initial high lung volumes (early forced expiration), it is a measure of the integrity and function of the large airways. This test is also a good indicator of patient effort. A reduced $FEF_{200-1200}$ will be observed in patients with significant obstructive lung disease and in many patients with severe restriction. The $FEF_{200-1200}$ is both independent of the FVC and most responsive to bronchodilator therapy.

The normal FEF_{25-75} is approximately 4 L/s (240 L/min). This test is a good measure of small or distal airway function. Since it measures lung function at lower lung

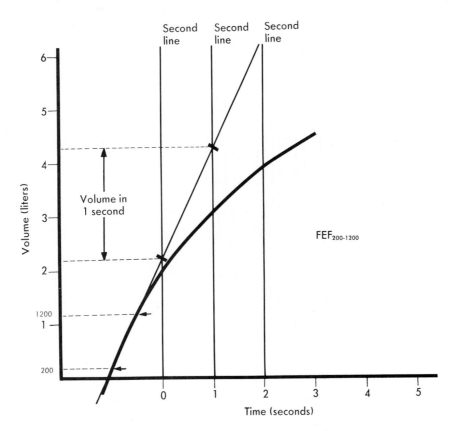

Fig. 17-9   Forced expiratory flow, 200-1200.

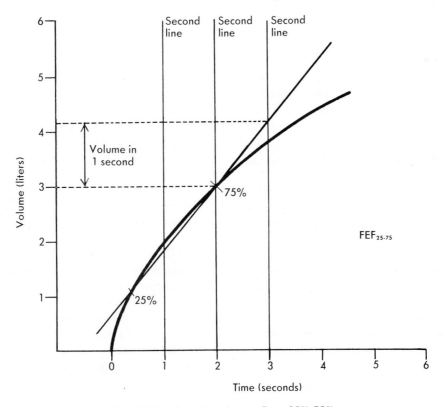

Fig. 17-10   Forced expiratory flow, 25%-75%.

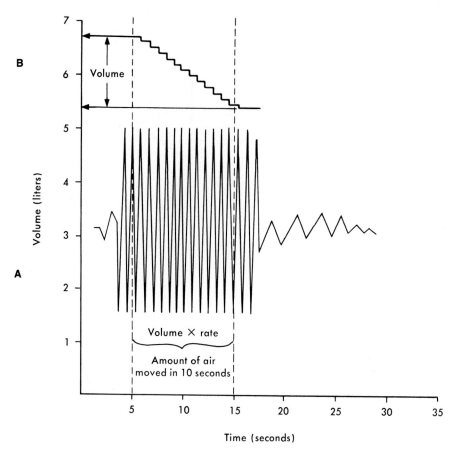

Fig. 17-11 Maximum voluntary ventilation tracing. **A,** Actual ventilations recorded during a 10-second period. **B,** Summation recording (addition of inspiratory volume) measured during the 10 seconds. Summation volume times correction factor (eg, 25 for Collins spirometer) equals actual volume.

volumes, it is relatively independent of patient effort. A reduced FEF_{25-75} will be observed in patients with obstructive lung disease. The test is also sensitive to the early changes that occur in the obstructive lung disease process. Because of this, the FEF_{25-75} may detect changes in the lung function that are not apparent from the $FEF_{200-1200}$.

Maximum voluntary ventilation. The maximum voluntary ventilation (MVV) test is an index of the integrity and function of the lung-thorax relationship. Test results reflect the influence of airway resistance, the status of the respiratory muscles, and the integrity of the lung parenchyma. This test is extremely dependent on patient effort.

The patient usually takes a standing position (with support, if necessary) and is instructed to breathe as rapidly and deeply as possible for 10, 12, or 15 seconds. The volumes are measured on a spirogram (Fig. 17-11) or electronically for the specific period of time. The volumes are then extrapolated to liters per minute. For example:

> Volume of air moved in 10 seconds: 30 L
> Correction factor to liters per minute: 60 s/10 = 6
> MVV = 30 × 6 = 180 L/min

The use of a ventilometer pen on many spirometers simplifies the measurement of the volume of gas moved in the specific time period. The ventilometer simply adds all inspiratory volumes in a period of time. Once corrected for the gear train reduction, it provides an easy way to measure the volume of gas moved (Fig. 17-11):

> Volume of air moved in 10 seconds: 1.2 L
> Correction factor to liters per minute: 60 s/10 = 6
> Gear reduction factor: 25
> MVV = 1.2 × 25 × 6 = 180 L/min

As with all volumes measured on a water-sealed spirometer, the recorded values are corrected to BTPS.

Predicted MVV values are based on sex, age, and body surface area. Normal values vary significantly (25% to 30%) in the population; therefore, only major reductions in the values are clinically significant. The MVV is greatly reduced in patients with moderate and severe airway obstruction. Generally, a measured value less than 75% of the predicted value is significant. The normal value for adult males is about 160 to 180 L/min; it is slightly lower in adult females. In restrictive lung disease the MVV value may be normal or only slightly reduced.

Peak expiratory flow. The peak expiratory flow (PEF) is the maximum flow that occurs at any point in time during the FVC. It is measured by means of a tangent drawn to the steepest portion of the FVC curve. Normal peak flows average 9 to 10 L/s. Because of such high flows, it is difficult to measure accurate peak flows from a spirogram. In this instance, the electronic measuring devices (pneumotachometers) are preferable because of their accuracy.

The reliability of PEF as a clinical tool for evaluation of lung mechanics is limited because of the initial high flows that can occur even in obstructive disorders. Decreased peak flows reflect nonspecific mechanical problems of the lung, patient cooperation, and effort. Table 17-4 summarizes spirometric values and airflow volume values in normal, obstructive, and restrictive states.

SUPPLEMENTARY PULMONARY FUNCTION TESTS

The pulmonary function tests discussed here are classified as supplementary because they do not constitute standard clinical spirometry. Supplementary testing provides the additional information sometimes necessary to better define a patient's pulmonary disease process.

Definitions

The following pulmonary function tests are used to provide additional information to help better define a patient's pulmonary disease process.

Table 17-4 Spirometric and Airflow Volume Measurements

Measurement	Normal*	Obstructive	Restrictive
V_T	500 ml	N ↑	N ↓
IVC	3500 ml	N ↓	N ↓
ERV	1000 ml	N ↓	N ↓
VC	4500 ml	N ↓	↓
FVC	4500 ml	N ↓	↓
RV	1500 ml	N ↑	N ↓
FRC	2500 ml	N ↑	N ↓
TLC	6000 ml	N ↑	↓
$FEV_{0.5}$	>50% FVC†	↓	N
FEV_1	>70% FVC†	↓	N
FEV_2	>83% FVC†	↓	N
FEV_3	>93% FVC†	↓	N
$FEF_{200-1200}$	>5 L/s (300 L/min)	↓	N ↓
FEF_{25-75}	>4 L/s (240 L/min)	↓	N ↓
MVV	160-180 L/min (±25%)	↓	N ↓
PEF	9-10 L/s	N ↓	N ↓

*Examples for young healthy male of average size.
†FVC = measured, *not* predicted.

airway resistance (Raw) the driving pressure necessary to move a volume of gas in a specific period of time. Mathematically, it is the ratio of the driving pressure to the flow and is expressed in centimeters of water per liter per second (cm H_2O/L/s).

compliance (C) a measure of the distensibility of the chest and/or lungs; that is, it is the volume change in the lung per unit of pressure change and is expressed in liters per centimeter of water (L/cm H_2O).

closing volume (CV) a measure of the volume of gas remaining in the lung when the small airways presumably begin to close during a controlled maximum exhalation.

closing capacity (CC) the sum of the closing volume and the residual volume (CC = CV + RV).

flow volume curve or loop the graphic relationship between flows and resultant volume during an FVC and subsequent forced inspiratory volume maneuver.

diffusing capacity of the lung (DL) the volume of a gas per minute that will transverse the alveolar-capillary membrane for a given partial pressure gradient.

ventilation and perfusion scans lung function studies in which radioactive materials are used to assess gas distribution and blood flow in the lungs.

Clinical test procedures

Airway resistance. The most common method for measurement of airway resistance is body plethysmography. Airway resistance is the ratio of the driving pressure to the airflow and can be represented with the following formula:

$$Raw = \frac{\Delta P}{\dot{V}}$$

Where Raw is airway resistance; ΔP is driving pressure; and $\dot{V}$ is airflow.

The driving pressure (ΔP) is equal to the airway pressure (P_{ao}) minus the alveolar pressure (P_{alv}). To measure the driving pressure, the body plethysmograph is used. The patient is placed in the sealed plethysmograph. Volume changes in the thorax will create volume changes in the chamber, which in turn are reflected by changes in the chamber pressure. During inspiration, the lung increases in size. This creates a subatmospheric pressure in the alveoli, and air moves into the lung because of the pressure gradient. At the same time, the increased size of the thorax is compressing the gas in the chamber, and a reciprocal increase in chamber pressure results (Boyle's law). During exhalation the opposite occurs. Recording the pressure in the plethysmograph (P_p) during this time provides a value for one variable in the formula used to calculate the airway resistance. In the absence of airflow, airway pressure at the mouth is equal to the alveolar pressure (P_{alv}). While the patient is breathing, an electronic shutter momentarily closes. This creates a no-flow situation, and the alveolar pressure can be determined. During this time, if one measures the airflow ($\dot{V}$) with a pneumotachometer, the airway resistance can be calculated by the following formula:

$$Raw = \frac{P_{alv}/P_p}{\dot{V}/P_p}$$

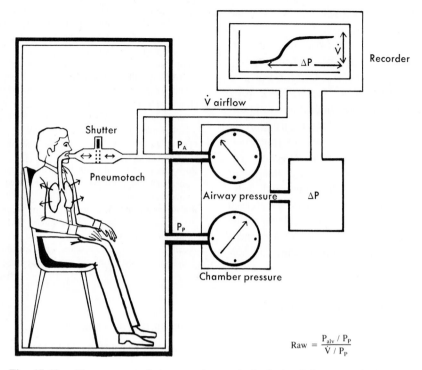

$$Raw = \frac{P_{alv} / P_P}{\dot{V} / P_P}$$

Fig. 17-12   Measurement of airway resistance in the body plethysmograph (see text).

where Raw is airway resistance; P_{alv} is alveolar pressure; P_p is plethysmograph pressure; and $\dot{V}$ is airflow. This formula actually describes the relationship between two sets of ratios: (1) changes in the alveolar pressure and pressure in the plethysmograph (P_{alv}/P_p) and (2) changes between flow and pressure in the plethysmograph ($\dot{V}/P_p$). For this test, the patient is usually instructed to pant at V_T of approximately 100 to 200 ml at high rates, usually greater than 100 breaths per minute. Panting reduces many of the artifacts that would otherwise interfere with the test results. Fig. 17-12 shows the technique for measuring airway resistance in the body plethysmograph.

Airway resistance is normally between 0.5 and 2.5 cm $H_2O/L/s$, measured at the standardized flow of 0.5 L/s. It is lower during inspiration and higher during exhalation. In addition, airway resistance decreases with increasing lung volumes, primarily because of the increasing airway caliber. Any factor that reduces the caliber of the airway will cause an increase in airway resistance. Such factors include edema, bronchial secretions, bronchoconstriction, and vascular congestion (inflammation). A loss of lung elastance (increased compliance) will also cause an increase in airway resistance because of the loss of parenchymal support surrounding the small airways. Therefore, disorders such as asthma, emphysema, and bronchitis will cause increases in airway resistance.

Compliance. Compliance is a measure of the distensibility of the lungs (C_L), the thorax (C_T), or both (C_{LT}). In essence, it measures the ease with which the lung volume

is changed. It is expressed in liters per centimeter of water (L/cm H_2O). Increased compliance means a greater increase in lung volume per centimeter of water pressure; likewise, a reduced compliance means a smaller change in lung volume per centimeter of water.

When one is determining the C_{LT}, it is necessary to know the transpulmonary pressure and the specific lung volumes at each pressure. In doing this, a pressure-volume curve is generated (Fig. 17-13). The transpulmonary pressure (P_L) is the difference between the intrapleural pressure (P_{pl}) and the alveolar pressure (P_{alv}): $P_L = P_{pl} - P_{alv}$. When compliance is measured under static conditions (static compliance), the alveolar pressure is equal to the atmospheric pressure (P_{atm}). In this case, the atmospheric pressure is assumed to be equal to zero by standard; therefore the transpulmonary pressure is equal to the intrapleural pressure: $P_L = P_{pl}$.

The formula for calculating static lung compliance (C_L) is

$$C_L = \frac{\Delta V}{\Delta P}$$

where ΔP is the pressure gradient or P_L. Since $P_L = P_{pl}$, $P_L = P_{pl}$. Therefore:

$$C_L = \frac{\Delta V}{\Delta P_{pl}}$$

For measurement of C_L, the patient is asked to swallow a balloon catheter. The catheter is positioned in the lower

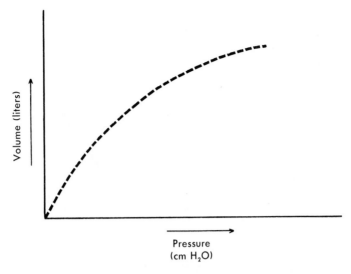

Fig. 17-13   Pressure-volume curve demonstrating compliance.

third of the esophagus and connected to a manometer for measurement of pressure. At this point, the esophageal pressure is equal to the intrapleural pressure. Pressure changes can be plotted against various lung volumes (Fig. 17-13). Normal C_L is approximately 0.2 L/cm H_2O.

The lung-thorax compliance (C_{LT}) can be measured with body plethysmography. By serial reduction of pressures within the chambers and measurement of the resulting changes in volume, a pressure-volume curve can be plotted. Normal C_{LT} is approximately 0.1 L/cm H_2O. Given these two values, thoracic compliance can be calculated as follows:

$$\frac{1}{C_T} = \frac{1}{C_{LT}} - \frac{1}{C_L}$$

$$\frac{1}{C_T} = \frac{1}{0.1} - \frac{1}{0.2 \text{ L/cm } H_2O}$$

$$C_{LT} = 0.2 \text{ L/cm } H_2O$$

The total C_{LT} is about one half of either the lung or thorax compliance alone. This is a result of the opposing forces of the lung and thorax.

When compliance measurements are made during the breathing cycle, dynamic compliance is measured. In the normal lung, the dynamic compliance (Cdyn) is equal to the lung compliance because of the opposing forces between the lungs and the thorax.

Changes in lung and chest wall compliance occur in several disease processes. C_L is most affected by bronchopulmonary diseases, whereas chest wall compliance is most affected by diseases of the thoracic nerves, joints, and muscles and by obesity. Restrictive lung diseases reduce C_L as a result of the stiffness of the lung tissue. In obstructive lung diseases such as pulmonary emphysema, the C_L is high because of destruction of the lung support tissues and parenchyma.

Closing volume. Closing volume (CV) measures the amount of gas that remains in the lung when the small airways presumably begin to close during exhalation. A modification of the single-breath nitrogen test is used to calculate this volume. CV is measured and often expressed as a ratio to VC (CV/VC). A second measurement often made is called the closing capacity (CC). CC is the sum of the closing volume and the residual volume (CC = CV + RV). CC is expressed as a ratio to the total lung capacity (CC/TLC).

The single-breath nitrogen washout procedure often used is also called the resident gas technique. The patient is allowed to sit quietly and breathe room air for several minutes. The patient then exhales completely to the RV level. At this point the patient is switched to a 100% oxygen gas source and inhales to the TLC. The patient then exhales slowly into a spirometer system, which measures the nitrogen content of the exhaled gas as well as exhaled volumes. Fig. 17-14 represents a typical recording for the single-breath nitrogen test to measure CV. As the patient exhales into the spirometer system, the larger airways (which now hold 100% oxygen) empty first, followed by the smaller distal airways. These airways tend to collapse in the basal regions of the lung, at which point the nitrogen percentage of the exhaled air rises abruptly. The volume expired after this rise is the CV (phase IV). The increase in nitrogen percentage results from the fact that when the basal airways close, exhaled gas will contain a large portion of alveolar gas from the apical lung regions (high nitrogen percentage).

Early obstructive airway disease, smoking, and increasing age increase the CV to more than the 15% to 20% of the VC found in normal young adults. The CV can also be increased in patients with moderate to severe restrictive disorders where the CV exceeds the FRC. The CC usually represents about 30% to 40% of the TLC in healthy adults. Unfortunately, the CV cannot be measured accurately in

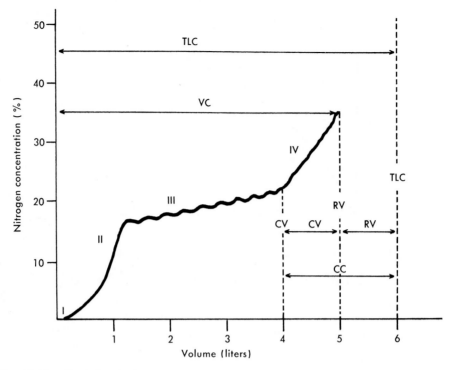

Fig. 17-14   Single-breath nitrogen test curve for measuring closing volume and capacity. *Phase I*, expired dead space gas; *phase II*, mixed dead space and alveolar gas; *phase III*, alveolar plateau; *phase IV*, airway closure.

the presence of disorders characterized by severe airway obstruction.

Flow volume loops. The flow volume loop or curve is not so much a new pulmonary function test as a different way of graphically representing the events that occur during forced inspiration and expiration. Rather than recording volume against time, the flow volume procedure simply records flow against volume.

Flow volume loops are made possible by simultaneous use of electronic flow and pressure transducers combined with an X-Y recorder. The patient is instructed to perform a forced expiratory vital capacity (FEVC) maneuver followed by a forced inspiratory vital capacity (FIVC) maneuver. The electronic transducers then measure flow and volume simultaneously (Fig. 17-15). The expiratory portion of the resulting graph—above the zero flow x-axis—is called the maximum expiratory flow volume curve (MEFV). The inspiratory portion of the graph—below the zero flow x-axis—is called the maximum inspiratory flow volume curve (MIFV).

The initial portion of the MEFV is effort dependent; however, after the first third of the expiratory curve, the curve is effort independent and reproducible. The effort-independent portion follows the peak expiratory flow and is altered in disease changes of both restriction and obstruction (Fig. 17-16).

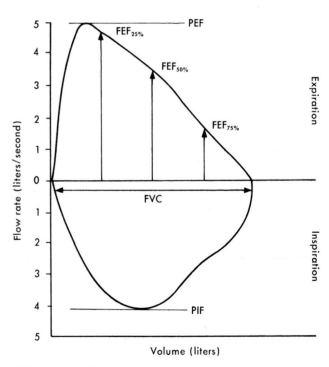

Fig. 17-15   Flow volume loop. *PEF*, Peak expiratory flow; *PIF*, peak inspiratory flow; *FEF%*, forced expiratory flow at x% of FVC; *FVC*, forced vital capacity.

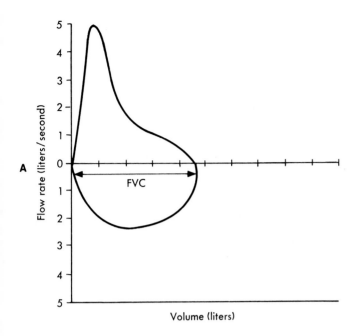

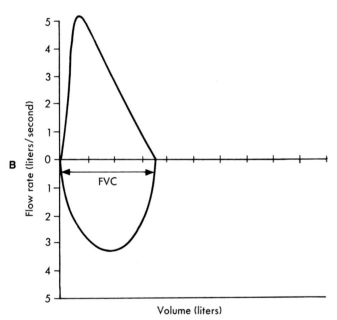

Fig. 17-16 Flow volume loops comparing, **A,** obstructive and, **B,** restrictive disorders.

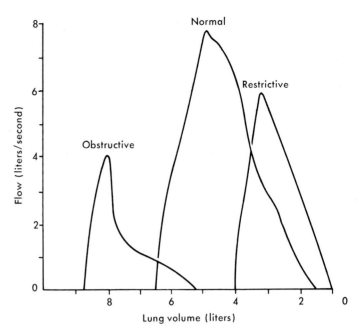

Fig. 17-17 Maximum expiratory flow volume curve example comparing normal with obstructive and restrictive disorders. Displayed as flows at actual lung volumes.

The predicted values for FVC, FEV_t, peak flow, and so on, are the same as with the conventional values. The expired flows increase rapidly to a peak and then decrease in a somewhat linear fashion.

Patients with obstructive lung disease show low flows. This is true in absolute terms as well as in percentage predicted. The inspiratory portion of the curve is more sensitive to central airway obstruction, whereas the expiratory portion of the curve is more sensitive to peripheral airway obstruction and restrictive disease processes. The restrictive lung disease processes will show near-normal peak ex-

piratory flow volume (FEV_t) when compared with the percentage of FVC (%FEV_t/FVC).

It is debatable whether maximum inspiratory/expiratory flow volume curves offer any diagnostic advantages over the FEV_t and FEF tests. The primary advantage is the graphic representation, which may promote an increased understanding of lung function and the related ease of superimposing measurements to evaluate bronchodilator therapy and progression of the disease process (Fig. 17-17).

Diffusing capacity of the lung (D_L). D_L provides a measure of the amount of functioning pulmonary capillary bed in contact with functioning alveoli. It is a clinical assessment tool for evaluation of the lung's gas exchange mechanism. This method of evaluating the movement of gas across the alveolar-capillary membrane into the pulmonary blood flow is more a measure of the integrity of the functional lung unit than of pulmonary mechanics. D_L is defined as the number of milliliters of a gas entering the pulmonary blood flow per minute for each millimeter of mercury of partial pressure difference between the alveoli and the pulmonary blood. D_L is expressed in millimeters per minute per millimeter of mercury. (ml/min/mm Hg).

The gas normally employed to measure D_L is carbon monoxide (CO). Carbon monoxide has a high affinity for hemoglobin and diffuses rapidly into the pulmonary blood flow. In fact, it has an affinity for hemoglobin nearly 210 times greater than that of oxygen. This high affinity keeps the capillary partial pressure of carbon monoxide low. As a result, its movement across the alveolar-capillary membrane is diffusion limited and not limited by a reduction in the Pco diffusion gradient. Clinically, a reduction in the diffusion of carbon monoxide will occur as a result of two major factors: (1) increased "thickness"* of the alveolar-capillary membrane and/or (2) decreased functional surface area available for diffusion. In addition, other factors should also be taken into consideration since these can also influence the DLco measurement:

1. $\dot{V}_A/\dot{Q}_c$ abnormalities;
2. Pa_{O_2};
3. Hemoglobin content;
4. Pulmonary capillary blood volume;
5. Pulmonary capillary blood flow.

The DLco is a measure of the transfer of carbon monoxide from the alveoli to the pulmonary blood flow and can be described by the following formula:

$$D_{LCO} = \frac{ml \ CO \ transferred/min}{A\text{-}a \ gradient \ of \ CO \ (mm \ Hg)}$$

Although several tests can be used to measure DL, the single-breath technique is most commonly used. The patient is required to inhale a deep breath of a 0.3% carbon monoxide and 10% helium gas mixture. The patient must inhale from the RV level, hold his or her breath for 10 seconds, and then exhale. The amount of carbon monoxide that diffuses into the patient's lungs is the difference in the concentration of carbon monoxide in the alveolar gas at the end of the 10-second interval and the beginning concentration. Normal diffusing capacity of carbon monoxide is about 25 to 30 ml/min/mm Hg. As stated before, several factors can alter the DLco above or below the normal value; such factors and their influence are summarized in Table 17-5.

Further study of the DLco and the relationship to alveolar volume (V_A) can provide interesting insights into gas exchange and pulmonary disease. For example, the DLco is usually reduced in pulmonary emphysema but not in chronic bronchitis. This is because of the loss of the alveolar-capillary bed that occurs in emphysema. In chronic bronchitis, the loss of lung parenchyma is minimal and does not alter the DLco.

Ventilation and perfusion scans. Various ventilation and perfusion studies ($\dot{V}/\dot{Q}$ scans) can be used to measure the gas distribution and pulmonary blood flow in the lungs. The radioxenon (^{133}Xe) method is used to measure regional distribution of ventilation. The patient performs the test in a supine or sitting position. The patient then inhales a normal V_T from a closed system containing a specific volume or concentration of ^{133}Xe. The patient holds his or her breath for a 10- to 20-second period of time,

during which photoscintigrams are made over the lung field (Fig. 17-18).

Serial photoscintigrams can also be made over a 10- to 15-minute period with the use of a rebreathing technique. This is helpful in determining the rate of equilibrium of gas in the lung. Finally, the patient may be returned to atmospheric breathing with serial photoscintigrams made to determine the washout of the ^{133}Xe.

Lung perfusion can be studied by means of microaggregated albumin particles tagged with radioactive iodine (^{131}I). The patient is injected with the iodine preparation, and serial photoscintigrams are made over the lung fields (Fig. 17-19) as the blood perfuses the lungs.

The $\dot{V}/\dot{Q}$ scans provide maximum information when used together. Scintillation counters can be used to quantify the $\dot{V}/\dot{Q}$ information. The information describes how the alveolar ventilation and pulmonary perfusion are matched in the patient. In the normal person, the $\dot{V}/\dot{Q}$ scans will show greater ventilation and perfusion in the bases of the lung and less ventilation and perfusion in the apices. The scans can identify areas of the lung that are not receiving ventilation and/or adequate perfusion.

GENERAL INTERPRETATION OF PULMONARY FUNCTION TESTS

When one is interpreting pulmonary function test results, it is imperative to relate the principle of the test to the normal physiology of the lung. For example, the FEF tests measure the maximum flows during a certain phase of the FVC maneuver. In essence, one is measuring how fast a gas is moving through a tube, or a series of tubes, during a specific time. Factors that would alter the flow of gas become critical to an understanding of how and why certain pulmonary disorders alter the results.

The FEF will always be reduced in significant obstructive disease processes and yet may be normal in many restrictive lung disorders, because those factors that nor-

---

*Whether actual thickening occurs is debated; however, the membrane does not transfer the gas normally, making it act as though it had an increased distance from one side to the other.

Table 17-5   Effect of Various Factors on the Diffusing Capacity of Carbon Monoxide

Factor	Diffusing capacity
↑ Hematocrit (↓)	↑ (↓)
↑ Pulmonary blood flow (↓)	↑ (↓)
↑ Exercise level	↑
↑ Alveolar volume (V_A)(↓)	↑ (↓)
Diffuse pulmonary fibrosis	↓
Emphysema	↓
Pulmonary embolism	↓
Pulmonary hypertension	↓
↑ Pa_{O_2}	↓
↑ Pa_{CO_2}	↑
Supine body position	↑

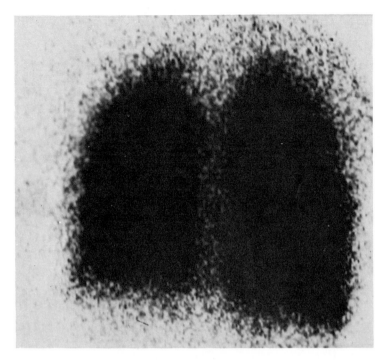

Fig. 17-18   Xenon 133 ventilation scan showing normal regional distribution of ventilation.

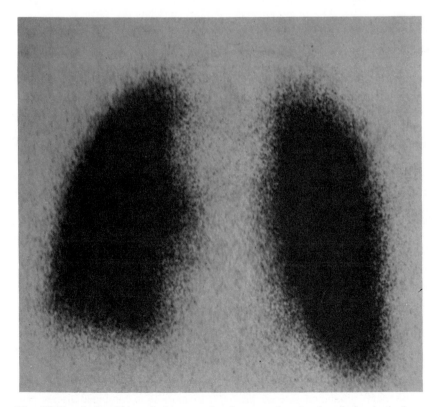

Fig. 17-19   Iodine 131 perfusion scan showing normal regional perfusion in the lung.

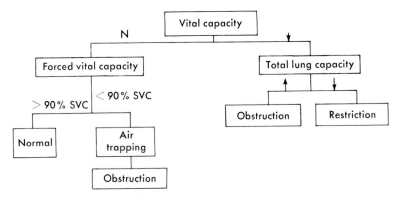

Fig. 17-20   Schema of lung volumes and capacities. N-Normal; $\downarrow$ = Decreased or less than normal; $\uparrow$ = increased or above normal.

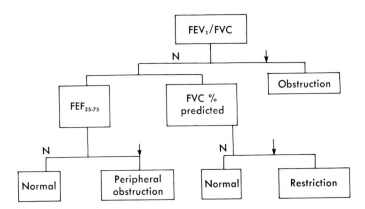

Fig. 17-21   Schema of forced expiratory volumes timed. N = Normal; $\downarrow$ = decreased or less than normal.

mally obstruct flow do not exist in many restrictive disorders. If the restrictive disease is severe, however, the patient may not be able to create sufficient force in the stiff lung to expel gas at a normal rate. Here the reduced FEF is not a result of obstruction but, rather, is caused by the restricted (stiff) lung. Unless one can determine why certain results are obtained, interpretation can become a confusing and frustrating process. Furthermore, one would not be able to evaluate the validity of the test results. The following section develops a logical format to provide an overall view of pulmonary function test interpretation and the reasoning process involved.

Lung volumes and capacities

In Fig. 17-20, the VC can be reduced in both restrictive and obstructive disease processes. Therefore, since the TLC is the differential diagnostic test, it is included. A normal VC does not rule out early obstructive processes; therefore the FVC will test for air trapping, which occurs in early airway disease. In this case, the VC, FVC, and TLC will establish either a normal lung or the primary disease process (obstruction, restriction). In addition, depending on the degree of alteration, combined disease processes can be present.

Forced expiratory volumes timed

The FEV_t helps measure the degree or severity of the lung malfunction caused by the underlying pulmonary disease. FEV_t describes the severity of obstructive defects whereas the VC, FVC, TLC, and DLCO measure the severity of restrictive processes.

In Fig. 17-21, a normal FEV_1/FVC ratio does not rule out either an early or a mild airway obstruction, whereas a decreased ratio does identify an obstructive process. The degree of obstruction depends on the percentage of FVC the FEV_1 measures. The FEF_{25-75} is specific for the middle to small (peripheral) airways; therefore reduction in the FEF_{25-75} when the FEV_1/FVC is normal signifies peripheral airway obstruction and disease. Remember that in restrictive disorders the FEV_t values often are within normal range; therefore the FVC percentage predicted becomes an important indicator. A normal FEV_1/FVC will usually rule out significant airway and large airway obstruction but not early airway disease or mild peripheral airway obstruction. In pulmonary function test interpretation the disease process is relatively easy to classify as primarily obstructive or restrictive. However, the role of each disease is difficult to appraise in combined disease processes. For this reason, the TLC, expressed as a percentage of predicted (TLC%

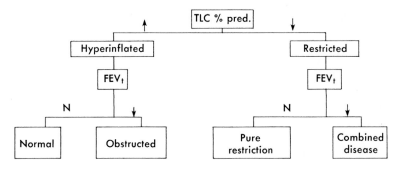

Fig. 17-22   Schema of total lung capacity as percent of predicted. N = Normal; $\downarrow$ = decreased or less than normal; $\uparrow$ = increased or above normal.

pred), is probably the most clinically powerful measure in pulmonary function testing.

In Fig. 17-22, the decreased TLC% pred identified the primary problem as restrictive but did not rule out an obstructive component. When the decreased TLC% pred and the decreased FEV_t are put together, an interpretation of a combined disease process is apparent.

SUMMARY

Pulmonary function testing provides valuable information on the mechanical and physiologic characteristics of the lung in health and disease. The use of conventional and supplementary tests of lung function can aid in the diagnosis of disease patterns and in the assessment of the need for and results of various therapeutic interventions.

Respiratory care practitioners can and must incorporate the results of pulmonary function testing into the planning, implementation, and evaluation of the care they provide to patients. Only in this manner can rational decisions be made regarding the status of the patient, the selection of appropriate therapy, and the objective evaluation of therapeutic outcomes.

BIBLIOGRAPHY

Ayers LN et al: A guide to the interpretation of pulmonary function tests, ed 2, Upper Montclair, NJ, 1978, Projects in Health, Inc.

Bates DV, Macklem PT, and Christie RV: Respiratory function in disease, ed 2, Philadelphia, 1971, WB Saunders Co.

Blair HT: Clinical indications and usefulness of pulmonary function testing, Medical Grand Rounds, Baylor College of Medicine, August 1975.

Cotes JE: Lung function: assessment and application in medicine, ed 4, Oxford, England, 1979, Blackwell Scientific Publications.

Craig DB et al: Closing volume and its relationship to gas exchange in seated and supine positions, J Appl Physiol 31:717, 1971.

Fishman A, editor: Assessment of pulmonary function, New York, 1980, McGraw-Hill Book Co.

Foster RE, Dubois AB, Briscoe WA, and Fisher AB: The lung: physiologic basis of pulmonary function tests, ed 3, Chicago, 1986, Year Book Medical Publishers.

Hunsinger DL et al: Respiratory technology: a procedure manual, ed 2, Reston, Va, 1976, Reston Publishing Co, Inc.

Morris JF et al: Prediction nomogram (BTPS), spirometric values in normal males and females, Am Rev Respir Dis 103:57, 1971.

Petty TL: Pulmonary diagnostic techniques, Philadelphia, 1975, Lea & Febiger.

Rarey KP and Youtsey JW: Respiratory patient care, Englewood Cliffs, NJ, 1981, Prentice-Hall, Inc.

Ruppel G: Manual of pulmonary function testing, ed 3, St Louis, 1982, The CV Mosby Co.

Seaton AN et al: Lung perfusion scanning in coal workers pneumoconiosis, Am Rev Respir Dis 103:338-348, 1971.

Slonim NB Hamilton LH: Respiratory physiology, ed 4, St Louis, 1981, The CV Mosby Co.

West JB: Pulmonary pathophysiology: the essentials, ed 3, Baltimore, 1985, Williams & Wilkins Co.

Wilson AF, editor: Pulmonary function testing: indications and interpretations, New York, 1985, Grune & Stratton, Inc.

18

Systematic Analysis of the Chest Radiograph

Richard L. Sheldon
Richard D. Dunbar

It is impossible to write a comprehensive discussion of chest radiology in one chapter. Entire lifetimes have been spent developing techniques, accumulating experience, and developing a sixth sense that would lead an experienced chest radiologist to identify an abnormal finding on an x-ray film of the chest. This chapter is not intended to make an expert radiologist of the practitioner, but it is worthwhile for the practitioner to recognize some of the basic areas of normality and abnormality. All the abnormal chest findings cannot be covered in one brief chapter, so it is our intent to introduce a systematic approach to reading the chest radiograph that will allow practitioners to develop a framework on which to build and refine their understanding of this important diagnostic tool.

achalasis	mesothelioma
anomaly	metastasis
asbestosis	pectus carinatum
benign	pectus excavatum
coccidiomycosis	pneumomediastinum
consolidation	pulmonary alveolar proteinosis
coarctation of the aorta	pulmonary hemosiderosis
fibrosis	sarcoidosis
Goodpasture's syndrome	scleroderma
hiatal hernia	situs inversus
histoplasmosis	subphrenic
infiltrate	tetralogy of Fallot
lordotic	tracheobronchomegaly

OBJECTIVES

After completion of this chapter, the reader will be able to:

1. Describe the technical basis by which an x-ray image is produced;
2. Differentiate the standard positions used for chest radiographs;
3. Describe the effect of tissue density on x-ray penetration and image projection;
4. Define the key characteristics of a normal chest radiograph;
5. Ascertain the presence of selected abnormalities on a chest radiograph and their clinical significance.

KEY TERMS

Most terms used in this chapter are defined in context. The following terms are introduced without explicit definition but may be found in the text glossary:

FUNDAMENTALS OF RADIOGRAPHY

X-rays are electromagnetic waves that radiate from a tube through which an electrical current has been passed. The tube is made of a cathode, which is attached to a low-voltage electron source called a transformer. The end of the cathode wire is inside the vacuum-sealed tube, and as the electrons flow through the wire they are "boiled off," accelerate across a short gap, and strike a positively charged tungsten plate called the anode. The electrons coming off the cathode wire are focused so that they hit a very small area on the anode. This area is called the "target" (Fig. 18-1).

When the electrons strike the target, physical changes occur, which result in the emission of x-rays. These rays are emitted in all directions but, because of the construction of the tube, only a few are allowed to escape through the window and are actually used. The rest are absorbed harmlessly into the wall of the x-ray machine.

X-rays are not reflected back like light rays but penetrate matter, and their ability to penetrate matter depends

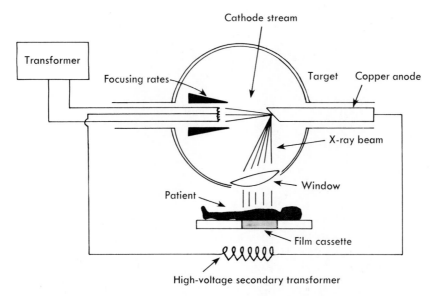

Fig. 18-1   The electrical current is generated by the transformer, *A*, passes through the focusing plates, *B*, and arrives at the cathode. The electrons are "boiled off," making a cathode stream, *C*. They then strike the anode target, *D*, and are transformed into "x-rays," *E*. The x-rays leave the sealed vacuum x-ray tube through a window, *F*, and strike the patient, *G*, pass through the patient, and cast a shadow on the film cassette, *H*, making an "x-ray picture."

on the density of the matter. Very dense objects such as bone will absorb (not allow penetration) more x-rays than air-filled objects such as lung tissue. The four main objects shown in chest radiographs are bone, air, soft tissue, and fat.

If a sheet of film is placed on the side of the patient opposite where the x-ray tube is located, the x-rays passing through the patient will be absorbed by some objects and "cast a shadow" on the film. X-rays that pass through the low-density (air-filled) objects strike the film full force and create a black image. X-rays that strike bone are partially absorbed, and less darkening of the corresponding area on the x-ray film is seen. This area is relatively unchanged and is seen as white on the film.

The standard chest film is taken in two directions. First, with the patient standing upright with his or her back to the x-ray tube, the chest is pressed against a metal cassette containing the film, and the arms are positioned out of the way. The x-ray beam leaves the tube and first strikes the patient's back (posterior), moves through the chest, exits through the front (anterior), and then strikes the film. Since the beam moves in a posterior-to-anterior direction, this is called a PA view. The patient is then turned sideways, and a lateral or side view is obtained. Thus two films—a PA and a lateral film—are routinely taken.

Other views are sometimes obtained when special problems are identified. If the patient is in an intensive care unit and cannot be moved, the film is placed in the bed, behind the patient's back, and the x-ray tube is positioned in front. Since the x-rays are moving from anterior to posterior, this is called an AP portable view. Oblique views

are taken, left and right lateral decubitus, with the patient lying on the right or left side to see if free fluid (pleural effusion or blood) is present in the chest. Also, an apical lordotic view is sometimes requested if it is necessary to look at the right middle lobe or the top (apical region) of the lung.

If an area of the lung consolidates because of pneumonia, tumor, obstruction, or collapse, it will show as a white patch on the film. Cavities will look like black holes. Diffuse patterns (interstitial markings) will appear fine and lacelike in the lung tissue.

Some densities that appear on the film are normal (eg, the heart and the lymph nodes). When they become abnormal they change shape, and, by developing a clear understanding of how the normal structure looks, one can make an accurate diagnosis of the disease process by observing how the shape of the structure is altered.

One of the most important of the x-ray technician's jobs is to make sure the patient is not rotated or turned. Even a slight rotation will distort normal structures to make them appear falsely abnormal.

SYSTEMATIC INTERPRETATION OF THE CHEST X-RAY FILM

Now we take a step-by-step approach to chest radiographs, thus forcing the practitioner to concentrate on certain areas of the film rather than letting his or her eye scan it in a random manner. Many of the findings on chest x-ray films are subtle and require the ability to collect many pieces of information that may suggest where the abnor-

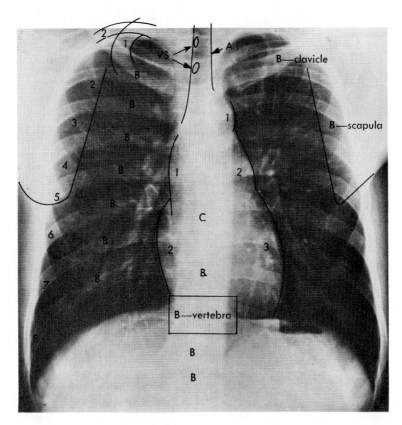

Fig. 18-2   *A,* Airways. Do the vertebral spinous processes seen end on *(VS)* go down the middle of the air column? In this case they do not. This patient is rotated slightly. *B,* Bones. Ribs numbered 1 through 8 on the right side where they swing anteriorly. Clavicles, scapula, and vertebrae are in the *B* category also. *C,* Cor. Cardiac shadow: *(right side) 1,* superior vena cava, *2,* right atrium; *(left side) 1,* aortic arch, *2,* pulmonary artery segment, *3,* left ventricle.

mality can be found. Even though the practitioner may be unable to identify what the abnormality is, attention can be directed to the fact that something is wrong with the film, and more expert help can be sought in delineating the precise nature of this problem.

We introduce here a systematic approach in which the alphabet is used to make the practitioner concentrate on specific areas of the film as suggested by the subsequent letters of the alphabet. This will ensure a thorough inspection of the film.

A: Airways (Figs. 18-2, 18-4, and 18-10)

Is the trachea midline? Do the vertebral spines go right through the middle of the tracheal air column? If not, the film has been rotated or the trachea may have been deviated to one side or the other because of fibrosis drawing it to one side, loss of volume in one lung drawing it to one side, or hyperinflation on one side forcing it to the opposite side.

Is the trachea the same width as the vertebral column? If not, tracheobronchomegaly, also known as Mounier-Kuhn syndrome, may be present. This is a rare disorder. Is the trachea buckling to the side opposite the aortic arch? This

is a common, normal finding. Are the larger bronchi, especially those just distal to the main carina or at the openings to the lobes, tapering? This may suggest the presence of a bronchogenic carcinoma invading carinal lymph nodes, which, in turn, are compressing the main bronchi.

B: Bones (Figs. 18-2 and 18-5)

The ribs should be an equal distance apart. If the space between the ribs is narrowed on one side more than on the other, this may suggest loss of muscle tone, as in a patient who has a paralysis involving that side of the chest. Notching of the ribs can be a significant finding that should be carefully examined. Bilateral notching of the superior aspect of the first rib is suggestive of scleroderma or rheumatoid arthritis (Fig. 18-15). Inferior notching of the third through the ninth ribs suggests coarctation (narrowing) of the aorta. Tetralogy of Fallot may cause inferior rib notching on the left side only. The ribs can be inspected for cough fractures, which may be seen on the sixth through the ninth ribs, usually the seventh in the posterior axillary line. Such anomalies as bifid ribs can be seen. These usually have no clinical significance. Pectus carinatum (pigeon breast) is associated with congenital atrial and ventricular septal defects or asthma from early childhood. The spine should also be inspected for such conditions as kyphoscoliosis, which, if severe enough, will result in loss of pulmonary volume and subsequently hypoventilation. Demineralization of the bones (washed-out bones on the x-ray film) may be seen with steroid therapy, aging, renal disease, or other metabolic diseases.

C: Cor (Figs. 18-2, 18-7, 18-18, 18-10, and 18-12)

The right border of the heart is composed of two bulges that should always be seen. Their obliteration may represent pectus excavatum, as suggested in the previous section. The bulges will be blurred or absent in the presence of right middle lobe collapse, pneumothorax (Fig. 18-12), or pneumonia involving the portion of the lung that comes in contact with the heart. Loss of superior bulge may be seen with an abnormal aortic arch.

The left border of the heart is composed of three bulges: the most superior is the aorta, followed by the main pulmonary artery segment, and then the most inferior of the three, the left ventricle. Pneumonias located next to these bulges will obliterate the edges of the bulges; this can be helpful in identifying the presence of pneumonia. There are multiple congenital cardiac lesions that will appear as abnormal cardiac shapes, and they will not be dealt with in this chapter.

If the width of the heart is greater than one half the distance across the lungs at the level of the diaphragms on the PA projection, the cardiothoracic (C/T) ratio is increased, and the heart is considered enlarged, usually from congestive heart failure. Other heart problems can also cause the heart to enlarge.

D: Diaphragm (Figs. 18-3, 18-8, 18-11, and 18-15)

The right side of the diaphragm is usually about one half a rib interspace higher than the left side. Scalloping can appear on the right side. This occurs in approximately 5% of all cases and is of no clinical significance (Fig. 18-3). One diaphragm may be elevated above the normal limits, in which case the following should be kept in mind: thoracic tumor with resultant paralysis of the phrenic nerve (Fig. 18-8); old surgery to the chest, which will result in fibrosis; scarring of the pleura and subsequent entrapment of the diaphragm and elevation. Subphrenic abscess will usually result in elevation of the right posterior portion of the diaphragm. This can best be identified from a lateral view. Some rare causes of hemidiaphragm elevation include trauma (Erb's paralysis), stroke, tumor or infection in the neck or cervical spine, pneumonia, and radiation therapy.

An interesting anomaly of the diaphragm is the accessory diaphragm, usually on the right side and associated with scimitar syndrome, a congenital cardiac defect composed of both heart and lung malformations. The accessory diaphragm is usually oriented upward and backward to the posterior wall and has a lower lobe between it and the true diaphragm.

E: Esophagus (Fig. 18-4)

The esophagus will be located behind the trachea. An air-fluid level would suggest certain disorders such as achalasia or stricture.

F: Fissures (Figs. 18-5, 18-6, 18-8, and 18-9)

The fissure lines divide the lung into various lobes. The two long (major) fissures or the oblique fissures (one each for the right and left lungs) are best seen on the lateral-view x-ray film. The inferior end of these fissures never runs into the anterior chest wall but ends in the diaphragm. Sometimes it is important to know which fissure is for the right lung and which is for the left. They usually run with the sixth rib, and on the lateral view the right fissure ends in the higher of the two sides of the diaphragm. The left fissure can be identified as the one that ends in the portion of the diaphragm that has a stomach bubble under it. If the stomach bubble is not well seen, this may cause some confusion. The heart will usually obliterate the anterior part of the left side of the diaphragm.

The short fissure, also called the minor or horizontal fissure, is seen on the right. It is absent in approximately 20% of normal chest radiographic films. Approximately one half of the normal films show a short fissure, and it is rarely seen projecting all the way across the right lung (Figs. 18-5 and 18-6).

The azygos lobe (Fig. 18-11) is visible in about 0.4% of normal chests. This fissure is distinctive in its appearance. It is almost always seen on the right, but left azygos lobes caused by an accessory hemiazygos vein have been identified. The azygos lobe is evidence of a pleural reflection from the azygos vein, which has descended during the embryologic period into its proper resting position, bringing with it a piece of pleura that remains radiographically evident. It looks like an upside-down comma.

There is also a superior accessory lobe, which is found in about 5% of the normal films and is seen below the horizontal fissure on the right. It separates the superior segment of the right lower lobe from the rest of the lobe. Inferior accessory lobes also occur in about 5% of normal films, and these separate the medial basilar segment of the right lower lobe from the rest of the right lower lobe. It therefore runs obliquely from the right border of the heart. The left minor fissure occurs rarely and represents a separate minor fissure.

G: Gastric bubble (Fig. 18-5)

It is important to make sure that the gastric bubble, if present, is seen on the left. If it is found on the right, mislabeling of the chest radiograph should be suspected, or the patient may have situs inversus. If the gastric bubble is absent, the possibility of achalasia should be considered.

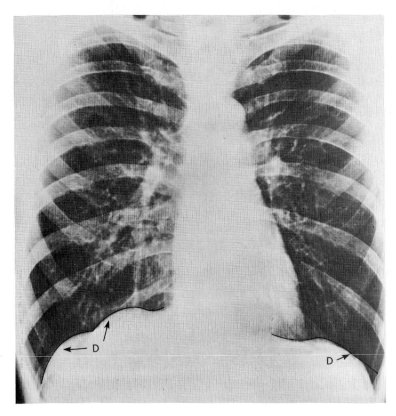

Fig. 18-3 *D*, Diaphragm. This example shows scalloping on the right, with the right side higher than the left. This is normal.

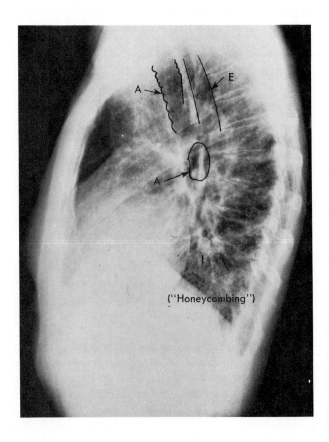

Fig. 18-4 *A*, Airway. This is the lateral view of the trachea and the right and left main stem bronchi. *E*, Esophagus. Its proper position is behind the trachea. The vertical lines seen in this area are the scapulae on end. *I*, Interstitial markings are increased with a big esophagus. The increased markings are due in this case to scleroderma. Note the "honeycombed" appearance of the lung markings.

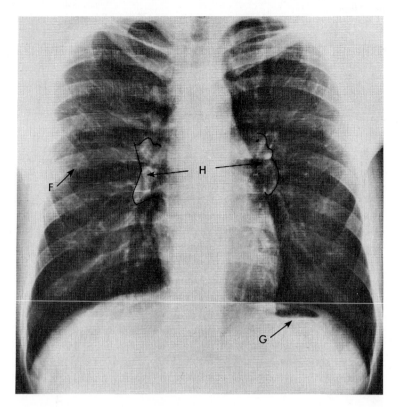

Fig. 18-5 *F,* The horizontal fissure line or "short" fissure is shown on the right. *G,* Gastric bubble. Note the thickness of the left diaphragm above it. This is normal. *H,* Hila. The left hilum is higher than the right. This is the proper relationship.

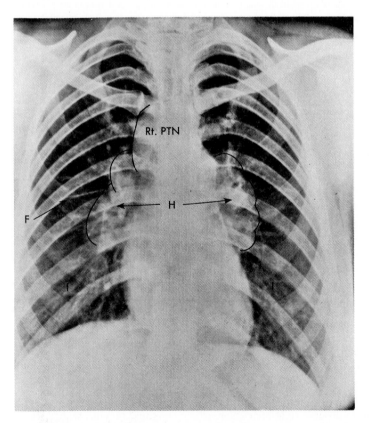

Fig. 18-6 *F,* Another example of a short fissure line. This horizontal fissure is a little thickened: *H,* Enlarged hila bilaterally and right paratracheal nodes *(Rt. PTN)* consistent with sarcoid. *I,* Note the diffuse, multidirectional lines in the lower portion of the lung. These lines are interstitial markings, and they are increased, consistent with interstitial disease. Sarcoidosis causes interstitial infiltrates and is the cause for the finding of hilar node enlargement and interstitial infiltrate in this patient.

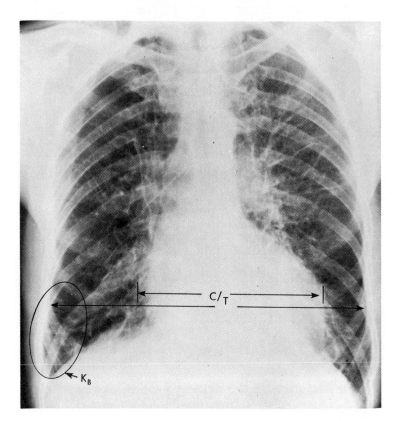

Fig. 18-7 K_B, Kerley B lines seen in their most common position. Note that the cardiothoracic ratio, which normally should be one half, is increased. This chest film is an excellent example of cardiogenic pulmonary edema.

A bubble behind the heart could indicate the presence of a hiatal hernia. The top of the gastric bubble should be no more than 2 cm from the top of the dome of the diaphragm.

H: Hila (Figs. 18-5 and 18-6)

The displacement of the hilar part of the chest anatomy constitutes the most important indirect sign of collapse of part of the lung. Ninety-seven percent of left hila are higher than right hila. The right hilum is never higher than the left one. The left should not be more than 3 cm higher than the right. If any of these rules are violated, the hilum is out of its proper position. This results from either hyperinflation of the lung on one side of the hilum, pushing it in the opposite direction, or collapse of an area of lung, which would pull the hilum in the direction of the collapse.

Enlargement of the hilar area is also an important finding. The hilar area can enlarge because of spreading cancer, infection somewhere in the lung, immunologic diseases, or sarcoid, to name a few. Enlarging left hila are hard to see; it is less difficult to observe right hilar enlargement.

I: Interstitium (Figs. 18-6, 18-8, 18-9, and 18-15)

Interstitial infiltrates are separated classically into alveolar and interstitial patterns. If there is an interstitial infiltrate, its presence can be confirmed by looking at the anterior air space, the area behind the sternum and in front of the heart. This is best seen on the lateral film. If an interstitial infiltrate is seen in the lateral view in the anterior air space, this is good evidence that, in fact, the patient does have a true interstitial infiltrate. Breast shadows overlying the lower portions of the lung will accentuate normal lung findings, and the practitioner should not be trapped into thinking that there is an abnormal interstitial pattern in female patients.

The alveolar pattern is caused by filling of the alveolus with water or material of near water density, such as pus, blood, or edema fluid. In the case of near drowning or congestive heart failure, the alveolar space fills with water. With Goodpasture's disease or idiopathic pulmonary hemosiderosis, these spaces fill with blood. In the case of pulmonary alveolar proteinosis, they fill with a proteinlike material. In the case of desquamative interstitial pneumonitis, they fill with cells. Sometimes this differential diagnosis can be narrowed if one has an idea of the type of material the patient is coughing up.

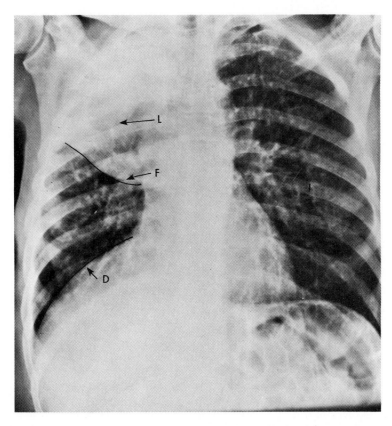

Fig. 18-8   *D*, The diaphragm is markedly elevated. Is the right phrenic nerve paralyzed? *F*, Fissure line. This horizontal fissure drifted up and is bulging. *L*, Lobe. This right upper lobe was full of tumor, which had blocked the bronchus. This resulted in collapse of the lobe. Forceful growth against the fissure line make it bulge, and growth of the tumor into the phrenic nerve caused paralysis of the right diaphragm. *I*, Interstitial marking. Another example of interstitial lines.

J: Junction lines

Junction lines are vertical lines in the mediastinum seen only on the PA projection. They include the right paraspinal line, left paraspinal line, right para-aortic line, left para-aortic line, posterior junctional line, anterior junctional line, right paratracheal line, and left paracardial line. These lines may be difficult to find, but if they are outlined or seen to bulge, a mass lesion may be displacing them.

K: Kerley's lines (Fig. 18-7)

Initially the Kerley B line was all that was observed, but now Kerley A and Kerley C lines have also been described. The Kerley B line is 1 mm thick and approximately 1 to 2 cm long and is found in the periphery of the lung, usually on the right at the base. The B line is a short, straight, horizontal line originating from the pleural surface. This is evidence of congestive heart failure. Kerley A lines are 1 mm thick and 2 to 4 cm long within the lung, midway between the hila and the pleura, and oriented in many directions. The actual length of the Kerley C lines is controversial, but they have been reported to be associated with engorgement of the pleural lymphatic vessels. These lines resemble an interstitial infiltrate, mentioned previously under "Interstitium." They have been called "everywhere lines."

L: Lobes (Fig. 18-8)

Collapse of a lobe is the result of obstruction of a bronchus from an intrinsic mass, narrowing from tuberculosis, traumatic fracture of the bronchus, extrinsic pressure from the lymph nodes or cardiac enlargement, or mucus plugging. There are certain tumors that have been known to metastasize to the large bronchi and cause collapse. These include tumor from kidney, breast, and skin.

Cardiac enlargement as a result of certain disease states has been reported to be associated with obstruction. The left lower lobe bronchus can be compressed by a large left atrium or left pulmonary artery.

Right middle lobe syndrome is a distinct clinical entity that results from collapse of the right middle lobe. It is sometimes seen in persons with asthma and other allergic disorders. The signs of collapse of a lobe include displaced fissure lines, loss of aeration, elevation of the diaphragm

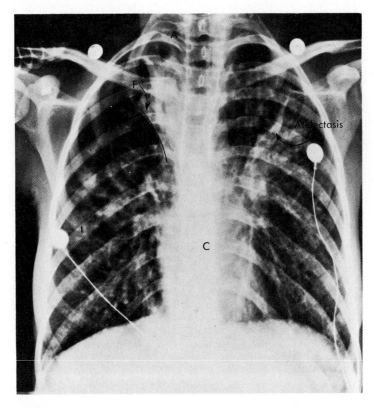

Fig. 18-9   *A,* Because of right upper lobe collapse the trachea is shifted to the right of the vertebral spines. *C,* The cardiac border on the left has been lost because of collapse of the lung on the left and because of several areas of atelectasis. *F,* The horizontal fissure line has been moved up and medially to the right. *I,* Interstitial markings are well seen. Several areas on the right upper-to-mid lung fields appear to be an alveolar infiltrate.

on the involved side, deviation of the trachea to the involved side, shifting of the heart to the right, narrowing of the trachea to the right, narrowing of the rib cage, compensatory overaeration, or hilar displacement.

It is helpful to know where each lobe goes when it collapses and how to find it. The right upper lobe is demonstrated by the horizontal fissure swinging up (Fig. 18-8) and, with complete collapse, swinging up to the right paratracheal mediastinum (Fig. 18-9). This is best seen on a PA view. The left upper lobe moves anteriorly, and on PA projection there is no sharp border to delineate the collapse. It is therefore best to see this form of collapse on a lateral film. The aortic knob can be obliterated.

The right middle lobe is seen best with a lateral or an apical lordotic view. On PA projection, the right heart border is obliterated when the right middle lobe collapses.

With collapse of the lingula, the left heart border is lost on the PA projection, with displacement of the lower half of the left major fissure. This displacement is usually forward. The collapse of the right lower lobe results in downward posterior and medial displacement of the lung toward the spine. The right heart border is usually seen well. This collapse is best seen on PA projection. The left lower lobe

has the same direction of collapse as the right lower lobe. The left border of the heart is seen well, but the "ivory heart" sign, as described by Felson,[1] may be seen. This constitutes loss of lung markings seen through the heart and results in a pure white heart shadow with no lung markings seen through it. This is best seen on the PA projection.

M: Mediastinum (Fig. 18-10)

The mediastinum is the part of the chest found between both lungs. It contains the heart, the great vessels, several important nerves (such as the vagus nerve and the phrenic nerve), hilar nodes, and other soft tissue such as fat pads. It is classically described as having an anterior compartment, a middle compartment, and a posterior compartment. Several organs come to rest in each of these compartments, and enlargements or mass lesions found in these compartments help determine the disease entity.

Sometimes air gets into the mediastinum, which is called a pneumomediastinum. It can best be seen on the lateral view, but the subtle findings of a small line around the heart in the PA view can be a tip-off that a pneumomediastinum has occurred.

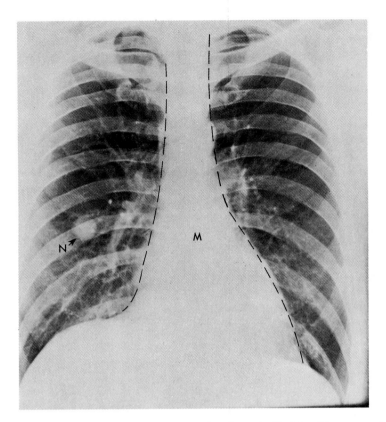

Fig. 18-10 *M*, Mediastinum is outlined with broken lines. *N*, Nodule with an area of calcium deposited in it—small white dot within the nodule at the 3- to 4-o'clock position. This means the nodule is benign; in this case it is a coccidiodomycosis scar.

N: Nodules (Fig. 18-10)

Nodules can be of two types: benign, not indicating a serious clinical problem, or malignant, which involves a serious diagnosis and prognosis. Nodules less than 1 cm are usually benign. Regardless of its size, a lesion that has calcium in it is most likely benign. If the nodule is 1 to 6 cm, it may be malignant. Nodules in the 1 to 6 cm size range are described as solitary coin lesions if they have clear areas of normal lung surrounding them.

If old films are available, it should be determined whether a nodule is growing. Malignancy is highly likely if the lesion is enlarging. However, nonmalignant lesions, such as old scars from histoplasmosis, can slowly enlarge.

Sometimes nodules cavitate so that they have hollow centers. This occurs with squamous cell carcinomas. It also occurs with tuberculosis, coccidiomycosis, and Wegener's granulomatosis. Sometimes one of these cavities will become the home of a colony of fungus. The fungus will form itself into a ball and actually be able to roll around inside the cavity. This should suggest a method to diagnose balls of fungus. If the patient lies on his or her side and a lateral decubitus film taken that shows the density inside the cavity moving to a more dependent position because of gravity, the diagnosis is confirmed. If possible, comparison should be made with old films to determine whether the nodule is growing.

O: Overaeration

A finding of overaeration on a chest radiograph can be extremely subtle. The film should be checked for an area that indicates more air in a part of the lung exceeding the aeration on the matching part of the opposite lung. This will be viewed as a much darker area on the film since air does not stop x-rays. Usually this will not have any distinct borders, so it will appear as a diffuse area of overaeration. It can be either an obstructed or nonobstructed area of the lung. Nonobstructed areas of overaeration usually suggest emphysematous blebs or bullae. Emphysema will occur with overaeration.

The obstruction form of overaeration is usually secondary to an inhaled foreign body or tumor. Another cause of overaeration is a pneumatocele, an area of lung destruction that follows a staphylococcal pneumonia. It usually has a distinct border caused by a thin wisp of tissue of overaeration in a tension pneumothorax. This occurs when rupture of the lung forces air into the pleural space, causing the lung to collapse. This will appear with overaeration throughout the entire side of the involved lung.

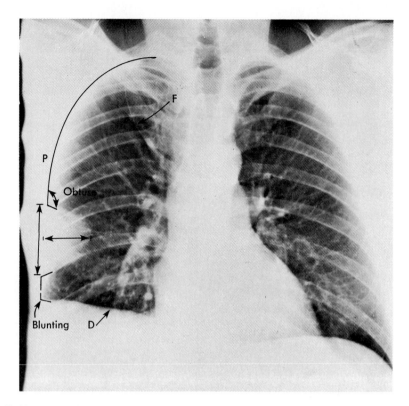

Fig. 18-11 *D,* Right diaphragm abnormally shaped. *F,* Fissured line showing an azygos lobe. Note the typical white, almost almond shape at the end of this fissure line. This is where the azygos vein came to rest. This is a normal, but uncommon, finding. *P,* Pleura with a typical pleural-based lesion showing an obtuse angle with the chest wall and vertical dimensions greater than horizontal. If it were reversed (acute angle with the chest wall and horizontal dimensions greater than vertical), then the lesion would be originating from lung tissue.

P: Pleura (Figs. 18-11 and 18-12)

The practitioner should run his or her eye all around the lung looking for thickening of the pleura, mass lesions, loss of marking in the lung next to the pleura, or blunting of the costophrenic (CP) angle. The CP angle is at the very bottom of the lung, where the diaphragm and the chest wall meet. Any blunting of the sharp angle formed by the diaphragm and the lateral portion of the chest wall suggests the presence of fluid, called pleural effusion.

Thickening of the pleura at the apex of the lung field is caused by old tuberculosis in about one half of patients. No cause for thickening is found in the other half.

Rare phrenic tumors called mesotheliomas are usually located along the lateral edge of the lung field. It should be determined whether the mass seen on the lung-pleural junction actually arises from pleural tissue or from the lung itself. This will make a difference in treatment and clinical course, depending on whether the lesion comes from the lung or from the pleura. There are two good rules of thumb to help. Pleura-based lesions tend to form an obtuse angle with the chest wall. In contrast, a tumor originating from the lung forms an acute angle. Another important differentiation is that if the vertical dimension of the lesion is greater than the horizontal dimension, then the lesion is based in the pleural. If the opposite is true (Figs. 18-11 and 18-12), then the lesion is based in the lung.

If a pneumothorax occurs (Fig. 18-12), the pleural edges will become visible when one looks through and between the ribs to see where the lung markings have pulled away from the chest wall. A thin line will be present just parallel to the chest wall. This can be easily missed if it is not carefully looked for. Pleural effusions have some specific findings on chest x-ray films. One that has been mentioned is blunting of the CP angle (Fig. 18-11). However, one form of pleural effusion is called the subpulmonic effusion. This type will spare the CP angle because the fluid is tucked under the lung and is not free to migrate down to the most dependent corner that makes up the CP angle. If this does occur, the diaphragm will tend to be flattened and go straight out laterally toward the chest wall, almost reaching it, then sharply drop off into the CP angle.

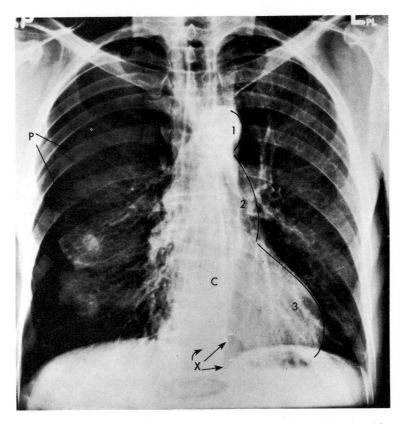

Fig. 18-12   *C*, Cardiac shadow shows the three bulges on the left, and bulge *1* and *2* are absent on the right. *P*, Pleural surface is displaced away from the chest wall, in this case because of a large pneumothorax. With the lung collapsing away from the chest wall, the right heart border has been obliterated. *X*, "X-tra" densities: surgical clips used to stop bleeding during surgery.

Q: "Quickly examine name plate"

Since there does not seem to be a good "Q" relationship to chest radiograph films, this would be an excellent time for the practitioner to quickly look at the name plate on the chest x-ray film and make sure that this film, in fact, belongs to the patient with whom the practitioner is concerned.

R: Respiration

Respiration affects the chest film. The lung makes obvious shifts with inspiration and expiration. A great deal can be determined about the nerve supply to the diaphragm via the phrenic nerve by the sniff test, a form of rapid respiration. In addition, the heart size has been described as changing with respiration. Whether this actually happens is debated.

If the chest radiograph has been taken properly and inspiration has been deep enough, the diaphragm will have descended to the bottom of the sixth rib anteriorly or the tenth rib posteriorly. Anything less than that will misrepresent some of the markings that are used to evaluate the film. Inspiration or expiration films are taken to accentuate and clearly define the presence of a small pneumothorax.

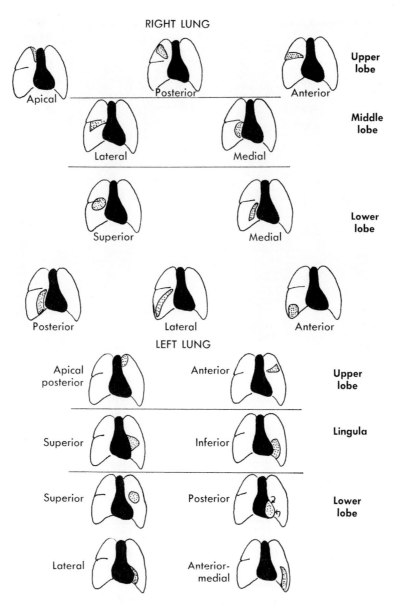

Fig. 18-13   The *dotted areas* show the approximate location of infiltrates should they occur in segments of the lung. Ten areas are shown for the right lung corresponding to the ten segments in the right, and eight areas are shown for the eight segments of the left lung.

S: Segments (Fig. 18-13)

It is sometimes important to determine which segment is involved with an infiltrative process. This requires understanding of the anatomy of the segments and of which structures sit next to them. The silhouette sign as described by Felson[1] has been a helpful technique used for identifying which segments are involved. The silhouette sign depends on the fact that an infiltrate will obscure the demarcating line of the structure it sits next to. We show some examples of this as we go through this section.

There are ten segments on the right and eight on the left. Fig. 18-13 demonstrates where each of these areas can be found.

T: Thoracic calcifications (Figs. 18-14 and 18-16)

Areas of calcification within the lung are frequent and represent benign lesions the majority of the time. However, there are a few that need to be identified and discussed. Eggshell calcifications have been described to occur in the hilar lymph nodes in patients who have silicosis, sarcoidosis, and other granulomatous diseases. Calcifications of the pulmonary artery, much like the calcification

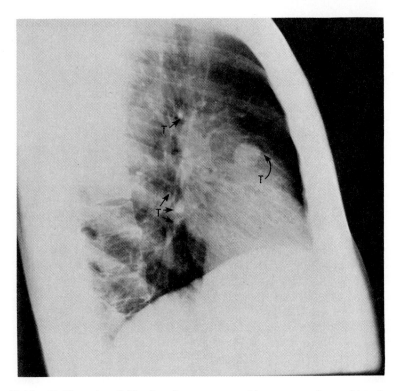

Fig. 18-14   *T*, Thoracic calcifications here represent old scars secondary to histoplasmosis.

seen in the aorta, can imply severe pulmonary hypertension. The most common causes of calcifications seen in the lung are healed infections caused by histoplasmosis, coccidiomycosis, or tuberculosis. Also described are calcifications seen in patients who have had chickenpox, pneumonia, and paragonimiasis. Paragonimiasis, caused by a parasitic worm that will reside in the lung, is commonly seen in patients who live in Asia.

The pneumoconioses (silicosis, asbestosis, etc) involve calcifications not only within the lung and the hilar lymph nodes, as noted, but also calcifications of the pleura.

A rare but interesting lung disease has been called alveolar microlithiasis, a familial disease that involves calcium phosphate deposits in the lung. With this disease, the lung resembles a snowstorm because of the myriads of calcifications within the alveolar sacs and ducts. An interesting pleural sign, called the "negative" pleural sign, has been described in this disease. It is a dark line running all the way around the outer border of both lungs. Lung tissue has been whited out because of the calcium phosphate deposits. The pleura, which does not absorb any of the calcium, appears as a thin dark line around the lung, making the chest radiograph look as though it were a negative made from a photograph.

U: Underperfusion

Underperfusion involves loss of blood vessels in a portion of the lung. When this occurs in association with pulmonary embolism, it is known as Westermark's sign. This is a subtle finding, and sometimes it is difficult to spot. It is the loss of vessel markings past where a pulmonary embolism has impacted. This same finding can be associated with the malpositioning of a Swan-Ganz catheter so that the catheter itself becomes an embolic device and blocks the flow of blood from the tip on out.

Another important disorder is MacLeod and Swyer-James syndrome. This is associated with loss of small peripheral vessels. There is no overinflation, and a normal to small hilum is associated with the syndrome. It is secondary to acute bronchopneumonia in infancy and may look like unilateral pulmonary agenesis.

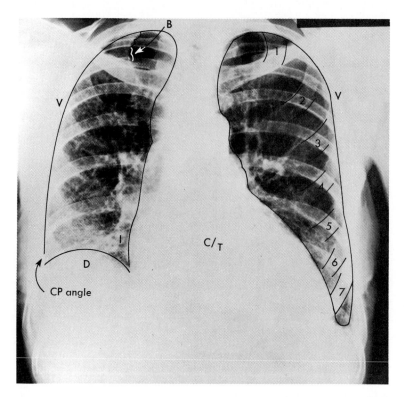

Fig. 18-15   *B,* Bone. The ribs on the left side are down by seven ribs anteriorly, so this is a good inspiration as far as the left side is concerned. The right side does not show as good an inspiration. Note the notching on the first rib on the right. *I,* Interstitial marking at both lung bases in this female patient show more "honeycombing." *V,* Volume. The right lung should be larger than the left. In this case the opposite is true and is therefore abnormal. *D,* Diaphragm. Why is the right diaphragm too high and the CP angle laterally is obscured? This is probably because of a pleural effusion. The *C/T* ratio is increased. The heart is therefore too large.

V: Volume (Fig. 18-15)

In evaluation of lung volume it is important to know that the right lung represents 55% of the total of both lungs and therefore should appear larger than the left lung. A problem is suggested in a lung that disrupts this relationship.

W: Women's breast shadows (Fig. 18-16)

The difference in women's and men's anatomy must be taken into account in the reading of chest radiographs. Women's breast shadows overlie the lower lung fields and will accentuate the lung markings behind them. This creates an impression of increased interstitial markings—a false impression. Absence of a breast shadow will make the chest film appear to be "overaerated" on the side where the breast is absent. It is a sign that the patient has undergone surgery to remove a breast, usually because of cancer.

Also, the nipples will appear as small coin lesions on chest x-ray films of women. Special techniques, such as x-ray–dense markers attached to the patient's nipples, are used. The film is then retaken, and the film with the nipple

markers is compared with the previous x-ray film to see whether these "coin lesions" correspond to the area in question.

X: "X-tra" densities (Fig. 18-12)

"X-tra" densities, such as bullets, other foreign bodies within the chest well, and radiopaque dyes, can sometimes be seen. In Fig. 18-12, surgical clips used in a previous operation to obtain control of bleeding can be observed.

SUMMARY

Chest radiography represents an important tool in the diagnosis and management of disorders of the pulmonary and cardiovascular systems. Under the guidance of a trained radiologist, interpretation of the chest x-ray film provides information that is essential in the identification and monitoring of disease processes. The respiratory care practitioner can and should understand the application of this key diagnostic tool and its appropriate use in the provision of comprehensive respiratory care.

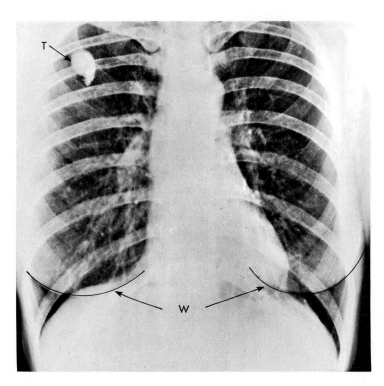

Fig. 18-16 *T*, Thoracic calcifications on this example are a result of old tuberculosis. *W*, Women's breast shadows. Note how the breast shadows accentuate the underlying tissue, making it appear as though there is an interstitial disease process present. As the lung tissue moves out beyond the breast shadow the increased interstitial pattern disappears.

REFERENCE

1. Felson B: Chest roentgenology, Philadelphia, 1973, WB Saunders Co.

BIBLIOGRAPHY

Felson B, Weinstein AS, Spitz HB: Principles of chest roentgenology: a programmed text, Philadelphia, 1965, WB Saunders Co.

Fraser RG and Pare JAP: Diagnosis of diseases of the chest, ed 2, vols I to IV, Philadelphia, 1977-1979, WB Saunders Co.

Lillington GA: In Burton GG, Gee GN, and Hodgkin JE, editors: Respiratory care, Philadelphia, 1977, JB Lippincott Co.

Lillington GA and Jamplis RW: A diagnostic approach to chest diseases, ed 2, Baltimore, 1976, Williams & Wilkins Co.

19

Synopsis of Cardiopulmonary Diseases

Craig L. Scanlan
Tarsem L. Gupta

One of the most challenging aspects of respiratory care is its involvement in a variety of respiratory and cardiopulmonary disorders. For the student or practitioner in this field, this broad scope of care demands a basic understanding of the causes, clinical features, and management approaches employed in a large number of disease entities and syndromes. Although a full treatment of pathology and pathophysiology is beyond the scope of this text, subsequent chapters assume a basic comprehension of common respiratory and cardiopulmonary disorders. To this end, we will provide a synopsis of the major disease categories most frequently encountered by the respiratory care practitioner, including brief descriptions of the etiology, clinical signs and symptoms, and current treatment approaches used in managing several of the most common disorders.

Our primary focus will be on disorders common in the adult patient requiring general respiratory care. More detail on patients requiring critical care and disorders specific to infants and children are provided in subsequent chapters.

OBJECTIVES

After completion of this chapter, the reader should be able to:

1. Differentiate the major respiratory infectious disorders according to etiology, clinical signs and symptoms, and treatment approaches;

2. Describe the normal immune mechanisms of the body and their relationship to both respiratory-related hypersensitivity reactions and decreased host defenses (with an emphasis on AIDS);

3. Compare and contrast the two primary disorders associated with chronic obstructive pulmonary disease (COPD);

4. Identify and describe the major inhalational lung diseases caused by: (1) organic or inorganic dusts and (2) noxious fumes and chemicals;

5. Differentiate the primary benign and malignant pulmonary neoplasms;

6. Identify the commonalities and differences between the various clinical disorders causing pulmonary restriction, including their cause, clinical features, and management;

7. Differentiate the major cardiovascular disorders affecting respiratory function, including their etiology, clinical signs and symptoms, and common treatment approaches;

8. Describe the major postoperative respiratory complications and the mechanisms useful in preventing and treating these problems.

KEY TERMS

Most terms used in this chapter are defined in context. The following terms are introduced without explicit definition, but may be found in the text glossary:

aerobic	exfoliate
agammaglobulinemia	extravasation
allographic	fibrinolysis
amyloidosis	hematogenous
anaerobic	laparotomy
angiography	lavage
ascites	leukocytopenia
autosomal	leukocytosis
demyelination	lupus erythematosus
diplegia	lymphadenopathy
diplopia	mucopurulent
dysarthria	myalgia
dysphagia	mycelium
embolectomy	myopathy
endorphin	neoplastic

neuropathy	ptosis
nocturia	pyogenic
nosocomial	rhinorrhea
nuchal	serotype
opsonin	strabismus
pandemic	syncope
paresis	thrombocytopenia
parotitis	thrombolysis
petechia	thrombophlebitis
platypnea	urticaria
pneumatocele	vasculitis

PULMONARY INFECTIONS AND RELATED DISORDERS

Infection is the most common cause of respiratory disease. The most common infections of the respiratory system seen in the hospital are the bacterial pneumonias. Tuberculosis, at one time extremely limited in prevalence, is again becoming a major health problem. Viral and fungal infections, the cause of many pneumonia-like illnesses, are also responsible for many respiratory disorders. Disorders commonly associated with respiratory infections include lung abscess and bronchiectasis.

Bacterial pneumonias

Pneumonia is an inflammatory process of the lung parenchyma. The most frequent cause of pneumonia is bacterial infection.

The most common bacterial pneumonias are caused by the gram-positive organisms *Streptococcus pneumoniae* and *Staphylococcus aureus.* Bacterial pneumonias caused by gram-negative organisms, such as *Klebsiella pneumoniae, Pseudomonas aeruginosa,* and *Haemophilus influenzae,* are less common in the community, but are a major cause of concern in the hospital (see Chapter 14). Conditions predisposing to bacterial pneumonias in general include viral respiratory infections, alcoholism, malnutrition, exposure to cold or noxious gases, depressed cerebral function, and cardiac failure.

Pneumococcal pneumonia. Two thirds to three fourths of all bacterial pneumonias are caused by *S pneumoniae,* an aerobic gram-positive diplococcal organism. The onset of pneumococcal pneumonia is usually sudden and marked by shaking chills, high fever, pleuritic chest pain, tachypnea, a cough with mucopurulent or blood-streaked ("rusty") sputum, and sometimes vomiting. Respirations may be accompanied by grunting and nasal flaring. On physical examination, chest excursions may be diminished on the involved side, breath sounds are diminished, fine inspiratory crackles (rales) are heard, and a pleural friction rub may be present. Signs of consolidation, if they occur, appear later.

In terms of laboratory testing, the sputum stains gram-positive and cultures out the pneumococcal organism.

Sometimes a good sputum specimen can be obtained only by transtracheal aspiration. Early in the infection, blood cultures may be positive for the pneumococci. Typically, the blood count shows leukocytosis. Blood gases usually reveal a moderate to severe hypoxemia on room air, with accompanying hyperventilation. The pH may be higher than normal because of the hypocapnea.

The chest radiograph may be unremarkable, except for a vague haziness in the involved part of the lung. Consolidation, if it develops, may be well defined either in a lobar or patchy distribution (see box on p. 414). Shadows in the costophrenic angles may appear in 10% to 20% of patients, indicating a pleural effusion (see subsequent section).

Treatment involves antibiotic therapy, usually with penicillin (Table 19-1), bed rest, analgesics for pain, adequate hydration, oxygen therapy, and pulmonary physical therapy as needed. Complications such as empyema, pleural effusion, and respiratory failure are treated as they arise.

Staphylococcal pneumonia. Staphylococcal pneumonia is caused by *S aureus,* an aerobic gram-positive cocci. Staphylococcal pneumonia often appears following viral infections of the respiratory tract, such as influenza. It is also common in debilitated patients and infants, especially after the administration of certain antibiotics.

Staphylococcal pneumonia often begins with a mild cough, headache, and generalized malaise. Depending on the host's resistance, it can abruptly change to a severe illness with high fever, chills, and a heavy cough productive of purulent or blood-streaked sputum. On physical examination, there may be signs of consolidation, pleural effusion, empyema, or even tension pneumothorax. Likewise, the chest radiograph shows a bronchial or lobar distribu-

Table 19-1 Common Antibiotics Used With Selected Bacterial Lung Infections

Infectious agent	Primary drug	Secondary drug
S pneumoniae	Penicillin	Erythromycin Cephalosporins
S aureus	Oxacillin Nafcillin	Vanomycin
K pneumoniae	Cephalosporins	Chloramphenicol
P aeruginosa	Gentamicin Carbenicillin	Cephalosporins
H influenzae	Ampicillin	Chloramphenicol Cephalosporins
Legionella pneumophila	Erythromycin	Tetracycline Rifampin
Mycobacterium tuberculosis	Isoniazid Rifampin Pyrazinamide Ethambutol	Capreomycin Kanamycin Ethionamide Cycloserine Para-aminosalicyclic acid

RADIOGRAPHIC FEATURES OF PNEUMONIAS

PATTERN	DESCRIPTION
Alveolar or acinar	Fluffy shadows that result from fluid accumulation in the distal airspaces of the lung; usually range from 0.5 to 1.0 cm in diameter and commonly are coalescent
Interstitial or reticular	Shadows that are a lacy network of linear markings that may reflect increased inflammatory material within the space surrounding the airspaces and/or vascular structures, but most commonly represent chronic changes such as fibrosis; linear changes may be the only abnormality or they may coexist with nodular shadows
Bronchopneumonia	Scattered fluffy shadows that tend to be patchy and follow the distribution of the central conducting airways; these may become confluent but rarely produce the "air-bronchogram" effect
Lobar pneumonia	Confluent shadows that usually terminate at pleural surfaces and usually but not always involve entire lobes or segments; a feature of lobar pneumonia is that the densities often surround the conducting airways to form a highly visible contrasting interface, the so-called "air bronchogram"
Necrotizing pneumonia	Pneumonia in which cavities are seen, that is, lung abscess; these lucencies may be apparent at the onset or may evolve as the inflammatory process advances; it is important not to confuse pneumonia in a patient with emphysema with necrotizing pneumonia

From Mitchell RS: Synopsis of clinical pulmonary disease, ed 4, St Louis, 1988, The CV Mosby Co.

tion and may reveal consolidation, pneumatoceles, abscesses, empyema, and pneumothorax (Fig. 19-1).

Diagnosis of staphylococcal pneumonia normally is confirmed by sputum smear and culture, although cultures of the pleural fluid and blood may also be positive. As with pneumococcal pneumonia, the white count is usually elevated. Blood gases usually reveal a severe hypoxemia on room air, which may manifest itself as a central cyanosis. Also as with pneumococcal pneumonia, the hypoxemia may cause hyperventilation, resulting in an elevated pH.

Initial therapy consists of full systemic doses of penicillinase-resistant antibiotics, such as oxacillin or nafcillin (see Table 19-1). As compared with pneumococcal pneumonia, staphylococcal pneumonia responds more slowly to an antibiotic regimen. Supportive therapy includes treatment of hypoxemia with oxygen, maintenance of adequate hydration and electrolyte balance, and pulmonary physical therapy. Despite these measures, complications are common, and the mortality rate associated with staphylococcal pneumonia is high.

Gram-negative pneumonias. Many important gram-negative infections occur during a hospital stay. Some gram-negative organisms, such as the Salmonelleae, are an important cause of illness outside of the hospital but only rarely cause nosocomial infections. Other gram-negative bacteria may cause disease after unusual environmental exposure. However, the most common gram-negative pathogens responsible for pneumonia are introduced through contaminated sources unique to the hospital setting. Once these organisms colonize the upper respiratory tract, the presence of impaired clearance mechanisms or compromised host immune responses allows infection of the lungs (Fig. 19-2).

The largest group of gram-negative bacilli is the Enterobacteriaceae. Organisms within this family vary widely in distribution and disease potential. *Escherichia coli* is responsible for most incidents of urinary tract infections and blood sepsis and is also a common cause of pulmonary and surgical wound infections. *K pneumoniae* is the next most frequent gram-negative pathogen, causing pneumonia both in the hospital and often in the community. As with E coli, *K pneumoniae* is also a frequent cause of nosocomial blood sepsis.

Less likely to cause bacteremia, but commonly identified as a source of nosocomial pneumonia are the *Enterobacter* and *Serratia* species. Like *Klebsiella*, these organisms grow well in infusion fluids and often appear in epidemic fashion in the hospital setting. *Proteus* infections most often involve the urinary tract but can also occur in other sites, including the lungs.

Among the gram-negative obligate aerobes, *P aeruginosa* is the most significant pathogen. Often associated

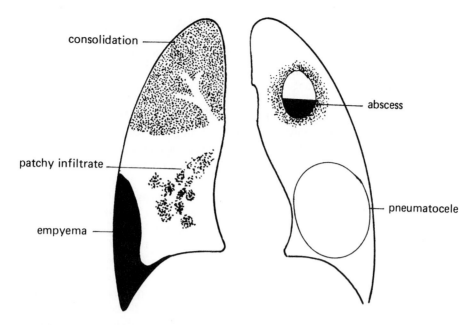

Fig. 19-1 Schema of various radiographic manifestations of staphylococcal pneumonia. (From Farzan S: A concise handbook of respiratory diseases, ed 2, East Norwalk, Conn, 1985, Appleton & Lange.)

Fig. 19-2 Pathogenesis of gram-negative pneumonia. (From Farzan S: A concise handbook of respiratory diseases, ed 2, East Norwalk, Conn, 1985, Appleton & Lange.)

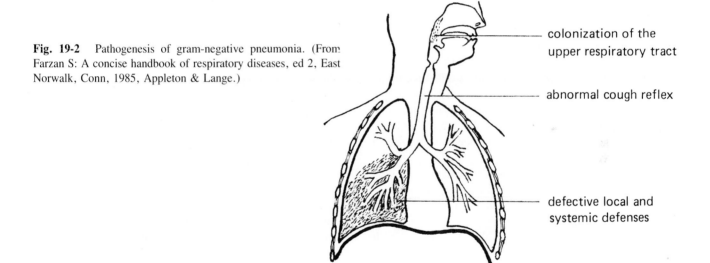

with contaminated respiratory equipment, *Pseudomonas* organisms can cause severe pneumonia, especially in immunosuppressed hosts. *Pseudomonas* organisms also have a tendency to infect highly susceptible tissues, such as burn wounds or lung parenchyma affected by cystic fibrosis.

H influenzae pneumonia is usually seen in children. However, the incidence of *H influenzae* in adults has increased in recent years and is associated with chronic conditions such as alcoholism, chronic obstructive pulmonary disease, lung cancer, and ischemic vascular disease. Physical findings associated with *H influenzae* in adults are

nondistinctive, resembling that of pneumococcal pneumonia.

With a few major exceptions, the clinical characteristics of the pulmonary infections produced by these organisms are similar. Typically, the patient is already suffering from a serious acute illness or chronic debilitating condition. For this reason, the onset of the pneumonia may be difficult to distinguish from a general deterioration caused by the underlying or primary disease process.

Physical findings are variable, but most similar to those exhibited in staphylococcal pneumonia. Because of the underlying or primary disease process, laboratory test results may not confirm the diagnosis. Since these organisms frequently colonize the airways of patients with chronic lung disease, their presence does not necessarily establish the cause of the pneumonia. Indeed, failure to culture these organisms is common. Radiographic findings range from patchy infiltrates to consolidation, often involving multiple lobes. Pleural effusion is common, especially with *H influenzae* pneumonia, with an incidence as high as 25%. Evidence of necrosis, such as cavity formation, is also common, especially with *K pneumoniae*.

Antibiotic treatment of most gram-negative pneumonias involves the use of a broad spectrum cephalosporin such as cefuoxime, cefoperazone, or cefotaxime (see Table 19-1). Aminoglycosides such as gentamicin, tobramycin, and amikacin are used for *P aeruginosa* infections, along with carbenicillin and ticarcillin, to delay the emergence of resistance. For *H influenzae* pneumonia, ampicillin is still the first-line drug of choice. Supportive therapy includes the maintenance of a patent airway, the provision of adequate oxygenation, and the correction of fluid and electrolyte imbalances. Despite aggressive intervention, the prognosis for patients with gram-negative nosocomial pneumonias generally is poor.

Legionellosis (legionnaires' disease). Legionnaires' disease is caused by *L pneumophila,* a bacterium that stains poorly, appears to be gram-negative, and does not biochemically resemble any known human pathogen. The organism is probably acquired by inhalation of aerosols or dust from air-conditioning equipment or soil excavation. The infection does not appear to be communicable among patients. During severe outbreaks, the mortality rate is as high as 10%. Death is attributed to respiratory failure or shock, often complicated by disseminated intravascular coagulation (DIC).

The initial symptoms of legionnaires' disease are comparable to influenza, that is, general malaise, diffuse myalgia, and headache. Typically, these symptoms are followed within 1 to 2 days by a high fever and chills. Nausea, vomiting, and diarrhea may also occur early in the disease. Within 72 hours, a dry cough begins that is nonproductive or produces scanty mucoid sputum, which is sometimes blood-streaked. Dyspnea and hypoxia become marked as signs of consolidation develop. Pleuritic chest pain occurs in about one in three patients. Severe confusion or delirium may occur.

Laboratory tests typically reveal leukocytosis, hyponatremia, and abnormal liver function. Radiographic examination usually shows patchy, often multilobar pulmonary consolidation and, occasionally, small pleural effusions. The illness usually worsens for 4 to 7 days before improvement begins in those who recover.

Erythromycin is the primary antibiotic used in the treatment of legionnaires' disease (see Table 19-1). Rifampin and tetracycline have been used to treat patients who cannot tolerate erythromycin. Supportive therapy includes maintenance of a patent airway, provision of adequate oxygenation, and correction of fluid and electrolyte imbalances. Assisted ventilation and management of shock may be necessary for patients who develop cardiopulmonary failure.

Pulmonary tuberculosis

Pulmonary tuberculosis is an infection caused by the acid-fast *Mycobacterium tuberculosis* and characterized by tubercle formation in the lung. Infection normally occurs by inhalation of organisms carried on droplet nuclei produced in the cough of an infected person.

The first, or primary, infection usually occurs in children, is self-limiting, and normally escapes detection. Without detection or treatment, the organism remains in the body, in most cases contained by various host defense mechanisms. However, about one in twenty individuals develop the progressive inflammation and tissue necrosis that characterize the postprimary or chronic infection. Malnutrition, diabetes, certain viral infections (including AIDS), chronic corticosteroid use, silicosis, and general debility all predispose development of the chronic infection.

The most frequent symptoms associated with chronic pulmonary tuberculosis are cough, malaise, weight loss, and a low-grade fever that tends to occur in the afternoon. Night sweats, pleuritic pain, and a productive cough may or may not be present. In the presence of these symptoms, the appearance of blood in the sputum strongly suggests tuberculosis.

On physical examination, fine persistent crackles (rales) may be heard over the upper lobes. These are best heard during inspiration after a slight cough. Advanced disease may lead to retraction of the chest wall, deviation of the trachea, wheezes, and signs of pulmonary consolidation.

A chest x-ray study helps disclose tuberculosis in many cases. Hilar lymph node enlargement associated with a small parenchymal lesion that heals with calcification is the usual picture of primary infection (Fig. 19-3). However, many primary infections do not show abnormalities on x-ray study. The postprimary or chronic progressive form of tuberculosis typically reveals upper lobe infiltrations with evidence of cavitation. However, this tendency for upper lobe involvement is not always the case. When tuberculosis occurs secondary to an immune disorder, such as AIDS, the organisms may invade both the middle and lower lobes.

Skin testing can reveal a past or present infection. The tuberculin skin test is based on a delayed hypersensitivity (type IV) reaction to a specific, bacterial protein antigen. The test may be administered intracutaneously (Mantoux) or by multiple puncture methods, such as the tine test. The Mantoux method, employing purified protein derivative (PPD), is the most reliable. A positive reaction is evident with induration of 10 mm or more in diameter.

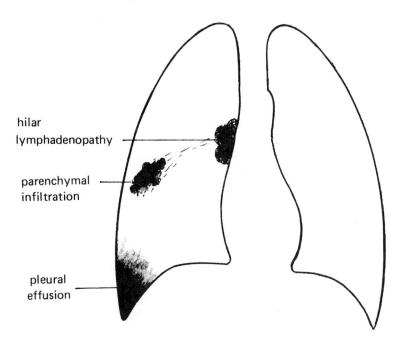

hilar
lymphadenopathy

parenchymal
infiltration

pleural
effusion

Fig. 19-3 Primary intrathoracic tuberculosis. (From Farzan S: A concise handbook of respiratory diseases, ed 2, East Norwalk, Conn, 1985, Appleton & Lange.)

Absolute confirmation of the diagnosis is by recovery of the tubercle bacillus from sputum, gastric washings, or tracheal washings. If there is no spontaneous sputum production, tracheal wash with saline or sputum induction by inhalation of a heated saline aerosol can produce a reliable specimen for bacteriologic examination. Cultures of pleural effusions or tissue biopsies may also confirm presence of the organism.

The treatment of tuberculosis has undergone substantial change in recent years. Any patient in whom tuberculosis is suspected should initially be isolated. Once diagnosis is established, appropriate antibiotic therapy is begun. Currently this therapy consists of prolonged administration of a combination of agents, principally isoniazid (INH), rifampin, pyrazinamide, and ethambutol. According to a joint statement promulgated by the American Thoracic Society and the US Centers for Disease Control in 1986, a 6-month regimen initially consisting of 2 months of isoniazid, rifampin, and pyrazinamide, followed by 4 months of isoniazid and rifampin, is usually effective in treating fully susceptible organisms (see Table 19-1). A 9-month program of isoniazid and rifampin is also highly successful. When isoniazid resistance is suspected, a 12-month regimen of rifampin and ethambutol, sometimes supplemented initially with pyrazinamide, is indicated. Second-line antituberculosis drugs include capreomycin, kanamycin, ethionamide, para-aminosalicylic acid (PAS), and cycloserine (see Table 19-1). The major factor determining the outcomes of tuberculosis treatment is patient compliance with the drug regimen. In promoting and monitoring

compliance, the physician, nurse, and respiratory care practitioner all play a major role.

In the past, it was common to hospitalize and isolate confirmed cases of tuberculosis until several successive negative sputum cultures were obtained. However, given the relatively low virulence of *M tuberculosis*, this approach is no longer deemed necessary. Patients with tuberculosis should be considered for discharge after (1) appropriate antibiotic therapy has been initiated and (2) successive sputum cultures yield low counts of acid-fast bacilli.

Nonetheless, epidemiologic studies have indicated that the greatest source of new infection and new cases of tuberculosis result from contact with patients having active disease. Especially prone to developing tuberculosis in these situations are very young children and adolescent members of the patient's family. For this reason, household members and individuals having close contact with such patients should be skin tested. All contacts exhibiting a 5 mm or greater induration on skin test who have no history of reaction in the past should be considered infected with *M tuberculosis* and immediately started on a preventive regimen, usually consisting of 6 months of isoniazid therapy.

A vaccine for tuberculosis has been developed. This bacille-calmette Guerin (BCG) vaccine is an attenuated strain of the bovine bacillus. BCG vaccination offers some protection to individuals with a negative skin test, although not complete immunity. Unfortunately, several factors limit the usefulness of the BCG vaccine. First, the risk of developing tuberculosis is already low among those who are tuberculin-negative. Second, once vaccinated, individuals will exhibit a positive reaction to the tuberculin derivative used for skin testing. This makes it difficult for the physician to discover early infections that can occur in these immunized individuals. For these reasons, BCG vaccination is recommended only where exposure to tuberculosis is great and the usual control measures are not possible.

Viral infections of the respiratory tract

Over 200 different viruses are responsible for infections of the respiratory system in humans. The five principal groups of viruses involved in infectious disorders of the lungs are the influenza viruses, rhinoviruses, adenoviruses, parainfluenza viruses, and respiratory syncytial viruses. Less frequently associated with respiratory disease are herpes simplex (type 1), the coxsackieviruses, the Epstein-Barr virus, the echoviruses, and the polioviruses.

In order of prevalence, the primary respiratory infections caused by viruses are rhinitis, pharyngitis, bronchiolitis, tracheobronchitis, laryngotracheobronchitis, and pneumonia. Many viruses can cause more than one type of infection, and several different viruses produce identical syndromes. Viruses may also cause asthmatic episodes, exacerbate the symptoms of chronic respiratory disease, and contribute to the development of some cases of bronchiectasis.

The development of a specific viral infection is often associated with factors such as the patient's age, the time of year, and the setting. In general, viral infections of the respiratory tract are more common in children than in adults. However, adults regularly exposed to young children often develop these infections. Moreover, special populations such as college students and military recruits often show a high incidence of unique viral infections.

Influenza. Influenza is an acute viral disease that produces fever, myalgia, headache, and malaise. The incidence of influenza varies widely, from sporadic occurrences during an interepidemic year to widespread pandemic outbreaks affecting millions. Influenza infections are usually self-limiting, lasting a week or less. However, influenza infections are commonly complicated by bacterial superinfections or the presence of chronic respiratory disease.

Influenza is an RNA virus. There are three serotypes of the influenza virus, designated as A, B, and C. The A virus is associated with pandemic influenza whereas the B type tends to cause more localized epidemics. Influenza C infection in humans is sporadic and mild, being manifested only as pharyngitis and common colds.

The principal method of controlling influenza infections is vaccination. Vaccines are developed for the particular serotype and strain of the virus. Most physicians recommend vaccination in epidemic or pandemic years for those with chronic respiratory or cardiopulmonary disorders.

Supportive management of influenza includes bed rest, fluids to maintain adequate hydration, and analgesics for pain. The antiviral agent amantadine can decrease the duration of fever and other systemic symptoms associated with influenza A when given within the first day or two of the illness. Patients who develop significant bacterial superinfections are generally hospitalized and started on a regimen of penicillinase-resistant penicillin. Thereafter, a gram stain, culture, and sensitivity of a sputum sample are used to identify the offending bacterial agent and to help select a more specific antibiotic.

Adenovirus infections. Most respiratory infections caused by adenoviruses occur in children, being responsible for about 5% of all lower respiratory tract illnesses in these patients. Childhood adenovirus infections can appear before the age of 6 months, but reach a peak incidence in the preschool years and decline in frequency after age 9. Adenoviruses also are an important cause of respiratory disease in special populations, such as college students and military recruits.

There are three primary types of adenovirus respiratory infections: (1) an acute, febrile, but generally self-limiting condition similar to influenza; (2) a pertussis-like syndrome similar to that caused by *H Influenzae;* and (3) pharyngoconjunctival fever. Overwhelming, fatal pneumonias have been reported in both children and adults infected with some strains of the adenovirus. Respiratory infections caused by adenoviruses are transmitted primarily by the fecal-oral route. These viruses also are isolated from at least half of all surgically removed tonsils.

The patient with a flu-like adenovirus infection typically exhibits a fever, cough, sore throat, rhinorrhea, mild chills, and headache. Pneumonia may complicate the condition in about one in ten cases. The pharyngoconjunctival form of the infection (sometimes called swimming pool conjunctivitis) involves acute unilateral conjunctivitis, preauricular adenopathy, and pharyngitis. As mentioned earlier, clinical signs and symptoms alone do not provide a sufficient basis for differentiating the pertussis-like adenovirus infection from bacterial whooping cough caused by *H influenzae.*

Occasionally, mixed infections of adenoviruses with measles, mumps, influenza, and parainfluenza viruses occur, resulting in more severe morbidity. *Mycoplasma pneumoniae* also has been isolated with adenoviruses in the respiratory tract.

As with other viral respiratory diseases, the management of adenovirus infections is largely supportive. In military populations, these infections are best managed by vaccination. Proper chlorination of swimming pools will prevent the spread of pharyngoconjunctival fever. As with influenza, the major complication is a secondary bacterial pneumonia.

Paramyxoviral infections. The paramyxoviruses mainly affect children and include the measles, mumps, parainfluenza, and respiratory syncytial viruses. Both the parainfluenza and respiratory syncytial viruses are transmitted by direct, person-to-person contact or by dispersal of droplet nuclei through the air.

There are three known serotypes of parainfluenza viruses, designated as types 1, 2, and 3. The most common specific illness caused by the parainfluenza viruses is childhood croup. Details on the clinical features and treatment of this illness are provided in Chapter 32.

Because the population is usually exposed to the parainfluenza viruses during childhood, most adults have developed antibodies to them. Nonetheless, these viruses occasionally cause adult respiratory infections, especially viral laryngitis and pharyngitis. In addition to the mumps virus, type 3 parainfluenza virus may cause parotitis.

Little is known about the pathogenesis of parainfluenza infections. The development of vaccines for the parainfluenza viruses has been complicated by the possibility that antibody production might worsen the severity of the natural infection. Indeed, the severe disease caused by these viruses in newborn infants may result from an immune response that occurs when natural infection appears in the presence of maternal antibodies.

Respiratory syncytial viruses infect infants and children more often than they do adults, with the most common specific disorder being bronchiolitis. Details on the clinical features and treatment of bronchiolitis are also provided in Chapter 32. In adults, respiratory syncytial viruses can cause colds and, less frequently, bronchopneumonia or bronchitis.

Fungal (mycotic) infections

The most common mycotic infections in the US are coccidioidomycosis, histoplasmosis, blastomycosis, and aspergillosis. These infections are caused, respectively, by *Coccidioides immitis, Histoplasma capsulatum, Blastomyces dermatitidis,* and *Aspergillus fumigatus* (Fig. 19-4). Coccidioidomycosis, histoplasmosis, and blastomycosis share the following common features:

1. Infections occur in circumscribed geographic areas where the infecting agents are found in the soil and can be aerosolized.
2. The fungal agent in each case is dimorphic; it exists in nature as a mycelium (mold) bearing infectious spores, which enter the host and then evolve to a yeastlike phase; the latter phase is the definitive tissue pathogen.
3. Although local skin or mucous membrane inoculation is theoretically a possible route of infection, the usual portal of entry of these infections is the respiratory tract.
4. Clinical manifestations and pathologic events closely resemble those in tuberculosis; asymptomatic or minimally symptomatic primary pulmonary infection is common. Chronic pulmonary, local metastatic, or disseminated infection is uncommon.

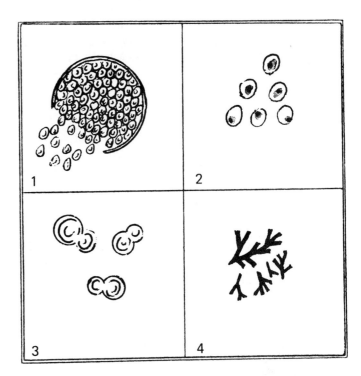

Fig. 19-4   Fungi commonly causing respiratory tract infection. *1, Coccidioides immitis; 2, Histoplasma capsulatum; 3, Blastomyces dermatitidis; 4, Aspergillus fumigatus.* (From Farzan, S: A concise handbook of respiratory diseases, ed 2, East Norwalk, Conn, 1985, Appleton & Lange.)

5. The pathologic responses to these organisms are similar and consist of variable amounts of suppuration and granuloma formation.
6. An intact, cell-mediated, immune response is critical to limitation and control; its absence is correlated with a high risk of disseminated disease.
7. Amphotericin B is the primary therapy for all three infections.

Unlike the other three mycotic agents, *A fumigatus* is distributed worldwide. For this reason, *A fumigatus* frequently colonizes the skin and mucous surfaces of the normal human host. Invasive disease caused by *A fumigatus* is therefore rare unless the physical barriers to infection are breached or some other specific defect of host defense is present.

Once established, *A fumigatus* infection may manifest itself in one of three forms: allergic aspergillosis, aspergilloma, or invasive aspergillosis. Allergic aspergillosis is a form of hypersensitivity pneumonitis, discussed later in the section on immune disorders. Aspergilloma, or fungus ball aspergillosis, is the result of colonization of *A fumigatus* in a preformed cavitary lung lesion, such as that caused by tuberculosis. In aspergilloma, an actual fungus ball, consisting of matted mycelia combined with fibrin and other cellular debris, develops. Invasive aspergillosis is the most serious form of infection, found most often in immunocompromised hosts. Fungal mycelia first invade the pulmonary parenchyma, followed by a blood-borne spread to other organs, especially the kidneys. Progressive systemic invasion of the organism results in death if not treated quickly, usually with amphotericin B.

Lung abscess

Lung abscess is an inflammatory lesion resulting in necrosis of lung tissue. It is characterized by the onset of pulmonary symptoms 10 to 14 days after disruptions of bronchopulmonary structure or function by any one of the following means: (1) suppression of the cough reflex, (2) aspiration of infected material, (3) bronchial obstruction, (4) pneumonias, (5) ischemia, as with pulmonary infarction, and (6) bacteremia or blood sepsis. Lung abscesses also commonly occur during immunosuppressive therapy, as in organ transplantation.

Infection with pyogenic or anaerobic bacteria in any of these situations causes lung abscess. Single lung abscesses are associated with inflammation behind an obstructed bronchus or after aspiration. The so-called "putrid lung abscesses" are caused mainly by aspiration of oral materials containing anaerobic streptococci, *Bacteroides* organisms, or fusospirochetes. Colonization of the oral cavity with these organisms is common in alcoholic patients with severe tooth decay and infected gums. Putrid abscesses are usually located in the posterior segments of the upper or superior segments of the lower lobes.

Multiple lung abscesses may be a feature of the blood-borne spread of *Staphylococcus* organisms, *K pneumoniae,* or other necrotizing organisms. Multiple abscesses are almost always nonputrid.

Early in the process, patients with a lung abscess exhibit signs and symptoms similar to those of any acute severe pneumonia: fever, chills, prostration, pleuritic chest pain, cough, and leukocytosis. Coughing is often nonproductive at onset. Consolidation resulting from pneumonitis surrounding the abscess is the most frequent finding.

In terms of laboratory findings, simple sputum cultures are usually inadequate in determining the bacterial cause of a lung abscess, necessitating transtracheal aspiration or bronchoscopy to obtain an appropriate sample. On the chest film, a lung abscess may be indistinguishable in its early stages from any localized pneumonitis. Later, a dense shadow may appear. Finally, after the abscess communicates with a bronchus and starts to drain, a central radiolucency, often with a visible air-fluid level appears.

If the abscess ruptures into a bronchus, the patient may suddenly begin to cough up copious amounts of sputum. Hemoptysis may also occur at this time. Foul-smelling brown or gray sputum indicates a putrid infection caused by a mix of organisms, including anaerobes. Green or yellow "musty" sputum without an offensive odor indicates a nonputrid infection with a single pyogenic organism. Rarely, a peripherally located abscess ruptures into the pleura, causing an empyema. When a lung abscess becomes chronic, severe debility, localized bronchiectasis, clubbing, and even secondary amyloidosis may occur.

In the past, lung abscesses were often treated by surgical drainage or resection. Today this approach is a last resort, with medical management by appropriate antibiotic the regimen of choice. In addition to antibiotic therapy, both postural drainage and therapeutic bronchoscopy can promote removal of abscess secretions. However, to avoid spread of the infection to healthy lung lobes or segments, postural drainage must be performed with extreme caution. In some patients, an artificial airway may be needed to facilitate clearance of abscess secretions. The prognosis for acute lung abscesses that are managed early is good. Chronic lung abscess responds more slowly to treatment. Patients with a chronic lung abscess complicated by severe hemoptysis generally have a poor prognosis.

Bronchiectasis

The term bronchiectasis means simply dilation of the bronchi, but in general usage it also implies the destruction of bronchial walls. Anatomically, there are three categories of bronchiectasis (Fig. 19-5). *Saccular* (cystic) bronchiectasis is the classic advanced form, characterized by irregular dilatations and narrowings. The term *fusiform* is used when the dilatations are especially large. *Cylindrical,* or tubular, bronchiectasis is simply the absence of normal bronchial tapering. Cylindrical bronchiectasis is usually a manifestation of severe chronic obstructive lung disease rather than of true bronchial wall destruction.

Bronchiectasis usually is caused by repeated or prolonged episodes of pneumonitis, especially those complicating pertussis or influenza during childhood. Bronchiectasis may also be associated with bronchial obstruction caused by neoplasms, or the aspiration of a foreign body.

Bronchiectasis that involves most or all of the bronchial tree is usually genetic or developmental in origin. Cystic fibrosis, Kartagener's syndrome (bronchiectasis with dextrocardia and paranasal sinusitis), and agammaglobulinemia are all examples of inherited or developmental diseases associated with bronchiectasis.

Most cases of bronchiectasis are accompanied by severe chronic bronchitis. More advanced cases of bronchiectasis are often associated with anastomoses between the bronchial and pulmonary vessels. These anastomoses cause substantial right-to-left shunting, resulting in hypoxemia, pulmonary hypertension, and cor pulmonale.

Clinically, bronchiectasis is characterized by a chronic, loose cough, usually productive of large amounts of mucopurulent, often foul-smelling sputum. In advanced cases the sputum settles out into three distinctive layers: cloudy mucus on top, clear saliva in the middle, and purulent solid material on the bottom. Hemoptysis occurs in at least half of all cases. Advanced, untreated bronchiectasis is ac-

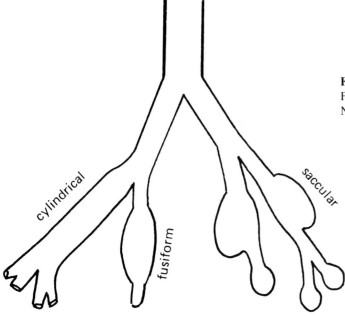

Fig. 19-5   Various morphologic types of bronchiectasis. (From Farzan S: A concise handbook of respiratory diseases, ed 2, East Norwalk, Conn, 1985, Appleton & Lange.)

companied by frequent bronchopulmonary infections, chronic malnutrition, sinusitis, clubbing, cor pulmonale, and right ventricular failure. Physical signs are variable and not always helpful in diagnosis. Likewise, simple chest radiographs generally are insufficient to establish diagnosis.

Bronchoscopy often reveals a deep velvety red mucosa, with pus welling up from the areas of involvement. Cultures of sputum often show a variety of organisms, including common mouth flora, fusospirochetes, and anaerobic streptococci, among others. Microscopic examination of the sputum may reveal necrotic elastic tissue, muscle fibers, and epithelial debris.

The diagnosis of bronchiectasis is confirmed by *bronchography*. Bronchography involves radiographic exposure of the lung after instillation of a contrast material, either iodized oil, iodine in water, or, more recently, powdered tantalum. Bronchography should only be performed after the use of vigorous bronchial hygiene, postural drainage, and a course of antimicrobial therapy for at least a week. Bronchography should include every lung segment, but both lungs should not be studied at one time in patients with significantly impaired pulmonary function.

The most important feature of the treatment of bronchiectasis is regular and vigorous bronchial hygiene, with postural drainage, generally continued for the rest of the patient's life. Antimicrobial therapy may be helpful in the management of acute exacerbations of bronchiectasis. However, prolonged antimicrobial therapy tends to allow drug-resistant organisms to multiply in the irreversibly ulcerated bronchi and thus should be avoided.

Surgical resection of affected segments or lobes should be considered only when irreversible involvement of localized areas is clearly demonstrated. Resection should be postponed until all efforts at medical management have failed.

Except for its congenital forms, bronchiectasis should be regarded as a preventable disease. A child who inhales a foreign body should have it immediately removed by bronchoscopy or surgery if necessary (see Chapter 32). Vigorous treatment of pneumonias also greatly reduces the incidence of complicating bronchiectasis. Timely vaccination against measles, pertussis, and other childhood diseases commonly complicated by pneumonia is another preventive measure.

CHRONIC OBSTRUCTIVE PULMONARY DISEASE

Chronic obstructive pulmonary disease (COPD) is a broad term used to describe a generalized airway obstruction that is not fully reversible with treatment. As shown in Fig. 19-6, COPD is almost always a mixture of emphysema and chronic bronchitis, at times with elements of asthma.

Classically, chronic bronchitis is defined by its symptoms: a history of a productive cough for at least 3 months a year for two consecutive years. Pathologically, there is hypertrophy of the bronchial glands and an increase in the number of the goblet cells lining the respiratory tract mucosa, which typically is chronically inflamed.

Emphysema, on the other hand, is defined mainly in anatomic terms as a destructive process of the lung parenchyma leading to permanent enlargement of the distal airspaces. Emphysema can be classified as either centrilobular (CLE), which mainly involves the respiratory bronchi-

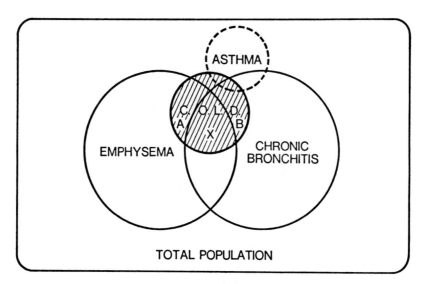

Fig. 19-6 Interrelationships among chronic bronchitis, emphysema, asthma, and chronic obstructive lung disease (COLD). The shaded area roughly indicates the proportions of symptomatic individuals with COLD. Patients with severe anatomic emphysema with little bronchitis are designated type A emphysema. Those with severe bronchial abnormalities with emphysema are designated type B bronchitis. The many patients with a mixed syndrome are depicted in the X zone. (From Burrows B, Knudson RJ, and Kettrl LG: Respiratory insufficiency, Chicago, 1975, Year Book Medical Publishers.)

oles, or panlobular (PLE), which can involve the entire terminal respiratory unit. CLE is predominantly a disease of bronchitic patients who smoke cigarettes, whereas PLE can occur in nonsmokers. PLE is also the type of emphysema associated with a hereditary deficiency of an enzyme inhibitor called alpha-1 antitrypsin. As CLE progresses, it becomes increasingly difficult to distinguish it from PLE, at which point it may be labeled mixed or endstage emphysema. In either case, *bullae,* or airspaces greater than 1 cm in size, may develop.

In chronic bronchitis, increased secretions and mucosal edema are the primary factors in airway obstruction. Airway obstruction in emphysema, on the other hand, is caused by the destruction of elastic tissues that normally maintain small airway patency. Physiologically, this results in a loss of elastic recoil (increased compliance), an increase in total lung capacity (TLC). O_2 diffusion is also impaired because of the decrease in available surface area. However, this loss of alveolar surface area tends to be balanced by the destruction of the capillary bed, so that $\dot{V}/\dot{Q}$ imbalances are slight.

In terms of radiographic examinations, the patient with bronchitis may have a normal chest x-ray film. Classically, the patient suffering from severe emphysema exhibits flattened diaphragms, an increased retrosternal airspace (evidence of lung hyperinflation), and attenuation of pulmonary vasculature toward the lung periphery. Although there are typical radiologic patterns, COPD cannot be diagnosed by a chest x-ray study alone.

In the pulmonary function laboratory, patients with chronic bronchitis and emphysema both tend to exhibit a decrease in expiratory flow rates, with little or no response to bronchodilator therapy. Blood gas measurements can vary widely in COPD. Pao_2 levels may range from normal to very low whereas the arterial Pco_2 may be normal, low, or high.

Only when pulmonary function testing includes measurement of TLC, diffusing capacity, and lung compliance (C_L) can a clear distinction be made between these two forms of COPD. Generally, the emphysematous patient will exhibit an increased TLC, reduced diffusing capacity, and increased compliance. By contrast, in the stable patient with chronic bronchitis, results of these tests tend to be normal or near normal. Table 19-2 summarizes the clinical and physiologic features that distinguish chronic bronchitis from emphysema.

Treatment for the individual patient with COPD is based less on the specific diagnosis than on the symptoms and their severity. First, patients must be encouraged to stop smoking and taught to avoid other respiratory irritants. Although the use of mucolytics and expectorants is common, their efficacy has yet to be proved. Bronchodilator therapy, either orally or by aerosol, is indicated only when an asthmatic component exists. Likewise, corticosteroids should be considered only when there is evidence of airway reactivity.

In addition, depending on the clinical situation, patients with COPD may be treated with antibiotics, supplemental oxygen, and other medications. Antibiotics are used to treat or prevent respiratory infections, since these are the primary factors in acute exacerbations of both chronic bronchitis and emphysema. As described in Chapter 27, breathing exercises (to increase efficiency of breathing) and aids to bronchial hygiene (such as postural drainage) are also frequently employed in severe cases of COPD. Given the chronic nature of these disorders, the best approach is a comprehensive pulmonary rehabilitation program that includes both patient education and physical conditioning activity. More details regarding pulmonary rehabilitation are provided in Chapter 34.

IMMUNOLOGIC DISORDERS

The body's immune system plays a critical role in the defense against both external substances, such as infectious agents, toxins, and foreign particles, and internal threats, such as malignant cells. Ironically, when the immune response is excessive or exaggerated, it may actually cause disease. Likewise, deficiencies in the body's immune response can result in an increased incidence of infectious disorders, especially those caused by the so-called "opportunistic" organisms. For this reason, it is essential that respiratory care practitioners have a basic understanding of the immune system in health and disease.

As shown in Fig. 19-7, the basic elements of the immune system are T lymphocytes, B lymphocytes (both derived from a hematogenous stem cell), and circulating macrophages. T lymphocytes have receptors for both antigen-antibody complexes and complement. In addition to these receptors, B lymphocytes also possess surface immunoglobulins. The basic body immune response involves interaction between these lymphocytes and the macrophages.

In both cases, the macrophage serves as a phagocytic and secretory cell. As a phagocytic cell, the macrophage is capable of binding antigens to its cell membrane receptors, engulfing and lysing this foreign material. As a secretory cell, the macrophage is capable of elaborating a variety of active agents and mediators. This "processing" of the antigen by the macrophage sensitizes both the T and B lymphocytes. Once sensitized by this process, these lymphocytes can thereafter respond to the antigen by producing a variety of chemical substances that aid in biologic defense.

Cell-mediated immunity (CMI) involves interaction between circulating macrophages and the T lymphocytes. Once sensitized to a specific antigen, T lymphocytes synthesize and release a variety of proteins called lymphokines, which stimulate the sensitization of additional T cells and increase macrophage activity in the area of antigen exposure. In turn, these activated macrophages secrete several chemical factors that recruit and activate additional

Table 19-2   Features That Distinguish Bronchial and Emphysematous Types of Chronic Obstructive Lung Disease

	Bronchial type B	Emphysematous type A
CLINICAL FEATURES		
History	Often recurrent chest infections	Often only insidious dyspnea
Chest exam	Noisy chest, slight overdistention	Quiet chest, marked overdistention
Sputum	Frequently copious and purulent	Usually scanty and mucoid
Weight loss	Absent or slight	Often marked
Chronic cor pulmonale	Common	Infrequent
Roentgenogram	Often evidence of old inflammatory disease	Often attenuated vessels and radiolucency
General appearance	"Blue bloater"	"Pink puffer"
PHYSIOLOGIC TESTS		
Lung volumes: TLC	Normal or slightly decreased	Increased
RV	Moderately increased	Markedly increased
RV/TLC	High	High
Lung compliance:		
Static	Normal or low	High
Dynamic	Very low	Normal or low
Airways resistance:		
Expiratory	Very high	High
Inspiratory	High	Normal
Diffusing capacity	Variable	Low
Chronic hypoxemia	Often severe	Usually mild
Chronic hypercapnia	Common	Unusual
Pulmonary hypertension	Often severe	Usually mild
Cardiac output	Normal	Often low

From Burrows B, Knudson RJ, and Kettrl LJ: Respiratory insufficiency, Chicago, 1975, Year Book Medical Publishers.

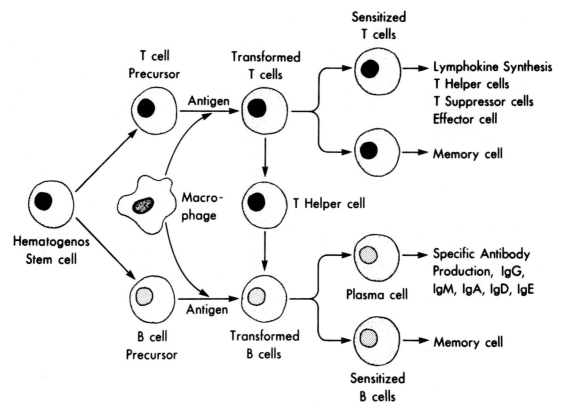

Fig. 19-7   Development of the humoral and cellular immune systems. Macrophage processing of antigen occurs prior to presentation to B lymphocytes and T lymphocytes, with T helper lymphocyte facilitation of immunoglobulin production. (From Kryger MH, editor: Pathophysiology of respiration, New York, 1981, John Wiley & Sons, Inc.)

lymphocytes to the site of the immune reaction. In addition, the T lymphocytes produce several chemical mediators that promote a direct cytotoxic effect. This cytotoxic effect is critical in protection against intracellular pathogens, such as viruses and *Pneumocystis carinii*. The cytotoxic effect also functions in both allographic tissue rejection and tumor resistance. Finally, sensitization of the T cells induces a subset of T lymphocytes called T helper cells. These T helper cells are critically important in the development of humoral immunity.

Humoral immunity involves interaction between circulating macrophages, the B lymphocytes, and the T helper cells. Once sensitized to a specific antigen, B lymphocytes synthesize proteins called *immunoglobulins*. Only one kind of immunoglobulin is produced by each lymphocyte, and each immunoglobulin is specific to the original sensitizing antigen.

Immunoglobulins play several key roles in host defense. Some immunoglobulins serve as opsonins, stimulating phagocytic cells to engulf antigenic material. Others can fix complement, thereby initiating a complex series of enzymatic reactions that result in recruiting more phagocytes and lymphocytes to the affected area. Still others simply inhibit bacterial multiplication.

Excessive immune response (allergic reactions)

Allergic reactions represent an excessive or exaggerated response of the immune system against environmental antigens that are not normally harmful. Although such *hypersensitivity* may involve any organ system in the body, we will focus solely on allergic responses of the respiratory system.

Categories of allergic reactions. Allergic or hypersensitivity reactions of the lung may be classified into one of four major types (Table 19-3). Of course, some hypersensitivity states may involve more than one of these categories.

Type I, or immediate-type hypersensitivity, is produced when IgE antibodies fixed to mast cells react with antigens such as pollens, molds, or animal danders (Fig. 19-8). Reexposure to the allergen causes the release of histamine and other mediators of inflammation. This response is characteristic of extrinsic asthma, hay fever, anaphylaxis, and contact dermatitis.

Type II, or cytotoxic hypersensitivity, is mediated by IgG or IgM antibodies. These antibodies react with antigen on target cells and activate complement, causing cellular lysis. Cytotoxic hypersensitivity occurs in Goodpasture's syndrome, poststreptococcal glomerulonephritis, and certain drug reactions.

Type III, or immune complex hypersensitivity, may also be mediated by IgG or IgM antibodies. These antibodies form complexes with antigen and complement and cause the release of mediators that cause local tissue inflammation. Hypersensitivity pneumonitis, rheumatoid arthritis, and certain collagen vascular disorders, such as systemic lupus erythematosus, are examples of this process. In type III allergic responses, prolonged exposure to antigen may result in a chronic inflammatory process and subsequent organ fibrosis.

Type IV hypersensitivity, also known as delayed type or cell-mediated hypersensitivity, is mediated by sensitized T lymphocytes. These T cells react directly with antigen, producing inflammation through the action of lymphokines. The delayed type or cell-mediated hypersensitivity reaction is thought to contribute to acute and chronic transplantation reactions, tuberculosis, sarcoidosis, and other granulomatous diseases.

Examples of allergic reactions. Common examples of hypersensitivity or allergic reactions associated with pulmonary disease are asthma (type I), Goodpasture's syndrome (type II), and hypersensitivity pneumonitis or extrinsic allergic alveolitis (type III). The tuberculin skin test, an example of the type IV hypersensitivity reaction, was previously discussed. Sarcoidosis, also an example of the type IV response, will be described under the section on restrictive disorders.

Asthma. Asthma is a hypersensitivity disorder characterized by reversible airway obstruction, which results from a combination of bronchospasm, mucosal edema, and excessive secretion of viscid mucus (Fig. 19-9). In chronic asthma, there may also be hypertrophy of the bronchial smooth muscle. In combination, these factors cause obstructions to airflow, a maldistribution of ventilation, and hyperinflation.

There are two primary forms of asthma: atopic, or extrinsic, and nonatopic, or intrinsic. Atopic, or extrinsic, asthma represents a type I or immediate-type hypersensitivity reaction to external antigenic material, such as pollens, molds, or animal danders. This form of the disease

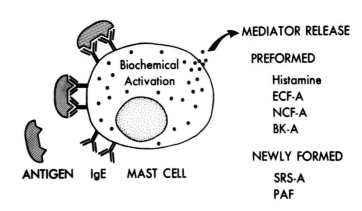

Fig. 19-8   Release of preformed and newly synthesized mediators of inflammation from mast cells. Interaction between antigen and membrane-bound IgE results in biochemical activation and release of mediators from mast cells and circulating basophils. (From Kryger MH, editor: Pathophysiology of respiration, New York, 1981, John Wiley & Sons.)

accounts for about 50% of all asthma cases. The antibodies produced are specific immunoglobulins of IgE. This antigen-antibody reaction releases both vasoactive and bronchoconstrictive chemical mediators, which cause the characteristic tissue changes.

The other half of asthmatic patients suffer from the nonatopic, or intrinsic, form of asthma. In this type of asthma the bronchial reaction occurs in response to nonimmunologic stimuli such as infection, irritating inhalants, cold air, exercise, and emotional upset. Unlike those with atopic asthma, these patients do not demonstrate elevated IgE antibodies in their serum. Apparently, reflex stimulation of the parasympathetic nervous system in susceptible individuals is the major mechanism for this form of asthma.

Regardless of origin, asthma is characterized by recurrent attacks of dyspnea, cough and expectoration of tenacious mucoid sputum, and wheezing. Symptoms may be mild and may occur only in association with respiratory infection, or they may be severe to the point of being life-

Table 19-3   Immunologic Respiratory Diseases

	Mechanism	Examples
Type I	IgE on cell reacts with allergen-releasing mediator	Asthma, hay fever
Type II	IgG or IgM directed against basement membrane; complement activated	Goodpasture's syndrome
Type III	Circulating antigen-antibody complexes deposited in lung; complement activated: inflammatory reaction	Hypersensitivity pneumonitis, collagen vascular diseases
Type IV	Cell-mediated (T lymphocyte) immunity: lymphokines: inflammatory reaction	Tuberculosis, granulomatous diseases

From Kryger MH, editor: Pathophysiology of respiration, New York, 1981, John Wiley & Sons, Inc.

Bronchospasm
Airway edema and infiltration
Mucus Hypersecretion

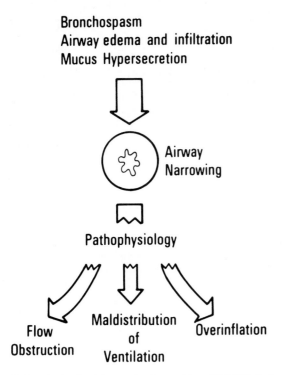

Fig. 19-9 Pathophysiology of asthma. (From Tisi GM: Pulmonary physiology in clinical medicine, ed 2, Baltimore, 1984, Williams & Wilkins Co.)

threatening. Classic atopic asthma usually begins in childhood and becomes progressively more severe throughout life. The acute attack is characterized by dyspnea usually associated with expiratory wheezing that may easily be heard with the naked ear. Cough may or may not be present. Prolonged asthma attacks that do not respond to standard therapeutic measures are known as *status asthmaticus.*

In terms of laboratory testing, the sputum is characteristically tenacious and mucoid, containing "plugs" and "spirals." On microscopic examination of the sputum, eosinophils are numerous. The differential blood count may also show eosinophilia.

Arterial blood gas results will vary, depending on the stage of the attack (Table 19-4). Early in an asthmatic attack, hyperventilation caused by anxiety may cause a slight hyperoxemia, accompanied by hypocapnea. As the attack progresses, the maldistribution of ventilation worsens, causing the arterial Po_2 to fall, despite a continued respiratory alkalosis. Should the attack progress still further, worsening airway obstruction (in combination with an increased work of breathing) causes a rise in the $Paco_2$ and a resulting respiratory acidosis. This last stage of respiratory acidosis is an ominous sign, indicating progression to status asthmaticus and the potential need for intubation and artificial ventilation.

The radiographic examination may show no abnormalities. In severe paroxysms, reversible hyperexpansion may occur. Severe attacks may also be complicated by pneumothorax.

Treatment for asthma may be divided into two phases: (1) treatment of the acute attack and (2) maintenance therapy, which is aimed at preventing further attacks. Drugs of choice for the emergency management of acute asthma include adrenergic agents such as terbutaline, along with the methylzanthines, such as aminophylline. However, for status asthmaticus or for acute attacks in epinephrine-resistant patients, adrenal corticosteroids may be necessary (more details on the drug management of asthma are provided in Chapter 20). Oxygen should be given in sufficient concentration to relieve hypoxemia. Dehydration, if present, must be corrected by intravenous fluid replacement. Arterial blood gases should be monitored every 30 to 60 minutes during the acute phases of an attack.

Depending on the category of asthma diagnosed, maintenance therapy may include corticosteroids, methylxanthines, mast cell inhibitors, or adrenergic agents (see Chapter 20). Desensitization to specific antigens may be useful in some forms of atopic asthma.

Goodpasture's syndrome. Goodpasture's syndrome consists of chronic, relapsing pulmonary hemosiderosis, often in association with fatal glomerulonephritis. Recent elucidation of a type II, or cytotoxic hypersensitivity, immunologic mechanism indicates that the same antibody affects both the alveolar and glomerular basement membranes.

Clinical features of this syndrome include a cough with recurrent hemoptysis, dyspnea, pulmonary infiltration, and iron deficiency anemia resulting from the breakdown of large amounts of hemoglobin into hemosiderin, which deposits in the lungs.

Transbronchial lung biopsy through a flexible fiberoptic bronchoscope (FFB) is a valuable diagnostic procedure. To distinguish this condition from idiopathic pulmonary hemosiderosis, one must demonstrate IgG deposits on the alveolar-capillary membrane by a technique called *immunofluorescence* staining. In addition to the pulmonary pathology, evidence of glomerulonephritis and progressive renal failure is common.

Table 19-4 Arterial Blood Gases in Asthma*

	Stages			
	1	2	3	4
Pao_2	↑	N	↓	↓
$Paco_2$	↓	↓	↓	↑
pH	↑	↑	↑	↓

* ↑, increase; ↓, decreases; N, normal
From Tisi GM: Pulmonary physiology in clinical medicine, ed 2, Baltimore, 1984, Williams & Wilkins Co.

Patients with Goodpasture's syndrome have a poor prognosis. Immunosuppressive treatment with prednisone and cyclophosphamide has been effective in some patients. There are several recent reports of patients with progressive respiratory and renal failure who improved after multiple plasma exchanges, a procedure called *plasmapheresis*. When the principal feature of the disease is renal failure, hemodialysis may be indicated.

Extrinsic allergic alveolitis. Extrinsic allergic alveolitis, or hypersensitivity pneumonitis, results from a type III, or immune complex antigen-antibody, reaction. IgG antibodies are usually present. As delineated in Table 19-5, hypersensitivity pneumonitis is caused by exposure to a variety of organic dusts. Exposure in sensitized individuals causes both an interstitial and alveolar inflammatory process.

Clinically, hypersensitivity pneumonitis is manifested by an acute onset of fever, dry cough, dyspnea, and malaise that occurs 5 to 6 hours after exposure to the offending antigen. Radiographic examination of the chest typically reveals a diffuse, fine granular infiltration. Unlike type I reactions, eosinophilia usually does not occur. A history of exposure is important in making the diagnosis.

Treatment for hypersensitivity pneumonitis consists of cessation of exposure and, if symptoms are severe, a course of corticosteroid treatment. Repeated exposure may result in severe pulmonary fibrosis.

Decreased immune response (immunodeficiency)

Deficiencies in the body's immune response, either humoral or cell-mediated, can compromise its ability to resist infection. Clinical conditions associated with a decreased immune response include alcohol intoxication, diabetes, uremia, hypogammaglobulinemia, and leukocytopenia. Many therapeutic interventions, such as radiation therapy and the use of immunosuppressive drugs, also decrease patients' immune responses. More recently, acquired immune deficiency syndrome (AIDS) has come to our attention as an immune disorder of significant concern and growing magnitude.

Acquired immune deficiency syndrome (AIDS). First recognized in 1981, AIDS is caused by infection with the human T lymphotropic retrovirus, now simply called the human immunodeficiency virus (HIV). HIV directly attacks the T lymphocytes (including the T helper cells) of the immune system. Thus HIV primarily compromises the cell-mediated component of the immune system. However, by virtue of its affect on the T helper cells, HIV also compromises the humoral (antibody) component of host defense.

As of 1989, more than 100,000 cases have been diagnosed in the US, with the number doubling every 12 months. Three population groups account for the vast majority of AIDS cases: homosexual or bisexual men (about 75%), heterosexual men or women who are intravenous drug abusers (about 20%), and hemophiliac adults and children who are not drug abusers (1% or less). AIDS has also been well documented in prison populations, central African immigrants to Europe, heterosexual partners of individuals of either sex who harbor the virus, and children of mothers who are at high risk for the syndrome. Concern over the association between AIDS and the transfusion of blood or blood products has been minimized since the inception of mandatory testing of whole blood and blood products for the HIV virus.

The clinical management of AIDS requires a combination of approaches: preventive, therapeutic, and supportive. Because no current cure exists and mortality currently averages 70% to 90% within 2 years of diagnosis, the main emphasis of management is currently on prevention.

A high priority has been given to the development of a vaccine against HIV, yet some formidable barriers must be

Table 19-5   Hypersensitivity Pneumonitis

Disease	Source of antigen	Precipitins
Air-conditioner and humidifier lung	Fungi in air conditioners and humidifiers	Thermophilic actinomycetes
Aspergillosis	Ubiquitous	*A fumagatis, A flavus, A niger, A nidulans*
Bagassosis (sugarcane workers)	Moldy bagasse	*Thermoactinomyces vulgaris*
Bird fancier's lung	Pigeon, parrot, hen droppings	Serum protein and droppings
Byssinosis	Cotton, flax, hemp workers	Unknown
Farmer's lung	Moldy hay	*Micropolyspora faeni, T vulgaris*
Malt worker's lung	Moldy barley, malt dust	*A clavatus, A fumigatus*
Maple-bark pneumonitis	Moldy maple bark	*Cryptostroma corticale*
Mushroom worker's lung	Mushroom compost	*M faeni, T vulgaris*
Sequoiosis	Moldy redwood sawdust	*Graphium aurea basidium pullalans*
Wheat weevil disease	Infested wheat flour	*Sitophilus granarius*

From Mitchell RS: Synopsis of clinical pulmonary disease, ed 4, St Louis, 1988, The CV Mosby Co.

overcome before this preventative approach can become a reality. Until this time, prevention must involve more traditional public health interventions. These methods include antibody testing to protect blood and organ recipients and education programs about the dangers of intravenous drug abuse and safer sexual practices. Recommendations for preventing the spread of HIV within the hospital are discussed in Chapter 14.

Therapy for patients with AIDS can be divided into two categories: treatment aimed at the HIV infection itself and treatment aimed at the secondary infections and malignant disorders. The first drug that directly treats HIV infection, AZT (azidothymidine, or zidovudine), has been approved by the FDA for treatment of AIDS patients who have a history of cytologically confirmed *Pneumocystis* pneumonia and of patients with AIDS or AIDS-related complex (ARC) who have a T4 lymphocyte count of less than 200 cells/mm^3. Unfortunately, as many as one third of all AIDS patients exhibit significant side effects (anemia and granulocytopenia) to AZT, necessitating reduction or discontinuation of the drug or blood transfusion. Investigations are under way on other drugs that have in vitro activity against the virus, such as dideoxycytidine, ribavirin, HPA23, and suramin.

The other therapeutic consideration in AIDS is the treatment of the secondary infections and malignant diseases, which account for most of the morbidity and mortality of AIDS. About 66% of adults with AIDS have *P carinii* pneumonia (PCP), about 25% have Kaposi's sarcoma, about 14% have *Candida* esophagitis, and 7% suffer from infection with the cytomegalovirus (CMV). Two key points underlie the treatment of these secondary problems: (1) prompt diagnosis and early institution of therapy are essential and (2) prolonged or indefinite therapy is usually required.

The pulmonary manifestations of AIDS are most commonly caused by PCP. The diagnosis of PCP is usually not made initially unless the patient comes from a group at risk for AIDS. The best diagnostic results are obtained by lung biopsy, in which the cysts typical of *P carinii* are revealed in impression smears of lung tissue stained with methenamine-silver. Bronchoalveolar lavage is also useful in this regard.

Symptoms of PCP may be insidious, with only exertional dyspnea. In children, however, PCP usually exhibits a fairly sudden onset with high fever, severe dyspnea, and cough. There may also be chest pain, a variable amount of sputum production, and lymphadenopathy. Although the chest radiograph may be normal, it usually reveals diffuse densities of alveolar or interstitial type. Arterial blood gas analysis will usually show a large $P(A-a)O_2$, indicating the presence of physiologic shunting.

Current drug treatment of PCP consists of either trimethoprim sulfamethoxazole or pentamidine isethionate, both by IV. In mid-1989, the FDA also gave final approval for pentamidine administration by aerosol.

Other pulmonary infections associated with AIDS include those of viral origin (CMV and the Epstein-Barr virus), fungal infections (cryptococcosis, aspergillosis, histoplasmosis, and coccidioidomycosis), and tuberculosis. A peculiar form of mycobacterial infection caused by *Mycobacterium avium intracellulare* is also seen in AIDS patients. Other lung infections seen in AIDS include those caused by *H influenzae* and *S aureus*. In addition, there have been isolated reports of *Nocardia, L pneumophila, Toxoplasma gondii,* and *Cryptospordium* organisms. In every case, the response to treatment of these infections is poor.

The final aspect of clinical management is social and supportive. Besides the economic cost, the personal and social costs of AIDS are immense. In an attempt to address these emerging problems, the Health and Public Policy Committee of the American College of Physicians (in conjunction with the Infectious Disease Society of America) has recently published a position paper of importance to all health professionals involved with AIDS patients (see Bibliography).

INHALATIONAL LUNG DISEASES

Inhalational lung diseases are caused by the inhalation of organic or inorganic dusts, or noxious fumes and chemicals. Diseases caused by exposure to organic dusts (hypersensitivity pneumonitis) were previously discussed. Our focus here will be on the lung's reaction to inorganic dusts and noxious fumes and chemicals.

Inhalation of inorganic dusts (pneumoconioses)

A pneumoconiosis represents any change in the lung caused by the inhalation of an inorganic dust. As indicated in the box on p. 429, a host of inorganic material may be inhaled into the lungs. Some of these, such as iron and tin, cause little or no tissue reaction and are thus categorized as "inert" pneumoconioses. Others, such as silica, provoke a tissue reaction and are classified as "active" pneumoconioses.

Silicosis. In most cases, the inhalation of free silica (silicon dioxide) is responsible for silicosis. Other silica-containing compounds, such as bauxite or the silicates, may also be responsible. Depending on the intensity of exposure, silicosis may become evident in as few as 18 months or take as long as 30 years to develop.

Clinically, symptoms may be absent. More commonly, the patient will exhibit a history of unusual susceptibility to upper respiratory tract infections, "bronchitis," and pneumonia. The most common complaint is dyspnea on exertion. Initially, the cough may be dry, but later becomes productive, frequently with blood-streaked sputum. Severe, occasionally fatal, hemoptysis may occur. Physical findings may be absent in patients with advanced sili-

---

COMMON PNEUMOCONIOSES

Inert pneumoconioses
  Iron: siderosis
  Tin: stannosis
  Barium: baritosis
  Cement
  Fiberglass
  Talc
Active pneumoconioses caused by silica or silica content
  (ie, fibrosis and other pathology producing)
  Silica
  Silicates, including kaolin
  Diatomaceous earth
  Asbestos
  Bauxite
Active pneumoconioses without silica
  Aluminum and aluminum oxide
  Coal
  Graphite
  Nickel carbonyl
  Tungsten carbide
  Beryllium
  Cadmium
  Cerium

From Mitchell RS: Synopsis of clinical pulmonary disease, ed 4, St Louis, 1988, The CV Mosby Co.

cosis. Lung biopsy is occasionally indicated to establish diagnosis for insurance compensation.

Although not firmly diagnostic, the radiographic exam can strongly suggest the diagnosis. Abnormalities are usually bilateral, symmetric, and predominantly in the hilar region. Small nodules tend to be of uniform density and size. Enlargement of hilar lymph nodes occurs early in the progression of the disease. Interstitial fibrosis is manifested by fine linear markings and reticulation.

Unfortunately, there is no definitive treatment available for silicosis or for any of the pneumoconioses. Prevention, by careful regulation of the workplace environment, is the only way to reduce the incidence of these disorders. Symptomatic or supportive treatment is indicated for chronic cough and wheezing.

Other representative pneumoconioses. Asbestosis and coal workers' pneumoconiosis (CWP) are among the most common pneumoconioses other than silicosis. Asbestosis is caused by the inhalation of hydrous silicates of various metals in fibrous form, whereas CWP is caused by exposure to coal dust, consisting mainly of carbon. Clinically, patients with these disorders exhibit symptoms similar to silicosis. Neoplastic complications of asbestosis include bronchogenic carcinoma and pleural mesothelioma. As with silicosis, both conditions can lead to a progressive, massive fibrosis.

Inhalation of noxious fumes and chemicals

Among the hundreds of noxious fumes or chemicals capable of producing a pathologic response in the lung, carbon monoxide, nitrogen dioxide, and sulfur dioxide are the most common. Accidental exposure to high concentrations of these gases can cause acute injury to the lung. A good example is silo-filler's disease.

Silo-filler's disease is a pulmonary disease caused by inhalation of nitrogen dioxide and sulfur dioxide fumes emanating from agricultural silos that have been freshly filled. These noxious fumes cause an increase in capillary permeability, resulting in a form of pulmonary edema.

The initial phase, appearing promptly after exposure, consists of cough, dyspnea, and weakness. This may progress or be followed by a decrease in symptoms, which may then reappear and become progressively worse. Diffuse crackles (rales) and rhonchi are heard, and the chest radiograph shows bilateral fluffy infiltrates that may coalesce into dense areas of pulmonary edema. Supplementary oxygen and ventilatory support may be necessary to correct the resulting hypoxemia. The mortality rate can be as high as 30%.

PULMONARY NEOPLASMS

Pulmonary neoplasms may be broadly divided into those that are benign and those that are malignant. The most common benign pulmonary neoplasm is bronchial adenoma, while the bronchogenic carcinoma is the most common malignancy of the respiratory tract.

Bronchial adenoma

Bronchial adenomas arise from the glandular structures of the bronchial mucous membranes and account for about 80% of all benign bronchopulmonary tumors.

The majority of bronchial adenomas arise in the proximal bronchi. The primary symptoms, cough and localized wheeze, are similar to those found in bronchogenic carcinoma. Bronchial adenomas typically are vascular, accounting for the high incidence (25% to 30%) of hemoptysis. Since bronchial adenoma does not tend to exfoliate, examination of the sputum is not helpful. Treatment is by resection, usually via lobectomy. The prognosis for patients with bronchial adenomas is good.

Bronchogenic carcinoma

Bronchogenic carcinoma is the most common intrathoracic malignancy, arising from the mucosa of the bronchial tree. It occurs predominantly in men and may appear at any age, although most cases occur in the cancer age group (over 40). The importance of hereditary and environmental factors in the etiology of bronchogenic carcinoma is not known. However, the disease is relatively rare in nonsmokers.

Bronchogenic carcinoma is characterized by a persistent

nonproductive cough, hemoptysis, and localized persistent wheeze. These clinical findings are associated with the bronchial irritation, erosion, and partial obstruction caused by the developing tumor. Some patients may be asymptomatic.

Pulmonary infections occurring distal to the bronchial obstruction, such as pneumonia or lung abscess, frequently dominate the clinical picture and can mask the underlying neoplasm. If the lesion is large enough, there may be physical and radiographic signs of partial or complete bronchial obstruction with associated atelectasis and infection.

Early detection and surgical removal before metastasis occur offer the only hope of cure. A positive diagnosis of bronchogenic carcinoma can be made in 40% to 60% of cases on the basis of sputum cytology. Ideally, several fresh specimens should be studied. More recently, forceps or brush biopsy obtained under fluoroscopic guidance through the flexible fiberoptic bronchoscope (FFB) provides the diagnosis in 75% to 80% of bronchial tumor cases. The American Cancer Society does not recommend routine chest x-ray studies as the basis for detection of early lung cancers.

RESTRICTIVE DISORDERS INVOLVING THE RESPIRATORY SYSTEM

Restrictive lung disease represents a broad category of disorders with widely variable causes that share a common denominator, that is, a reduction in lung volume. As summarized in the box below, there are five major categories of restrictive lung disease: skeletal/thoracic, neuromuscular, pleural, interstitial, and alveolar. In addition, a number of commonly used drugs can interfere with neuromuscular transmission.

CATEGORIES OF RESTRICTIVE PULMONARY DISORDERS

CATEGORY	EXAMPLES
Skeletal/thoracic	Kyphoscoliosis
	Ankylosing spondylitis
CNS/neuromuscular	Cord transection
	Amyotrophic lateral sclerosis
	Guillain-Barré syndrome
	Myasthenia gravis
Pleural	Effusion/empyema
	Pneumothorax
	Hemothorax
Interstitial	Sarcoidosis
	Pneumoconiosis
Alveolar	Pneumonia
	Pulmonary edema

Fig. 19-10 depicts the major pathophysiologic features of these categories of restrictive lung disease. As is evident, all restrictive disorders lower lung volumes; however, only the interstitial and alveolar forms result in a decrease in lung compliance. A decrease in lung compliance, in turn, causes a maldistribution of ventilation, increased work of breathing, increased airway caliber, and increased expiratory flow rates.

Skeletal and thoracic disorders

Among the most common restrictive conditions in this category are kyphoscoliosis, ankylosing spondylitis, and severe obesity.

Kyphoscoliosis. Kyphosis is a condition in which the normal posterior curve of the spine is exaggerated. Scoliosis represents abnormal lateral curvature of the spine. Patients with kyphoscoliosis can develop pulmonary problems because of lung compression inside a distorted rib cage (Fig. 19-11). Chronic pulmonary compression can lead to recurrent bronchial infections and, in extreme cases, respiratory failure.

Depending on the severity of the condition, patients may have normal lung function or show varying degrees of pulmonary restriction. Blood gas measurements are variable, but the Pao_2 may be reduced from lung compression and the resulting low $\dot{V}/\dot{Q}$ ratios, especially at the lung bases. $Paco_2$ levels are frequently not elevated, except in the terminal stages of the condition, as with frank respiratory failure.

Treatment is directed at preventing or minimizing recurrent infections and relieving any clinically significant hypoxemia. Periodic hyperinflation, using intermittent positive pressure breathing, has proven successful in the short term in increasing lung compliance. In selected patients, surgery may help to reverse the abnormal spine curvature.

Ankylosing spondylitis. Ankylosing spondylitis is a condition occurring mainly in men in which the vertebral bodies and the costovertebral joints become fused, causing a dramatic decrease in thoracic wall compliance. However, because good, uniform diaphragmatic movement is retained, TLC and VC are only slightly reduced, and the effects on ventilation are minor. Fibrocystic changes in the upper portions of the lung are apparent in some patients with ankylosing spondylitis.

Obesity. For many years, severe obesity was considered a pure mechanical restriction to ventilation, caused by the greatly increased mass of the thorax and abdomen. However, as shown in Fig. 19-12, we now know that obesity can be but a component of a more general syndrome, consisting of chronic hypercapnia and hypoxemia in combination with sleep apnea and decreased respiratory center responsiveness to CO_2. Common complicating factors, attributable mainly to chronic hypoxemia, include polycythemia, pulmonary vascular hypertension, and cor pulmonale. Because of its similarity to Charles Dickens'

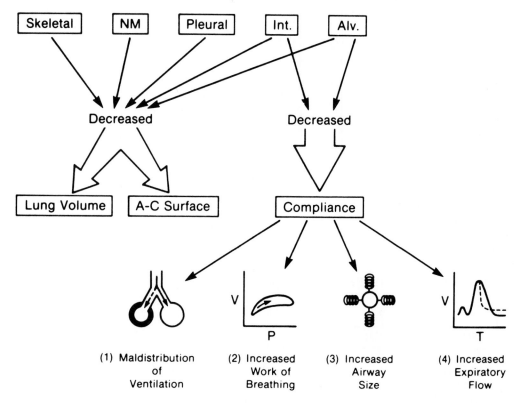

Fig. 19-10   Pathophysiology of restrictive lung disease. (From Tisi GM: Pulmonary physiology in clinical medicine, ed 2, Baltimore, 1984, Williams & Wilkins Co.)

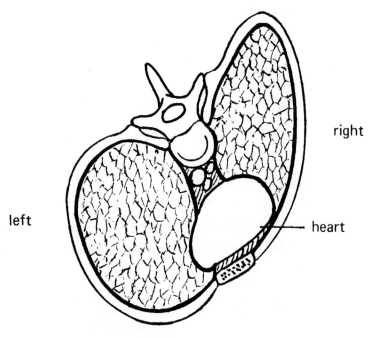

Fig. 19-11   Changes in the thorax resulting from scoliosis. Scoliosis results in rotation of the spine along its longitudinal axis, which in turn causes marked deformity of the rib cage. (From Farzan S: A concise handbook of respiratory diseases, ed 2, East Norwalk, Conn, 1985, Appleton & Lange.)

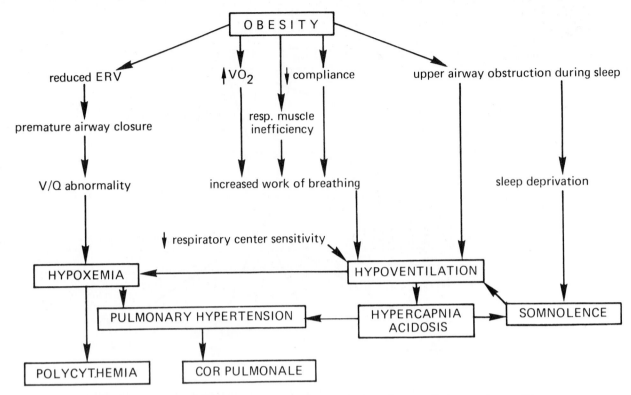

Fig. 19-12   Pathogenesis and pathophysiology of obesity—hypoventilation syndrome. (From Farzan S: A concise handbook of respiratory diseases, ed 2, East Norwalk, Conn, 1985, Appleton & Lange.)

description of the fat boy in the Pickwick Papers, this condition is often referred to as the "pickwickian syndrome."

Weight reduction appears to reverse the abnormality. Oral progesterone therapy has been reported to stimulate ventilation in some patients. Rarely, if weight reduction cannot be accomplished and episodes of sleep apnea are severe, tracheostomy may be necessary. More recently, continuous positive airway pressure (CPAP) by nose has been used to alleviate nocturnal airway obstruction (see Chapters 28 and 35).

Neuromuscular conditions

Processes that interfere with the transmission of central neural output to the respiratory muscles can also result in restrictive impairments. Included in this category are disorders of the spinal cord, peripheral nerves, neuromuscular junctions, and respiratory muscles themselves. Some diseases in this category, such as poliomyelitis, can involve both the central respiratory control mechanism and the peripheral neuromuscular apparatus. Characterizing all these abnormalities is an inability to generate normal respiratory pressures, either automatically or intentionally.

These neuromuscular disorders have several characteristics in common. Although the FRC is maintained near normal levels, inspiratory muscle weakness causes a decrease in both the IRV and TLC. On the other hand, expiratory muscle weakness results in an increased RV. Both the VC

and the maximum inspiratory force (MIF; also called maximum inspiratory pressure, or P_{Imax}) are diminished.

Because muscle strength and VC can diminish substantially before producing respiratory failure, the presence of severe hypoxemia and hypercapnia in these conditions indicates either extreme progression of the primary process or the effects of complications such as atelectasis. In the presence of reasonable inspiratory muscle function, the existence of hypoxemia and/or hypercapnia suggests the presence of a complication rather than progression of the primary restrictive process. In acute neuromuscular disorders, this latter distinction makes monitoring of MIF superior to serial VC measurements, because VC may be diminished in either case (see Chapter 31).

Neuromuscular disorders that persist for long periods of time are associated with chronic decreases in the compliance of both the lung and thorax. Decreases in lung compliance may be caused by microatelectasis, altered surfactant activity, or mild fibrotic changes resulting from recurrent infections. These secondary disorders cause a mismatching of $\dot{V}/\dot{Q}$ and may lead to a hypoxemia greater than that expected from hypoventilation alone. Decreases in the compliance of the chest wall are probably a result of gradual stiffening of the costochondral and costovertebral joints and to fibrotic changes or spasticity of the respiratory muscles.

The decrease in lung volume that occurs in chronic neuromuscular disorders is caused by the combined effects of muscle weakness and secondary alterations in the mechanical properties of the lung and chest wall. Hence, for chronic disease, measurement of VC is a more important indicator of the total effect of the disorder than is the assessment of MIF.

In contrast with the mechanical disorders of the thoracic cage, in which an effective cough is usually well preserved, the expiratory muscle weakness characterizing neuromuscular disorders precludes development of a forceful cough. In cervical spinal cord injuries, paralysis of the abdominal and intercostal muscles prevents spontaneous coughing altogether. Because such patients are unable to produce an effective cough, even minor causes of increased airway secretions may result in major respiratory complications. For this reason, pneumonia is a common problem in patients suffering from neuromuscular disorders, and respiratory failure resulting from pneumonia is a frequent cause of death in this group.

In the absence of major complications, the patient with neuromuscular involvement often breathes substantially faster than the decrease in V_T would demand. Sometimes this results in an increase in minute ventilation. Thus, early in the course of the illness, the $Paco_2$ may be lower than normal. The basis for the tachypnea is probably microatelectasis, which also accounts for the mild arterial hypoxemia commonly observed in these patients. Microatelectasis is probably the result of the patient's inability to sigh, which results in changes in alveolar surface forces and an increased tendency for alveolar collapse.

In progressive disorders, as muscle weakness worsens, V_T decreases and dead space ventilation per minute increases. This results in alveolar hypoventilation and a worsening hypoxemia. At this point, the decision whether to provide artificial ventilatory support must be made. Ultimately, the long-term outcome of this approach will depend on the nature of the neuromuscular process and on the potential for specific treatment.

Diaphragmatic paralysis. In the absence of pulmonary complications, neuromuscular disorders rarely progress to the point of respiratory failure unless diaphragmatic weakness or paralysis is present. Because diaphragmatic paresis, or paralysis, represents the end result of all neuromuscular disorders, it is not usually considered a separate clinical entity. However, certain forms of diaphragmatic paralysis have unique clinical features. For this reason, we will discuss these problems separately.

Bilateral diaphragmatic paralysis. Bilateral phrenic nerve interruption can result in complete diaphragmatic paralysis. The most prominent clinical symptom of complete diaphragmatic paralysis is orthopnea. In the supine posture, the weight of the abdominal contents pushes the patient's diaphragm up into the thorax. Negative pressure generated by the intercostal muscles pulls the diaphragm further into the thorax during inspiration, producing a paradoxic inward motion of the upper abdomen with thoracic expansion. This paradoxic motion impairs the normal distribution of ventilation to the lung bases, resulting in gas exchange abnormalities that predispose to atelectasis and hypoxemia.

In the upright position, patients often experience a dramatic increase in VC, improvement in gas exchange, and alleviation of most symptoms. In this position, the weight of the abdominal contents offsets the negative intrapleural pressures, and the diaphragm no longer rises with inspiration.

Unilateral diaphragmatic paralysis. Most cases of unilateral diaphragmatic paralysis are the result of tumors invading the phrenic nerve. This condition may also be caused by compression or destruction of the phrenic nerve by surgery, trauma, or thoracic aneurysms. Isolated phrenic neuropathy or an acute infectious neuritis may also cause diaphragmatic paralysis, which in these cases is usually permanent. There is no effective treatment for permanent unilateral diaphragmatic paralysis. Reversible unilateral diaphragmatic paralysis is a rare complication of acute pneumonias, but may commonly occur following cardiac surgery.

Patients with unilateral diaphragmatic paralysis typically exhibit a 15% to 20% reduction in both VC and TLC in the upright posture, with greater impairment in the supine position. Nonetheless, in the absence of other disease, most patients with unilateral diaphragmatic paralysis remain asymptomatic.

Since patients with unilateral diaphragmatic paralysis normally have no major symptoms, this condition is most often diagnosed by x-ray film. Typically, the paralyzed side maintains its normal contour but is displaced upward. On fluoroscopy, the paralyzed hemidiaphragm may descend somewhat on inspiration, mimicking normal muscle contraction. However, with a sudden forceful inspiration (the so-called "sniff" test), the paralyzed side rises further into the thorax, opposite to the direction of the normal side. This paradoxical motion is caused by the sudden increase in intraabdominal pressure and the sudden fall in intrapleural pressure that occurs during the sniff.

Spinal disorders. The two most common restrictive conditions involving the spinal column are functional transection and disorders of the anterior horn cells.

Functional transection. Functional transection of the spinal cord is most often caused by motor vehicle trauma or diving accidents. Transection at or above the level of the fourth cervical nerve segment (C-4) results in complete cessation of all respiratory muscle activity. Transection below this level still allows for use of the diaphragm, but only the diaphragm.

In patients whose respiration depends solely on diaphragmatic activity, as with some quadriplegics, the expulsive phase of the cough (which requires contraction of the expiratory muscles) cannot be generated. Moreover, lacking the stabilizing influence of the contracting intercostal muscles, the upper rib cage of the patient breathing solely with the diaphragm moves inward during inspiration, instead of expanding outward. The result is a diminished VT. Should portions of the lower cervical segments remain intact, there will be some accessory muscle activity and less paradoxic motion. Paradoxic motion will also diminish over time as the condition becomes chronic from stiffening of the thorax.

When the quadriplegic patient is in the upright posture, the weight of the abdominal contents pulls downward on the diaphragm. The abdominal muscles, having lost their tone, cannot oppose this action, and the diaphragm shortens. Thus, in the upright posture, the effectiveness of the quadriplegic's diaphragm is markedly diminished and platypnea may result. Abdominal binders can be used to offset this loss of abdominal muscle tone and should be considered whenever the patient's VT falls when moved to the upright position.

Anterior horn cell involvement. Poliomyelitis used to be the most common cause of impaired anterior horn cell function. Although sporadic cases of poliomyelitis still occur in the US, amyotrophic lateral sclerosis (ALS) is now the most common cause of anterior horn cell dysfunction and its resultant respiratory muscle weakness.

Respiratory symptoms generally do not occur until late in the course of ALS. Respiratory failure may not be anticipated until an episode of bronchitis or aspiration pneumonia produces an acute complication. Supportive measures during the acute incident often return the patient to a stable condition. However, in most patients, respiratory failure caused by diaphragmatic involvement proves fatal within 3 to 4 years of diagnosis.

Diseases affecting the peripheral motor nerves. The peripheral nerves may be affected by a variety of toxic agents, inflammatory processes, vascular disorders, malignancies, and assorted metabolic and nutritional imbalances.

Polyneuritis. Polyneuritis is the general term denoting the widespread sensory and motor disturbances of peripheral nerves associated with these disorders. It may appear at any age, although it is most common in young or middle-aged men. Clinically, polyneuritis is characterized by the slow development of pain, tenderness, paresthesia, weakness, fatigability, and sensory impairment over a period of weeks. Typically, muscular weakness is greatest in the distal portions of the extremities. Tendon reflexes are usually depressed or absent. Flaccid weakness and muscular atrophy of affected parts may occur.

Guillain-Barré syndrome. In Guillain-Barré syndrome, patients often develop polyneuritis 1 to 2 weeks after a mild upper respiratory infection or episode of gastroenteritis. Less frequently, Guillain-Barré syndrome may occur in patients recently immunized against viral infections. The etiology of this disorder is unknown. However, recent research suggests that either a hypersensitivity or autoimmune response of the nerves may be responsible. This response is believed to lead to demyelination of the nerves and a mononuclear inflammatory reaction.

Clinically, early lower extremity weakness progresses within a few days to the upper extremities and face. Facial diplegia, dysphagia, or dysarthria may occur. Sensory changes usually are not present, but muscle tenderness and nerve sensitivity to pressure may occur. Weakness of trunk and extremity muscles may be severe, including flaccid paraplegia and marked respiratory muscle weakness. At the height of the disorder, the cerebrospinal fluid usually shows a very high protein content with few or no white cells, an anomaly called "albuminocytologic dissociation."

The treatment of patients with Guillain-Barré syndrome is usually symptomatic. Recently, plasmapheresis has been used, but with limited success. Respiratory insufficiency that requires ventilatory support develops in about one in four of all patients with Guillain-Barré syndrome. The duration of ventilatory support averages 6 to 8 weeks, but periods of up to 30 months have been reported in the literature. Approximately 30% of patients receiving ventilatory support can be extubated within two weeks. The mortality rate for the Guillain-Barré syndrome is less than 5%, with the majority of survivors recovering completely. A minority have persistent weakness and continue susceptible to recurring episodes of respiratory failure in association with respiratory infections.

Abnormalities of neuromuscular transmission. Abnormalities of neuromuscular transmission affect respiration by impairing the chemical activity occurring between the motor end-plate and skeletal muscle cells. Myasthenia gravis is the classic example of this type of abnormality in neuromuscular transmission. Botulism and tetanus also affect the chemical activity occurring between the motor end-plate and skeletal muscle, thereby impairing respiratory muscle activity.

Myasthenia gravis. Myasthenia gravis is the most common disorder impairing neuromuscular transmission, affecting mainly women between the ages of 20 to 30. Although almost any muscle group in the body may be affected, the disease tends to have a special affinity for muscles innervated by the bulbar nuclei, including those of the face, lips, eyes, tongue, throat, and neck. The cause of myasthenia gravis is unknown. However, current evidence suggests that the primary mechanism is an autoimmune process resulting in rapid inactivation of acetylcholine at the myoneural junction.

Clinically, the patient with myasthenia gravis exhibits pronounced fatigability of muscles, with consequent weakness and paralysis. Weakness of the extraocular muscles is apparent as diplopia and strabismus. Ptosis of the eyelids may become evident, especially late in the day. Speech and swallowing difficulties can occur after prolonged exercise of these functions. In patients with long-standing myasthenia, myopathy with severe diaphragmatic paresis may develop and lead to chronic respiratory failure.

In most cases the diagnosis of myasthenia gravis is obvious from the history and physical findings. The diagnosis may be confirmed using the tensilon (edrophonium) test. Tensilon is a quaternary ammonium salt that exerts a direct stimulant effect on the neuromuscular junction. Intravenous injection of 10 mg tensilon relieves weakness caused by myasthenia gravis within 20 to 30 seconds of administration.

In most patients, initial treatment consists of anticholinesterase drug therapy with neostigmine methylsulfate. Subcutaneous or IM injection of neostigmine methylsulfate results in prompt relief of symptoms within 10 to 15 minutes, which lasts up to 4 hours. Encouraging short-term results have also been reported with the use of large amounts of adrenocorticotropic hormone (ACTH). Long-term ACTH injections and long-term oral prednisone have also been used with some success in chronic myasthenia. Beneficial effects in some patients have been reported upon surgical removal of the thymus gland.

A sudden onset of respiratory failure may occur as a result of an acute episode of the basic disease process (myasthenic crisis) or the excessive use of anticholinergic drugs (cholinergic crisis). Respiratory failure may also follow initiation of ACTH or corticosteroid therapy. In the myasthenic crisis, mortality may be reduced by withdrawing anticholinesterase medications for approximately 72 hours after onset of respiratory difficulty and instituting positive pressure ventilatory support through an artificial airway.

Botulism. Botulism is a type of food poisoning caused by ingestion of the toxin produced by *Clostridium botulinum,* an anaerobic spore-forming bacillus that habitates the soil. In humans, the source of the toxin is usually vacuum-packed foods that spoil, especially home-canned vegetables, smoked meats, and vacuum-packed fish.

The botulism toxin blocks the release of acetylcholine at the motor end-plate of skeletal muscle, causing muscular paralysis. Clinically, the patient begins to exhibit visual disturbances, a dry throat and mouth, dysphagia, and dysphonia within 12 to 36 hours after ingestion of the toxin. Nausea and vomiting may occur with some types of toxin. Progressive muscle weakness responds to the tensilon (edrophonium) test in a manner similar to myasthenia. Left untreated, the progressive muscle weakness leads to respiratory failure, with a mortality rate between 30% and 70%. Dysphagia may also result in aspiration pneumonia, with its associated high mortality.

Diagnosis is by identification of the toxin in the patient's sera or in suspected foods. Once diagnosed, the US Centers for Disease Control can assay the toxin type and provide a type-specific antitoxin. Supportive measures include maintenance of adequate ventilation and oxygenation, usually by mechanical ventilatory support.

Tetanus. Tetanus is an acute disorder of the nervous system caused by fixation of the *Clostridium tetani* endotoxin. Like *C botulinum, C tetani* is an anaerobic spore-forming bacillus found in the soil. It may also be recovered from the feces of animals. Typically, the organism enters the body through puncture wounds, although it may also infect purulent necrotic lesions. The tetanus endotoxin acts on both the motor end-plate and the anterior horn cells of the spinal cord and brainstem.

The average incubation period for *C tetani* is 8 to 12 days after exposure. Early symptoms may be limited to pain and tingling at the wound site, with some spasticity of the local muscles. Progressive stiffness of the jaw and neck muscles usually follows, accompanied by dysphagia and irritability. Later, the patient exhibits hyperreflexia, with spasms of the muscles of the jaw (trismus), face, neck, abdomen, and back. Painful tonic convulsions, with glottic and respiratory muscle spasms, are frequently seen. These convulsions can cause complete airway obstruction and asphyxia.

Tetanus is readily prevented by immunization. Once diagnosed, tetanus is treated with tetanus immune globulin or tetanus antitoxin. Supportive measures for mild cases include bed rest with minimal stimulation and sedative and anticonvulsant drug therapy (chlorpromazine or diazepam). More severe cases require the establishment of an artificial airway, preferably via tracheotomy. Mechanical ventilatory support may also be necessary, with some patients requiring muscle paralysis with curare. Overall mortality with tetanus averages about 40%; however, patients surviving the acute episode usually exhibit full recovery.

Disorders of the muscles. The two most common disorders of the muscles causing pulmonary restriction are muscular dystrophy and polymyositis.

Muscular dystrophy. Muscular dystrophies represent a group of hereditary disorders characterized by progressive degeneration of the skeletal muscles, resulting in severe muscle weakness. The most common form is pseudohypertrophic, or Duchenne's muscular dystrophy. Because Duchenne's muscular dystrophy occurs primarily as a result of an X-linked recessive trait, this disorder predominantly affects males. Other forms have an autosomal mechanism of inheritance and are therefore seen in both sexes.

Patients with muscular dystrophy are predisposed to pulmonary complications; respiratory failure is a frequent cause of death. Inspiratory muscle weakness, which typically develops late in the progression of the disease, results in chronic alveolar hypoventilation. Chronic alveolar hypoventilation may also appear in patients with adequate muscle strength, suggesting that their disease may involve a defect in the central respiratory control mechanism. Expiratory muscle weakness may impair coughing in some patients; the accompanying weakness of the muscles used to swallow can lead to aspiration and recurrent pneumonias.

Polymyositis. Polymyositis is a chronic inflammatory disease that affects the striated muscles. If associated with involvement of the skin, the disorder is known as dermatomyositis. In addition to the striated muscles and skin, other organs may be affected, including the lung and heart. A type IV (delayed type or cell-mediated) hypersensitivity reaction may be responsible for this disorder.

Clinically, the patient with polymyositis exhibits progressive weakness of the skeletal muscles of the extremities, as well as the cervical, pharyngeal, and trunk muscles. Direct involvement of the lungs in the disease process may result in inflammation and fibrosis. However, the primary respiratory complications are caused by respiratory muscle weakness and difficulties in swallowing. For this reason, pneumonia is the most common cause of death in these patients. Corticosteroids and immunosuppressive drugs appear to slow progression of the disease but increase the incidence of pulmonary infections by opportunistic organisms.

Drugs. A number of commonly used drugs interfere with neuromuscular transmission, thereby causing pulmonary restriction. Three different mechanisms may be involved. Anesthetic-like action at the presynaptic level may be caused by drugs such as clindamycin or propranolol. Postsynaptic, or curare-like, action has been observed with lincomycin, polymyxin B, chloroquine, and procainamide. Also, stabilization of the postsynaptic membranes may occur with antibiotics such as gentamicin, streptomycin, or neomycin.

Delayed recovery from anesthesia or difficulty in withdrawing a patient from ventilatory support suggests a possible drug effect. Patients affected by these drugs often have mild or latent myasthenia. Concurrent electrolyte disturbances, especially hypokalemia, hypocalcemia, or hypomagnesemia, can enhance these drug effects and contribute to muscle weakness in myasthenic patients. Respiratory failure is especially likely in patients with antibiotic-induced postoperative muscle weakness. Treatment of these patients involves maintenance of the artificial airway, positive pressure ventilatory support, correction of associated electrolyte disturbances, and withdrawal of the offending drug agent.

Pleural disorders

Pleural disorders can result in restriction either through direct pathologic involvement of the pleural membranes themselves or as a result of space-occupying lesions. Pleurisy is an example of the former; pleural effusion, empyema, pneumothorax, and hemothorax are examples of the latter.

Pleurisy. Pleurisy is a condition characterized by abnormal deposits of a fibrinous exudate on the pleural surface. Pleurisy is seldom a disease process itself, but rather a complicating factor of other disorders, such as pneumonia, pulmonary infarction, and pulmonary neoplasms. Pleurisy may also precede the development of some pleural effusions. "Pleuritic" chest pain, or pain that intensifies during inspiration, is the primary symptom. Referred pain may also occur. A pleural friction rub, with its characteristic grating sound, is usually heard on auscultation. Splinting

of the involved side of the chest is also common and usually accompanied by shallow respirations. Often, the patient will lie on the painful side. Treatment is aimed at resolving the underlying disease process.

Pleural effusion. A pleural effusion is defined simply as the abnormal collection of fluid in the pleural space. As shown in Fig. 19-13, the normal balance of oncotic and hydrostatic forces between the systemic and pulmonary microcirculations in the pleural space favors the continuous movement of fluid from the parietal to the visceral pleural capillaries. Abnormal amounts of plasma fluid may accumulate in the pleural space when either hydrostatic pressures increase or oncotic pressures decrease. Abnormal fluid originating in this manner is called a *transudate*.

Alternatively, inflammatory processes, infiltrative diseases, or tumors may cause fluid accumulation in the pleural space without upsetting the balance of oncotic and hydrostatic forces. Abnormal pleural fluid originating in this manner is called an *exudate*. Exudates may be distinguished from transudates by their higher protein content. The box below differentiates between the common disease

---

DISEASES ASSOCIATED WITH EXUDATIVE AND TRANSUDATIVE PLEURAL EFFUSIONS

EXUDATES	TRANSUDATES
Malignancy	Congestive heart failure
Carcinoma	Hypoproteinemic states,
Mesothelioma	including
Lymphoma	Nephrotic syndrome
Infection	Liver cirrhosis
Parapneumonic	Pneumothorax
Tuberculosis	Atelectasis
Fungal	Pulmonary embolism
Viral	(some cases)
Collagen-vascular	Peritoneal dialysis
Systemic lupus	Meigs' syndrome (benign
Rheumatoid arthritis	ovarian tumor)
Pulmonary embolism	
(some cases)	
Pancreatitis	
Subphrenic abscess	
Uremia	
Asbestosis	
Chylothorax	
Traumatic hemothorax	
Esophageal rupture	
Drug-induced effusion	
Postradiation therapy	
Sarcoidosis	
Idiopathic (undiagnosed)	

From Martin L: Pulmonary physiology in clinical practice: the essentials for patient care and evaluation, St Louis, 1987, The CV Mosby Co.

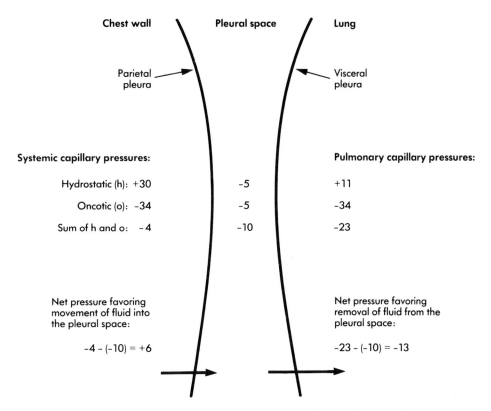

Fig. 19-13   Normal pleural fluid movement. A physiologic balance between the systemic and pulmonary capillaries provides for continuous movement of fluid from parietal pleura capillaries into the pleural space and then into visceral pleura capillaries. All pressures are in cm H_2O. Pressures that tend to force fluid out of the capillaries are shown by a plus sign (+); pressures that act to hold fluid in the capillary or pleural space are assigned a minus sign (−). There is a net +6 cm H_2O pressure favoring fluid movement into the pleural space. In this diagram the surfaces are shown apart, but in healthy people they touch, separated only by a thin (and radiologically invisible) film of pleural fluid. (From Martin L: Pulmonary physiology in clinical practice: the essentials for patient care and evaluation, St Louis, 1987, The CV Mosby Co.)

processes causing either of these two primary types of pleural effusions.

Clinically, the patient with a pleural effusion may be asymptomatic. In other cases, chest or referred shoulder pain may be present. Depending on the severity of the effusion, dyspnea may range from mild to severe. Based on the underlying cause, fever, sweat, cough, and expectoration may also be present. On physical examination, decreased motion of the chest, decreased to absent breath sounds, decreased to absent vocal fremitus, a flat percussion note, and egophony may be noted on the affected side. With large effusions, the mediastinum may shift away from the fluid, as indicated by displacement of the trachea and the cardiac apex. However, underlying atelectasis may cause a shift toward instead of away from the fluid.

In general, the fluid volume must be at least 300 ml before a pleural effusion becomes evident on normal x-ray study. Obliteration of the costophrenic angle is the earliest sign of pleural effusion. Movement of the fluid shadow, which "pours" into dependent areas of pleural space when the patient is placed on the involved side, may be helpful in demonstrating small effusions.

Definitive diagnosis of pleural effusion is made by thoracentesis (Fig. 19-14). In addition to providing a definitive diagnosis of pleural effusion, thoracentesis also provides samples for study, which are useful in identifying the underlying cause.

Treatment of pleural effusion must be directed at resolution of the primary disease process. When necessary, a small amount of fluid can be removed by therapeutic thoracentesis. However, when the amount of fluid is large, or it continues to accumulate despite treatment of the primary disease process, chest tube drainage may be necessary. A typical three-bottle chest drainage system is shown in Fig. 19-15. The amount of suction (usually −20 cm H_2O) is controlled by the depth to which a tube open to the atmosphere is inserted in the suction control bottle, which is connected to a negative pressure source. The middle bottle provides a water seal, which prevents air from "backtracking" in the system, should it fail. The third bottle is used for collection of pleural fluid. Commercially avail-

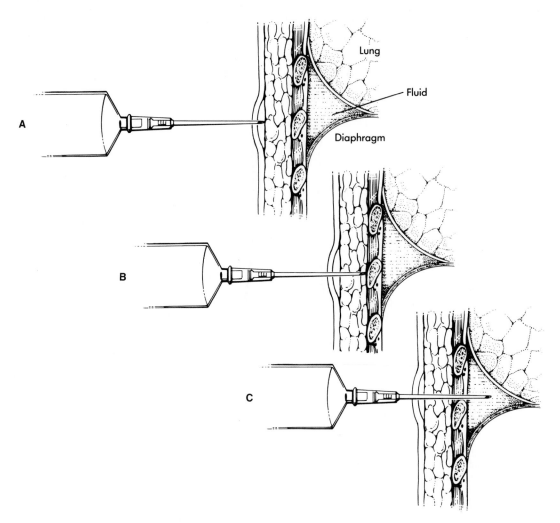

Fig. 19-14   Technique of thoracentesis. **A,** Using a small-bore needle (0.25 gauge), the skin is injected with local anesthetic. **B,** With a larger needle (0.22 gauge), local anesthetic is injected into the periosteum of the rib. **C,** With the aspirating needle (0.22 gauge or larger), the pleural space is entered, and fluid is removed. (From Martin L: Pulmonary physiology in clinical practice: the essentials for patient care and evaluation, St Louis, 1987, The CV Mosby Co.)

able systems incorporate all these components, but do so in a single, disposable apparatus.

Pleural empyema.   When pleural fluid is purulent or contains pyogenic organisms, the term pleural empyema applies. Pleural empyema may result from the (1) direct spread of a bacterial pneumonia, (2) rupture of a lung abscess into the pleural space, (3) invasion from a subdiaphragmatic infection, or (4) traumatic penetration. The most common infectious agents are anaerobic bacteria, *Staphylococcus, Streptococcus,* and certain gram-negative bacteria. Although the clinical findings may be obscured by the underlying disease process, pleural pain and fever, in conjunction with the physical and x-ray signs of pleural effusion, are characteristic. Thoracentesis reveals a purulent exudate from which the causative organism may be cultured. As with lung abscess, empyema may become chronic.

Pneumothorax.   Pneumothorax is a condition in which air enters the pleural space. This air may originate either from inside the lungs (through the airways) or from outside the lungs (through the chest wall). The box on p. 439 summarizes the major causes of pneumothorax.

Clinically, a small pneumothorax may go unnoticed. Pain may be experienced when the pneumothorax occurs, especially if parietal pleural irritation accompanies the air leak. With a large pneumothorax, the patient may appear acutely dyspneic. On physical examination, chest expansion is reduced, the percussion note is increased in resonance, breath sounds are absent, and tactile fremitus is absent over the pneumothorax. The diagnosis can be confirmed by chest radiograph.

In tension pneumothorax, positive pressure develops in the pleural space, causing compression of the affected lung. In this case, the trachea and mediastinal contents

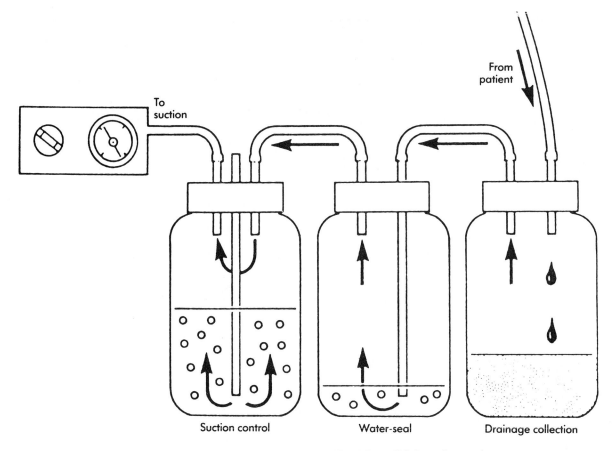

Fig. 19-15   Three-bottle pleural drainage system. (From Luce JM: Intensive respiratory care, Philadelphia, 1984, WB Saunders Co.)

POTENTIAL CAUSES OF PNEUMOTHORAX

1. Air in the pleural space from the airways
   a. Idiopathic—occurs spontaneously without apparent reason: presumably caused by rupture of clinically inapparent bleb, cyst, or bulla
   b. Rupture or tear of esophagus or other mediastinal structure into the pleural space.
   c. Chronic lung disease (most commonly from severe emphysema, asthma, or interstitial fibrosis)
   d. Positive pressure ventilation, particularly with use of positive end-expiratory pressure (see Chapter 10)
   e. Infection, tumor, or foreign body causing a bronchopleural connection
2. Air in the pleural space from outside the chest wall
   a. Trauma
   b. During thoracentesis or pleural biopsy
   c. During insertion of central venous catheter

From Martin L: Pulmonary physiology in clinical practice: the essentials for patient care and evaluation, St Louis, 1987, The CV Mosby Co.

---

shift away from the affected side. Compression of the mediastinum can disrupt cardiac filling, resulting in a rapid fall in blood pressure and shock.

Because the gas pressure in a pneumothorax is greater than that in the pleural venous system, reabsorption of air in the pleural space can occur spontaneously. For this reason, many small pneumothoraces resolve without treatment. Reabsorption of pleural air can be expedited by administration of oxygen. By removing nitrogen from the blood, oxygen administration dramatically lowers total venous gas pressures, thereby enhancing gas movement from the pleural space into the pleural capillaries. Large pneumothoraces, particularly those resulting in pressure build-up in the pleural space, are usually treated by chest tube drainage, as previously described.

Hemothorax. Hemothorax is a condition characterized by pooling of blood in the pleural space. Although most commonly associated with thoracic trauma, hemothorax may also occur with tumors, tuberculosis, and pulmonary infarction. The physical findings of hemothorax are the same as those described for pleural effusion. Experience with military casualties has shown that early removal of all blood from the pleural space is desirable. Although this may be accomplished by thoracentesis, chest tube drainage is usually necessary.

ETIOLOGIES OF THE INTERSTITIAL AND ALVEOLAR RESTRICTIVE LUNG DISEASES

Infectious	Gram-negative and -positive pneumonias; tuberculosis; coccidioidomycosis; viral pneumonias; opportunistic pneumonia secondary to *P carinii* or cytomegalic inclusion virus
Neoplastic	Lymphangitic carcinoma; bronchoalveolar carcinoma; leukemic infiltration; Hodgkin's
Thromboembolic	Fat emboli; Lipoidal embolization
Cardiovascular	Cardiogenic and non-cardiogenic pulmonary edema
Mixed connective tissue	Rheumatoid lung; lupus erythematosus; scleroderma
Inhalational	*Organic dusts*—farmer's lung; bagassosis; pigeon breeder's disease; maple bark disease
	Inorganic dusts—silicosis; asbestosis; coal worker's pneumoconiosis; siderosis; berylliosis
	Toxic—smoke inhalation; oxygen toxicity; aspiration pneumonia
Airway disease	Bronchiolitis obliterans (small airway disease)
Idiopathic granulomas	Sarcoidosis; eosinophilic granuloma; Wegener's granulomatosis; Goodpasture's syndrome
Drug toxicity	Busulfan; methotrexate; oxygen; nitrofurantoin
Idiopathic interstitial fibrosis	Usual interstitial pneumonia; desquamative interstitial pneumonia

From Tisi GM: Pulmonary physiology in clinical medicine, ed 2, Baltimore, 1984, Williams & Wilkins Co.

Interstitial and alveolar restrictive disorders

The last major category of restrictive disorders are those caused by interstitial or alveolar disease processes. Interstitial pulmonary disease processes predominantly involve inflammatory or fibrotic changes in the connective tissue of the lungs. Alveolar disease processes, on the other hand, affect primarily the alveolar-capillary epithelial region. Given the fact that portions of the terminal respiratory unit contain connective tissue, many of these disorders functionally affect both the alveolar epithelium and its surrounding connective tissue. The box above summarizes the ten major categories of interstitial and alveolar disorders that can result in pulmonary restriction. Many of these processes, such as those associated with infections, neoplasms, and the inhalation of organic or inorganic dusts, have already been discussed. The contribution of thromboembolic and cardiovascular disorders to pulmonary restriction will be addressed in the next section.

CARDIOPULMONARY VASCULAR DISORDERS

Although the respiratory care practitioner is primarily responsible for the treatment of disorders of the respiratory system, the physiologic interrelationship between the heart, vasculature, and lungs often necessitates an integrated clinical approach to disorders characterizing these organ systems. For this reason, we will look first at cardiac failure in general, followed by a discussion of pulmonary disorders associated with the cardiovascular system. Next, we will investigate the origin, pathophysiology, and management of one of the most severe manifestations of

cardiovascular failure—shock. Finally, we look at cardiopulmonary diseases associated with various embolic disorders.

Cardiac failure

Cardiac failure initially may involve failure of either the left or right ventricle alone. However, combined failure of both ventricles of the heart is generally the rule, especially after salt and water retention occur.

As indicated in the box on p. 441, there are two primary categories of disorders associated with ventricular failure: (1) those caused by myocardial weakness or inflammation and (2) those caused by excessive ventricular work load.

Left ventricular failure. Left ventricular failure is most commonly caused by hypertension, coronary heart disease, or cardiac valve disorders, specifically those associated with the aortic valve. Although less common, left ventricular failure may also be caused by disorders of the mitral valve, hypertrophic cardiomyopathy, congestive cardiomyopathy, left-to-right shunts, congenital heart defects, and certain drugs. Finally, infectious endocarditis may directly cause left ventricular failure or may simply aggravate the problems associated with other valve diseases.

Left ventricular failure is characterized predominantly by its symptoms: exertional dyspnea, cough, fatigue, and nocturia. Exertional dyspnea is caused by pulmonary venous congestion and the resultant decrease in lung compliance. This exertional dyspnea typically worsens when the patient assumes a recumbent position, resulting from increased pulmonary vascular engorgement. Paroxysmal nocturnal dyspnea (PND), often with a dry cough, may ap-

---

ETIOLOGY OF VENTRICULAR FAILURE

MYOCARDIAL WEAKNESS OR INFLAMMATION
Coronary artery disease
Myocarditis
Congestive cardiomyopathies
Drugs

EXCESSIVE WORK LOAD
Increased resistance to ejection (afterload)
    Hypertension
    Stenosis of aortic or pulmonary valves
    Hypertrophic cardiomyopathy
Increased stroke volume
    Aortic insufficiency
    Mitral insufficiency
    Tricuspid insufficiency
    Congenital left-to-right shunts
Increased body demands
    Hypoxemia
    Anemia
    Thyrotoxicosis
    Pregnancy
    Arteriovenous fistula

---

pear at any time. PND is best associated with left ventricular failure caused by severe hypertension, aortic stenosis or insufficiency, or myocardial infarction. Of course, the dyspnea of left ventricular failure must be differentiated from other common conditions causing shortness of breath on exertion or positional change. These conditions include chronic pulmonary disease, obesity, severe anemia, ascites, abdominal distention caused by gastrointestinal disease, and the advanced stages of pregnancy.

When present, nocturia is attributed to the enhanced excretion of accumulated edema fluid that occurs as renal perfusion increases in the recumbent position. Nocturia may also reflect the decreased work of the heart at rest and the delayed effects of diuretics given during the day.

Besides the symptoms of the underlying disease process, physical examination of the patient with left ventricular failure usually discloses signs of left ventricular hypertrophy, specifically an increased strength and leftward and downward displacement of the apical impulse. A gallop rhythm, pulsus alternans, and an accentuated pulmonary component of the second sound (P_2) may or may not be present. Likewise, physical signs of pleural effusion, though common, may not always be present.

The chest radiograph usually will reveal evidence of pulmonary venous congestion, such as increased blood flow to the upper lobes, and Kerley B lines. Left ventricular enlargement will normally be apparent on x-ray film, except when the left ventricular failure is a result of acute myocardial infarction or a cardiac arrhythmia. Left atrial enlargement is apparent in the case of mitral stenosis.

Right ventricular failure. The most common causes of right ventricular failure are mitral stenosis, pulmonary vascular hypertension, stenosis of the pulmonary valve, and right ventricular myocardial infarction (in association with inferior myocardial infarction). Less common causes of right ventricular failure are tricuspid valve disease and infectious endocarditis involving the right side of the heart.

Right ventricular failure is characterized predominantly by its signs. Anorexia, bloating, and right upper abdominal pain are common, reflecting hepatic and visceral congestion secondary to elevated venous pressure. Often, one can observe an elevated jugular venous pressure, sometimes accompanied by an abnormal systolic pulsation. The jugular venous pressure can be estimated by noting the extent of jugular filling during expiration above the clavicles with the patient sitting up at a 45-degree angle.

The liver is enlarged (hepatomegaly) and may be tender. Dependent edema usually subsides overnight in the early stages of this disorder, but eventually persists and worsens in severity. Pleural effusion, if it occurs, is more common on the right side. Coolness of the extremities and peripheral cyanosis of the nail beds, caused by reduced peripheral blood flow, may be noted. Sinus tachycardia is usually present, and a right ventricular S_3 sound may be heard.

In pure right ventricular failure, the ECG indicates right ventricular hypertrophy. On radiographic examination of the chest, both right atrial and right ventricular enlargement may be seen. However, specific chamber enlargement on x-ray film is difficult to define when the right ventricular failure is secondary to left ventricular failure.

General treatment of ventricular failure. Treatment of ventricular failure is directed at the underlying cause. Supportive therapy usually includes concurrent efforts to decrease myocardial work load, increase the force and efficiency of myocardial contraction, and reduce the retention of sodium and water.

Decrease myocardial work load. Rest (either in bed or sitting in a chair) decreases the work of the heart and promotes diuresis. Oxygen therapy can also reduce myocardial work load, especially when hypoxemia is present. When left ventricular failure is associated with both a high left ventricular filling pressure (more than 20 mm Hg) and low cardiac output, vasodilator therapy can improve myocardial performance by reducing the impedance to left ventricular output, or afterload.

Increase myocardial contractility. In patients with atrial fibrillation and a rapid ventricular rate, digitalis or one of its derivatives may be used to slow AV conduction, thereby prolonging diastolic filling time and increasing cardiac output. Digitalis is less effective in hypertrophic states such as cardiomyopathy. In acute myocardial infarc-

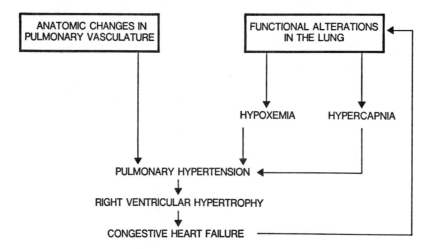

Fig. 19-16   Mechanisms of pulmonary hypertension and congestive heart failure from cor pulmonale. (From Burrows B, Knudson RJ, and Kettrl LJ: Respiratory insufficiency, Chicago, 1975, Year Book Medical Publishers.)

tion, more potent inotropic agents, such as dobutamine, are indicated (see Chapter 22).

Remove sodium and water. Dietary restriction of sodium may be useful but depends on the severity of the failure. Sodium diuresis is most easily accomplished with diuretics. Furosemide (Lasix) and ethacrynic acid, potent diuretics with a short duration of action, may be necessary in acute conditions. Unfortunately, these agents, especially the thiazide diuretics, can cause significant potassium loss. For this reason, aldosterone antagonists such as spironolactone, which causes sodium diuresis without potassium loss, are useful. Spironolactone can be combined with thiazides to neutralize their potassium-wasting effect.

Cardiopulmonary and pulmonary vascular disorders

Distinct from pure cardiac failure, a number of disorders clearly involve the lung, heart, and pulmonary vasculature together. These conditions include cor pulmonale, pulmonary edema, and pulmonary vascular hypertension.

Cor pulmonale. Cor pulmonale refers to right ventricular failure caused by pulmonary parenchymal or vascular disease. Typically, the patient has pre-existing chronic bronchitis or pulmonary emphysema, with their characteristic signs and symptoms. Less common causes include pneumoconiosis, pulmonary fibrosis, kyphoscoliosis, and the pickwickian syndrome. Singly or in combination, obliteration of the pulmonary capillary bed, interstitial or alveolar fibrosis, and chronic hypoxemia increase pulmonary artery pressure, leading to right ventricular hypertrophy and, eventually, right ventricular failure (Fig. 19-16).

Cor pulmonale may be acute, subacute, or, most commonly, chronic. Thus the clinical features of cor pulmonale depend on both the primary disease and its effects on the heart. The dominant symptoms of chronic cor pulmonale are respiratory and include chronic productive cough, exertional dyspnea, wheezing, and fatigability. As with

right ventricular failure in general, dependent edema and right upper quadrant pain may appear. Signs of chronic cor pulmonale include cyanosis, clubbing, distended neck veins, right ventricular heave or gallop, prominent lower sternal or epigastric pulsations, and hepatomegaly. However, unless the patient is in shock, pulses are full and the extremities warm.

As with right ventricular failure in general, the electrocardiogram will typically indicate right ventricular hypertrophy, including tall, peaked P waves with right axis deviation and deep S waves in lead V_6. However, left axis deviation and low voltage may be noted in patients with pulmonary emphysema. Arrhythmias are frequent and nonspecific.

The chest x-ray film will show an enlarged right ventricle, often accompanied by an engorged pulmonary artery circulation. Depending on the cause, interstitial or alveolar disease may also be apparent on the chest film.

In terms of laboratory findings, polycythemia is common. Typically, arterial blood gas analysis reveals an arterial oxygen saturation below 85%, with an elevated P_{CO_2}.

Right ventricular failure may be differentiated from left ventricular failure by its history (of respiratory disease), the absence of orthopnea, the greater severity of cyanosis, the presence of bounding pulses, and the observation of warm extremities in the presence of edema.

Pulmonary edema. Pulmonary edema represents a condition in which excessive amounts of plasma enter the pulmonary interstitium and alveoli. Because acute pulmonary edema is normally accompanied by severe respiratory distress, tachypnea, and hypoxemia, it is considered a medical emergency. Appropriate treatment of pulmonary edema depends on proper identification of the underlying cause.

As in the pleural space, there normally exists a balance of oncotic and hydrostatic forces at the alveolar-capillary region that prevents fluid accumulation in the interstitial

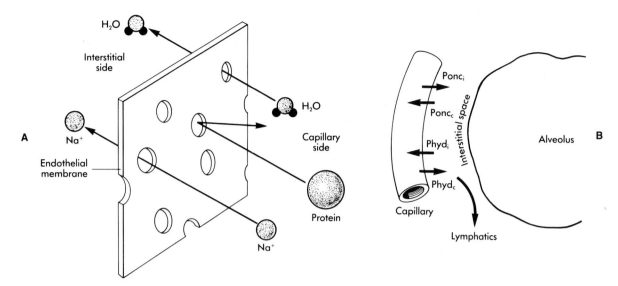

Fig. 19-17   **A,** Fluid transport from capillary to interstitial space. The intact endothelial membrane is permeable to water and to small solutes (eg Na^+) but is impermeable to protein. In noncardiogenic pulmonary edema, proteins leak through the damaged membrane, flooding the interstitium and alveolar spaces. **B,** Balance of colloid and hydrostatic forces in pulmonary capillary. Colloid osmotic pressure is normally closely balanced against capillary hydrostatic pressure. Capillary hydrostatic pressure favors movement of fluid out of the capillary and is opposed by the hydrostatic pressure in the interstitial fluid. Colloid osmotic pressure of the plasma proteins tends to keep fluid in the capillary and is opposed by the osmotic pressure of proteins in interstitial fluid. The exact pressures (oncotic and hydrostatic) within the pulmonary capillary are not known for sure, but the net result is a slight and continuous leak of fluid out of the capillaries and into the pulmonary interstitium, where it is picked up by interstitial lymphatics. It is estimated that lymph flow from the lung is approximately 10 to 20 m/min. When this balance of forces is upset so that fluid movement overwhelms lymphatic drainage, pulmonary edema results. $Phyd_c$, Hydrostatic pressure in pulmonary capillary; $Phyd_i$, hydrostatic pressure in pulmonary interstitium; $Ponc_o$, oncotic pressure in pulmonary capillary; $Ponc_i$, oncotic pressure in pulmonary interstitium. (Redrawn from Martin L: Pulmonary physiology in clinical practice: the essentials for patient care and evaluation, St Louis, 1987, The CV Mosby Co.)

Table 19-6   Mechanisms in the Pulmonary Capillary That Influence Movement of Fluid into the Pulmonary Interstitium

Mechanism	Normal	Factor favoring excess fluid movement	Common clinical cause	Type of pulmonary edema
Hydrostatic pressure	6 to 12 mm Hg*	Increased value	Left ventricular failure	Cardiac
Oncotic pressure	20 to 25 mm Hg†	Decreased value	Liver cirrhosis	Noncardiac
Membrane permeability	—	Increased permeability	ARDS	Noncardiac

*Measured as pulmonary artery wedge pressure.
†Oncotic pressure can be qualitatively assessed by measurement of serum total protein or albumin, each of which correlates with the measured oncotic pressure. A low oncotic pressure is rarely, if ever, a sole cause of pulmonary edema; however, it is definitely a contributor factor in presence of another mechanism.
From Martin L: Pulmonary physiology in clinical practice: the essentials for patient care and evaluation, St Louis, 1987, The CV Mosby Co.

area (Fig. 19-17). Pulmonary edema occurs when this balance is upset, either by an increase in hydrostatic pressure, a decrease in oncotic pressure, or an increase in the permeability of the capillary endothelial membrane (Table 19-6). Pulmonary edema caused by an increase in pulmonary hydrostatic pressures is classified as *cardiogenic* pulmonary edema. Pulmonary edema caused by either a decrease in oncotic pressure or an increase in the permeability of the capillary endothelial membrane is categorized as *noncardiogenic* pulmonary edema.

Cardiogenic pulmonary edema. Cardiogenic pulmonary edema may be caused by any disorder that elevates pulmonary capillary hydrostatic pressure sufficiently to cause fluid transudation into the alveolar interstitium or alveoli.

Acute left ventricular failure is the most common cause of cardiogenic pulmonary edema. For this reason, both the causes and clinical manifestations of cardiogenic pulmonary edema are similar to those previously described for left ventricular failure in general. However, the respiratory signs and symptoms in acute cardiogenic pulmonary edema are more severe. Typically, the patient is extremely dyspneic and tachypneic. Hypoxemia is usually evident on visual inspection as central cyanosis. Diffuse crackles and wheezes may often be so prominent as to make cardiac auscultation difficult.

The treatment of cardiogenic pulmonary edema aims at decreasing left ventricular and pulmonary vascular pressures. Elevating patients to the semi-Fowler's position or placing them in a chair decreases venous return to the heart. Morphine sulfate, given either intravenously or intramuscularly, relieves anxiety, increases venous compliance, and decreases left ventricular preload. Oxygen, administered in as high a concentration as possible, relieves dyspnea and, by alleviating hypoxemia, lowers pulmonary vascular resistance. Tourniquets, applied with sufficient pressure to obstruct venous but not arterial flow and rotated every 15 minutes, also decrease venous return. As much as 700 ml of blood may be trapped in the extremities by this method.

Diuresis via furosemide (Lasix) or ethacrynic acid is useful because of the potent and prompt diuretic action of these drugs. If abnormally high left ventricular afterload is a contributing factor, vasodilator therapy should be employed, using agents such as hydralazine (Apresoline) or prazosin (Minipress). Rapid digitalization is also of value in most patients.

Noncardiogenic pulmonary edema. Pulmonary edema, in the absence of underlying cardiac disease and arising in previously healthy individuals, can be caused by (1) certain drugs, such as nitrofurantoin or heroine, (2) the inhalation of smoke and other toxic substances, and (3) rapid ascent to a high altitude. Pulmonary edema may also occur in some patients after severe central nervous system trauma. This so-called *neurogenic* pulmonary edema is probably caused by a reflex stimulation of the adrenergic portion of the autonomic nervous system, causing a rapid shift of blood from the systemic to the pulmonary circulation.

However, the most common cause of acute noncardiogenic pulmonary edema is damage to the alveolar-capillary membrane and the resultant increase in permeability of this membrane to both water and serum proteins. Damage to the alveolar-capillary membrane can be caused by a host of factors, all resulting in a severe disturbance in oxygen transfer from the alveoli into the pulmonary capillaries. These conditions, characterized by massive pulmonary capillary leakage with normal hydrostatic pressure, are grouped together under the rubric of the adult respiratory distress syndrome (ARDS). Details on the causes, clinical manifestations, and treatment of ARDS are provided in Chapter 28.

Pulmonary hypertension. Pulmonary hypertension is a condition characterized by abnormally high pulmonary artery pressures. Clinically, pulmonary hypertension exists when the mean pulmonary artery pressure exceeds 22 mm Hg.

Table 19-7 summarizes the major causes of pulmonary hypertension and their underlying mechanisms. Lung and heart disease, in conjunction with hypoxemia, are the primary causes. Treatment of pulmonary hypertension is directed at the underlying cause; for example, reversal of left ventricular failure or relief of hypoxemia.

However, one form of this disorder, called idiopathic or primary pulmonary hypertension, occurs in the absence of any other disease of the lungs or heart. Pathologically, primary pulmonary hypertension is characterized by diffuse narrowing of the pulmonary arterioles without obvious reason. The clinical picture is similar to that of pulmonary

Table 19-7 Causes of Pulmonary Hypertension

Disease or condition	Underlying mechanism(s)
Lung diseases, including all forms of restrictive and obstructive lung conditions	Hypoxemia: loss of pulmonary blood vessels; acidosis
Heart disease, including left ventricular heart failure, mitral valve disease, congenital heart disease	Increased pulmonary capillary hydrostatic pressure
Pulmonary thromboembolic disease	Pulmonary artery narrowing; loss of pulmonary blood vessels
Pulmonary arteritis	Pulmonary artery narrowing: loss of pulmonary blood vessels
High altitude	Hypoxemia
Hypoventilation	Hypoxemia; acidosis
Chest wall deformity	Hypoxemia, acidosis: pulmonary artery narrowing
Idiopathic	Loss of pulmonary blood vessels: pulmonary artery narrowing

From Martin L: Pulmonary physiology in clinical practice: the essentials for patient care and evaluation, St Louis, 1987, The CV Mosby Co.

hypertension from any other cause. Patients exhibit evidence of progressive right ventricular failure and low cardiac output with weakness and fatigue. Edema and ascites become evident as the disorder progresses. Peripheral cyanosis is present, and syncope may occur with exertion. Late in the course of the disease, thrombi may develop as a result of the chronic low output failure, predisposing the patient to pulmonary embolism.

Previously, there was no effective treatment for primary pulmonary hypertension. However, recent studies using a variety of oral vasodilators have shown promising results. These agents include phentolamine, nitrates, hydralazine, and selected calcium channel blockers. Of these agents, hydralazine and the calcium channel blocker, niphedipine (Procardia), are probably the most effective.

Shock

Shock is a condition in which perfusion to vital organs is inadequate to meet their metabolic needs. There are five general types of shock: hypovolemic, cardiogenic, septic (both hyperdynamic and hypodynamic), anaphylactic, and neurogenic. Table 19-8 differentiates these categories according to their typical cardiopulmonary manifestations.

Although these states differ substantially in terms of underlying cause and cardiopulmonary response, all shock states, at least in their severe forms, have common features.

Common features of shock. Features common to most forms of shock are certain endocrine and organ system responses. Typically, these are protective responses designed to assure continued perfusion to the vital organs.

Endocrine responses. Typically, the catecholamines, both epinephrine and norepinephrine, are elevated during shock. Elevation of catecholamine levels represents a protective response designed to assure continued perfusion to the vital organs. In the case of hemorrhagic shock, increased catecholamine levels also promote hemostasis by facilitating blood coagulation. Although the catecholamines dominate the other hormones released during shock, their effects may be overcome by other factors.

All forms of shock also stimulate the release of ACTH from the pituitary gland, thereby increasing plasma levels of the glucocorticoids. The glucocorticoids may have a mild inotropic effect on the heart and may stabilize cell membranes, thereby decreasing the movement of fluid from the intravascular space into the interstitium.

In most forms of shock, aldosterone levels are also elevated. Increased levels of aldosterone occur because of both the increased ACTH levels and the increased activity of the renin-angiotensin system. Decreased renal blood causes the release of renin from the kidneys, with the eventual production of angiotensin II. Angiotensin II causes vasoconstriction and stimulates the synthesis and release of aldosterone from the adrenal cortex. Aldosterone causes the kidneys to conserve sodium and water, while facilitating the excretion of both potassium and hydrogen ions. Water conservation in shock is also enhanced by release of an antidiuretic hormone (ADH) via stimulation of the baroreceptors.

Organ system responses to shock. In response to shock the kidneys conserve both sodium and water, via both the hormonal mechanisms just described and by the intrinsic regulatory properties of the tubules themselves. The brain responds to shock with release of hormones such as ACTH, ADH, and the endorphins. In shock states the heart exhibits a decrease in myocardial contractility, caused by both decreased concentrations of calcium and increased levels of endorphins. Cardiac function during shock is further compromised by either (1) decreased venous return (as in hypovolemic, hypodynamic septic, and neurogenic shock), (2) increased afterload (as in hypovolemic, hypodynamic septic, and cardiogenic shock), and (3) decreased coronary blood flow in all but hyperdynamic septic shock.

The lungs respond to shock with increased extravasation of protein and water into the interstitium, which may cause interstitial and alveolar pulmonary edema. As previously discussed, the increased extravasation of fluids in cardiogenic shock is caused by increased pulmonary vascular hydrostatic pressures. On the other hand, the increased extravasation of protein and water in septic and neurogenic shock is caused by increased capillary permeability.

Pulmonary edema, caused by cardiogenic or hypovolemic shock, is easily cleared once the underlying problem is resolved. However, the pulmonary edema occurring with septic and neurogenic shock is less readily cleared. In these cases the lungs stiffen and compliance decreases. Since perfusion of flooded alveoli continues, $\dot{V}/\dot{Q}$ becomes mismatched, resulting in a decreased Pao_2, an increased shunt fraction, and an increased $P(A-a)o_2$.

Other responses. Shock can lead to disseminated intravascular coagulation (DIC), a condition characterized by platelet aggregation and fibrin deposition, with formation

Table 19-8   Cardiopulmonary Response in Shock

Type of shock	Pulmonary artery pressure	Systemic vascular resistance	Cardiac output
Hypovolemic	Decreased	Increased	Decreased
Septic (hyperdynamic)	Increased or decreased	Decreased	Increased
Septic (hypodynamic)	Decreased	Increased	Decreased
Cardiogenic	Increased	Increased	Decreased
Neurogenic	Decreased	Decreased	Increased or decreased
Anaphylactic	Decreased	Decreased	Increased or decreased

of thrombi throughout the microvasculature. Thrombi in the microvasculature further complicate the patient's microcirculatory status and may worsen the supply of oxygen and other nutrients to the tissues.

Hypovolemic shock. Hypovolemic shock is caused by a decrease in intravascular fluid volume, with a resultant decrease in both cardiac output and tissue perfusion. The decreased intravascular fluid volume may be caused by hemorrhage, vomiting, diarrhea, or fluid sequestration (functional loss) in the bowel, peritoneal cavity, or interstitium.

In the early stages of hypovolemic shock, blood is diverted from organs that withstand ischemia well (such as the skin and skeletal muscle) to organs that withstand ischemia poorly (such as the kidneys, brain, and heart). At this early stage of hypovolemic shock, the patient's mental status, pulse, blood pressure, and respiratory rate may all be normal. However, careful examination typically will reveal postural changes in blood pressure, skin temperature (cool and clammy), neck vein size (flattened), and concentrated urine.

As hypovolemia worsens, blood flow to the brain and heart eventually becomes insufficient to meet their metabolic needs. The patient may be anxious, agitated, confused, combative, or obtunded. Even in the supine position the blood pressure is below normal. Typically, the pulse is rapid, weak, and irregular, and the breathing pattern is deep and rapid.

Cardiogenic shock. Cardiogenic shock may be caused by myocardial disease, valvular disease, increased afterload, mechanical obstruction to venous return, or arrhythmias. Clinical signs and symptoms are essentially those of severe acute left ventricular failure. As with hypovolemic shock, the patient may be anxious, agitated, confused, combative, or obtunded. Typically, the patient has a rapid pulse, low blood pressure, and is tachypneic. Pulsus paradoxus may be present if the cause of the problem is pericardial tamponade. Unlike all other forms of shock, the neck veins are distended. Urine output is characteristically low.

Septic shock. Septic shock is caused by bacteria in the blood stream (bacteremia). The most common offenders are the gram-negative organisms associated with nosocomial infections. Among the most frequent events predisposing to gram-negative bacteremia and septic shock are urinary tract infections, artificial tracheal airways, IV-related thrombophlebitis or contamination, postoperative infections, infected burns, and severe neutropenia, as may occur with cancer. The mortality rate for gram-negative sepsis is often over 50%.

Sepsis may result in one of two forms of shock: hyperdynamic or hypodynamic. Often, hyperdynamic shock occurs first, followed by the more severe state of hypodynamic septic shock.

Hyperdynamic septic shock. In hyperdynamic septic shock, the patient may be agitated or somnolent. Typical signs include a fever; a rapid, bounding, and strong pulse; a normal or slightly decreased blood pressure; and tachypnea. The skin usually is flushed, warm, and dry; the neck veins are normal. Urine output is adequate, but if the pathologic process continues, fluid is lost from the blood compartment into the interstitial and cellular spaces, resulting in progression to hypodynamic septic shock.

Hypodynamic septic shock. Hypodynamic septic shock represents a severe state of sepsis that manifests itself much like hypovolemic shock. The patient may be disoriented, agitated, or somnolent. The patient exhibits a normal or subnormal temperature, a rapid and weak pulse, a low blood pressure, and a rapid respiratory rate. The skin is cold and clammy, neck veins are flat, and urine output is low. There may be evidence of metabolic acidosis or respiratory alkalosis and DIC. Left untreated, hypodynamic septic shock greatly impairs organ perfusion to the kidney, brain, and heart, resulting in anuria, nitrogen retention, acidosis, circulatory collapse, and, eventually, death.

Anaphylactic shock. An anaphylactic reaction is an immediate and frequently fatal shock-like response that occurs within minutes after administration of foreign sera or drugs, especially penicillin and aspirin. Other drugs that can induce anaphylaxis are immune antisera such as tetanus antitoxin; protein-based drugs such as chymotrypsin and streptomycin; water-soluble iodine radiographic contrast media; and certain vaccines.

Symptoms of anaphylactic shock include apprehension, paresthesias, generalized urticaria or edema, choking, cyanosis, wheezing, coughing, incontinence, low blood pressure, fever, dilation of pupils, loss of consciousness, and convulsions. Death may occur within 5 to 10 minutes.

Neurogenic shock. Neurogenic shock is caused by generalized loss of vasomotor tone, as may occur in spinal cord trauma, severe gastric dilatation, sudden pain, or the administration of a high spinal anesthetic. This leads to inadequate cardiac output and poor tissue perfusion. Typically, a patient suffering from neurogenic shock has a rapid pulse and low blood pressure. The respiratory rate may be normal as may the patient's mental status. Usually, the skin is warm and dry, and the neck veins are flat.

Treatment of shock. The general management of shock involves fluid resuscitation, ventilatory and cardiac support, and drug therapy. Specific measures aim at correction of the underlying problem causing the inadequate perfusion. Special considerations are warranted in septic and anaphylactic shock.

Fluid resuscitation. The goal of fluid resuscitation in shock is to restore perfusion pressure to the vital organs. Typically, fluid resuscitation is accomplished by IV administration of plasma volume expanders such as blood plasma, dextran, or isotonic electrolyte solutions in sufficient quantity to restore blood pressure, peripheral perfusion, and urine output. Ideally, central venous pressure

(CVP) or pulmonary artery wedge pressure is monitored to prevent fluid overload. Whole blood may be necessary in hypovolemic shock due to hemorrhage.

Ventilatory and cardiac support. In terms of ventilatory and cardiac support, the first step is to establish an artificial airway and provide appropriate ventilatory support. Oxygen should be administered in as high a concentration as possible. In cases involving cardiac arrest, basic and advanced cardiac life support measures are implemented, as described in Chapter 22. Support for a failing ventricle in cardiogenic shock may be provided by intra-aortic balloon counterpulsation.

Drug therapy. Hypovolemic shock and septic shock do not usually require drug therapy, although inotropic agents, such as calcium, may increase cardiac output in some patients. In cardiogenic and neurogenic shock, drug therapy is usually necessary. In cardiogenic shock, agents that reduce afterload on the left ventricle and increase its contractility are beneficial. In neurogenic shock, vasopressor agents may be of value. Diuretics, which reduce circulating fluid volume and thereby decrease ventricular afterload, are useful mainly in cardiogenic shock.

In septic shock, large doses of corticosteroids have been administered, but their efficacy remains uncertain. The best treatment for septic shock is early and aggressive intervention with appropriate antimicrobial drugs. For this reason, blood cultures should be taken whenever sepsis is suspected. In addition, a survey of potential sources of infection, such as Foley catheters or IV infusions, must be carried out as soon as possible. Quick elimination of these sources of bacteremia is often the most important step in the management of septic shock.

In anaphylactic shock, epinephrine is administered immediately, usually followed by aminophylline. Hydrocortisone may also be useful in anaphylactic shock. Otherwise treatment is similar to neurogenic shock.

Embolic disorders

Embolic disorders occur when a portion of the vasculature becomes blocked by abnormal material in the circulation. Given the pulmonary circulation's function as a "filter" for the vascular system, such disorders represent a frequent cause of respiratory problems. Although there are many types of embolic disorders, we will focus on the three most common in the management of patients receiving respiratory care: pulmonary thromboembolism, fat embolism, and DIC.

Pulmonary thromboembolism. Seventy-five percent of pulmonary thromboemboli arise from clots occurring in the deep veins of the lower extremities. This event is so common in older, bed-ridden patients and those having undergone extensive abdominal or pelvic surgery that any sudden occurrence of pulmonary or cardiac distress in such patients should immediately suggest this diagnosis.

The clinical and laboratory features of pulmonary thromboembolism often depend on the level at which the obstruction occurs, hence on the size of the embolus. If obstruction occurs in a small terminal artery, clinical findings may be minimal or absent. Embolization of a medium-sized artery results in predominantly pulmonary symptoms and signs. Obstruction of a large artery is manifested predominantly by cardiac signs of acute right ventricular failure, with neck vein distention and liver engorgement, often progressing to shock, syncope, and sudden death.

Sudden dyspnea is the most frequent symptom of pulmonary thromboembolism. In fact, sudden dyspnea in any high-risk patient strongly suggests embolization of the pulmonary circulation. On physical examination, the patient with a pulmonary thromboembolism often exhibits crackles (rales) and wheezing on auscultation, and signs of consolidation or pleural effusion may be present. If present, signs of consolidation are caused by congestive atelectasis and infarction, which occur in only about 10% of the cases. Pleuritic pain occurs mainly in those with severe embolization, with about one in three of these patients exhibiting hemoptysis. Many of these respiratory signs and symptoms are similar to those occurring in pneumonia. As delineated in Table 19-9, however, there are several key differences in the clinical presentation of these two disorders.

Cardiovascular signs may include tachycardia, accentuation of the second pulmonary sound, splitting of the second sounds of the aortic and pulmonary valves, diastolic gallop, cyanosis, and elevated central venous pressure. Pulmonary signs, which may be transient, include tachypnea.

Arterial blood gas analysis usually reveals hypoxemia in the presence of respiratory alkalosis. A normal Po_2 generally excludes massive embolism. Other laboratory studies are unreliable.

The chest radiograph is usually negative. Following large emboli, an area of decreased pulmonary vascularity may be observed. Enlargement of a main pulmonary artery, elevation of a hemidiaphragm, and pleural effusion may be noted. Pulmonary densities, caused by congestive atelectasis or infarction, may appear, but usually not until several days after the initial event.

When ordinary x-ray studies are negative, lung scans may be helpful in establishing the diagnosis (see Chapter 17). A normal perfusion scan generally rules out pulmonary embolism. On the other hand, the demonstration of normal ventilation of an area of lung in the absence of perfusion strongly suggests pulmonary embolism. When either a major embolism is suggested or scanning is not definitive, pulmonary angiography can confirm the diagnosis.

Treatment of pulmonary thromboembolism depends on its severity. In general, the hypoxemia should be treated with oxygen, ideally 100%. Shock, if present, is managed with vasopressors. Intravenous heparin may be helpful in preventing further embolization. Thrombolysis, using urokinase or streptokinase, may help dissolve massive emboli of recent origin. Where cardiac bypass surgery is available, pulmonary embolectomy may be the only life-saving measure for massive embolization.

Fat embolism. Fat embolism was originally described in trauma victims suffering from long bone fractures and was therefore thought to result from bone marrow embolization. However, we now know that bone fractures are just one of many potential types of trauma that can cause this disorder. Clinically, the fat embolism syndrome manifests itself in neurologic dysfunction, respiratory insufficiency, and petechiae of the axilla, chest, and arms.

Following trauma, the blood concentration of fat macroglobules, which are approximately 20 μm in diameter, increases and peaks at about 12 hours, returning to normal within a few days. The increase in fat macroglobule concentrations is greatest after fracture of the femur shaft, but also occurs after other types of fractures and has even been observed after laparotomy. Other potential sources of fat macroglobules are (1) coalescence of chylomicrons in response to stress or prolonged hypotension and (2) mobilization of subcutaneous fat. The fat globules are filtered by the lung, and if present in large enough amounts, may block the pulmonary circulation and lead to right ventricular failure. Fat embolization may also occur in the brain, skin, and kidney. Brain embolization results in confusion, nuchal rigidity, and, occasionally, deep coma. Microembolization of the capillaries in the skin produces the characteristic petechiae.

In the lung, breakdown of the trapped fat globules releases free fatty acids. These free fatty acids, in turn, cause an increase in the level of kinins, which provoke local inflammatory reactions. Fatty acids may also cause vasculitis and destroy pulmonary surfactant. The end result is pulmonary edema, decreased alveolar-capillary oxygen transfer, and a severe hypoxemia. Free fatty acids may also cause thrombocytopenia and inhibit fibrinolysis, resulting in DIC.

Diagnosis of the fat embolism syndrome is difficult. Fat globules in the sputum and urine and elevated serum lipase values are common after many forms of trauma not specific to fat embolization. Patients with fat embolism syndrome do exhibit a decrease in the hematocrit and platelet count and may show changes in coagulation tests. Biopsy of the skin petechiae usually shows fat globules in the capillaries.

Once symptoms of the fat embolism syndrome develop, treatment is limited to supportive measures. Respiratory failure is managed in a manner similar to that used to treat noncardiogenic pulmonary edema. Steroids in high doses may be beneficial. Heparin can clear fat from the plasma, but its overall benefits are questionable.

Disseminated intravascular coagulation (DIC). DIC is a thrombohemorrhagic disorder that accompanies a variety of clinical conditions. Among the possible causes of DIC are endothelial injuries, such as vasculitis; conditions

Table 19-9 Pulmonary Thromboembolism Contrasted with Bacterial Pneumonia

	Thromboembolism	Pneumonia
SYMPTOMS		
Pain: Onset	Usually sudden	Sudden or gradual
Character	Often pleuritic	Usually pleuritic
Location	Usually lateralized	Usually lateralized
Severity	Variable	Variable
Cough	Uncommon until infarction	Usually present
Dyspnea	Mild to severe	Mild to severe
Sputum	More bloody	More purulent or rusty
Fever	None to moderate	Usually high
Chills	Rare	Common
Collateral history	Immobilization; previous phlebitis; postoperative, especially leg, hip, and pelvis; birth control medication; malignancy; CHF; prior PTE	Chronic alcoholism, COPD, bronchiectasis, diabetes, immunodeficient states
SIGNS		
Respiratory rate*	Rapid	Rapid
Pulse*	Rapid	Rapid
Chest examination	Often normal, especially early	Usually consolidated
Heart examination	Normal to frank failure	Usually normal
Extremities	Calf tenderness, + cuff test in 50%	Normal

From Mitchell RS: Synopsis of clinical pulmonary disease, ed 4, St Louis, 1988, The CV Mosby Co.

causing the release of thromboplastic material into the circulation, as in head trauma, massive tissue injury, and abruptio placenta; challenges to the immune system; infections; neoplasms; shock; and miscellaneous factors, such as stroke.

DIC involves activation of the clotting cascade, which generates thrombin in amounts that far exceed the circulatory system's ability to neutralize this clot material. Excess thrombin leads to intravascular coagulation. Intravascular coagulation, in turn, causes (1) deposition of fibrin in the microvasculature, (2) consumption of coagulation factors and platelets, and (3) secondary activation of fibrinolysis. Occlusion of capillaries and arterioles with fibrin causes tissue ischemia.

Strangely, bleeding is also a characteristic of DIC. Bleeding in DIC is a secondary phenomenon caused by the inhibitory effects of fibrinogen and fibrin degradation products (FDP) on hemostasis, thrombocytopenia, and the consumption of clotting factors.

In fact, bleeding is the primary sign in patients with acute DIC. Such bleeding usually occurs at multiple sites, such as surgical wounds, venipuncture sites, and the nose. Evidence of tissue ischemia may also be present. Bleeding and tissue ischemia are associated with marked abnormalities of coagulation tests, including prolongation of prothrombin time, partial thromboplastin time, and thrombin time. On the other hand, plasma levels of clotting factors tend to decrease during DIC. However, the underlying clinical condition causing DIC may mask the expected decrease in clotting factors.

DIC may also occur chronically. Chronic DIC is more difficult to recognize than the acute version. Active bleeding may not be present, and only a few laboratory tests may be abnormal. As a general rule, acute DIC is usually associated with bleeding, whereas chronic DIC is more often present with tissue ischemia and thrombosis, particularly involving the fingers and toes.

DIC is not a disease itself, but only occurs in the presence of other processes that trigger intravascular coagulation. Management of DIC involves aggressive treatment of the underlying disease. In conditions such as malignancy, however, control of the underlying disease may be difficult. In these situations, management of DIC often includes administration of clotting factors, platelets, and packed red cells. Correction of shock and tissue ischemia must be a high priority. Initial enthusiasm for heparin therapy in DIC has waned because of the lack of uniform benefit and increased possibility of secondary bleeding. Recent studies using antithrombin III and other synthetic antithrombins in the management of DIC are encouraging.

RESPIRATORY COMPLICATIONS OF SURGERY

Respiratory complications are the primary cause of morbidity after major surgical procedures and the second most important cause of postoperative death in elderly patients. Patients undergoing chest and upper abdominal operations are particularly prone to develop pulmonary complications. Moreover, surgery and anesthesia represent special hazards to those with pre-existing chronic lung disease.

The three most common respiratory complications associated with surgery are atelectasis, pulmonary aspiration, and postoperative pneumonia.

Atelectasis

Atelectasis is the most common postoperative pulmonary complication, affecting nearly one in four patients recovering from abdominal surgery. Atelectasis normally develops during the first or second postoperative day and accounts for over 90% of the febrile episodes during this time period. With most patients, the course of postoperative atelectasis is self-limiting, and their recovery is uneventful.

The development of atelectasis involves both obstructive and nonobstructive factors. Obstruction may result from an increase in the amount or tenacity of secretions, as caused by COPD, intubation, or anesthetic agents. Nonobstructive factors that contribute to atelectasis include shallow breathing and a transient decrease in surfactant production. Shallow breathing, a failure to take deep breaths, results in a progressive decrease in functional residual capacity and may lead to alveolar collapse, particularly in the basal or dependent portions of the lung. Since perfusion remains unchanged, a $\dot{V}/\dot{Q}$ mismatch results, causing arterial hypoxemia. Moreover, regions of atelectasis are especially prone to infection. In general, if an area of the lung remains atelectatic for over 72 hours, pneumonia is almost certain.

Clinically, patients with atelectasis usually exhibit a fever of unknown origin and tachypnea. Physical examination may demonstrate elevation of the diaphragm on the affected side, scattered crackles (rales), and decreased breath sounds. However, these physical signs are not always present.

The best treatment for postoperative atelectasis is prevention. The likelihood of postoperative atelectasis can be minimized by early mobilization of the patient, frequent positional changes, and a vigorous regimen of deep breathing and coughing.

Should atelectasis develop, treatment consists of airway clearance by chest percussion, coughing, and, if necessary, nasotracheal suction. Hyperinflation techniques, including incentive spirometry and intermittent positive pressure breathing (IPPB) are also useful in facilitating deep breathing and re-expansion of atelectatic areas (see Chapter 26). Atelectasis caused by obstruction of a large airway may require therapeutic bronchoscopy, a procedure that can usually be performed at the bedside with moderate sedation.

Pulmonary aspiration

Two thirds of all aspiration events follow thoracic or abdominal surgery. Of these, about one half result in pneumonia. Nearly one in three patients with gross aspiration that progresses to pneumonia will die as a result of this condition.

In conscious and alert patients, protective mechanisms in the esophagus and pharynx normally prevent aspiration of oropharyngeal or gastric contents. Insertion of nasogastric or endotracheal tubes and depression of the central nervous system by drug agents interferes with these defense mechanisms and increases the likelihood of aspiration. Other factors increasing the likelihood of aspiration include gastroesophageal reflux, food in the stomach, and supine or head down positioning. Also, some 80% of all patients with tracheostomies show evidence of one or more incidents of aspiration. This fact helps account for the high incidence of pulmonary infections among these patients.

Clinically, the patient who suffers an aspiration episode typically exhibits tachypnea, crackles (rales), and signs of hypoxemia soon after the incident. Because of the architecture of the lung, the superior basal segments of the lower lobe are infected most often. Massive aspiration may progress quickly to cardiopulmonary arrest.

The extent of pulmonary injury caused by aspirated gastric contents is determined by the amount aspirated, the pH of the aspirate, and the frequency of the event. Aspirates with pH levels of 2.5 or less cause immediate chemical pneumonitis. This chemical pneumonitis results in local edema and inflammation and increases the likelihood of a secondary infection.

As with atelectasis, the best treatment for aspiration is prevention. The most important measures in the prevention of aspiration are to (1) avoid general anesthesia in patients who have recently eaten; (2) properly position the patient before, during, and after surgery; and (3) maintain a cuffed endotracheal tube in place until pharyngeal reflexes have completely returned.

Once it has occurred, treatment of aspiration involves reestablishing patency of the airway by vigorous suctioning, using bronchoscopy as necessary. Corticosteroids may inhibit the inflammatory response of the lung parenchyma following massive aspiration of stomach contents.

Postoperative pneumonia

Some three fourths of all hospital-acquired pneumonias occur in postoperative patients. In such patients, impairment of normal swallowing and respiratory clearance mechanisms allow bacteria to enter and remain in the lower respiratory tract. Atelectasis, aspiration, and copious secretions are important predisposing factors. Instrumentation of the respiratory tract, anesthesia, surgical pain, and use of narcotics-analgesics and sedatives all increase the susceptibility of the host (see Chapter 14).

The risk of pneumonia is not the same for all surgical patients. Patients at highest risk include the elderly, the severely obese, those with chronic obstructive pulmonary disease or a history of smoking, and those with an artificial airway in place for prolonged periods of time.

Occasionally, infecting bacteria originate from respiratory therapy equipment, such as ventilators. Organisms such as *P aeruginosa* and *K pneumoniae* can thrive in the moist reservoirs of these machines and have been the source of epidemic infections in intensive care units.

The clinical manifestations of postoperative pneumonia are essentially those associated with the causative organism. However, fever, tachypnea, increased secretions, and physical changes characteristic of pulmonary consolidation are common findings. Moreover, the chest x-ray film usually shows localized parenchymal consolidation.

Treatment of postoperative pneumonia consists of measures to aid the clearing of secretions and the administration of antibiotics specific to the infecting organism.

Efforts to prevent postoperative pneumonia should start in the preoperative period and include a careful evaluation of the patient's disease and risk factors. Concerted efforts should be made before elective surgery to have the patient stop smoking, improve nutrition, and correct gross obesity. To reduce exposure to antibiotic-resistant microorganisms, the preoperative hospital stay should be as short as possible. Ideally, training in hyperinflation methods and coughing should be included as part of the preoperative regimen.

After surgery, early mobilization, vigorous respiratory care, and careful fluid and electrolyte balance are critical. Should evidence of infection develop, measures to facilitate clearance of secretions and the administration of antibiotics specific to the offending organism should be instituted immediately.

SUMMARY

Respiratory care is provided to patients with a wide variety of respiratory and cardiopulmonary disorders. Of course, the physician holds primary responsibility for the diagnosis and management of these conditions. However, to effectively participate in this process and to provide quality respiratory care, the practitioner must have a basic understanding of the causes, clinical features, and management approaches employed in these disorders. Only by developing such knowledge can the practitioner expect to assume a key role in patient management.

BIBLIOGRAPHY

Acquired immunodeficiency syndrome (AIDS) among blacks and Hispanics—United States, MMWR 35:655, 1986.

AMA Council on Occupational Health: The pneumoconioses: diagnosis, evaluation, and management, Arch Environ Health 7:131-171, 1963.

American Thoracic Society and the Centers for Disease Control: Treatment of tuberculosis and tuberculosis infection in adults and children, Am Rev Respir Dis 134:355-363, 1986.

American Thoracic Society: Diagnostic standards and classification of tuberculosis and other mycobacterial diseases, Am Rev Respir Dis 123:343-351, 1981.

American Thoracic Society: The tuberculin skin test, Am Rev Respir Dis 124:356-342, 1981.

American Thoracic Society: The diagnosis of nonmalignant diseases related to asbestosis, Am Rev Respir Dis 134:363-368, 1986.

Arnow PM et al: Nosocomial legionnaires' disease caused by aerosolized tap water from respiratory devices, J Infect Dis 146:460, 1982.

Barnes DM: Strategies for an AIDS vaccine, Science 233:1149, 1986.

Bartlett JG et al: Bacteriology and treatment of primary lung abscess, Am Rev Respir Dis 109:510, 1974.

Bartlett RH et al: Studies on the pathogenesis and prevention of postoperative pulmonary complications, Surg Gynecol Obstet 137:925, 1973.

Bennett JV and Brachman PS, editors: Hospital infections, ed 3, Boston, 1986, Little, Brown & Co.

Berk SL et al: *Escherichia coli* pneumonia in the elderly: with reference to the role of *E. coli* K1 capsular polysaccharide antigen, Am J Med 72:899, 1982.

Blaisdell FW and Lewis FR: Respiratory distress syndrome of shock and trauma: post-traumatic respiratory failure, Philadelphia, 1977, WB Saunders Co.

Bodey GP et al: Infections caused by *Pseudomonas aeruginosa,* Rev Infect Dis 5:279, 1983.

Burrows B, Knudson RJ, and Kettrl LJ: Respiratory insufficiency, Chicago, 1975, Year Book Medical Publishers.

Centers for Disease Control: Nosocomial infection surveillance, 1984, CDC Surveillance Summaries—1986, MMWR 35(1SS):17SS, 1986.

Chanock RM et al: Respiratory syncytial virus. In Evans AS, editor: Viral infections of humans: epidemiology and control, New York, 1976, Plenum Publishing.

Chusid JG: Nervous system. In Krupp MA and Chatton MJ: Current medical diagnosis and treatment, Los Altos, Calif, 1981, Lange Medical Publications.

Coolfont report: a PHS plan for prevention and control of AIDS and the AIDS virus, Public Health Rep 101:341, 1986.

Coombs RRA and Gell PGH: Classification of allergic reactions responsible for clinical hypersensitivity and disease. In Coombs RRA, Gell PGH, and Lachmann PJ, editors: Clinical aspects of immunology, ed 3, Oxford, England, 1975, Blackwell Scientific.

Curran JW et al: The epidemiology of AIDS: current status and future prospects, Science 229:1352, 1985.

De Troyer A and Deisser P: The effects of intermittent positive pressure breathing on patients with respiratory muscle weakness, Am Rev Respir Dis 124:132, 1981.

Diagnosis and management of mycobacterial infection and disease in persons with human T-lymphotropic virus type III lymphadenopathy-associated virus infection, MMWR 35:448, 1986.

Donath J and Kahn FA: Pulmonary infections in AIDS, Comp Therapy 13:49-58, 1987.

Drachman DB: Myasthenia gravis (2 parts), N Engl J Med 298:136, 185, 1978.

Elliott JL et al: The acquired immunodeficiency syndrome and *Mycobacterium avium-intracellulare* bacteremia in a patient with hemophilia, Ann Intern Med 98:290, 1983.

Farzan S: A concise handbook of respiratory diseases, ed 2, East Norwalk, Conn, 1985, Appleton & Lange.

Fauci AS et al: The acquired immunodeficiency syndrome: an update, Ann Intern Med 102:800, 1985.

Foy HM and Grayston JT: Adenoviruses. In Evans AS, editor: Viral infections of humans: epidemiology and control, New York, 1976, Plenum Publishing.

Glezen WP, Loda FA, and Denny FW: The parainfluenza viruses. In Evans AS, editor: Viral infections of humans: epidemiology and control, New York, 1976, Plenum Publishing.

Goedert JJ: Testing for human immunodeficiency virus, Ann Intern Med 105:609, 1986.

Gossling HR and Donahue TA: The fat embolism syndrome, JAMA 241:2740, 1979.

Gottlieb MS et al: The acquired immunodeficiency syndrome, Ann Intern Med 99:208, 1983.

Gracey DR, Divertie MB, and Howard FM Jr: Mechanical ventilation for respiratory failure in myasthenia gravis: two year experience with 22 patients, Mayo Clin Proc 58:597, 1983.

Guttman L and Pratt L: Pathophysiologic aspects of human botulism, Arch Neurol 33:175, 1976.

Hardy AM et al: The economic impact of the first 10,000 cases of acquired immunodeficiency syndrome in the United States, JAMA 255:209, 1986.

Health and Public Policy Committee, American College of Physicians, and the Infectious Disease Society of America: Acquired immunodeficiency syndrome (position paper), Ann Intern Med 104:575, 1986.

Holcroft JW: Shock. In Dunphy JE and Way LW: Current surgical diagnosis and treatment, ed 5, Los Altos, Calif, 1981, Lange Medical Publications.

Influenza—United States, MMWR 29:615, 1981.

Ingram RH Jr and Fanta CH: Neuromuscular processes. In Scientific American medicine, New York, 1988, Scientific American.

Inkley SR, Oldenburg FC, and Vignos PJ Jr: Pulmonary function in Duchenne muscular dystrophy related to stage of disease, Am J Med 56:297, 1974.

Jackson GG and Muldoon RL: Viruses causing common respiratory infections in man, Chicago, 1975, University of Chicago Press.

Jaffee HJ and Katz S: Current ideas about bronchiectasis, Am Family Phys 7:69-76, 1973.

Johanson WG Jr et al: Nosocomial respiratory infections with gram-negative bacilli: the significance of colonization of the respiratory tract, Ann Intern Med 77:701, 1972.

Kilbourne ED, editor: The influenza viruses and influenza, New York, 1975, Academic Press, Inc.

Kryger MH, editor: Pathophysiology of respiration, New York, 1981, John Wiley & Sons, Inc.

Landesman SH, Ginzburg HM, and Weiss SH: Special report: the AIDS epidemic, N Engl J Med 312:521, 1985.

Larson EL: Persistent carriage of gram-negative bacteria on hands, Am J Infect Control 9:112, 1981.

Lopez M and Salvaggio JE: Hypersensitivity pneumonitis: current concepts of etiology and pathogenesis, Ann Rev Med 27:453, 1976.

Luelmo F: BCG vaccination, Am Rev Respir Dis 125(part 2):3, 70, 1982.

Manson RM and Rushing JL: Respiratory tract and mediastinum. In Krupp MA and Chatton MJ: Current medical diagnosis and treatment, Los Altos, Calif, 1981, Lange Medical Publications.

Markand ON et al: Postoperative phrenic nerve palsy in patients with open-heart surgery, Ann Thorac Surg 39:68, 1985.

Marron RW: Human T-cell lymphotrophic virus type III (HTLV-III) embryopathy, Am J Dis Child 140:638-640.

Martin L: Pulmonary physiology in clinical practice: the essentials for patient care and evaluation, St Louis, 1987, The CV Mosby Co.

McGowan JE Jr: Antimicrobial resistance in hospital organisms and its relation to antibiotic use, Rev Infect Dis 5:1033, 1983.

Merigan TC: Respiratory viral infections. In Scientific American medicine, New York, 1988, Scientific American.

Mitchell RS: Synopsis of clinical pulmonary disease, ed 4, St Louis, 1988, The CV Mosby Co.

Montgomerie JZ: Epidemiology of *Klebsiella* and hospital-associated infections, Rev Infect Dis 1:736, 1979.

Moore P and Owen J: Guillain-Barré syndrome: incidence, management and outcome of major complications, Crit Care Med 9:549, 1981.

Morgan WKC and Seaton A: Occupational lung diseases, Philadelphia, 1975, WB Saunders Co.

Moser KM: Pulmonary embolism, Am Rev Respir Dis 115:829, 1977.

Moylan J et al: Fat embolism syndrome, J Trauma 16:341, 1976.

Newsome-Davis J et al: Diaphragm function and alveolar hypoventilation, Q J Med 45:87, 1976.

Oh WH and Mital MA: Fat embolism: current concepts of pathogenesis, diagnosis, and treatment, Orthop Clin North Am 9:769, 1978.

Pellegrini CA: Postoperative complications. In Dunphy JE and Way LW: Current surgical diagnosis and treatment, ed 5, Los Altos, Calif, 1981, Lange Medical Publications.

Peterman TA and Curran JW: Sexual transmission of human immunodeficiency virus, JAMA 256:2222, 1986.

Qureshi GD: The blood and spleen: disseminated intravascular coagulation. In Rakel RE, editor: Conn's current therapy, Philadelphia, 1987, WB Saunders Co.

Reinarz JA et al: The potential role of inhalation therapy equipment in nosocomial pulmonary infection, J Clin Invest 44:831, 1965.

Riley EA: Idiopathic diaphragmatic paralysis: a report of eight cases, Am J Med 32:404, 1962.

Robin ED, Cross CE, and Zelis R: Pulmonary edema, N Engl J Med 288:239-246, 292-304, 1973.

Rosenthal S and Tager IB: Prevalence of gram-negative rods in the normal pharyngeal flora, Ann Intern Med 83:355, 1975.

Rothstein RJ et al: Tetanus prevention and treatment, JAMA 240:675, 1978.

Rubin RH: Mycotic infections. In Scientific American medicine, New York, 1988, Scientific American.

Sanders CV Jr et al: *Serratia marcescens* infections from inhalation therapy medications: nosocomial outbreak, Ann Intern Med 73:15, 1970.

Sasahara AA, Sonnenblick EM, and Lesch M, editors: Pulmonary emboli, New York, 1975, Grune & Stratton.

Snider DE et al: Standard therapy for tuberculosis, Chest 87:1175, 1985.

Snider DE, Caras GJ, and Koplan JP: Preventive therapy with isoniazid, JAMA 244:2736, 1986.

Spray SB, Quidema GD, and Cameron JL: Aspiration pneumonia: incidence of aspiration with endotracheal tubes, Am J Surg 131:701, 1976.

Staub NC: State of the art review: pathogenesis of pulmonary edema, Am Rev Respir Dis 109:358-372, 1974.

Stoddart JC: Postoperative respiratory failure: an anaesthetic hazard?, Br J Anaesthesiol 50:695, 1978.

Swartz MN: Clinical aspects of legionnaires' disease, Ann Intern Med 90:492, 1979.

Swift TR: Disorders of neuromuscular transmission other than myasthenia gravis, Muscle Nerve 4:334, 1981.

Tarhan S et al: Risk of anesthesia and surgery in patients with chronic bronchitis and chronic obstructive pulmonary disease, Surgery 74:720, 1973.

Tisi GM: Pulmonary physiology in clinical medicine, ed 2, Baltimore, 1984, Williams & Wilkins Co.

Urmey W et al: Upper and lower rib cage deformation during breathing in quadriplegics, J Appl Physiol 60:618, 1986.

Wagenvoort CA and Wagenvoort N: Pathology of pulmonary hypertension, New York, 1977, John Wiley & Sons, Inc.

Weinstein MP et al: The clinical significance of positive blood cultures: a comprehensive analysis of 500 episodes of bacteremia and fungemia in adults. I. Laboratory and epidemiologic observations, Rev Infect Dis 5:35, 1983.

Wenzel RP, editor: Prevention and control of nosocomial infections, Baltimore, 1987, Williams & Wilkins Co.

Williams DM et al: Pulmonary infection in the compromised host (2 parts), Am Rev Respir Dis 114:359, 593, 1976.

Wray NP and Nicotra MB: Pathogenesis of neurogenic pulmonary edema, Am Rev Respir Dis 118:783, 1978.

Yu VL: *Serratia marcescens:* historical perspective and clinical review, N Engl J Med 300:887, 1979.

Ziskind M, Jones RN, and Weill H: Silicosis, Am Rev Respir Dis 113:643-665, 1976.

Basic Therapeutics

Section VI

Basic Therapeutics

20

Pharmacology for Respiratory Care

James A. Peters
Barbara A. Peters

Respiratory pharmacology is concerned with the use of chemical agents or drugs that affect the pulmonary system. Generally, drugs are useful to the extent that they can maintain, enhance, or alter some physiologic function when a patient's normal mechanisms are insufficient to cope with a particular disease process. Determining when drugs are necessary is the responsibility of the physician. Administering and monitoring the effect of selected drugs is the responsibility of the respiratory care practitioner.

Although competent respiratory care practitioners must have general knowledge of *all* common drugs used in the care of their patients, it is in the area of airway pharmacology that in-depth understanding must be demonstrated. These drugs include bronchodilators, mucolytics, expectorants, steroids, and selected antimicrobial agents. Additionally, local anesthetics, such as xylocaine, may be nebulized before bronchoscopy.[1] Only by the intelligent and careful application of these potent chemicals can the desired therapeutic objectives be achieved without undo risk or hazard.

OBJECTIVES

After completion of this chapter, the reader should be able to:

1. Apply the general principles of pharmacology and nervous system pharmacodynamics to drug usage in respiratory care;

2. Differentiate the three major goals of respiratory care pharmacology;

3. Compare and contrast the mechanism(s) of action, indications for, and side effects of the various pharmacologic agents used for bronchodilation;

4. Differentiate the various mucokinetic drug agents, including their clinical usage and limitations;

5. Explain the appropriate role of anti-inflammatory agents in respiratory care, including the adrenocorticosteroids and cromolyn sodium;

6. Discuss the indications for and limitations of aerosolized antimicrobial therapy, including selected antibiotic, antiviral, and antiprotozoal agents.

KEY TERMS

Most terms used in this chapter are defined in context. The following terms are introduced without explicit definition, but may be found in the text glossary:

absorption	in vivo
adhesion	isomer
alkaloid	lysis
anorexia	mucopolysaccharide
antibody	nucleotide
antigen	ocular
atrophy	osmolarity
biofeedback	palpitation
Cheyne-Stokes' breathing	parenteral
diuresis	pathogenic
effector	pharmacopoeia
emulsification	polarity
exacerbation	purulent
expectorant	refractory
genitourinary	rhinitis
hydrolysis	seminal vesicles
hypnotic	serous
insomnia	subcutaneous
intrabursal	suppurative
intractable	synaptic cleft
intramuscular	systemic
intravenous	threshold response
in vitro	vasopressor

PRINCIPLES OF PHARMACOLOGY

A drug is a chemical substance that exerts a biologic effect.[2] Medically, a drug can be defined as a substance that is used for the treatment, diagnosis, or prevention of disease.[3] Pharmacology is the study of how drugs affect the body and how the body acts upon drugs.

Specifically, pharmacology concerns six basic areas: (1) the chemical and physical properties of drugs; (2) the physiologic effects and site of action of drugs; (3) how drugs exert their effects or the "mechanism of action"; (4) what the body does with drugs, ie, the absorption, distribution, metabolism, and excretion of drugs; (5) dosages and routes of administration of drugs; and (6) side effects and toxicity. Only by understanding all of these key elements for each drug used can the respiratory care practitioner ensure the safe and effective application of the pharmacologic agents prescribed.

Drug nomenclature

Practitioners will encounter many different drug names. To minimize confusion, Table 20-1 lists the system of nomenclature of pharmacologic agents. Most frequently, the generic name or the trademark or brand name is used. In this book the generic name will be used; if the brand name is mentioned, it will be in parentheses following the generic name.

Routes of administration

For a drug to exert a therapeutic effect, it must become available for absorption. Availability of a drug agent to the body depends on both its form (solid, liquid, etc) and its route of administration.

There are three major routes available for the administration of therapeutic drug agents: (1) gastrointestinal (oral or rectal), (2) parenteral, and (3) topical. Selection of the "best" route for the administration of a drug depends on the following considerations:

1. The available form(s) of the drug;
2. The desired rate of onset and duration of action of the drug;
3. The safety of the available route(s);
4. Whether a local or systemic (body-wide) effect is desired;
5. Whether the patient can swallow and retain an oral preparation;
6. The stability of the agent in gastrointestinal fluids;
7. The relative amount of the drug needed; and
8. The convenience of the available route(s).

In general, the gastrointestinal route, specifically oral administration, is the safest, most convenient, and most economical route of drug administration. Drug forms available for oral administration include pills, capsules, water solutions, alcohol elixirs, and emulsions. Rectal administration methods include suppositories and liquid solutions.

Parenteral routes are those involving drug administration by injection. The most common methods of parenteral drug administration are the subcutaneous, intramuscular, and intravenous routes.

Topical routes include those methods where a drug agent is applied directly to a body area, such as the skin or mucous membranes. Lotions and ointments applied to the skin usually exert only a local effect. However, the application of a drug agent to highly vascularized mucous membranes, such as the mouth or nose, can result in rapid absorption and systemic (as opposed to local) effects.

The inhalation route represents a special case of topical drug administration. To administer a drug agent by the inhalation route, it must first be either vaporized or placed in an aerosol suspension. Generally, this approach requires special equipment, such as vaporizers or aerosol generators (see Chapter 23). Moreover, because of the nature of the respiratory tract mucosa, administration of drugs by inhalation can result in rapid absorption and strong systemic effects. Also, because some portion of all drugs administered by this route is lost on exhalation, it is impossible to know for certain exactly how much of a given agent actually reaches the patient.

Table 20-2 compares and contrasts these various routes of drug administration according to their relative advantages and disadvantages.

Table 20-1   Naming of Drugs

Name	Explanation	Example
Chemical name	Name based on chemical structure	1-(3,5-dihydroxyphenyl)-2-isopropylaminoethanol
Generic name	Common name; may reflect chemical name	Metaproterenol, orciprenaline
Official name	The name that is used in an official drug publication; may be the same as generic name	Alupent, Metaprel

Modified from Ziment I: Respiratory pharmacology and therapeutics, Philadelphia, 1978, WB Saunders Co.

Drug administration

The safe use of drugs requires awareness of many different factors, including the following:
1. Mode of action,
2. Side effects,
3. Toxicity,
4. Range of common dosages,
5. Rate and route of excretion,
6. Individual differences in response,
7. Interaction with other drugs or food, and
8. Contraindications.

As with any drug agent, the administration of respiratory care related medications can result in untoward patient reactions. Moreover, drugs administered via the inhalation route increase the risk of contamination to the lungs, possibly resulting in infection. When preparing medications, the practitioner must observe proper techniques of handling and cleaning of the aerosolizing equipment.

The following list identifies the minimum requirements for a proper prescription for respiratory care related drugs. The practitioner should seek clarification from the physician if the order does not specify the necessary information.
1. Prescription should be complete with:
   a. Patient's name,
   b. Drug name,
   c. Dose,
   d. Frequency it is to be given,
   e. Duration of administration (for some aerosol treatments),
   f. Route of administration, and
   g. Signature of physician.
2. Before administering the prescribed drug the practitioner should double check:
   a. Patient's chart for order,
   b. Patient's name band,
   c. Medication labels,
   d. Dates on medication,
   e. Dosage, and
   f. Charted response to previous drug administration.

When administering a medication, nothing should be taken for granted. The practitioner should habitually double check all information. If an error is suspected or a question arises, the practitioner should not proceed until satisfied that all is proper.

Although there are "standard" dosages routinely prescribed for patients, drug administration should always be individualized according to the patient's needs. Very young and very old patients generally have a more difficult time with drugs because of the body's decreased ability to handle drugs at the extremes of age. Accumulation of a drug can ensue, and, as drug levels build up in the body, adverse effects become more common.

Basic pharmacokinetics

It is well recognized that some drugs work better than others. The *efficacy* of a drug represents its peak, or maximum, biologic effect. On the other hand, the *potency* of a drug represents its biologic activity per unit weight, or the amount of drug required to produce a given effect.

Fig. 20-1 illustrates the concepts of drug potency and efficacy for two different drugs, labeled X and Y. Relative dosage is plotted on a horizontal logarithmic axis, with effect (measured as percent response) plotted on the vertical axis. Both drug agents exhibit the typical S-shaped dose-response curve and exert a comparable maximum effect (R_{max}). However, drug X achieves this maximum effect at a dosage some ten times lower than that required by drug Y. Thus drug X is said to be more potent than drug Y. Nonetheless, both drugs are capable of producing the same maximum effect and, therefore, have the same efficacy.

Fig. 20-2 illustrates differences in efficacy between two

Table 20-2 Routes of Administration of Drugs

Route	Advantages	Disadvantages
Oral (or rectal)	Convenience, economy	Absorption may be variable and erratic; requires patient cooperation
Subcutaneous	Ease of administration; rapid absorption of aqueous solutions	Only limited volumes of solution can be given; irritating solutions may cause sloughs
Intramuscular	Ease of administration; more rapid absorption than subcutaneous route	Unsuitable if patient is on anticoagulants
Intravenous	Immediate action permits titration of dosage; large volumes can be given; irritating substances may be administered if well diluted	Increased risk of overdose or untoward side effects; occasional difficulty of venipuncture
Inhalation	Immediate action permits titration of dosage; direct delivery to site of action	Requires special equipment; risk of overdose or untoward side effects; requires patient cooperation

From Mathewson HS: Pharmacology for respiratory therapists, ed 2, St Louis, 1981, The CV Mosby Co.

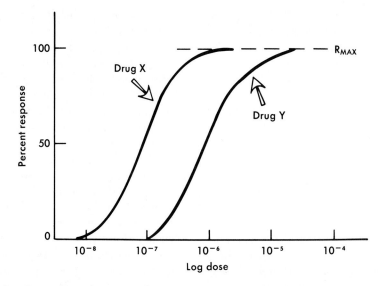

Fig. 20-1 Comparison of potency of two drug agents. (From Lehnert BE and Schachter EN: The pharmacology of respiratory care, St Louis, 1980, The CV Mosby Co.)

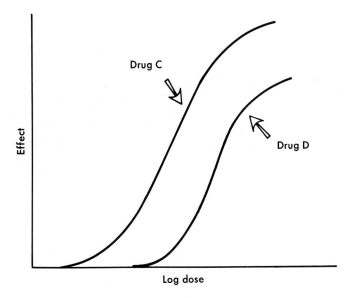

Fig. 20-2 Comparison of efficacy of two drug agents. (From Lehnert BE and Schachter EN: The pharmacology of respiratory care, St Louis, 1980, The CV Mosby Co.)

drugs, labeled C and D. Clearly, drug C is more potent than drug D, producing its effect at a substantially lower dose. In addition, the maximum effect of drug C (indicated by the highest portion of the dose-response curve) is greater than that of drug D. This indicates that drug C also has a greater efficacy than drug D. Although potency is important in determining the dosage of a particular agent, our primary goal is to use that drug or combination of drugs that produce the desired effect with minimal side effects.

A *side effect* represents any effect produced by a drug other than its desired effect. Every drug has side effects. A "drug of choice" is that drug that best achieves the desired response with minimal side effects. An example of a side effect is a respiratory drug that exerts effects on the heart, such as increasing heart rate. This is an undesired response since a drug that was given for pulmonary purposes is producing a cardiovascular effect. Typically, the dose that can be given a patient is limited by the side effects it produces. Unfortunately, side effects may occur even when the amount of drug given is less than the normal or prescribed dose. Therefore, careful monitoring of the patient is essential.

Also related to the body's response to chemical agents is the concept of *half-life*. Half-life is a measure of how rapidly a drug is inactivated or excreted from the body. Specifically, half-life refers to how much time it takes the body to decrease a given concentration of a drug to half its initial level. Half-life varies according to the chemical makeup of the pharmacologic agent and helps determine how often a drug should be given to maintain a therapeutic level.

Half-life also varies according to the patient's condition. For example, the half-life of a drug administered to a geriatric patient may be prolonged because of compromised liver function. Likewise, a drug given to a premature infant may stay in the body longer because necessary enzyme systems are not yet fully developed.

The liver is responsible for the metabolism and inactivation of most drugs. Typically, enzymatic processes in the liver convert a drug to a less active form. Enzymes capable of inactivating drugs are also found in other organ systems. For example, the stomach contains an enzyme capable of inactivating the bronchodilator isoproterenol, while an enzyme in the blood plasma can hydrolyze and inactivate the neuromuscular blocking agent succinylcholine.

The absorption, activity, and excretion of drugs are affected by both the chemical nature of the drug itself and the characteristics of the body fluids in which they act. For example, only lipid-soluble drugs can readily diffuse across cell membranes. Since chemical agents that ionize are not lipid soluble, the degree of ionization of a drug also will affect its cellular absorption and activity.

For agents that form ions in solution, the degree of ionization is determined by both the surrounding pH and the dissociation constant of the drug, or its pKa. The pKa of a drug agent is the pH at which it is 50% ionized. Drugs that are weak acids, such as salicylic acid (aspirin), have low dissociation constants (the pKa for salicylic acid is 3.5). On the other hand, drugs that are weak bases, such as quinine, have high dissociation constants (the pKa for quinine is 8.2).

In general, when the pH of the body fluids equals the pKa of the drug, we can expect 50% ionization. With weak acids, less ionization (and therefore greater absorption across cell membranes) will occur when the pH is lower (more acidic) than the pKa. In contrast, drugs that are weak bases tend to dissociate less in environments more alkaline (higher pH) than their pKa values. For example, in the stomach (with a pH of about 1.0), salicylic acid remains mostly unionized and is therefore readily absorbed through the gastric mucosa. However, at this pH, quinine is almost completely ionized and poorly absorbed in the stomach.

For these reasons, the acid-base status of patients also plays a role in their response to drugs. In patients with an acid-base imbalance, the absorption, activity, and excretion of drug agents may be substantially different from that expected in patients with a normal pH.

Since the kidneys are the major route of excretion for most drugs, the plasma and urine pH, by their effect on drug ionization and lipid solubility, are important determinants of the rate of drug clearance from the body. In contrast to cellular absorption, urinary excretion is enhanced when a drug or drug metabolite is in ionized form. Ionization of the agent minimizes its reabsorption through the renal tubular cells, thereby facilitating its clearance in the urine. Of course, any compromise in renal function can impair drug excretion and thereby lead to toxic drug levels.

Weight, and more specifically, the percentage of body fat, as well as the size of a person, represents another influence on response to a given dose of a drug. A person with more body fat has greater storage sites for fat-soluble drugs, and the larger a person is, the more potential there is for fluid volume diluting a given dose to a level that is less than effective. However, the size and amount of fat are less of a concern with drugs that are topically applied, such as those administered directly to the lungs by inhalation of aerosol.

Repeated use of a specific drug may result in a decreased response to the same dose. This phenomenon is known as tolerance, or *tachyphylaxis,* and is seen occasionally in asthmatic patients who have become "trigger happy" with their aerosol cartridge inhalers. Tolerance in such patients is addressed best through proper patient education. Alternatively, a combination of different drugs that work by different mechanisms can be employed, thus minimizing the likelihood of tolerance to a specific drug.

Another factor that can alter the expected response to a given drug is interaction with other drugs. Since the average patient receives about ten different drugs while in the hospital, the potential for undesired interactions resulting in adverse effects is very real.[4] It is difficult to predict the effect various drugs will have when combined together, hence the danger of multiple drug usage.

Drug interactions can result in *additive* effects, where the action of two drugs together equals the sum of their individual effects. Alternatively, administration of two or more drugs together can result in *potentiation*, where each increases the effect of the other.[5] This is also referred to as synergism or a multiplicative effect. On the other hand, one drug may block or *antagonize* the action of another agent.

Additional factors that affect the response a patient has may be the time of administration, the pathologic state of the patient, genetic factors, and psychologic factors.[6] When a drug is given may influence the drug's effect, since many body processes vary in a cyclic manner throughout the day. There may be times at which a drug has greater effect than at other times. The pathologic condition of the patient is important because certain body systems such as the liver or kidneys may not allow inactivation or excretion of the drugs as expected, possibly leading to cumulation. Genetically, a person may lack certain enzymes that a particular drug requires to exert its effect. Finally, the psychologic state of the patient can play an important part in the effectiveness of the drug. Belief that a drug will work typically results in a better therapeutic outcome. The practitioner's attitude and confidence are of definite benefit and may make the difference between a good or marginal response to a given drug regimen.

Receptor theory of drug action

Drugs are thought to produce their effects either (1) by acting discretely at some specific receptor site or (2) by acting diffusely at many tissues. Those acting diffusely are termed saturation-dependent, or nonreceptor, drugs and include alcohol, hypnotics, anesthetics, and mucus-diluting agents such as water and saline. However, the majority of drugs act at receptor sites.

A receptor is a special location where specific molecules on cells form reversible bonds with a specific drug. Receptor-drug interaction has been likened to action between a lock and key. Receptors (the lock) are very specific as to what drugs (keys) will bond there. The shape, the size, and the polarity of the drug molecule must be within the range of the receptor's specifications or no drug effect will occur. *Affinity* is the tendency a drug has to combine with a receptor.[5] If a drug has affinity and produces an effect, it is termed an *agonist*. A partial agonist is a drug that has affinity but cannot produce the full effect.

In contrast, an *antagonist* is a drug that has affinity but produces no effect. An antagonist is capable of blocking any effect that an agonist would produce if the antagonist gets to the receptor first. This would be analogous to putting a toothpick in a lock, thus not allowing the key to work. The toothpick fits inside the lock but is not able to open it. An antagonist can be competitive (forms reversible bond with receptor) or noncompetitive (forms irreversible bond), depending on the type of chemical bonds formed between the receptor and the drug.

Pharmacodynamics of the nervous system

The nervous system and the endocrine system are the body's internal communication network. The nervous system is capable of rapid response and discrete control, while the endocrine system is slower and typically more diffuse in its response. Both systems help regulate the body's internal environment; this process of regulation is referred to as homeostasis. Both systems are similar in that pharmacologic agents can interact with them at receptor sites and thereby modify function at selected tissue locations.

Looking closer at the nervous system, we can classify it into several major divisions, as follows:

A. Central nervous system
B. Peripheral nervous system
   1. Somatic nervous system
   2. Autonomic nervous system
      a. Sympathetic nervous system
      b. Parasympathetic nervous system

The central nervous system (CNS) consists of the brain and spinal cord, and the peripheral nervous system consists of those nerve pathways outside of the CNS. These pathways can be functionally divided into the afferent pathways, those that conduct information to CNS, and the efferent pathways, those that conduct information away from the CNS.

The somatic nervous system, which is under conscious control, conducts impulses from the CNS to the skeletal muscles. The autonomic nervous system, in contrast, functions beyond the level of our conscious control, although biofeedback techniques can control some of its functions. The autonomic system derives its name from the fact that it performs its many duties, minute by minute, whether we are awake or asleep, in an automatic fashion. Among other things, the autonomic nerves govern the activities of the cardiac muscle, the smooth or involuntary muscles of all body systems (such as the genitourinary and cardiovascular systems), the sweat glands, and certain endocrine glands. Functioning of the autonomic nervous system (ANS) is vital for maintaining homeostasis.

The autonomic division is itself divided into two competitive subdivisions, sympathetic and parasympathetic (Fig. 20-3). Most of the structures listed above are innervated by both divisions. Balance between these two opposing divisions provides precise control of organ function.

Generally, the effects of each subdivision of the autonomic nervous system on a given receptor organ are antagonistic to the other; inactivity of one allows the action of the other to dominate the organ response. Each exerts a constant action against the other, like two forces maintaining a steady pull on each end of a rope. This action is called *tone*, and it establishes a balance of influence on receptor function, ensuring fine control and rapid response. The sympathetic division is designed mainly to protect the integrity and maintain the safety of the organism, which involves the expenditure of energy. The parasympathetic division, on the other hand, is less dynamic in its response and is more concerned with conservation and restoration of function. Table 20-3 summarizes the major differences be-

Table 20-3   Differentiation Between Sympathetic and Parasympathetic Systems

	Sympathetic nervous system	Parasympathetic nervous system
Origin	Thoracolumbar	Craniosacral
Preganglionic fibers	Short	Long
Postganglionic fibers	Long, with many branches	Short, with few branches
Transmitter at ganglia	Acetylcholine	Acetylcholine
Receptor at ganglia	Nicotinic	Nicotinic
Transmitter at effector organ	Norepinephrine (acetylcholine at sweat glands, blood vessels of skeletal muscles)	Acetylcholine
Receptor at effector organ	Alpha, beta	Muscarinic
Major effect	Fight or flight	Feed or breed

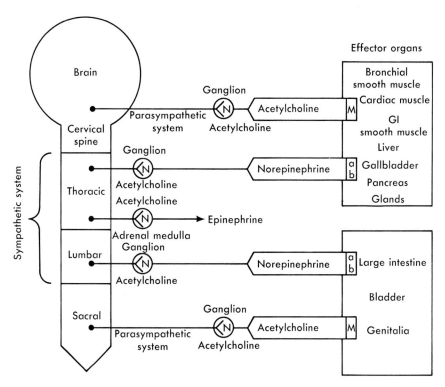

Fig. 20-3 Sympathetic and parasympathetic nervous system innervation. Note that there is dual innervation to effector organs. *Acetylcholine* is the transmitter at all ganglia and at parasympathetic sites. Their receptors are labeled *N* for nicotinic and *M* for musarinic. The transmitters for the *sympathetic system* at the *effector organs* are labeled *a* and *b* for alpha and beta respectively (see text).

tween the sympathetic and parasympathetic components of the autonomic system.

Anatomy. Sympathetic fibers arise in the thoracic and lumbar spinal cord segments, traveling uninterrupted until they reach a ganglion. A ganglion is simply a relay point where many interconnections (synapses) are possible. The preganglionic sympathetic fibers are short and terminate at ganglia, whereas postganglionic fibers are long and terminate at various effector organs. The ratio of preganglionic to postganglionic fibers varies between 1:11 to 1:17. Therefore, an impulse coming in on a preganglionic fiber results in impulses going out on many postganglionic fibers. This phenomenon tends to produce multiple effects at many different locations. In addition, sympathetic innervation results in endocrine action via release of epinephrine from the adrenal gland into the blood. Thus, stimulation of the sympathetic system results in a diffuse response throughout the body.

The parasympathetic fibers originate from the brain and the sacral spinal cord segment and travel without synapsing until they reach the ganglia, which are located near the effector organs. The preganglionic fibers are long, and the postganglionic fibers are short; their ratio is about 1:2, resulting in a more specific and localized response.

Chemical transmitters. The location where nerve fibers synapse, such as at the ganglia or at the effector or-

gan, is called the *neuroeffector junction*. At these special sites, nerve impulses are passed along by a chemical transmitter or mediator, rather than by electrical depolarization (Fig. 20-4). The chemical transmitter is released when a nerve impulse arrives and depolarizes the membrane that contains the transmitter. The transmitter then flows across the synaptic cleft, where it combines with the receptors of the ganglionic fibers or those of the effector organ. When the receptors are activated by the right chemical transmitter, the membrane depolarizes, producing a new impulse or resulting in a response at the effector organ. It is at these locations that autonomic-active drugs exert their effects.

The chemical transmitter at the ganglia of both the sympathetic and parasympathetic systems is acetylcholine. At effector organs, the sympathetic fibers release norepinephrine, whereas the parasympathetic fibers release acetylcholine. As long as the chemical transmitter is present, it will exert its influence. For a drug to have the desired effect, it must be similar to the chemical transmitter at the ganglia or effector organ we want to influence. The nature of the chemical transmitter and its receptor identifies the type of nerve and its response.

Since nerve stimulation must be temporary, something must happen to the transmitter soon after it is released. In fact, there are specific enzymes that destroy the transmit-

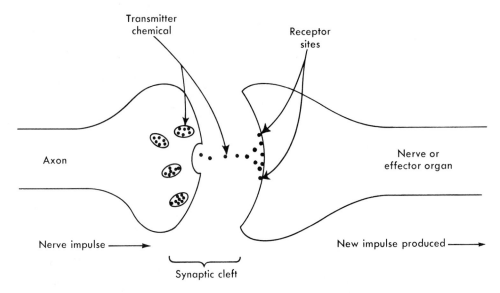

Fig. 20-4   The *nerve impulse* releases a chemical transmitter that flows across the *synaptic cleft* at the ganglion and effector organ. The chemical transmitter attaches to a receptor and initiates a new electrical impulse. Drugs can attach to the receptor sites, producing a response that is similar to the natural chemical transmitter released from the axon terminal.

ters as soon as they have exerted their effect. Norepinephrine (as well as epinephrine) is either (1) reabsorbed into the axon terminal that secreted it, (2) deactivated by a catechol-o-methyl transferase (COMT) enzyme, or (3) deactivated by a monoamine oxidase (MAO) enzyme. The parasympathetic transmitter, acetylcholine, is deactivated by acetylcholinesterase. The removal or deactivation of the transmitter makes it possible for the receptor sites to be stimulated again and again.

Sympathetic nerves that act through the release of norepinephrine (or epinephrine) are called *adrenergic,* deriving their name from the fact that the medulla of the adrenal gland releases adrenaline or epinephrine. Drugs that act like adrenaline are known as adrenergic agents. Since these drugs mediate the effects of the sympathetic nervous system, they are also frequently called sympathomimetic drugs, or drugs that mimic the sympathetic system. Another common term for these drugs is catecholamine. This name is derived from the plant *Mimosa catechu,* which has a chemical agent with a ring structure that is called a catechol. Drugs that resemble the chemical structure from this catechu plant and have an amino group are called catecholamines.[7] Epinephrine and norepinephrine have this same basic structure so they are often referred to as catecholamines.

Cholinergic nerves release and produce their effects via acetylcholine. Drugs that have acetylcholine-like effects are called cholinergic agents. Since acetylcholine is the mediator in the parasympathetic nervous system, agents with its effects are also called parasympathomimetic drugs.

Drugs that block the above effects can be referred to as adrenergic blockers or cholinergic blockers (or anticholin-

ergic). Alternatively, the terms sympatholytic or parasympatholytic may be used to refer to drugs having antagonist effects on these two components of the autonomic nervous system.

Receptors.   The receptors for these chemical transmitters are very specific. The ganglia receptors are called nicotinic receptors, named after the drug nicotine, which was found to exert a stimulating effect here. (Nicotinic receptors are also found at skeletal muscles in the somatic nervous system.) The receptors at the parasympathetic effector site are called muscarinic receptors, named after a mushroom poison (muscarine), which was found to exert its stimulating effects here.

It is interesting to note that acetylcholine is the transmitter at both of these locations, but the receptors are slightly different. This can be understood with our lock and key explanation. In this case, the locks (receptors) are slightly different, but the key (acetylcholine) is a master key that can "unlock" both the nicotinic and muscarinic sites. However, drugs exist that selectively work only at one site or the other, allowing us to achieve a more specific effect. Table 20-4 summarizes the effects observed when nicotinic and muscarinic receptors are stimulated.

The sympathetic system receptors at the effector sites are of two basic types, alpha and beta. The characteristic effects of stimulating these two receptor sites are shown in Table 20-5. Beta receptors can be further differentiated into two groups according to their abilities to (1) hydrolyze fatty acids, (2) stimulate the heart, (3) dilate bronchi, and (4) relax arterioles. Some beta stimulators primarily produce hydrolysis of fatty acids and cardiac stimulation, while others produce bronchodilation and arteriole relaxation. Receptors that affect primarily the heart are called beta$_1$ receptors, and those that primarily dilate bronchi are called beta$_2$ receptors. Drugs that primarily stimulate beta$_2$ receptors are the desired drugs to use for bronchodilation since fewer cardiac side effects accompany their use.

Alpha receptor stimulation in the cardiopulmonary system results in vasoconstriction, slight bronchoconstriction, and a reflex decrease in heart rate (see Chapter 7). As with beta receptors, alpha receptors can be further categorized according to their specific actions. Alpha$_1$ receptor stimulation results in contraction of innervated smooth muscle. Alpha$_2$ stimulation inhibits the release of norepinephrine from the presynaptic area. Drugs can be chosen that will selectively stimulate either or both of these alpha recep-

tors. Generally, the predominant alpha effect is that associated with alpha$_1$ stimulation. Alpha$_1$ stimulating drugs have been used in respiratory care for decreasing mucosal congestion of the airways and nasal passages.

Cellular action. At the level of the smooth muscle cells, specific biochemical reactions occur in response to the release of chemical transmitters or pharmacologic agents (Fig. 20-5). Beta$_2$ adrenergic drugs bind to the receptor, adenylate cyclase, which is an enzyme that catalyzes the conversion of adenosine triphosphate (ATP) to cyclic adenosine monophosphate (cAMP). The level or concentration of cAMP is important in mediating the effect of the drug that is bound to the receptor. cAMP exerts its effects through various enzyme systems (kinases), which result in the primary effect, bronchial smooth muscle relaxation. Any drug that promotes an increase in cAMP levels will result in smooth muscle relaxation; any drug that causes a decrease in cAMP levels will result in smooth muscle constriction.

The level of cAMP is increased via activation of the cellular adenylate cyclase receptor mechanism. Beta$_2$ adrenergic drugs increase cAMP via this mechanism. However, cAMP levels can also be increased by blocking its inactivation. Normally, the enzyme phosphodiesterase hydrolyzes cAMP into an inactive form (5'AMP), thereby decreasing its concentration. Therefore, any drug that interferes with the action of phosphodiesterase will also increase cAMP levels. Stimulation of the alpha receptor also results in decreased levels of cAMP.

The action at the cholinergic receptors of smooth muscle is similar; only the nucleotides are different. In this case, guanosine triphosphate (GTP) is converted to cyclic guanosine monophosphate (cGMP). An increase in the level of cGMP results in an increase in bronchial smooth muscle constriction. As shown in Fig. 20-5, the bronchial smooth muscle tone is a function of the amount of cAMP and cGMP present at any given time. The level of cAMP and cGMP is a result of the sympathetic and parasympathetic nervous system activities as well as the action of any drugs that may be present.

Table 20-4 Effects of Nicotinic and Muscarinic Stimulation on Various Organ Systems

Organ system	Nicotine effects	Muscarinic effects
Autonomic ganglia	Stimulated	—
Airways in lung	*	Constriction
Heart rate	*	Decreased
Blood pressure	*	Decreased
Blood vessels	*	Dilation
Gastrointestinal		
Tone	Increased	Increased
Motility	Increased	Increased
Sphincters	—	Relaxed
Salivary gland	First increase,	Increase
secretions		
Sweat glands	then decrease	Increase
Bronchial gland		Increase
secretions		
Eye	—	Pupil constriction; decreased accommodation
Skeletal muscle	Stimulated	—

Modified from Bergersen BS: Pharmacology in nursing, ed 14, St Louis, 1979, The CV Mosby Co.
*Stimulation of nicotinic receptors at ganglia produces both sympathetic and parasympathetic effects. If muscarinic effects are blocked with atropine, then nicotinic stimulation results in sympathetic-like results.

Table 20-5 Alpha and Beta Receptor Effects in the Cardiopulmonary System and Elsewhere

	Alpha	Beta$_1$	Beta$_2$
Cardiopulmonary	Vasoconstriction	—	Vasodilation
	Slight bronchoconstriction	—	Bronchodilation
	Decrease in heart rate (reflex)	Increase in heart rate	—
	—	Increase in heart contraction	—
Other effects	Enhancement of histamine release		Inhibition of histamine release
	Constriction of GI sphincters	Lypolysis	Skeletal muscle tremor
	Contraction of ureters	Relaxation of GI system	
	Dilation of pupils	Relaxation of uterus	
	Contraction of pilomotor muscles		
	Hepatic glycogenolysis		
	Contraction of uterus		

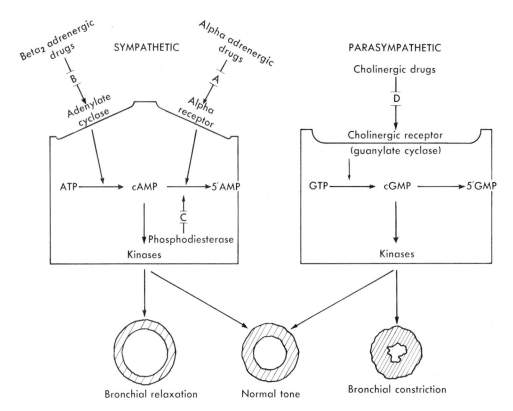

Fig. 20-5   Model of drug mechanism of action for adrenergic and cholinergic drugs. Note that drugs act at specific receptor sites, which then influences cAMP or cGMP levels. The amount of cAMP to cGMP determines the outcome on the bronchial smooth muscle. At *A, B, C,* and *D,* blocking agents can inhibit the function of the specific enzyme system.

Obviously, antagonists can block these reactions at several key points. At point A, alpha effects can be blocked by drugs like phentolamine. Beta blockers, like propranolol, act at point B, whereas xanthines, such as theophylline, block phosphodiesterase at point C. Anticholinergic drugs, like atropine, block cholinergic stimulation at point D.

Goals of respiratory pharmacology

The primary purpose of respiratory pharmacology is to relieve or prevent the pathologic triad, bronchospasm, mucosal edema, and retained secretions. The agents used to relieve these symptoms can be called the treatment triad and consist of bronchodilators, decongestants, and mucokinetic agents. The pathologic triad and treatment are outlined below:

Pathologic Condition	Treatment
Bronchoconstriction	Bronchodilator (eg, isoproterenol, isoetharine)
Airway edema	Decongestant (eg, phenylephrine)
Retained secretions	Hydration (eg, water); mucolytics (eg, acetylcysteine)

Fig. 20-6 shows the specific sites of action of the various categories of pharmacologic agents employed to re-

lieve the pathologic triad. Bronchodilators increase the lumen of the airways by relaxing the spasm of the bronchial muscle, which is triggered by disease or irritation. Most decongestants (agents that relieve congestion) act by contracting the muscle fibers of the arterioles and small arteries, thereby reducing blood flow to the affected area and lowering the hydrostatic pressure that permits fluid to move into the tissues. Mucokinetic agents are used to loosen and mobilize secretions. Mucokinetic action may involve (1) simple dilution of the mucus by direct application of liquid agents, (2) stimulation of serous secretion within the airways, thereby decreasing mucus viscosity, or (3) actual chemical breakdown of secretion components. Bronchodilators and mucokinetic agents are discussed in detail in this chapter. The decongestants are most often combined with bronchodilators for aerosol therapy either as a separate drug or simply as a secondary action of the primary bronchodilator agent. Decongestants are discussed as applicable.

Prevention of the symptoms associated with the pathologic triad is directed at minimizing or blocking the underlying causes. Inflammatory responses caused by immune reactions or infection are the primary causative factors in the development of the pathologic triad. Preventative treatment therefore includes selected anti-inflammatory or anti-

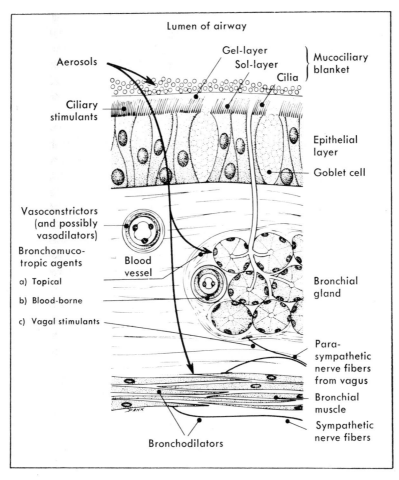

Lumen of airway

Aerosols

Gel-layer
Sol-layer
Cilia

Mucociliary blanket

Ciliary stimulants

Epithelial layer

Goblet cell

Vasoconstrictors (and possibly vasodilators)

Bronchomuco-tropic agents

a) Topical

b) Blood-borne

c) Vagal stimulants

Blood vessel

Bronchial gland

Para-sympathetic nerve fibers from vagus

Bronchial muscle

Sympathetic nerve fibers

Bronchodilators

Fig. 20-6   Schema of anatomy showing important components of mucokinetic system. (From Ziment L: Secretions of the respiratory tract: physiology and pharmacology, New York, 1976, Projects in Health, Inc.)

microbial agents. Both of these categories of drugs have become a vital part of the current respiratory care pharmacopoeia and will no doubt assume a growing role in the future.

BRONCHODILATORS

Bronchodilation is most commonly achieved via the use of adrenergic agents. Supplementing this approach in the pharmacopoeia of respiratory care are selected anticholinergic drugs, the xanthines, and, more recently, the prostaglandins.

Adrenergic bronchodilators

Adrenergic bronchodilators are the most widely used of all pharmacologic agents in respiratory care. Although our major focus will be on their relative efficacy in relieving bronchial smooth muscle contraction, adrenergic bronchodilators are potent drugs with multiple side effects. For this reason, the clinician must have full knowledge of the range of action of these agents and be able to recognize

and respond to any untoward effects associated with their administration.

Some preparations of these drugs are administered orally, others by inhalation, and some are effective given by either route. The general effects that adrenergic agents exhibit on the body as a whole were summarized in Table 20-5. Table 20-6 summarizes the common adrenergic agents in current use, providing information on their commercial preparations, dosages, and quantitative estimation of their effects. This table can be referred to as each agent is discussed.

In addition to their effects on the bronchial smooth muscle and vasculature, some adrenergic bronchodilators facilitate the transport of airway mucus. Studies following the parenteral use of the beta stimulant, terbutaline, showed up to 110% of average tracheal mucus velocity in patients with chronic obstructive airway disease.[8] There was no apparent increase in flow in normal subjects. It is therefore possible that the effectiveness of catecholamines in the treatment of obstructive disease is a result of the dual action of bronchodilation and increased mucus transport. Although the mechanism for the latter is not apparent, it may account for instances of subjective evidence of increased mucus removal even though tests of airway patency show no improvement.

It also has been observed that some beta$_2$ adrenergic compounds, specifically fenoterol, can decrease lung recoil pressure.[9] In principle, this effect could result in a decrease in breathing work for some patients. The decrease in lung recoil pressure appears related to the systemic action of the drug on the parenchyma of the lung, via absorption into the circulation. However, this action is of short duration (30 minutes).

It is well recognized that many of the effects of bronchodilators, especially side effects and possibly some bronchodilator effects, occur as a result of the aerosolized drug being absorbed into the circulation. Studies indicate that only about 10% of the aerosolized drug actually deposits in the lung, the remainder either being exhaled or deposited in the mouth or oropharynx and swallowed.[10] Thus plasma levels of the drug may be responsible for some of the drug action via absorption in the gastrointestinal tract, if not metabolized, or via bronchial absorption.[11,12]

It is important to reiterate the commonly experienced side effects with adrenergic bronchodilators, as summarized as follows:

Side effect	Cause
Increased heart rate	Beta$_1$ stimulation
Arrhythmias, palpitation	Beta$_1$ stimulation
Skeletal muscle tremor	Beta$_2$ stimulation
Anxiety, nervousness, insomnia, nausea	Beta$_2$ CNS stimulation
Decreased Pao$_2$ (occasional)	Beta$_2$ vasodilation in lung producing altered $\dot{V}/\dot{Q}$

All patients will experience one or more of these side effects while using adrenergic bronchodilators. Some patients will be more sensitive to adverse effects than others, and the dose that is necessary to achieve adequate bronchodilation may result in excessive side effects. Thus termination of treatment occurs before therapeutic effects are achieved. Careful monitoring of respiratory patients is always essential, especially for those patients who are receiving heart medication or using other adrenergic drugs.

Proper monitoring by a respiratory care practitioner should include the following: assessment of pulse and respiratory rate before, during, and after the treatment; bedside measurement of pulmonary function values before and after treatment; auscultation of lung fields before and after treatment; and continual observation for systemic symptoms of unwanted side effects, such as tremor, sweating, or fatigue.[13] A treatment should be terminated if the pulse rate becomes excessive (increases more than 20 beats/min)

Table 20-6   Adrenergic Bronchodilators

Generic name	Brand name(s)	Available preparations	Single dose		Action			Duration (hours)
			Inhalation	Oral	alpha	beta$_1$	beta$_2$	
Epinephrine	Adrenalin Asthmanephrin	1:100 (1%) 10 mg/ml	0.25-0.5 ml	NA	+3	+4	+3	0.5 to 2 (Short)
Racemic epinephrine	Vaponefrin Micronephrin	1:44 (2.25%) 22 mg/ml	0.25-0.5 ml	NA	+2	+3	+2	0.5 to 2 (Short)
Ephedrine	Tedral Bronkotabs	15, 25, 50 mg tabs	NA	15-50 mg	+2	+3	+3	3 to 4 (Medium)
Isoproterenol	Isuprel	1:200 (0.5%) 5 mg/ml	0.25-0.5 ml	NA	—	+4	+4	0.5 to 2 (Short)
Metaproterenol	Alupent Metaprel	1:20 (5%) 50 mg/ml MDI (0.65 mg) 20 mg tabs	0.2-0.3 ml 2-3 puffs	20 mg	—	+2	+2	3 to 4 (Medium)
Isoetharine	Bronkosol Dilabron	1:100 (1%) 10 mg/ml	0.25-0.5 ml	NA	—	+1	+3	3 to 4 (Medium)
Salbutamol	Ventolin Proventil Albuterol	1:200 (0.5%) MDI (90 µg) 2, 4 mg tabs	0.5 ml 1-2 puffs	2 or 4 mg	—	+1	+4	4 to 6 (Long)
Terbutaline sulfate	Bricanyl Brethine Brethaire	2.5, 5 mg tabs 1:1000 IV/SC MDI (0.2 mg)	0.5 ml* 2 puffs	2.5 or 5 mg	—	+1	+4	3 to 7 (Long)
Bitolterol mesylate	Tornalate	MDI (0.37 mg)	2 puffs	NA	—	+3	+4	5 to 8 (Long)
Fenoterol	Berotec (Europe)	5, 10 mg tabs	NA	5 or 10 mg	—	+1	+4	8 to 10 (Long)

*Use of the parenteral form of terbutaline for inhalation under FDA investigation.

or should not even be started if a patient is experiencing tachycardia. Attaining the desired respiratory rate usually requires no more than simple coaching of the patient to breathe in a manner that is slow, relaxed, and of proper volume to ensure maximum therapeutic effect (see Chapter 23). All of the above monitored parameters should be charted, as well as any other patient response to the treatment. There are many individual variations that may modify these general recommendations, and specific problems or questions should be discussed with the patient's physician.

Epinephrine. Epinephrine is the standard against which most sympathomimetics are judged. Epinephrine is a potent drug, and since it stimulates all three adrenergic receptors, its use carries with it the risk of serious, unwanted side effects. It performs important functions in regulating the body's metabolism and maintaining a state of alertness to cope with the environment. The practitioner sees this drug used frequently in the hospital for its effect on the circulation and to combat allergic reactions, for which it is administered by injection under the skin, into muscle, or into superficial veins. It is almost completely inactivated in the stomach; thus oral use is not feasible. However, it has been used parenterally for many years for the relief of acute bronchial asthma.

Epinephrine is one of the most powerful bronchodilators and decongestants, whether given by injection or by aerosol. Its action by aerosol is both topical and systemic. Thus, inhalation generally affords quicker response than does subcutaneous or intramuscular injection, although not exceeding the intravenous route.

There are two major hazards to aerosolized epinephrine. First, the unwanted side effects may be a danger as well as a nuisance, and the effect on the cardiovascular system may outweigh its benefits. This is especially true in elderly patients or in those with known heart or vascular disease. Second, repeated use of epinephrine often leads to tolerance, necessitating dangerously larger doses to achieve the desired therapeutic effect. A patient exhibiting this phenomenon is considered to be *epinephrine-fast*. Less commonly seen is a paradoxical response in which the symptoms of acute airway obstruction actually are made worse by these aerosols. It is believed that this adverse effect is a result of the development of an allergy to some of the metabolic end products of the drugs.[14]

If epinephrine is to be used as a bronchodilator-decongestant aerosol, nothing stronger than a 1% aqueous solution (1:100) should be considered safe. Two effective inhalations from 30 to 60 seconds apart are sufficient, and treatments should be spaced at least 4 hours apart. Because of the development of safer preparations, some of which are described later in this chapter, the use of epinephrine aerosol has rapidly declined in recent years.

l-**Norepinephrine; levarterenol.** This major sympathetic nerve stimulus mediator, when administered therapeutically, is limited in its action and, although not a bronchodilator, is included here for completeness. Levarterenol is exclusively an alpha receptor stimulant, with its primary effector the cardiovascular system. Given intravenously, its only clinical use is the support of blood pressure in certain types of shock.

Racemic epinephrine (Micronephrin, Vaponefrin). This drug is a mixture of two isomers (chemical formula is identical but atoms arranged differently) of epinephrine. It is a little less potent in its effects than epinephrine and, therefore, exerts fewer side effects, yet can achieve reasonable bronchodilation. It serves the purpose of relaxing bronchial smooth muscle and decreasing mucosal congestion by its alpha action. It has been recommended for laryngotracheobronchitis[15] and may be of value in recently extubated patients because of its decongestant action. The use of racemic epinephrine also has shown to be effective for the acute signs of croup.[16]

Ephedrine. Although ephedrine is not used as an aerosol, its close similarity to the action of epinephrine and its frequency of use warrants its mention at this time. Ephedrine is an alkaloid derived from the plant *Ephedra vulgaris,* an herb used by the Chinese for over 5000 years. Ephedrine has a less intense, but longer lasting, bronchodilating effect than epinephrine. Its longer duration of action is attributable to the fact that it is not inactivated by COMT or MAO. Also unlike epinephrine, it is a strong cerebral stimulant. A major advantage of ephedrine is its oral effectiveness; it is used commonly in over-the-counter preparations with other bronchodilators, expectorants, or sedatives. Excessive use, as by patient self-administration, can cause serious mental excitation.

Isoproterenol (Isuprel). A powerful beta stimulator with negligible alpha effects, isoproterenol has enjoyed wide use as an aerosol bronchodilator. Although more selective in its effects than are epinephrine and ephedrine, its role as a bronchodilator is limited by its stimulation of beta$_1$ receptors. The rise in cardiac output associated with its beta$_1$ effects can increase pulmonary perfusion in excess of ventilation, especially in poorly ventilated areas of the lung. This effect will reduce the $\dot{V}/\dot{Q}$ ratio in these areas and can actually worsen arterial hypoxemia. Further, strong beta$_1$ stimulation can increase the risk of cardiac arrhythmias, especially in the presence of hypoxemia.[17]

However, clinical experience with isoproterenol is extensive enough that it can still be used effectively as an inhalant, with a wide range of safety. A major advantage of this aerosol is its somewhat better bronchodilating effect than that of epinephrine, with nearly complete absence of vasopressor action. In contrast to epinephrine, isoproterenol produces vasodilation and, thus, has negligible decongestant value. This vasodilatory action tends to lower diastolic blood pressure, thereby encouraging an increase in heart rate. Other side effects are infrequent and mild. These include nausea, excitement, and tremors.[18]

Although available in aqueous concentrations of 1:100 and 1:200, for routine aerosol use the 1:200 strength is recommended. For intermittent short-term therapy, as in self-administration, two to four well-spaced inhalations at 4-hour intervals is a conservative program, although the general safety of the drug allows for considerable flexibility according to clinical need. Since all aerosols are, in a sense, foreign bodies, overuse of them often causes severe pharyngeal and laryngeal irritation, further aggravating the very condition being treated. Warning of this possibility should be included in instructions given to all patients who are to treat themselves. For prolonged bronchodilation, especially as administered with mechanical ventilators, the isoproterenol should be further diluted to concentrations of 1:400 or 1:600.

Metaproterenol (Alupent, Metaprel). A derivative of isoproterenol, metaproterenol has many of the same effects.[19,20] It can be taken orally, inhaled as an aerosolized powder from a pressurized cartridge, or a liquid form can be nebulized. It has $beta_1$ side effects when given by inhalation and comparable $beta_2$ effects when compared with isoproterenol but with significantly increased duration of action.

Isoetharine (Bronkosol). Isoetharine is a commonly used bronchodilator with a lesser effect than isoproterenol. The cardiovascular side effects of isoetharine have also been noted to be less intense.[21] It is claimed to be mostly a $beta_2$ stimulator, with clinically insignificant $beta_1$ activity. In one test of cardiovascular responses to a strong exposure to the drug, intravenous administration of isoetharine to anesthetized patients caused a decrease in systolic and diastolic blood pressures ($beta_2$ effect) and an increase in heart rate ($beta_1$ effect) but not arrhythmias.[22] Isoetharine can be administered orally as well as by aerosol, and it is reportedly more effective in conditions characterized by diffuse bronchospasm, as in bronchial asthma, than in those with obstructing secretions, as chronic bronchitis.[23]

Salbutamol (Proventil, Ventolin). Salbutamol is a selective $beta_2$ stimulant that has fewer side effects than isoproterenol.[24,25] Nebulized salbutamol appears to take longer to achieve bronchodilation but has a longer-lasting effect because it is not metabolized by COMT.[26] A major asset is its effectiveness, whether given by mouth, intravenously, or in aerosol form. However, for many conditions the administration of the aerosolized drug appears to offer fewer side effects, and there are some indications that better results are achieved by this route in acute asthma.[27]

Terbutaline sulfate (Bricanyl, Brethine, Brethaire). Terbutaline is available in oral, parenteral, and MDI preparations. Use of the parenteral form as a nebulized aerosol is currently undergoing investigation. Terbutaline is a very specific $beta_2$ adrenergic with minimal $beta_1$ effects. It is twice as potent as metaproterenol and has a longer duration of action.[28]

Bitolterol mesylate (Tornalate). Bitolterol mesylate is a *pro-drug,* that is, a chemical compound metabolized to an active form upon administration. Bitolterol mesylate is hydrolyzed in the tissues and blood into the beta adrenergic bronchodilator colterol, an agent that in animal studies exhibits preferential $beta_2$ effects. As a pro-drug, bitolterol mesylate has both a rapid onset of action and a comparatively longer duration of action (up to 8 hours in some patients) than other comparable agents.[29] It is currently available only in an MDI preparation.

Fenoterol. Fenoterol is not yet available for general clinical use in the US. Studies indicate that it is an effective $beta_2$ stimulant, whether given orally or by inhalation. Its duration of effect appears to be persistent (about 8 hours) and is accompanied by minimal $beta_1$ effects. However, a recent study using aerosolized fenoterol versus terbutaline reported a better overall clinical effect for terbutaline.[30] More clinical studies will determine its overall usefulness.

It should be emphasized that adverse effects, or at least failure to achieve or sustain benefit, are commonly seen with most of the adrenergics now in use. Although unsatisfactory results may represent side effects, local airway irritation or the actual blockade of beta receptors by accumulated adrenergic metabolites may also be involved.[31] Isoproterenol is especially susceptible to the latter reaction, particularly if used too frequently or over too long a period of time. Metabolic products of the breakdown of isoproterenol can accumulate faster than enzymatic degradation can destroy them. Some of the metabolites block the beta receptor from bronchodilator action, and further administration of isoproterenol actually can increase bronchospasm.

Anticholinergic (parasympatholytic) bronchodilators

Anticholinergic or parasympatholytic bronchodilators act at the muscarinic receptors of the parasympathetic nervous system.[32] Normally, acetylcholine acts as the chemical transmitter at these postganglionic sites. Agents that competitively block the action of acetylcholine will decrease intracellular levels of cGMP, thereby favoring smooth muscle relaxation.

Atropine sulfate. Atropine is the model anticholinergic bronchodilator agent. An alkaloid found in the plants *Atropa belladonna* and *Datura stramonium,* atropine has been used for many years in the treatment of airway disease. Inhalation of the smoke of stramonium leaves was a favorite remedy for asthma, but the increased use of adrenergic drugs has gradually displaced atropine as a bronchodilator. Yet, recent evidence suggests that anticholinergic bronchodilators may have a useful place in the pharmacopoeia of respiratory care, especially in the treatment of reflex bronchoconstriction caused by increased vagal tone.[33,34]

Related to other drugs such as scopolamine and hyoscyamine, atropine blocks the effect of parasympathetic stimuli by increasing the threshold of response of effector cells to acetylcholine. In principle, such action will elicit a response resembling stimulation of adrenergic receptors, since these are freed of competing and counteracting cholinergic stimulus.

Although other parasympathetic nerves are affected, atropine inhibits vagal stimulation of the heart and respiratory tract, thereby elevating blood pressure and cardiac rate and dilating bronchi. In addition, atropine may act on the central nervous system, stimulating the cerebral respiratory centers to generate rapid, deep breathing.[34] Relative to the patient with airway obstruction, the two most important actions of atropine can be summarized as follows:

1. Reduction of secretions. Atropine inhibits secretions of nose, mouth, pharynx, and bronchi by reducing their fluid volumes and increasing their viscosities. This property made atropine and related derivatives popular in compounds prescribed to relieve symptoms of the common cold and in preoperative medication to reduce the mucus-producing stimulus of anesthetics and airway instrumentation. However, this effect of atropine poses a potential threat to patients already handicapped by thick, bronchial exudates, subjecting them to the risk of serious aggravation of their obstruction. This hazard has probably been the major impediment to the continued use of atropine in respiratory problems.

2. Bronchodilation. By blocking cholinergic influences on bronchial muscle, atropine potentiates beta-adrenergic dilation and widens the airways. Because there is no evidence that acetylcholine plays an active role in generating bronchospasm, atropine is a less effective dilator than either epinephrine or isoproterenol. Yet the beneficial effect of atropine on bronchoconstriction has been well demonstrated in airways that were subjected to dust inhalation and protected by the drug parenterally administered.[35] Aerosol studies have employed 1% and 0.2% concentrations of atropine in equal parts of propylene glycol and water.[36]

With the proper administration of atropine aerosol, airway resistance can be significantly reduced in normal subjects as well as in obstructed patients. Bronchi are also protected against the induced bronchospasm of inhaled irritants such as carbachol and aluminum dust. Results were equally satisfactory with the 0.2% as with the 2% solution. It has been suggested that atropine in small amounts be added to sympathomimetic mixtures, and one study demonstrated that an aerosol of isoproterenol and atropine methonitrate gave better bronchodilation than either alone, combining the rapid onset and short duration of isoproterenol with the slower but more prolonged effect of atropine.[37]

Ipratropium bromide (Sch 1000, Atrovent). Ipratropium bromide (chemically N-isopropyl-nortropine) is an atropine-like agent originally developed in the 1960s. Like atropine, ipratropium bromide probably acts by antagonizing the action of acetylcholine and inhibiting increases in intracellular cyclic guanosine monophosphate (cGMP).[38,39]

Ipratropium bromide is available currently only in MDI form, with a usual dosage of approximately 36 μg (two inhalations) four times per day. At these dosage levels, it produces bronchodilation almost as effectively as isoproterenol. Onset of its action is three to six times as long as that of isoproterenol, but its duration is four times greater.

In contrast to atropine, ipratropium bromide does not elicit any subjective drying of oral or ocular secretions. One study has suggested that atropine-like products acted predominantly on receptors in the larger airways, whereas beta$_2$ adrenergics favored the smaller airways.[40] Other investigators have found no difference in the pattern or apparent site of response of ipratropium bromide to fenoterol or metaproterenol.[41,42]

Besides its centrally mediated anticholinergic effects,[43] ipratropium bromide also appears to lessen the effects of cell mediators that initiate bronchospasm (serotonin, histamine, PGF$_2$ alpha and bradykinin), and even potentiates the smooth muscle relaxation effects of adrenergics.[44,45] It was observed that if ipratropium bromide was followed by metaproterenol in allergic asthmatics, there was significantly greater airway improvement over either agent used alone.[46] Ipratropium bromide may also be useful in patients for whom adrenergic bronchodilators are contraindicated.[47] Moreover, the response to this bronchodilator is even greater in those asthmatics with a major psychogenic component to their asthma.[48]

Xanthines

Xanthines are a group of organic vegetable compounds related to a naturally occurring precursor of uric acid. The three most important xanthines are caffeine, theophylline, and theobromine. We are all familiar with caffeine as an important ingredient of coffee, tea, cola drinks, and cocoa, but the xanthine group as a whole has some specific physiologic actions that make them valuable as pharmacologics. Although the relative effects of these three agents vary, all produce the following responses:

1. CNS stimulation,
2. Bronchodilation,
3. Pulmonary vasodilation,
4. Smooth muscle relaxation,
5. Diuresis,
6. Coronary artery dilation,
7. Cardiac stimulation, and
8. Skeletal muscle stimulation.

Although caffeine and theobromine were used in the past for cardiac stimulation and diuresis, they have been replaced by more effective agents. Theophylline, on the other hand, still plays an important role in clinical therapeutics. In addition to its use for bronchodilation, theophylline is employed in certain types and stages of congestive heart failure and is especially valuable in correcting Cheyne-Stokes' breathing. It has more recently received attention from its ability to decrease the frequency of apneic episodes in premature infants.[49-51]

The value of theophylline can be appreciated from reviewing Fig. 20-5. Unlike the adrenergics, which increase cyclic adenosine monophosphate (cAMP) by stimulating its production, theophylline is thought to maintain cAMP levels by inhibiting phosphodiesterase, thereby decreasing its destruction. Theophylline may also competitively antagonize the prostaglandin PGF_2, a potent bronchoconstricting agent, and appears to have an effect on calcium movement across the cellular membranes of smooth muscle.

In concept, the action of theophylline should allow patients to alter medications between beta$_2$ adrenergics and xanthines, thereby decreasing the likelihood of developing tolerance to the adrenergics, as well as minimizing their adverse effects. For this reason, the practitioner will see theophylline, or its various derivatives, frequently used for patients with diffuse bronchospasm and in cases of intractable bronchial asthma, especially when there is refractoriness to the sympathomimetics.

Acute exacerbations of bronchospasm are commonly treated with intravenous administration of theophylline derivatives. Intramuscular and rectal routes are sometimes used, but these are less effective. For overall treatment of patients prone to bronchospasm, oral theophylline or its derivatives are frequently part of the drug regimen along with adrenergic agents. The goal is to maintain therapeutic levels of theophylline in the plasma, which is approximately 10 to 20 μg/ml of serum. However, the therapeutic dose is close to the toxic dose, and adverse effects are more likely. For this reason, prescribing physicians periodically monitor serum theophylline levels on their patients to accurately adjust the dosage and to minimize side effects.[52] The most common side effects, occurring at plasma levels of 20 to 30 μg/ml, are anorexia, nausea, and vomiting. Cardiovascular effects such as tachycardia, palpitations, and arrhythmias may be seen at plasma levels in excess of 30 μg/ml. CNS effects, which include nervousness, insomnia, and tremulousness, may be seen at and above therapeutic levels, with seizures possible when plasma levels reach 40 to 50 μg/ml. Variables that affect the half-life of the drug and, therefore, alter the dosage or frequency of administration of theophylline are listed in the box opposite.

Patients who smoke cigarettes have a shorter half-life of theophylline and require greater frequency of administration.[53] It has also been reported that certain upper respiratory tract viral infections can increase the half-life of theophylline in a significant manner.[54]

As an aerosol, aminophylline has not enjoyed as widespread use as the sympathomimetic agents. The aerosol is irritating to the pharynx and can cause substantial wheezing and coughing. Moreover, most evidence indicates that aminophylline by aerosol has a minimal effect on forced expiratory flow rates in patients with acute obstructive disorders.[55,56]

VARIABLES AFFECTING HALF-LIFE OF THEOPHYLLINE

SITUATIONS REQUIRING INCREASED DOSAGE	INCREASE*
Cigarette smoking	25-75%
Exposure to smog or hydrocarbons	10-25%
High caffeine intake	10-20%
Barbiturate or phenytoin use	10-15%
High-protein diet	10-15%
Suboptimal blood levels	—
Patients known to have high tolerance to theophylline	—
Children 2 months to 16 years	—

SITUATIONS REQUIRING DECREASED DOSAGE	DECREASE*
Hepatic congestion or insufficiency	20-50%
Marked obesity	20-50%
Overt heart failure	20-30%
Marked hypoxemia	10-25%
Febrile illness	10-20%
Antibiotic use of erythromycin, troleandomycin, lincomycin, or clindamycin	10-20%
Cimetidine use	10-20%
Patients exhibiting toxic symptoms	—

*Approximate guidelines for dosage adjustments. Serum levels provide more accurate guidance. (Modified from information supplied by Irwin Ziment, MD. Used by permission.)

Prostaglandins

Prostaglandins are naturally occurring, 20-carbon, unsaturated fatty acids synthesized mainly in the seminal vesicles, kidneys, and lungs. Of the 14 known prostaglandins, three are of substantial interest in respiratory pharmacology: PGE_1, PGE_2, and PGF_{2a}. PGE_1 and PGE_2 cause relaxation of bronchial smooth muscle; prostaglandin PGF_{2a} causes contraction of bronchial smooth muscle.

Unlike the adrenergic or anticholinergic drugs previously discussed, prostaglandins do not act through autonomic neural control or mediator release. Instead, they appear to act directly on smooth muscle.[57] PGE_1 and PGE_2 increase cellular adenyl cyclase and therefore cAMP, but via a pathway that cannot be blocked by sympathetic antagonists. PGF_{2a} is thought to act via direct stimulation of cGMP production.

Prostaglandins are produced in vivo during anaphylactic reactions and with pulmonary edema and embolism. Their synthesis is also increased with hypoxia, hypocapnea, and mechanical stimulation of the lung. This latter effect may help explain the hypotension sometimes associated with positive pressure ventilation.[57]

Because of the experimental nature of prostaglandins, a

detailed description of their therapeutic actions is unjustified in this text. The interested student can find many good references in the literature.[58-65] In general, aerosolized PGE$_1$ has been shown to decrease airway resistance in asthmatic patients to a greater degree than isoproterenol, and PGE$_2$ has an additive effective to beta-adrenergic stimulation. Approaching the problem from a different direction, bronchodilation can also be achieved experimentally by the action of a substance known as polyphloretin phosphate, which inhibits the constrictor effect of PGF$_{2a}$. It is expected that the future will show the prostaglandins revealing previously unknown mechanisms in the production of bronchospasm and at the same time increasing our arsenal against airway obstruction.

MUCOKINETIC DRUGS

The mucociliary system represents the primary clearance and defense mechanism of the conducting zone of the lung (see Chapter 6). Mucokinetics is concerned with the movement of mucus in the respiratory tract and the overall effectiveness of the mucociliary system.

The effectiveness with which the mucociliary system fulfills its important role in clearance and defense depends on complex interactions between the mucus "blanket" itself and the cilia. The blanket consists of a high-viscosity mucopolysaccharide gel layer that "floats" on top of a low-viscosity serous sol layer. Interestingly, although consisting mainly of water, the gel component of the mucus is relatively impervious to water (which is its primary constituent). This suggests that the gel layer serves not only to facilitate surface transport, but also to prevent dehydration.[66]

In health, the composition of the mucus blanket represents a delicate balance between the production of the goblet cells and the bronchial glands. The goblet cells are primarily responsible for production of the mucopolysaccharide gel layer, whereas the bronchial glands probably produce most of the serous-like secretions. Goblet cells are under local control, increasing their production mainly in response to irritant factors such as noxious gases or infectious agents. Although the bronchial glands can respond locally, they are primarily under central control, being stimulated to increase production mainly by vagal (parasympathetic) innervation.

The bronchial glands therefore can be affected by drugs that act either locally or systemically. They can be stimulated directly by topical cholinergic drugs or systemically by agents that evoke a vagal response. Because cholinergic drugs (such as pilocarpine) have strong muscarinic side effects, their use as mucokinetic agents is limited. However, oral expectorants, such as glyceryl guaiacolate or the iodides, are commonly used as systemic agents, evoking a vagal response by irritating the lining of the stomach.

Ciliary activity also is affected by chemical and physical agents, being increased by both adrenergic and cholinergic drugs and the methylxanthines.[57] Ciliary activity is reduced by dehydration, cigarette smoke, alcohol, and anticholinergics such as atropine.

Normal mucokinesis, then, depends on the proper composition of the gel and sol layers as well as optimum functioning of the cilia. Impairment of either of these systems can hinder both pulmonary clearance and defense, increasing the likelihood of obstruction or infection. Mucokinetic therapy aims to maintain or improve functioning of the mucociliary mechanism, thereby promoting effective clearance of respiratory tract secretions and minimizing the possibility of infection. Aerosolized agents used to facilitate mucokinesis fall into four major categories: (1) diluting or hydrating agents, (2) wetting agents, (3) mucolytics, and (4) proteolytics.

Diluting or hydrating agents

Water. Of all the agents used to modify the character of respiratory tract secretions, none is more important than water. Although water can be aerosolized or vaporized (see Chapter 23), there is no substitute for adequate systemic hydration. Generous consumption of water is necessary for optimum functioning of the respiratory system as well as the body in general. Water is one of the few agents that has no side effects unless taken in extremely large quantities. Only in those small infants or patients with congestive heart failure or excessive fluid retention is water restriction considered. Water is the first and most important agent to be considered when patients have difficulty mobilizing bronchial secretions.

Saline. Saline (NaCl) is one of the most commonly used aerosols, either alone or with bronchodilators. Normal saline can be nebulized for diluting the mucus and enhancing clearance, or it can be instilled directly into the airway to increase the effectiveness of suctioning.

Normal saline (0.9% NaCl) is considered a bland aerosol since its osmolarity approximates that of body fluids. However, as aerosolized normal saline particles enter the respiratory tract, the water in the droplets evaporates, resulting in a hypertonic solution (greater than 0.9%). Because of this increased tonicity, a normal saline aerosol can provoke bronchospasm in certain patients, particularly those with reactive airways. For these patients, the use of a supplementary bronchodilator may be necessary.

Half-normal saline (0.45% NaCl) is also used for mucosal hydration. Clinicians that prefer half-normal saline argue that evaporation of water from droplets of this hypotonic solution during its passage into the respiratory tract ultimately results in a solute concentration like that of normal saline. For this reason, half-normal saline is also often preferred with ultrasonic nebulization, since these small particles can face significant evaporation (see Chapter 23).

Hypertonic saline (1% to 15% NaCl) is the agent of choice for sputum induction. Its increased osmolarity is thought to result in increased movement of fluid into the mucosal blanket (bronchorrhea), Moreover, its irritant properties promote coughing, which helps mobilize secretions. Since absorption of saline from the lungs into the circulation does occur, frequent use of the hypertonic saline in sodium-restricted patients is contraindicated.

Propylene glycol. Propylene glycol is both a solvent and hygroscopic agent. As a solvent for bronchodilators, it helps stabilize aerosol droplets and can act as a mild preservative, inhibiting bacterial growth. In concentrations less than 5%, it has a demulcent (soothing) effect on the respiratory mucosa. In concentrations of greater than 5%, it is used to induce sputum. Its hydrating action is probably associated with its hygroscopic activity, that is, by attracting water it dilutes the mucus. It should be noted that, since it inhibits the growth of fungi and mycobacteria, it should not be used for sputum inductions when the goal is to culture these organisms. In low concentrations, aerosolized propylene glycol appears to be safe.

Oral expectorants. Oral expectorants are included in our discussion of diluting agents because they promote dilution of mucus indirectly. Examples of oral mucokinetic agents are potassium iodide, commonly referred to as SSKI (saturated solution of potassium iodide), glyceryl guaiacolate (Guaifenesin), and more common home remedies such as spices. These agents work by irritating the lining of the stomach, thereby stimulating the afferent fibers of the vagus nerve. Impulses sent to the CNS cause a vagal efferent response, stimulating bronchial glands to secrete a watery, serous discharge. In concept, this action dilutes respiratory tract secretions, particularly the sol portion of the mucus blanket. This vagal activity occurs with apparently little or no bronchial constriction.

Wetting agents

Wetting agents are chemical substances designed to lower the surface tension of respiratory tract fluids. Some agents represent true detergents, interacting with the mucus to produce emulsification of the hydrophobic bonds between water and the mucopolysaccharide molecules. In concept, these agents should disperse the mucus into smaller particles, thereby improving water penetration and facilitating transport and removal. Other chemicals, such as ethyl alcohol, act by destabilizing the alveolar plasma exudates common in acute pulmonary edema. While the action of ethyl alcohol is generally well documented in the literature, the in vivo effects of detergents are less well substantiated. For the sake of completeness, however, we discuss both categories of wetting agents.

Detergents. Although no detergent solutions designed for aerosol administration to the respiratory tract are currently on the market, two agents are of both historical and scientific note: (1) Alevaire, an aqueous solution of 0.125% tyloxapol (Superinone), 2% sodium bicarbonate, and 5% glycerine, and (2) Tergemist, an aqueous solution

of 0.125% sodium ethasulfate and 0.1% potassium iodide. Since the surface-active constituents of these agents, tyloxapol and sodium ethasulfate, both have similar detergent properties, we will use tyloxapol as the model for discussion.

In vitro studies of the action of tyloxapol on homogenized specimens of sputum clearly demonstrated its detergent action.[67] Sputum, with a measured surface tension of 52 dynes/cm, was not altered by the addition of water. However, when subjected to the action of tyloxapol, the surface tension dropped by 20%. In addition to lowering the surface tension of the sputum, it was observed that the wetting agent decreased adhesion between the mucus and the glass surface to which it was attached. If applied in vivo, this would allow the mucoid layer to be separated easily from the bronchial wall and then readily expelled by cough.

Although the detergent effect of tyloxapol on mucoid specimens in the laboratory is unquestioned, its true clinical effectiveness was never demonstrated.[68] For this reason, the FDA removed it from the market in the 1970s. Clinical observations on the value of Alevaire in specific patients may have been associated with the simple humidifying effects of its water-glycerin solvent or, alternatively, with the mucolytic properties of the sodium bicarbonate in the mixture.[69]

As an example of a "failure" in respiratory pharmacology, the events associated with the introduction and withdrawal of Alevaire from the market should prove useful to the respiratory care practitioner in understanding the critical difference between the results of in vitro and in vivo testing. Moreover, the fact that this agent exhibited significant physical effects on sputum in the laboratory should encourage further investigation into drugs having comparable in vivo actions.

Ethyl alcohol. Whereas the detergent agents were developed to act directly on the mucus of the respiratory tract, ethyl alcohol is applied to destabilize the alveolar plasma exudates that can occur in cardiogenic pulmonary edema.

Cardiogenic pulmonary edema can be characterized by the accumulation of a thin, watery exudate in the alveoli and bronchioles. The commonly observed "frothing" of this exudate is attributable, in part, to its surfactant content. The surfactant lowers the surface tension of the exudate, facilitating the formation of stable bubbles that can obstruct ventilation. Contrary to popular opinion, ethyl alcohol does not lower the surface tension of this froth; this would only increase its stability. Instead, it probably denatures the lecithin component of the surfactant, raising surface tension, and thereby destabilizing the froth.[70] Normally, 5 to 15 ml of 30% to 50% ethyl alcohol is nebulized, usually by positive pressure (to impede venous return and lower pulmonary vascular pressures). A minor and temporary side effect is irritation of the airway mucosa.

Mucolytics

N-Acetylcysteine (Mucomyst). In the continuing search for agents effective in disrupting the mucoproteins responsible for the high viscosity of sputum in certain respiratory diseases, the action of the naturally occurring amino acid, L-cysteine, was studied. Although it was found to be a potent mucolytic, it had substantial irritating properties. These were minimized by modifying the acid into an acetyl form, as it is now employed.

The chemical reaction between acetylcysteine and bronchial mucus has been extensively studied.[71] Acetylcysteine chemically replaces the disulfide bonds of mucoproteins with weaker sulfhydryl bonds. This action disrupts the molecular structure and lowers the viscosity of the mucus.

Mucolysis is as effective with a 10% as with a 20% concentration, and while the stronger preparation can induce bronchospasm in some patients, the lesser strength is a negligible hazard.[72] Other studies have found both 10% and 20% to be harmless, neither producing significant bronchospasm.[73] One can now obtain commercial preparations of acetylcysteine premixed with selected beta-adrenergic bronchodilators. This combination can help minimize the bronchospasm that may occur in susceptible patients.

The possibility of damage to alveolar surfactant has been of concern with the inhalation of microaerosols of any kind and especially with one of potent lytic qualities. Examination of both human and animal lung tissue after use of 10% acetylcysteine aerosol showed no change in surface activity.[74] Serious complications are rare. A burning sensation in the upper passages is occasionally reported, and nausea may be experienced. Some patients complain of the "rotten egg" odor, but most quickly adjust to it and ignore it.

In general, the clinical response to this aerosol for the removal of mucoid secretions has been favorable. Indications for its use cover a wide range from the cystic fibrosis of childhood (in which it seems to have scored considerable success), through the suppurative lung diseases, to the chronic bronchitis-emphysema of late adulthood.[75,76] Nevertheless, a minority have felt that acetylcysteine, though effective in vitro, has not shown any benefit in patients and is of no clinical value.[77]

A practical point to note is the chemical reactivity between acetylcysteine and certain component parts of nebulization equipment, especially iron, copper, and rubber. To avoid the loss of potency of such reactions, parts coming in contact with the amino acid (liquid or aerosol) should be made of glass, plastic, aluminum, chromed metal, silver, or stainless steel.

There is no critical dosage schedule for administering acetylcysteine aerosol; it is used according to individual needs. However, when using the premixed acetylcysteine and beta-adrenergic solution, one must limit the frequency of administration with respect to the bronchodilator. It can be administered by hand nebulizer, compressor, or aerosol mask and in positive-pressure breathing devices, but the drug itself should not be put in a heated nebulizer. In addition to the aerosol route, acetylcysteine is often effectively used by direct instillation, especially to facilitate bronchial aspiration through tracheostomy or endotracheal tubes.

Sodium bicarbonate. Reference was made to the mucolytic effect of this common household commodity, baking soda, in the preceding discussion of the action of tyloxapol. Large mucoid molecular chains tend to break as the pH of their environment rises, and local bronchial alkalinity can reach a pH of 8.3 without irritation or damage.[78] With the availability of more potent mucolytics, such as acetylcysteine, and the proteolytics (discussed next), sodium bicarbonate aerosol is seldom used. However, it is common to encounter patients in whom mucolysis from the usually effective agents lessens. For such patients, it is occasionally beneficial to switch to aerosolized 2% sodium bicarbonate to see whether mucus flow can be stimulated. For home use, a teaspoonful of the soda in a cup of sterile water makes a readily available solution.

Proteolytics

As the name indicates, members of this group lyse the protein material found in purulent sputum. Although there are no commercial aerosol preparations currently on the market, a brief description of the development of this type of therapy is pertinent.

Trypsin. Because the effectiveness of mucolytics decreases with increasing purulency of bronchial secretions, the early efforts to find a proteolytic agent centered on trypsin, a proteinase (enzyme active against protein) of the pancreas. Trypsin plays an important role in the natural digestion of ingested protein, but it is most effective on protein that is already partially digested. It also acts on respiratory and intestinal mucin and fibrin. Its use is strictly contraindicated in patients with an alpha-l-antitrypsin deficiency.

Early use of aerosolized trypsin demonstrated its effectiveness in cleansing the upper airways of proteinaceous accumulations, apparently without damage to living cells or impairment of ciliary function.[79-81] However, many investigators were disappointed with its results, feeling that it sometimes worsened the obstruction. Hoarseness was a frequent and troublesome complication because of too high concentrations of the drug or too rapid administration. Other side effects include chills, fever, dyspnea, nausea, and vomiting.

More recently, trypsin has shown promise in the treatment of pulmonary alveolar proteinosis.[82] In this particular disorder, trypsin acts to lyse the proteinaceous material that accumulates in the alveolar region, facilitating its removal by expectoration or bronchoscopy.[83] Dosage schedules for effective treatment of pulmonary alveolar proteinosis require a minimum of 100,000 units a day for at least 3 weeks.

Deoxyribonuclease (dornase; Dornavac). Pancreatic deoxyribonuclease is more specific in its action than is trypsin, since it depolymerizes (breaks long chains into smaller ones) deoxyribonucleic acid (DNA).[84] Therapeutically, this is most important, since it has been determined that from 30% to 70% of the solid matter of purulent secretions is composed of DNA.[85] The principal source of dornase is beef pancreas, but dornase is also produced by the pathogenic bacterium hemolytic *Streptococcus*. The filtrate of a culture of hemolytic *Streptococcus* contains two active enzymes, streptococcal fibrinolysin (streptokinase) and streptococcal deoxyribonuclease (streptodornase). We might infer from its name that streptokinase acts mostly on fibrous tissue and as such is not particularly relevant to our present discussion. A combination of these two enzymes is commercially prepared as Varidase, and although it is rather widely used for local application and intracavitary instillation, it has had limited use as an aerosol.[86,87]

Clinically, dornase has been indicated in any bronchopulmonary condition in which the accumulation of purulent sputum interferes with ventilation or with the resolution of an infection. It was indicated in pneumonia, pulmonary abscess, bronchiectasis, cystic fibrosis, and especially in an acute respiratory infection superimposed on chronic lung disease.[88]

Dornase was considered effective only against infected sputum. No significant side reactions were noted, and the only common patient complaint was burning of the mouth following treatment, which was easily prevented by a vigorous mouthwash immediately following therapy. Inhalation of 100,000 units two to three times daily for no more than four consecutive days was the normal dosage schedule.

As might be expected, some researchers believe that enzyme aerosols have no useful role in clinical medicine.[89] Moreover, prolonged use of dornase was associated with the appearance of inhibiting antideoxyribonuclease, which inactivates proteolytic action.[90] Formal approval of dornase by the FDA for clinical use was withdrawn in 1977 because of insufficient evidence to support its effectiveness.

ADRENOCORTICOSTEROIDS

Adrenocorticosteroids have assumed a position of great importance in clinical therapeutics. Although we are interested in a relatively limited aspect of their use at present, some general background knowledge of them is essential.

For the sake of convenience, we use the commonly employed abbreviated expression "steroid," with the understanding that we mean adrenocorticosteroid. We must understand also that, like many familiar terms, it is not really correct, for steroids comprise a large group of organic compounds, many of which have other physiologic properties than those in which we are interested. The steroids that concern us are potent hormones secreted by the cortex (outer layer) of the adrenal glands, as opposed to the sympathomimetic products of the adrenal medulla, already described. There are five general groups of complex organic compounds produced in the adrenal cortex, of which the only group important to this discussion are the glucocorticoids. The name of this group derives from its involvement in carbohydrate metabolism; its two most clinically useful members are cortisol and cortisone. Many commercial preparations and modifications of these two are available, with variable potencies and supposed specific responses.

Actions

The adrenal steroids exert a tremendous influence on the body physiology, touching all organ systems. They have been referred to as "stress hormones" because they are secreted in excessive amounts when the body is put under stress, and severe trauma or prolonged grave illness may cause a depletion of their supply. In a complex way the steroids give support to the body to aid it through a crisis, and if they are acutely depleted or if their production is interrupted by abrupt destruction of the adrenals, the body functions deteriorate rapidly. On the other hand, a slow, chronic increase of cortical function does not produce a catastrophic picture but rather a multiplicity of signs and symptoms described as Cushing's syndrome.

A patient beginning to show evidence of excessive steroid action is often referred to as "Cushinoid." We describe some of the more common and important effects of hyperadrenalism to illustrate the wide range of steroid action. The glucocorticoids have the following effects.[91-93]

Formation of glucose from body protein. When excessive, the formation of glucose from body protein can raise the blood glucose level high enough to produce "steroid diabetes" or to activate a latent, subclinical true diabetes. There can be associated protein loss with muscle wasting and weakness.

Depletion of bone calcium. Through a process of resorption, calcium is removed from bone. Structural thinning is such that fractures are frequent. This state of the bone is called osteoporosis.

Increase of fat production. Excessive amounts of fat are produced, also from body protein, and are characteristically deposited in the subcutaneous tissues of the head and trunk. This results in a rounding of the facial contour, referred to as moon face, and an accumulation of fat at the base of the neck and upper back, called buffalo hump. These are two of the most prominent visible signs of a Cushinoid state.

Impairment of immunologic response. Steroids inactivate circulating antibodies and thus can protect the body against the harmful effects of severe allergies. However, this function also lowers the body's resistance to infection, a significant point in the therapeutic use of steroids.

Reduction of inflammatory response. Steroids decrease the local vascular congestion and cellular infiltration that is the natural response to injury or infection. In addition, the deposition of fibrous tissue as part of the reparative process is inhibited. Of use in controlling the adverse effects of inflammation, this function also facilitates the spread of infection, since it interferes with the usual process of localization. This is a serious threat to the patient with quiescent tuberculosis.

Elevation of blood pressure. Steroids, through the mediation of certain electrolytes and other hormones, elevate the blood pressure. Of therapeutic significance, when the cardiovascular system no longer responds to sympathomimetics, such as in certain states of shock, steroids often aid the vasoconstrictors to regain their pressor effects on the arterioles.

To complete the review of steroid action, the pituitary gland should be discussed. The adrenal cortex is directly controlled by the anterior division of the pituitary gland, through a pituitary hormone called adrenocorticotropic hormone (ACTH). The name itself describes a substance that stimulates (-tropic) the adrenal cortex. Administration of ACTH elicits the same response as cortisol and cortisone by stimulating the adrenal production of these substances. This presupposes that the adrenal cortex is in a functioning state, able to respond. Because the adrenals are likely to slacken in their activity during the therapeutic administration of steroids (the body is receiving adequate hormone from its outside source), there is risk of adrenal atrophy with prolonged loss of function. Under such circumstances, ACTH may be given for periods of time to stimulate the adrenals to function and to prevent their atrophy.

Use in respiratory care

In the treatment of respiratory diseases, steroids usually are administered orally and by inhalation. They are used for their potent anti-inflammatory and antifibrogenic effects already mentioned, for their ability to inhibit production and release of histamine (histamine produces bronchospasm), and to make beta$_2$ receptors more responsive to beta$_2$ adrenergics.[94,95] Thus, steroids not only help decrease the frequency of acute bronchospasm but also increase the effectiveness of adrenergic bronchodilators, especially in conditions where some tolerance has developed to them.[96]

Steroids are of particular value in the treatment of persons with asthma and with resistant allergies of the respiratory tract. The practitioner will witness dramatic responses to steroid therapy, but because of the diffuse action of the drug, various undesired effects can frequently accompany its use. Unlike the other respiratory agents, which typically exert their side effects during or soon after the treatment, steroid side effects are typically insidious and develop over a period of time (days to months).

One common side effect is a fungal infection, candidiasis, of the oropharynx or larynx, which can occur with the aerosol administration of steroids. Using the proper dosage can greatly minimize this complication. Having patients rinse their mouth out after treatments is also helpful in preventing this complication. Fortunately, for some of the more recently introduced steroids, candidiasis may be the only real side effect, since systemic absorption from the lung is minimal.

A summary of the steroids currently used in respiratory therapy is provided in Table 20-7. The following discussion highlights the major agents in this category.

Dexamethasone sodium phosphate (Decadron, Turbinaire). Dexamethasone is available in metered dose inhaler (MDI) preparations and can be used alone or mixed with isoproterenol. The consensus of its users is that this steroid is therapeutically active and effective throughout the entire respiratory tract from the nose to the bronchioles in the treatment of nasal allergies, allergic asthma, and some chronic obstructive states.[97,98] However, with no doubt concerning its local effects, dexamethasone has been found to have definite systemic effects, readily detected by special urinary excretion tests. The systemic side effects have limited the use of aerosolized dexamethasone in the lungs in favor of some newer products to be mentioned.

Beclomethasone dipropionate (Vanceril, Beclovent). After several years of use in Europe, the inhalant steroid beclomethasone became available in the US in 1976. This drug was a significant step forward in the treatment of patients with bronchospasm. It is indicated in patients over 6 years of age with intrinsic, extrinsic, or mixed asthma who need chronic steroid therapy. Overall, the use of beclomethasone appears to be an effective aerosolized steroid with minimal adverse effects that is of great therapeutic value to many patients.

Studies show that asthmatic symptoms decrease in about

Table 20-7 Commonly Used Steroids

Drug	Dose	Route
Beclomethasone (Vanceril, Beclovent)	2 inhalations tid/qid (42 µg/puff)	Aerosol
Flunisolide (AeroBid)	2 inhalations bid (250 µg/puff)	Aerosol
Triamcinolone acetonide (Azmacort)	2 inhalations tid (100 µg/puff)	Aerosol
	4-48 mg/day	Oral
Prednisone (Deltasone, Meticorten, Orasone)	5-60 mg/day	Oral
Dexamethasone (Dalalone, Decadron, Decaject, Hexadrol)	0.75-9 mg/day	Oral
	3 puffs tid/qid (84 µg/puff)	Aerosol
Methylprednisone (Solu-Medrol)	4-48 mg/day	Oral
	10-40 mg (initially)	IV
	40-120 mg (initially)	IM

80% of the cases concomitant with an improvement in pulmonary function. This occurs without the systemic side effects of oral steroids,[99-101] although candidiasis may occur in a few. Most patients who have been dependent on oral steroids can switch to beclomethasone aerosol and maintain control of the asthmatic symptoms.[102,103] However, during acute exacerbation, oral steroids may be needed in previously steroid-dependent patients,[104] as well as in patients with pulmonary infiltration with eosinophilia.[105] Beclomethasone also has been reported to be of value in cases of perennial rhinitis to minimize the symptoms that develop in people susceptible to various antigens such as pollen.[106-108]

Triamcinolone acetonide (Azmacort). The steroid triamcinolone is a poorly soluble compound with good local and negligible systemic effects, which can be aerosolized for respiratory tract action. It is packaged as a suspension for intramuscular, intraarticular, or intrabursal injection and has recently become available in an MDI preparation. Studies show that in inhalation dosages of about 100 μg each, four times per day, this agent allows most steroid-dependent asthmatics to stop oral steroids.[109,110] However, there are no studies indicating superiority of this steroid to any other when aerosolized. The majority of patients who are dependent on oral steroids can achieve a therapeutic effect with minimal side effects by using aerosolized triamcinolone.[111,112]

Flunisolide (AeroBid). Flunisolide is a recent addition to the group of aerosolizable steroids, also prepared in the MDI form. It has also been shown to be well tolerated and effective in the treatment of steroid-dependent asthma.[113] The recommended dosage for adults and children is two inhalations (250 μg each) twice a day, for a total daily dosage of 1 mg.[114]

No matter which steroid is aerosolized, the determination of the actual dose of steroid aerosol to be administered is a matter of professional judgment and is the responsibility of the attending physician. By and large, since steroid aerosols are usually packaged in MDIs for home use, the physician gives directions for use directly to the patient. However, if the practitioner is assigned to supervise the patient's treatment program, the patient should ensure that the physician gives specific orders. Whereas this should be the practice for any treatment, there are many instances in which established routines can be used, allowing the practitioner some flexibility to adjust techniques to individual needs. The great potency of the steroids and the possibility of adverse reactions mitigate against their administration with anything less than specific instructions for each patient. The many variables that influence the efficiency of aerosol treatment, such as function of the nebulizer, depth of ventilation, and ventilatory rate, make it impossible to precisely predict the systemic absorption of the drug. For this reason, astute clinical observation, in conjunction with more objective indicators such as pulmonary function tests, should be used to monitor and adjust the therapeutic dosage schedule. Details on the proper use of metered dose inhalers are provided in Chapter 23.

CROMOLYN SODIUM

Cromolyn sodium has proven effective for many years as an agent that helps prevent bronchospasm. It is an integral part of the treatment program for many asthmatics but is not considered useful in acute asthmatic attacks. It has been beneficial to many people in preventing exercise induced asthma (EIA) as well.[115,116] It recently has been suggested that it might prevent EIA by minimizing airway cooling that occurs during rapid breathing, such as with exercise. This might be mediated by action on the bronchial vasculature.[117]

The primary action of cromolyn sodium is one of blocking the release of mediators such as histamine and leukotrienes $C_4 D_4 E_4$, which can cause bronchospasm (leukotrienes are the active agents in what was formerly called the slow-reacting substance of anaphylaxis, SRS-A).[118] These mediators are normally stored in special white blood cells called mast cells. When specific antibody receptors on the cells come in contact with specific antigens (pollen, dust, etc), stored mediators are released (Fig. 20-7).

For most of us this response merely attracts more white blood cells, dilates the local blood vessels, and results in a few more secretions at the site of irritation, all to help protect the body against the invasion of the foreign antigen. But people who are hypersensitive (allergic) have exaggerated responses to these antigens. The result is excessive bronchospasm and secretions with a marked increase in airway resistance.

As explained previously, steroids can decrease the immune response and help prevent this from occurring, but their side effects can be profound, especially if large doses are used over long periods of time. Cromolyn sodium, on the other hand, can help inhibit this mast cell response with minimal side effects. However, it does not appear to work on everyone.

It must be emphasized that cromolyn sodium is only of value in preventing or moderating asthmatic attacks and is not effective once bronchospasm is established. However, a recent study stands alone in demonstrating some bronchodilatory effect of cromolyn sodium in asthmatic patients.[119] More studies will undoubtedly further explore this new finding.

The regular use of cromolyn sodium inhalations during remission of symptoms can reduce the frequency and severity of attacks and lessen the amount of adrenocorticosteroids previously needed to control symptoms.[120-122] Studies are now showing cromolyn sodium to be as effective as theophylline in the prophylactic treatment of asthmatics, when used on a regular basis. Cromolyn sodium has the additional advantage of decreasing bronchial hy-

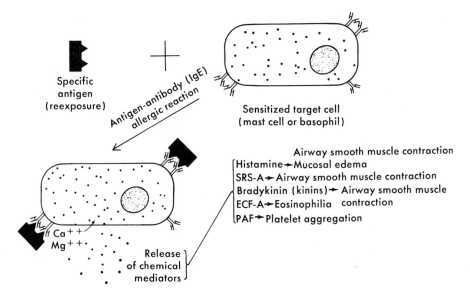

Fig. 20-7 Release of mediators from sensitized target cell in type I, IgE-mediated, immunologic reaction. (From Lehnert BE and Schachter EN: The pharmacology of respiratory care, St Louis, 1980, The CV Mosby Co.)

perreactivity, thereby decreasing the frequency of asthmatic exacerbations.[123,124]

For the prevention of bronchospasm, cromolyn sodium (Intal) is packaged as a 1% dry powder aerosol (administered by a SpinHaler rotary dispersion device) or in a 1% solution form for nebulization. Cromolyn sodium has also demonstrated clinical effectiveness in the reversal of histologic changes that occur with perennial rhinitis.[125-127] A liquid nasal spray has been marketed for this purpose (Nasalcrom). Also available now is a 4% solution (Opticrom) for allergic conjunctivitis. Currently under investigation is the oral use of cromolyn sodium to prevent severe food allergies.[128]

ANTIBIOTICS

When it became apparent that aerosol therapy was an effective route for the administration of drugs, interest soon developed in treating resistant respiratory tract infections, especially such localized bronchopulmonary diseases as lung abscess, necrotizing pneumonia, and bronchiectasis, which were especially resistant to conventional therapy.

In the mid-1940s sulfonamides were aerosolized, but the advent of penicillin and subsequent antibiotics stimulated extensive use of aerosols and the accumulation of a significant background of experience.[129-134] The rationale for aerosol therapy was based on the speculation that even with adequate blood levels of systemically administered antibiotics, the diffusion of the drug from blood into infected tissue for its direct antibacterial action was blocked by tissue reaction to the infection. It was believed that the presence of thick bronchial and alveolar exudates composed a formidable diffusion barrier, especially in local-

ized lesions. Also, it was thought that interstitial edema and fibrosis of the diseased area were additional factors in preventing therapeutic antibiotic tissue levels. These observations were borne out by the frequent observation of active microbial growth in sputum while intensive systemic therapy was being administered.

The ideal antibiotic for aerosol use has effective topical action and is poorly absorbed. Further, the infection being treated must be accessible from the respiratory tract surface. From a practical point of view it can be generalized that aerosolized antibiotics play their greatest role in the treatment of stubborn, gram-negative respiratory tract infections, where the nature of the infection and the frequently accompanying airway obstruction require long-term therapy. Large doses of effective antibiotics can be used, self-administered at home if desired, with minimal hazard of untoward reactions. In the interest of economy, antibiotics should be aerosolized during inhalation only, using either a simple pump or gas-powered hand nebulizer or an ultrasonic nebulizer. Table 20-8 lists those antibiotics that have been found suitable for aerosolization, with suggested doses for their use.[135]

Recently, particularly encouraging results have followed the use of aerosolized antibiotics in cystic fibrosis patients. Those using nebulized gentamicin over a 2-year period showed significantly less lung deterioration compared to those who received only nebulized saline.[136] Another study of cystic fibrosis patients used a nebulized dose of carbenicillin and gentamicin. After a 4-month daily treatment regimen, there was significant improvement of pulmonary function values and a dramatic drop in required hospitalizations.[137] These studies indicate that nebulized antibiotics appear to be an effective supplement to oral or

IV antibiotic therapy in carefully selected patient categories.

However, aerosol application of antibiotics is not a substitute for the systemic route. Although some patients respond dramatically, others show little or no benefit from this approach.[138,139] In view of the modifying factors listed previously and with variability of bacterial susceptibility encountered in systemic therapy, this is not surprising. However, the efficacy of aerosolized antibiotics can be significantly increased by using a technique that deserves special mention.[140] The same exudates and secretions that impair drug diffusion from blood to tissue are able to interfere with the action of aerosolized particles, and they are probably responsible for many instances of therapeutic failure. The prior or concomitant use of bronchodilators will aid penetration of antibiotic particles but will not bring them into bacterial contact in the presence of thick secretions. Often, extensive therapy with heated water aerosol and chest physical therapy are essential to clear the airways for penetration and deposition of antibiotic aerosols.

In summary, aerosolized antibiotics are not intended to supplant the systemic route; rather, they should be considered as a supplement in treating resistant, localized infections of the lung in selected patient categories. When used in conjunction with techniques designed to enhance pulmonary clearance, aerosolized antibiotic agents may help reduce the amount of secretion and inhibit further bacterial growth. However, we must remember that the risk of distant spread of infection to other parts of the body can best be controlled by maintaining therapeutic blood levels by systemic administration of antibiotics.

ANTIVIRAL AGENTS

Antibiotics are not effective against viral illness. Recently, agents that are effective against some viruses, particularly those responsible for small airway infections (bronchiolitis) in children, have been studied.

A significant threat to a pediatric patient is an infection with the respiratory syncytial virus (RSV). Studies with a new synthetic nucleoside agent, ribavirin (Virazole), are demonstrating its effectiveness in the treatment of RSV, as well as influenza A and B.[141-145]

Ribavirin appears to be the first broad-spectrum antiviral agent showing antiviral properties against both DNA and RNA viruses, the two major groups of viruses. Studies of ribavirin's effectiveness against other viral infections such as viral hepatitis, Lassa fever, genital herpes, and herpes zoster, have demonstrated promising but inconclusive results. Further studies are needed to justify ribavirin therapy for these indications.[146]

For the treatment of children with respiratory syncytial virus, ribavirin is supplied as a powder for reconstitution with sterile water. Administration is via a specialized microaerosol generator called the Small Particle Aerosol Generator-2 (SPAG-2), commercially available from the drug manufacturer. Treatment is carried out via an oxyhood, face mask, or mist tent for 12 to 18 hours per day over a period of at least 3 days. Using the recommended dosage and diluent in the aerosol generator, the average aerosol concentration of the drug is about 190 µg per liter of carrier gas. Adverse effects are relatively minor and include rash and conjunctivitis.

As a result of precipitation of the drug in the ventilator circuitry, attempts to apply the aerosol to children undergoing mechanical ventilation has posed serious problems, including jamming of the expiratory valve mechanisms. Recently, several clinicians have reported success in ribavirin administration during mechanical ventilation with special circuitry designed for this purpose.[147-148]

Despite these problems, ribavirin clearly shows promise in the treatment of specific viral infections of the lung in children and may lead to more widespread use of similar agents in other viral disorders.

ANTIPROTOZOAL AGENTS

Among the opportunistic infections common in immunosuppressed patients, none has received more attention recently than *Pneumocystis carinii* pneumonia, or PCP. *Pneumocystis* is considered a protozoan organism, occurring in a wide variety of animals as a saprophyte. Latent infection is common in humans, but manifest symptoms tend to occur mainly in those whose immune systems are suppressed by steroids, cytotoxic drugs, radiotherapy, or leukemia. Treated conventionally, patients with PCP exhibit mortality rates between 30% and 50%.

Recently, the incidence of PCP has dramatically increased. This increase is directly associated with the spread of the acquired immune deficiency syndrome (AIDS).[149] Although PCP is only one of many opportunis-

Table 20-8 Antibiotics for Aerosol Use

Antibiotic	Aerosol dose
Carbenicillin	1-3 g
Neomycin*	50-400 mg
Bacitracin*	5000-200,000 units
Streptomycin	750-1000 mg
Chloramphenicol	200-400 mg
Kanamycin*	100-400 mg
Colymycin-M	25-150 mg
Polymyxin*	10-50 mg
Gentamicin*	40-120 mg
Amphotericin*	5-20 mg
Mycostatin*	100,000-400,000 units

From Miller WF: Fundamental principles of aerosol therapy, Respir Care 17:295, 1972.
*Poor or nonabsorbed in aerosol state.

tic infections associated with AIDS, it is among the most common. In fact, recent guidelines from the Centers for Disease Control recommend that patients with PCP for whom no other cause of immunodeficiency can be identified be treated as AIDS cases.

The first agent proven to be of value in treating PCP was pentamidine isethionate (Pentam 300).* Pentamidine isethionate is an aromatic diamide compound that has been used extensively in the tropics for treatment of *Trypanosoma* and *Leishmania* infections. In the management of PCP infections in immunosuppressed children and adults, pentamidine can reduce mortality rates to about 3% in infants and 25% or less in children and adults.[149] Pentamidine probably interferes with the synthesis of DNA and RNA, but its actual mode of action is not fully understood.

Traditionally, pentamidine was administered via the intramuscular or intravenous route, at dosages of about 4 mg/kg/day. The usual length of therapy is 14 to 21 days. Approximately 50% of patients started on pentamidine require changing to another agent because of adverse effects. These adverse effects include anemia, neutropenia, azotemia, hypotension, and hyponatremia.[150] Pentamidine is also associated with alterations in blood glucose levels (both hyperglycemia and hypoglycemia). Hypoglycemia usually occurs early during the course of therapy and may occur precipitously. Hyperglycemia may not be noted until several months after treatment is completed. Appreciable quantities of pentamidine concentrate in the urine, and drug levels are detectable for up to 6 to 8 weeks after cessation of therapy.

Partly because of these potent side effects, recent research has focused on the clinical efficacy of aerosolized pentamidine.[151,152] After aerosol administration, the drug is almost exclusively recovered from the lung, with little extrapulmonary distribution. Moreover, aerosol administration delivers significantly higher concentrations of pentamidine to the air spaces than does intravenous delivery, especially in patients with diffuse alveolar infiltrates.[153] Adverse effects of aerosolized pentamidine include bronchial irritation, with little evidence of systemic toxicity. Based on these findings, the FDA gave full approval to the use of pentamidine via the aerosolized route in mid-1989.

Pentamidine has emerged as a mainstay of therapy in the management of *Pneumocystis carinii* pneumonia in AIDS patients, especially in those who are allergic to trimethoprim-sulfamethoxazole.[154] Although success in the treatment of PCP will not affect current long-term outcomes in AIDS patients, the high incidence of this disorder in other selected patient categories, including newborn infants, demands continuing research on the use of this and other antiprotozoal agents.

*A newer agent, trimethoprim-sulfamethoxazole (TMP-SMX), is considered the first-line drug of choice in the treatment of PCP.

SUMMARY

The primary purpose of respiratory pharmacology is to relieve or prevent the pathologic triad of bronchospasm, mucosal edema, and retained secretions. Bronchoconstriction and mucosal edema are addressed directly via autonomic-active agents, or by anti-inflammatory drugs that block or prevent certain immunologic responses. Still in the experimental stage, prostaglandins may be of potential use in the relief of bronchospasm.

The clearance of retained secretions is approached using hydrating and wetting agents, mucolytics, and (historically) proteolytics. Associated with poor clearance and altered defense mechanisms, resistant infections of the lung may be treated with aerosolized antibiotic, antiviral, and antiprotozoal agents as a supplement to the systemic route.

Effective use of these various drug categories demands that the respiratory care practitioner possess a sound background in the general principles of pharmacology and an in-depth knowledge of the mechanism of action, appropriate use, hazards, and side effects of all specific agents commonly applied in clinical practice. With an increasing emphasis on the self-administration of aerosolized drugs, practitioners must also develop the skills necessary to ensure patient compliance and understanding of proper use and dosage schedules.

REFERENCES

1. Hodgkin JE, Johnson L, and Lopez B: An improved method for aerosolizing anesthetic for flexible bronchoscopy, Respir Care 21:134-137, 1976.
2. Goodman LS and Gilman A: The pharmacological basis of therapeutics, ed 6, New York, 1980, The MacMillan Co.
3. Meyers FH, Jawetz E, and Goldfien A: Review of medical pharmacology, ed 5, Los Altos, Calif, 1976, Lange Medical Publications.
4. Issellbacher KJ et al: Harrison's principles of internal medicine, ed 9, New York, 1980, McGraw-Hill Book Co.
5. Goth A: Medical pharmacology: principles and concepts, ed 11, St Louis, 1984, The CV Mosby Co.
6. Bergersen BS: Pharmacology in nursing, ed 14, St Louis, 1979, The CV Mosby Co.
7. Harper HA, Rodwell VW, and Mayes PA: Review of physiological chemistry, ed 16, Los Altos, Calif, 1977, Lange Medical Publications.
8. Santa Cruz R et al: Tracheal mucus velocity in normal man and patients with obstructive lung disease: effects of terbutaline, Am Rev Respir Dis 109:458, 1974.
9. DeTroyer A, Yernault JC, and Rodenstein D: Influence of beta-2 agonist aerosols on pressure-volume characteristics of the lungs, Am Rev Respir Dis 118:987, 1978.
10. Ziment I: Why are they saying bad things about IPPB? Respir Care 18:677-689, 1973.
11. Davies DS: In Junod AE and DeHaller R, editors: Lung metabolism, New York, 1975, Academic Press, Inc.
12. Blackwell EW et al: Metabolism of isoprenaline after aerosol and direct intrabronchial administration in man and dog, Br J Pharmacol 50:587, 1974.
13. Smoker JM et al: A protocol to assess and administer aerosol bronchodilator therapy, Respir Care 31:780-785, 1987.
14. Keighley JF: Iatrogenic asthma associated with adrenergic aerosols, Ann Intern Med 65:985, 1966.

15. Singer OP and Wilson WJ: Laryngotracheobronchitis: 2 years' experience with racemic epinephrine, Can Med Assoc J 115:132-134, 1976.

16. Wesley CR, Cotton EK, and Brooks JG: Nebulized racemic epinephrine by IPPB for the treatment of croup: a double-blind study, Am J Dis Child 132(5):484-487, 1978.

17. Sympathomimetic bronchodilators (editorial), Lancet 1:535, 1971.

18. Sollman R: A manual of pharmacology, Philadelphia, 1957, WB Saunders Co.

19. McEvoy JDS, Vall-spinosa A, and Paterson JW: Assessment of orciprenaline and isoproterenol infusions in asthmatic patients, Am Rev Respir Dis 108:490-500, 1973.

20. Sobol BJ and Reed A: The rapidity of Alupent and isoproterenol, Ann Allergy 32:137-141, 1974.

21. Lands AM et al: The pharmacologic actions of the bronchodilator drug isoetharine, J Am Pharm Assoc 47:744, 1958.

22. Shulman M et al: Cardiovascular effects of isoetharine administered to surgical patients during cyclopropane anesthesia, Br J Anaesthesiol 42:439, 1970.

23. El-Shaboury AH: Controlled study of a new inhalant in asthma and bronchitis, Br Med J 5416:1037, 1964.

24. Kelman GR et al: Cardiovascular effects of solbutamol, Nature 221:1251, 1969.

25. Owen JA: A bronchodilator well-known in Europe, Hosp Formulary, Aug 1975, pp 386-388.

26. Snider GL and Laguanda R: Albuterol and isoproterenol aerosols: a controlled study of duration of effect in asthmatic patients, JAMA 221:682-685, 1972.

27. Bloomfield P et al: Comparison of solbutamol given intravenously and by intermittent positive-pressure breathing in life-threatening asthma, Br Med J 1(6167):848-850, 1979.

28. Brogden RN, Speight TM, and Avery GS: Terbutaline: a preliminary report of its pharmacological properties and therapeutic efficacy in asthma, Drugs 6:324-332, 1973.

29. Pinnas JL et al: Multicenter study of bitolterol and isoproterenol nebulizer solutions in nonsteroid-using patients, J Allergy Clin Immunol 79:768-775, 1987.

30. Trembath PN et al: Comparison of four weeks' treatment with fenoterol and terbutaline aerosols in adult asthmatics: a double-blind crossover study, J Allergy Clin Immunol 63(6):345-400, 1979.

31. Eisenstadt WS and Nichols SS: Adverse effects of adrenergic aerosols in bronchial asthma, Ann Allergy 27:283, 1969.

32. Mathewson HS: Anticholinergic aerosols, Respir Care 28:467-469, 1983.

33. Siminsson BG, Jonson B, and Strom B: Bronchodilatory and circulatory effects of inhaling increasing doses of an anticholinergic drug, ipratropium bromide (SCH 1000), Scand J Respir Dis 56:138, 1975.

34. Davison FR: Handbook of materia medica, toxicology, and pharmacology, St Louis, 1949, The CV Mosby Co.

35. Nadel JA and Widdecombe JG: Mechanism of bronchoconstriction with dust inhalation, Clin Res 10:91, 1962.

36. Dautreband L et al: Effects of atropine microaerosols on airway resistance in man, Arch Int Pharmacodyn 139:198, 1962.

37. Chamberlain DA et al: Atropine methonitrate and isoprenaline in bronchial asthma, Lancet 2:1019, 1962.

38. Storms WW et al: Aerosol Sch 1000, Am Rev Respir Dis 111:419, 1962.

39. Gross NJ: Sch 1000: a new anticholinergic bronchodilator, Am Rev Respir Dis 112:823, 1975.

40. Ingram RH and McFadden ER Jr: Localization and mechanisms of airway responses, N Engl J Med 297(11):596-600, 1977.

41. Pare PD, Lawson LM, and Brooks LA: Patterns of response to inhaled bronchodilators in asthmatics, Am Rev Respir Dis 127(6):680-685, 1983.

42. Villate-Navarro JE et al: Comparative effects of terbutaline sulphate and ipratropium bromide on the respiratory system, Med Clin (Barc) 74(7):275-279, 1980.

43. Scano G, Stendardi L, and Sergysels R: Lung mechanics after aerosol and intravenous SCH 1000 in normal humans, Int J Clin Pharmacol Ther Toxicol 20(10):454-457, 1982.

44. Kitamura S et al: Effect of ipratropium bromide on the action of bronchoactive agents, Arzneimittelforsch 32(2):128-130, 1982.

45. Nadel JA: Parasympathetic regulation of lungs and airways: chairman's summary, Postgrad Med J 51(suppl 7):86-90, 1975.

46. Bruderman I, Cohen-Aronovski R, and Smorzik J: A comparative study of various combinations of ipratropium bromide and metaproterenol in allergic asthmatic patients, Chest 83(2):208-210, 1983.

47. Yeung R, Nolan GM, and Levison H: Comparison of the effects of inhaled SCH 1000 and fenoterol on exercise-induced bronchospasm in children, Pediatrics 66(1):109-114, 1980.

48. Rebuck AS and Marcus HI: SCH 1000 in psychogenic asthma, Scand J Respir Dis (Suppl) 103:186-191, 1979.

49. Gerhardt T, McCarthy J, and Bancalari E: Aminophylline therapy for idiopathic apnea in premature infants: effects on lung function, Pediatrics 62(5):801-804, 1978.

50. Brazier JL et al: Plasma xanthine levels in low birthweight infants treated or not treated with theophylline, Arch Dis Child 54(3):194-199, 1979.

51. Aranda JV and Turmen T: Methylxanthines in apnea of prematurity, Clin Perinatol 6(1):87-108, 1979.

52. Iwainsky H and Sehrt I: Theophylline therapy—foundations and possibilities, Z Erkr Atmungsorgane 152(1):21-36, 1979.

53. Powell JR et al: The influence of cigarette smoking and sex on theophylline disposition, Am Rev Respir Dis 116:17-23, 1977.

54. Chang KC et al: Altered theophylline pharmacokinetics during acute respiratory viral illness, Lancet 1(8074):1132-1133, 1978.

55. Segal MS: Aminophylline: a clinical overview, Adv Asthma Allergy, 2:17, 1975.

56. Stewart BN and Block AJ: A trial of aerosolized theophylline in relieving bronchospasm, Chest 69:718, 1976.

57. Rau JL: Respiratory therapy pharmacology, ed 2, Chicago, 1984, Year Book Medical Publishers.

58. Parker CW and Snider DE: Prostaglandins in asthma, Ann Intern Med 78:963, 1973.

59. Seth RV et al: Effect of propranolol on the airway response to prostaglandin E$_2$ in normal man, Br J Clin Pharmacol 12:731, 1981.

60. Brown R, Ingram RH, and Mcfadden RR: Effects of prostaglandin F$_{2a}$ on lung mechanics in nonasthmatic and asthmatic subjects, J Appl Physiol 44:150, 1978.

61. Cuthbert MF: Bronchodilator activity of prostaglandins E$_1$ and E$_2$ in asthmatic subjects, Proc R Soc Med 64:15, 1971.

62. Fanberg BL: Prostaglandins and the lung, Am Rev Respir Dis 108:482, 1973.

63. Hyman AL, Spannhake EW, and Kadowitz PJ: Prostaglandins and the lung, Am Rev Respir Dis 117:111, 1978.

64. Katz RI and GJ: Prostaglandins—basic and clinical considerations, Anesthesiology 40:471, 1974.

65. Said SI et al: Pulmonary alveolar hypoxia release of prostaglandins and other humoral mediators, Science 185:1180, 1974.

66. Dulfano JJ, Adler KB, and Wooten O: Physical properties of sputum. IV. Effects of 100 per cent humidity and water mist, Am Rev Respir Dis 107:130, 1973.

67. Tainter ML et al: Alevaire as a mucolytic agent, N Engl J Med 253:764, 1955.

68. Paez PN and Miller WF: Surface active agents in sputum evacuation: a blind comparison with normal saline solution and distilled water, Chest 60:312, 1971.

69. Palmer KNV: The effect of an aerosol detergent in chronic bronchitis, Lancet 1(272):611, 1957.

70. Helmholz HF, MD: Personal communication,

71. Sheffner AL: The mucolytic activity, mechanisms of action, and metabolism of acetylcysteine, Pharmacotherapy 1:47, 1964.

72. Hirsch SR and Kory RC: An evaluation of the effect of nebulized N-acetylcysteine on sputum consistency, J Allergy 39:265, 1967.

73. Moser KM and Rhodes PG: Acute effects of aerosolized acetylcysteine upon spirometric measurements in subjects with and without obstructive pulmonary disease, Dis Chest 49:370, 1966.

74. Thomas PA and Treasure RI: Effect of N-acetyl-L-cysteine on pulmonary surface activity, Am Rev Respir Dis 94:175, 1966.

75. Webb WR: New mucolytic agents for sputum liquefaction, Postgrad Med 36:449, 1964.

76. Mucolytic agents, Br Med J 2:603, 1966.

77. Anderson G: A clinical trial of mucolytic agent—acetylcysteine in chronic bronchitis, Br J Dis Chest 60:101, 1966.

78. Tainter ML et al: Alevaire as a mucolytic agent, N Engl J Med 253:764, 1955.

79. Limber CR et al: Enzymatic lysis of respiratory secretions by aerosol trypsin, JAMA 149:816, 1952.

80. Unger L and Unger AH: Trypsin inhalations in respiratory conditions with thick sputum, JAMA 152:1109, 1953.

81. Prince HE et al: Aerosols of pancreatic dornase in broncho-pulmonary disease, Ann Allergy 12:71, 1954.

82. Riker JB and Wolinsky H: Trypsin aerosol treatment of pulmonary alveolar proteinosis, Am Rev Respir Dis 108:108, 1973.

83. Lehnert BE and Schachter EN: The pharmacology of respiratory care, St Louis, 1980, The CV Mosby Co.

84. Salomon A et al: Aerosols of pancreatic dornase in bronchopulmonary disease, Ann Allergy 12:71, 1954.

85. Sherry S et al: Presence and significance of deoxyribose nucleotide in purulent exudate, Proc Soc Exp Biol Med 68:179, 1948.

86. Meunster JJ et al: Treatment of unresolved pneumonia with streptokinase and streptodornase, Am J Med 12:357, 1942.

87. Craven JF: Treatment of obstructive atelectasis by aerosol administration of proteolytic enzymes, J Pediatr 42:228, 1953.

88. Clifton EE: Pancreatic dornase aerosol in pulmonary, endotracheal, and endobronchial disease, Chest 30:1, 1956.

89. Lyons HA: Use of therapeutic aerosols, Am J Cardiol 12:461, 1963.

90. Miller WF: In Kagan BM, editor: Antimicrobial therapy, Philadelphia, 1970, WB Saunders Co.

91. Forsham PH: The adrenal gland, Clin Symp 15:3, 1963.

92. Kleiner IS and Orten JM: Biochemistry, ed 7, St Louis, 1966, The CV Mosby Co.

93. Williams RH, editor: Textbook of endrocrinology, Philadelphia, 1962, WB Saunders Co.

94. Aviado DM and Carrillo LR: Antiasthmatic addition and corticosteroids: a review of the literature on their mechanism of action, J Clin Pharmacol 10:3-11, 1970.

95. Ellul-Micallef R and Fenech FF: Effect of intravenous prednisolone in asthmatics and diminished adrenergic responsiveness, Lancet 2:1269-1270, 1975.

96. Mathewson HS: Risks and benefits of aerosolized steroids, Respir Care 28:325-326, 1983.

97. Norman PS et al: Adrenal function during the use of dexamethasone aerosols in the treatment of ragweed hay fever, J Allergy 40:57, 1967.

98. Fisch BR and Grater WC: Dexamethasone aerosol in respiratory tract disease, J New Drugs 2:298, 1962.

99. Clark TJ: Corticosteroid treatment of asthma, Schweiz Med Wochenschr 110(6):215-218, 1980.

100. Chambers WB and Malfitan VA: Beclomethasone dipropionate aerosol in the treatment of asthma in steroid-independent children, J Int Med Res 7(5):415-422, 1979.

101. Datau G and Rochiccioli P: Corticotropic testing during long-term beclomethasone dipropionate treatment in asthmatic children, Poumon Coeur 34(4):247-453, 1978.

102. Richards W et al: Steroid-dependent asthma treated with inhaled beclomethasone dipropionate in children, Ann Allergy 41(5):247-277, 1978.

103. Kass I, Vijayachandra Nair S, and Patil KD: Beclomethasone dipropionate aerosol in the treatment of steroid-dependent asthmatic patients: an assessment of 18 months of therapy, Chest 71(6):703-707, 1977.

104. Lee-Hong E and Collins-Williams C: The long-term use of beclomethasone dipropionate for the control of severe asthma in children, Ann Allergy 38(4):242-244, 1977.

105. Hudgel DW and Spector SL: Pulmonary infiltration with eosinophilia: recurrence in an asthmatic patient treated with beclomethasone dipropionate, Chest 72(3):359-360, 1977.

106. Neuman I and Toshner D: Beclomethasone dipropionate in pediatric perennial extrinsic rhinitis, Ann Allergy 409(5):346-348, 1978.

107. Brown HM, Storey G, and Jackson FA: Beclomethasone dipropionate aerosol in treatment of perennial and seasonal rhinitis: a review of five years' experience, Br J Clin Pharmacol 3:283S-286S, 1977.

108. Girard JP, Cuevas M, and Heimlich EM: A placebo controlled double-blind trial of beclomethasone dipropionate in the treatment of allergic rhinitis, Allergol Immunopathol 6(2):109-116, 1978.

109. Bernstein IL, Chervinsky P, and Falliers CJ: Efficacy and safety of triamcinolone acetonide aerosol in chronic asthma: results of a multicenter short-term controlled and long-term open study, Chest 81:20-26, 1982.

110. Grieco MH et al: Clinical effects of aerosol triamcinolone acetonide in bronchial asthma, Arch Intern Med 138:1337-1341, 1978.

111. Golub JR: Long-term triamcinolone acetonide aerosol treatment in adult patients with chronic bronchial asthma, Ann Allergy 44(3):131-137, 1980.

112. Chervinsky P and Petraco AJ: Incidence or oral candidiasis during therapy with triamcinolone acetonide aerosol, Ann Allergy 43(2):80-82, 1974.

113. Slavin RG et al: Multicenter study of flunisolide aerosol in adult patients with steroid-dependent asthma, J Allergy Clin Immunol 66(5):379-385, 1980.

114. Corticosteroid aerosols for asthma, Medical Letter 27:5-6, 1985.

115. Poppius H et al: Exercise asthma and disodium cromoglycate, Br Med J 4:337-339, 1970.

116. Chan-Yeung M: The effect of SCH 1000 and disodium cromoglycate on exercise-induced asthma, Chest 71:320-323, 1977.

117. Pichurko BM et al: Influence of cromolyn sodium on airway temperature in normal subjects, Am Rev Respir Dis 130(6):1002-1005, 1984.

118. Woenne R, Kattan M, and Levison H: Sodium cromoglycate-induced changes in the dose-response curve of inhaled methacholine and histamine in asthmatic children, Am Rev Respir Dis 119(6):927-932, 1979.

119. Weiner P et al: Bronchodilating effect of cromolyn sodium in asthmatic patients at rest and following exercise, Ann Allergy 53(2):186-188, 1984.

120. Mathison DA et al: Cromolyn treatment of asthma, JAMA 216:1454, 1971.

121. Smith JM: Prolonged use of disodium cromoglycate in children and young persons—ten years experience, Schweiz Med Wochenschr 110(6):183-184, 1980.

122. Turner-Warnick M: Clinical practice with regard to management of the adult asthmatic with cromoglycate, Schweiz Med Wochenschr 110(6):181-183, 1980.

123. Furuwaka CT et al: A double-blind study comparing the effectiveness of cromolyn sodium and sustained-release theophylline in childhood asthma, Pediatrics 74(4):453-459, 1984.

124. Bernstein IL: Cromolyn sodium, Chest 87(1-Suppl):68S-73S, 1985.

125. Liern Caballero M, Alberola Carbonell C, and Climent P'erez JL: Clinical and histological study to assess changes in the nasal mucosa in patients with chronic perennial rhinitis comparing sodium

cromoglycate and placebo, Scand J Respir Dis 59(3):160-166, 1978.

126. Goodman ML and Irwin JW: Disodium cromoglycate in anaphylaxis and pollinosis, Ann Allergy 40(3):177-180, 1978.

127. Frostad AB: The treatment of seasonal allergic rhinitis with a 2% aqueous solution of sodium cromoglycate delivered by a metered dose nasal spray, Clin Allergy 7(4):347-353, 1977.

128. Jones EA Jr: Oral cromolyn sodium in milk induced anaphylaxis, Ann Allergy 54(3):199-201, 1985.

129. Olsen A: Streptomycin aerosol in the treatment of chronic bronchiectasis: preliminary report, Proc Staff Meet Mayo Clin 21:53, 1946.

130. Garthwaite B and Barach AL: Penicillin aerosol therapy in bronchiectasis, lung abscess, and chronic bronchitis, Am J Med 3:261, 1947.

131. Eastlake C Jr: Aerosol therapy in sinusitis, bronchiectasis, and lung abscess, Bull NY Acad Med 26:423, 1950.

132. Christie HE et al: Aerosol therapy for lung abscess, Can Med Assoc J 62:478, 1950.

133. Melica A et al: Oxytetracycline inhalation in the treatment of acute and chronic bronchial infection, G Clin Med 47:416, 1962.

134. Naumov GP: Pathologic changes in upper respiratory passages and lungs following use of antibiotic electroaerosols, Fed Proc 25:654, 1966.

135. Stout SA and Derendorf H: Local treatment of respiratory infections with antibiotics, Drug Intell Clin Pharm 21:322-329, 1987.

136. Kun P, Landau LI, Phelan PD: Nebulized gentamicin in children and adolescents with cystic fibrosis, Aust Paediatr J 20(1):43-45, 1984.

137. Battistini A et al: Aerosol administration in antibiotic therapy of cystic fibrosis, Pediatr Med Chir 5(4):161-169, 1983.

138. Pines A et al: Gentamicin and colistin in chronic purulent bronchial infections, Br Med J 2:543, 1967.

139. Bilodeau M et al: Studies of absorption of kanamycin by aerosol, Ann NY Acad Sci 132:870, 1966.

140. Spier R et al: Aerosolized pancreatic dornase and antibiotics in pulmonary infection, JAMA 178:878, 1961.

141. Hall CB et al: Ribavirin treatment of experimental respiratory syncytial viral infection: a controlled double-blind study in young adults, JAMA 249:2666-2670, 1983.

142. Knight V et al: Ribavirin small-particle aerosol treatment of influenza, Lancet 2:945-949, 1981.

143. Knight V: Aerosol treatment of influenza, Cardiovasc Res Center Bull 19:118-127, 1981.

144. McClung HW et al: Ribavirin aerosol treatment of influenza B virus infection, JAMA 249:2671-2674, 1983.

145. Rimar JM: Ribavirin for treatment of RSV infection, MCN 11:413, 1986.

146. Eggleston M: Clinical review of ribavirin, Infect Cont 8:215-218, 1987.

147. Tiffin NH, Warren JB, and Lee RJ: Administration of ribavirin to a mechanically ventilated infant, RRT 23(1):10-12, 1987.

148. Demers RR et al: Administration of ribavirin to neonatal and pediatric patients during mechanical ventilation, Respir Care 31:1188-1196, 1986.

149. Salamone FR and Cunha BA: Update on pentamidine for the treatment of *Pneumocystis carinii* pneumonia, Clin Pharm 7:501-510, 1988.

150. Wharton JM et al: Trimethoprim sulfamethoxazole or pentamidine for *Pneumocystis carinii* pneumonia in the acquired immunodeficiency syndrome, Ann Intern Med 105:37-44, 1986.

151. Haverkos HW: Assessment of therapy for *Pneumocystis carinii* pneumonia: PCP therapy project group, Am J Med 76:501-508, 1984.

152. Corkery KJ, Luce JM, and Montgomery AB: Aerosolized pentamidine for treatment and prophylaxis of *Pneumocystis carinii* pneumonia: an update, Respir Care 33:676-685, 1988.

153. Montgomery AB et al: Selective delivery of pentamidine to the lung by aerosol, Am Rev Respir Dis 137:477-478, 1988.

154. Wordell CJ and Hauptman SP: Treatment of *Pneumocystis carinii* pneumonia in patients with AIDS, Clin Pharm 7:514-527, 1988.

21

Airway Care

Kim F. Simmons

Respiratory care practitioners spend a great deal of time working with patients who have diseased lungs and impaired gas exchange. It is important to remember that adequate gas exchange is not possible if a patent airway is not provided, even with normal lungs. The importance of an adequate airway is demonstrated in the sequencing of cardiopulmonary resuscitation procedures, where the airway is given first priority (see Chapter 22). Airway care procedures are the responsibility of respiratory care practitioners in many areas of the hospital setting, including on the general medical and surgical floors, in the critical care areas, as well as in the emergency room.

There are two broad areas of airway care in which respiratory care practitioners must develop skills. First, the respiratory care practitioner must be proficient in the techniques of airway clearance, including those methods designed to ensure patency of the patient's airway, natural or artificial. Second, the respiratory care practitioner must be skilled in the placement and use of artificial airways used to support patients whose own natural airways are inadequate. This chapter explores each of these areas.

OBJECTIVES

Specifically, after completion of this chapter, the reader will be able to:

1. Describe the hazards and complications and outline the procedure used in nasotracheal suctioning;

2. Compare and contrast rigid and flexible fiberoptic bronchoscopy, as used for both therapeutic and diagnostic purposes;

3. Differentiate the four primary indications for insertion of an artificial airway;

4. Differentiate the advantages, disadvantages, and methods of establishing tracheal airways via the oral, nasal, and tracheostomy routes;

5. Describe the role and responsibilities of the respiratory care practitioner in the maintenance of artificial

tracheal airways, including procedures for airway clearance and cuff care;

6. Identify the appropriate course of action in common artificial airway emergencies, including tube obstruction, cuff leaks, and accidental extubation;

7. Differentiate the methods and procedures used to extubate patients with orotracheal or nasotracheal tubes versus those employed to remove a tracheostomy tube.

KEY TERMS

Most terms used in this chapter are defined in context. The following terms are introduced without explicit definition, but may be found in the text glossary:

bacteremia	nonresectable
biopsy	otorhinolaryngologist
debridement	pneumomediastinum
duodenum	pneumothorax
electrocautery	polymorphonuclear cells
endoscopy	precursor
extrathoracic	pulmonologist
iridium	stylet
ligate	tincture of benzoin
maxillofacial	tomography
methylene blue	tracheitis
mucopolysaccharide	

AIRWAY CLEARANCE TECHNIQUES

Obstruction of the airway occurs secondary to retained secretions, foreign objects such as tumors and aspirated food, and structural changes within the airway such as edema or traumatic injuries. The first technique described in this section will allow the practitioner to remove secretions by mechanical aspiration known as suctioning. Removal of foreign objects and suctioning below the carina are often done by bronchoscopy, which is performed by a physician. This technique often requires the assistance of respiratory care practitioners. Management of the structural changes and injuries will be discussed subsequently in the section on artificial airways.

Airway aspiration (suctioning)

Retention of secretions causes an increase in airway resistance, increased work of breathing, and may result in hypoxemia, hypercapnea, atelectasis, and infection. As described in Chapter 6, secretions of normal consistency and quantity are handled by the mucociliary escalator mechanism and swallowing. Difficulty in clearing secretions may result from their tenacity, amount, or to the patient's inability to generate an effective cough. Difficulty in clearing secretions is the primary indication for suctioning. Disease processes that may require suctioning include infectious disorders, COPD, cystic fibrosis, and conditions impairing the cough mechanism, such as central nervous system depression or neuromuscular disease.

Complications. Despite the benefits of airway aspiration, there are several significant complications associated with suctioning. These complications, ranging from mucosal damage to sudden death, are summarized in the box opposite.

Hypoxemia is the most common complication of suctioning. It should be remembered that air as well as secretions are being removed during the suctioning procedure. In fact, greater decreases in oxygenation have been reported after suctioning than after an equivalent period of apnea. Moreover, hypoxemia has been suggested as a precursor to some of the other complications.

To prevent this complication, it is recommended that patients always be preoxygenated prior to suctioning with 100% O_2 and, where indicated, hyperinflated with a manual resuscitator. Of course, the respiratory care practitioner should use caution in preoxygenating patients with chronic hypercapnea, since this technique could decrease their stimulus to breathe. Limiting the amount of time suction is applied also minimizes the likelihood of hypoxemia.

Cardiac arrhythmias occur mainly as a result of hypoxemia. Mechanical stimulation of the airway, particularly the area around the larynx, will also cause arrhythmias. If the patient is connected to a cardiac monitor, the respiratory care practitioner should check it often for the appearance of this complication. Bradycardia may result from vagal stimulation as the catheter enters the larynx or touches the carina. Tachycardia may result from patient agitation and hypoxemia. If any major change is seen in the heart rate or rhythm, suctioning should be stopped, and the respiratory care practitioner should immediately administer oxygen to the patient, providing manual ventilation as necessary.

Hypotension can occur secondary to cardiac arrhythmias that cause a decrease in cardiac output or to severe coughing episodes that decrease venous return. If any signs of

---

COMPLICATIONS ASSOCIATED WITH ENDOTRACHEAL SUCTIONING

Hypoxemia
Cardiac arrhythmias
Hypotension
Atelectasis
Mucosal trauma
Contamination/infection
Increased intracranial pressure

---

hypotension are noted, the suctioning procedure should be stopped and oxygenation and ventilation restored.

Atelectasis occurs secondary to removing air from the lungs as the secretions are removed. This complication can be minimized by limiting the amount of negative pressure used, the duration of suctioning, and by providing hyperinflation before and after the procedure. Another factor associated with atelectasis is the use of too large a suction catheter. As long as the catheter is smaller than the airway, some of the air drawn into the catheter will come from the upper airway. On the other hand, if the catheter completely occludes the airway, then the negative pressure will be applied to only the airway below the catheter. Therefore, it is recommended that the external diameter of the catheter should never exceed one half to two thirds of the internal diameter of the airway.

Mucosal trauma can occur as the tube is passed through the upper airway and the trachea. This trauma is caused, in part, by the rigidity of the catheter as it touches the walls of the airway. It is therefore essential to avoid excessive force when advancing the catheter. Lubrication of the catheter will also help facilitate its passage.

The amount of negative pressure used may also contribute to trauma, by causing the catheter to adhere to the wall of the airway. It is recommended that the suction pressure be limited to -100 to -120 cm H_2O for adults, -80 to -100 cm H_2O for children, and -60 to -80 cm H_2O for infants. These settings may be altered, depending on the consistency of the secretions. Thicker secretions may require more negative pressure and thinner secretions less.

Mucosal trauma may also be associated with adherence of the catheter to the wall of the airway during application of negative pressure. As the catheter is withdrawn, mucosal tissue may literally be torn away from the underlying basement membrane or submucosa. Again, limiting the amount of negative pressure can minimize this problem. Moreover, a variety of catheter designs are now available that decrease the likelihood of catheter adherence to the airway wall (Fig. 21-1).

Contamination of the lungs with bacteria is possible as the catheter is passed through the upper airway. Transient

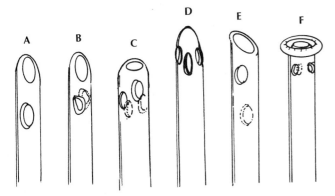

Fig. 21-1 Suction catheter tips.

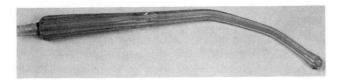

Fig. 21-2 Yankauer-type tonsil suction.

bacteremia has been reported with nasotracheal suctioning secondary to mucosal damage. Immunosuppressed patients are likely to develop more serious complications. Sterile technique and gentle insertion should help minimize this complication.

Increased intracranial pressures have been reported during the suctioning procedure, secondary to an increase in the mean arterial pressure or coughing. These changes are only transient, with values normally returning to baseline within 1 minute. However, in patients with elevated intracranial pressures, these changes could be significant.

Procedure. Access to the trachea for suctioning can be gained through the nose, mouth, or an artificial airway. Nasotracheal suctioning will be discussed at this time. Tracheal suctioning through the mouth should be avoided as this will cause gagging. Oropharyngeal secretions can be removed using a rigid tonsillar, or Yankauer, suction tip (Fig. 21-2). Suctioning through an artificial airway will be discussed in the section on airway maintenance.

Step 1: Assess the need for suctioning. Routine suctioning of a patient should be discouraged. The decision to suction a patient should be based on current physical assessment findings, including coarse rhonchi, tactile fremitus, and an ineffective cough.

Step 2: Assemble and check the equipment. Most suction catheter packages include the catheter, gloves, and a cup that is used for rinsing the catheter. Additional equipment needed includes water-soluble lubricating jelly, sterile water, suction apparatus (tubing, collection container, and regulator), and an oxygen delivery device or manual resuscitator connected to an oxygen source (see the box below). The practitioner should check the level of suction pressure. If no vacuum is generated at the thumbport, check for leaks in the tubing, at the collection container, or the regulator.

Step 3: Preoxygenate the patient. For alert and cooperative patients capable of a spontaneous deep breath, apply the oxygen therapy device and instruct them to take a few large breaths. For those not capable of a spontaneous deep breath, a manual resuscitator connected to an oxygen source should be used. Caution should be taken with chronically hypercapneic patients breathing on a hypoxic drive.

Step 4: Insert the catheter. After the catheter has been lubricated, insert it gently through the nostril, without applying negative pressure. If any resistance is met in the nose, gentle twisting of the catheter should help. If twisting does not permit insertion, withdraw the catheter and attempt to insert it in the other nostril.

As the catheter moves into the lower pharynx, have the patient assume a "sniffing" position by flexing the neck and extending the atlanto-occipital joint (Fig. 21-3). This position helps align the opening of the larynx with the lower pharynx, making catheter passage through the larynx more likely. Forward displacement of the tongue, which pulls the epiglottis upward and forward, may also increase the likelihood of catheter passage into the trachea (see Fig. 21-3). Continue to insert the catheter until the patient coughs or a resistance is felt much lower in the airway.

Step 5: Apply suction. When the patient coughs, apply suction while withdrawing the catheter using a rotating motion. If an obstruction is felt, pull the catheter back a few centimeters before applying suction. This maneuver will minimize mucosal damage. Since oxygenation has been shown to decrease after 5 seconds of suctioning, total application time should not exceed 10 to 15 seconds. If any cardiac disturbances result, remove the suction catheter immediately.

Step 6: Reoxygenate and hyperinflate the patient. Apply the oxygen device and proceed as in Step 3. Patients un-

---

**EQUIPMENT NEEDED FOR AIRWAY
ASPIRATION (ENDOTRACHEAL
SUCTIONING)**

Sterile suction catheter with thumb port
Sterile glove(s)
Sterile basin
Sterile water or saline
Sterile water-soluble lubricating jelly
Adjustable suction source
Oxygen delivery system (mask and manual resuscitator)

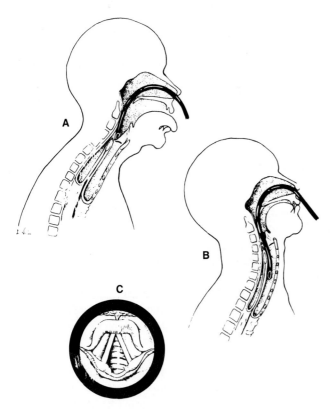

Fig. 21-3 Technique of nasotracheal suctioning. **A,** Optimal position of head in order to direct catheter tip anteriorly into the trachea. The neck is flexed and the head is extended. The tongue is protruded (and held there by a gauze 4 × 4). **B,** After the catheter has been advanced into the trachea, the tongue is released and the patient's head may be more comfortably positioned. **C,** View of the vocal cords from above. The cords are most widely separated during inspiration. (From Sanderson RG: The cardiac patient: a comprehensive approach, Philadelphia, 1972, WB Saunders Co.)

able to voluntarily take a deep breath must be hyperinflated and reoxygenated with the manual resuscitator. Assuming no serious complications occur, the procedure should be repeated from Steps 3 to 6 until the patient's breath sounds have cleared or improved.

Bronchoscopy

Bronchoscopy may be used for both therapeutic and diagnostic purposes. The therapeutic uses of bronchoscopy include removal of foreign objects, aspiration of secretions, and endobronchial surgery. Diagnostic testing includes biopsy, obtaining sputum samples for culture, and quantification of structural airway changes.

There are two types of bronchoscopes in use: rigid and flexible. The rigid bronchoscope is an open metal tube with a distal light source and a port for attaching oxygen or ventilating equipment (Fig. 21-4). The rigid bronchoscope is used most often by otorhinolaryngologist or thoracic surgeons. The tube is passed through the mouth,

down into the trachea, and as far as the bronchi. A telescoping tube with mirrors can be used to view the segmental bronchi. Suctioning is accomplished by passing a metal suction tube through the bronchoscope. The large internal diameter of this suction tube allows for aspiration of thick inspissated secretions and large mucous plugs. By passing a grasping forceps through the device, removal of foreign bodies and biopsies of tumors within the airway can also be accomplished. The primary problems with the rigid bronchoscope are patient discomfort and limited access to the smaller airways.

The flexible fiberoptic bronchoscope, or FFB, has gained popularity over the years because of its multifunctionality and ability to access very small airways. Only two areas of the lung are relatively inaccessible to the FFB: the superior segment of the posterior lobe and the medial portions of the upper lobes.

The typical FFB has a light transmission channel, a visualizing channel, and a multipurpose open channel that may be used for aspiration, tissue sampling, or oxygen administration (Fig. 21-5). This type of bronchoscope is most often used by the pulmonologist, often with the assistance of a respiratory care practitioner. The practitioner prepares the patient by explaining the procedure and administering an aerosolized local anesthetic to the patient's upper airway (to minimize gagging). The physician then inserts the bronchoscope orally or nasally, using the head control to direct the tip to the location desired.

Patient monitoring during the procedure is often done by the practitioner and should include ongoing assessment of the pulse, respiratory rate, and ECG. In addition, pulse oximetry can be used to monitor changes in arterial oxygen saturations. In some settings, the practitioner may also collect the sputum or tissue samples obtained by the physician and prepare them for the laboratory. Practitioners may also be responsible for cleaning and maintenance of the bronchoscope.

FFB is one of the most definitive diagnostic tools for lung cancer. Moreover, as compared with transthoracic biopsy, FFB carries a much lower risk of pneumothorax. Biopsy of tumors in the airway or in the parenchyma can often be obtained by using a brush or forceps inserted through the bronchoscope. Endobronchial washings also can be used to check for cancerous cells. Diagnosis of airway changes such as granulomas, stenosis, fistulas, or tears can also be done with fiberoptic bronchoscopy.

Aspiration of secretions to treat atelectasis is possible, but the fiberoptic bronchoscope channel is relatively small and may become plugged if secretions are thick. Removal of foreign objects from the airway can be done using a variety of tools. Forceps are used for small, solid objects. Large objects and organic material such as food can be retrieved with a "basket." This bronchoscope accessory has been used to remove objects as large as tweezers (9 cm) from mainstem bronchi.

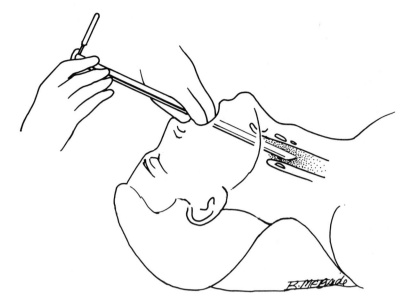

Fig. 21-4   Rigid tube bronchoscope.

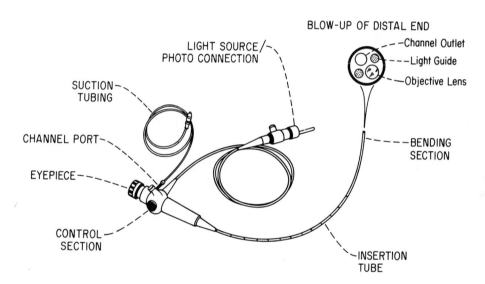

Fig. 21-5   Flexible fiberoptic bronchoscope.

Acute complications of bronchoscopy include damage to the mouth and/or nose (lacerations and minor bleeding), laryngospasm, transient changes in pulmonary function, hypoxemia, cardiac arrest, and pneumothorax (with transbronchial biopsy). The most common late complication is pulmonary infection, as manifested by fever and the signs and symptoms of pneumonia.

Laser therapy via bronchoscopy is a new palliative procedure for nonresectable lung cancer. The primary indication of bronchoscopic laser therapy are endobronchial tumors causing large airway obstruction. After the tumor is visualized, the laser energy is directed through a fiberoptic cable and fed into the bronchoscope. The laser then can be set on low power to cause thermal necrosis and coagulation or high power for vaporization.

Complications of laser therapy via the fiberoptic bronchoscope include hypoxemia, cardiac arrhythmias, hemorrhage, paroxysmal cough, and bronchial perforation. Effectiveness of therapy can be evaluated by improved pulmonary function studies, especially in flow rates. Other improvements, such as decreased dyspnea and orthopnea, have been reported. As laser therapy via the fiberoptic bronchoscope is a relatively new procedure, techniques and applications vary greatly from institution to institution. More research and clinical experience will help define future standards for this new technique.

Another therapeutic application of FFB is endobronchial radiotherapy, or brachytherapy. The bronchoscope is used to guide a catheter to the site of the tumor. The catheter is then left in place and attached to a source of iridium 192. Endobronchial radiotherapy may be used in combination with laser therapy. In this approach, the bronchoscope is passed to the area of the tumor. If the tumor is endobronchial and totally occlusive, the laser may be used to partially open the airway before insertion of the endobronchial catheter. If the airway is partially occluded, or the tumor is extrabronchial, the endobronchial catheter is put into position. As with bronchoscopic laser therapy, only additional research and clinical experience will determine the long-term efficacy of this new technique.

In summary, airway clearance techniques are important aspects of airway care from both a diagnostic and therapeutic perspective. Suctioning can be done alone by the respiratory care practitioner, who must take care to avoid complications such as hypoxemia and cardiac arrhythmias. The practitioner may also serve as a valuable assistant to the pulmonologist in therapeutic or diagnostic bronchoscopy procedures and should become familiar with the technique and complications of this useful tool.

INDICATIONS FOR ARTIFICIAL AIRWAYS

A variety of situations can occur in which a patient's own airway is not adequate, necessitating placement of an artificial airway. Four basic indications for placement of an artificial airway include:
1. To relieve airway obstruction;
2. To facilitate removal of secretions;
3. To protect the lower airways from aspiration; and
4. To facilitate application of positive pressure ventilation.

Relieving airway obstruction

Airway obstruction can occur at any point in the airway, but it is usually classified as either upper or lower in origin. Upper airway obstruction occurs above the glottis and includes the area of the nasopharynx, oropharynx, and larynx. Lower airway obstruction occurs below the vocal cords and includes the area of the trachea, mainstem bronchi, and the conducting airways.

Airway obstruction may also be classified by degree as either partial or complete. Partial airway obstruction varies in severity from a slight impairment to ventilation, with mild increases in the work of breathing, to almost complete obstruction, with associated stridor and marked respiratory difficulty. Complete airway obstruction results in no air flow, although exaggerated respiratory efforts, including retractions and the use of accessory muscles, may occur.

The causes of airway obstruction include crushing injuries secondary to trauma, edema, tumors, and anatomic or

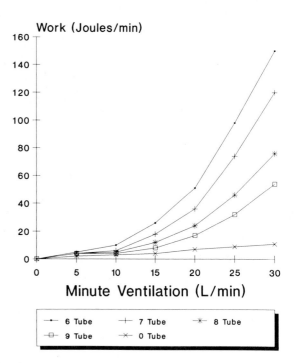

Fig. 21-6   Relationship between work of breathing, artificial airway size, and minute ventilation demonstrated in healthy volunteers. (Redrawn from Respiratory Care 33(2), 1988.)

physiologic changes in muscle tone or tissue support. Decreased muscle tone in the upper airway results in collapse, whereas increased muscle tone in the larynx may lead to closure.

Artificial airways can be used to bypass an airway obstruction and provide a clear passage for airflow. Such airways can bypass upper airway obstructions, laryngeal obstructions, and some extrathoracic tracheal obstructions. Normally, airway obstructions beyond the level of the trachea must be dealt with using other means.

Although they may be used to relieve acute airway obstruction, all artificial airways increase airway resistance above normal. The smaller the inner diameter of the airway, the greater will be the increase in airway resistance, and the resulting work of breathing for a given minute ventilation. Fig. 21-6 clearly demonstrates these relationships for four different-sized endotracheal tubes, as compared with normal ("O tube"). As can be seen, the work of breathing through a given size of tube (measured in joules/ min) increases exponentially with increasing minute ventilations. Moreover, smaller tubes are associated with dramatic increases in work, especially at higher minute ventilations. Clearly, artificial airways can impose an additional work load on the respiratory muscles, especially in patients with high ventilatory demands. Thus it is essential that the additional work load imposed by an artificial airway must be considered when its initial or continuing need is considered.

Facilitating secretion removal

As described in Chapter 6, normal airway secretions function to humidify inspired air and clear small, inhaled particles from the respiratory tract. If these secretions cannot be cleared, airway obstruction may result, causing increased work of breathing, hypoxemia, and hypercapnea. Moreover, stagnant secretions present an ideal medium for bacterial growth, which may ultimately result in pulmonary infection. Artificial airways facilitate secretion removal mainly by providing more direct access to the airway.

Protecting the airway

Four reflexes that help prevent aspiration of foreign material into the lower airway are the pharyngeal, laryngeal, tracheal, and carinal reflexes. The pharyngeal reflex produces a gag and swallowing response. The laryngeal response to stimulation is to close the glottis. Stimulation of tracheal and carinal reflexes result in coughing. The innervation for all these reflexes arises from the cranial nerves. The pharyngeal reflex is the only reflex innervated by two nerves: the glossopharyngeal (ninth cranial) and the vagus (tenth cranial). The remaining three reflexes are innervated by the vagus nerve.

Patients with CNS depression have varying degrees of decreased reflex response to stimulation. The loss of reflexes generally proceeds from the pharynx to the trachea, receding in the reverse order. For example, during the induction of anesthesia, the first response to disappear is the gag reflex, with the last being the cough (carinal) reflex. This same sequence of reflexes can be used to evaluate the level or severity of coma. For example, the patient with only a carinal cough reflex is more obtunded than one who still exhibits a pharyngeal gag.

Some artificial airways placed into the trachea have a small cuff (a balloon-like structure) that may be inflated to seal the space between the sides of the tube and the walls of the trachea. These cuffs are designed to prevent liquid or particulate matter from the pharynx or larynx from being aspirated into the lower trachea and lungs. The use of cuffs and their effectiveness will be discussed in detail later in this chapter.

Facilitating positive pressure ventilation

Long-term positive pressure ventilation can only be accomplished if a seal is maintained between the patient's airway and the device providing the driving pressure. With short-term intermittent positive pressure breathing (IPPB) treatments, a temporary seal can usually be maintained by the alert and cooperative patient via a mouthpiece and, if necessary, noseclips. Obviously, this arrangement is not practical for long-term mechanical ventilation, which may last for hours, days, or months. For this purpose, a cuffed artificial airway is placed into the trachea, and the cuff inflated to provide a seal.

SELECTING AND ESTABLISHING AN ARTIFICIAL AIRWAY

In general, artificial airways can be divided into those that are inserted into the pharynx and those that are inserted into the trachea.

Pharyngeal airways

Pharyngeal airways are designed to prevent airway obstruction by keeping the tongue pulled forward and away from the posterior pharyngeal wall. This type of obstruction is common in the unconscious patient because of a loss of muscle tone. By providing a clear passage into the lower oropharynx, pharyngeal airways also can facilitate suctioning. Since pharyngeal airways are used extensively in emergency life support, further details on their application, and the use of other emergency airway procedures, are provided in the next chapter.

Tracheal airways

Tracheal airways extend beyond the pharynx into the trachea. There are two basic types of artificial airways that can be inserted into the trachea: endotracheal and tracheostomy tubes. Endotracheal tubes are inserted either via the mouth (orotracheal) or nose (nasotracheal), through the larynx, and into the trachea. Tracheostomy tubes, however, are inserted through a surgically created opening in the trachea.

Endotracheal tubes are semi-rigid tubes, most often made from polyvinyl chloride or related plastic polymers. Fig. 21-7 portrays a typical endotracheal tube and its key components. The proximal end of the tube, *1*, is attached to a standard adapter with a 15 mm external diameter. The curved body of the tube, *2*, usually has length markings, indicating the distance (in cm) from the beveled tube tip, *3*. Other markings may include the designation "IT" and Z-79. IT is an abbreviation for implantation tested, meaning the tube material has been shown nontoxic to living tissue. Z-79 means the tube meets the design standards of the Z-79 Committee of the American National Standards Institute (ANSI).

In addition to the beveled opening at the tip, there should be an additional side port or "Murphy eye," *3A*, which ensures gas flow if the main port should become obstructed. The angle of the bevel, *4*, minimizes mucosal trauma during insertion. The tube cuff, *5*, is permanently bonded to the tube body and provides the capability to seal the airway for protection, or to provide positive pressure ventilation. A small filling tube, *6*, leads from the cuff to a pilot balloon, *7*, used to monitor cuff integrity and pressure once the tube is in place. Finally, a spring-loaded valve, *8*, with a standardized attachment for a syringe allows inflation and deflation of the cuff. Not shown, but incorporated into most modern endotracheal tubes, is a radiopaque indicator that is imbedded in the distal end of the tube body. This indicator allows for easy identification of tube position on x-ray film.

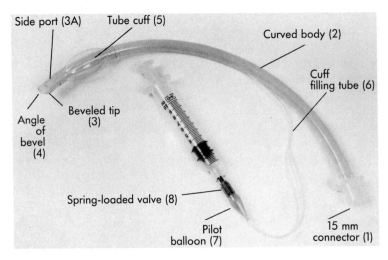

Fig. 21-7   Typical endotracheal tube.

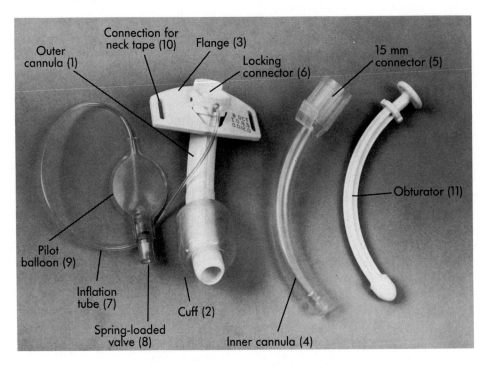

Fig. 21-8   Parts of a tracheostomy tube.

As with endotracheal tubes, tracheostomy tubes are generally manufactured from plastic polymers, although some are still made from silver. Fig. 21-8 portrays a typical plastic polymer tracheostomy tube and its key components. The outer cannula, *1,* forms the primary structural unit of the tube, to which is attached the cuff, *2,* and a flange, *3.* The flange prevents tube slippage into the trachea and provides the mechanism for attachment at the neck. A removable inner cannula, *4,* with standard 15 mm adapter, *5,* is normally kept in place within the outer cannula, but can be removed for routine cleaning, or if it becomes obstructed. To prevent its accidental removal, the inner cannula can be locked in place at the proximal end of the outer cannula, *6.* As with the endotracheal tube, an in-

flation tube, *7,* leads from the cuff to a pilot balloon, *9,* and spring-loaded valve, *8.* The tube is stabilized at the stoma site by cotton tape, *10,* which attaches to the flange and is tied around the neck. An obturator with a rounded tip, *11,* is used for tube insertion. Prior to insertion, the obturator is placed within the outer cannula, with its tip extending just beyond the distal end of the tube. This minimizes mucosal trauma during insertion, particularly the "snowplowing" effect that a rough tube edge can exert on the posterior tracheal wall. Finally, as with endotracheal tubes, a radiopaque indicator in the distal end of the tube provides confirmation of tube position on x-ray film.

Placement of a tracheal tube can be used to achieve any one or all four primary indications for artificial airways.

Airway obstruction above the level of the glottis can be bypassed through the use of endotracheal tubes, assuming there is no crushing injury of the larynx. If such an injury exists, a tracheostomy tube can be placed. The direct access to the trachea and lower airways provided by these tubes makes suctioning most efficient. Aspiration of pharyngeal contents into the lower airways can be minimized by inflating the cuff on the distal end of endotracheal and tracheostomy tubes. Tracheal tubes also provide an efficient airway for positive pressure ventilation, again by virtue of the cuff seal.

Orotracheal, nasotracheal, and tracheostomy tubes differ in regard to their appropriate use and methods of insertion. Since the respiratory care practitioner shares primary responsibility for airway management, a clear understanding of the indications, advantages, disadvantages, and hazards associated with the use of these devices is essential.

Oral endotracheal tubes. The oral endotracheal, or orotracheal, tube is the airway of choice in an emergency. This is because oral intubation, as compared with the nasal route or surgical tracheotomy, is the quickest and easiest means of establishing a tracheal airway.

Despite this important advantage, there are several disadvantages to the use of orotracheal tubes, especially for prolonged periods. Patient discomfort and gagging are common in conscious patients. For this reason, orotracheal tubes are used mainly for short-term airway management of unconscious patients, such as during general anesthesia. Accidental extubation, or removal, of an orotracheal tube is also a common problem. Extubation may occur when an unrestrained patient dislodges the tube or when the patient's oral secretions loosen the tape used to secure the tube. Dislocation of the tube, up or down in the trachea, may be related to the loosening of the tape or motion of the cheeks to which the tube is taped. Provision of oral hygiene is difficult because of the securing tape and the space occupied by the tube. Nutrition via oral intake is impossible for these patients. Damage to the lips, teeth, gums, and oropharynx may occur during the intubation procedure or later because of pressure necrosis from the tube.

Oral intubation procedure. Placement of an orotracheal tube, called orotracheal intubation, is a skill that can be accomplished by properly trained physicians, respiratory care practitioners, and nurses. Familiarity with the structures in the upper airway and proper selection of equipment are essential parts of this training. Following is a description of the basic steps in orotracheal intubation. Proficiency in this technique can only be developed by extensive training, mannequin practice, and application on anesthetized patients under the guidance of an anesthesiologist or other appropriately skilled individual.

Step 1: Assemble and check equipment. The box above, right lists the equipment necessary for intubation. Attach the laryngoscope blade to the handle and check the light source for secure attachment and brightness. Assemble suction equipment and check suction pressure prior to

---

EQUIPMENT NECESSARY FOR ENDOTRACHEAL INTUBATION

Oxygen flowmeter and tubing
Suction apparatus
    Flexible suction catheters
    Yankauer (tonsillar) tip
Manual resuscitation bag and mask
Oropharyngeal airway(s)
Laryngoscope (2) with assorted blades
Endotracheal tubes (3 sizes)
Tongue depressor
Stylet
Stethoscope
Tape
Syringe
Lubricating jelly
Magill forceps
Local anesthetic (spray)
Towels (for positioning)

---

intubation, since vomitus or secretions may obscure the pharynx or glottis.

Select an appropriate size tube, but have available one size larger and one size smaller. Table 21-1 provides guidelines for selection of orotracheal tubes according to patient age and includes recommended maximum suction catheter sizes to be used with each tube size. Note that endotracheal tube sizes are normally expressed in metric units, corresponding to the internal diameter of the tube. The French scale, still common with suction catheters, is based on the external circumference of tubes and catheters. To convert French to metric, simply divide the French size by 3.14. For example, a no. 12 French suction catheter is approximately 4 mm in external diameter.

Table 21-1   Pediatric to Adult Endotracheal Tube Sizes

Age	Tube size (mm)	Suction catheter (size French)
Premature	2.5	5
Newborn	3.0	6
6 mo	3.5	6
18 mo	4.0	8
3 yr	4.5	8
5 yr	5.0	10
6 yr	5.5	10
8 yr	6.0	10
12 yr	6.5	12
16 yr and small adult females	7.0	14
Adult females (average)	8.0	14
Adult males	9.0	14

From Eubanks DH and Bone RC: Comprehensive respiratory care, St Louis, 1985, The CV Mosby Co.

After selecting the appropriate size tube, check the cuff for leaks, being sure to deflate it prior to insertion. Insert a stylet into the tube to add rigidity and shape for easier insertion. Lubricate the stylet to facilitate its removal later.

Step 2: Position the patient. Align the mouth, pharynx, and larynx to facilitate visualization of the glottis and insertion of the tube. The larynx, pharynx, and mouth can be aligned by combining moderate cervical flexion with

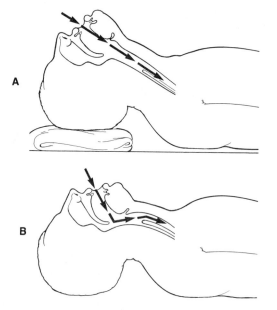

Fig. 21-9   **A,** Correct preintubation head position. **B,** Incorrect preintubation head position.

extension of the atlanto-occipital joint. This position may be accomplished by placing one or more towels under the patient's head, flexing the neck, and then tilting the head backward with the hand (Fig. 21-9).

Step 3: Preoxygenate the patient. Prior to intubation, the patient is often apneic or in respiratory distress. Restore adequate ventilation and oxygenation by bag and mask prior to attempting intubation. Use 100% oxygen to provide a reserve during the intubation procedure. No longer than 30 seconds should be devoted to any intubation attempt. If intubation fails, immediately ventilate and oxygenate the patient for 3 to 5 minutes before another attempt is made.

Step 4: Insert the laryngoscope. Use the left hand to hold the laryngoscope; with the right hand, open the mouth (Fig. 21-10). Insert the laryngoscope into the right side of the mouth, and move toward the center, displacing the tongue to the left. Then advance the tip of the blade along the curve of the tongue until the epiglottis is visualized.

Step 5: Visualize the glottis. The arytenoid cartilage and epiglottis should come into view as the blade reaches the base of the tongue (Fig. 21-11). If these structures are not visible, it is likely that the blade has advanced too far and may be in the esophagus. If this is the case, maintain upward force on the laryngoscope, slowly withdrawing it until the larynx comes into view.

Step 6: Displace the epiglottis. The technique used to move the epiglottis depends on the type of blade used (Fig. 21-12). The curved or MacIntosh blade lifts the epiglottis indirectly as the tip of the blade is advanced into the

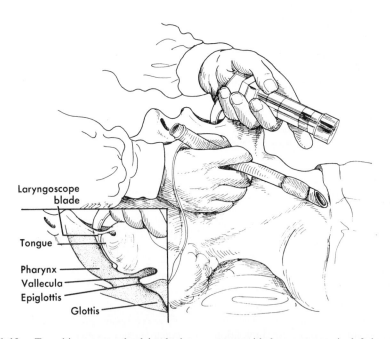

Laryngoscope blade
Tongue
Pharynx
Vallecula
Epiglottis
Glottis

Fig. 21-10   To achieve orotracheal intubation, rescuer, with laryngoscope in left hand, introduces blade into right side of mouth, displacing tongue to the left. (From Ellis PD and Billings DM: Cardiopulmonary resuscitation: procedures for basic and advanced life support, St Louis, 1980, The CV Mosby Co.)

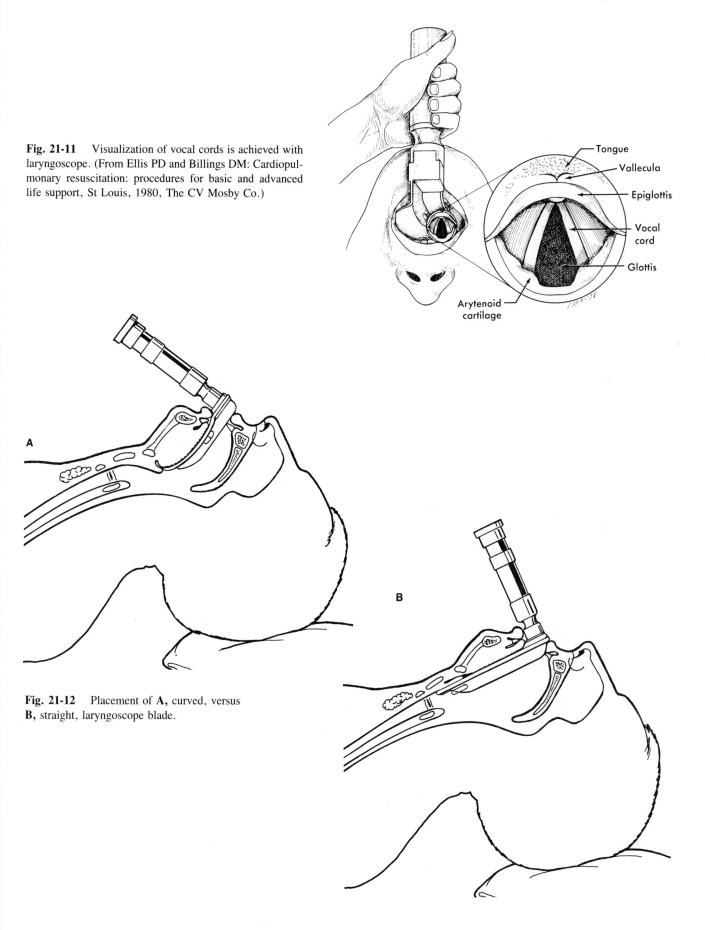

Fig. 21-11 Visualization of vocal cords is achieved with laryngoscope. (From Ellis PD and Billings DM: Cardiopulmonary resuscitation: procedures for basic and advanced life support, St Louis, 1980, The CV Mosby Co.)

Tongue

Vallecula

Epiglottis

Vocal cord

Glottis

Arytenoid cartilage

A

B

Fig. 21-12 Placement of **A,** curved, versus **B,** straight, laryngoscope blade.

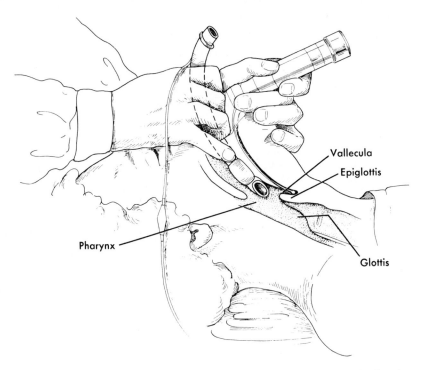

Fig. 21-13 Insertion of endotracheal tube. (From Ellis PD and Billings DM: Cardiopulmonary resuscitation: procedures for basic and advanced life support, St Louis, 1985, The CV Mosby Co.)

vallecula and the laryngoscope is lifted up and forward (Fig. 21-12, *A*). The straight or Miller blade lifts the epiglottis directly as the tip of the blade is advanced beyond it and the laryngoscope is lifted up and forward (Fig. 21-12, *B*).

In lifting the tip of the blade, avoid levering the laryngoscope against the teeth, as this can cause damage to the teeth and gums. Avoid this problem by keeping the wrist fixed and moving the handle of the laryngoscope in the direction it is pointing when the epiglottis is visualized.

Step 7: Insert the tube. Once the glottis is visualized and the epiglottis moved, insert the tube from the right side of the mouth and advance without obscuring the glottic opening (Fig. 21-13). The tip of the tube should be seen passing between the cords and then advanced until the cuff has passed the cords by 2 to 3 cm. The average depth of tube insertion for an adult is 23 cm from the teeth.

Once the tube is in place, stabilize the tube with the right hand, using the left hand to remove the laryngoscope and the stylet. Then inflate the cuff to seal the airway and immediately ventilate and oxygenate the patient.

Step 8: Confirm tube placement. The first technique used to assess proper placement is auscultation. Listen for equality of breath sounds as the patient is being manually ventilated with oxygen. Air movement or gurgling sounds over the epigastrium indicate possible esophageal intubation. Observe the chest wall for adequate and equal chest expansion. These movements, combined with auscultation, are often reinforcing. For example, decreased breath sounds on the left and decreased chest wall movement on the same side would indicate intubation of the right mainstem bronchus, which can be rectified by slowly withdrawing the tube while listening for restoration of breath sounds on the right.

Capnography, or end-tidal CO_2 analysis, may be used to supplement auscultation as a means of determining proper tube placement. Since inspired air contains about 0.04% CO_2, and end-tidal gas about 6% of this gas, proper placement of an endotracheal tube in the respiratory tract will cause carbon dioxide levels to abruptly rise during end expiration. If, on the other hand, the tube is misplaced in the esophagus, the "end expired" CO_2 levels will remain near zero. Unfortunately, capnography cannot warn the clinician of tube misplacement in a mainstem bronchus.

Proper tube placement in the trachea can be confirmed without a chest x-ray study using a fiberoptic laryngoscope. After assuring patient reoxygenation, insert a fiberoptic laryngoscope directly into the endotracheal tube (Fig. 21-14). Visualization of the carina distal to the tip of the endotracheal tube assures proper placement in the trachea. More precise placement can be accomplished by moving the laryngoscope from the tube tip to the carina, while measuring this distance.

Step 9: Stabilize the tube. Secure the tube to the skin above the lip and on the cheeks using tape while holding the tube in position. Do not secure the tube until placement is confirmed by auscultation. Use a bit block, oropharyngeal airway, or similar device to prevent the patient from compressing the tube between the teeth (Fig.

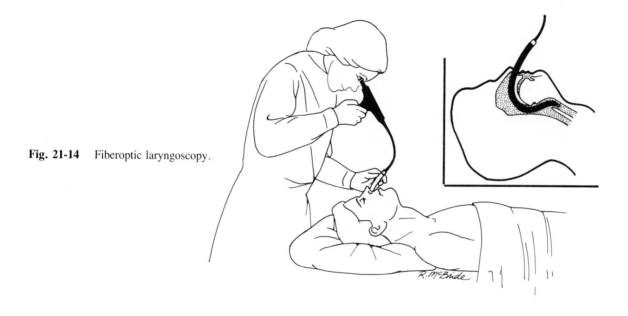

Fig. 21-14   Fiberoptic laryngoscopy.

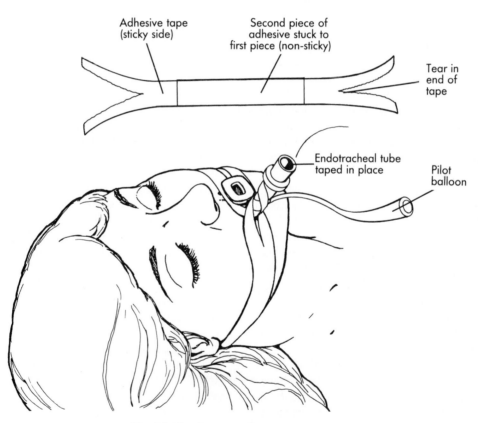

Fig. 21-15   Securing the endotracheal tube.

21-15). After the tube is stabilized, have a chest radiograph taken to ensure that the tube is above the carina.

Complications of oral intubation include damage to the teeth and gums and laceration of the lips, tongue, pharynx, larynx, and esophagus. The most serious complications are acute hypoxemia, hypercapnea, bradycardia, and cardiac arrest. Proper technique, adequate prior ventilation and ox-

ygenation of the patient, and adherence to strict time limits in intubation attempts will help minimize these hazards.

Nasal endotracheal tubes. Nasal endotracheal, or nasotracheal, tubes generally are considered more difficult to insert than orotracheal tubes. Nonetheless, nasotracheal insertion is the route of choice in many clinical situations, including patients with cervical spine or maxillofacial injuries who are in need of a short-term artificial airway.

Once in place, nasotracheal tubes offer several distinct advantages over orotracheal tube placement. Since the tape that holds the tube in place is positioned mainly on the nose and upper cheeks, tube stability is enhanced and oral hygiene is facilitated. Also, the nasotracheal tube is better tolerated by the conscious and semi-conscious patient.

However, there are several disadvantages to the nasal route for intubation. Since a tube one size smaller than an orotracheal tube may be needed to pass through the nose, airway resistance will be higher. Necrosis of the nasal septum and external nares also may occur, since regular switching between nares is not always practical. Sinusitis and otitis media may result from the tube blocking drainage from the sinuses and the eustachian tubes, respectively. Nosebleed is not usually a problem until extubation. Oral feedings are still difficult, but patients may be allowed to sip water in small quantities.

Nasal intubation procedure. Nasotracheal intubation may be accomplished using either a direct visualization or blind intubation method. The direct visualization approach may employ a fiberoptic or bronchoscope laryngoscope. Successful application of the blind technique requires that the patient be awake or at least capable of spontaneous breathing. Direct visualization will be discussed first.

The equipment needed for nasotracheal intubation by direct visualization is the same as for oral intubation, with the addition of Magill forceps. Sprays of 0.25% racemic epinephrine and 2% lidocaine are also suggested by many for local anesthesia and vasoconstriction of the nasal passage.

Equipment assembly, patient positioning, and preoxygenation are carried out as with oral intubation. The tube should be lubricated to facilitate passage. Insertion, with the bevel directed toward the septum, proceeds inferiorly and posteriorly. When the tip of the tube is in the oropharynx, the practitioner should open the mouth, insert the laryngoscope, and visualize the glottis. With the right hand, the practitioner uses the Magill forceps to grasp the tube just above the cuff and directs it between the cords (Fig. 21-16). Flexion of the neck will help advance the tube past the cords. The average depth of insertion is 25 cm from the external naris. Confirmation of position and stabilization follow, as with the oral route.

Alternatively, the practitioner may use a fiberoptic bronchoscope or laryngoscope to guide tube passage. With the bronchoscopic method, the distal end of the bronchoscope is passed through the endotracheal tube and directed into the trachea. Once placement is assured, the endotracheal tube slides down over the bronchoscope into its position within the trachea. The procedure is similar with a fiberoptic laryngoscope, except manipulation of the tube is accomplished mainly by positioning of the head and neck.

Blind nasal intubation may be accomplished with the patient supine or sitting up. As with the direct visualization, the tube is inserted through the nose. As the tube ap-

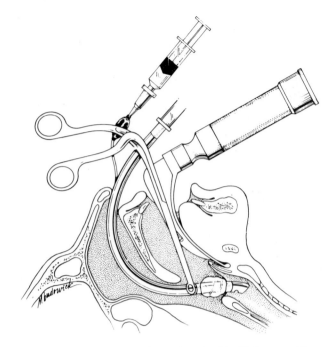

Fig. 21-16 Nasal intubation using the Magill forceps. (From Finucane BT and Santora AH: Principles of airway management, Philadelphia, 1988, FA Davis Co.)

proaches the larynx the practitioner listens through the tube for air movement. The breath sounds become louder and more tubular when the tube passes through the larynx. Successful passage of the tube through the larynx usually is indicated by a harsh cough, followed by vocal silence. If the sounds disappear, the tube is moving toward the esophagus. Failure to advance the tube through the larynx can be corrected by tube, head, and neck manipulations. Confirmation of tube placement and stabilization should follow.

A recently developed aid to facilitate blind nasotracheal intubation is the flexible light wand. The light wand is a battery-powered stylet with a bulb at its distal tip. The wand is passed through the nose to the laryngopharynx. Once passed beyond the glottis, the wand light is visible through the neck, confirming its placement in the trachea. An endotracheal tube is then passed over the light wand, which serves as a stent.

Complications associated with nasotracheal intubation include damage to the nasal septum resulting in bleeding, or trauma to the nasopharynx, oropharynx, or larynx. Hypoxemia, hypercapnea, bradycardia, and cardiac arrest are also possible, but generally less likely than with oral intubation. The decreased incidence of serious problems reported with nasotracheal intubation (as opposed to the oral route) does not necessarily indicate that this approach is inherently safer. It may simply mean that the nasal route is commonly applied electively to patients who are generally more stable than those undergoing oral intubation.

Tracheostomy tubes. Because it enters the trachea directly, a tracheostomy tube is considered to be the most efficient artificial airway and is the device of choice for overcoming upper airway obstruction or trauma. As compared with orotracheal or nasotracheal tubes, tracheostomy tubes offer the advantages of lower airway resistance, less movement of the tube within the trachea, greater patient comfort, and the ability to provide oral feedings. Moreover, since a tracheostomy tube is shorter than either an orotracheal or nasotracheal tube, deeper and more efficient suctioning is possible.

Nonetheless, tracheostomy tubes have several disadvantages. First, the use of a tracheostomy tube requires a surgical procedure (tracheotomy) that carries an overall mortality rate ranging from 0% to 5%. Incisional hemorrhage occurs in 5% to 10% of all tracheotomy procedures. Approximately 13% of patients undergoing tracheotomy also develop subcutaneous emphysema, or air between the interstitial spaces of the muscles and skin. Dissection of air into the pleural space or mediastinum (pneumothorax or pneumomediastinum, respectively), is more serious, but less common, occurring in about 5% of the cases. However, neither the incidence rate nor potential seriousness of these complications should deter tracheotomy when it is indicated.

The primary indication for tracheostomy is the prolonged need for an artificial airway. The amount of time that constitutes "prolonged" is an area of great controversy, ranging anywhere from 3 days to 3 weeks. The primary concern in this debate is how long an endotracheal tube can remain in place before laryngeal and/or tracheal damage occurs. Some authors report a correlation between the length of intubation and the development of complications. Others report complications in patients who were intubated just 1 day longer than those that did not develop complications. Still others report a correlation between the duration of intubation and the development of tracheal, but not laryngeal, lesions. The specific types of airway damage will be discussed later in this chapter.

At present, the best advice regarding the optimal time to change from endotracheal intubation to tracheostomy is that the decision must be individualized. Factors to be considered in making this decision are (1) the estimated length of time the patient will need an artificial airway; (2) the patient's tolerance of the endotracheal tube; (3) the patient's overall condition, including nutritional, cardiovascular, and infection status; (4) the patient's ability to tolerate a surgical procedure; and (5) the relative risks of continued endotracheal intubation versus tracheostomy.

In regard to relative risk, the early complications and undesirable consequences of tracheostomy tend to be more severe than those of endotracheal intubation, especially among patients having pre-existing bleeding disorders. However, endotracheal tubes can also cause bleeding from the gums and nose in such patients, resulting in clot formation in the posterior oropharynx. For this reason, tracheotomy with electrocautery is considered by some the procedure of choice for airway management of patients prone to bleeding or hemorrhage.

Tracheotomy procedure. Tracheotomy should be performed by a skilled surgeon as an elective procedure when the patient's airway is already stabilized. It is believed that the mortality rate and morbidity associated with this surgical procedure are reduced when done electively.

The patient can be taken to surgery if other procedures are to be done or can remain in ICU. The respiratory care practitioner may be asked to assist in the procedure, especially if performed at the bedside. Therefore the procedure will be briefly described.

Local anesthesia is used and the patient mildly sedated, conditions permitting. If an endotracheal tube is in place, it should not be removed until just prior to the insertion of the tracheostomy tube, since this ensures a patent airway and provides additional stability to the trachea during the procedure. Entrance into the trachea is made through either a horizontal incision between rings, or a vertical one through the second and third rings (Fig. 21-17). The vertical incision requires opening of fewer tissue planes and affords easier insertion and removal of the tracheostomy tube. The vertical incision also may allow for more movement of the tracheostomy tube with swallowing. The horizontal incision causes less cosmetic disfigurement, but can result in improper angulation of the tracheostomy tube at its distal end.

Once the skin and subcutaneous tissue have been incised, the platysma muscles are divided and the thyroid gland is located. The thyroid isthmus, which overlies the second and third tracheal rings, must be divided and ligated. Careful surgical technique is required as the thyroid is a highly vascular structure. As little cartilage as possible should be removed to promote better closure after extubation.

Once the stoma is created and the tracheostomy tube is selected and prepared for insertion, the endotracheal tube may be removed. The lumen of the trachea can be evaluated to ensure that the tracheostomy tube is of the correct size, which will occupy approximately two thirds to three quarters of the internal tracheal diameter. Table 21-2 delineates the various tracheostomy tube sizes by Jackson size, internal diameter, external diameter, and French size. The traditional use of the Jackson system is a holdover from the days of silver tracheostomy tubes. Table 21-3 provides guidelines for the selection of tracheostomy tubes according to a patient's age, using the Jackson size for reference. Within an age category, the exact size tube chosen depends on the patient's size and weight.

Insertion of the tube, inflation of the cuff, and securing of the tube follow. Wound edges should not be excessively tight, since this will promote the development of subcutaneous, or mediastinal, air. Traction sutures on the lower edge will help in opening the stoma in case of accidental extubation.

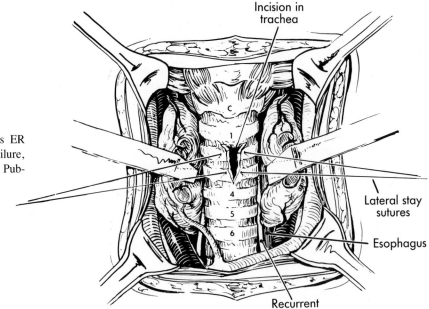

Fig. 21-17 Tracheal incision. (From Crews ER and Lapuerta L: A manual of respiratory failure, Springfield, IL, 1972, Charles C Thomas, Publisher.)

Table 21-2   Approximate Tracheostomy Tube Sizes*

Jackson size	Internal diameter	External diameter	French size
00	2.5	4.5	13
0	3.0	5.0	15
1	3.5	5.5	16.5
2	4.0	6.0	18
3	4.5-5.0	7	21
4	5.5	8	24
5	6.0-6.5	9	27
6	7.0	10	30
7	7.5-8.0	11	33
8	8.5	12	36
9	9.0-9.5	13	39
10	10.0	14	42
11	10.4-11.0	15	45
12	11.5	16	48

From Eubanks DH and Bone RC: Comprehensive respiratory care, St Louis, 1985, The CV Mosby Co.
*Tube sizes are approximate.

Table 21-3   Pediatric to Adult Tracheostomy Tube Sizes

Age	Jackson reference
Premature	000-00
Birth-6 mo	0
6-18 mo	1
18 mo to 4-5 yr	1-2
4-5 yr to 10 yr	2-3
10 to 14 yr	3-5
14 yr to adult	5-9

From Eubanks DH and Bone RC: Comprehensive respiratory care, St Louis, 1985, The CV Mosby Co.

AIRWAY TRAUMA ASSOCIATED WITH TRACHEAL TUBES

Depending on the type of airway used, damage to the patient's own airway may occur anywhere from the nose down into the lower trachea. Nasal and oral damage were discussed in the section related to nasal and orotracheal tubes. In this section, laryngeal and tracheal changes will be discussed in terms of etiology, symptoms, and treatment. The types and location of laryngeal and tracheal damage associated with the use of tracheal airways is shown in Fig. 21-18.

Four areas of the airway most commonly affected are the posteromedial portion of the vocal cords, the posteromedial portion of the arytenoid cartilages, the posterolateral aspect of cricoid cartilages, and the trachea from rings two through seven. Occasionally the anterior tracheal wall also may be affected. These areas receive the greatest pressure and friction because of the inability of the artificial airway to conform to the patient's own anatomic airway.

The severity of damage may range from swelling, edema, and minor bleeding to permanent anatomic airway changes. The reported incidence with which these complications are reported in the literature may vary because of the method of evaluation and the time elapsed before follow-up. For example, slight changes in the mucosa may not present symptoms but can be detected by fiberoptic bronchoscopy. Therefore, if bronchoscopy is used, the reported incidence will be higher. Some forms of airway damage may take weeks, months, or years to develop. If patient follow-up is done sooner than the damage becomes evident, the reported incidence will be lower.

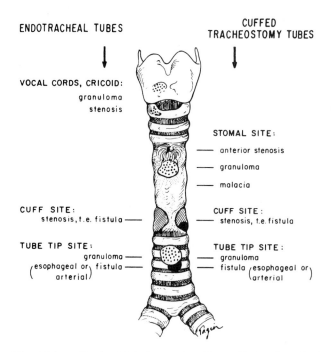

ENDOTRACHEAL TUBES

CUFFED
TRACHEOSTOMY TUBES

VOCAL CORDS, CRICOID:
granuloma
stenosis

STOMAL SITE:
— anterior stenosis
— granuloma
— malacia

CUFF SITE:
stenosis, t.e. fistula —

CUFF SITE:
— stenosis, t.e. fistula

TUBE TIP SITE:
granuloma —
(esophageal or) fistula —
arterial

TUBE TIP SITE:
granuloma —
fistula (esophageal or) arterial

Fig. 21-18   Tracheal injuries produced by cuffed endotracheal and tracheostomy tubes. (From Grillo HC: Surgery of the trachea, Curr Probl Surg, July 1970.)

It is important to realize that the damage to the airway often cannot be assessed while an artificial airway is in place. It is therefore essential that the patient's airway be evaluated carefully after extubation. Techniques commonly used to diagnose airway damage include physical examination, simple neck radiography, air tomography, fluoroscopy, laryngoscopy, and bronchoscopy.

Laryngeal lesions

The etiology of these changes is the interaction between an endotracheal tube and the patient's airway. Trauma during intubation, movement of the tube, and reaction to the material of the tube are some of the risk factors. It is generally believed that the longer the endotracheal tube is in place, the more severe will be the resulting complications. It is also reported by some that the nasotracheal intubation results in fewer complications as compared with the oral route because of smaller tubes, better tube stability, and less pressure on the glottis.

Glottic edema and vocal cord inflammation are transient changes that occur secondary to pressure from the endotracheal tube or trauma during intubation. The reported incidence varies from 20% to 30% and may occur after only a few hours of intubation. Symptoms most often associated with edema and inflammation are hoarseness and stridor. Hoarseness is the most common symptom, exhibited by nearly three fourths of extubated patients. Generally, hoarseness is benign and, depending on its severity, resolves over a few hours to days.

Stridor is a high-pitched noise heard during inspiration. When heard in the adult, stridor indicates that the lumen of the anatomic airway is reduced to 5 mm or less in diameter. This is a more serious symptom because it is associated with increased airway resistance and increased work of breathing. Stridor is often treated with racemic epinephrine (2.25% Vaponephrine) via aerosol. The goal of the treatment is to reduce glottic or airway edema by mucosal vasoconstriction. A steroid may also be added to the aerosol to further reduce the inflammation.

To reduce the development of edema in patients who have had prolonged intubation or those who have failed prior extubation because of glottic edema, steroids may be given intravenously 24 hours prior to extubation. It is important to realize that swelling may worsen over 24 hours after extubation and patients should be evaluated periodically for the development of glottic edema. If stridor continues and is unresponsive to treatment, structural changes that narrow the airway should be considered.

Laryngeal and vocal cord ulcerations have been reported in 20% to 50% of extubated patients. These changes have been reported after as few as 7 hours of intubation and are generally acute in nature. The primary symptom is hoarseness, which usually resolves spontaneously. No therapy is indicated.

Vocal cord polyps and granulomas may occur as the epithelium heals after ulceration. Polyps and granulomas may take weeks to months to form. Some authors report these changes as uncommon, while others report incidence rates as high as 42%. Early symptoms include difficulty in swallowing, hoarseness, and stridor. Case reports indicate that these symptoms tend to resolve spontaneously in most patients. Long-term complications include dry cough, difficulty in raising sputum, orthopnea, and lower respiratory tract infections. Depending on the severity of these complications, surgical intervention to remove established granulomas may be indicated.

Vocal cord paralysis secondary to endotracheal tubes has been reported, most often affecting both cords. Incidence varies from about 3% to 5% of previously intubated patients. The primary symptom is a stridor that does not resolve with racemic epinephrine treatments. However, obstructive symptoms may resolve within 24 hours, and full movement of the cords can return over several days. If the obstructive symptoms do not resolve, tracheotomy may be indicated.

Laryngeal web is the result of necrotic tissue forming fibrin and incorporating cellular debris. This "membrane" may occupy varying amounts of the glottic lumen. Formation of laryngeal webs often takes days or months. Symptoms include stridor or abrupt total airway obstruction. Treatment consists of aspirating the web with a suction catheter if the web is pliable. Laryngoscopy may otherwise be indicated.

Laryngeal stenosis has been reported secondary to tracheotomy, when performed too close to the first tracheal ring. As the tracheostomy stoma heals, the area near the cricoid cartilage is narrowed. The symptoms associated with laryngeal stenosis are similar to those of vocal cord paralysis, namely, stridor and hoarseness. This obstruction usually does not resolve spontaneously, necessitating surgical intervention for correction.

Tracheal lesions

Whereas laryngeal lesions occur only with orotracheal and nasotracheal tubes, tracheal lesions may result from the use of any tracheal airway. The most common tracheal lesions caused by artificial airways are tracheal granulomas, tracheomalacia, and tracheal stenosis. Less common but more serious complications are tracheoesophageal and tracheoinnominate fistulas.

Tracheal granulomas are reported to form in the trachea in proximity to the tip of the tracheal tube and are probably related to movement of the tube. Case reports indicate a 30% acute incidence of tracheal granulomas, with 10% of the patients going on to demonstrate chronic changes associated with tracheal stenosis.

Tracheomalacia and tracheal stenosis are two complications that may occur either separately or together. Tracheomalacia is the softening of the cartilaginous rings, which results in the collapse of the trachea during inspiration. Processes similar to those that cause mucosal ulceration may lead to debridement of the epithelium and exposure and necrosis of the cartilaginous rings. The extent of tracheomalacia depends on the degree of cartilaginous damage.

Tracheal stenosis is a narrowing of the lumen of the trachea, which can occur as the tracheal rings start to heal. Fibrous scarring causes the airway to narrow. In patients with endotracheal tubes, this type of damage most often occurs at the point in the trachea that was in contact with the inflated cuff. However, tracheal stenosis has been reported to affect segments of the trachea larger than those normally in contact with the tube cuff. In patients with tracheostomy tubes, stenosis may occur at the cuff site or the tip of the tube, but most often at the stoma site. The etiology of the changes at the cuff site and tip of the tube are the same as with endotracheal tubes. The stenosis at the stoma site may be caused by too large a stoma, infection of the stoma, movement of the tube, or frequent tube changes.

Signs of possible tracheal damage prior to extubation include difficulty in sealing the trachea with the cuff and evidence of tracheal dilatation on chest x-ray film. Post-extubation signs and symptoms depend on the severity of the damage. These signs and symptoms may develop acutely within minutes, but more commonly become evident over a 2- to 3-month period. Difficulty with expectoration may be observed in mild cases. Dyspnea at rest indicates more severe damage than dyspnea on exertion. Stridor will occur if the tracheal lumen is less than 5 mm in diameter.

Pulmonary function studies, especially flow volume loops, may be helpful in quantifying the severity of the damage, as well as in distinguishing between tracheomalacia and tracheal stenosis (see Chapter 17). Tracheomalacia will appear as a variable obstruction with different inspiratory and expiratory patterns. Tracheal stenosis will appear as a fixed obstructive pattern, with flattening of both the inspiratory and expiratory limbs of the flow volume loop.

Treatment depends on the severity, especially the length and circumference of the damage. Laser therapy may be useful if the lesion is small. Resection and end-to-end anastomosis may be indicated when the damage involves less than three tracheal rings. More involved damage may require staged repair.

Tracheoesophageal and tracheoinnominate fistulae are communications between the trachea and esophagus and the trachea and innominate artery. Tracheoesophageal fistula may occur in infants as a developmental defect. As a complication of artificial airways, tracheoesophageal fistula has an incidence of between 1% and 5% and has been reported with both tracheostomy and endotracheal tubes. If it occurs soon after tracheotomy, incorrect surgical technique may be the cause. Later development is related to sepsis, malnutrition, tracheal erosion from the cuff and the tube, and esophageal erosion from nasogastric tubes. Diagnosis can be made by a history of recurrent aspiration and abdominal distention as air is forced into the esophagus during positive pressure ventilation. Direct examination of the trachea and esophagus by bronchoscopy and endoscopy will confirm the diagnosis. Treatment involves the closure of the defect in the trachealis muscle and the wall of the esophagus.

Tracheoinnominate fistula is a rarer complication, but is the most common cause of delayed hemorrhage after tracheotomy. This potentially life-threatening complication occurs if the tracheal tube is placed too low, thereby rubbing against and eroding into the innominate artery. Diagnosis may be made by pulsation of the tracheostomy tube prior to the onset of hemorrhage. Once hemorrhage begins, the patient should be taken to surgery. Even with proper corrective action, only 25% of patients who develop this serious complication survive.

Prevention

Damage to the larynx and the trachea ranges from acute inflammation to chronic structural changes such as stenosis. Not all patients develop long-term sequelae, and the reasons for these differences are not clearly understood. The amount of time before intubation causes damage also varies greatly from patient to patient. Despite these discrepancies, some precautions can be taken to minimize the development of airway damage.

Many studies suggest that movement of the tube may be a primary causative factor. Several methods can be used to limit tube movement. Sedation to keep patients comfortable may prevent them from trying to extubate themselves.

Nasotracheal tubes are easier to stabilize and may move less than orotracheal tubes. Patients with tracheostomy tubes should have respiratory therapy equipment attached through the use of swivel adapters so the tubing may move without moving the airway. If the tracheostomy patient requires oxygen therapy, tracheostomy collars are preferred to T-tubes or Briggs adapters.

Once in place, endotracheal and tracheostomy tubes should not be changed unless necessary. Selection of the correct size airway is also important. Some authors suggest that an endotracheal tube one size smaller than can be fit through the opening of the glottis should be used. The patient should be discouraged from unnecessary coughing or efforts to talk, which prevent the cords from closing around the tube. Pressure necrosis from the cuff on endotracheal or tracheostomy tubes may be reduced by limiting cuff pressure to that needed to minimize aspiration or provide ventilation. If the airway has been placed to provide access for suctioning or to bypass an obstruction, it may not be necessary to inflate the cuff at all.

Infected secretions have been implicated in the development of tracheitis and mucosal destruction, and infection of the tracheotomy stoma has been linked to tracheal stenosis. Therefore, sterile techniques should be used when working with these tubes. Good tracheostomy care, including aseptic cleaning of the stoma with hydrogen peroxide, should be carried out routinely. Soiled tracheostomy dressings should also be changed as needed.

It should be realized that the most serious complications of tracheal airways occur in less than 10% of the patients requiring intubation. This relatively small risk should never deter action when a tracheal airway is needed. However, once the airway is established, only sound techniques of airway management and maintenance can minimize the possibility of serious complications.

AIRWAY MAINTENANCE

Once a tracheal airway is in place, the respiratory care practitioner must attend to several aspects of airway maintenance. Among the critical responsibilities in this area are (1) securing the tube and maintaining its proper placement, (2) providing for patient communication, (3) assuring adequate humidification, (4) minimizing the possibility of infection, (5) facilitating clearance of secretions, (6) providing appropriate cuff care, and (7) troubleshooting airway-related problems. Although each of these topics will be discussed in a separate section, it is important to realize that certain aspects of airway maintenance are interrelated. For example, not checking to see if the patient needs to be suctioned could result in an obstructed tube, which may, in turn, require troubleshooting.

Securing the airway and confirming placement

Endotracheal tubes, nasal or oral, are often secured by using tape. The tape is secured to one side of the face then wound around the tube and airway once or twice before securing the end to the skin again (see Fig. 21-15). Silk tape is adequate if the period of intubation is short, such as during surgery. However, this type of tape is easily loosened by oral secretions, which may result in movement of the tube. Cloth tape seems to be better for longer use and may adhere better to the skin by applying tincture of benzoin. Some practitioners recommend applying benzoin to the tube itself so the tape will be more securely attached to the tube. Disadvantages of taping tubes in place include allergic reactions to the tape and damage to the skin when removing soiled or loose tape.

Alternatively, some manufacturers have developed tube holder systems that use straps and plastic adapters to stabilize the tube. Case reports demonstrate that the incidence of skin damage, tube movement, and self-extubations with these stabilizing devices are less than with traditional taping methods. However, of and by themselves, these devices cannot prevent airway trauma.

Tracheostomy tubes may be held in place through the use of cloth ties that are threaded through the flanges of the tube. Two separate pieces may be used and tied together on the side of the patient's neck. Another method uses one long piece of cloth tie that goes through one flange and around the patient's neck, and threads through the other flange before being tied. An alternative to cloth ties is a strip of foam rubber with Velcro attachments that are threaded through the flanges. This system is easier to change and does not cause skin necrosis as often as cloth ties. Whichever material is used, the ties should be loose enough to fit one finger's width between the ties and the patient's neck. This will also help minimize damage to the skin.

Proper placement of endotracheal tracheostomy tubes may be checked on chest x-ray film. The tip of the tube should be 3 to 7 cm above the carina. This position will minimize the chance of the tube moving down into the mainstem bronchi or up into the larynx. There are two important points to remember when assessing tube position on x-ray film. First, on an AP film, the esophagus is behind the trachea. Therefore, esophageal intubation may be missed. If a tube is suspected of being located in the esophagus, a lateral film will help. Second, the position of an endotracheal tube will change with head and neck position. Flexion of the neck will move the tube toward the carina, and extension will pull the tube toward the larynx. Therefore, when reviewing a film for tube placement, the practitioner should check the position of the head and neck. If the tube is malpositioned, the practitioner should remove the old tape and reposition the tube using the markings on the tube as a guide. This often requires two people to prevent extubation.

As an alternative to using chest films to confirm tube placement, a practitioner trained in fiberoptic laryngoscopy may confirm the position of the tube visually. In this method, the fiberoptic laryngoscope is inserted into the tube and the carina directly visualized. By moving the laryngoscope from the tube tip to the carina and measuring the distance of laryngoscope displacement, the exact distance of insertion can be determined.

Providing for patient communication

One of the most frustrating aspects of providing care to a patient with a tracheal tube is their impaired ability to communicate. Phonation requires moving vocal cords and airflow between them. Endotracheal tubes prevent vocal cord movement and do not allow for exhaled air to pass between the cords. Standard tracheostomy tubes allow for vocal cord movement but no airflow.

The experienced practitioner may use lip reading, but this technique is difficult in patients with orotracheal tubes because of the tape around the mouth that is used to secure the tube. Alternatively, the alert patient may write messages on paper or some other writing surface. This sounds simple, but may be made difficult by restricted hand movement resulting from restraints and arterial or intravenous line placement in the hand or forearm. Moreover, it is often difficult for critically ill patients to hold up their heads to see a writing pad. A better solution is a letter, phrase, or picture board. These communication adjuncts allow patients to communicate simply by pointing. The use of large but simple drawings are particularly important for patients who cannot clearly see print.

In conscious patients for whom long-term tracheostomy is indicated, consideration should be given to a "talking" tracheostomy tube (Fig. 21-19). These specialized airways provide a separate inlet for compressed gas, which escapes above the tube, thereby allowing phonation.

Assuring adequate humidification

Endotracheal and tracheostomy tubes provide an airway to conduct gas to and from the lungs, but they do not function as well as our natural airways. Specifically, artificial tracheal airways bypass the normal humidification, filtration, and heating functions of the upper airway. It has been shown that decreased humidity in the inspired air will cause secretions to thicken. Cool air may also decrease ciliary function. Singly or in combination, these conditions may impair the mucociliary escalator and result in retention of secretions. If a patient is intubated to facilitate secretion clearance, failure to provide adequate humidification will compound the problem. Tenacious secretions may plug the tracheal tube and render it useless. In fact, a plugged tracheal tube constitutes an emergency situation, the management of which will be discussed later in this chapter.

To prevent these problems, inspired air should be provided to the airway as near to body temperature and body humidity as possible. The device chosen to provide saturated gas at or near body temperature may be a heated hu-

Fig. 21-19   Pitt speaking tracheostomy tube.

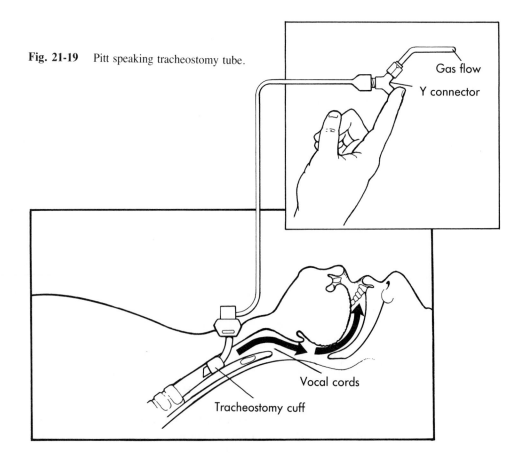

Gas flow

Y connector

Vocal cords

Tracheostomy cuff

midifier designed for high flows, or a heated jet-type neb- ulizer. These devices should be heated to a temperature between 32 and 36°C at the proximal end of the airway. The air may need to be heated to a higher temperature at the humidification device, since it will lose heat as it moves toward the patient (see Chapter 23).

Minimizing nosocomial infections

Patients with tracheal airways are among the most sus- ceptible group to developing nosocomial infections (see Chapter 14). Entrance of infectious organisms into the lower airway can occur through the lumen of the tube or around its outer border. Endotracheal intubation introduces pharyngeal organisms into the lower airway as the tube is passed through the mouth or nose. Pathogenic bacteria may be found in the mouth, especially if the patient is re- ceiving antibiotics that have eliminated the normal flora. It has also been suggested that patients on antacid therapy have a high incidence of pathogenic organisms since rais- ing of the gastric pH allows more bacterial growth. Aspi- ration of the pharyngeal contents around the tube may oc- cur in up to 70% of intubated patients.

Anything that is passed through the tube, such as suc- tion catheters, saline, or aerosolized medications, may carry bacteria into the lower airway. Bacteria may be found adhering to the inner walls of the tubes within a sub- stance called *gylcocalyx*. This material, composed of polysaccharides and the bacteria that produce it, forms a film on the surface of artificial devices such as tracheal air- ways. This material seems to protect the bacteria from an- tibiotics and phagocytosis by macrophages. Common pathogens of pulmonary infections such as *Pseudomonas aeruginosa Staphylococcus aureus, Staphylococcus epi- dermis,* and *Acinetobacter* organisms are excellent produc- ers of gylcocalyx. Polyvinyl chloride appears to be a ma- terial to which bacteria most easily colonize. These two factors, in combination with mucopolysaccharides nor- mally contained in sputum, make tracheal airways a pri- mary site for the development of gylcocalyx.

Although the presence of gylcocalyx has been demon- strated, its role in the development of pneumonia is still not well understood. It is possible that pieces of this film may be broken off as suction catheters are passed through the tube and down into the lungs.

The presence of pathogenic organisms in the lower air- way is only one factor in the development of pulmonary infection. Retained secretions also play a role. Impaired mucociliary clearance may occur secondary to the pres- ence of the tube, which blocks the mucociliary escalator proximal to the cuff. Also responsible for impaired clear- ance may be improperly humidified air or damage to the epithelium from an improper suctioning technique.

Impaired clearance may also result from the patient's in- ability to develop an effective cough. The ability to gener- ate an effective cough may be impaired for two reasons.

First, pain, sedation, muscle fatigue, or impaired neuro- muscular reflexes may compromise thoracic compression, thereby lowering the velocity of the expired air. Likewise, the inability to close the glottis means less intrathoracic pressure can be generated for a given compression, thus further compromising the expulsive force needed to pro- duce an effective cough. Despite these factors, many pa- tients with endotracheal tubes can generate an effective "huff." Patients with tracheostomy tubes seem better able to accomplish this maneuver, possibly because the airway is shorter.

Bacteria introduced into the lower airways should be handled by the normal defense mechanisms, including an- tibodies, alveolar macrophages, and polymorphonuclear cells. However, the patient's own defense mechanism may not be adequate because of chronic illness, malnutrition, or immunosuppression. To minimize the development of contamination and/or pneumonia, practitioners should try to prevent introducing organisms into the airway by (1) ad- hering to sterile technique during suctioning, (2) ensuring that only aseptically clean or sterile respiratory equipment is used for each patient, and (3) consistently washing hands between patient contacts (see Chapter 14). Retention of secretions may be minimized by appropriate suctioning techniques, chest physiotherapy when indicated, and ade- quate humidification. Routinely changing the inner can- nula on tracheostomy tubes also has been suggested as a means of minimizing bacterial contamination and infec- tion.

Facilitating clearance of secretions

The primary means to facilitate secretion clearance in patients with tracheal airways is tracheobronchial aspira- tion or tracheal suctioning. The indications, hazards, and equipment needed for suctioning through tracheal tubes are essentially the same as those described earlier for nasotra- cheal suctioning. A review of that section may be useful before proceeding with the following description of trache- obronchial aspiration.

Alterations in the procedure for tracheobronchial aspira- tion are as follows:

Step 1: Assess the patient. If breath sounds are clear, periodically perform one pass of the suction catheter to en- sure the tip of the tube does not become plugged. Tena- cious secretions may not move with airflow and, therefore, not create adventitious sounds.

Step 2: Assemble the equipment. The equipment used for tracheobronchial aspiration is the same as for nasotra- cheal suctioning, with the addition of sterile saline for in- stillation into the airway to thin secretions and facilitate their removal. If the secretions are tenacious, instillation of acetylcysteine or sodium bicarbonate (2%) tends to be more effective than normal saline. This may require a phy- sician's order.

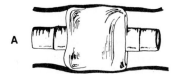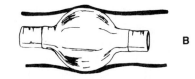

Fig. 21-20 Diagram comparing shapes of high residual volume, low-pressure cuff, **A,** and low residual volume, high-pressure cuff, **B.** (From McPherson SP: Respiratory therapy equipment, ed 4, St Louis, 1989, The CV Mosby Co.)

Step 3: Preoxygenate and hyperinflate the patient. To accomplish hyperinflation in these patients, use manual resuscitators. Patients with COPD may need to be hyperinflated without increasing the F_{IO_2}. Other patients should receive 100% oxygen.

Step 4: Insert the catheter. Insert the catheter carefully. When an obstruction is felt or a strong cough elicited, withdraw the catheter and apply suction.

Step 5: Apply suction as was done with nasotracheal suction.

Step 6: Reoxygenate as was done with nasotracheal suction.

Given their already compromised pulmonary status, patients receiving ventilatory support are especially prone to develop hypoxemia during tracheobronchial aspiration. Much research has been done to find better methods of preventing this complication. The current literature is controversial, but following are some suggestions. Hyperoxygenation and hyperventilation have been reported to be more effective when accomplished through the ventilator, as opposed to manual resuscitators. This appears to be especially true for patients on high levels of support, such as positive end-expiratory pressure (PEEP). Insertion of the suction catheter through an adapter that does not require disconnection of the ventilator circuit from the airway may also be helpful in preventing hypoxemia. This technique is recommended for patients receiving high levels of support, especially PEEP levels greater than 10 cm H_2O.

Related to this technique are two new catheter designs. The first, a multiuse suction catheter incorporated directly into the ventilator circuit, allows suctioning without disconnecting the patient from the circuit. When changed every 24 hours, this type of catheter does not increase bacterial contamination. The second design is a double-lumen catheter that can provide both suction pressure and oxygen delivery. When the valve on this double-lumen catheter is closed, suction pressure is delivered to the airway; when the valve is opened, oxygen is delivered. Ongoing research on these new approaches will ultimately determine their relative utility in minimizing hypoxemia during tracheobronchial aspiration.

Providing cuff care

Cuff inflation is used to provide a sealed airway for mechanical ventilation and to prevent or minimize aspiration.

As previously mentioned, tracheal stenosis and tracheomalacia may be induced by the cuff. The pathogenesis of these problems is related to the amount of cuff pressure transmitted to the tracheal wall. If cuff pressure exceeds the perfusion pressure of the mucosa, ischemia, ulceration, necrosis, and exposure of the cartilage may result.

The amount of pressure transmitted from the cuff to the tracheal wall depends on the diameter, thickness, and compliance of the cuff. Inflated cuffs were the major cause of airway damage in the 1960s when small-volume, high-pressure cuffs were commonly used. Since the 1970s, high residual-volume, low-pressure cuffs have been used (Fig. 21-20). The diameter of these cuffs is greater than the diameter of the trachea, meaning the cuff can be inflated to seal the airway without being fully inflated and with less internal pressure. Thus, when properly used, these cuffs should transmit less pressure to the tracheal wall than their small-volume, high-pressure counterparts. The use of these cuffs has lessened the incidence of tracheal damage, not eliminated it.

One of the most important aspects of airway care is the measurement of cuff pressure. The perfusion pressure of the tracheal mucosa ranges from 30 mm Hg at the arterial side to 18 mm Hg at the venous side. Maximum recommended levels of cuff pressures thus range from 20 to 25 mm Hg.

Measurement of cuff pressure can be done with a three-way stopcock, syringe, and pressure manometer (Fig. 21-21). With the stopcock opened to the syringe, manometer, and cuff, air is added or removed while the practitioner observes the pressure changes on the manometer.

It is important to realize most manometers are calibrated in centimeters of water (cm H_2O) and not mm Hg. Thus the "acceptable range" is 27 to 33 cm H_2O. It is not necessary to inflate the cuff to these levels if the trachea can be sealed with less. Overinflation of a high-volume, low-pressure cuff changes its performance to a high-pressure cuff. This problem is common if the tube chosen is too small for that patient's trachea.

In terms of inflation techniques, two alternative procedures are used: the minimal occluding volume (MOV) and the minimal leak technique (MLT). Periodic deflation of the cuff for 5 to 10 minutes every hour has also been suggested, although the adequacy of this method remains questionable.

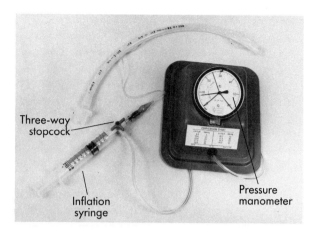

Fig. 21-21   Measuring cuff pressure by way of in-line pressure monitor.

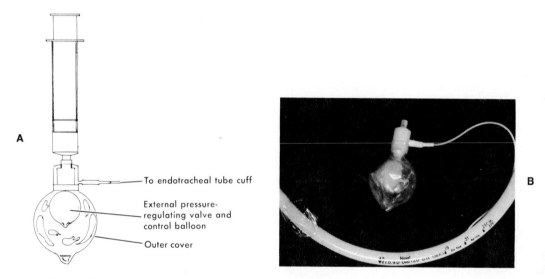

Fig. 21-22   **A,** Lanz external pressure-regulating valve and control balloon regulate cuff pressure. **B,** Endotracheal tube with pressure-regulating valve. (From McPherson SP: Respiratory therapy equipment, ed 4, St Louis, 1980, The CV Mosby Co.)

In the MOV technique, the practitioner slowly inflates the cuff to the point where the air heard escaping around the cuff during positive pressure ventilation ceases. Because the airways expand during the application of positive pressure, pressure on the trachea during inspiration is less than during expiration. The amount of ischemia that may result using the MOV technique depends on both the intracuff pressure used and the rate of the positive pressure breaths.

The MLT method is similar to the MOV method in that air is slowly injected into the cuff until the leak stops. However, once a seal is obtained, the practitioner removes a small amount of air, allowing a slight leak at peak inflation pressure. Because this leak occurs during the application of positive pressure, pharyngeal secretions tend to be blown upward at peak inflation, minimizing the likelihood of aspiration.

Some authors suggest that the MLT approach negates the need for pressure monitoring. However, clinical research has shown that a minimal leak is obtained only at cuff pressure in excess of 25 mm Hg in some patients. For this reason, cuff pressure measurements should still be conducted, regardless of the cuff inflation method used.

Alternatives to cuff pressure measurements include different types of cuffs and inflation techniques. The Lanz tube incorporates an external pressure regulating valve and control reservoir designed to limit the cuff pressure to 16 to 18 mm Hg (Fig. 21-22). The Kamen-Wilkinson foam cuff (Fig. 21-23) is another alternative designed to seal the trachea with atmospheric pressure in the cuff. Prior to insertion, the foam cuff must be deflated. Once in position, the pilot tube is opened to the atmosphere, and the foam allowed to expand against the tracheal wall. Expansion of the cuff stops when the tracheal wall is encountered.

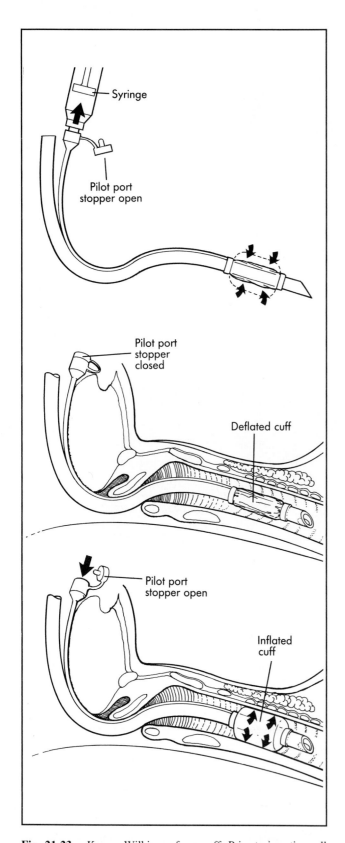

Fig. 21-23   Kamen-Wilkinson foam cuff. Prior to insertion, all air is removed and foam compressed (top). Tube is then inserted normally (middle). After insertion and stabilization, cuff port is open to atmosphere to allow inflation (bottom).

The adequacy of a tracheal seal must also take into account the potential for aspiration. The use of minimal leak technique and high-volume cuffs does not absolutely preclude aspiration of pharyngeal contents. Also, aspiration is reported to be more common in spontaneously breathing patients than in those receiving positive pressure ventilation. This may be because of the movement of pharyngeal secretion around the cuff during the negative pressure phase of a spontaneous inspiration. Aspiration has also been reported to be a more common occurrence with tracheostomy tubes than with endotracheal tubes.

The methylene blue test can help determine whether this "leakage" type of aspiration is occurring. Methylene blue may be added to the patient's feedings or, alternatively, swallowed by the patient in a small amount of water solution. Once the dye is introduced, the patient's trachea is suctioned through the artificial airway. If blue-tinged secretions are obtained when performing suctioning, aspiration is occurring.

Once aspiration is confirmed, efforts must be made to minimize its occurrence and prevent its progression. Oropharyngeal suctioning (above the tube cuff) should be performed as needed. To decrease the possibility of aspiration associated with feedings, the head of the bed should be elevated (where possible). Also, the feeding tube can be inserted into the duodenum, with its position confirmed by x-ray film. The use of slightly higher cuff pressure during and after feeding may also help minimize aspiration.

Thus the proper method of maintaining a cuff depends, in part, on the purpose(s) for which the artificial airway was originally inserted. Moreover, each patient has individual needs to which care should be adjusted accordingly.

Troubleshooting

The areas discussed so far are routine aspects of airway care. Three emergency situations that may occur include obstruction of the tube, cuff leaks, and inadvertent extubation. Symptoms frequently encountered under these circumstances include various degrees of respiratory distress, changes in breath sounds, and air movement through the mouth. Each condition presents somewhat differently and is associated with different approaches to management.

Tube obstruction. Obstruction of the tube is one of the most common causes of airway emergencies. Tube obstruction can be caused by (1) kinking of or biting on the tube, (2) herniation of the cuff over the tube tip, (3) impingement of the tube orifice against the trachea, and (4) mucus plugging (Fig. 21-24).

Depending on whether the tube obstruction is partial or complete, different clinical signs will be present. If partial airway obstruction occurs with the spontaneously breathing patient, decreased breath sounds and decreased air flow through the tube will be noticed. If the patient is receiving intermittent positive pressure ventilation via a volume ventilator, peak inspiratory pressures will rise, often

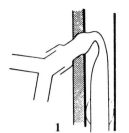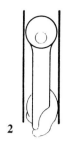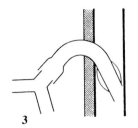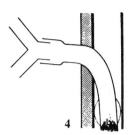

Fig. 21-24   Causes of tube obstruction. See text for details. (From Sykes MK, McNichol MW, and Campbell EJM: Respiratory failure, Philadelphia, 1969, FA Davis Co.)

causing the pressure limit alarm to sound. With complete tube obstruction, the patient will exhibit severe distress, no breath sounds will be heard, and no gas flow through the tube will be discernible.

Kinking of the tube or its impingement against the trachea can be relieved by movement of the head and neck, which results in movement of the tube. If these methods do not relieve the obstruction, a herniated cuff may be blocking the airway, and the practitioner should attempt to deflate the cuff. If these steps fail to overcome the obstruction, the practitioner should try to pass a suction catheter through the tube. How far one can insert the catheter helps determine the site of obstruction. If a catheter is inserted near to or just past the end of the tube and does not elicit a cough, a herniated cuff or mucus plugging is the likely problem. In the case of mucus plugging, the practitioner should attempt to aspirate the plug before considering more drastic action.

In situations involving tracheostomy tubes with an inner cannula, the practitioner should remove the inner cannula and check to see if the plug is lodged in the tube. If it is, the patient can be ventilated through the outer cannula with a bag and mask, or the inner cannula can be replaced with a backup one.

If the obstruction cannot be cleared using the above techniques, the airway must be removed and replaced. In patients having undergone recent tracheotomy (4 or 5 days), the stoma may not be well established and may close when the tube is removed. Ideally, suture ties left in place by the surgeon can be used to pull open the stoma.

Regardless of the ease with which a new airway can be reestablished, once an obstructed airway has been removed, first priority must be given to restoring adequate ventilation and oxygenation. For patients with a tracheotomy stoma, this may require sealing the wound with a gauze pad, like that used to temporarily close chest wounds in the field. Only after adequate ventilation and oxygenation are assured should airway reinsertion be undertaken.

Cuff leaks. A leak in the cuff, pilot tube, or one-way valve is a problem usually for the patient receiving mechanical ventilation. This will cause a leak in the system, a loss of volume delivered to the patient, and a decrease in peak inspiratory pressure and delivered volume.

A small leak in the cuff system can be detected by decreasing cuff pressures over time. A large leak, such as would occur with a blown cuff, will have a more rapid onset. Breath sounds will be decreased, but the spontaneously breathing patient will have air movement through the tube. With positive pressure breaths, air flow can often be felt at the mouth. Under such circumstances, the practitioner should try to reinflate the cuff while checking the pilot tube and valve for leaks. Leaks at the valve or in the pilot tube can be bypassed using a needle and stopcock placed in the pilot tube distal to the leak. This will allow the cuff to be reinflated and avoid emergency reintubation. A blown cuff requires extubation and reintubation.

Accidental extubation. Accidental displacement of the tube out of the trachea is often detected by decreased breath sounds, decreased air flow through the tube, and the ability to pass a suction catheter to its full length without meeting an obstruction or eliciting a cough. With positive pressure ventilation, air flow through the mouth or into the stomach may be heard and peak inspiratory pressures may be lowered. The practitioner should completely remove the tube and provide ventilatory support as needed until the patient can be reintubated.

Decreased breath sounds are a common finding in airway emergencies, but the practitioner should attempt to identify specific indicators for each of these problems, such as the inability to pass a suction catheter (obstruction), the ability to fully pass a catheter (extubation), or air flow around the tube (leaky cuff). Replacement equipment should be kept at the bedside, as well as a manual resuscitator, mask, and gauze pads (for tracheostomized patients).

EXTUBATION

For most patients, endotracheal intubation is a temporary measure, which means extubation can be done at some point in time. Patients who are not candidates for extubation are those with permanent tracheostomies and those requiring permanent ventilatory support.

Extubation is indicated when the reason(s) for establishing the artificial airway no longer pertain. Specifically, if instituted to overcome an airway obstruction, the airway should be removed when the obstruction has been cleared. Alternatively, if instituted to facilitate secretion clearance, the airway should be removed when the patient can handle his or her own secretions. Likewise, in terms of protecting the lower airway, if the patient is conscious and the pharyngeal reflex has returned to normal, an artificial airway is no longer indicated. Finally, if the purpose of airway insertion was to facilitate positive pressure ventilation, the airway should be removed when the patient no longer needs ventilatory support.

Since the respiratory care practitioner plays a key role in extubation, and because the techniques differ, we will review the procedures for removing orotracheal, nasotracheal, and tracheostomy tubes separately.

Endotracheal extubation

The following procedure is recommended for orotracheal or nasotracheal extubation:

Step 1: Assemble equipment needed for the procedure, including suctioning apparatus, suction kits, oxygen and aerosol therapy equipment, manual resuscitator and mask, aerosol nebulizer with racemic epinephrine and normal saline (if ordered), and an intubation tray.

Step 2: Suction the endotracheal tube and through the pharynx to above the cuff. This will minimize the likelihood of aspirating secretions into the trachea after the cuff is deflated. Dispose of this kit and prepare another for use, or prepare a rigid tonisillar (Yankauer) suction tip. Patients will often cough after the tube is pulled and may need help with clearance.

Step 3: Oxygenate the patient well after suctioning. Extubation is a stressful procedure that can otherwise cause hypoxemia.

Step 4: Deflate the cuff. Remove all the air possible. Some practitioners then cut the valve off the pilot tube to ensure that any remaining air is easily displaced during removal.

Step 5: Remove the tube. Two techniques are used to remove the tube. In the first method, give a large breath with the manual resuscitator, removing the tube at peak inspiration (when the cords are maximally abducted). In the second method, have the patient cough, pulling the tube during the expulsive expiratory phase. This will also result in maximal abduction of the cords.

Step 6: Apply appropriate oxygen and humidity therapy, if ordered. Patients who have been receiving mechanical ventilation may still require some oxygen therapy, usually at a higher F_{IO_2}. Other patients may require some oxygen, since this is a stressful procedure. If humidity therapy is indicated, most clinicians suggest a cool (as opposed to heated) mist during the post-extubation phase of airway management. This is because a heated mist may potentiate the mucosal swelling that normally occurs after extubation, thereby worsening airway obstruction.

Step 7: Assess the patient. Check for good air movement by auscultation, looking for stridor or decreased air movement, which indicate upper airway problems. Assess the patient's respiratory rate, heart rate, color, and blood pressure. Check for nose bleeding following nasotracheal extubation. Encourage the patient to cough; assist as needed.

Step 8: Reassess the patient often. Edema may worsen with time. Arterial blood should be sampled and analyzed as needed.

The major complication associated with extubation is laryngospasm. Post-extubation laryngospasm is usually a transient event, lasting a matter of seconds. Should this occur, oxygenation may be maintained with a high F_{IO_2} and application of positive pressure. If the spasm persists, a neuromuscular blocking agent may have to be administered, which will necessitate manual ventilation or reintubation.

Another complication common after extubation is glottic edema. When stridor is heard immediately upon extubation, the practitioner should be wary of further problems, because the swelling can worsen dramatically. If stridor is present, a racemic epinephrine treatment may be given to lessen the swelling. In children, post-extubation edema is often subglottic and may require re-establishment of the airway.

Tracheostomy decannulation

There are several approaches to removing tracheostomy tubes. In most situations, a weaning process is used. Weaning may be accomplished using fenestrated tracheostomy tubes, tracheostomy buttons, or progressively smaller tubes.

Fenestrated tracheostomy tubes. A fenestrated tracheostomy tube is a double-cannulated tube that has an opening in the posterior wall of the outer cannula above the cuff (Fig. 21-25). Removal of the inner cannula opens the fenestration. Plugging of the proximal opening of the tube's outer cannula, accompanied by deflation of the cuff, allows for assessment of upper airway function. Removal of the plug allows access for suctioning. If the need for mechanical ventilation occurs, the inner cannula can be reinserted.

One problem associated with this type of tracheostomy tube is malposition of the fenestration, such as between the skin and the stoma, or against the posterior wall of the larynx. Customizing the fenestration may avoid this problem. This can be done by measuring the distance from the skin to the anterior inside wall of the trachea for the proximal end of the fenestration, and then from the anterior wall to the posterior wall for the distal end of the fenestration. Proper fenestration placement can be confirmed using fiberoptic bronchoscopy in situ.

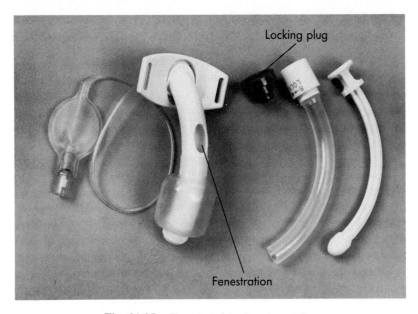

Fig. 21-25   Fenestrated tracheostomy tube.

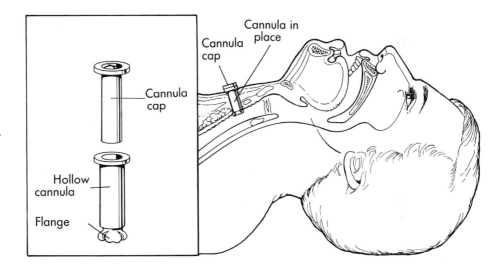

Fig. 21-26   Tracheostomy button.

Case reports have demonstrated granular tissue formation in some patients using a fenestrated tracheostomy tube. This granular formation tends to occur on the anterior tracheal wall above the proximal opening of the fenestration. Granulation tissue may result in occlusion of the fenestration, bleeding (especially with tube changes), and airway obstruction upon decannulation. Given the reported relative positions of the fenestration and the granulation tissue, this problem may relate to poor positioning of the fenestration within the airway.

Tracheal buttons. The tracheal button may also be used to maintain a tracheotomy stoma. Unlike the fenestrated tube, the tracheal button fits from the skin to just inside the anterior wall of the trachea (Fig. 21-26). Since the tracheal button does not provide a cuff, its use is limited to relieving airway obstructions and facilitating the removal of secretions. Adapters can be used that will allow for suctioning through the button. An optional one-way valve on

the proximal end of the button allows for inspiration with less dead space and expiration with speech.

Progressively smaller tubes. A third airway weaning technique is the use of smaller and smaller tracheostomy tubes. As with fenestrated tubes, this approach maintains the airway but allows for increasing use of the upper airway. This technique is also indicated in patients whose airway is too small for the fenestrated tubes that are currently available. The use of progressively smaller tubes also is believed to allow for better healing of the stoma.

Prior to decannulation of a tracheostomy tube, fiberoptic assessment of the upper airway should be done to ensure a patent airway. After removal of the tube, fenestrated or not, the stoma will close on its own in a matter of days. The particular technique used for decannulation will depend on the patient's needs and the experience and preferences of the patient's attending physician.

SUMMARY

The maintenance of a patent airway is one of the most important functions of the respiratory care practitioner. Airway clearance, including suctioning and assisting with bronchoscopy, is the most common responsibility of respiratory care personnel. Proficiency in airway clearance methods requires a working knowledge of the indications and complications associated with these procedures.

The ability to recognize the need for an artificial airway, to select the most appropriate airway, and to insert or assist in the insertion of the selected airway are equally important skills. Maintenance of inserted artificial airways is also a major responsibility of respiratory care personnel. In this role, the respiratory care practitioner must ensure that the patient's needs are addressed on an individual basis and that any immediate or long-term risks to the patient are minimized.

Finally, respiratory care practitioners assume an important role in deciding when and how best to remove an artificial airway. It is toward this goal, that is, restoration of normal airway function, that the practitioner must always strive.

BIBLIOGRAPHY

Ackerman MH: The use of bolus normal saline instillation in artificial airways: is it useful or necessary? Heart Lung 14:505-506, 1985.

Allen MD et al: Combined laser therapy and endobronchial radiotherapy for unresectable lung carcinoma with bronchial obstruction, Am J Surg 150:71-77, 1985.

Appel-Hardin SJ: Communicating with intubated patients, Crit Care Nurs Nov/Dec 1984.

Arens JF, Lejume FE, and Webre DR: Maxillary sinusitis: a complication of nasal tracheal intubation, Anesthesiology 40:415, 1974.

Baker PO, Baker JP, and Koen PA: Endotracheal suctioning techniques in hyoxemic patients, Respir Care 28:1563-1568, 1983.

Barnes CA and Kirchoff KT: Minimizing hypoxemia due to endotracheal suctioning: a review of the literature, Heart Lung 15:164-176, 1986.

Bekoe S, Magovern GJ, and Shively JG: Prolonged cuff intubation without tracheal injury, CVP 3(4): 1975.

Berlauk JF: Prolonged endotracheal intubation vs tracheostomy, Crit Care Med 14:742-745, 1986.

Blanc VF and Tremblay NA: The complications of tracheal intubation: a new classification and review of the literature, Anesth Analg 53:202, 1974.

Bostick J and Wendelgass ST: Normal saline instillation as part of the suctioning procedure: effects on Pao₂ and amount of secretions, Heart Lung 16:532-537, 1987.

Brooks R, Bartlett RH, and Gazzaniga AB: Management of acute and chronic disorders of the trachea and subglottis, Am J Surg 150:24-31, 1985.

Bugge-Asperheim B, Birkel S, and Storen G: Tracheoesophageal fistula caused by cuffed tracheal tubes, Scand J Cardiovas Surg 15:315-319, 1981.

Cabal L et al: New endotracheal tube adapter reducing cardiopulmonary effects of suctioning, Crit Care Med 7:552, 1979.

Carroll PF: Artificial airways equal real risks, Nursing 86 16(8):56-59, 1986.

Carroll RG: Evaluation of tracheal tube cuff designs, Crit Care Med 1:45, 1973.

Carroll RG and Grenvik A: Proper use of large diameter, large residual volume cuffs, Crit Care Med 1:153-156, 1973.

Chew JY and Cantrell RW: Tracheostomy complications and their management, Arch Otolaryngol 96:538, 1972.

Ching NPH and Nealon TF: Clinical experience with new low-pressure high-volume tracheostomy cuffs, NY State J Med 74:2379, 1974.

Conardy PA et al: Alternation of endotracheal tube position: flexation and extention of the neck, Crit Care Med 4:8, 1976.

Conley JM and Smith DJ: Emergency endotracheal intubation by respiratory care personnel in a community hospital, Respir Care 26:336, 1981.

Cooper JD and Grillo HC: The evolution of tracheal injury due to ventilatory assistance through a cuffed tube, Ann Surg 169:334, 1969.

Coppolo DP et al: A role for the respiratory therapist in flexible fiberoptic bronchoscopy, Respir Care 30:323-327, 1985.

Craig KC, Benson MS, and Pierson DJ: Prevention of arterial oxygen desaturation during closed airway endotracheal suction: effect of ventilator mode, Respir Care 29:1013-1018, 1984.

Credle WF, Smiddy JF, and Elliott RC: Complications of fiberoptic bronchoscopy, Am Rev Respir Dis 109:67-72, 1974.

Daly SM et al: Unrecognized aspiration of an oropharyngeal airway, Ped Radiol 13:227-228, 1983.

Dane TEB and King EG: A prospective study of complications after tracheostomy for assisted ventilation, Chest 67:398, 1975.

Darvich-Kodjouri C: Care of the patient with a new tracheostomy, Curr Rev Respir Crit Care 10(6):43-47, 1987.

Demers RR: Complications of endotracheal suctioning procedures, Respir Care 27:453-457, 1982.

Demers RR: Management of the airway in the perioperative period, Respir Care 29:529-539, 1984.

Demers RR, Sullivan MJ, and Paliotta J: Airflow resistances of endotracheal tubes, JAMA 237:1362, 1977.

Deutschman CS et al: Paranasal sinusitis associated with nasotracheal intubation: a frequently unrecognized and treatable source of sepsis, Crit Care Med 14:111, 1986.

Dobrin P and Canfield T: Cuffed endotracheal tubes: mucosal pressures and tracheal wall blood flow, Am J Surg 133:562, 1977.

Douglas S and Larson EL: The effect of a positive end-expiratory pressure adapter on oxygenation during endotracheal suction, Heart Lung 14:396-400, 1985.

Downs JB: Who should intubate? (editorial), Respir Care 26:331, 1981.

El-Naggar M et al: Factors influencing choice between tracheostomy and prolonged translaryngeal intubation in acute respiratory failure: a prospective study, Anesth Analg 55:195, 1976.

Elpern EH, Jacobs ER, and Bone RC: Incidence of aspiration in tracheally intubated adults, Heart Lung 16:527-531, 1987.

Evaluation: Artificial airways, Health Devices 7:76, 1978.

Finch JS: Intubation tracheal injury, Curr Rev Respir Ther 7(17):131-135, 1985.

Finucane BT and Santora AH: Principles of airway management, Philadelphia, 1988, FA Davis Co.

Fluck RR: Suctioning-intermittent or continuous? Respir Care 30:836-837, 1985.

Galoob HD and Toledo PS: Comparison of five types of tracheostomy tubes in the intubated trachea, Ann Otol Rhinol Laryngol 87:99, 1978.

Garson AA et al: Influence of cannula size on resistance to breathing through tracheostomies, Surg Forum 14:219, 1963.

Goodman LR et al: Radiographic evaluation of endotracheal tube position, Am J Roetgenol 127:433-434, 1976.

Goodnough SK: The effects of oxygen and hyperinflation on arterial oxygen tension after endotracheal suctioning, Heart Lung 14:11-17, 1985.

Green NM: Fatal cardiovascular and respiratory failure associated with tracheostomy, N Engl J Med 261:846, 1959.

Grossbach I: Troubleshooting ventilator and patient related problems. Part II, Crit Care Nurs 6:64-74, 1982.

Hand RW et al: Inadvertent transbronchial insertion of narrow bore feeding tubes into pleural space, JAMA 251:2396-2397, 1984.

Harada RH and Repine JE: Pulmonary host defense mechanisms, Chest 87:247-252, 1985.

Heffner JE, Miller KS, and Sahn SA: Tracheostomy in the intensive care unit. Part 1. Indications, technique, management, Chest 90:269-274, 1986.

Heffner JE, Miller KS, and Sahn SA: Tracheostomy in the intensive care unit. Part 2. Complications, Chest 90:430-436, 1986.

Herbert RC and De Sessa PC: Compression of an endotracheal tube lumen by its cuff: a case report, Respir Care 26:653, 1981.

Herranz MF: Individualized fenestration of tracheostomy tubes, Respir Care 29:1246, 1984.

Holley HS and Gildea JE: Vocal cord paralysis after tracheal intubation, JAMA 214:281, 1971.

Jackson CV, Savage PL, and Quinn DL: Role of fiberoptic bronchoscopy in patients with hemoptysis and a normal chest roentgenogram, Chest 87:142-144, 1985.

Jago RH: Resuscitation following trauma, Clin Anesthesiol 4:605, 1986.

Kamen JM and Wilkinson CJ: A new low-pressure cuff for endotracheal tubes, Anesthesiology 34:482, 1971.

Kastanos N et al: Laryngotracheal injury due to endotracheal intubation: incidence, evolution, and predisposing factors: a prospective long-term study, Crit Care Med 11:362-367, 1983.

Knipper J: Evaluation of adventitious sounds as an indicator of the need for tracheal suctioning, Heart Lung 13:292, 1984.

Kvale PA et al: YAG laser photoresection of lesions obstructing the central airways, Chest 87:283-288, 1985.

Lake KB and Van Dyke JJ: Prolonged nasotracheal intubation, Heart Lung 9:93-96, 1980.

Latto IP and Rosen M: Difficulties in tracheal intubation, London, 1985, Bailliere-Tindall.

Lechman MJ, Donahoo JS, and Macvaugh H: Endotracheal intubation using percutaneous retrograde guidewire insertion followed by antegrade fiberoptic bronchoscopy, Crit Care Med 14:589-590, 1986.

Lederman IS et al: A comparison of foam and air-filled endotracheal cuffs, Anesth Analg 53:521, 1974.

LeFrock JL et al: Transient bacteremia associated with nasotracheal suctioning, JAMA 236:1610-1612, 1976.

Lewis FR, Schlobohm RM, and Thomas AN: Prevention of complications from prolonged tracheal intubation, Am J Surg 135:452, 1978.

Light RW: Other diagnostic techniques. In George R, Light R, and Matthay R, editors: Chest medicine, New York, 1983, Churchill-Livingstone.

Lindholm CE et al: Flexible fiberoptic bronchoscopy in critical care medicine, Crit Care Med 2:250, 1974.

Lindholm CE et al: Cardiorespiratory effects of flexible fiberoptic bronchoscopy in critically ill patients, Chest 74:362, 1978.

Lockhart JS and Griffin C: Occluded trach tube, Nursing 87 17(4):33, 1987.

Lowy FD et al: The incidence of nosocomial pneumonia following urgent endotracheal intubation, Infect Control 8(6):245-248, 1987.

Magovern GJ et al: The clinical and experimental evaluation of a controlled-pressure intratracheal cuff, J Thorac Cardiovas Surg 64:747, 1972.

MacMahon H, Courtney JV, and Little AG: Diagnostic methods in lung cancer, Sem Oncology 10:20-33, 1983.

McCullough P: Wire basket removal of a large endobronchial foreign body, Chest 87:270-271, 1985.

McLaughlin AJ and Scott W: Training and evaluation of respiratory therapists in emergency intubation, Respir Care 26:333, 1981.

McPherson SP: Respiratory therapy equipment, ed 3, St Louis, 1985, The CV Mosby Co.

Milam MG: Aspiration of a nasopharyngeal airway, Chest 93:223-224, 1988.

Miller JD and Kapp JP: Complications of tracheostomies in neurosurgical patients, Surg Neurol 22:186-188, 1984.

Mohsenifar Z, Jasper AC, and Koerner SK: Physiologic assessment of lung function in patients undergoing laser photoresection of tracheobronchial tumors, Chest 93:65-69, 1988.

Neff TA and Clifford D: A new monitoring tool — the ratio of the tracheostomy tube cuff diameter to the tracheal air column (C/T ratio), Respir Care 28:1287-1290, 1983.

Off D et al: Efficacy of the minimal leak technique of cuff inflation in maintaining proper intracuff pressures for patients with cuffed artificial airways, Respir Care 28:1115-1120, 1983.

Orens D et al: Therapeutic use of laser systems in pulmonary medicine: a case report, Respir Care 31:202-206, 1986.

Ovassapian A: Fiberoptic nasotracheal intubation: incidence and causes of failure, Anesth Analg 62:692, 1983.

Paegle RD and Bernard WM: Squamous metaplasia of tracheal epithelium associated with high-volume, low-pressure airway cuffs, Anesth Analg 54:340, 1975.

Pavlin EG, VanNimwegan D, and Hornbein TF: Failure of a high compliance low-pressure cuff to prevent aspiration, Anesthesiology 42:216-219, 1975.

Pereira W et al: Fever and pneumonia after flexible fiberoptic bronchoscopy, Am Rev Respir Dis 112:59-64, 1975.

Pierce JB and Piazza DE: Differences in postsuctioning arterial blood oxygen concentration values using two postoxygenation methods, Heart Lung 16:34-45, 1987.

Poe RH et al: Utility of fiberoptic bronchoscopy in patients with hemoptysis and a nonlocalizing chest roentgenogram, Chest 92:70-75, 1988.

Quie PG: Lung defense against infection, J Pediatr 108:813-816, 1986.

Rindfleisch SH and Tyler ML: Duration of suctioning: an important variable, Respir Care 28:457-459, 1983.

Ritz R et al: Contamination of a multiple-use suction catheter in a closed-circuit system compared to contamination of a disposable single-use suction catheter, Respir Care 31:1086-1091, 1986.

Roberts JT: Fundamentals of tracheal intubation, New York, 1983, Grune & Stratton.

Rudy EB et al: The relationship between endotracheal suctioning and changes in intracranial pressure: a review of the literature, Heart Lung 15:488-494, 1986.

Sackner MA, Wanner A, and Landa J: Applications of bronchofiberoscopy, Chest 62(suppl):70s, 1972.

Sackner MA: Bronchofiberoscopy, state of the art, Am Rev Respir Dis 111:62, 1975.

Sanderson PJ: The sources of pneumonia in ICU patients, Infect Control 7:104-106, 1986.

Shapiro BA and Kacmarek RM: Airway care, Curr Rev Respir Care 2(19):147-151, 1980.

Shapiro BA, Harrison RA, and Trout CA: Clinical applications of respiratory care, ed 3, Chicago, 1985, Year Book Medical Publishers.

Shekleton ME and Nield M: Ineffective airway clearance related to artificial airway, Nurs Clin North Am 22:167-178, 1987.

Siddharth P and Mazzarella L: Granuloma associated with fenestrated tracheostomy tubes, Am J Surg 150:279-280, 1985.

Sills J: An emergency cuff inflation technique, Respir Care 31:199-201, 1986.

Smith RM, Benson MS, and Schoene RB: Efficacy of oxygen insufflation in preventing arterial oxygen desaturation during endotracheal suctioning of mechanically ventilated patients, Respir Care 32:865-869, 1987.

Sosenko M and Glassroth J: Fiberoptic bronchoscopy in the evaluation of lung abscesses, Chest 87:489-494, 1985.

Sottile FD et al: Nosocomial pulmonary infection: possible etiologic significance of bacterial adhesion to endotracheal tubes, Crit Care Med 14:265-270, 1986.

Stark P: Inadvertent nasogastric tube insertion into the tracheobronchial tree, Radiology 142:239-240, 1982.

Stauffer JL, Olson DE, and Petty TL: Complications and consequences of endotracheal intubation and tracheotomy: a prospective study of 150 critically ill adult patients, Am J Med 70:65-76, 1981.

Stauffer JL and Silvestri RC: Complications of endotracheal intubation, tracheostomy, and artificial airways, Respir Care 27:417-434, 1982.

Stock C: Perioperative complications of elective tracheostomy in critically ill patients, Crit Care Med 14:861-863, 1986.

Sunderrajan EV et al: Potentially lethal complications of artificial airways: case reports, Missouri Med 77:299, 1980.

Suratt PM, Smiddy JF, and Gruber B: Death and complications associated with fiberoptic bronchoscopy, Chest 69:747, 1976.

Synder GM: Individualized placement of tracheostomy tube fenestration and in situ examinations with the fiberoptic laryngoscope, Respir Care 28:1294-1298, 1983.

Tasota FJ et al: Evaluation of two methods used to stabilize oral endotracheal tubes, Heart Lung 16:140-146, 1987.

Tobin MJ and Grenvik A: Nosocomial lung infection and its diagnosis, Crit Care Med 12:191-197, 1984.

Toledo LW: Laser bronchoscopy, J Post Anesth Nurs 3:171-177, 1987.

Treanor S, Benitez WD, and Raffin TA: Respiratory therapists as fiberoptic bronchoscopy assistants, Respir Care 30:321-327, 1985.

Treloar DM and Stechmiller J: Pulmonary aspiration in tube-fed patients with artificial airways, Heart Lung 13(6):667-671, 1984.

Turnbull AD and Carlon G: Airway management in the thrombocytopenic cancer patient with acute respiratory failure, Crit Care Med 7:76-77, 1979.

Via-Reque E and Rattenborg C: Prolonged oro- or nasotracheal intubation, Crit Care Med 9:637-639, 1981.

Weber AL and Grillo HC: Tracheal stenosis: an analysis of 151 cases, Radiol Clin North Am 16:291-308, 1978.

Wen-Hsien Wu et al: Pressure dynamics of endotracheal and tracheostomy cuffs, Crit Care Med 1:197, 1973.

Whited RE: A prospective study of laryngotracheal sequelae in long-term intubation, Laryngoscope 94:367-377, 1984.

Wissing DR, Romero MR, and Payne K: An unusual complication of prolonged intubation, Respir Care 32:359-360, 1987.

Zmora E and Merritt TA: Use of side-hole endotracheal tube adapter for tracheal aspiration: a controlled study, Am J Dis Child 134:250, 1980.

22

Emergency Life Support

Craig L. Scanlan

Emergency life support involves a variety of methods and procedures designed to deal with sudden, life-threatening events caused by failure of the cardiovascular or respiratory system. Respiratory care practitioners play a vital role in providing emergency life support. In the hospital setting, respiratory care practitioners normally serve as key members of the resuscitation team. In addition to providing skills essential in managing the airway, practitioners often participate in circulatory support, drug and electrical therapy, and postresuscitative care.

In the community, respiratory care practitioners frequently serve as certified cardiopulmonary resuscitation instructors, extending their knowledge to lay personnel through organizations such as the American Heart Association or American Red Cross.

Both roles require mastery of an extensive knowledge base and the development and maintenance of an array of sometimes difficult manual skills. Although no substitute for supervised practice under simulated conditions, this chapter will provide the foundation knowledge necessary to apply effectively both basic and advanced life support techniques in a variety of setting and with various patient groups.

OBJECTIVES

After completing this chapter, the reader will be able to:

1. Identify the major categories of sudden death, including specific causes of respiratory and cardiac arrest;

2. Differentiate the goals, methods, procedures, and personnel resources of basic and advanced cardiac life support;

3. Describe the procedures used to determine unresponsiveness, breathlessness, and pulselessness in a vic-

tim suspected to have suffered respiratory or cardiac arrest or both;

4. Outline the basic life support procedures used to restore the airway and provide ventilatory and circulatory support to adults, children, and infants under both normal and special circumstances;

5. Describe the procedures used to evaluate the effectiveness of basic life support measures;

6. Distinguish the single and double rescuer protocols used in basic life support;

7. Compare and contrast the key adjunctive equipment and procedures used in advanced cardiac life support to maintain and restore respiratory and cardiac function;

8. Differentiate the common cardiac arrhythmias and their clinical significance;

9. Describe the appropriate use of pharmacologic and electrical therapies in advanced cardiac life support;

10. Identify the role of the respiratory care practitioner in postresuscitative patient care;

11. Describe the common complications, hazards, and pitfalls associated with basic and advanced cardiac life support equipment and procedures.

KEY TERMS

Most terms used in this chapter are defined in context. The following terms are introduced without explicit definition but may be found in the text glossary:

aspiration	hyperkalemia
barotrauma	hyperosmolarity
bigeminy	hyperthyroidism
BUN	hypocalcemia
cannulation	intermammary
cardiac tamponade	intra-abdominal
extrathoracic	laryngectomy
hemodialysis	mesenteric
hemothorax	multifocal

Portions of the section on basic life support excerpted with permission from Ellis PD and Billings DM: Cardiopulmonary resuscitation: procedures for basic and advanced life support, St Louis, 1980, The CV Mosby Co.

nephrotoxic
percutaneous
pneumothorax
regurgitation
sublingual

supraventricular
tracheostomy
trigeminy
trismus
xiphisternal

CAUSES AND PREVENTION OF SUDDEN DEATH

Sudden death is a common event both inside and outside the hospital setting. Among adults, coronary heart disease is the primary cause of sudden death, accounting for some 500,000 fatalities annually.[1]

Accidents are the second leading cause of sudden death in the US.[2] Trauma from motor vehicle accidents, drowning, electrocution, burns, suffocation, and drug intoxication are among the major factors involved in accidental death among adults.[3]

Among children, accidents are the leading cause of sudden death, causing some 44% of the fatalities in the 1- to 14-year-old age group.[1] A particularly serious cause of sudden death in children is obstruction of the airway by foreign bodies.[4,5] Foreign body obstruction accounts for over 3000 deaths annually, most of which occur in children under 5 years of age.[6]

Among neonates, nearly 6% require special life support in the delivery room. This figure rises to over 80% for infants with birth weights less than 1500 g.[3]

Although not all these deaths are preventable, early use of both basic and advanced resuscitation methods can reduce this alarming toll of sudden death. Indeed, comprehensive implementation of resuscitation methods on a community-wide basis throughout the nation could save between 100,000 and 200,000 lives per year.[3,7-9]

Emergency life support involves a variety of methods and procedures designed to deal with sudden, life-threatening events caused by failure of the cardiovascular or respiratory system.[8-12] Emergency life support traditionally consists of two related phases: basic life support (BLS) and advanced cardiac life support (ACLS).[3]

BLS aims to (1) prevent circulatory or respiratory arrest through prompt identification and intervention or (2) support failed circulation and respiration through application of cardiopulmonary resuscitation methods.[13,14] BLS should be initiated by any person present when the incident occurs. Trained individuals should begin cardiopulmonary resuscitation (CPR) as soon as possible; if no trained individual is present, the local emergency medical system must be activated immediately.[3]

ACLS includes the essential elements of BLS but provides additional measures beyond those normally available to lay personnel. These include using adjunct equipment to support oxygenation and ventilation, establishing an intravenous route for drug administration, administering selected pharmacologic agents, cardiac monitoring, defibril-

lation, arrhythmia control, and providing postresuscitative care.[3] Whereas BLS can be initiated and conducted by lay personnel, ACLS requires the supervision of a physician, either in person or through appropriate alternative means.

DETERMINING THE NEED FOR EMERGENCY LIFE SUPPORT

Indications

The primary indications for emergency life support are respiratory or cardiac arrest. Among the most common causes of respiratory arrest are drug overdose, drowning, suffocation, stroke, electrocution, smoke inhalation, acute airway obstruction by a foreign body, and airway obstruction resulting from unconsciousness or coma (see box below).[3]

Like respiratory arrest, cardiac arrest has many potential causes. Clinically, the most frequently occurring causes of primary cardiac arrest are electrical disturbances or ar-

---

CAUSES OF RESPIRATORY ARREST

DEPRESSION OF RESPIRATORY CENTER IN THE MEDULLA OBLONGATA

General anesthesia
Barbiturates
Narcotics
Muscle relaxants
High-intensity electrical shock
Overadministration of oxygen if hypoxia stimulates ventilation (chronic obstructive lung disease)
Head trauma
Brain lesions

INTERFERENCE WITH VENTILATION OR RESPIRATION CAUSING ALTERATIONS IN OXYGEN AND CARBON DIOXIDE EXCHANGE

Airway obstruction by foreign object
Airway obstruction by blood, pus, vomitus, mucus, or other fluid
Respiratory distress syndrome
Airway obstruction by space-occupying lesion
Chest trauma
Edema of the airways (infection, surgery, trauma, or burns)
Anaphylactic reactions (bronchospasm or laryngospasm)
Carbon monoxide poisoning
Suffocation

INTERFERENCE WITH NEUROMUSCULAR TRANSMISSION TO VENTILATORY MUSCLES

Myasthenia gravis
Guillain-Barré syndrome
Some types of spinal cord trauma

rhythmias associated with acute myocardial infarction. Additional causes of cardiac arrest are listed in the box below.

If the primary incident is respiratory arrest, the heart will normally continue to function for a few minutes. However, without ventilation, body stores of oxygen are rapidly depleted. The resulting tissue hypoxia quickly impairs both cardiac and neural function. For this reason, rapid recognition of respiratory arrest, combined with appropriate intervention, can prevent a secondary cardiac arrest and minimize the likelihood of permanent cerebral damage.

If, on the other hand, the primary event is cessation of cardiac function, no oxygen is circulated and tissue hypoxia occurs almost immediately. A secondary respiratory arrest quickly ensues as the brain stem is deprived of its oxygen supply.

When ventilation and circulation both cease, a condition of clinical death is said to exist.[12] With early recognition and intervention, clinical death is a potentially reversible phenomenon. However, should tissue hypoxia be prolonged, irreversible cell damage will occur, resulting in biologic death.

Exactly how much time can elapse before clinical death becomes biologic death is unknown. Generally, biologic death ensues within 4 to 6 minutes after ventilation and circulation cease. However, many factors may extend this time period, including hypothermia and certain pharmacologic agents. In fact, many organs can sustain periods of anoxia of 15 minutes or more. The primary exception is the brain. Although other organ systems may be successfully resuscitated after prolonged periods of oxygen lack, brain death may occur rapidly, resulting in total and irreversible loss of cerebral function.

Thus, the goal of emergency life support is to reverse clinical death by restoring ventilation and circulation before either morbid neurologic impairment or brain death can occur. Emergency life support should be initiated whenever the signs and symptoms of clinical death are recognized. However, emergency life support never should be continued beyond the point at which brain death is likely to have occurred. Since firm evidence regarding brain death is seldom available during resuscitation efforts, the decision to discontinue emergency life support is as much a moral and ethical judgment as a clinical one.

Assessment

Prompt and accurate recognition of the status of a victim or patient in a life-threatening situation is an essential component in the provision of effective emergency life support. Since time is critical under such circumstances, assessment procedures must be simple and easily performed.

Each of the three major steps involved in the provision of basic life support includes a quick and simple assessment component.[3,13] Before initiating airway management techniques, the practitioner should first determine that the victim is unresponsive. Before proceeding with artificial ventilation, the practitioner must determine that the victim is not breathing. Before initiating circulatory support, the practitioner must confirm that the victim has no palpable pulse.

Determining unresponsiveness. The basic life support sequence is initiated when an otherwise conscious patient or victim is found in an unresponsive or collapsed state. Since many patients in the hospital setting exhibit decreased levels of consciousness, practitioners can avoid needless intervention by being fully aware of their patient's degree of responsiveness (see box on p. 516).

When approaching a collapsed victim outside the hospital setting who appears unconscious, the practitioner should first look for any obvious head or neck injuries. If such injuries are apparent, great care should be taken in subsequent manipulation of the neck and in any effort to move the individual.[3,13]

Whether outside or inside the hospital setting, the practitioner then quickly assesses the individual's level of consciousness by tapping or gently shaking the shoulder and shouting "Are you OK" or an equivalent verbal stimulus. If these methods fail to arouse the victim, the practitioner should call for help and activate the emergency medical system.[3]

CAUSES OF CARDIAC ARREST

INTERFERENCE WITH THE HEART'S CONTRACTILE FORCE

Heart failure
Cardiac rupture
Myocardial infarction
Cardiac tamponade
Hemorrhage

INTERFERENCE WITH ELECTRICAL IMPULSE FORMATION AND CONDUCTION IN THE HEART

Hypokalemia
Hyperkalemia
Electrical shock
Trauma (cardiac surgery)
Severe acidosis
Hypothermia
Idiopathic dysrhythmia
Cardiac pacemaker dysfunction
Hypoxia
Myocardial infarction

INTERFERENCE WITH BLOOD FLOW IN THE HEART

Pulmonary embolus
Air embolus

LEVELS OF CONSCIOUSNESS

Level 1	Normally aware; responding to person, date, time, place
Level 2	Confused (lethargic, obtunded), drowsy, delirious, agitated
Level 3	Stuporous, aroused only by strong stimuli; combative, irritable
Level 4	Semicomatose (semiconscious); responding only to strong or painful stimuli; coughing, swallowing reflexes usually present; vomiting and incontinence likely
Level 5	Comatose (unconscious), unarousable, unresponsive; most reflexes absent; pupil response and reflex eye movements may be present

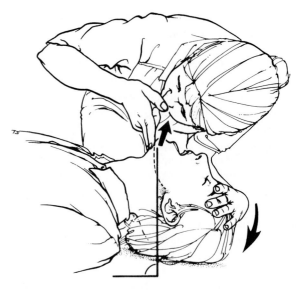

Fig. 22-1 Determining breathlessness. (From American Heart Association: Standards for cardiopulmonary resuscitation and emergency cardiac care, JAMA (suppl) 255:2843-2989, 1986. Copyright 1986, American Medical Association.)

Determining breathlessness. Assessment of the ventilatory status of the victim or patient should precede initial attempts to provide artificial ventilation. To determine breathlessness, the practitioner places the ear over the victim's airway while simultaneously observing for spontaneous chest movement (Fig. 22-1). Breathlessness is confirmed if no chest movement is observed and no breath sounds are heard or felt.[13] This procedure should take no longer than 3 to 5 seconds.

Determining pulselessness. The patient's circulatory status is assessed before circulatory support measures are initiated. This is accomplished by palpating the carotid pulse with two or three fingers placed lightly between the trachea and sternocleidomastoid muscle of the neck (Fig. 22-2). Because the pulse may be slow, weak, or irregular, the practitioner should allow about 5 to 10 seconds to confirm the presence or absence of a pulse.[3] In the hospital setting, the practitioner may alternatively palpate the femoral pulse if it is readily accessible.

In hospital critical care settings, bedside monitoring equipment may provide supporting or confirming information regarding a patient's respiratory or circulatory status. However, information obtained from these devices should never substitute for careful manual assessment of the patient.

BASIC LIFE SUPPORT

Basic life support involves activities instituted without adjunctive equipment to restore ventilation and circulation to victims of airway obstruction, respiratory arrest, or car-

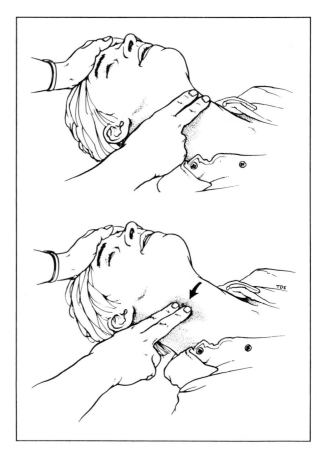

Fig. 22-2 Determining pulselessness. (From American Heart Association: Standards for cardiopulmonary resuscitation and emergency cardiac care, JAMA (suppl) 255:2843-2989, 1986. Copyright 1986, American Medical Association.)

diac arrest.[3,14] These skills, alone or combined, can be used by a single practitioner to restore ventilation and circulation until the victim is revived or until advanced life support equipment and personnel are available.

Restoring ventilation

Airway restoration procedures. Initial action for restoration and maintenance of adequate ventilation involves securing an open airway. Before attempting any airway maneuver, the practitioner must quickly inspect the victim to ascertain that there is no trauma or potential trauma to the neck and face. In the presence of spinal cord trauma, the practitioner must carefully position the neck in vertical alignment and modify any procedure that requires neck hyperextension.[3,13] If a victim is not found in the supine position necessary for airway maneuvers, the practitioner should employ the log-roll technique to obtain a proper orientation.[13]

The most common airway obstruction is caused by the tongue falling into the pharyngeal passage, thereby blocking air flow.[15-17] Extension of the neck pulls the tongue from the posterior pharyngeal wall and creates an open airway. This may be accomplished by one of two procedures. The head-tilt–chin-lift method is the primary airway restoration maneuver recommended for the lay public.[3,18] An additional method, generally limited to use by trained clinicians, is the jaw thrust technique.[19] In most cases, one of these maneuvers alone may be sufficient to restore an open airway.

Head-tilt–chin-lift. For most situations, the head-tilt–chin-lift approach is the most effective airway restoration maneuver. This method also allows loose dentures to remain in place, thereby making mouth-to-mouth ventilation easier.[18] The head-tilt–chin-lift technique is also the least fatiguing method to maintain an open airway. The procedure is as follows (Fig. 22-3):

1. Position the victim on his or her back.
2. Place the fingers of one hand under the victim's chin and then bring the mandible forward. Place the other hand on the victim's forehead to maintain backward tilt. Place the fingers on the anterior portion of the mandible to avoid pressure on the soft tissues under the tongue. Except when using mouth-to-nose ventilation, do not completely close the victim's mouth, since a passage for air escape on exhalation is necessary.

Jaw-thrust maneuver. The jaw-thrust maneuver is also called the mandible thrust, anterior displacement of the mandible, or triple airway maneuver. The jaw-thrust maneuver is an effective technique for opening the airway but is more fatiguing and technically more difficult than the head-tilt–chin-lift method.[19]

The jaw-thrust maneuver should be used when the victim has suspected or confirmed spinal cord trauma, since the neck can be supported and the airway opened with

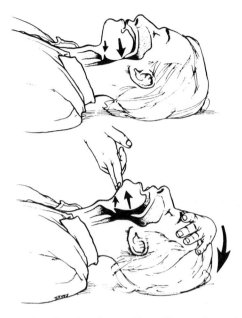

Fig. 22-3 Opening the airway. *Top:* Airway obstruction produced by tongue and epiglottis. *Bottom:* Relief by head tilt–chin lift. (From American Heart Association: Standards for cardiopulmonary resuscitation and emergency cardiac care, JAMA (suppl) 255:2843-2989, 1986. Copyright 1986, American Medical Association.)

minimal movement, thus preventing further spinal cord damage.[3] However, the position assumed by the practitioner in the jaw-thrust maneuver is not appropriate for single rescuer mouth-to-mouth ventilation or external cardiac compression. The jaw-thrust maneuver is therefore useful only when two or more trained rescuers are involved in the resuscitation effort. The procedure is as follows (Fig. 22-4):

1. Place the victim on his or her back and kneel or stand at the victim's head.
2. Place the finger tips behind the angles of the victim's jaws in front of the earlobes and displace the mandible forward and upward while at the same time tilting the head backward. Hold the thumbs on the victim's lower lip to keep the victim's mouth open for air exchange. The carotid sinus lies directly under the sternocleidomastoid muscle inferior to the angle of the mandible. Do not compress this area, since carotid pressure may cause bradycardia.

Evaluating the effectiveness of airway restoration. One of these two airway maneuvers may be the only lifesaving measure required; the practitioner should therefore evaluate the effectiveness of the maneuver before proceeding with other emergency life-support measures. As previously described, the practitioner should look for the rise and fall of the victim's chest and listen for breathing efforts, which should be audible. The practitioner can also feel the air exchange by placing a cheek near the victim's mouth and nose. If the victim is not breathing after at-

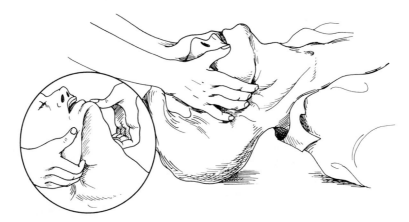

Fig. 22-4   Jaw-thrust maneuver. (From Ellis PD and Billings DM: Cardiopulmonary resuscitation: procedures for basic and advanced life support, St Louis, 1980, The CV Mosby Co.)

tempts to establish an open airway, the practitioner should immediately proceed with efforts to restore ventilation.

Providing artificial ventilation. In situations of respiratory arrest, the practitioner must provide oxygen within 4 to 6 minutes to prevent biologic death. The practitioner can restore the oxygen supply by exhaling into the victim's mouth, nose, or tracheal stoma. These procedures can be used for any victim, with appropriate modification for the victim's size, age, and respiratory rate.

Mouth-to-mouth ventilation. The practitioner can restore oxygenation through mouth-to-mouth ventilation by inflating the victim's lungs with exhaled air. The practitioner doubles his or her tidal volume by taking deep breaths and breathing into the victim's mouth; the practitioner's exhaled air provides approximately 18% oxygen and 2% carbon dioxide, sufficient to achieve an arterial oxygen tension (Pao_2) of between 50 to 60 mm Hg.[11]

Two slow deep breaths at the onset of mouth-to-mouth ventilation can restore alveolar volume and maintain adequate body oxygenation for as long as 15 seconds. Continued expired air ventilation usually is sufficient to maintain life until advanced life-support equipment and personnel are available.

Before beginning mouth-to-mouth ventilation, the practitioner should verify the absence of breathing. The practitioner should log-roll the victim to the supine position and use the head-tilt–chin-lift method to establish the airway. If the victim has dentures, the practitioner should not remove them because the seal of the victim's mouth is easier to maintain if the dentures are in place. If spinal trauma is present or suspected, the neck should not be hyperextended, and the practitioner should instead use the jaw-thrust maneuver. Practitioners who are concerned with the aesthetics of this procedure may place a handkerchief (not tissue) over the victim's mouth. The procedure for adults is as follows (Fig. 22-5):

1. Place the victim on his or her back.

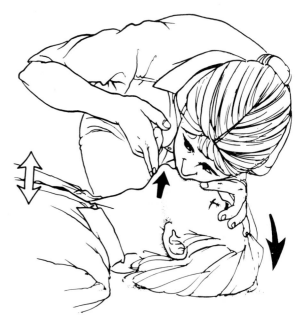

Fig. 22-5   Adult mouth-to-mouth ventilation. (From American Heart Association: Standards for cardiopulmonary resuscitation and emergency cardiac care, JAMA (suppl) 255:2843-2989, 1986. Copyright 1986, American Medical Association.)

2. Kneel at the victim's shoulder and maintain the head-tilt–chin-lift position, except when contraindicated. Pinch the victim's nose with the thumb and index finger close to the nares to prevent air escape during ventilation.

3. Take a deep breath, doubling the tidal volume (about 800 to 1200 cc), and, while making a seal over the victim's mouth, exhale slowly but forcibly for 1 to 1½ seconds.[20] Sealing the lips is important to prevent air escape during exhalation; however, excess pressure can obstruct the airway. If a seal cannot be

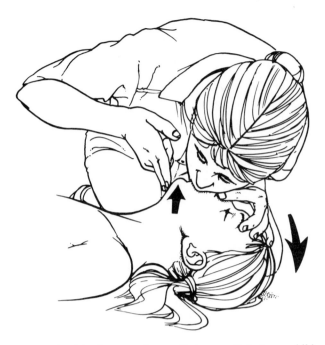

Fig. 22-6 Mouth-to-mouth ventilation applied to a child. (From American Heart Association: Standards for cardiopulmonary resuscitation and emergency cardiac care, JAMA (suppl) 255:2843-2989, 1986. Copyright 1986, American Medical Association.)

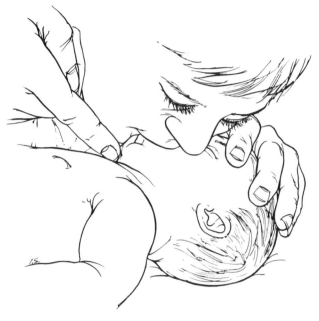

Fig. 22-7 Mouth-to-mouth and nose seal for infants. (From American Heart Association: Standards for cardiopulmonary resuscitation and emergency cardiac care, JAMA (suppl) 255:2843-2989, 1986. Copyright 1986, American Medical Association.)

maintained using this method, attempt mouth-to-nose ventilation.

4. Remove the mouth to allow the victim to exhale passively. A second breath is provided after this deflation pause.[20]

5. Should the initial attempt to ventilate fail, reposition the victim's head and repeat the effort.[13] If a second attempt at ventilation fails, assume that the airway is obstructed and proceed with methods to alleviate this cause of respiratory arrest.

6. Assuming successful mouth-to-mouth ventilation can be achieved, continue the effort at a rate of one breath every 5 seconds to maintain the minimum adult respiratory rate of 12 breaths per minute.[12]

The procedure for children and infants is as follows (Figs. 22-6 and 22-7):

1. Children 3 to 12 years old usually can be resuscitated in a manner similar to that used for adults (see Fig. 22-6).[21-23] A smaller volume of air will be needed to inflate the lungs; however, the practitioner can still judge the effectiveness of ventilation by observing chest excursions.[3,13] The respiratory rate for this age group should be maintained at 15 breaths per minute.[12]

2. In children younger than 3 years, it may be more effective to ventilate the victim by covering both the nose and mouth and using smaller breaths of air (see Fig. 22-7).[21-23] Small puffs of air from the cheek are sufficient. The volume of air needed can be judged by the effectiveness of the ventilation and, of course, depends on the size of the infant or neonate.

3. A respiratory rate of 15 breaths per minute (one breath every 4 seconds) is sufficient for children, whereas infants should be ventilated 20 times per minute (one breath every 3 seconds).[3]

Mouth-to-nose ventilation. There are times when mouth-to-mouth ventilation cannot be accomplished effectively. These situations include trismus (involuntary contraction of the jaw muscles) or traumatic injury to the jaw or mouth. There are also times when a tight seal with the lips simply cannot be maintained with the mouth-to-mouth method. In these situations, the mouth-to-nose method of ventilation should be used.[15,24] The procedure is as follows (Fig. 22-8):

1. Place the victim on his or her back.

2. Use the head-tilt–chin-lift maneuver to establish the airway, being sure to completely close the victim's mouth.

3. Inhale deeply and exhale into the victim's nose. Greater force may be needed than with mouth-to-mouth ventilation because the nasal passageways are smaller.

4. Remove the mouth from the victim's nose to permit the victim to exhale passively through the nose. If

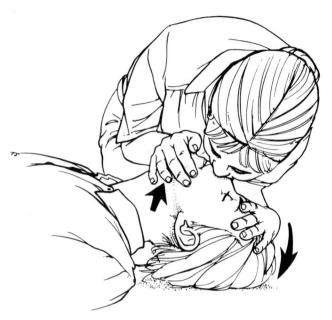

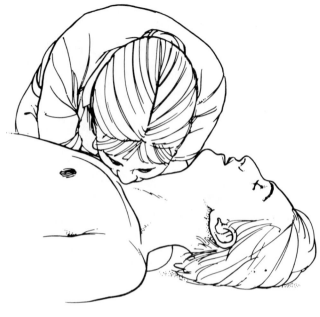

Fig. 22-8   Mouth-to-nose ventilation. (From American Heart Association: Standards for cardiopulmonary resuscitation and emergency cardiac care, JAMA (suppl) 255:2843-2989, 1986. Copyright 1986, American Medical Association.)

Fig. 22-9   Mouth-to-stoma ventilation. (From American Heart Association: Standards for cardiopulmonary resuscitation and emergency cardiac care, JAMA (suppl) 255:2843-2989, 1986. Copyright 1986, American Medical Association.)

the victim is unable to exhale through the nose because of nasopharyngeal obstruction from the soft palate, the victim's mouth may need to be opened or the lips separated to facilitate exhalation.

5. Maintain ventilation at the appropriate rate for the victim's age.

Mouth-to-stoma ventilation. Victims with tracheostomies or laryngectomies can be ventilated directly through the stoma or tube.[3,13] These victims can be identified by an obvious stoma or a tracheostomy or laryngectomy tube in place. Some victims wear an identifiable Medic Alert tag or bracelet. If no chest expansion occurs during mouth-to-mouth ventilation, the practitioner may suspect the presence of a stoma. The procedure is as follows (Fig. 22-9):

1. Place the victim on his or her back with the neck in vertical alignment. It is usually unnecessary to extend the neck or seal the victim's nose or mouth, since oropharyngeal structures are bypassed by the presence of the stoma.

2. Breathe directly into the stoma (or tube). If the victim has a cuffed tracheostomy tube in place, inflate the cuff to prevent air escape around the tube. If using an uncuffed tube, it may be necessary to seal the victim's mouth and nose with a hand or, if available, a tight-fitting face mask.

3. The respiratory rate depends on the victim's age.

Evaluating the effectiveness of ventilatory efforts. The practitioner can determine adequate ventilation by observing the rise and fall of the victim's chest or abdomen,

by feeling resistance as the victim's lungs expand, or by hearing and feeling air escape during exhalation. The practitioner should also note the skin color; a return of normal color, particularly in the nail beds and mucous membranes, indicates effective oxygenation. The practitioner should momentarily terminate ventilation efforts approximately every minute to observe the victim for spontaneous breathing.

Hazards and complications. The most common complications associated with the emergency restoration of ventilation are aggravation of existing injuries to the neck or spine and gastric distention and vomiting.

Aggravating neck and spine injuries. As previously described, it is possible to worsen injuries of the neck or spine by inappropriately moving the head or extending the neck. This pitfall can be avoided by carefully preassessing the victim for potential head, neck, or spine injuries. Should this assessment indicate the possibility of this type of injury, the head should be carefully supported and side-to-side motion avoided. Moreover, the airway should be opened using the jaw thrust maneuver rather than the head-tilt–chin-lift. If the jaw-thrust maneuver is unsuccessful in establishing an airway, a slight head tilt should be tried.[3]

Gastric distention and vomiting. During prolonged mouth-to-mouth ventilation it is likely that some air will enter the esophagus and stomach.[25] Some gastric distention during mouth-to-mouth ventilation is usual, particularly in children. However, severe gastric distention may cause pressure on the diaphragm, thereby restricting lung

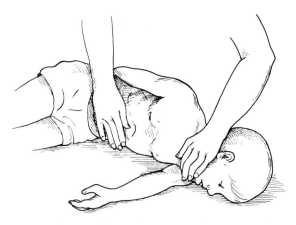

Fig. 22-10   Relieving gastric distention with gentle pressure on abdomen. (From Ellis PD and Billings DM: Cardiopulmonary resuscitation: procedures for basic and advanced life support, St Louis, 1980, The CV Mosby Co.)

expansion during inspiration. Gastric distention can also increase vagal tone and cause reflex bradycardia and hypotension.[12]

Most important, however, is that severe gastric distention promotes regurgitation and vomiting. In the unconscious patient lacking normal protective reflexes, regurgitated stomach contents may easily be aspirated into the lungs. Massive aspiration of stomach contents into the lungs is almost always fatal.

The practitioner can minimize gastric distention by breathing smoothly and avoiding rapid bursts of air into the victim's mouth.[20,25] Use of the least amount of exhaled air necessary to produce lung expansion, as evaluated by the rise and fall of the chest, may prevent excess air from entering the stomach. Mouth-to-nose ventilation also appears to lessen the probability of gastric distention, probably because the high resistance passages of the nose allow less of the inflation pressure to reach the hypopharynx.[15] Last, downward pressure applied to the cricoid cartilage may effectively compress the esophagus between the larynx and vertebral column, thereby preventing regurgitation.[26] Of course, this last technique should only be performed by trained health care professionals and is limited to situations involving two or more rescuers.[3]

If and only if gastric distention is impairing ventilation should efforts be made to expel the accumulated air manually.[3] To perform this procedure, all rescue efforts (including external cardiac compression) should be temporarily halted. The victim should be turned to the side, facing away from the practitioner. The practitioner can apply gentle pressure with the flat of the hand between the umbilicus and lower rib cage to expel air and gastric contents (Fig. 22-10).

Ideally, suction equipment should be available during this procedure. If advanced life-support equipment and

personnel are available, stomach contents may also be removed through a nasogastric tube.

Occasionally the victim may vomit during rescue attempts. If vomiting occurs, the practitioner should immediately turn the victim onto the side, wipe out the mouth, and resume the resuscitation effort.[3]

Addressing an obstructed airway

If attempts to open an airway are unsuccessful or, if on inspection of the mouth, a foreign body can be observed, the practitioner can use several procedures to obtain a clear passageway.

For adults and children, the procedure of choice is the abdominal thrust or Heimlich maneuver.[27-32] For infants with an obstructed airway, back blows are combined with chest thrusts.[3] Chest thrusts may also be used with female victims in the advanced stages of pregnancy and in markedly obese individuals.[3] Both procedures normally are followed by a manual check and removal of any obstructing foreign material.

Abdominal thrusts. Abdominal thrusts applied to the epigastrium can dislodge an obstruction caused by a food bolus, vomitus, or other foreign body. Quick thrusts to the abdomen rapidly displace the diaphragm upward, thereby increasing the intrathoracic pressure and creating expulsive expiratory airflow. Like a normal cough, this expulsive expiratory airflow may be sufficient to expel the foreign body from the airway. The procedure is as follows (Fig. 22-11):

1. If the victim is sitting or standing, stand behind him or her and wrap the arms around the victim's waist. Make a fist with one hand and place the thumb side between the victim's umbilicus and xiphoid (see Fig. 22-11, *A*). Grasp the fist with the other hand and deliver a quick upward and inward thrust. Deliver the thrust with the fist, not the arms. Each thrust should be separate and distinct and can be repeated six to ten times or as necessary.

2. When the victim has collapsed or is unconscious, the abdominal thrust can be delivered with the victim in the lying position. Place the victim on the back, face upward, so that the foreign body can be easily expelled. If the victim vomits, quickly turn the victim's head to the side and wipe out the mouth. Kneel astride the victim's hips and place the heel of one hand on the abdomen between the umbilicus and xiphoid and the other hand on top. Rock forward to give a quick forward and downward thrust (see Fig. 22-11, *B*), repeating it six to ten times or as necessary. An alternative approach is to kneel near the victim's hips with the shoulders over the victim and, using the same hand position, to press on the epigastrium. This position is preferred if mouth-to-mouth ventilation or external cardiac compression might be necessary, since the practitioner can easily change position to perform these procedures. If two practi-

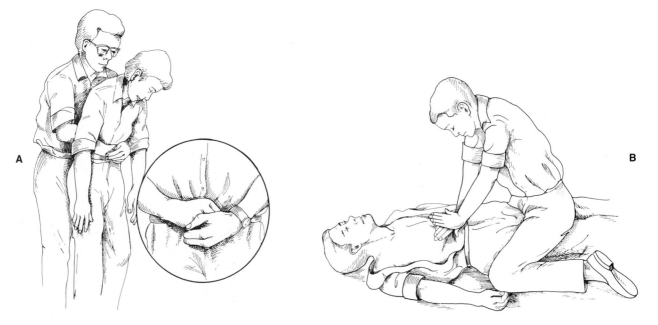

Fig. 22-11   Abdominal thrusts. **A,** Adult victim standing. **B,** Adult victim lying. (From Ellis PD and Billings DM: Cardiopulmonary resuscitation: procedures for basic and advanced life support, St Louis, 1980, The CV Mosby Co.)

tioners are available, one can give the abdominal thrusts and the other can manage the airway and retrieve the foreign body.

3. A victim who is alone can attempt to dislodge the foreign body with self-administered abdominal thrusts. He or she may be able to press a fist into the abdomen or push the abdomen against a firm surface such as a countertop, sink, chair back, railing, or tabletop.

Back blows. Because the Heimlich maneuver has a greater potential for intra-abdominal injury when applied to infants and neonates, the procedure of choice for clearing a foreign body from the upper airway of these victims is a combination of back blows with chest thrusts.[3] Back blows alone may create sufficient force to dislodge trapped objects.[31,32] Chest thrusts normally follow back blows when the airway remains obstructed.[3,13] The procedure is as follows:

1. Back blows to infants and neonates can be administered more efficiently if the practitioner holds the child straddled over the arm (Fig. 22-12).
2. Use the flat portion of the hand gently but quickly to deliver four back blows between the shoulder blades.

Chest thrusts. If the back blows do not clear the infant's airway, the practitioner should turn the infant over and institute a series of four chest thrusts. Like the abdominal thrust, the chest thrust creates a rapid rise in intrathoracic pressure, thereby facilitating expulsion of the foreign body from the airway. Chest thrusts for infants are performed in the same manner and at the same location as

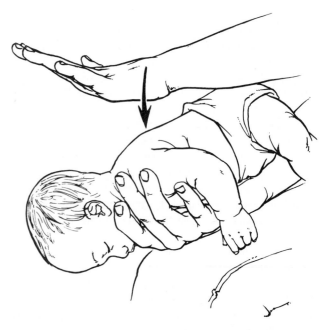

Fig. 22-12   Back blow in infant. (From American Heart Association: Standards for cardiopulmonary resuscitation and emergency cardiac care, JAMA (suppl) 255:2843-2989, 1986. Copyright 1986, American Medical Association.)

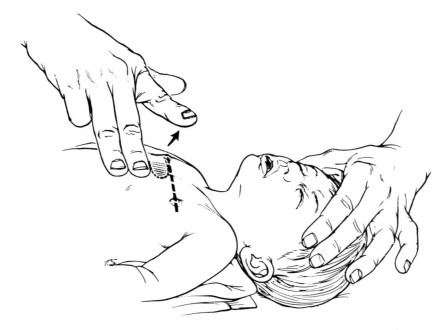

Fig. 22-13   Position for chest thrusts in infant. (From American Heart Association: Standards for cardiopulmonary resuscitation and emergency cardiac care, JAMA (suppl) 255:2843-2989, 1986. Copyright 1986, American Medical Association.)

those used for external cardiac compression (Fig. 22-13) but are done at a slower rate. Chest thrusts may also be used with female victims in the advanced stages of pregnancy and in markedly obese individuals.

Manual removal of foreign material. If successive abdominal thrusts, back blows, or chest thrusts do not clear the airway, the practitioner should attempt to remove the obstructing foreign body manually. Manual removal of an obstructing foreign body is normally limited to unconscious victims and is accomplished using the tongue-jaw lift technique combined with a finger sweep.[3,13]

The victim's mouth is opened by simultaneously grasping the tongue and lower jaw between the thumb and fingers and lifting the mandible (Fig. 22-14). Then the practitioner inserts the index finger of the opposite hand along the inside of the cheek, down past the base of the tongue into the throat. A hooking action with the tip of the finger will usually dislodge the foreign body into the mouth for grasping and removal. Great care must be taken to avoid blind probes and to ensure that the object is not forced deeper into the throat or into the trachea or below the epiglottis. Occasionally it is useful to push a foreign body to the opposite side of the throat to dislodge it and remove it as it is grasped.

If the victim's mouth cannot be opened easily, the practitioner can use the cross-finger technique to wedge the mouth open and maintain an opened position (Fig. 22-15). Alternatively, the practitioner can attempt to wedge the index finger behind the last molars and twist the finger in

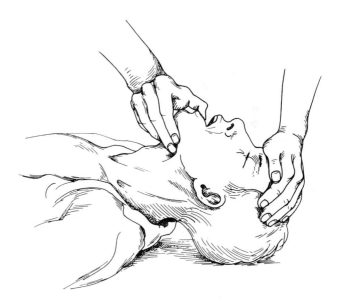

Fig. 22-14   Jaw-lift maneuver. (From Ellis PD and Billings DM: Cardiopulmonary resuscitation: procedures for basic and advanced life support, St Louis, 1980, The CV Mosby Co.)

this space to open the jaw, while using the other hand to retrieve the foreign body or remove the fluid.

Evaluating the effectiveness of foreign body removal. The practitioner must ascertain after each maneuver whether the foreign body has been expelled and the obstructed airway cleared. If the victim is unable to expel the

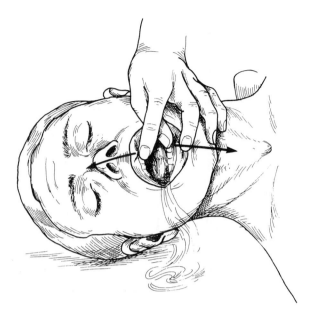

Fig. 22-15 Crossed-finger technique. (From Ellis PD and Billings DM: Cardiopulmonary resuscitation: procedures for basic and advanced life support, St Louis, 1980, The CV Mosby Co.)

foreign body, the practitioner should repeat the appropriate sequence (abdominal thrusts for adults and children; back blows and chest thrusts for infants) until successful.[3,13]

Successful removal of an obstructing body is indicated by (1) confirmed expulsion or removal of the foreign body, (2) clear breathing and ability to speak, (3) a return of consciousness, and (4) a return of normal color.

Hazards and complications. The major hazard associated with the Heimlich maneuver is possible damage to internal organs, such as laceration or rupture of abdominal or thoracic viscera.[33,34] This possibility can be avoided by ensuring proper placement of the arms and fist below the xiphoid and lower margin of the ribs.[3,13]

The major complication associated with manual removal of foreign material from the airway is the possibility of forcing the object deeper into the airway.[3] This hazard can be minimized by attempting to remove only those objects actually within reach. The use of Kelly clamps or Magill-type forceps to remove foreign bodies should be limited to trained personnel.

Restoration of circulation

External cardiac compression. In situations in which no adjunct equipment is available, it is possible for a single practitioner to restore circulation by means of external cardiac compression (ECC). In this procedure the practitioner manually compresses the victim's ventricles between the sternum and thoracic spine. Compression can provide one third to one fourth of the normal cardiac output and can maintain a systolic blood pressure of 100 mm Hg.[3]

Exactly how external cardiac compression works is still a matter of debate.[35] The conventional "cardiac pump theory" is based on the assumption that compression of the heart between the sternum and spine increases pressure in the ventricles sufficiently to close the atrioventricular valves, thereby directing blood into the systemic and pulmonary circulations. The "thoracic pump theory" assumes that the pressure generated by chest compression is transmitted mainly to the arterial side of the circulation, with the pressure in the extrathoracic veins increasing little if at all. According to this theory, it is this arteriovenous pressure gradient that is responsible for blood flow, not the valve action of the compressed heart. Both mechanisms may be involved in circulatory support by external cardiac compression.[3]

ECC can be delivered to any victim; however, the practitioner must modify the position, rescue technique, and compression rate according to the victim's age and size. The practitioner should judge the need for modifications of rescue technique by the victim's size and the effectiveness of the cardiac compression as determined by palpating the pulse. The procedure for adults is as follows (Fig. 22-16 to 22-18):

1. Place the victim on his or her back on a firm surface. Since cerebral blood flow is difficult to achieve when the victim is upright, make every attempt to move the victim to a horizontal position before initiating ECCs. Compression of the heart is more effective when the victim is on a firm surface; therefore place the victim on the ground or floor. If the victim is in bed or on a litter, place a board or tray underneath to provide a firm surface. A cardiac arrest board or spine board can be used, but use of items such as bedboards, removable heads of beds, and trays can be improvised. Some suggest that elevating the legs 30 to 40 degrees for 5 to 15 seconds before initiating ECC improves circulatory efficiency.[12] It is theorized that this "Woodward maneuver" initiates spontaneous cardiac activity in some instances because the rush of venous blood depresses vagus tone and thus vagal inhibition to the heart, which allows an increased heart rate. Additionally, elevating the legs causes a 20% increase in blood volume (as much as 1000 ml) to return to the heart, which increases cardiac output.

2. Expose the victim's chest to identify landmarks for correct hand position. If the victim is fully clothed, open the jacket or shirt and, if time allows, remove any underwear.

3. Choose a position close to the victim's upper chest so that the weight of the body can be used for compression. If the victim is on a bed or litter, stand next to the bed or litter with the victim close to that side of the bed. If the bed is high or the practitioner short, it may be necessary to lower the bed, stand on a stool or chair, or kneel on the bed next to the vic-

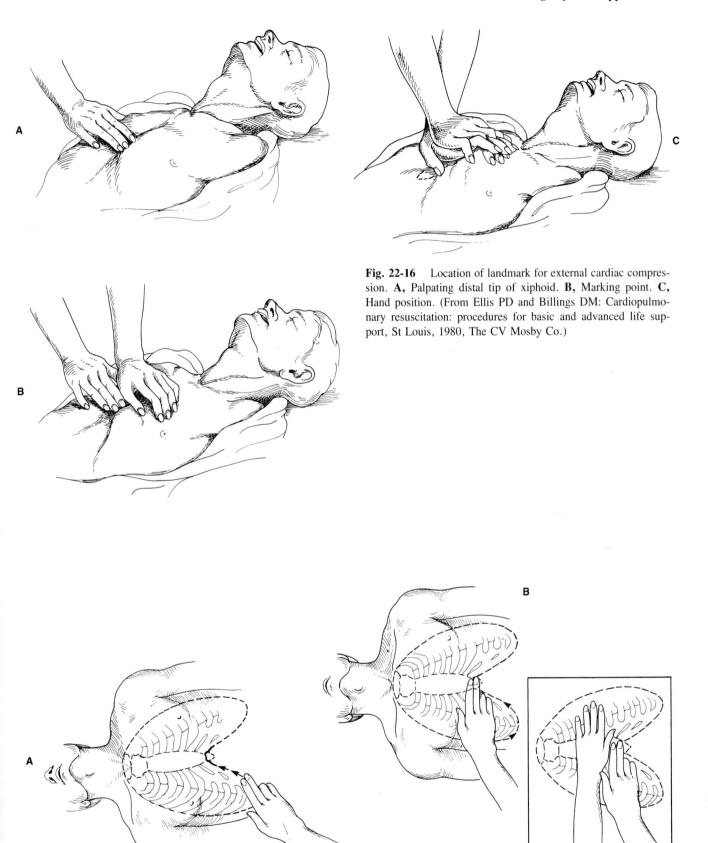

Fig. 22-16 Location of landmark for external cardiac compression. **A,** Palpating distal tip of xiphoid. **B,** Marking point. **C,** Hand position. (From Ellis PD and Billings DM: Cardiopulmonary resuscitation: procedures for basic and advanced life support, St Louis, 1980, The CV Mosby Co.)

Fig. 22-17 Xiphisternal junction. **A,** Locating junction. **B,** Hand position. (From Ellis PD and Billings DM: Cardiopulmonary resuscitation: procedures for basic and advanced life support, St Louis, 1980, The CV Mosby Co.)

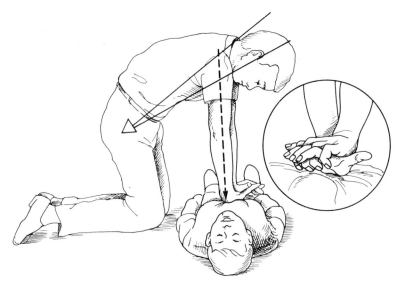

Fig. 22-18   Practitioner's position for external cardiac compression. Note interlocked fingers to prevent pressure on rib cage. (From Ellis PD and Billings DM: Cardiopulmonary resuscitation: procedures for basic and advanced life support, St Louis, 1980, The CV Mosby Co.)

tim. If the victim is on the ground, kneel at the victim's shoulders.

4. Next identify the lower third of the sternum, since this is the point where the ventricles are most effectively compressed between the sternum and the thoracic spine. This landmark can be located in two ways. First, palpate the distal tip of the xiphoid (see Fig. 22-16, *A*). Mark this point with three fingers of one hand while placing the heel of the other hand next to the fingers (see Fig. 22-16, *B*). This should be about 1 to 1½ inches (3.3 cm) from the xiphoid. The heel of the hand on the sternum should be parallel to the midline of the sternum; slight ulnar deviation may be required to achieve this position. Place the other hand on top of the hand on the sternum with the elbows straight. The fingers should not touch the rib cage because this increases the likelihood of fracture; many find that interlocking the fingers is a comfortable way to keep the fingers off the chest (see Fig. 22-16, *C*). An alternative approach is to identify the lower margin of the portion of the victim's rib cage that is closest to the practitioner and to palpate the rib cage to the midline to locate the notch where the ribs meet the sternum (see Fig. 22-17, *A*). This notch is the xiphisternal junction and can be used as a landmark for hand position. Place two fingers on the junction and the heel of the other hand proximal to the fingers (see Fig. 22-17, *B*). Once the landmark is found, place the other hand on top of the hand on the sternum and lock the elbows.

5. ECC is accomplished with the weight of the body exerting force on the outstretched arms, elbows held straight. Normally, this requires that the practitio-

ner's hips be positioned above the patient. Keep the shoulders over the victim and use a rocking motion from the hips to create downward pressure (see Fig. 22-18). Do not let the hands leave the chest and compress the sternum 1½ to 2 inches (3.8 to 5.0 cm), which requires 80 to 100 pounds of pressure. Apply compression regularly, rhythmically, and without bouncing. The compression phase of the cycle should be at least equal in duration to the relaxation phase. Some even recommend that the compression phase consist of 60% of the cycle to increase cardiac output and stroke volume.[36] The rate of compression for adults is 80 to 100 beats per minute. This rate is consistent with both the cardiac and thoracic pump theories of circulatory support and accommodates, as necessary, any additional time that may be required for ventilation.[37] If it is necessary to terminate CPR effort for transportation or advanced life-support measures, compressions must be resumed as quickly as possible. ECC should not be interrupted for more than 5 seconds (30 seconds if intubating the victim).[38] This is particularly important if drugs are being administered.

The procedure for children is as follows (Fig. 22-19)[21-23,39,40]:

1. Place the victim on the back on a firm surface. Small children may require additional support under the upper body. This is particularly true when ECCs are given with mouth-to-mouth ventilation, since extension of the neck raises the shoulders.

2. Use the lower third of the sternum as a landmark for hand position in children over 5 years of age. In smaller children, the midsternal position is used. The

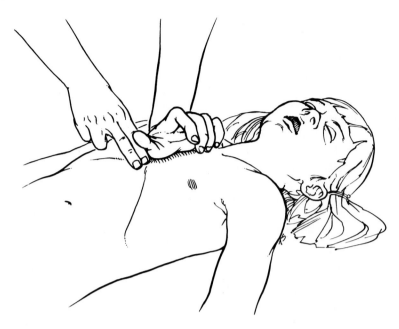

Fig. 22-19   Locating hand position for chest compressions in child. (From American Heart Association: Standards for cardiopulmonary resuscitation and emergency cardiac care, JAMA (suppl) 255:2843-2989, 1986. Copyright 1986, American Medical Association.)

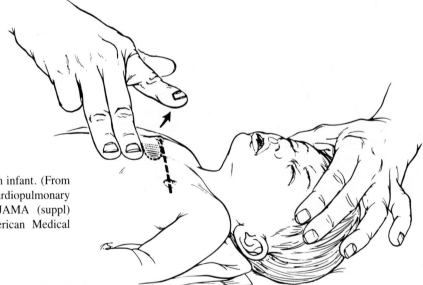

Fig. 22-20   Position for chest compressions in infant. (From American Heart Association: Standards for cardiopulmonary resuscitation and emergency cardiac care, JAMA (suppl) 255:2843-2989, 1986. Copyright 1986, American Medical Association.)

liver and spleen of younger children lie higher in the abdominal cavity, and chances of trauma are greater if the sternum is compressed at a lower point. The heel of one hand is sufficient to achieve compression in these young children (See Fig. 22-19).

3. Judge the rate and depth of compression by the size of the child and effectiveness of the compression. For children over 5 years, or large toddlers, compress the sternum with the heel of one hand 1 to 1½ inches at a rate of 80 to 100 beats per minute.

The procedure for infants and neonates is as follows (Fig. 22-20)[21,39,40]:

1. Recent evidence demonstrates that the heart of the neonate and infant is located lower in the chest than was previously thought. To achieve proper positioning for ECC in this group, use a point on the sternum one fingerbreadth below the intermammary line.

2. Apply compressions with the middle and index fingers on the sternum. Compression should be ½ to 1 inches at the rate of at least 100 beats per minute.

Evaluating the of effectiveness of ECC. It is important to make ongoing evaluation of ECC to judge the effectiveness of the compressions as well as the victim's response. It is ultimately the hemodynamic consequences that determine successful CPR, and it is imperative that an effective technique be developed for compression depth, rhythm, and rate. If external cardiac compressions are not effective, cardiac emptying is incomplete and decreased cardiac output and heart failure will ensue. If the compression cycle does not allow an adequate relaxation phase, venous return and stroke volume may be decreased, creating a situation similar to cardiac tamponade. Compression rates should be appropriate for the victim's age. If possible, the practitioner should make a quick appraisal of the effectiveness of the ECC every minute and a more comprehensive assessment every 4 to 5 minutes.

The presence of a pulse is the most reliable indicator of effective ECC. In adults and children the practitioner can use the carotid or femoral pulse; in infants and neonates, the practitioner can more easily palpate the brachial pulse.[3] The pulse should be palpable with each compression. If one practitioner is present, he or she can palpate the pulse every minute; if two or more practitioners are available, they can monitor the pulse continuously.

Skin color is a parameter that is readily observed but imprecise in judging effectiveness of CPR maneuvers. However, if normal color returns, the practitioner can assume that oxygenation has improved.

The practitioner may use pupil response to estimate the effectiveness of cerebral oxygenation. Pupil response may be altered by drugs and diseases. Therefore, unless the victim's medical history is known, interpretation of this response may be invalid. The practitioner should open the eyelids and observe the pupils for size and response to light. Pupils that are constricted and that respond to light indicate adequate cerebral oxygenation; pupils that are dilated but react to light indicate inadequate oxygenation; dilated and nonreactive pupils are an ominous sign. The likelihood of irreversible brain death is high if pupils have been dilated and fixed for 15 to 30 minutes or longer.

Cerebral blood flow and oxygenation can also be evaluated by return of consciousness and the presence of tears. The lacrimal glands are supplied by the internal carotid artery, and, if blood supply is adequate, tears will be present. Additionally, reflexes such as swallowing or vomiting may return.

External cardiac compression in special circumstances. Several unique circumstances exist that require modification of the normal procedures for applying external cardiac compressions. These situations include near drownings, electrical shock, and patients with pacemakers or prosthetic heart valves.

Drowning. When cardiac arrest occurs as a result of drowning, the practitioner should move the victim as quickly as possible to a firm surface. ECC cannot be given while the practitioner and victim are in the water unless the victim is on a firm surface (such as a small boat or surfboard) and the practitioner can maintain correct rescue position.

Electrical shock. During electrical shock, cardiac or respiratory arrest can occur as a result of ventricular fibrillation or secondary to tetany or paralysis of the muscles of respiration. Initially, the practitioner should remove the victim from contact with the source of electricity to assess the victim's cardiopulmonary status. If cardiac arrest has occurred, the practitioner should administer ECC immediately.

Pacemakers. Cardiac arrest may occur in victims with cardiac pacemakers as a result of battery failure or other mechanical difficulties. CPR for these victims is similar to the procedure previously described. If mechanical failures cannot easily be identified and remedied, the practitioner should administer ECC.

Prosthetic valves. If the practitioner administers ECC to a victim who has a recently implanted prosthetic valve (particularly mitral or tricuspid), it may lacerate the area and cause irreparable damage to the heart. It is recommended, therefore, that the practitioner use ECC only for several minutes and that internal cardiac compression be attempted if a qualified surgeon and appropriate equipment are available.

Contraindications to ECC. There are several instances in which ECC is not usually effective. These include flail chest, chest deformities, massive air or pulmonary emboli, bilateral pneumothorax, or cardiac tamponade. The practitioner must assess each victim carefully and weigh the alternatives of further injury and possible death against potential life saving when initiating CPR for these victims. If facilities and personnel are available, the chest can be opened and internal cardiac compression attempted in these instances (discussed in the section on advanced cardiac life support).

Hazards and complications. Administering ECC is not without hazards, and the practitioner must make every attempt to minimize these by using correct technique. The practitioner must weigh the risks of complications, however, against the alternative of certain death if no CPR efforts are initiated. Complications can include laceration of the liver; contusion of the lung; fractured ribs, sternum, or spine; pneumothorax; hemothorax; fat emboli; cardiac tamponade; and ruptured heart.[41-44]

The most common cause of complications is incorrect hand placement on the sternum.[3] If the hands are placed too far on the victim's left chest, it is likely to result in fractured ribs and laceration of the heart or lungs. If the practitioner places the hands too far to the victim's right chest, the chances of fractured ribs or lacerations of the lung are increased. If the practitioner places the hands too high on the sternum, it can cause a fractured sternum, while hands too low can cause a fractured xiphoid or lacerations of the liver. The practitioner's correct identification of landmarks and hand placement cannot be overemphasized.

Cardiopulmonary resuscitation

Although artificial ventilation and ECC may be used singly, it is more likely that respiratory and cardiac arrest occur together. In fact, respiratory arrest is most certainly followed by cardiac arrest if oxygen supplies are not restored. Since ventilation without circulation or circulation of unoxygenated blood is futile, it is often necessary for the practitioner to combine artificial ventilation and ECC, performing CPR. CPR can be administered by one, or preferably two, practitioners.

Single-practitioner CPR. If only one person is available for rescue, the practitioner must assess the situation, initiate CPR, and evaluate the effectiveness of CPR alone. The practitioner initially determines unresponsiveness, calls out for help, positions the victim, and opens the airway. If the victim is not breathing, the practitioner administers two initial breaths. Next, the practitioner establishes pulselessness and begins external chest compressions. When the practitioner combines ECC with artificial ventilation for adults, he or she administers them in a cycle of 15 compressions at a rate of 80 to 100 per minute, interspersed with two breaths. After four cycles of 15 compressions and two breaths, the victim or patient should be reassessed. With infants and children, the cycle consists of five compressions to one breath.

Two-practitioner CPR. When two persons are available, assessment, rescue, and evaluation can be shared. One practitioner gives mouth-to-mouth ventilation and evaluates the effectiveness of CPR; the other administers ECC. To facilitate movement, each practitioner should assume the appropriate rescue portion on opposite sides of the victim.

When two people provide support, one breath is interposed during the relaxation phase after every fifth compression, necessitating a pause of 1 to 1.5 seconds. The compression rate is maintained at 80 to 100 per minute. The efforts of CPR should be evaluated every minute, and all efforts should be interrupted every 4 to 5 minutes to observe spontaneous pulse and breathing.

To provide rest for the practitioner who is delivering ECC and to prevent hyperventilation in the practitioner giving mouth-to-mouth ventilation, the practitioners may change positions. The practitioner doing ECC calls for the change, saying in sequence with compression rate, "We will change next time" or words to this effect. The practitioner performing mouth-to-mouth ventilation gives a breath at the end of the next compression cycle and moves quickly into position for cardiac compression, identifies the landmarks, and prepares to initiate a new cycle of compressions. The first practitioner completes the fifth compression of the cycle and moves to the victim's head to begin delivery of ventilation.

Rescue attempts should continue until advanced life support is available, until the practitioner(s) note spontaneous pulse and breathing, or until a physician pronounces the victim dead. A cardiopulmonary emergency presents a crisis for the victim and family, and appropriate support and intervention should be provided for both. Victims who survive CPR should be transported quickly to facilities for continued life support.

ADVANCED CARDIAC LIFE SUPPORT

ACLS extends BLS capabilities by providing additional measures beyond immediate ventilatory and circulatory assistance. These measures include using adjunct equipment to support ventilation and oxygenation, using electrocardiographic (ECG) monitoring, establishing an intravenous route for drug administration, and using selected pharmacologic agents and electrical therapies. Successful intervention during this phase is normally followed by an individualized regimen of postresuscitative care.[3]

The initiation of BLS methods should never be delayed while awaiting advanced capabilities. Quick intervention is the primary factor associated with success in any resuscitation effort. Moreover, the application of ACLS measures should never interfere with or delay continuity in the provision of basic ventilatory and circulatory assistance. Last, any adjunctive equipment employed in a resuscitation effort must be in good working order. Assurance of proper equipment functions requires periodic performance testing according to prescribed standards and regulations.[3]

Support for oxygenation, airway control and ventilation

During advanced cardiac life support efforts in the hospital setting, the respiratory care practitioner assumes primary responsibility for the skilled use of adjunctive methods to support oxygenation, maintain and enhance airway access, and provide more effective ventilation. For this reason, practitioners must demonstrate high levels of proficiency in these ACLS skills.

Oxygenation

Although appropriately applied expired-air ventilation provides an acceptable level of alveolar oxygenation, the low cardiac output and high intrapulmonary shunting that characterizes resuscitation of patients with cardiac arrest enhances the likelihood of tissue hypoxia. Tissue hypoxia can result in metabolic acidosis, which, in turn, can impede the action of certain drugs or thwart effective use of electrical therapies. For this reason, supplemental oxygen, preferably at a concentration of 100%, should be applied as soon as possible.[3]

During ACLS, supplemental oxygen normally will be administered concurrently with and through adjunctive devices designed to support ventilation. Therefore, the ability of these devices to provide a high concentration of oxygen is a key factor in judging their performance. The performance of these devices will be discussed in a subsequent section.

Artificial airways

Artificial airways are adjunctive devices designed to alter and enhance the normal passageway available for ventilation and oxygenation. After appropriate use of BLS methods to secure the airway, the practitioner may employ an artificial airway to achieve one or more of the following goals: (1) to assist in restoring airway patency, (2) to help maintain adequate ventilation, (3) to isolate and protect the airway from aspiration, and (4) to provide access for clearance of secretions and foreign material by aspiration techniques.[12]

Which artificial airway, if any, should be used in a given situation depends on careful assessment of the victim's status in conjunction with an in-depth knowledge of the capabilities and limitations of the equipment at hand.

Masks. A well-fitting mask, used in conjunction with expired-air ventilation, has been shown effective in helping to maintain adequate ventilation during resuscitation efforts.[45] Mask-to-mouth ventilation is generally easier to accomplish and provides higher tidal volumes than the bag-valve-mask technique discussed later.[46]

Used for this purpose, an ideal mask should be made of transparent material, be capable of tightly sealing against the face, provide an inlet for supplemental oxygen, and employ a standard 15/22 mm connection.[3] Moreover, it should be available in various sizes to accommodate adults, children, and infants. One-way valves, if provided, should be simple, dependable, and jam-free.

The use of masks as an adjunct method to support ventilation presumes that the airway can be maintained by conventional BLS techniques. Application of the mask-to-mouth technique is best accomplished with the practitioner positioned at the head of the victim, using the jaw thrust maneuver to maintain the airway (Fig. 22-21). Obviously, this approach can only be applied when a second person is available to provide chest compressions.

Mask-to-mouth ventilation with supplemental oxygen represents a viable alternative to bag-valve-mask methods of airway maintenance and ventilation. For this reason, in the absence of highly trained personnel, mask-to-mouth ventilation should be considered the adjunct procedure of choice until an esophageal airway or endotracheal tube can be properly placed.[3]

Pharyngeal airways. Pharyngeal airways are designed to assist in restoring airway patency and maintaining adequate ventilation, particularly when a bag-valve-mask combination or gas-powered resuscitator is used. A properly placed pharyngeal airway also may help provide access for suctioning.

Pharyngeal airways restore airway patency by separating the tongue from the posterior pharyngeal wall. Two types of pharyngeal airways are commonly used in clinical prac-

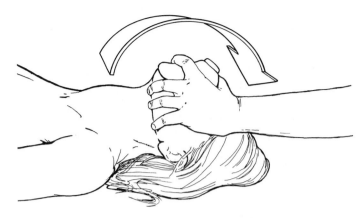

Fig. 22-21　Proper placement of hands to hold resuscitator mask to patient's face and perform head-tilt maneuver.

tice: the oropharyngeal airway and the nasopharyngeal airway.

Oropharyngeal airways. Oropharyngeal airways come in many different designs and are available for adults, children, and infants. Fig. 22-22 shows the two most common oropharyngeal airway designs: the Guedel airway (see Fig. 22-22, *A*) and the Berman airway (see Fig. 22-22, *B*). Both are characterized by an external flange, *1,* a curved body, *2,* that conforms to the shape of the oral cavity, and one or more channels, *3.* The Guedel airway has a single center channel, whereas the Berman type uses two parallel side channels.

Because placement of an oropharyngeal airway may provoke a gag reflex, vomiting, or laryngeal spasm, these devices generally are contraindicated in conscious or semiconscious patients.[3] The use of oropharyngeal airways to maintain airway patency is also contraindicated when there is trauma to the oral cavity or to the mandibular or maxillary areas of the skull. Moreover, oropharyngeal airways should never be placed when either a space-occupying lesion or foreign body is already obstructing the oral cavity or pharynx.

Two techniques may be used to insert an oropharyngeal airway.[12] In the first method the practitioner uses a tongue blade to displace the tongue away from the roof of the mouth. The curved portion of the airway is then slipped over the tongue, following the curve of the oral cavity.

In the second approach, the practitioner applies the jaw-lift technique to help displace the tongue. The oropharyngeal airway is rotated 180 degrees before insertion. In this manner the airway itself helps separate the jaws and further displace the tongue. As the tip of the airway reaches the uvula, the practitioner rotates it by 180 degrees, aligning it as in the pharynx.

In either approach, incorrect placement can displace the tongue further back into the pharynx, thereby worsening the obstruction. For this reason, oropharyngeal airways must be inserted carefully and only by trained personnel.

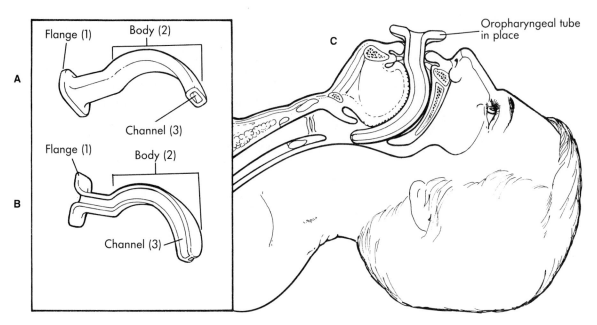

Fig. 22-22   Oropharyngeal airways. **A,** Guedel airway. **B,** Berman airway. **C,** Airway in place.

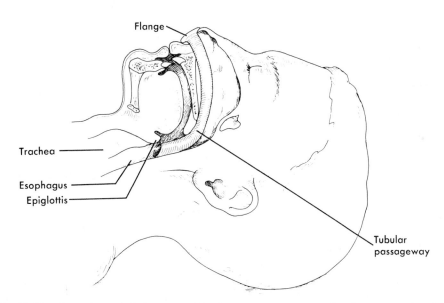

Fig. 22-23   Nasopharyngeal airway provides long passageway extending from external naris to base of tongue just above epiglottis. (From Ellis PD and Billings DM: Cardiopulmonary resuscitation: procedures for basic and advanced life support, St Louis, 1980, The CV Mosby Co.)

As shown in Fig. 22-22, *C,* the tip of a properly inserted oropharyngeal airway lies at the base of the tongue above the epiglottis, with its flange portion extending outside the teeth. Only in this position can the airway help maintain airway patency and assist the practitioner in providing ventilation.

Nasopharyngeal airways. As shown in Fig. 22-23, a properly inserted nasopharyngeal airway provides a passageway from the external nares to the base of the tongue, at a point just behind the epiglottis. Like the oropharyngeal airway, the nasopharyngeal airway helps restore airway patency by separating the tongue from the posterior pharyngeal wall.

Generally, the nasopharyngeal airway is indicated in those situations in which placement of an oropharyngeal airway is not possible. The nasopharyngeal airway is also the adjunct of choice when it is impossible to separate the jaws of a victim, as may occur with seizures.

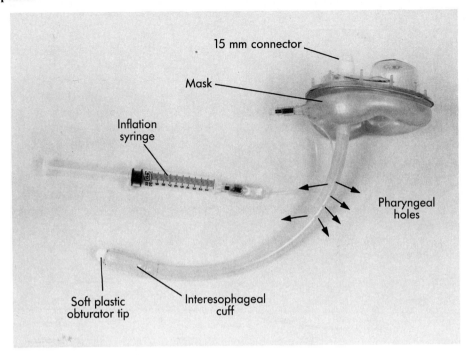

Fig. 22-24 Parts of esophageal obturator airway.

A nasopharyngeal airway should not be used when there is trauma to the nasal region or when the nasal passages are blocked by space-occupying lesions or foreign objects. Moreover, because of the higher position of the epiglottis in children and infants and the increased likelihood of its displacement, the use of nasal airways is generally limited to adults.[3]

Nasal airways are typically manufactured from either rubber or plastic polymers and sized by external diameter in French units, with 26 to 32 French being the common size range for adults. Anatomically, the length of the airway is more critical than its diameter. The practitioner may estimate the appropriate length by measuring the distance from the patient's earlobe to the tip of the nose.

To insert a nasopharyngeal airway, the practitioner should tilt the patient's head slightly backward. Ideally, the selected airway should be lubricated with a water-soluable agent to ease insertion. Once lubricated, the airway is positioned perpendicular to the frontal plane of the face and slowly advanced through the inferior meatus of either the right or left nasal cavity. If an obstruction to insertion is felt, the most likely cause is a deviated nasal septum. In this case the practitioner should simply attempt passage through the other naris.[12]

Once the airway is inserted, the practitioner should attempt to quickly visualize and confirm its correct positioning, using a tongue depressor if necessary. A properly positioned nasopharyngeal airway may be stabilized by its own flange or, alternatively, by a large safety pin.

Esophageal obturator airway. As shown in Fig. 22-24, the esophageal obturator airway (EOA) consists of a cuffed hollow tube tipped with a soft plastic obturator at its distal end. The tube, which passes through a mask, has

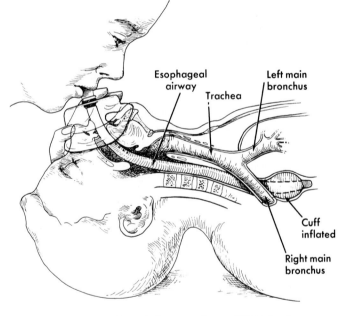

Fig. 22-25 Esophageal obturator airway (EOA) in place.

several holes in its upper portion. Some EOAs are modified to include a gastric tube that can be extended beyond the distal tip into the stomach. This modified version is called the esophageal gastric tube airway (EGTA).[3]

In concept, the EOA is inserted blindly into the esophagus, thereby blocking off this passageway. With the esophageal cuff inflated and the mask tightly sealed to the victim's face, air under pressure is diverted out the pharyngeal holes in the tube and into the trachea and lungs (Fig. 22-25).[47]

In practice, the effectiveness of the EOA is determined

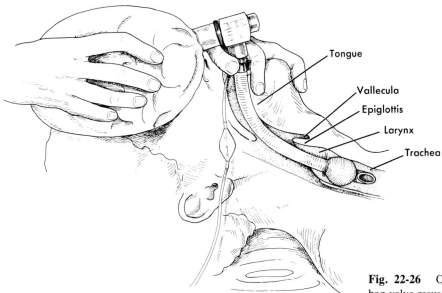

Tongue

Vallecula

Epiglottis

Larynx

Trachea

Fig. 22-26   Orotracheal tube in place being used with bag-valve resuscitator.

by the adequacy of the seal obtained between the mask and victim's face. Even among highly trained personnel an adequate seal is difficult to obtain; thus the level of oxygenation and ventilation that can be achieved with the EOA tends to fall short of that realized with endotracheal intubation.[47]

Moreover, the EOA has been associated with several potentially life-threatening complications. The most common complication of EOA use is inadvertent insertion into the trachea.[3] Obviously, if not immediately recognized, this complication will quickly result in asphyxia. Also reported in the literature as complications of EOA use are esophageal laceration and rupture.[48]

The EOA is contraindicated in conscious individuals or in those with spontaneous respirations.[3] Also, because of the increased likelihood of displacing the epiglottis in children and infants, the EOA is not used with victims under 16 years of age. Last, the EOA should never be used in patients with known esophageal disease or those who have ingested caustic substances.

Since the EOA is used mainly in field situations when endotracheal intubation is not available, the respiratory care practitioner will most likely encounter this type of airway adjunct already placed in patients being admitted to the emergency room. For this reason, emphasis here is on proper removal, rather than insertion, of the device.

Removal of the EOA is almost always followed by immediate regurgitation of stomach contents.[3] Use of the EGTA decreases the likelihood of regurgitation but does not eliminate its possibility.

In unconscious or semiconscious patients, the EOA should not be removed until a cuffed endotracheal tube is in place.[3] In this manner, the lower airway can be protected from the possible aspiration of stomach contents that can occur with regurgitation.

In patients who are alert and breathing spontaneously, the EOA should be removed as soon as is practical. In these situations, the patient should be placed in a lateral or side-lying position to minimize the likelihood of aspiration. Suction equipment should also be available to assist in clearance of vomitus, should regurgitation occur.[12]

Endotracheal intubation. Endotracheal intubation is indicated during resuscitation efforts when (1) conventional methods fail to provide adequate ventilation to the unconscious patient, (2) the risks of aspiration are high, and (3) prolonged artificial ventilation is necessary.[3]

Once positioned properly, an endotracheal tube can maintain a patent airway, prevent aspiration of stomach contents, permit suctioning of the trachea and mainstem bronchi, facilitate ventilation and oxygenation, and provide a route for drug administration.[3] For this reason, endotracheal intubation is the preferred method of securing the airway during resuscitation efforts. However, attempts to intubate the trachea must never interfere with the provision of adequate ventilation and oxygenation by alternative means. Therefore, endotracheal intubation should be performed only by highly trained personnel. Moreover, no attempt at intubation of the trachea during resuscitation should last more than 30 seconds.[3]

Fig. 22-26 shows a cuffed orotracheal tube properly positioned in the trachea, being used in conjunction with a manual resuscitation device to provide ventilation and oxygenation. With this arrangement, ventilation no longer need be synchronized with chest compressions. Instead, adequate ventilation and oxygenation can be provided with 12 to 15 asynchronous breaths per minute.[49]

Respiratory care practitioners can and should be trained in endotracheal intubation techniques, as applied in both emergency life support and prolonged mechanical ventilation situations. Details on the necessary equipment, proce-

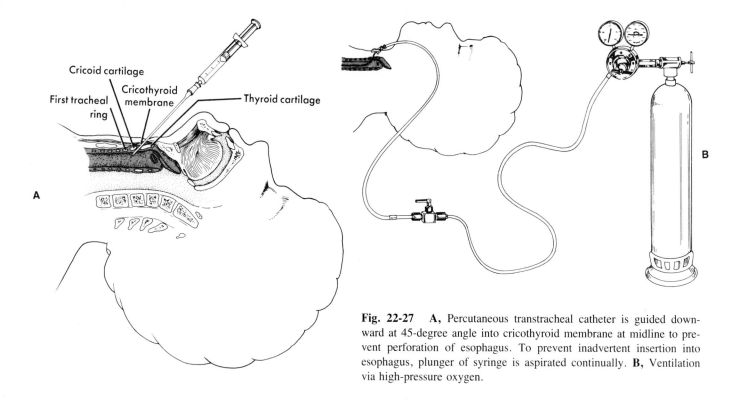

Fig. 22-27   A, Percutaneous transtracheal catheter is guided downward at 45-degree angle into cricothyroid membrane at midline to prevent perforation of esophagus. To prevent inadvertent insertion into esophagus, plunger of syringe is aspirated continually. **B,** Ventilation via high-pressure oxygen.

dure, and short- and long-term complications of endotracheal intubation are provided in Chapter 21.

Percutaneous routes. Situations sometimes arise in which the airway cannot be secured by endotracheal intubation. These include, but are not limited to, upper airway or laryngeal trauma, foreign body obstruction, and laryngospasm. In such cases, restoration of ventilation and oxygenation may depend on establishing an alternative airway route, one below the site of obstruction. Typically, these methods establish direct access to the trachea through a percutaneous route, that is, through the skin of the anterior neck.

The two most common methods of percutaneous airway access in emergencies are transtracheal catheterization and cricothyrotomy. Obviously, because such methods carry significant risks, they should be performed only by skilled personnel and then only after all other methods have failed.

Transtracheal catheterization. As shown in Fig. 22-27, *A,* transtracheal catheterization involves puncture of the cricothyroid membrane with a 12- to 16-gauge needle surrounded by a plastic catheter. Alternatively, the membrane immediately below the first tracheal ring may be used as the point of entry. In either case, the needle is guided at a 45-degree angle caudally into the trachea. Aspiration of air into the attached syringe confirms proper placement.

Once positioned in the trachea, the catheter is advanced over the needle until the hub reaches the puncture site, where it is stabilized. Ventilation is provided by connecting the catheter to a high-pressure (50 psi) oxygen source with a manual or automatic valving mechanism (Fig. 22-27, *B*).[50] In the "on" position, oxygen flows through the valve into the trachea under positive pressure, causing lung inflation. In the "off" position, the valve closes and the patient exhales normally through the nose and mouth.

Transtracheal catheterization is an extremely delicate procedure. Misplacement of the catheter into the esophagus can result in inadequate ventilation, not to mention gastric insufflation and regurgitation. Puncture of one of the many arteries in the region can result in hemorrhage. Subcutaneous and mediastinal emphysema are also possible results of incorrect placement. Nonetheless, when performed by appropriately trained personnel, transtracheal catheterization is a quick and effective means of providing oxygenation and ventilation when other methods fail.

Cricothyrotomy. A cricothyrotomy is a surgical procedure that opens a passageway through the cricothyroid membrane (Fig. 22-28). Once the opening is established, an endotracheal tube can be inserted directly into the trachea. As with transtracheal catheterization, cricothyrotomy represents a procedure of last resort in attempting to secure an obstructed airway.

Since cricothyrotomy establishes a larger opening than that possible with transtracheal catheterization, suctioning of the lower airway is possible with this method. On the other hand, even when performed by skilled personnel, cricothyrotomy can be more time-consuming than transtracheal catheterization. Moreover, incorrectly performed cricothyrotomy can cause permanent damage to the vocal cords. For these reasons, cricothyrotomy has generally been replaced by transtracheal catheterization as the preferred emergency method of dealing with persistent upper airway obstruction.

Fig. 22-28   Cricothyroidotomy.

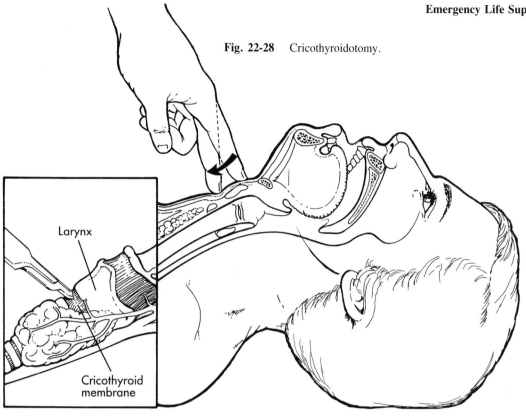

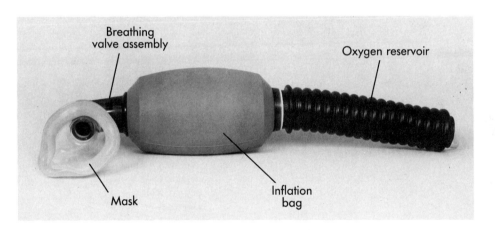

Fig. 22-29   Typical bag-valve-mask manual resuscitator.

Ventilation

Adjunctive equipment used to support ventilation in ACLS includes manual- and gas-powered resuscitators. Manual resuscitators, also called bag-valve devices, are available for adults, children, and infants. Gas-powered resuscitators, on the other hand, are strictly limited to adult application.[3]

Manual resuscitators. Manual resuscitators are devices that combine a self-inflating bag with a nonrebreathing valve mechanism.[51] Manual resuscitators may be used in conjunction with a face mask, endotracheal tube, or esophageal obturator airway. All provide ventilation with ambient air. When supplied with a supplementary oxygen source, up to 100% oxygen concentrations may be pro-

vided. Although initially designed as adjuncts for emergency life support, manual resuscitators are used extensively in other respiratory care settings, particularly in the areas of airway management and continuous mechanical ventilation.[51]

An ideal manual resuscitator should have a true nonrebreathing valve system capable of 15 L/min input flow without jamming and be able to provide up to 100% oxygen at high delivered stroke volumes and ventilation rates without limiting delivered pressure. Additionally, it should consist of materials that are easy to clean, have standard 15/22 mm connections, and be available in adult and pediatric sizes.[3,52,53] A typical manual resuscitator meeting these criteria is shown in Fig. 22-29. A comparison of the

Table 22-1   Summary of Characteristics of Self-Inflating Manual Resuscitators

Resuscitator	Type of patient valve	Type of bag inlet valve	Approximate volume of full bag
AMBU (early models)	Spring disk	Spring disk	2000 ml
Hope	Spring disk	One-way leaf valve	Adult, 2000 ml; pediatric, 730 ml
Penlon	Cupped disk	Spring disk	300 ml
Air Viva	Spring disk	—	2000 ml
Hope II	Spring ball	One-way leaf valve	Adult, 2000 ml; pediatric, 730 ml
AMBU E-2	Diaphragm	One-way leaf valve	Adult Mark II, 1300 ml; infant, 400 ml
Laerdal RFB-II, adult	Diaphragm and duck bill	One-way leaf valve	RFB-II, 1800 ml; adult, 1600 ml
Laerdal Child	Diaphragm and duck bill	One-way leaf valve	500 ml
Laerdal Infant	Diaphragm and duck bill	One-way leaf valve	240 ml
PMR	Diaphragm and leaf valve	Diaphragm	2000 ml
High Oxygen PMR	Diaphragm and leaf valve	Diaphragm and one-way leaf valve (air) or oxygen inlet	2000 ml
AIRbird	Diaphragm and leaf valve	One-way leaf valve	Adult, 2000 ml; pediatric, 500 ml
Hudson Lifesaver and Robertshaw Bag Resuscitators	Diaphragm and leaf valve	Leaf valve	Adult, 1800 ml; child, 600 ml
Hudson Lifesaver II, adult	Duck bill	One-way leaf valve	1600 ml
Hudson Lifesaver II, pediatric	Duck bill	One-way leaf valve	450 ml

From McPherson SP: Respiratory therapy equipment, ed 3, St Louis, 1985, The CV Mosby Co.

Maximum suggested oxygen flow rate	Type of oxygen reservoir	Maximum oxygen percentage expected with optimum conditions (%)	Type of pressure relief	Spontaneous breathing opens valve for oxygen (inhalator)
Less than 10 to 15 L/min to avoid valve jamming	Tube or bag with inlet one-way valve such as Laerdal's reservoir assembly	Up to 100	None	No
Less than 15 L/min to avoid valve sticking or chattering	Sleeve with tube or bag	Up to 100	Optional magnetic ball set to open at 40 cm H_2O	No
High oxygen flow rates will not affect proper function	Tube	Up to 100	Leak in cupped disk	No
5 L/min may cause chattering; 10 to 15 L/min may cause jamming of valve	None	Up to 80	Spring ball set to open near 40 cm H_2O bag pressure	No
High oxygen flows will not affect proper function	"Elephant" bore tube	Up to 100	Optional magnetic ball set to open at 40 cm H_2O	No
High flows may be used when unit is equipped with valve without affecting proper function	Tube or bag with inlet one-way valve such as Laerdal's reservoir assembly	Up to 100	Adult bag stretches at 70 cm H_2O; infant at 50 cm H_2O	Yes
High oxygen flows will not affect proper function	Tube or oxygen reservoir assembly	Up to 100	None	Yes
High oxygen flows will not affect proper function	Tube or oxygen reservoir assembly	Up to 100	Spring-loaded valve set to open near 35 cm H_2O bag pressure	Yes
High oxygen flows will not affect proper function	Tube or oxygen reservoir assembly	Up to 100	Spring-loaded valve set to open near 35 cm H_2O bag pressure	Yes
Oxygen flows up to 20 L/min will not affect proper function; flows from 20 to 50 L/min may cause some resistance to patient's exhalation	None commercially available	Up to 80	None	Yes
High oxygen flows will not affect proper function; low oxygen flows less than 12 L/min decrease bag refill and available breathing rates (high or low oxygen flows will not affect operation on modified unit)	None (tube on modified unit;)	Up to 100	None	Yes
High oxygen flows will not affect proper function	Tube or tube with bag and safety one-way valve inlet	Up to 100	Fixed orifice leak	Yes
With oxygen reservoir system, high flows will not affect proper function	Tube or tube with bag assembly may be added as modification; demand valve can also be attached	Up to 100	None	Yes
High flows will not affect proper function	Hudson's reservoir assembly with safety-inlet and outlet valves	Up to 100	None	Yes
High flows will not affect proper function	Hudson's reservoir assembly with safety-inlet and outlet valves	Up to 100	Spring-loaded valve set to open at 35 cm H_2O ± 5 cm H_2O	Yes

Fig. 22-30   Ventilation using bag-valve-mask and head-tilt/chin-lift method.

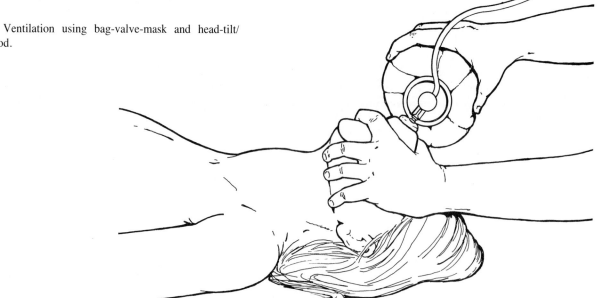

commonly available manual resuscitators in current use appears in Table 22-1.

Although all contemporary manual resuscitators listed can deliver 100% oxygen, the actual concentration provided depends on the interaction of several factors. These factors include oxygen input flow, reservoir volume, delivered stroke volume and rate, and bag refill time.[54-56]

Given the importance of delivering as high a concentration of oxygen as possible in cardiac or respiratory arrest situations, the respiratory care practitioner must be aware of the specific capabilities, appropriate use, and limitations of the manual resuscitator(s) normally used in emergency and critical care. As a general guideline, the practitioner should always use an oxygen reservoir, provide the highest acceptable oxygen input flow, and use the longest refill time that conditions allow.[51]

These guidelines notwithstanding, research shows that when manual resuscitators are used with masks, ventilation is less effective than when delivered by the mouth-to-mouth or mouth-to-mask technique.[46] This problem is due to the difficulty in maintaining an effective seal with the bag-valve-mask combination. Successful application of a manual resuscitator with a face mask requires practitioners to position themselves at the head of the patient, maintain extension of the patient's head and neck, keep the lower jaw elevated, and secure a tight seal all with one hand, while using the other hand to compress the bag (Fig. 22-30).

Obviously, extensive practice and training are required to apply this method effectively, and some individuals with small hands simply may not be able to achieve good ventilation with an appropriate seal. In such circumstances, the victim should immediately be ventilated by the mouth-to-mouth or mouth-to-mask technique or (if available) with a gas-powered resuscitator.

The major hazard associated with the use of manual resuscitators is the potential for pulmonary barotrauma.[57] Given that the full bag volume of the adult versions of these devices is generally no more than 2000 ml, the potential for barotrauma when applied to an adult is small. However, application of an adult manual resuscitator to a small child or infant is contraindicated. Moreover, some "pediatric" manual resuscitators have bag capacities in excess of 500 ml, clearly enough to cause barotrauma if applied to small children or infants. Ideally, to minimize the possibility of barotrauma when ventilating infants and small children, a pressure manometer should be used with the manual resuscitator.[3]

Gas-powered resuscitators. Gas-powered resuscitators are manually cycled, pressure-limited valves that are driven by a high-pressure compressed oxygen source.[51] Those incorporating a pressure-sensitive valve that responds to patient inspiratory effort are commonly called demand valves (Fig. 22-31). Like manual resuscitators, gas-powered resuscitators may be used in conjunction with a face mask, endotracheal tube, or esophageal obturator airway. Also like manual resuscitators, the use of these devices should be restricted to trained personnel. However, even when used by trained personnel, gas-powered resuscitators used in conjunction with a mask tend to cause gastric insufflation.[3]

An ideal gas-powered resuscitator should be able to provide 100% oxygen at instantaneous and constant flow of at least 40 L/min and incorporate a 60 cm H_2O inspiratory pressure relief valve with audible alarm. In addition, the trigger mechanism should allow both hands to be used to maintain the airway position and mask seal, and connections should employ the 15/22 mm standard.[58,59] Gas-powered resuscitators should never be used with children or infants.[3]

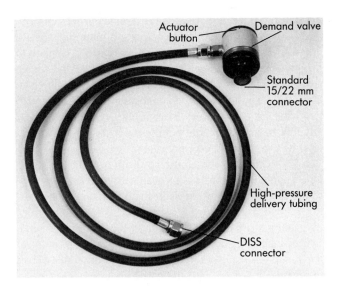

Fig. 22-31 Gas-powered resuscitator.

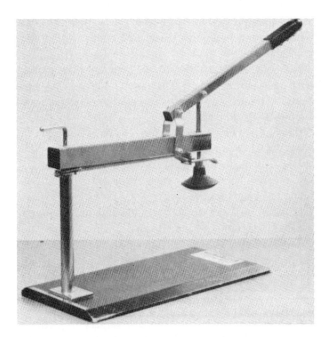

Fig. 22-32 Portable hand pump for external cardiac massage designed by Dr. James J. Lally. The plunger can be adjusted according to the individual's size. (From Stephenson HE Jr: Cardiac arrest and resuscitation, ed 4, St Louis, 1974, The CV Mosby Co.)

Perfusion support

The primary adjunctive equipment used to support perfusion in ACLS is the mechanical chest compressor. Additional approaches to perfusion support include internal cardiac compression, cardiopulmonary bypass, and intra-aortic balloon counterpulsation.

Mechanical compressors. Several types of mechanical compressors are available for use as an adjunct to manual chest compression. Properly applied, these devices can provide an optimum pattern of chest compression and eliminate the rapid fatigue that occurs with manual techniques.[60] Although models for children and infants have been marketed, the AHA currently recommends that manual compressors be used only with adults.[3]

The hazards of mechanical compressors are essentially the same as those common to manual chest compression, including the potential for separation of the ribs at the costochondral junction, sternal fractures, and organ lacerations. The major drawback in their use is the potential for delay or interruption in the application of manual chest compression while setting up or adjusting the apparatus.

The manually operated chest compressor consists of a simple, reliable, and low-cost lever device that is easy to set up and use (Fig. 22-32). Ideally, the user should be able to adjust the movement of the plunger head from 1.5 to 2.0 inches.[3]

The pneumatic mechanical chest compressor is powered by compressed gas and provides user-adjustable rates, plunger displacements, and compression-to-relaxation ratios (Fig. 22-33). Most pneumatic mechanical chest compressors can provide ventilation through an automatically cycled, pressure-limited valve similar to the gas-powered

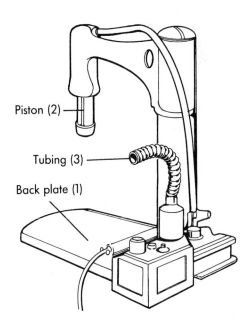

Fig. 22-33 Pneumatically powered chest compressor.

resuscitators previously described. These compressor-ventilators are most effective when used with a cuffed endotracheal tube.[3]

The bulk of these automatic devices can limit mobility when the victim must be transported, and constant monitoring by trained personnel is essential to maintain correct position of the plunger.

Internal cardiac compression. In some situations, external cardiac compression cannot be accomplished effectively. As indicated in the box below, these situations usually involve one or more abnormalities of the thorax, lungs, heart, or great vessels.[11]

In these cases, restoration of circulation may require internal cardiac compression. Internal cardiac compression, performed only by a skilled surgeon, requires exposure of the pericardium by thoracotomy and direct manual compression of the heart by the surgeon's hand (Fig. 22-34).

Because it requires a major surgical procedure, internal cardiac compression carries with it all the risks common to both surgery in general and thoracic surgery in particular. These risks include operative trauma, hemorrhage, and infection. However, such risks are small compared with the likely outcome if internal cardiac compression is not performed. Of course, internal cardiac compression is performed only in the hospital setting by a qualified surgeon.

Cardiopulmonary bypass (extracorporeal circulation). Cardiopulmonary bypass, using a pump-oxygenator or "heart-lung machine," has been successfully applied to restore circulation after cardiac arrest caused by certain specific conditions such as massive pulmonary embolism. Obviously, application of this approach is limited to centers where it is available. Even in these centers, the time required to institute cardiopulmonary bypass tends to prohibit its use as an emergency support measure.

Intra-aortic balloon counterpulsation. Intra-aortic balloon counterpulsation is a mechanical procedure designed to increase mean aortic pressures and coronary blood flow to the myocardium during diastole. This is accomplished by placing a gas-actuated balloon in the descending aorta. Synchronous inflation of the balloon after left ventricular contraction provides a forceful counterpulsation that boosts retrograde flow back into the aortic arch and coronary arteries (Fig. 22-35). Since this counterpulsation only augments existing left ventricular function, the intra-aortic balloon cannot, by itself, provide adequate perfusion during true cardiac arrest.

INDICATIONS FOR INTERNAL CARDIAC COMPRESSION

ABNORMALITIES OF THORAX AND LUNG

Pectus excavatum
Pectus carinatum
Flail chest
Intrathoracic hemorrhage
Bilateral pneumothorax
Tension pneumothorax

ABNORMALITIES OF GREAT VESSELS AND HEART

Massive air embolism
Massive pulmonary embolism
Cardiac tamponade
Failure of external chest compression
Severe mitral stenosis
Ventricular aneurysm
Refractory ventricular fibrillation
Myocardial laceration
Tetanic heart
Position of heart not in midline

OTHER

Open-chest surgery
Lack of defibrillator during episodes of ventricular fibrillation
Pregnancy (third trimester)

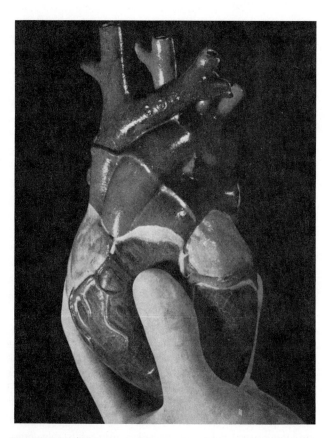

Fig. 22-34   With apex of heart cupped in practitioner's palm, fingers are extended toward base of heart posteriorly and thumb is extended toward base of heart anteriorly for internal cardiac compression. (From Stephenson HE Jr: Cardiac arrest and resuscitation, ed 4, St Louis, 1974, The CV Mosby Co.)

Currently, this device is used mainly to provide interim support for (1) patients with mechanical failure of the left ventricle that is surgically correctable or (2) patients exhibiting poor ventricular function after coronary bypass surgery.

Restoration of cardiac function

Perfusion support techniques are designed to restore circulation only on an interim basis. ACLS must go beyond simple perfusion support and attempt to identify, remove, or alleviate the underlying cause of cardiac failure. This is

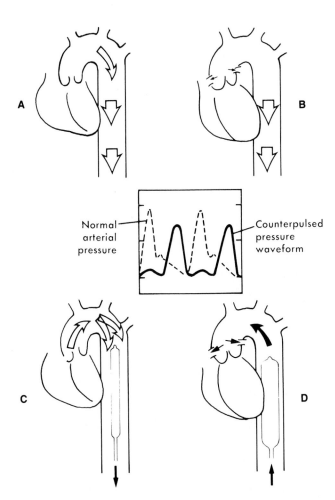

Fig. 22-35 Physiology of counterpulsation. Diagram of normal cardiac cycle pressure flow sequence compared with counterpulsed pressure flow sequence. **A,** Normal systole, characterized by antegrade volume flow and peak intra-aortic pressures. **B,** Normal diastole, showing continued antegrade volume flow and adequate intra-aortic pressure for coronary perfusion. **C,** Balloon deflation before systole, allowing antegrade volume flow from the aortic arch (systolic unloading). **D,** Counterpulsed diastole, mechanically boosting volume flow retrograde to the aortic arch, heightening diastolic pressure and coronary perfusion. (From Schroeder JS and Daily EK: Techniques in bedside hemodynamic monitoring, St Louis, 1976, The CV Mosby Co.)

accomplished by combining ECG monitoring with drug administration and selected electrical therapies.

Electrocardiographic monitoring. Because most sudden deaths of cardiac origin are caused by electrical abnormalities, or arrhythmias, of the heart, ECG monitoring should be initiated as soon as the appropriate equipment and personnel are available.[3] This may be accomplished with standard ECG equipment or the sensing paddles now available on many defibrillators.

Given their important role in ACLS, it is essential that respiratory care practitioners be skilled in arrhythmia recognition. Although the experienced practitioner will become adept at quick visual interpretation of gross arrhythmias appearing on ECG monitors at the bedside, these skills only develop after much practice with actual rhythm "strips."

Comprehensive examination of ECG rhythm strips proceeds through four systematic steps. First, the heart rate is calculated, using the number of RR intervals in a given time span (usually at least 6 seconds). Then, again using the RR interval, the regularity of the rhythm is determined. Next, the presence or absence of P waves, their shape, and the duration of the PR interval are determined. Last, the QRS complex is inspected and its duration measured.

Without attempting an exhaustive analysis, we will provide an overview of the most common arrhythmias encountered in clinical practice, emphasizing the life-threatening examples. Table 22-2 provides a brief summary of these common arrhythmias and their key features, categorized by the site at which they originate.[61,62] We will limit our discussion of these key features to the following rhythm disturbances: sinus arrhythmia, sinus bradycardia, sinus tachycardia, sinoatrial arrest, premature atrial contractions, paroxysmal supraventricular tachycardia, atrial flutter, atrial fibrillation, atrioventricular block, premature ventricular contractions, ventricular tachycardia (including the variant called torsade de pointes), and ventricular fibrillation.

Sinus arrhythmia (Fig. 22-36). Sinus arrhythmia is the most frequent and least harmful of all arrhythmias, occurring most frequently in the young but found at almost any age. Its distinguishing characteristic is simply an irregular but rhythmic change in cardiac rate synchronous with the respiratory cycle.[61,62] Typically, the heart rate is observed to increase during inspiration and decrease during expiration. Otherwise the overall rate, P wave, PR interval, and QRS complex are normal. Sinus arrhythmia can be exaggerated by inspiratory breath holding and eliminated by exercise. Presumably, sinus arrhythmia is caused by alterations in the strength of vagal (parasympathetic) tone on the sinus node. This condition has no pathologic implications, and no treatment is indicated.

Sinus tachycardia (Fig. 22-37). In sinus tachycardia, the sinus node discharges at rates between 100 to 160 per

Table 22-2   Summary of Common Cardiac Arrhythmias

Arrhythmia	Category	Rate	Rhythm	P waves	PR interval	QRS complex	Treatment	Comments
Sinus arrhythmia	Benign	60–100/min	Irregular	Normal	Normal	Normal	None	Heart rate periodically increases and decreases
Sinus tachycardia	Minor	100–160/min	Regular	Normal	Normal	Normal	Remove underlying cause; digitalis or beta blockers	May result from sympathetic stimulation or parasympathetic inhibition; also increased metabolic rates, hypoxemia
Sinus bradycardia	Minor	40–60/min	Regular	Normal	Normal	Normal	Remove underlying cause; atropine	May result from excessive parasympathetic stimulation
Sinoatrial arrest	Minor	60–100/min; lower with missed beats	Regular except missed beat	Normal	Normal	Normal	None unless frequent; treat underlying cause	May result from excessive parasympathetic stimulation
Premature atrial contractions	< 6 min/minor > 6/min major	60–100/min	Regular except PAC	PAC p-wave abnormal	PAC PR may be <0.12	Normal	<6/min none; >6/min antiarrhythmics such as lidocaine	Caused by atrial irritability; no compensatory pause (compare with PVCs)
Paroxysmal supraventricular tachycardia	Major	160–250/min	Regular	May be hidden or abnormal	Difficult to assess	Normal; some may be widened	Carotid artery massage; tranquilizers, adrenergic antagonists, digitalis, procainamide; synchronous cardioversion	Caused by atrial irritability; may compromise ventricular filling
Atrial flutter	Major	atrial: 200–400/min ventricular: 60–150/min	Depends on conduction (regular or irregular)	"F" waves sawtooth pattern	Difficult to assess	Normal	Carotid artery massage; tranquilizers, adrenergic antagonists, digitalis, procainamide; synchronous cardioversion	Ratio of blocked to transmitted impulses may be constant at 2:1, 3:1, or 4:1

Arrhythmia	Severity	Rate	Rhythm	P wave	PR interval	QRS	Treatment	Comments
Atrial fibrillation	Major	atrial: > 350/min ventricular: variable	Markedly irregular	Indistinguishable; uneven baseline	Indistinguishable;	Normal	Synchronous cardioversion; digitalis, propranolol	May compromise ventricular filling, resulting in pulse deficit
First degree atrioventricular block	Major	60–100/min	Regular	Normal	PR > 0.20	Normal	Isoproterenol, atropine	Delayed AV nodal conduction; may be caused by ischemia or digitalis
Second degree atrioventricular block (Mobitz type 2)	Major	60–100/min	Regular	Normal; some not conducted	Normal or prolonged; fixed PR	Normal; some dropped at regular ratio (3:2, 4:3, etc)	Electrical pacemaker	Most often caused by ischemia; may progress to 3rd degree
Second degree atrioventricular block (Wenckebach type)	Major	60–100/min	Irregular	Normal; some not conducted	Progressive increase in PR time	Normal; some dropped at regular ratio (3:2, 4:3, etc)	Isoproterenol, atropine; electrical pacemaker	Most often caused by ischemia; may progress to 3rd degree
Third degree atrioventricular block	Major; can be lethal	atrial may be normal ventricular: < 40/min	Regular but AV separate	Normal	Cannot be determined	Usually normal; may be widened	Electrical pacemaker	May result in episodes of cerebral ischemia
Premature ventricular contractions	< 6/min minor > 6/min major	60–100/min	Regular except PVC	Normal; none with PVC	Normal; none with PVC	>0.12 sec; distorted	Antiarrhythmics such as lidocaine	indicates ventricular irritability; compensatory pause is normal RT wave leads to ventricular tachycardia
Ventricular tachycardia	Major; can be lethal	140–200/min	Usually regular	Absent or hidden	Absent or hidden	Continuous PVCs; same amplitude	Antiarrhythmics; countershock	May compromise ventricular filling & cause shock; can resolve itself
Torsade de pointes	Major; can be lethal	140–200/min	Usually regular	Absent or hidden	Absent or hidden	Continuous PVCs; changing axis and amplitude	Antiarrhythmics; countershock	A more serious form of ventricular tachycardia
Ventricular fibrillation	Lethal	Cannot be determined	Cannot be determined	Absent	Absent	Chaotic; no defined pattern	Countershock; defibrillation	No cardiac output

II

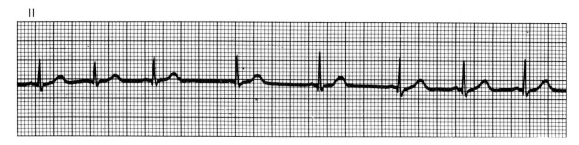

Fig. 22-36 Sinus arrhythmia. (From Conover MH: Cardiac arrhythmias: exercises in pattern interpretation, ed 2, St Louis, 1978, The CV Mosby Co.)

V_1

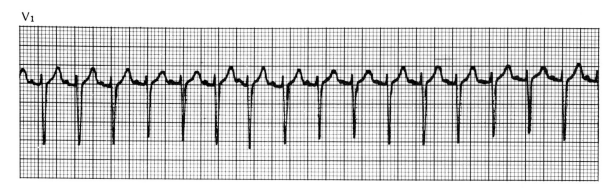

Fig. 22-37 Sinus tachycardia. (From Conover MH: Cardiac arrhythmias: exercises in pattern interpretation, ed 2, St Louis, 1978, The CV Mosby Co.)

II

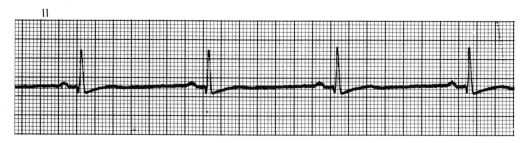

Fig. 22-38 Sinus bradycardia. (From Conover MH: Cardiac arrhythmias: exercises in pattern interpretation, ed 2, St Louis, 1978, The CV Mosby Co.)

minute. Typically, the rhythm is regular, and the P waves, PR interval, and QRS complex are normal.[61-62]

Alone or combined, physiologic, pharmacologic, or pathologic factors may contribute to the sinus node's increased rate of impulse formation. Sympathetic stimulation (fear, anxiety, pain, adrenal release of epinephrine, adrenergic drugs) is the most common cause of sinus tachycardia. Parasympathetic inhibition, like that caused by atropine and its derivatives, will have a similar effect. Increased metabolic demand, such as may occur with fever, severe burns, or hyperthyroidism, can also contribute to an increase sinus node discharge rate. Sinus tachycardia can also be caused by hypoxemia, hypercapnea, and any condition that results in a decrease in arterial blood pressure,

such as shock, congestive heart failure, acute myocardial infarction, and pulmonary embolism.

Treatment of sinus tachycardia is directed at removing the underlying cause. Among the drug agents that may be used to slow the heart rate when other approaches fail are digitalis preparations and beta-adrenergic blocking agents such as propranolol.

Sinus bradycardia *(Fig. 22-38).* In sinus bradycardia, the sinus node discharges at rates less than 60 per minute. Typically, the rhythm is regular, and the P waves, PR interval, and QRS complex are normal.[61]

As with sinus tachycardia, various physiologic, pharmacologic, or pathologic factors may contribute to the sinus node's decreased rate of impulse formation. Indeed, heart

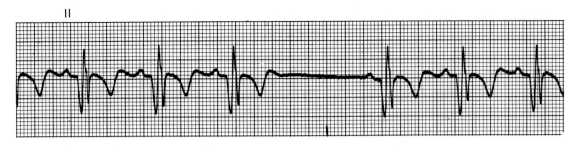

Fig. 22-39 Sinus arrest. (From Conover MH: Cardiac arrhythmias: exercises in pattern interpretation, ed 2, St Louis, 1978, The CV Mosby Co.)

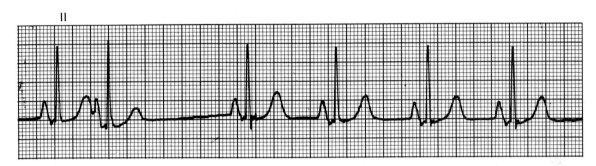

Fig. 22-40 Premature atrial contraction. (From Conover MH: Cardiac arrhythmias: exercises in pattern interpretation, ed 2, St Louis, 1978, The CV Mosby Co.)

rates less than 60 per minute are not uncommon in highly conditioned athletes. In the clinical setting, however, sinus bradycardia is most often associated with an increased level of parasympathetic tone, as may be produced by vagal stimulation or adrenergic blocking agents. Hypothermia and increased intracranial pressure may also contribute to a decreased rate of sinus impulse formation.

Normally, treatment of sinus bradycardia is directed at removing the underlying cause. Pharmacologic agents that increase the heart rate (positive chronotropic agents) may be used to reverse a sinus bradycardia. These include adrenergic drugs such as isoproterenol and anticholinergics such as atropine.

Sinoatrial arrest (Fig. 22-39). Although sinoatrial arrest can result in sudden cardiac standstill, more commonly it manifests itself simply as an infrequent dropped beat.[61,62] Thus the rate is normal (unless beats are dropped frequently), the rhythm is regular except for the missing beat, and P waves, PR intervals, and QRS complexes (where they appear) are all normal.

The basic defect of sinoatrial arrest is the failure of the sinus node to initiate an impulse, such as may occur when overwhelming vagal impulses suppress the node. Usually this is a transient phenomenon, but under certain pathologic conditions, failure of the sinoatrial node to generate an action potential can result in cardiac arrest. Death is obvious unless excitation can be resumed.

Sinus arrest is likely to accompany the early stages of anesthesia or certain bodily manipulations that elicit a strong vagal reflex. These include instrumentation during such examination of body cavities as cystoscopy, bronchoscopy, or pharyngeal probing and occasionally traction on thoracic organs during surgery. Prolonged sinus arrest is normally reversed with appropriate electrical therapy (see next section). Although controversial, mechanical stimulus, such as that provided by a sharp blow to the sternum (precordial thump) may also reverse asystole.[3,63]

Premature atrial contractions (Fig. 22-40). As described in Chapter 7, any area of the heart can initiate an action potential. Localized areas of the atria, atrioventricular node, and ventricular myocardium are the most common source for such independent excitation. Because they occur away from the normal focus of stimulation, they are referred to as *ectopic foci.*

The underlying cause of premature atrial contractions (PACs) is an increased excitability of the affected area of the myocardium or conducting system.[61,62] Although strong sympathetic stimulation is a prime offender in causing premature contractions, the presence or release of a variety of chemical or humoral agents can contribute to the development of an ectopic focus.

A premature atrial contraction typically occurs at normal cardiac rates. Because the action potential arises from other than the sinus node, the P wave often differs in shape from that of the normal sinus rhythm. Although a normal QRS follows the abnormal P wave, there may be a

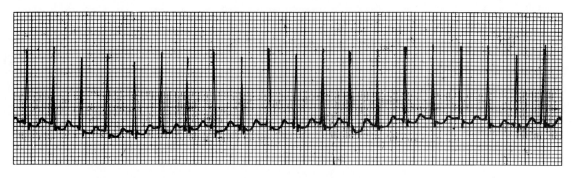

Fig. 22-41   Paroxysmal supraventricular tachycardia. (From Conover MH: Cardiac arrhythmias: exercises in pattern interpretation, ed 2, St Louis, 1978, The CV Mosby Co.)

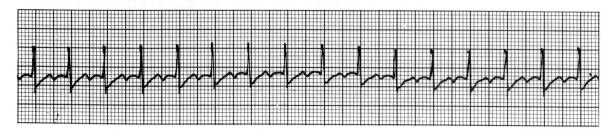

Fig. 22-42   Atrial flutter with 2:1 atrioventricular conductions. (From Conover MH: Cardiac arrhythmias: exercises in pattern interpretation, ed 2, St Louis, 1978, The CV Mosby Co.)

slight delay before the next normal sinus discharge, but this delay is substantially shorter than the compensatory pause associated with a premature ventricular contraction (PVC).[61] Thus, except for the PAC itself, the rhythm is essentially regular. In general, PACs occurring at rates of less than six per minute are not treated; frequencies above this usually demand intervention with an antiarrhythmic drug (see following section). More ominous are multifocal PACs, represent the frequent discharge of several different ectopic foci in the atrial myocardium.

Paroxysmal supraventricular tachycardia (Fig. 22-41). Bursts or sustained chains of premature contractions originating from above the atrioventricular (AV) node constitute paroxysmal supraventricular tachycardia (PSVT). During an attack, the cardiac rate may range from 160 to 250 per minute.[61] The rhythm is usually regular, is not affected by breathing or exercise, and may terminate abruptly. Because of the frequency of atrial discharge, P waves may be hidden in the QRS complex or T wave. Those visible are usually abnormal in shape. However, a QRS complex usually follows each atrial discharge; some of these may be widened (longer than 0.10 second).

At the high range of PSVT rates, there may be insufficient time for ventricular filling during diastole, thereby compromising cardiac output and potentially causing congestive failure. Vagal stimulation by carotid artery massage may halt this arrhythmia, but often pharmacologic intervention is necessary. Sedatives, adrenergic antagonists,

cholinergic stimulators, or direct cardiac suppressors may be used to convert PSVT to a normal sinus rhythm. PSVT resistant to drug treatment is usually treated by applying synchronous electrical stimulation to the myocardium, a procedure called *cardioversion* (subsequently described).[61]

Atrial flutter (Fig. 22-42). Atrial flutter is named for the flutterlike or sawtooth pattern seen on the ECG. It is caused by either a rapid circular movement of a stimulus or a repetitive single ectopic focus exciting the atria with a clocklike regularity at rates between 200 to 400 beats per minute. True P waves are absent, being replaced by the characteristic "F" or flutter waves.

Because the AV node cannot usually transmit more than 180 impulses per minute, many of the atrial signals are blocked. The ratio of blocked to transmitted impulses may be constant in a given instance, such as 2:1, 3:1, or 4:1.[61] Actual ventricular rates vary with the degree of block, ranging from 60 to 150 per minute, and can be irregular with variable block.

Flutter is usually caused by disease, and, even with a partial block, the ventricular rate may be high enough to compromise cardiac filling and emptying. Treatment, directed at the underlying cause, is similar to that employed to convert paroxysmal atrial tachycardia.

Atrial fibrillation (Fig. 22-43). Atrial fibrillation is the most common of the significant abnormal rhythm disturbances and is the usual end point of a preexisting flutter, although a flutter is not a prerequisite. The atria are subject

V₁

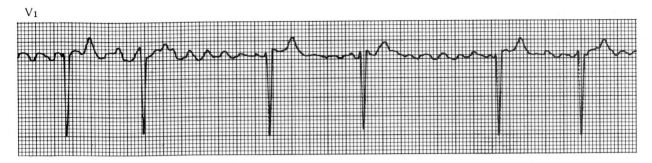

Fig. 22-43 Atrial fibrillation. (From Conover MH: Cardiac arrhythmias: exercises in pattern interpretation, ed 2, St Louis, 1978, The CV Mosby Co.)

to a completely uncontrolled, randomly irregular barrage of impulses at rates above 350 per minute, effectively precluding a coordinated contraction. P waves and PR intervals are indistinguishable, being replaced by irregular undulations of the isoelectric baseline. The AV node transmits as many of these as it can, resulting in a chaotic and irregular ventricular response. Some ventricular contractions are too weak to be palpated in the peripheral pulses, causing a discrepancy between the cardiac rate as counted over the chest and the rate of arterial pulsations. This phenomenon, called a *pulse deficit,* is a cardinal clinical sign of atrial fibrillation.[62]

Fairly normal activity is not incompatible with atrial fibrillation, as long as the ventricular rates remain controlled. However, fibrillation of the atrial walls can result in ineffective ejection of blood from their chambers. Retention of blood in these chambers raises the risk of blood clotting or thrombus formation and subsequent embolization. For this reason, attempts are usually made to convert atrial fibrillation to normal sinus rhythm by drug intervention or cardioversion.

Atrioventricular block *(Figs. 22-44 to 22-46).* Disorders of the myocardium caused by inflammation, infarction, or arteriosclerotic ischemia can reduce or destroy the ability of the AV node or the bundle of His to transmit sinus impulses to the ventricles.[61] A similar effect is caused by the toxic reaction of the myocardium to digitalis or its derivatives. Depending on the severity of the conduction impairment, three levels of AV block are recognized. In order of their relative severity, these are termed first-degree, second-degree, and third-degree heart block.

If the only abnormality is a prolonged PR interval (greater than 0.20 seconds), the block is considered first degree (see Fig. 22-44). If some atrial impulses are conducted but others are dropped—resulting in two or three times as many P waves as QRS complexes—the block is termed second degree (see Fig. 22-45). If no atrial impulses are conducted to the ventricles, the block is considered third degree or "complete" (see Fig. 22-46).[61]

If not for the ability of the ventricles to develop their own pacemaker, third-degree heart block would always be

fatal. Normally, an area of the ventricles does develop a pacemaker potential. However, this ventricular pacemaker tends to discharge at much slower rates than the normal sinus node, typically between 25 to 40 beats per minute. Under conditions of stress, or in the presence of other arrhythmias, this bradycardia may be inadequate for cerebral blood flow. Acute unconsciousness may occur without warning, resulting in Stokes-Adams syncope (fainting). Convulsions and death may accompany such episodes.

First- and second-degree AV block are generally managed with pharmacologic agents, specifically adrenergic stimulators or anticholinergic agents. When ventricular rates fall below 60 beats per minute, as in advanced second- and third-degree block, an electronic pacemaker may be indicated.[62] However, pacemakers are generally ineffective in cardiac arrest situations and are therefore not recommended as a component of ACLS.[3]

Premature ventricular contractions *(Fig. 22-47).* A premature ventricular contraction (PVC) occurs when an ectopic focus in the ventricular myocardium initiates a spontaneous depolarization. Since a PVC starts at the opposite end of the conduction chain, its path through the ventricular muscle is grossly abnormal. The result is a widened and distorted QRS complex and often an irregular T wave. Rates are generally normal and the rhythm regular except for the premature beat. P waves and PR intervals are normal in sinus beats but missing during the premature depolarization.

The distinguishing characteristic of PVCs is the longer than normal refractory period they impart to myocardial fibers.[61,62] Because the extra ectopic stimulus occurs out of phase, it interferes with the usual sequence of excitability and refractoriness and causes a lag before the next following contraction. This is called a *compensatory pause.* The interval between the premature beat and the next normal one is usually twice as long as the interval between two normal beats.

PVCs are caused by an increased excitability of the ventricles, due either to increased sympathetic stimulation or to local factors causing increased myocardial irritability. Symptoms may be absent, or the patient may complain of

V₁

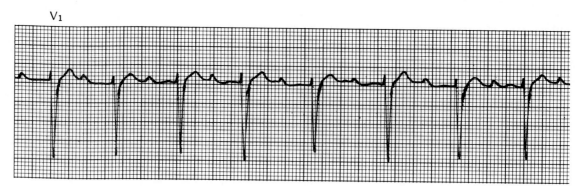

Fig. 22-44 First-degree heart block. (From Conover MH: Cardiac arrhythmias: exercises in pattern interpretation, ed 2, St Louis, 1978, The CV Mosby Co.)

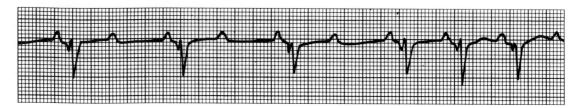

Fig. 22-45 Second-degree heart block (Mobitz type II). (From Conover MH: Cardiac arrhythmias: exercises in pattern interpretation, ed 2, St Louis, 1978, The CV Mosby Co.)

V₁

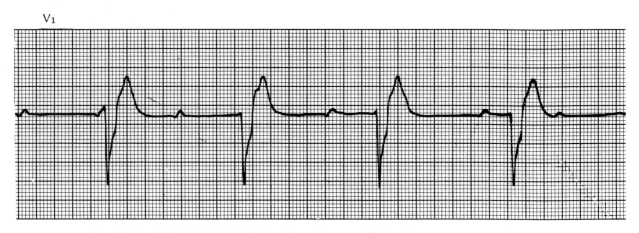

Fig. 22-46 Third-degree heart block. (From Conover MH: Cardiac arrhythmias: exercises in pattern interpretation, ed 2, St Louis, 1978, The CV Mosby Co.)

II

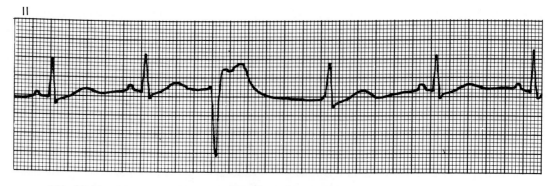

Fig. 22-47 Premature ventricular contraction. (From Conover MH: Cardiac arrhythmias: exercises in pattern interpretation, ed 2, St Louis, 1978, The CV Mosby Co.)

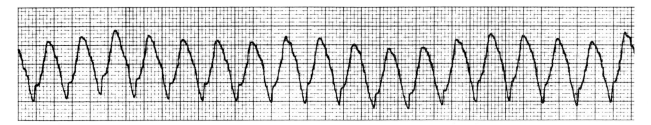

Fig. 22-48 Ventricular tachycardia. (From Conover MB: Exercises in diagnosing ECG tracings, ed 3, St Louis, 1984, The CV Mosby Co.)

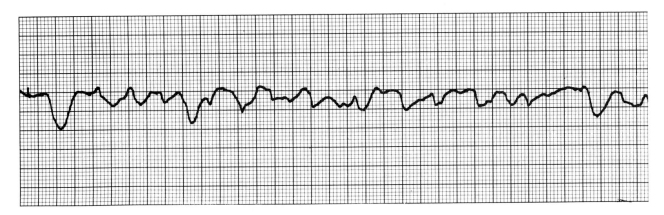

Fig. 22-49 Ventricular fibrillation. (From Conover MH: Cardiac arrhythmias: exercises in pattern interpretation, ed 2, St Louis, 1978, The CV Mosby Co.)

"palpitations" or a "thumping" in the chest. The patient may actually be aware of the absence of heart action during the compensatory pause as well as the difference in contractile force between normal and some abnormal beats.

The clinical significance of PVCs generally depends on the patient's tolerance of them, their frequency, and the presence or absence of underlying disease. Infrequently occurring unifocal PVCs are commonly observed in clinical practice and may not require treatment. Aggressive treatment is called for if the PVCs (1) are frequent (greater than six per minute), (2) originate from multiple foci, (3) occur close to the T wave, or (3) alternate with normal sinus beats, producing coupled rhythms called bigeminy or trigeminy.[62]

Treatment of PVCs includes the use of antiarrhythmic agents.[61] Ventricular ectopic foci are generally not responsive to parasympathetic stimulation, as are those arising from the atria. This is because the ventricles have little or no parasympathetic innervation.

Ventricular tachycardia (Fig. 22-48). Ventricular tachycardia occurs when one or more irritable foci within the ventricular myocardium discharge at rapid rates, creating the appearance of a prolonged chain of PVCs. Rates

typically range from 140 to 200 beats per minute and may be regular. Because of the dissociation of atrial and ventricular conduction, P waves may be buried in the QRS complex and therefore not easily discernible.[61] A variant of ventricular tachycardia, called *torsade de pointes,* is characterized by gradual alteration in the amplitude and direction of the electrical activity of the ventricles.[64]

Although it may occur in brief paroxysms and spontaneously end, ventricular tachycardia is always a sign of a serious underlying pathologic condition requiring aggressive and immediate treatment. Initial treatment of recurrent paroxysms of ventricular tachycardia is generally similar to the drug management of PVCs.[62] Torsade de pointes, on the other hand, is best treated by electrical pacing.[3] If pharmacologic management fails, or if the patient exhibits signs of circulatory failure, unsynchronized countershock may be necessary.

Ventricular fibrillation (Fig. 22-49). So grave as to be imminently fatal if not quickly corrected, ventricular fibrillation represents a rapid, sustained, and uncontrolled depolarization of the ventricular myocardium. The ECG is characterized by irregular, widened, and poorly defined QRS complexes. Rather than exhibiting coordinated contractions, the ventricles quiver in a totally disorganized manner, effectively reducing cardiac output to zero.

Frequently preceded by persistent or recurring ventricular paroxysmal tachycardia, fibrillation can be caused by many conditions, among which are electric shock, anesthesia, mechanical irritation of the heart, severe hypoxia, myocardial infarction, and large doses of digitalis or epinephrine. The rapid drop in cardiac output produces an acute cerebral hypoxia, often manifested by convulsions. Death ensues within a few minutes.

From a functional viewpoint, ventricular fibrillation may be considered a form of "cardiac arrest," for although there is some ventricular activity, it is of no value. This abnormality, like prolonged sinus arrest, constitutes a true emergency, with survival dependent on immediate initiation of ACLS measures, including appropriate electrical therapy.

Drug intervention. Although the full scope of drug usage in ACLS is beyond the scope of this chapter, respiratory care practitioners must have general knowledge of both the various drug categories and specific agents used in emergencies. To this end, we will summarize current pharmacologic management of emergency cardiovascular problems.

Routes of administration. Unless a central vein is already cannulated, the ideal route for drug administration in emergency life support situations is a peripheral intravenous (IV) line, preferably achieved through cannulation of an antecubital fossa vein.[3] Epinephrine, lidocaine, and atropine may also be administered through an endotracheal tube. Direct intracardiac injection is indicated only for epinephrine, and then only if the IV or endotracheal route is unavailable.

Major drug categories and agents. Table 22-3 summarizes the major drug categories and primary agents currently used in ACLS. These include analgesics, antiarrhythmics, chronotropics, inotropics, vasoactive agents, and buffers.

Analgesics. Morphine sulfate is the primary analgesic agent employed in ACLS. Besides being effective against the pain and anxiety common with myocardial infarction, morphine sulfate increases venous capacitance, decreases venous return, and causes a mild dilation of the arterial vasculature.[65] These secondary actions of morphine are particularly useful in the treatment of acute pulmonary edema and pulmonary vascular congestion.[3]

Antiarrhythmics. Antiarrhythmic drugs are used mainly to control ventricular arrhythmias caused by ectopic foci, such as frequent PVCs and ventricular tachycardia. They may also be useful in increasing the heart's response to electrical therapy (discussed later).[3]

The primary agents in this category are lidocaine, procainamide hydrochloride, and bretylium tosylate. Based on its proven safety and efficacy, lidocaine is the antiarrhythmic drug of first choice. Procainamide hydrochloride is recommended when lidocaine is contraindicated or is inef-

fective in controlling ventricular ectopic beats.[3] Bretylium tosylate is a newer agent with complex cardiovascular effects. In addition to its antiarrhythmic effects, bretylium tosylate causes catecholamines to be released into the circulation, followed by blockage of the postganglionic adrenergic receptors, potentially causing hypotension.[66] For these reason, bretylium tosylate generally is recommended only if lidocaine, procainamide, and defibrillation have already been used without success.[3]

Chronotropic and inotropic agents. Chronotropics are drugs that effect a change in heart rate. Inotropics affect the contractility of the myocardium. Positive "tropics" tend to increase heart rate or contractility, while negative "tropics" have the opposite effect. Most of these agents work by stimulating or inhibiting the autonomic nervous system, as described in Chapter 20. For this reason, their effects often extend beyond direct action on the myocardium to include vasomotor effects.

The primary positive chronotropic agent used in ACLS is atropine, a parasympatholytic drug used to treat sinus bradycardia, AV nodal block, and ventricular asystole. Epinephrine hydrochloride has a comparable effect but acts mainly through alpha-adrenergic stimulation. Epinephrine also has positive inotropic and vasomotor activity and enhances the fibrillating heart's response to electrical countershock.

Propranolol hydrochloride, a beta-adrenergic blocking agent effective against supraventricular tachycardia, is the model negative chronotropic drug. Verapamil also has negative chronotropic effects but works by blocking the calcium channels in the myocardial fibrils. Verapamil can cause hypotension and worsen congestive heart failure.

Isoproterenol hydrochloride is a sympathomimetic amine with powerful positive inotropic and chronotropic effects. Because it tends to increase myocardial work, worsen preexisting ischemia, and increase the occurrence of certain arrhythmias, isoproterenol hydrochloride is generally contraindicated in ACLS. The exception to this rule is a significant bradycardia unresponsive to atropine.[3]

Like isoproterenol hydrochloride, dobutamine hydrochloride is a beta-adrenergic catecholamine. Unlike isoproterenol, it is primarily a positive inotropic agent and is therefore useful in stimulating increased myocardial contractility. It can, however, induce a reflex vasodilation and, in sufficient dosage, cause tachycardia and worsen preexisting ischemia.

Calcium (chloride or gluconate) tends to exert a positive inotropic effect on isolated myocardial tissue, but its role in enhancing heart contractility in cardiac arrest is not proven.[67] Calcium is therefore indicated only in the presence of confirmed hyperkalemia or when toxicity to calcium channel blockers, such as verapamil, is evident.

Vasoactive agents. Vasoactive agents are employed in ACLS for their effect on peripheral vascular tone. Vaso-

Table 22-3 Drug Agents Used in Advanced Life Support

Drug	Indications	Contraindications	Preparation	Route	Dosage	Pharmacologic effects
Lidocaine HCl	Ventricular tachycardia, hyper-excitable myocardium, multi-focal PVCs, ventricular fibrillation	Heart block, asystole, EMD	Variable	IV bolus IV drip Intracardiac Endotracheal	1 mg/kg bolus 20–60 µg/kg/min	Raises electrical stimulation threshold Depresses ventricular electrical activity
Procainamide HCl	Ventricular tachycardia, hyper-excitable myocardium, multi-focal PVCs, ventricular fibrillation	Heart block, asystole, EMD	100 mg/ml (10 ml unit)	IV bolus IV drip	50 mg bolus (every 5 min) 1–4 mg/min drip	Raises electrical stimulation threshold Depresses ventricular electrical activity May cause hypotension
Bretylium tosylate	Ventricular tachycardia, hyper-excitable myocardium, multi-focal PVCs, ventricular fibrillation	Heart block, asystole, EMD	50 mg/ml (10 ml unit)	IV bolus	5 mg/kg in 50 to 100 ml diluent over 5–10 min	Raises electrical stimulation threshold Depresses ventricular electrical activity May cause hypotension
Atropine sulfate	Idioventricular rhythms, nodal bradycardia, electromechanical dissociation (EMD), escape ryhthms, sinus arrest, asystole	Sinus, atrial, and ventricular tachycardia	0.1 mg/ml (10 ml unit)	IV bolus Endotracheal	0.01 mg/kg (0.4–0.6 mg for adults)	Increased heart rate Increased force of contractions (mainly affects atrial activity)
Epinephrine HCl	Cardiac standstill, ventricular fibrillation, asystole, EMD, sinus arrest, idioventricular rhythm	Ventricular tachycardia, frequent PVCs	0.1 mg/ml (1:10,000)	IV bolus Intracardiac Endotracheal	0.1 ml/kg every 5 min 10 ml maximum	Increased heart rate Increased force of contractions Vasoconstriction Increased coronary perf pressures Increased myocardial irritability Increased myocardial O$_2$ consumption
Propranolol HCl	Angina pectoris, myocardial infarction (MI), supraventricular arrhythmias, ventricular tachycardia	Hypotension, CHF, reactive airway disease	1 mg/ml	IV bolus	1–5 mg (not to exceed 1 mg/min)	Decreased heart rate Decreased stroke volume Decreased myocardial O$_2$ consumption Increased LVEDP

Continued.

Table 22-3   Drug Agents Used in Advanced Life Support—cont'd

Drug	Indications	Contraindications	Preparation	Route	Dosage	Pharmacologic effects
Verapamil HCl	Angina pectoris, MI, supraventricular arrhythmias, mild hypertension	Hypotension, CHF, 2nd- or 3rd-degree heart block	2.5 mg/ml (5 ml unit)	IV bolus	0.075–0.15 mg/kg over 2-3 min	Decreased heart rate Prolonged atrioventricular conduction Decreased myocardial contractility Coronary artery vasodilation Peripheral vasodilation
Isoproterenol HCl	Idioventricular rhythms, bradycardia, heart block	Ventricular tachycardia, frequent PVCs	0.2 mg/ml (1:5000)	IV drip with dextrose	0.02–0.2 µg/kg/ min	Increased heart rate Increased force of contractions Vasodilation Possible decrease coronary perfusion
Dobutamine HCl	Depressed myocardial contractility	Hypertension, PVCs, atrial fibrillation, hypertrophic aortic stenosis	250 mg powder (reconstitute)	IV drip	2.5–10 µg/kg/min	Increased force of contractions Increased heart rate Enhanced atrioventricular conduction
Calcium salts (gluconate, chloride)	Hypocalcemia hyperkalemia	Concurrent digitalis use (relative)	100 mg/ml (10% solution)	IV (not to be mixed with other drugs)	chloride: 0.2 ml/kg gluconate: 0.3–1.0 ml/kg	Increased force of contractions Increased ventricular excitability May suppress sinus node
Dopamine HCl	Hypotension	Ventricular tachycardia, frequent PVCs	40 mg/ml (5 ml unit)	IV drip	2–30 µg/kg/min	Increased renal, splanic flow at low doses (4 to 6 µg/kg/min) beta-Adrenergic effects at moderate doses (6 to 10 µg/kg/min) alpha-Adrenergic effects at high doses (above 10 µg/kg/min)
Sodium nitroprusside	Hypertension	Hypotension CHF	50 mg powder (reconstitute)	IV drip only	0.5–10 µg/kg/min	Direct peripheral vasodilation

pressors that increase peripheral vascular tone (thereby raising blood pressure) include epinephrine hydrochloride, norepinephrine, and dopamine hydrochloride. Vasodilators that decrease peripheral vascular tone include the nitrites and nitrates, specifically nitroglycerin and sodium nitroprusside.

Although used primarily for its direct stimulatory effect on the myocardium, epinephrine hydrochloride may also be used as a vasopressor in continuous IV infusions. In patients with severe hypotension, norepinephrine has a more potent vasopressor action but is contraindicated in patients with hypovolemia. Norepinephrine may also increase myocardial oxygen consumption.

Dopamine hydrochloride is an alpha- and beta-active sympathomimetic amine with dose-dependent action. Low doses of this potent agent act primarily to dilate the renal and mesenteric circulations. Moderate doses increase cardiac output mainly by stimulating myocardial beta receptors. High doses exert a strong alpha effect, causing potent peripheral vasoconstriction.[3] Dopamine administration may cause tachycardia and, in high doses, can "overconstrict" the peripheral circulation.

Nitroglycerin and sodium nitroprusside act by relaxing vascular smooth muscle. Nitrogylcerin administered sublingually is highly effective in treating coronary artery spasms resulting in angina but may also be administered by IV in emergencies to treat unstable angina and congestive heart failure. In the absence of congestive heart failure, sodium nitroprusside is the preferred agent for the treatment of hypertensive cardiovascular emergencies.[3]

Buffers. Until recently, standard protocols in ACLS included administering alkalyzing buffer agents, specifically sodium bicarbonate ($NaHCO_3$). Earlier work with an organic buffer called tris(hydroxylmethyl)-aminomethane (THAM) failed to demonstrate its advantages over the inorganic buffer, $NaHCO_3$.

In concept, buffering agents such as $NaHCO_3$ can reverse the metabolic acidosis that commonly occurs with hypoxemia and shock. However, recent clinical studies demonstrate that $NaHCO_3$ administered during cardiopulmonary resuscitation may have deleterious effects that outweigh potential benefits. Among these negative effects are decreased oxygen unloading (caused by a left shift of the oxyhemoglobin curve), hyperosmolarity, hypernatremia, depression of myocardial and cerebral function, and inactivation of simultaneously administered catecholamines.[68] For these reasons, the routine use of sodium bicarbonate in cardiac arrest is no longer recommended.[3,68] Sodium bicarbonate should be considered only after rigorous efforts to restore adequate ventilation and perfusion have been attempted.

Electrical therapy. When an electrical shock of appropriate strength is applied to the myocardium, all myocardial fibers are simultaneously depolarized. In concept, this should "restart" the heart and allow its normal conduction mechanism to take over. Arrhythmias that can be success-

fully managed with electrical shock include paroxysmal atrial tachycardia, atrial flutter, atrial fibrillation, certain types of heart block, ventricular tachycardia, and ventricular fibrillation.

Unfortunately, electrical shock can also cause cardiac arrhythmias and damage myocardial tissue. An electrical current applied to a normal heart during the relative refractory period of ventricular repolarization (see Chapter 7) can cause fibrillation of the ventricular myocardium.[3] Actual myocardial damage may occur to either a normal or diseased heart if too much current is applied.[69]

To minimize the possibility of an electrical shock causing a cardiac arrhythmia, the electrical discharge can be synchronized to occur during ventricular depolarization (the QRS complex of the ECG). The application of a synchronous shock to the myocardium is called *cardioversion.* Cardioversion is the electrical therapy of choice whenever the arrhythmia is characterized by distinct QRS complexes. Conduction disorders characterized by distinct QRS complexes include all supraventricular arrhythmias and ventricular tachycardia.

To avoid damage to myocardial tissue, cardioversion should apply the minimum amount of energy necessary to convert the arrhythmia. Generally, a direct current discharge of between 25 to 100 joules (watt-sec) is sufficient to effect myocardial depolarization and restore a normal cardiac rhythm in adults. For children and infants, between 0.2 and 1.0 joule/kg is recommended.[3]

If, on the other hand, the conduction disorder exhibits no distinct QRS complexes (as with ventricular fibrillation), synchronous shock is not necessary. Unsynchronized electrical countershock is called *defibrillation.* In addition to its use with ventricular fibrillation, defibrillation may also be used to manage ventricular tachycardia that results in pulselessness, unconsciousness, or hypotension.[3]

Defibrillation typically requires higher energy levels than that needed for cardioversion. Currently, the American Heart Association recommends that an initial energy level of 200 joules be used for defibrillation of adult victims, with 2 joules/kg for children and infants.[3,70,71] If this level is ineffective in restoring orderly ventricular depolarization, the energy level of the second shock should be raised to between 200 and 300 joules. Third and subsequent shocks should never exceed 360 joules in the adult or about 4 joules/kg in children and infants.[70,71]

The success of defibrillation as an ACLS technique depends on a number of physiologic and procedural factors. Myocardial hypoxia and acidosis are among the primary physiologic factors that can thwart efforts to convert ventricular fibrillation. For this reason, defibrillation should be initiated as soon as ventricular fibrillation is identified. Administration of epinephrine and lidocaine may facilitate defibrillation. When monitoring equipment is not available or the underlying arrhythmia cannot be identified, "blind" defibrillation should be instituted immediately.[3]

Procedurally, electrode paddle size and placement are

important in ensuring that the full energy of the counter-shock is appropriately applied. For adults, paddles should be 10 cm in diameter, with 8 cm being adequate for older children. Electrode paddles for infants should be 4.5 cm.

Normally, one electrode is placed below the clavicle and just to the right of the upper portion of the sternum, with the other positioned on the midaxillary line to the left of the left nipple. Alternatively, one paddle may be placed on the left precordium, with the other positioned posteriorly under the patient, behind the heart. Paddles should be prepared with conducting gel and applied with firm pressure (about 25 lb).

Since defibrillation can cause damage to permanent pacemakers, care should be taken to place the electrode paddles no closer than 5 inches to these devices. Patients with permanent pacemakers who have undergone either cardioversion or defibrillation should have the function of these devices regularly checked for at least 6 weeks after the original event.[3]

Postresuscitative patient care

Care of a patient after a successful resuscitation effort involves careful monitoring and, where indicated, special supplemental support of various organ systems.[3,11,73]

If the patient is conscious and breathing spontaneously following the resuscitation effort, supplemental oxygen, maintenance of an IV infusion, and continuous cardiac and hemodynamic monitoring may be all that is necessary to ensure recovery. A 12-lead ECG, chest x-ray film, arterial blood gases, and a clinical chemistry profile should be obtained at the earliest possible convenience.[3] Ideally, the patient should be placed under close supervision and observation, preferably in an intensive or coronary care unit, as appropriate.

If, on the other hand, the patient remains unconscious, is apneic, or has an unstable cardiovascular status, placement in a special care unit is mandatory. Only in this context can underlying organ system insufficiency or failure be properly identified and managed. The organ systems most likely to exhibit failure in the postresuscitative stage of patient management are the respiratory, cardiovascular, and renal systems. CNS "failure" is an ominous sign and generally indicates a failed resuscitation attempt.

Respiratory management. If the patient remains apneic or exhibits irregular breathing after the resuscitation effort, mechanical ventilation should be instituted through a properly positioned endotracheal tube, with an initial oxygen concentration of 100%. Arterial blood gases, preferably obtained through an arterial line, should be analyzed as needed until the patient's oxygenation and acid-base status are stabilized. Arterial blood gas analysis will also help differentiate between pulmonary and nonpulmonary (or cardiac) causes of hypoxemia and tissue hypoxia, if present.[3] Details on the selection and use of mechanical ventilators and appropriate patient monitoring procedures are provided in Section VII of this text.

Cardiovascular management. A 12-lead ECG, chest x-ray film, clinical chemistry profile, and cardiac enzyme results should be reviewed, along with current and past drug histories obtained at the earliest possible convenience. Where feasible, a flow-directed, balloon-tipped pulmonary artery catheter should be inserted and connected to a thermal dilution cardiac output computer.[3] In this manner, the adequacy of circulating fluid volumes, left ventricular performance, and overall perfusion can be quickly and accurately assessed. On this basis, sound judgments can be made regarding the need for fluid therapy and the selection and titration of appropriate pharmacologic agents.

Renal management. Ideally, the bladder should be catheterized and fluid input and output carefully monitored. Renal function tests, including urine sediment, electrolytes, blood urea nitrogen (BUN), and creatinine, should be carefully monitored. If this evidence suggests renal failure, care should be taken with the administration of nephrotoxic drugs or agents normally excreted through the kidneys. If the problem is confirmed as renal in origin (as opposed to cardiovascular), hemodialysis may be indicated.[11]

Central nervous system management. Although significant advances are being made in limiting CNS damage associated with poor cerebral perfusion and oxygenation, current nonexperimental approaches to CNS postresuscitative care are limited to maintaining arterial perfusion pressures while simultaneously lowering intracranial pressures and preventing seizures.[11,72,73] Elevation of the head facilitates cerebral vascular drainage, while drug agents such as phenobarbital can decrease the occurrence of seizures. Since tracheobronchial suction and mechanical ventilation can both elevate intracranial pressures, respiratory care practitioners responsible for these components of management must exercise care in their use.[3] Special mechanical ventilation techniques may be necessary to minimize both the cardiovascular and cerebrovascular consequences of this mode of therapy.

SUMMARY

The prompt action of a respiratory care practitioner can restore ventilation and circulation to victims of respiratory or cardiac arrest. All practitioners should be skilled in the basic methods of airway maintenance, foreign body removal, artificial ventilation, and external cardiac compressions. The practitioner must be able to modify and evaluate the effectiveness of these procedures, taking into consideration the victim's age and the circumstances of the emergency.

In addition to providing BLS, respiratory care practitioners are key members of the in-hospital ACLS team. In this role the practitioner plays a vital part in managing the airway and providing effective oxygenation and ventilation. Practitioners may also participate in elements of circulatory support, drug and electrical therapy, and postresuscitative care.

By applying this expertise in an appropriate, proficient, and systematic manner—and sharing it through the education of lay personnel—respiratory care practitioners can help reduce the alarming toll of sudden death currently affecting our population.

REFERENCES

1. Statistical Resources Branch, Division of Vital Statistics: Final Mortality Statistics, 1981, Hyattsville, Md, 1984, National Center for Health Statistics.
2. US Department of Health and Human Services: Health, United States, 1985, Washington, DC, 1985, US Government Printing Office.
3. American Heart Association: Standards for cardiopulmonary resuscitation and emergency cardiac care, JAMA (suppl) 255:21, 2843-2989, 1986.
4. Singer J: Cardiac arrest in children, J Am Coll Emerg Phys 6:198-205, 1977.
5. Eisenberg M, Bergner L, and Hallstrom A: Epidemiology of cardiac arrest and resuscitation in children, Ann Emerg Med 12:672-674, 1983.
6. National Safety Council: Accident facts, Chicago, 1984, The Council.
7. Committee on Trauma, American College of Surgeons: Early care of the injured patient, ed 2, Philadelphia, 1976, WB Saunders Co.
8. Goldberger E: Treatment of cardiac emergencies, ed 2, St Louis, 1977, The CV Mosby Co.
9. Grant H and Murray R: Emergency care, Bowie, Md, 1971, Robert J Brady Co.
10. Huszar R: Emergency cardiac care, Bowie, Md, 1974, Robert J Brady Co.
11. Stephenson HE: Cardiac arrest and resuscitation, ed 4, St Louis, 1974, The CV Mosby Co.
12. Ellis PD and Billings DM: Cardiopulmonary resuscitation: procedures for basic and advanced life support, St Louis, 1980, The CV Mosby Co.
13. American Heart Association: A manual for instructors in basic life support, Dallas, 1985, The Association.
14. Shapter R, editor: Cardiopulmonary resuscitation: basic life support, Clin Symp 26:7, 1974.
15. Ruben H, Elam JO, Ruben AM et al: Investigation of upper airway problems in resuscitation, Anesthesiology, 22:271-279, 1961.
16. Boidin MP: Airway patency in the unconscious patient, Br J Anaesth 57:306-310, 1985.
17. Morikawa S, Safar P, and Decarlo J: Influence of head position upon airway patency, Anesthesiology 22:265, 1961.
18. Guildner C: Resuscitation: opening the airway, a comparative study of techniques for opening an airway obstructed by the tongue, J Am Coll Emerg Phys 5:558-590, 1976.
19. Safar P and Lind B: Triple airway maneuver, artificial ventilation and oxygen inhalation by mouth-to-mask and bag-valve-mask techniques. In Proceedings of the 1973 National Conference on CPR, Dallas, 1975, American Heart Association.
20. Melker R: Recommendations for ventilation during cardiopulmonary resuscitation—time for change? Crit Care Med 13:882-883, 1985.
21. Melker R: CPR in neonates, infants and children, Crit Care Q 1:49-65, 1978.
22. Ludwig S, Kettrick RG, and Parker M: Pediatric cardiopulmonary resuscitation, Clin Pediatr 23:71, 1984.
23. Torphy DE, Minter MG, and Thompson BM: Cardiorespiratory arrest and resuscitation of children, AJDC 138:1099, 1984.
24. Safar P and Redding J: "Tight jaw" in resuscitation, Anesthesiology 20:701-702, 1959.
25. Ruben H, Knudsen EJ, and Carugati G: Gastric inflation in relation to airway pressure, Acta Anaesth Scand 5:107-114, 1961.
26. Sellick BA: Cricoid pressure to control regurgitation of stomach contents during induction of anesthesia, Lancet 2:404-406, 1961.
27. Heimlich HJ et al: Food choking and drowning deaths prevented by external subdiaphragmatic compression, Ann Thorac Surg 20:188, 1975.
28. Heimlich H: A life saving maneuver to prevent food choking, JAMA 234:398, 1975.
29. Heimlich H: Death from food-choking prevented by a new life-saving maneuver, Heart Lung 5:755-758, 1976.
30. Heimlich H: The Heimlich maneuver: where it stands today, Emerg Med 10:89-93, 1978.
31. Day RL, Crelin ES, and DuBois AB: Choking: the Heimlich abdominal thrust vs back blows: an approach to measurement of inertial and aerodynamic forces, Pediatrics 70:113-119, 1982.
32. Day RL and DuBois AB: Treatment of choking, Pediatrics 71:300, 1983.
33. Visintine RE and Baick CH: Ruptured stomach after Heimlich maneuver, JAMA 234:415, 1975.
34. Palmer E: The Heimlich maneuver misused, Curr Prescrib 5:45-49, 1979.
35. Babbs CF: New versus old theories of blood flow during CPR, Crit Care Med 8:191-195, 1980.
36. Rudikoff M et al: Importance of compression rate during external cardiac massage in man, Circulation Suppl 54:II-225, 1976.
37. Taylor G et al: Importance of prolonged compression during cardiopulmonary resuscitation in man, N Engl J Med 296:1515-1517, 1977.
38. Vaagenes P et al: On the technique of external cardiac compression, Crit Care Med 6:176-180, 1978.
39. Orlowski JP: Optimum position for external cardiac massage in infants and children, Crit Care Med 12:224, 1984.
40. Ludwig S, Kettrick RG, and Parker M: Pediatric cardiopulmonary resuscitation, Clin Pediatr 23:71, 1984.
41. Nagel EI, Fine EG, Krischer JP et al: Complications of CPR, Crit Care Med 9:424, 1983.
42. Bjork RJ, Snyder BD, Campion DC et al: Medical complications of cardiopulmonary arrest, Arch Intern Med 142:500-503, 1982.
43. Atcheson SG and Fred HL: Complications of cardiac resuscitation, Am Heart J 89:263-264, 1975.
44. Enarson D et al: Flail chest as a complication of cardiopulmonary resuscitation, Heart Lung 6:1020-1022, 1977.
45. Safar P: Pocket mask for emergency artificial ventilation and oxygen inhalation, Crit Care Med 2:273-276, 1974.
46. Harrison RR, Maull KI, Keenan RL et al: Mouth-to-mask ventilation: a superior method of rescue breathing, Ann Emerg Med 12:765-768, 1982.
47. Donen N, Tweed WA, Dashfsky S et al: The esophageal obturator airway: an appraisal, Can Anaesth Soc J 30:194-200, 1983.
48. Pilcher DB and DeMeules JE: Esophageal perforation following use of esophageal airway, Chest 69:377-380, 1976.
49. Melker R and Cavallaro D: Synchronous and asynchronous ventilation during cardiopulmonary resuscitation, Ann Emerg Med 12:142, 1983.
50. Attia RR, Battit GE, and Murphy JD: Transtracheal ventilation, JAMA 234:1152-1153, 1975.
51. McPherson SP: Respiratory therapy equipment, ed 3, St Louis, 1985, The CV Mosby Co.
52. Evaluation: manually operated infant resuscitators, Health Devices 3:164, 1974.
53. Evaluation: manual resuscitators, Health Devices 8:133, 1979.
54. Barnes TA and Watson ME: Oxygen delivery performance of four adult resuscitation bags, Respir Care 27:139, 1982.
55. Steinbach RB and Carden E: Assessment of eight adult resuscitator bags, Respir Care 20:69, 1975.
56. White RD, Gilles BP, and Polk BV: Oxygen delivery by hand-oper

ated emergency ventilation devices, J Am Coll Emerg Phys 2:105-108, 1973.

57. Klick JM, Bushnell LS, and Bancroft ML: Barotrauma as a potential hazard of manual resuscitators, Anesthesiology 49:363, 1978.

58. Evaluation: gas-powered resuscitators, Health Devices 8:24, 1978.

59. Evaluation: oxygen-powered resuscitators, Health Devices 3:207-221, 1974.

60. Taylor GJ, Rubin R, Tucker M et al: External cardiac compression: a randomized comparison of mechanical and manual techniques, JAMA 240:644-646, 1978.

61. Goldberger AL and Goldberger E: Clinical electrocardiography, ed 2, St Louis, 1981, The CV Mosby Co.

62. Phillips RE and Feeney MK: The cardiac rhythms: a systematic approach to interpretation, Philadelphia, 1973, WB Saunders Co.

63. Miller J, Trech D, Horwitz L et al: The precordial thump, Ann Emerg Med 13:791, 1984.

64. Fontaine G, Frank R, and Grosgogeat Y: Torsades de pointes: definition and management, Mod Concepts Cardiovasc Dis 51:103-108, 1982.

65. Zelis R, Mansour EJ, and Capone RJ: The cardiovascular effects of morphine, J Clin Invest 54:1247-1258, 1974.

66. Koch-Weser J: Drug therapy: bretylium, N Engl J Med 300:473-477, 1979.

67. Dembo DH: Calcium in advanced life support, Crit Care Med 9:358, 1981.

68. Bishop RL and Weisfeldt ML: Sodium bicarbonate administration during cardiac arrest, JAMA 235:255-260, 1976.

69. Warner ED, Dahl C, and Ewy GA: Myocardial injury from transthoracic defibrillator countershock, Arch Pathol 99:55, 1975.

70. Adgey AA: Electrical energy requirements for ventricular defibrillation, Br Heart J 40:1197-1199, 1978.

71. Chameides L, Brown GE, Raye JR et al: Guidelines for defibrillation in infants and children, Circulation 56(suppl):502A-503A, 1977.

72. Safar P, Bleyaert A, and Nemoto EM: Resuscitation after global brain ischemia-anoxia, Crit Care Med 6:203-214, 1978.

73. Safar P and Bircher NG: Cardiopulmonary cerebral resuscitation, ed 3, Philadelphia, 1988, WB Saunders Co.

23

Humidity and Aerosol Therapy

Craig L. Scanlan

Humidity and aerosol therapy represents integral components of comprehensive respiratory care. Yet many of the approaches in current use are based on untested assumptions or subjective reports of patient benefits. Recent analyses of the scientific basis of both inpatient and outpatient respiratory care have found certain aspects of aerosol and humidity therapy to be lacking in hard scientific data to support their beneficial use.[1,2] Clearly, continuing research into both the safety and the efficacy of these therapeutic modalities must be conducted.[3] In the interim, respiratory care practitioners are obliged to apply the most current knowledge available in the selection and application of techniques of humidity and aerosol therapy.

Consistent with this approach, we will critically examine current concepts in humidity and aerosol therapy, emphasizing both accepted practices and areas of continuing controversy.

OBJECTIVES

After completion of this chapter, the reader should be able to:

1. Differentiate the two primary indications for humidity therapy and state quantitative standards for each;
2. Identify the factors that affect the performance of humidification devices;
3. Compare and contrast the major categories of humidification devices according to their principles of operation and clinical capabilities and limitations;
4. Identify the major hazards associated with the humidification of inspired gases and ways to minimize these risks;
5. Relate the physical properties of aerosols to their penetration and deposition in the human lung;
6. Differentiate the three major goals of aerosol therapy;
7. Compare and contrast the major categories of aerosol generators according to their principles of operation and clinical capabilities and limitations;

8. Identify the major hazards associated with the delivery of therapeutic aerosols to the respiratory tract and ways to minimize these risks.

KEY TERMS

Most terms used in this chapter are defined in context. The following terms are introduced without explicit definition but may be found in the text glossary:

absorption	insensible water loss
agglomeration	in situ
amplitude	inspissated
anhydrous	laryngitis
bronchoscopy	MHz
BTPS	malignant
coalescence	nosocomial
colonization	oscillation
cystic fibrosis	osmolarity
cytologic	pathogenic
desquamate	rheostat
heterogeneous	solute
homogeneous	solvent
hypernatremia	thermostat
hyperpyrexia	viscous resistance
inoculum	watt

HUMIDITY THERAPY

Indications

The general goal of humidity therapy is to ensure that the water vapor content of inspired gases is sufficient to meet patients' physiologic needs.[4] Under this general goal are two specific clinical indications: (1) to increase the water vapor content of dry therapeutic gases to approximate ambient conditions and (2) to provide inspired gases near BTPS for patients with artificial airways.

Humidifying therapeutic gases. By far the most common use for humidity therapy is the addition of water vapor to oxygen being administered to patients with normally functioning upper airways. Supplemental humidity may also be provided for anesthetic gases, for gases in the pulmonary function laboratory, or for therapeutic gas mixtures such as oxygen-carbon dioxide or helium-oxygen mixtures.

Regardless of the gas being used, purity standards require that it be supplied in the dry or anhydrous state (see Chapter 24). Although we have seen that the normal upper respiratory tract provides an efficient mechanism for heat and water exchange, prolonged exposure to dry gas can pose significant problems, even among normal persons. Among hospitalized patients, especially those with systemic dehydration, the humidification process of the nose and upper airway actually may be inadequate. Under these circumstances, water is drawn from the entire mucosal surface of the respiratory tract, rather than from just its upper portion. This depletion of mucosal moisture can increase the viscosity of surface secretions and adversely affect ciliary action, thereby compromising effective mucociliary clearance.

Compounding this problem is the fact that many patients who require gas therapy already have increased amounts of abnormal secretions. These secretions can become inspissated, covering the mucosal surface with a dry and crusted coat. Impervious to normal amounts of moisture, this inspissated layer can block the normal humidification process from the underlying mucosa. Further desiccation may be caused by the inhalation of therapeutic gases that are inadequately humidified.

Therefore the basic aim in humidifying therapeutic gases is to equal or exceed the water vapor content commonly found in room air. The American National Standards Institute (ANSI) has identified a 10 mg/L water vapor content as the minimum level of absolute humidity necessary to avoid mucosal damage to the upper airway.[5] This equates with approximately 50% relative humidity at a room temperature of 72°F. Common unheated humidifiers are generally capable of providing at least this level of moisture and often more.[6] Since patients using these simple systems are breathing through intact upper airways, the remainder of the water vapor needed for body humidity is supplied in the usual fashion.

Providing saturated gas near body temperature. Normally, inspired air is warmed to near body temperature and saturated with water vapor by the time it reaches the level of the carina.[7,8] Heat and moisture are supplied mainly by the respiratory mucosa of the upper airways. If the upper airways are bypassed by means of an endotracheal or tracheostomy tube, this mechanism is temporarily lost. If inadequate humidification is supplied to inspired gases through these tubes, the patient's secretions will become thick, inspissated, and difficult to remove.[9-13] Because the upper airways are bypassed, the heat and water vapor needed for body humidity in the lung will have to be supplied by the lower airways or by artificial means.

To prevent this large humidity deficit from drying the patient's secretions, heated humidification systems are used.[6,13] These systems are capable of controlling the temperature and humidity levels of inspired air and of providing saturated gases at or near the normal body temperature. The primary goal is to match the output of the humidifying device to the normal inspiratory conditions occurring at the level of the trachea.[4]

There is some controversy concerning the optimum levels of humidity and temperature for patients with artificial airways. Traditionally, the recommendation has been to keep the air 100% saturated at 37°C.[6,10-13] However, animal and human research has presented conflicting data regarding the actual minimum level of heart and moisture needed to maintain normal airway function.[14-21] Moreover, the clinical significance of providing all heat and moisture needs artificially (thereby preventing the natural evaporative heat and water vapor losses from the respiratory tract) is not well understood.

We do know that mucociliary clearance of secretions can be impaired when water vapor content drops to between 50% and 75% body humidity.[14] Mucociliary clearance is less affected as long as the temperatures are between 32° and 42°C and the absolute humidity exceeds 33 mg/L.[15] On the other hand, evidence of microscopic lung damage and alterations in surface tension has been reported in dogs with tracheostomies that have been breathing saturated gas at 35°C for 3 to 24 hours.[18] Recently ANSI has recommended an absolute humidity level of 30 mg/L as the minimum output of devices used to humidify gases delivered to patients with bypassed upper airways.[5] On the basis of this knowledge, a reasonable approach is to ensure that inspired gases for intubated patients are kept at 100% RH at temperatures between 32° and 34°C.[4]

Less is known about the humidity needs of patients with high body temperatures or abnormal secretions.[4] For patients with abnormal amounts of secretions, many recommend the application of aerosol generators capable of delivering particulate water to the respiratory tract.[11,22-24] Although still controversial and fraught with additional hazards, this approach is discussed in more detail later in this chapter.

Methods of humidification

Various types and brands of humidifier have been described and evaluated elsewhere.[6,25-27] Our discussion here is limited to a general overview of humidifier categories and their performance characteristics.

Factors affecting performance. Three key factors determine the efficiency with which a humidifier vaporizes liquid water: (1) the surface area between the water and the gas to be humidified, (2) the length of time the gas and water are in contact, and (3) the temperature of both the water and the gas.

Surface area exposure. The larger the surface area available for evaporation, the greater will be the amount of water vapor added to a gas in a given time period. The most common method of increasing the area of contact between the water and the gas is dispersal of the gas through the water in the form of small bubbles. Newer wick humidifiers employ a porous hygroscopic material to increase surface area. Similar material is used in hygroscopic condenser humidifiers (also called heat and moisture exchangers). Alternatively, water may be nebulized into the gas as small droplets.[6] This latter method involves the production of an aerosol and is discussed later in this chapter.

Time of contact. In general, the longer a gas is in contact with water, the greater the chance for that gas to become saturated with water vapor. In some humidifiers, higher gas flows lower the level of humidity obtained, indicating that the time of contact may not be sufficient for full saturation.[26] However, as long as a large surface area is maintained and the temperature of the water is sufficiently high, saturation occurs very rapidly, and the time of contact and the flow rate of the gas are less important.[6,28]

Temperature. The single most important factor contributing to a humidifier's overall performance is temperature. In all humidifiers, heat is lost as a result of evaporative cooling. Evaporative cooling lowers the temperature of a gas and, therefore, its ability to carry water vapor. Therefore, if a humidifier is not heated from some external source, as water vaporizes into the gas heat is lost and both the gas and the water are cooled. Since the gas leaving the humidifier is cooler than room air, the humidity output is limited to less than that of saturated air at ambient temperature.

The simple solution to this problem is to heat the humidifier. The most common approach involves the use of an electrical heating element to raise the temperature of the water reservoir. Alternatively, the patient's own body heat may be used, as with hygroscopic condenser humidifiers. In either case, heating can ensure that even humidifiers with a relatively small gas-water surface area can fully saturate the delivered gas at their working temperatures. Moreover, heating is the only way to ensure high levels of humidity at the high flow rates required with some oxygen delivery systems and mechanical ventilators.[29]

Types of humidifiers. By manipulating surface area, time, and/or temperature, engineers have developed a variety of humidifier designs. Decisions regarding the selection and appropriate use of these various types of humidifier demand general knowledge of their characteristics and limitations. We will discuss five major humidifier classes: (1) the pass-over humidifier, (2) the bubble-diffusion humidifier, (3) the cascade humidifier, (4) the wick humidifier, and (5) the hygroscopic condenser humidifier.

Pass-over humidifier. The pass-over or "blow-by" humidifier is the simplest of all devices that add water vapor to gas. Generally, gas entering the device simply passes over a large water surface. Evaporation supplies humidity to air directed across its surface. Baffles may be added in the gas stream to lengthen the time of contact, or the water reservoir may be heated to increase efficiency. Simple baf-

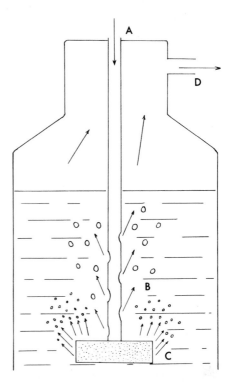

Fig. 23-1 The bubble-diffusion humidifier bubbles therapeutic gas, *A*, through a perforated tube, *B*, or a porous diffusion head, *C*. The larger the number of small bubbles, the greater the evaporation area to humidify the gas leaving outflow port, *D*.

fled pass-over humidifier are found in most infant incubators (see Chapter 32). A simple heated pass-over humidifier is found in the original Emerson postoperative ventilator. Although simple and moderately useful when heated, this type of humidifier generally has been replaced by more effective designs.

Bubble-diffusion humidifier. One of the oldest methods of humidifying gases consists of simply bubbling them through a reservoir of water. Fig. 23-1 illustrates two commonly employed techniques. Gas enters the unit at *A* and passes through a tube immersed nearly to the bottom of a jar containing water. Sometimes the tube contains multiple perforations, *B*, through which the gas escapes as bubbles. Instead of the holes, the immersed oxygen tube may be fitted with a porous stonelike diffusion head, *C*, at its lower tip. The size of the bubbles is determined by the size of the openings and the gas flow rate. The smaller the bubbles and the greater their number, the more surface area will be available for evaporation. Once the gas rises to the surface of the reservoir, it leaves the outflow port, *D*, and proceeds to the delivery system.

These units are generally capable of supplying dry gases with 60% to 100% relative humidity (RH) at their operating temperatures. As mentioned previously, evaporative cooling in unheated humidifiers results in operating temperatures that are several degrees cooler than room conditions. Since the humidifier gases are usually carried to the

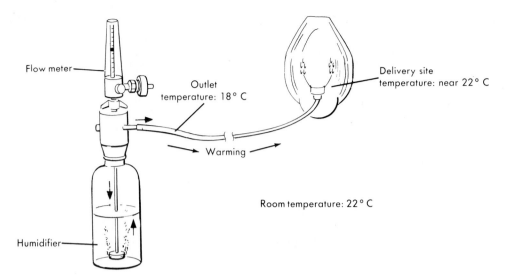

Flow meter

Outlet
temperature: 18° C

Delivery site
temperature: near 22° C

Warming

Room temperature: 22° C

Humidifier

Fig. 23-2   Gases leaving outlet of the simple humidifier are cooler than room temperature because of evaporation. Warming toward room temperature occurs en route to patient delivery site.

patient by a small-diameter tube 6 to 8 feet in length, some
warming of these gases occurs before they are inspired by
the patient. If no liquid water is available for evaporation
in the tubing or gas stream, then the relative humidity of
the gas will drop as its temperature rises toward room temperature. For these reasons, gases leaving an unheated
bubble-diffusion humidifier at 100% RH generally can
supply only about 35% to 40% of the water vapor needed
to saturate gas at body temperature. Fig. 23-2 portrays a
typical system that uses a simple unheated humidifier for
therapeutic gas administration, illustrating the effect of
temperature differences between the humidifier and the delivery site.

Large-reservoir heated humidifiers. When body humidity levels are needed, heat must be applied to either the
water in the humidifier, the gas, or both. Typically, most
heated humidifiers warm the water reservoir. Some also
maintain the heat leaving the unit by means of heating elements applied to the delivery tubing.[6] Although heated
humidifiers may employ the pass-over or blow-by design,
most modern systems use a modification of the bubble-
diffusion method, called a "cascade." More recently, a
"wick" design has been introduced.

Cascade humidifier. The cascade design is depicted in
Fig. 23-3. Dry gas enters the device at the inlet, *1,* causing
a pressure rise in the tower assembly, *2.* This pressure
opens a one-way valve at the base of the tower, *3,* displacing water downward, *4.* As the gas is dispersed upward
through a grid, *5,* displacement causes the level of the reservoir to rise, and water to "cascade" over the grid through
an orifice, *6.* This cascade effect creates a fine froth of
bubbles at the grid, facilitating quick evaporation. Water
temperature is controlled by a rheostat, *7,* connected to a
temperature sensor or thermostat, *8,* and a heating element, *9.* A metal connection between the temperature sen-

sor and the heating element, called a *shunt, 10,* will cause
direct heat transfer to the sensor when the water level becomes low, thereby turning off the heating element and
preventing delivery of heated dry gas to the patient.

Humidified gas leaves the device through a 22 mm outlet, *11,* via large-bore corrugated tubing, *12.* A thermometer, *13,* measures the temperature at or near the patient's
airway. Alternatively, the thermometer incorporates an
electronic sensor that automatically controls the rheostat,
keeping airway temperatures within a preset range. Called
a *servocontroller,* this type of mechanism may also include a warning alarm to alert clinicians to undesired temperature variations.

Wick humidifiers. Wick humidifiers were originally
developed to vaporize liquid anesthetic agents. A wick
humidifier incorporates a porous hygroscopic material,
or wick, that is partially submerged in the water reservoir (Fig. 23-4). The wick increases surface area and
enhances evaporation.[6] Capillary action causes water to
continually rise in the wick as it evaporates into the gas
stream (see Chapter 4). As compared to the cascade type,
the wick humidifier offers two major advantages: (1) saturation can be maintained even at continuous high flows
and (2) there is considerably less flow resistance through
the device.[6]

Both types of large-capacity heated humidifiers may incorporate reservoir feed systems that automatically maintain appropriate water levels. In addition to the obvious
advantage of saving personnel time, closed-feed systems
minimize the likelihood of bacteria contamination of the
water reservoir.

The most common use for these large-reservoir heated
humidifiers is to provide saturated gas at or near body temperature to patients receiving mechanical ventilatory support (see Chapter 30). Indeed, the original cascade design

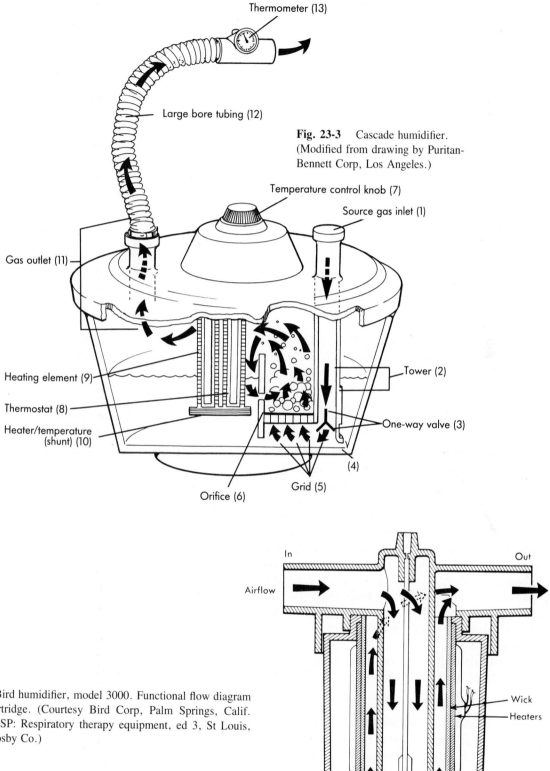

Thermometer (13)

Large bore tubing (12)

Fig. 23-3   Cascade humidifier. (Modified from drawing by Puritan-Bennett Corp, Los Angeles.)

Temperature control knob (7)

Source gas inlet (1)

Gas outlet (11)

Heating element (9)

Thermostat (8)

Heater/temperature (shunt) (10)

Tower (2)

One-way valve (3)

(4)

Orifice (6)

Grid (5)

Fig. 23-4   The Bird humidifier, model 3000. Functional flow diagram for humidifier cartridge. (Courtesy Bird Corp, Palm Springs, Calif. From McPherson SP: Respiratory therapy equipment, ed 3, St Louis, 1985, The CV Mosby Co.)

In

Out

Airflow

Wick

Heaters

Float

Constant water level

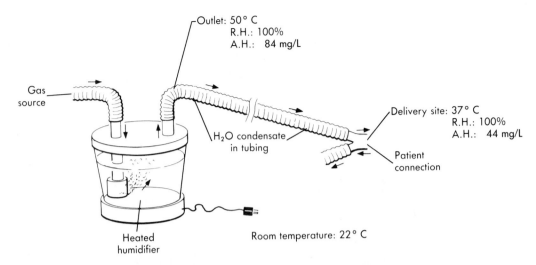

Fig. 23-5   Gases leaving outlet of heated humidifier are hot and saturated with water vapor. As cooling occurs in tubing, vapor condenses and absolute humidity, *A.H.*, decreases while relative humidity, *R.H.*, remains 100% (saturated). Note that almost half the original water vapor is "lost" to condensate in this example.

is optimally effective only when intermittent pressure variations cause the reservoir level to fluctuate. With the introduction of specialized high-flow oxygen delivery and CPAP systems (see Chapters 25 and 30), large-reservoir heated humidifiers have now been developed specifically for patients who are breathing spontaneously.[6,29,30] Regardless of design or application, these systems cannot meet body humidity requirements unless they are heated.

When heating is provided solely at the humidifier, significant cooling will occur throughout the delivery system. Since the gases leaving the humidifier are hot and saturated with water vapor, this cooling causes water vapor to condense in the tubing. Such condensation would quickly occlude small-diameter tubing; therefore large-bore (22 mm) corrugated tubing is used instead. However, even large-bore tubing can become occluded with condensate. To prevent this from occurring, water traps should be placed at low points in the delivery system to collect the condensate, with provisions made to check and drain the tubing periodically.

The magnitude of this cooling and condensation problem is illustrated in the following example (Fig. 23-5). In a typical hospital room, temperatures may be between 22° and 24°C. For the delivery of gases at near body temperature to the patient, temperature at the humidifier outlet may have to be in the 48° to 50°C range. At this temperature, saturated gas holds approximately 84 mg/L of water vapor. As these warm, water-laden gases transverse the delivery system, the temperature falls to near 37°C at the delivery site. At 37°C, the capacity of saturated gas is only 44 mg/L. Therefore, the cooling process will cause about half of the original water vapor leaving the humidifier to condense or "rain out" into the delivery tubing. Despite this drop in absolute humidity, relative humidity remains

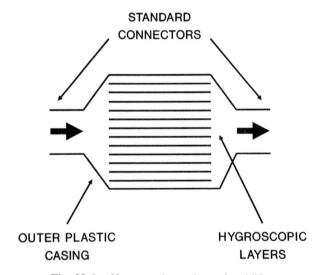

Fig. 23-6   Hygroscopic condenser humidifier.

at 100%. Of course, the actual numbers in this example are used to illustrate the concept; varying conditions will require different humidifier outlet temperatures and cause varying amounts of condensation. Should the delivery tubing be heated, the temperature gradient between the humidifier and the delivery site can be eliminated, allowing the humidifier to operated at lower temperatures and preventing or minimizing condensation in the tubing circuit.

Hygroscopic condenser humidifier. The hygroscopic condenser humidifier (HCH) is a specialized humidification apparatus designed solely for warming and humidifying the inspired gas in ventilator or anesthesia circuits.[27] Compared with other types of humidification device, the HCH employs a unique method to accomplish this function. As shown in Fig. 23-6, the HCH consists solely of a small disposable chamber containing either a honeycomb or layers of hygroscopically treated material (usually cellulose, synthetic felt, or polypropylene). There is no water reservoir or heating element. The HCH simply is placed between the patient's artificial airway and the connector of the ventilator or anesthesia circuit. Once in place, moisture in the patient's exhaled gases condenses on the surfaces of the hygroscopic material inside the HCH. As described in Chapter 4, condensation reverses the evaporation process. When the water vapor molecules condense, their internal (kinetic) energy is given up to the surroundings in the form of heat. During the subsequent inspiration, the condensed water evaporates from the hygroscopic material, thereby humidifying the dry gas delivered by the ventilator system. Although cooling does occur during this evaporative stage, its effects are mostly offset by the heat previously retained in the HCH during expiration.

Because of the nature of this process and its similarity to the function of the nasal cavity, hygroscopic condenser humidifiers are also referred to as heat and moisture exchangers (HMEs), or "artificial noses."[27] However, controlled laboratory studies of these devices indicate that hygroscopic condenser humidifiers fall short of the performance of the human nose. Specifically, most commercially available HCHs are capable of providing between 22 and 28 mg/L water vapor to the airway, or between 50% and 65% body humidity.[27,31-34]

As previously discussed, the ANSI standard for devices used to humidify gases delivered to patients with bypassed upper airways is an absolute humidity of 30 mg/L (about 70% body humidity).[5] However, this standard (based on large-reservoir heated humidifiers) does not take into account heat and humidity losses that typically occur between the humidification device and the patient's airway.[27] Since these losses are minimal with a properly placed HCH, and since the range of water vapor output of these devices appears minimally sufficient to prevent tracheo-bronchial damage,[17] their use may be appropriate under selected conditions. Specifically, current knowledge supports the use of HCHs for short-term use (24 to 48 hours) to warm and humidify the inspired gas in ventilator circuits when the patient (1) is normothermic, (2) is adequately hydrated, and (3) does not require therapeutic humidity for retained secretions.[27]

When properly applied to patients who meet these criteria, the HCH offers significant advantages over traditional humidification devices, particularly in minimizing the hazards associated with large-reservoir heated humidifiers. The hazards associated with humidity therapy in general, and with large-reservoir heated humidifiers in particular, are the subject of the next section.

Hazards of humidity therapy

Although humidity therapy generally is considered to present minimal hazards to the patient, its application is not without risk. Among the potential risks of humidity therapy are (1) alterations in normal heat and water exchange, (2) infection, and (3) electrical shock.[35,36]

Alterations in heat and water exchange. Normally, some 7% to 8% of body heat loss and approximately 6% of body water loss (called insensible water loss) occur through the lungs.[35] Airway temperatures substantially greater than 37°C can result in hyperpyrexia.[37,38] Moreover, negation of the normal mechanism of evaporative water loss can disrupt fluid balance, resulting in overhydration.[39] However, only electrically heated humidification devices have the ability to affect these normal mechanisms of heat and water exchange, and then only among certain categories of patient.[35,36] As previously discussed, hygroscopic condenser humidifiers cannot cause either hyperpyrexia or overhydration.

Clearly, caution should be observed in the use of electrically heated humidification devices for patients who are already feverish, and fluid balance should be carefully monitored in those with water retention. Either problem is compounded in pediatric and neonatal care, in which heat and water exchange may be more easily disrupted.[40-42] Preterm infants in particular are thermal-sensitive, and in this group high airway temperatures can be just as dangerous as insufficient ambient heat.

A clearly avoidable hazard is direct thermal injury to the respiratory tract.[43] Although the exact temperature at which such damage can occur is not known, long-term delivery of gas directly to the lower respiratory tract at temperatures above 50° to 60°C has the potential to cause at least temporary damage. Although the risk of thermal injury has been minimized with the temperature control and monitoring systems built into newer humidifying equipment, such devices can cause the practitioner to become complacent with regard to bedside observation and assessment. Automated monitoring or control systems are no substitute for astute and ongoing clinical observation; human and mechanical errors are frequent enough that the practitioner must rely on ongoing verification of proper function.

Infection. The infection potential of respiratory care equipment has typically focused on aerosol generators as the primary source for the spread of bacteria. On the assumption that they do not generate particulate water suspensions, true vaporizing humidifiers were considered incapable of transmitting bacteria through the air.

However, it has been clearly demonstrated that bubble-diffusion humidifiers can produce aerosols capable of carrying bacteria.[44,45] A recent study of the cascade-type humidifier has confirmed its potential to transmit pathogenic organisms through the production of particulate water aerosols.[46] Interestingly, the same study revealed that the wick-type humidifier did not produce either detectable aerosol or bacterial carryover. This apparent discrepancy is explained by the mechanism involved in humidifier aerosol generation. Humidifiers of the bubble-diffusion and cascade types produce particulate water through the collapse of unstable bubbles.[46] Since wick humidifiers do not produce water bubbles, they do not generate aerosolized water. In regard to hygroscopic condenser humidifiers, clinical research has demonstrated that the hygroscopic material in these devices can become grossly contaminated with pathogens from the patient within 4 hours of initial application.[47-49] However, these studies present conflicting results with respect to transmission of pathogens to the patient through aerosolization.

The actual magnitude of the infection hazard posed by humidifiers is not entirely clear. Whereas HCHs can become contaminated soon after application (because of their proximity to the patient's airway), most heated humidifiers in ventilator circuits remain sterile after 24 to 48 hours of use. This observation is probably due to a combination of factors, including (1) prior HEPA filtration of the gas entering these humidifiers, (2) the distance of the humidifier from the patient's airway, and (3) the poor survival of most nosocomial organisms at the 50°C temperature typically found in humidifier reservoirs.[50] Also, most organisms that do contaminate humidifier reservoirs arise from the patients who are receiving therapy, thereby simply reexposing them to a low inoculum.[46] Regular changes of the humidifier and circuitry with sterile replacements (every 24 hours), the use of prepackaged sterile disposables or wick humidifiers, closed-feed reservoir systems, and careful drainage of condensate *away* from the humidifier and the patient all minimize the likelihood of humidifier contamination and the spread of infection. Nonetheless, the hazard of infection with humidification devices, especially bubble or cascade types used on a long-term basis, is a real one. All appropriate safeguards should be employed, especially for patients at high risk.

Electrical hazards. Since heated humidifiers use an electrical source to power their heating elements (and their accompanying monitoring and alarm systems, if present), electrical shock is a potential hazard. Modern equipment standards and hospital preventive maintenance programs have lowered this risk, but faulty equipment can cause sufficient current leakage to pose a hazard, especially to patients with indwelling catheters or other conduits through which current may enter the body.[51] General guidance on minimizing of shock hazards with electrical equipment is provided in Chapter 13. With regard to heated humidifiers, the following minimum guidelines apply: (1) Only devices that have been certified to fall below the maximum current leakage standards should be placed in service, (2) devices in service should always be connected to appropriately grounded receptacles, and (3) any electrical malfunction, however slight, should be grounds for taking the equipment out of service immediately.

AEROSOL THERAPY

An aerosol is defined as a suspension of liquid or solid particles in a gas. Aerosol therapy represents the application of liquid or solid particle suspensions to the airway to achieve specific clinical objectives. The major objectives of aerosol therapy are (1) to provide humidification to the respiratory tract, (2) to serve as an adjunct for mobilization of bronchial secretions, and (3) to provide a route for direct administration of drugs to the respiratory tract.

The rational use of aerosols in the care of patients with respiratory disorders requires that clinicians understand both the general properties of these unique mixtures and the factors that determine their therapeutic effectiveness.

Physical properties of aerosols

Aerosol terminology. Several terms are used to describe the general properties of aerosol suspensions.[52,53] *Stability* refers to the ability of an aerosol to remain in suspension over time. Aerosol stability depends on a number of characteristics, including (1) the size and nature of the particulate matter, (2) the concentration of particles present, (3) the ambient humidity, and (4) the mobility of the carrier gas. Of course, instability is the opposite of stability, that is, the tendency of suspended particles to fall out of suspension.

Aerosol *density* refers to the number of aerosol particles per unit of carrier gas. Since direct clinical measurement of this particulate density is not practical, aerosol density is often equated with the actual weight of aerosol carried in a given volume of gas, called the *weight density*. Two units of weight density are common: grams of aerosol per square meter (g/m^3) or milligrams of aerosol per liter (mg/L). Given that one m^3 equals 1000 liters, and that 1 gram equals 1000 milligrams, a given weight density value is the same, regardless of units (eg, 44 g/m^3 = 44 mg/L). Although weight density is a useful measure, it may not always reflect the true particulate density of the aerosol. This is because most of an aerosol's mass (weight) typically is contained in a relatively small number of large particles.

From a therapeutic point of view, the clinical effectiveness of an aerosol is related to both its stability and its density. Unfortunately, aerosols, especially liquid suspensions, are dynamic mixtures. Not only is the size range of particulate matter usually great, but interaction among the particles and the suspending gas results in continual changes in the characteristics of the aerosol. Particles can shrink or disappear by evaporation, be "reborn" by condensation, grow by absorption, coalescence, or agglomeration, or leave the suspension altogether by settling as a result of gravity.

A large population of particles actually undergoes a process of *aging*, whereby there is a gradual increase in the number of particles of optimum size and concentration for

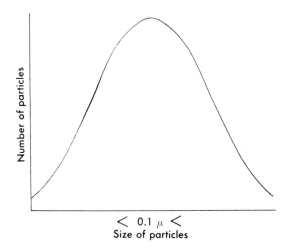

Fig. 23-7 Distribution curve of aerosol particle sizes. If a population of particles of many sizes is allowed to settle, the largest number will have diameters somewhere around 0.1μm, with decreasing frequency of sizes larger and smaller. (Modified from Lovejoy FW and Morrow PE: Anesthesiology 23:460, 1962.)

maximum stability, with a reduction in the range of sizes. This "ideal" state consists of particles that range from 0.01 to 3.0 μm in diameter, with a density in the range of 100 to 1000 particles per milliliter of gas.[53] Fig. 23-7 shows a distribution of particulate diameters according to size in a stable aerosol suspension. The median point on the distribution curve represents that particle size above and below which 50% of the aerosol mass lies. This point is called the *mass median diameter* (MMD) and, together with the relative "spread" of the curve, is a good measure of aerosol stability.

Related to the characteristic of stability are the concepts of penetration, deposition, retention, and clearance.[52] These terms describe the fate of particles once they come into contact with the respiratory tract. *Penetration* refers to the maximum depth to which suspended particles can be carried into the respiratory tract by the inhaled tidal air.

Deposition is the result of the eventual instability of an aerosol, which permits it to "fall out" on a nearby surface, whereas *retention* implies the deposition of particles at a specific location within the respiratory tract.

Aerosol *clearance* is the opposite of retention and, depending on its specific use, may have one of two meanings. Most authors use the term clearance to mean the process whereby deposited particles are removed from the site of deposition by one of several biologic mechanisms to be considered later. A less common but still appropriate use of the term clearance refers to the removal of still suspended particles in the exhaled air.

Penetration and deposition of aerosols. Exactly where inhaled particles deposit in the respiratory tract is of substantial clinical significance. For example, if our aim is to reach the smaller airways of the conducting system but the particles deposit mainly in the nose or mouth, it is unlikely that the aerosol will have the desired effect. In general, the penetration of aerosol particles into the respiratory tract is inversely related to their size. Thus, the smaller the particle size, the greater the depth of penetration.

In fact, only the smallest particles normally gain entrance to the respiratory tract at all. Nasal filtration is so effective that particles greater than 10 μm in diameter deposit in this portion of the upper airway. Particles below this size range gain entry but penetrate to varying depths according to their size.

Table 23-1 shows the deposition of aerosol particles in the 1 to 8 μm range for a normal subject breathing steadily through the mouth at a rate of 15 breaths per minute and at a tidal volume of 1500 ml.[54] Note that the larger particles tend to deposit in the upper airway (oropharynx), with few reaching the alveoli. As particle size decreases down to 3 to 4 μm, there is increasing penetration to the tracheobronchial (conducting) zone and alveolar region. However, as particle size drops below 3 to 4 μm, total deposition decreases and a larger percentage of the aerosol is exhaled. It is important to note that these data are for a normal sub-

Table 23-1 Deposition of Aerosols in the Human Lung

Particle size (μm)	Percent deposition in			% Total deposition	% Cleared (exhaled)
	Upper airway (oropharynx)	Conducting zone	Alveolar region		
1	0	0	16	16	84
2	0	2	40	42	58
3	5	7	50	62	38
4	20	12	42	74	26
5	37	16	30	83	17
6	52	21	17	90	10
7	56	25	11	92	8
8	60	28	5	93	7

Adapted from Stahlhofen W, Gebhart J, and Heyder J: Experimental determination of the regional deposition of aerosol particles in the human respiratory tract, Am Ind Hyg Assoc J 41:385-398, 1980.

ject, with an ideal ventilatory pattern, breathing an aerosol with a narrow dispersion of particle sizes. Results in clinical practice will obviously differ according to variation from these conditions. Nonetheless, the data demonstrate the general penetration pattern that is to be expected.

Other than particle size, five major factors determine the penetration and deposition of aerosols in the lung: (1) the actual physical nature of the particles, (2) the force of gravity, (3) the kinetic activity of the carrier gas molecules, (4) inertial forces, and (5) the pattern of ventilation.[55,56]

Physical nature of particles. Of the many physical and chemical characteristics of aerosols related to deposition and retention, the most important is the affinity of the suspended particles for water. Particles that tend to absorb water are said to be *hygroscopic*.

Initially small, a hygroscopic particle may absorb relatively large amounts of water from either the ambient air or the respiratory tract. As the particle absorbs water, it increases in diameter, sometimes manyfold. This change in size and mass will, of course, alter the site of eventual deposition.

The solubility and chemical nature of particles also may play important roles in determining penetration and deposition. Very small particles may dissolve in or chemically react with aerosolized water or other solvents of a larger size and thus eventually deposit at levels different from those dictated by their original sizes.

Finally, particle contour can influence deposition. Although we speak of aerosol particles as though they were all regular spheres of liquid, some solid substances produce particles with many angulations and irregular surfaces. Such particles may exhibit patterns of movement and deposition that are considerably different from those predicted on the basis of the physical laws we have been discussing.

Force of gravity. The speed with which a particle will "settle" is one measure of its tendency to deposit. This *sedimentation rate* is related to the force exerted by gravity on the particle mass and to the buoyancy provided by the carrier gas (see Chapter 4). The greater the mass of any body, the greater the influence of gravity. Conversely, the greater the density of the carrier gas, the greater the influence of buoyant forces.

Suspended particles of between 0.1 μm and 70 μm generally follow the prediction of Stokes' law of sedimentation. In its entirety, Stokes' law relates the velocity at which a small particle settles to several factors, including the particle volume, the particle density, the acceleration of gravity, and the density and viscous resistance of the carrier gas. For clinical purposes, we may simplify Stokes' law to state that the rate at which a particle settles is proportional to its density times the square of its diameter. Thus:

$$\text{Sedimentation rate} \propto \text{Density} \times \text{diameter}^2$$

Table 23-2 compares the relative velocities with which three hypothetical particles would settle under the influence of gravity. Particle x, with a density of 1 unit and a diameter of 2 units, will settle with a velocity of 4 units. Particle y, of the same density but with twice the diameter, will settle four times as fast, whereas particle z, with the same diameter but twice the density, will settle twice as fast.

Kinetic activity of gas molecules. The kinetic activity of carrier gas molecules affects mainly the smallest particles in a suspension, generally those with diameters of 0.1 μm or less. Because such particles approach the size of large molecules, they are minimally influenced by gravity. Rather, their motion is determined by the kinetic activity of the carrier gas molecules surrounding them. The suspended particles are constantly bombarded by these gas molecules and are thus impelled into high-speed random movements for very short distances, called *Brownian motion*. The smaller the particles, the greater their velocities.

This random movement of suspended matter, called Brownian diffusion, causes many of the particles to come into contact with nearby surfaces. Impaction on a surface as a result of such motion is called *diffusion deposition*. How much of a particulate suspension will deposit by this method is a function of its diffusion coefficient. The diffusion coefficient of an aerosol is calculated as the volume of particles that can diffuse a distance of 1 μm over an area of 1 cm² at a pressure of 1 atm. The diffusion coefficient of an aerosol is inversely proportional to its MMD and directly proportional to the temperature (kinetic activity) of the carrier gas.

The fraction of a given volume of aerosol particles that will fall out of suspension also is determined by the distance to the nearest surface. Therefore, the probability of diffusion deposition is a function of both the diffusion coefficient and the time available to impact on the nearest surface. Fig. 23-8 illustrates the difference between sedimentation due to gravity and diffusion deposition.

Inertial forces. Inertial mass is a property of all matter, including the smallest aerosol particles. According to Newton's first law of motion, inertial mass causes a body at rest to stay at rest unless acted on by an external force. Conversely, a body in motion will continue at constant velocity in a straight line unless acted on by an external force. For a body in motion, the greater its inertial mass, the greater will be the force needed to change its velocity or direction.

Table 23-2   Gravity Deposition

Particle	Density	Diameter	Velocity
x	1	2	4
y	1	4	16
z	2	2	8

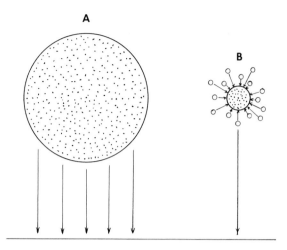

Fig. 23-8   The mass of the larger aerosol particle, **A**, makes it susceptible to the settling force of gravity. The smaller particle, **B**, is more affected by the bombardment of surrounding carrier gas molecules, eventually impinging on a nearby surface; this is called diffusion deposition.

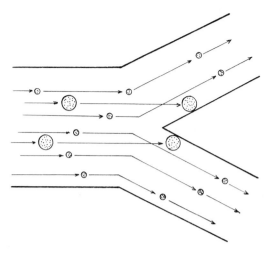

Fig. 23-9   Inertial impaction of large aerosol particles whose masses tend to maintain their motion in straight lines. As airway direction changes, the particles deposit on nearby walls. Smaller particles are carried around corners by the airstream and fall out less readily.

As applied to homogeneous aerosols, the inertial mass of a particle is proportional to the cube of its radius. A particle 2 μm in diameter will therefore have eight times (2^3) the inertial mass of a similar particle 1 μm in diameter and thus will require eight times as much force to alter its velocity or direction.

Fig. 23-9 illustrates the difference in behavior of small and large aerosol particles moving in an airstream. Inertial forces tend to keep the particles flowing at constant velocity in a straight line. Frictional forces, especially those associated with changes in direction of flow, tend to alter the direction of particle movement.

For the larger particles, when the stream undergoes a sudden change in direction, the forces of inertia exceed those of frictional resistance, and they continue on a straight course, impacting on the surface of the airway.[55,56] The amount of particle deposition caused by this inertial impaction is directly proportional to the mass of the aerosol particles and their mean velocity.

On the other hand, the inertial forces acting on the smaller particles in Fig. 23-9 are insufficient to overcome frictional resistance, making possible a change in direction with the airstream. Impaction of low-mass particles can occur but only at high velocities or under conditions of turbulent flow.

Ventilatory pattern. In general, the deposition and retention of aerosol particles is directly related to inhaled volume and inversely related to respiratory rate.[55] Moreover, because bulk gas flow in the respiratory zone is minimal, the effect of ventilatory pattern on particle behavior is significant mainly in the conducting zones of the lung. Thus the depth and frequency of ventilation have little influence on the deposition of particles once they have

reached the alveolar level,[57,58] although breath holding at end inspiration can increase alveolar deposition.[55]

The pattern of ventilation higher in the respiratory tract does help determine the volume of particles reaching the alveoli and thus exerts an indirect influence on deposition in this region. Deposition of particles is increased with both increasing tidal volume and decreasing frequency, and the effects of both are additive. Shallow breathing carries a reduced volume of aerosols per tidal volume, and rapid breathing rates reduce the time available for particle deposition by sedimentation or diffusion. High flows associated with rapid breathing do increase inertial impaction but mainly in the nose and large upper airways, thereby further limiting aerosol penetration.

As with many principles of aerosol therapy, disagreement and conflicting data persist concerning the optimum ventilatory pattern for maximum penetration and retention of mists.[59] If the objectives of the aerosol therapy require maximum penetration and deposition, the ideal ventilatory pattern appears to consist of slow, moderately deep breathing through the mouth, with breath holding at the end of inspiration.[55] This facilitates the introduction into the respiratory tract of a significant volume of particles and allows adequate time for larger particles to deposit by sedimentation and for the smallest to enter the alveoli and settle by diffusion. It also minimizes inertial impaction in the larger airways due to turbulent flow. Moreover, for patients with poor distribution of inspired air, increased tidal volumes may improve the distribution of aerosols to otherwise poorly ventilated areas.[22] This is a practical point that will be reiterated in our discussion of aerosol drug administration.

Clearance of aerosols

We now concern ourselves with the removal of particles from the respiratory tract by means other than exhalation. For clarity, we will discuss clearance from the conducting and respiratory zones separately. Moreover, because liquid aerosol particles are generally absorbed by the respiratory tract mucosa at the site of deposition, we will limit our focus to clearance of solid particles. Mucociliary transport is the primary mechanism for clearance of solid particles from the conducting zones; several mechanisms help clear the alveolar region of foreign particulate matter.

Mucociliary transport. As described in Chapter 6, the mucosa of the conducting zones of the lung consists of ciliated epithelium. The cilia continually propel an overlying thin gel layer of mucus toward the larynx at rates of up to 13.5 mm/min. Produced by goblet cells, this mucus layer is, on average, about 5 μm thick.[60] Its function is to entrap foreign particles and, with the aid of the cilia, to remove them from the respiratory tract.

The system is extremely efficient as long as both cilia and mucus are normal. Should a pathologic process increase the depth or viscosity of the mucous layer, its upward movement will gradually slow. Indeed, when the thickness of the fluid approaches four to five times the height of the cilia, surface transport effectively stops. Similarly, function will be impaired after damage to or destruction of the cilia themselves.

Respiratory zone clearance. Particles in the respiratory zones of the lung are removed by several mechanisms. Some particles (such as silica) may be considered functionally removed in situ through encapsulation and immobilization by a deposit of fibrous tissue, although they remain for the duration of the subject's life. (This response can result in the pathologic changes referred to as pulmonary fibrosis.) Other solid aerosols are picked up by the alveolar macrophages. The mobility of these phagocytic cells permits them to gather at sites of foreign matter deposition. After engulfing the particles within their own protoplasm, the macrophages can transport them for removal by the mucociliary mechanism or via the interstitial lymphatic vessels for transport to regional lymph nodes. Depending on solubility, some particles may dissolve in tissue fluid and diffuse into the general circulation, to be metabolized by the liver or other organ systems.

The preceding discussion of the properties of aerosols includes many generalizations and assumptions that are still under investigation.[59] The current interest in aerosols has led to many changes and refinements in research methods, making it difficult to correlate data from one source to another. These differences in technique account for much of the variance found in the literature, especially with respect to effective particle sizes and to the degree of penetration by aerosols. Nevertheless, we have reviewed the most widely accepted behavioral characteristics of aerosols as they apply to clinical medicine, and we can only be alert to new developments in this important field of study.

Indications for aerosol therapy

Although some indications for aerosol therapy are still controversial and much needs to be learned regarding the efficacy of certain treatment approaches, current knowledge supports its use to achieve selected clinical objectives.[3,59] As previously delineated, currently accepted objectives of aerosol therapy include the following:

1. To provide humidification to the respiratory tract.
2. To serve as an adjunct for mobilization of bronchial secretions.
3. To provide a route for direct administration of drugs to the respiratory tract.

Humidification of the respiratory tract. Aerosolized water serves a double function. Its principal duty is to deliver liquid water, in minute particle form, to the mucosal surface. The water that "rains out" in the airways is intended to help thin secretions and ease their removal through coughing or mechanical aspiration.

In addition to this local effect of water particles on the airway surfaces, aerosols provide an important source of moisture for humidifying the inspired carrier gas. As the gas enters the warmth of the body and its vapor capacity increases, suspended water particles evaporate into the gas, raising its vapor tension toward that of body humidity. Humidification can be increased by heating the water to be aerosolized so that when it reaches the respiratory tract it is at or near BTPS conditions.

Often heated water aerosol is used in lieu of a heated humidifier, described earlier. Again, for patients with artificial airways, the primary aim is to supply near body humidity levels to the inspired gases. However, only an aerosol can supply additional water (beyond BTPS) to the airway. In principle, this additional particulate water should aid in keeping the artificial airway cleared by not allowing respiratory tract secretions to accumulate or become inspissated. Of course, in order to avoid occlusion of the airway, secretions must be removed by coughing or suctioning (see Chapter 21).

Although the usefulness of aerosols in providing adequate humidification for patients with artificial airways is well accepted, its benefit to patients whose upper airways are intact is yet to be proved.[1,3,59] Traditionally, cool (unheated) water aerosols are used for their soothing effect on inflamed tissues of the upper airways of patients immediately after removal of an artificial airway (extubation), following fiberoptic bronchoscopy, and in treatment of the inflammatory obstruction that characterizes laryngitis or croup.[24,61,62] The lower temperature of these aerosols is thought to help decrease the swelling and tissue edema that may occur in these situations. On the other hand, heated water aerosols are considered preferable when the aim is to help mobilize secretions in patients with intact upper airways.

Aiding in mobilization of secretions. Aerosols may be used to facilitate the mobilization of secretions for either therapeutic or diagnostic purposes. Therapeutically, aerosol therapy has been used in patients with retained secretions that are difficult to mobilize. Diagnostically, aerosols may be applied to facilitate coughing and expectoration of sputum specimens for either cytologic or microbiologic examination.

Therapeutic use. Patients with acute and chronic respiratory diseases are often given various types of aerosol therapy to facilitate the removal of secretions.[24] These aerosols usually consist of bland solutions that are thought to have little pharmacologic activity. More controversial is the use of aerosols containing pharmacologically active mucolytic agents to aid in the mobilization of secretions.[3] The actions and uses of these mucolytic agents were described in Chapter 20.

Bland aerosols include chemically inactive solutions such as water, saline solution, propylene glycol, and (historically) detergents.[22,24,63] A recent review of the literature on bland aerosols failed to find substantial objective evidence of enhanced respiratory or mucociliary function.[61] However, subjective observations of improved efficiency of cough and ease of expectoration following bland aerosol inhalation suggest that this form of therapy can be a useful adjunct to other forms of bronchial hygiene.[11,24,62,63] Indeed, the lack of hard evidence that the inhalation of bland aerosols can cause measurable improvements in respiratory and mucociliary function may attest only to the inadequacy of available testing methods and measurements.[3]

When bland aerosols are indicated to facilitate the removal of secretions, several practical factors should be kept in mind. Since only a portion of the inhaled aerosol is retained, large-volume, high-density mists involving heated aerosols or ultrasonically produced mists have been recommended.[24] Both of these methods produce a greater weight of aerosol per liter of carrier gas than do conventional cool aerosol devices. Such aerosols are best administered by a mouthpiece system, with the patient's head and tongue positioned to minimize obstruction to flow. If a mask is used, the patient should be instructed in proper mouth breathing. In either case, slow, moderately deep breaths are recommended. Occasional sigh-like breaths at near inspiratory capacity may help open poorly ventilated areas and aid in the subsequent distribution of the mist.

The duration of therapy may vary according to individual need and tolerance. Generally, if significant amounts of liquid are to be deposited, treatment periods may range from 30 to 60 minutes several times a day; continuous administration may be necessary for patients with significant clearance problems.[24] To minimize or prevent the increase in airway resistance often seen with inhalation of high-density aerosols, prior treatment with bronchodilators should be considered.[24,64]

The patient's ability to clear mobilized secretions should also be monitored. Bland aerosols should be considered adjunct therapy, and other methods that help evacuate se-

cretions, such as proper coughing techniques and postural drainage, should also be used (see Chapter 27).

Sputum induction. Sputum induction represents a special application of aerosol therapy to help gather sputum specimens for diagnostic examination. Such examinations are conducted for either cytologic or microbiologic diagnosis.

In the cytologic sputum examination, specimens are prepared by cytotechnologists and carefully examined under the microscope for the presence of malignant cells signifying a cancerous lesion in the respiratory tract. Often, if the lesion is in communication with the airway, cells from the surface of the tumor will desquamate, mix with bronchial secretions, and be expectorated. Although the absence of malignant cells does not eliminate the possibility of cancer, their presence is strong evidence of the existence of cancer somewhere in the bronchi or lungs. Over the last decade the use of sputum induction to obtain cytologic specimens has been largely replaced with diagnostic fiberoptic bronchoscopy. However, since the "reach" of diagnostic bronchoscopy is limited to the larger airways, sputum-induction methods should still be available to assist clinicians in the diagnosis of pulmonary tumors.

On the other hand, the use of sputum-induction methods to assist in microbiologic diagnosis is still well established. Indeed, sputum induction has recently been demonstrated as a safe and effective alternative to diagnostic fiberoptic bronchoscopy in the diagnosis of *Pneumocystis carinii* pneumonia, an atypical respiratory infection that is seen in patients with AIDS and is caused by a parasitic organism.[65]

Microbiologic sputum examination attempts to determine the presence or absence of pathogenic organisms in the secretions and to identify those that are present. Initially the specimen is smeared on a glass slide, stained with an appropriate dye, and examined microscopically for organisms. This often gives a good idea of the general type of organism present and permits initiation of appropriate antibiotic therapy. During the search for specific identification of bacterial pathogens, the rest of the specimen is mixed with several kinds of culture medium and incubated to allow maximum growth. Subsequent examination of these cultures usually leads to identification of the organisms that are present.

Most of the patients treated by the respiratory care practitioner will have little trouble providing sputum specimens for analysis, and no special procedures will be required. However, patients with suspected cancer or chronic infections, such as tuberculosis, may have very scanty sputum or none at all, and obtaining specimens from them may be crucial. For these patients, the induced-sputum technique may be the best means of securing a specimen.

Because the bronchial mucosa responds to almost any inhaled irritant with increased secretions and a reflex cough, many methods of sputum induction have been tried. These include distilled water, hypertonic saline solution (3% to 10%), acetylcysteine, and even sulfur dioxide gas.[66] Sulfur dioxide gas, although effective, is simply too irritating and is no longer recommended. Moreover, the mucolytic agents have little value in the absence of secretions.

The saline aerosols are preheated to 140° to 185°F by an immersion heating unit in the aerosol generator.[66-68] This "superheated" aerosol is well saturated with humidity as the patient inhales it, and it also contains large numbers of particles for deposition throughout the bronchial tree. Because of their high osmolarity, hypertonic saline solutions draw fluid out from the mucosal layer into the bronchial lumen, increasing the volume of secretions available for expectoration.

Distilled water particles, on the other hand, condense on the bronchial mucosa, where they mix with and increase the volume of the normal thin layer of mucus present. The abundance of fine particles also has an irritant effect, stimulating a cough that facilitates expectoration. In concept, both the saline and water aerosols stimulate a cough that, in turn, mobilizes secretions, superficial mucosal cells, and any bacteria close to the bronchial lumen. Cells and bacteria, which the subject would be unable to produce by voluntary cough, can thus be examined.

When the technique of sputum induction was first introduced, it was customary to use a 20% solution of propylene glycol as the saline solvent because of the stabilizing properties attributed to this agent. It was believed that the inclusion of propylene glycol in the mixture ensured the penetration and deposition of a maximum number of particles in the respiratory tract. However, further experience demonstrated that propylene glycol itself had an inhibiting effect on *Mycobacterium tuberculosis,* destroying it or preventing its growth in culture.[66] This was a serious handicap, since the recovery of tubercle bacilli is an important function of sputum induction. Today, the use of propylene glycol for sputum induction is rare; hypertonic saline solution and distilled water are the agents of choice.

At some hospitals ultrasonic aerosol generators, which are described later, have been found to be useful in inducing cough for collection of sputum. Using distilled water at room temperature, these generators produce finely uniform particles that stimulate a heavy cough, usually after only a few breaths. Unfortunately, there are no available data comparing the relative amounts of secretions produced by ultrasonic aerosols as against the standard heated hypertonic saline aerosols.

When used to aid in the production of a sputum sample, the duration of aerosol therapy can be varied to suit each individual patient. The patient is instructed to inhale the aerosol through the mouth in an easy and comfortable manner, resting as often as necessary. Sputum should be collected over the ensuing 30 minutes, and care should be taken to avoid gathering oral or nasal secretions in the sample. Sterile containers should be available for all specimens. If sputum is to be examined for malignant cells, it must be free of foreign particles. This is best assured by having patients wash their teeth and thoroughly rinse their mouths before collection.

Drug administration. Drug administration by aerosol is a well-established component of comprehensive respiratory care. These actions are best documented for agents that affect airway caliber by relaxing the bronchial smooth muscle, that is, the bronchodilator drugs. The efficacy of certain other aerosolized agent is more controversial. Details on the use of pharmacologic agents in respiratory care were provided in Chapter 20.

The aerosol route has several advantages and disadvantages when compared with other methods of administration (see the box on p. 571).[69,70] Of course, the aerosol route is always available. Moreover, aerosols provide direct deposition of the agent at the desired site of action, thereby minimizing the requisite dose, the response time, and systemic side effects.[55]

However, there are several disadvantages.[3,24,55] The dosage of drugs delivered to the airways by the aerosol route is often difficult to estimate.[3,55,59,69] Individual patients may not adhere to the prescribed routine, either underutilizing or overutilizing the drug. Also, the dosage required for the desired effect may change significantly for a patient during acute exacerbations of airway obstruction and infection.

Still, objective test data indicate that these agents, when properly prescribed and administered, can dramatically improve pulmonary function. For this reason, selective administration of drugs directly to the airway is one of the best substantiated current uses of aerosol therapy.

Techniques of aerosol administration

Instruments used to generate suspensions of liquid or solid particles for deposition in the respiratory tract are called nebulizers (from "nebula," meaning a cloud or mist). Some devices designed to provide airway or room humidification also produce an aerosol suspension, but they generate water particles only to facilitate evaporation and not to maintain the water in suspension. Nonetheless, because these devices employ nebulization principles, we will consider them here.

The most common way to categorize nebulizers is according to their source of power. Gas-powered nebulizers are pneumatically driven by a gas source at pressures above atmospheric pressure and normally use a high-velocity jet to disperse the liquid or solid. Electrically powered nebulizers, on the other hand, employ electrical current in various indirect ways to disperse liquid solutions into an aerosol suspension.

Gas-powered nebulizers. Although gas-powered nebulizers are used for both aerosol generation and humidification, for the sake of simplicity we will refer to them as nebulizers and differentiate between their specific uses when indicated.

All gas-powered nebulizers used to generate liquid par-

ADVANTAGES AND DISADVANTAGES OF AEROSOL THERAPY

ADVANTAGES

Permits chemotherapeutic targeting in respiratory tract

Onset of therapeutic effect is usually rapid

Allows individual dose titration

Only small doses of potent drugs are usually required for therapeutic results

Extrapulmonary drug effects are usually minimized

Permits use of drugs that cannot be administered by other routes

Respiratory tract route is usually available for drug delivery

Simultaneous humidification and demulcent aerosol therapy is beneficial for intubated and tracheostomized patients

Self-administration by metered devices is convenient and generally is inexpensive

In clinical setting, patients receive close attention, supervision, monitoring, and breathing instructions by respiratory therapists during aerosol administration

DISADVANTAGES

Sophisticated, expensive equipment is often employed for aerosol generation and delivery

Under normal circumstances, aerosol retention and therefore precise drug dosage received by patient is unknown; overdosage and underdosage are common

Small percentage of aerosolized drug is deposited along respiratory tract

Patient cooperation is required in establishing breathing pattern that favors aerosol penetration and deposition

Aerosol particles may not reach site of need in presence of distal airway obstruction

Deposition in oropharynx leads to systemic absorption and increases possibility of extrapulmonary effects

Oropharyngeal irritation in some patients leads to gag reflex, nausea, vomiting, or aerophagia

Tracheobronchial mucosal irritation may lead to bronchospasm and coughing

Propellant, mixture of fluorocarbons (Freon), in pressurized nebulizers may cause detrimental side effects, for example, increases in airway resistance and possibly cardiac arrhythmias

Use of high concentrations of oxygen as carrier gas in sustained aerosol therapy may lead to oxygen toxicity

Aerosol generating and delivering equipment have been implicated as sources of nosocomial infection

Respiratory therapists involved in delivery of aerosol therapy and individuals in immediate vicinity of patient receiving aerosol therapy are exposed to airborne drugs

From Lehnert BE and Schachter EN: The pharmacology of respiratory care, St Louis, 1980, The CV Mosby Co.

ticulate aerosols employ a jet or restricted orifice to disperse the liquid into the gas. Because it functions without moving parts, the jet nebulizer is versatile, simple, and dependable. Although jet nebulizers come in many shapes and sizes, they all have the same fundamental features, as depicted in Fig. 23-10.

Pressurized gas, provided by a simple hand-operated bulb, a motorized compressor, or bulk gas, is the power source. The gas enters the nebulizer chamber through a restricted orifice, providing a jet stream of high velocity, *A.* The jet is directed across the end of a fine capillary tube, *B,* the other end of which is immersed in the solution to be nebulized. The high velocity of the gas produces a local drop in pressure immediately adjacent to the capillary tube opening (the Bernoulli effect). Because the reservoir surface is subject to atmospheric pressure, liquid is forced up the capillary tube *(solid arrows).* As it reaches the top of the tube, the liquid is sheared off into particles of varying sizes by the gas escaping from the jet. In general, the greater the gas velocity at the jet, the greater will be the production of aerosol particles.

These particles are then impelled against one or more

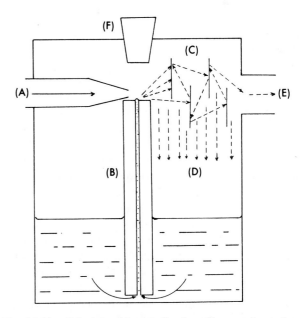

Fig. 23-10 Principle of jet nebulization. (See text for explanation.) (Modified from Egan DF: Conn Med 31:353, 1967.)

barriers called *baffles, C.* A baffle is simply a surface on which larger particles may impact, causing either further fragmentation or removal from the suspension by condensation back into the reservoir, *D.* Although baffles can be of many shapes and sizes, none is necessarily more effective than another; indeed, the configuration of the nebulizer chamber itself may function as an effective baffle. However, the more baffling that occurs throughout the nebulizer system, the smaller will be the MMD of the particles that evolve. In fact, sequential baffling makes possible the production of extremely fine aerosols of uniform and small particle size, called microaerosols. The MMD of such microaerosols can be as small as 0.5 μm.[71]

The outflow gas to the patient, *E,* thus contains aerosol particles in a size range determined, in part, by the design of nebulizer. Many nebulizer chambers provide an optional port for the introduction of air into the gas-particle mixture, *F.* When this port is opened, the forces at the jet entrain room air into the chamber, providing an increased flow through the nebulizer in direct proportion to the size of the opening. This increase in total output flow generally increases total aerosol output (in grams of liquid per liter per minute) but actually lowers the density of the aerosol delivered to the patient. This lower density is the result of the proportionately greater increase in carrier gas flow over aerosol production and an increase in particle evaporation.

Gas-powered nebulizers used in respiratory care include (1) the large-reservoir air-entrainment jet nebulizer, (2) the hydronamic (Babbington) nebulizer, (3) the small-volume jet medication nebulizer, (4) the metered-dose inhaler (MDI), and (5) the evaporative small-particle aerosol generator, or SPAG.

Large-reservoir air-entrainment jet nebulizer. The large-reservoir air-entrainment jet nebulizer is the primary gas-powered aerosol generator used to provide humidification to the respiratory tract. As the name implies, these large-reservoir jet nebulizers have a relatively large solution capacity (ranging from 0.5 to 3.0 L), and are intended for either intermittent or continuous use. Devices in this category also incorporate a variable air-entrainment system. When driven by oxygen to the jet, these units can entrain room air to dilute the oxygen to various levels. Common reusable reservoir jet nebulizers can reduce the 100% oxygen driving the jet to near 40% oxygen by entrainment and mixing of room air. Newer disposable units can produce oxygen concentrations below 30%. Dilution of oxygen or jet gas in these nebulizers functions on principles that are described further in Chapter 25.

The jets used in all gas-powered nebulizers are restricted orifices. Most nebulizers used in respiratory care operate with oxygen or compressed air from a source supplying 50 psig pressure. Because the jets are so small and create such high resistance, there is an upper limit of flow for each nebulizer when operated at the maximum available pressure of 50 psig. Generally, this upper flow limit in most air-entrainment nebulizers ranges between 12 and 15 L/min. Obviously, if a source pressure less than 50 psig is used (as will be the case with some air compressors), the maximum flow through the jet will be less. Because total airflow from an entrainment nebulizer is partly influenced by its jet flow capability, practitioners should know the maximum flow limit through the nebulizers they commonly use. Certain systems, such as oxygen hoods and tents, require minimum flows that are substantially greater than some nebulizers can provide (see Chapter 25).

Air entrainment increases both aerosol and total gas flow output from these reservoir nebulizers, but not necessarily in similar proportions. Although aerosol output may increase by one and one half to two times with the addition of air entrainment, there may be a 4- to 20-fold increase in total flow output, depending on the amount of air entrainment available. Therefore, while total aerosol output per minute increases with air entrainment, the particle density of the aerosol may actually decrease, resulting in a like decrease in the percent body humidity delivered. Although recent studies have generally confirmed this relationship, differences in humidity output of a given device at varying F_{IO_2} levels are not always significant.[72]

Of more importance in determining the humidity output of large-reservoir jet nebulizers is the operating temperature of the unit (Fig. 23-11). From our previous discussions of humidifiers, we already know how temperature affects humidity; these principles also apply to nebulizers. Some reservoir entrainment nebulizers can be heated to provide temperature control of the delivered mist.[6] Heating the water reservoir raises the temperature of gas leaving the nebulizer, thereby increasing the humidity-carrying capacity. This significantly increases both the total water output per minute and the percent body humidity delivered by the nebulizer. Laboratory studies of large-reservoir heated jet nebulizers demonstrate that these devices are capable of providing humidity outputs equivalent to 75% to 95% relative humidity at body temperature.[72] This level is sufficient for humidification of the respiratory tract, even in patients whose upper airways have been bypassed. However, this level of humidity will not provide significant additional water in particulate form for the mobilization of secretions. In light of this knowledge, normally heated jet nebulizers are not the devices of choice when the objective is to deposit additional particulate water in the respiratory tract. Alternative methods for delivering additional particulate water to the respiratory tract will be discussed subsequently.

If the unit is not heated, cooling as a result of evaporation occurs, and the delivered absolute humidity will be even lower. It has been demonstrated that, with unheated jet nebulizers driven by oxygen, the reservoir water temperature drops significantly.[73] At flows of up to 12 L/min, the temperature of the water may drop up to 13°C below its starting ambient temperature within 1 hour. Even the

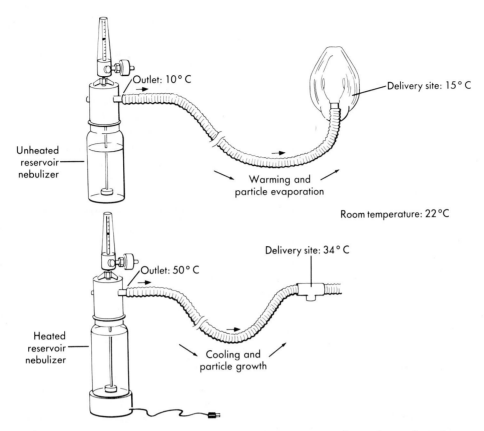

Fig. 23-11   Comparison of unheated versus heated reservoir nebulizers. Output from the unheated (cool) nebulizer is cooler than room temperature because of evaporation of aerosol in the nebulizer. As the aerosol warms on the way to the patient delivery site, further evaporation of particles occurs. Output from the heated nebulizer is hot and humid. Cooling occurs as the aerosol travels through tubing exposed to cooler room and water vapor condenses on aerosol particles, causing them to "grow" larger.

small-volume nebulizers used in ventilator circuits shows a temperature drop of up to 5°C in 10 minutes.

The effects of temperature on aerosols after they have left the nebulizer are also significant.[37] Unheated large-volume reservoir nebulizers will produce aerosols at temperatures less than that of room air. As the aerosol travels to the patient, warming occurs and increases the water vapor capacity of the carrier gas. Although this warming increases the evaporation of water particles, the increase in capacity exceeds the increase in actual water vapor content, resulting in an actual decrease in relative humidity at body temperature. Unheated large-reservoir jet nebulizers are capable of providing humidity outputs equivalent to 60% to 75% relative humidity at body temperature, insufficient to fully overcome a humidity deficit.[72]

Heated reservoir nebulizers produce warm, humid aerosols that will cool as they travel through tubing toward the patient. As with heated humidifiers, this drop in temperature causes condensation of water vapor. The vapor will condense directly on the walls of the tubing and on the aerosol particles themselves (a process called coales-

cence), increasing their size (MMD) and decreasing the stability of the aerosol as a whole.

Table 23-3 presents representative findings regarding the changes in gas temperature that occur at various distances from a heated nebulizer reservoir with large-bore tubing.[73] Measurements were made at 1-foot intervals from the res-

Table 23-3   Influence of Tubing on Vapor Temperature*

Distance from reservoir		Temperature in tube (°C)
cm	ft	
30.5	1	48.5
60.9	2	40.5
91.4	3	37.0
121.9	4	35.0
152.4	5	34.5

From Wells RE Jr et al: Humidification of oxygen during inhalation therapy, N Engl J Med 268:644, 1963.
*Reservoir temperature = 53°C; tube length = 153 cm; internal diameter = 1.9 cm.

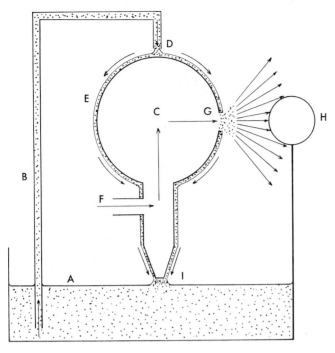

Fig. 23-12   Hydro-Sphere nebulizer. (See text for description.)

ervoir. Note that at a distance of 1 foot from the nebulizer the gas temperature was 48.5°C; at a distance of 3 feet the temperature had dropped to 37°C (body temperature). With this temperature drop, only about half the original water vapor (assuming saturation) can be carried at 37°C. The condensation will cause the particles to increase in size, and some will fall out of the airstream. "Rain out" of water in the tubing will be increased, as compared to the same nebulizer operated without reservoir heating.

It should also be noted in Table 23-3 that the drop in temperature at 1 to 2 feet is 8°C, whereas at 4 to 5 feet the drop in temperature is only 0.5°C. This illustrates the difference in heated and unheated reservoir nebulizers with respect to temperature effects and output.

Although heated all-purpose jet nebulizers can be employed to assist in the mobilization of secretions, their limited humidity output at normal working temperatures minimizes the delivery of substantial amounts of particulate water to the respiratory tract. Additional heating (discussed previously under "Sputum Induction") could rectify this problem but would limit application to intermittent use, because of the potential for hyperpyrexia or thermal injury. The hydronamic, or Babbington, nebulizer (to be discussed next) represents a modification of the jet principle designed, in part, to overcome these limitations.

Hydronamic (Babbington) nebulizer. Rather than using a jet and capillary tube to generate the aerosol, the hydronamic nebulizer uses gravity flow over a glass sphere, as demonstrated in Fig. 23-12. A pumping mechanism (not shown) carries solution from the reservoir, *A,* through a

tube, *B,* to the top of a hollow glass sphere, *C.* The solution is continuously "poured" onto the upper pole of the sphere at *D,* where it distributes itself by gravity as a very thin film, *E,* over the spherical surface. (For illustration purposes, the film depth is greatly exaggerated.)

A gas source, at pressures between 10 and 50 psi, enters the hollow sphere at *F,* pressurizing the interior of the sphere, *G,* rupturing the overlying liquid film, and dispersing it as small particles. An impactor baffle, *H,* removes the large droplets, permitting the outflow only of those within the therapeutic range. Excess unnebulized fluid flows down the sphere and is directed by the sphere's tapered base back into the reservoir for recirculation, *I.*

Among the advantages of the hydronamic aerosol generator are the following: (1) an absence of moving parts; (2) an aerosol particle size distribution within the 1 μm to 10 μm diameter range (MMD of 5 μm); (3) operating temperatures 6° to 10°F below ambient; and (4) a consistent aerosol density over a wide range of flows.[25,74,75] In combination, these characteristics make the hydronamic nebulizer an ideal device for delivery of high-density aerosols to the respiratory tract to aid in mobilization of secretions. Moreover, its ability to provide high-density aerosols at high flows below ambient temperatures make it particularly well suited for use with enclosures.

Small-volume jet medication nebulizers. Administration of drugs by aerosol is usually accomplished with small-volume jet nebulizers especially suited for this task. The prototype medication nebulizer is the so-called hand nebulizer, which combines a simple glass or plastic air jet powered by a manually operated rubber squeeze bulb (Fig. 23-13). Designed originally for the administration of small quantities of bronchodilator agents, the hand nebulizer has been largely replaced by the metered-dose inhaler (see below).

For the administration of mucolytic or antibiotic aerosols (see Chapter 20), or for longer therapy with dilute bronchodilators, small-volume nebulizers can be adapted to a power source. A small compressor is most practical, since it does not need the pressure regulator or flowmeter required for cylinder gas and is safe for home use. For treatments that may last up to 30 or 60 minutes, the use of an aerosol mask is advisable. Not only is the patient spared the nuisance and fatigue of holding a nebulizer to his or her face, but the design of such a mask holds a mass of aerosol particles about the mouth as a reservoir from which the patient can inhale. Since nebulization during the exhalation wastes medication, a simple Y connector can be inserted in the tubing that drives the nebulizer. Obstruction of one arm of the Y by the finger during inhalation permits nebulization; release during exhalation shunts compressor flow into the atmosphere. Commercial versions of these compressor-nebulizer combinations with built-in finger valves to control flow are available for home use.

Small-volume jet-powered medication nebulizers are

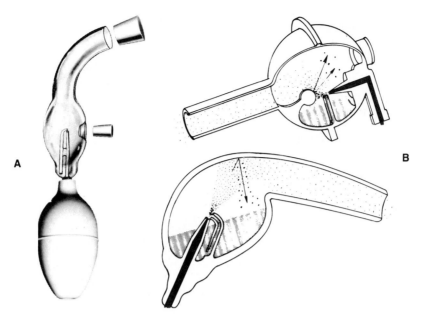

Fig. 23-13   A, The first medical nebulizer. **B,** Hand-bulb compression supplies sufficient pressure to power jet. Lateral negative pressure at jet causes liquid entrainment from capillary tube. (Courtesy Puritan-Bennett Corp, Los Angeles, Calif. From McPherson SP: Respiratory therapy equipment, ed 3, St Louis, 1985, The CV Mosby Co.)

also incorporated into breathing circuits for IPPB devices and mechanical ventilators. In these systems, the relationship between the output of the jet nebulizer and the main flow of gas in the circuit determines the characteristics of the aerosol produced.

As shown in Fig. 23-14, two different approaches are employed in breathing-circuit nebulizers: (1) sidestream nebulization and (2) mainstream nebulization.[6,22] In sidestream nebulization, the aerosol generator is injected into the gas stream. In mainstream nebulization, the entire gas flow to the patient passes through the chamber of the nebulizer. Some small nebulizers can be used in either a sidestream or a mainstream fashion.[6] Generally the sidestream method produces a fine, "dry" aerosol of small droplet size, ideal for deposition of bronchodilator drugs in the smaller airways. On the other hand, with mainstream nebulizers, less evaporation occurs, particle size is larger, and the additional flow passing through the device increases total aerosol output.[6,76] This method is preferable when greater volumes of a drug (for example, a mucolytic or local anesthetic) must be delivered to the larger airways.

The metered-dose inhaler. Popular because of its compactness and simplicity, the metered-dose inhaler (MDI) has become a mainstay in aerosol drug administration. As shown in Fig. 23-15, this device consists of a small vial containing the solution (or powder) to be nebulized and a propellant consisting of a physiologically inert gas that is liquefied under pressure. With the supplied mouthpiece in place, a slight squeeze releases a small valve, allowing the

pressurized gas to nebulize the medication and deliver it in self-limited, premeasured doses.

Just how inert the propellant gases of MDIs are is still a matter of controversy.[77,78] The gases are of a chemical group known as fluorocarbons, of which Freon 11 is the most widely used. Animal experiments suggest that fluorocarbons may cause cardiac arrhythmias and death if inhaled in the presence of hypoxemia, and rhythm disturbances in human beings have been reported. It is speculated that instances of sudden or unexpected death in asthmatic patients may be a result of fluorocarbon-induced cardiac arrest. This view is by no means unanimous, and some investigators question the evidence on which the claims of propellant hazards are based. Despite the unsettled question of safety, MDIs are very popular, and as long as they continue to be used patients should be instructed in their proper application and advised strongly not to exceed the prescribed daily dose limits.

The spray released from an MDI consists of large droplets of the propellant within which the drug is enclosed as either a solid crystal or a liquid. Although the drug particles themselves are in the ideal range for pulmonary penetration (MMDs between 2 and 5 μm), the effective MMD at the orifice of the device may be as large as 40 μm.[55] Although these large droplets shrink as the propellant evaporates, the process can take several seconds. Moreover, the initial velocity of the aerosol particles is high (approximately 30 m/sec). In combination, these factors contribute to substantial inertial impaction of the droplets

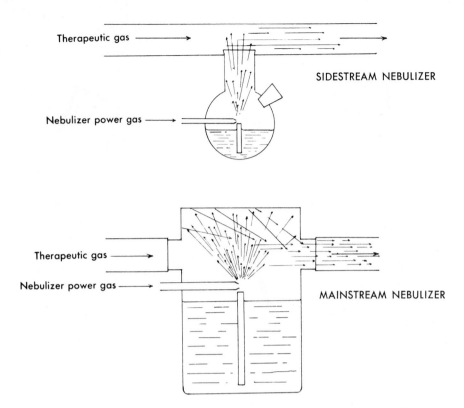

Fig. 23-14   Diagrammatic comparison of sidestream and mainstream nebulizers. The aerosol of the sidestream unit is considerably diluted by the large volume of dry therapeutic gas and provides limited humidity. It is used primarily to administer medication. The entire therapeutic gas flow passes through the mainstream nebulizer chamber and is able to pick up significant moisture. The effectiveness of this nebulizer can be increased by heating the fluid reservoir.

in the oropharynx, with 10% or less of the dose actually penetrating into the lower respiratory tract.[55]

Achievement of adequate deposition in the lung and the desired therapeutic effect can be maximized by (1) activation of the MDI during the course of a slow (less than 30 L/min) inhalation and (2) breath holding at end-inspiration for at least 10 seconds.[79] Unfortunately, the majority of patients using MDIs either do not properly coordinate aerosol discharge with inhalation or exhibit a pattern of breathing that is inconsistent with this ideal.[80]

Clearly, as simple as the MDI is, good results can be expected only with proper technique. In this regard, the respiratory care practitioner can assume a primary role in educating patients in the proper application of these important devices. At a minimum, all patients should be carefully instructed in the use of the MDI and given a demonstration by the practitioner until they exhibit satisfactory proficiency in its application on themselves. Under no circumstances should patients be permitted to rely solely on the manufacturer's directions.

In teaching patients how to use the MDI, some major points should be emphasized. First, the patient should be instructed to open the mouth wide so that the lips and teeth will not obstruct the aerosol flow. Second, the patient

should hold the nebulizer so that its delivery port is directed toward the mouth but is about 1 inch away from the lips. This allows the aerosol to be entrained in the inspiratory airflow. If the nebulizer tube is inserted into the mouth and the lips are tightly pursed about it, much of the aerosol will be deposited in the mouth. Third, the patient should be taught to inhale as slowly and deeply as possible and to deliver the first charge of aerosol just after starting an inhalation. The practitioner will observe that many patients release the aerosol at, or even before, the start of inhalation, depositing much of it outside the respiratory tract. Depending on the length of inhalation and the prescription, two or three aerosol doses may be delivered in one breath. Finally, the patient should be encouraged to hold his or her breath at end-inspiration for at least 5 to 10 seconds, thus allowing maximum aerosol distribution and deposition.

Recently two techniques have been introduced to facilitate proper application of the MDI: extension devices (spacers and holding chambers) and demand systems.[81,82] The extension devices minimize aerosol loss and maximize propellant evaporation, thereby increasing the stability of the suspension and its likelihood of deeper penetration. Demand systems simply synchronize MDI discharge with

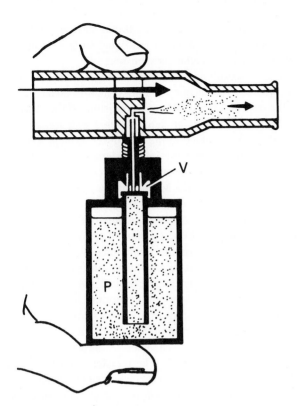

Fig. 23-15 Diagram of a metered-dose inhaler (MDI). The material to be delivered is dissolved in fluid with a boiling point below room temperature, confined in a pressurized container, *P*. A valve is designed to release a measured volume of fluid, *V*. Boiling liquid escapes and evaporates; particles of the active material continue in the airstream as a fine aerosol. (From Burton GG and Hodgkin JE, editors: Respiratory care: a guide to clinical practice, ed 2, Philadelphia, 1984, JB Lippincott Co.)

inspiration, thereby obviating the need for the patient to coordinate this action. The respiratory care practitioner should be well versed in and prepared to teach both of these adjunct methods for improving MDI use and should recommend their application where indicated.

Evaporative small-particle aerosol generator. The evaporative small-particle aerosol generator (SPAG) is a gas-powered jet nebulizer specially designed for the administration of the antiviral agent ribavirin (Virazole) to infants with bronchiolitis.[83] Available commercially from the pharmaceutical corporation that produces the drug, the SPAG incorporates a unique system to ensure an aerosol distribution of small and relatively uniform MMD, as required for penetration into the fine bronchioles of infants. As shown in Fig. 23-16, this is accomplished by having the aerosolized drug pass through a glass drying chamber, which is supplied with a separate source of anhydrous gas. The introduction of anhydrous gas into this chamber causes further shrinking and evaporation of the particles generated by the jet, so that 95% of the suspended particles are below 5 μm in size. As previously discussed, this low MMD further stabilizes the aerosol and provides for maximum pulmonary penetration.

Electrically powered nebulizers. Electrically powered nebulizers disperse liquid into particulate suspensions by converting electrical energy into physical energy. The two types of electrically powered nebulizers in common use are the centrifugal or spinning-disk nebulizer and the ultrasonic nebulizer. Centrifugal nebulizers are used exclusively for purposes of humidification, whereas ultrasonic nebulizers can be used both for humidification and to facilitate mobilization of secretions.

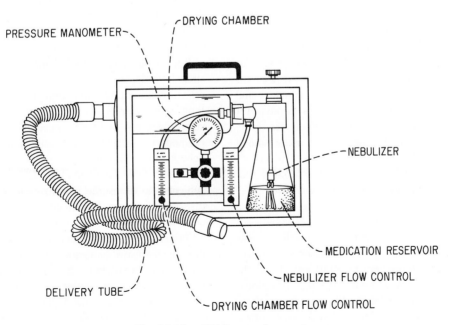

Fig. 23-16 SPAG aerosol generator.

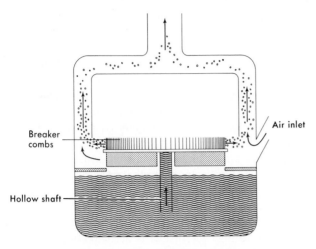

Fig. 23-17 Hollow shaft of centrifugal nebulizer draws water upward. Once water reaches spinning disk, it is thrown outward by centrifugal force through breaker combs and aerosol is produced. Fan blades on bottom of disk draw air in and blow it out top port, carrying aerosol out of unit. (From McPherson SP: Respiratory therapy equipment, ed 3, St Louis, 1985, The CV Mosby Co.)

Centrifugal nebulizers. As depicted in Fig. 23-17, the centrifugal nebulizer employs a rapidly rotating disk to break liquid water into fine particles. Driven by an electric motor, the disk draws water up from a large reservoir and impels it by centrifugal force against encircling breaker combs. The droplets produced in this manner are carried out of the device in an airstream generated by blades on the disk. The resulting aerosol tends to have a wide dispersion of particle sizes, most of which evaporate in the ambient air.

The centrifugal nebulizer was originally used both for room humidification and to "power" aerosol tents. However, because of the wide dispersion of particle sizes produced, the device causes substantial "rain out" in enclosures. For this reason, its use has been limited to supplemental room humidification. Because there is no need for a compressed gas source and the units are compact and easy to operate, the centrifugal nebulizer is popular for home use. Unfortunately, whether used in the home or the hospital, this device has been identified as a major source for the colonization and spread of pathogenic bacteria.[84] For this reason, centrifugal nebulizers are no longer recommended for either clinical or in-home use.

Ultrasonic nebulizers. The ultrasonic nebulizer is a complex electronic instrument that has been adequately described elsewhere, and here we review only briefly its major features and applications.[85-87] The ultrasonic nebulizer employs a piezoelectric transducer to convert electrical energy in the physical energy of high-frequency vibrations. When electrical energy is applied to the transducer, it responds by rapidly oscillating. These vibrations are transmitted to the solution being nebulized, creating a "foun-

tain" or "geyser" effect at the liquid surface. Continuous cavitation and disruption of the liquid surface of this geyser create the particulate suspension.

In a typical ultrasonic nebulizer (Fig. 23-18), an electrical module, *1,* transmits radiolike high-frequency signals to the transducer assembly, *2,* consisting of the transducer itself, *3,* and a couplant chamber filled with water, *4.* The signals are transmitted to the transducer through a shielded coaxial cable, *5,* that minimizes signal leakage. The frequency of the signal determines particle size and is preset to between 1.3 and 1.4 MHz (million cycles per second). The amplitude of the signal is set manually by adjustment of an output control, *6.* The amplitude of the signal determines the amount of energy applied to the transducer and thus the magnitude of its oscillations. The magnitude of transducer oscillations, in turn, determines the aerosol output of the device. Depending on the make and model of the nebulizer, adjustment of the amplitude control provides an aerosol output ranging from 0 to 6 ml/min.

Oscillations are transmitted through the couplant compartment to a nebulizer chamber, *7,* through a thin, flexible, plastic membrane, *8.* The transfer of energy through the couplant water and into the nebulization chamber is accompanied by the production of a small amount of heat, varying from 3° to 10°C above ambient. The solution to be nebulized is placed in the nebulization chamber, either directly or through a continuous-feed system, *10,* connected to an external reservoir, *11.* The aerosol particles are carried to the patient by a small blower that is provided with the instrument, *12,* or, alternatively, by connecting the chamber to a source of metered oxygen. Depending on the carrier gas flow, aerosols with as much as 0.5 g/L (500 mg/L) water content can be produced, some ten times the absolute humidity of saturated gas at body temperature. The MMD of the aerosol suspension produced by this method is approximately 6 μm, with an effective particle size range between 1 and 10 μm.[88-90]

Because ultrasonic nebulization is capable of producing such high-density aerosols, legitimate concern has been raised regarding possible damage to the lung. Washing the lung with water or saline solution is known to disrupt its surface tension stability, presumably by the removal of pulmonary surfactant. To determine whether ultrasonic nebulization could have a similar effect, several animal experiments have been conducted.[91,92] The lungs of dogs subjected to ultrasonic nebulization of isotonic saline and distilled water were examined, and no evidence of interference with surface tension stability was detected, even after 72 hours of exposure to aerosols. On the other hand, after prolonged aerosol exposure all animals that received saline mist and a few of those to whom water was administered showed microscopic pulmonary changes consistent with bronchopneumonia. The deposition of hypertonic saline, caused by the evaporation of water from the normal saline solution, was judged responsible. It was concluded that

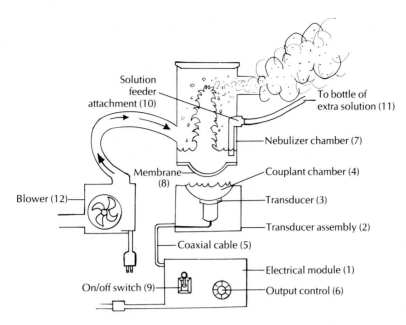

Solution feeder attachment (10)

To bottle of extra solution (11)

Nebulizer chamber (7)

Couplant chamber (4)

Membrane (8)

Blower (12)

Transducer (3)

Transducer assembly (2)

Coaxial cable (5)

Electrical module (1)

On/off switch (9)

Output control (6)

Fig. 23-18 Components of ultrasonic nebulizer. (From Eubanks DH and Bone RC: Comprehensive respiratory care, St Louis, 1985, The CV Mosby Co.)

continuous wetting of the lung with ultrasonic saline mist for long periods of time might be deleterious, although no time-limit safety guides were suggested.

On the basis of this knowledge, use of the ultrasonic nebulizer probably should be limited to intermittent application to facilitate mobilization of bronchial secretions. It may also be effective in stimulating cough for both therapeutic and diagnostic purposes. Water aerosol is usually more irritating than saline for this purpose and is valuable in inducing a sputum specimen for laboratory examination, but it appears equally useful in wetting thick bronchial secretions and stimulating expectoration. In general, the availability of safer, simpler, and less expensive techniques obviates the need for the ultrasonic nebulization except in unusual circumstances. However, if mobilization of secretions by other methods is unsatisfactory, and if the clinical situation suggests that the problem can be addressed by an increase in the density of inhaled water particles, then ultrasonic nebulization may be considered.

Ultrasonic nebulization also was once used extensively in the treatment of pediatric obstructive disorders, especially cystic fibrosis. In these conditions, inhalation of aerosolized water was considered standard therapy, either on an intermittent basis when secretions developed acutely or as a regular regimen of a prescribed number of hours daily in a mist tent. On the basis of current knowledge, however, there is insufficient evidence to support the regular application of water aerosols in general and ultrasonically produced mists in particular to these patients.[1-3,93]

Although indicated primarily as an adjunct in the mobilization of bronchial secretions, the ultrasonic nebulizer also has been applied as a vehicle for delivery of aero-

solized drugs. In this regard, there has been concern that the vibrational energy of ultrasonic nebulization might degrade or disrupt the structure of chemical substances and either destroy their specific action or produce harmful byproducts.[94] Studies of the complex relationships between high-frequency vibrations and mist production confirm this possible effect. In general, instruments with acoustic power outputs of less than 20 watts/cm^2 and an aerosol production of less than 2 ml/min will not degrade aerosolized drugs. However, power outputs in excess of 50 watts/cm^2 can disrupt the chemical structure of some nebulized medications.[95] In view of this knowledge, and with the availability of simpler and more cost-effective devices for the administration of aerosolized drug agents, there is no sound basis for using the ultrasonic nebulizer for drug administration.

With the use of ultrasonic nebulizers strictly delimited in the hospital setting, it is interesting to note their increased availability for use in the home. By and large, the cost and complexity of these devices have dropped substantially, and they are now offered to the consuming public as alternatives to the earlier steam vaporizers and centrifugal nebulizers. Certainly, their use as room humidifiers has merit, especially when centralized hot-air heating in cold climates creates uncomfortably low levels of ambient humidity. However, their potential as vehicles for the spread of infection should not be overlooked, especially in the home care of patients at high risk of pulmonary infections. For this reason, respiratory care practitioners responsible for the home care of such patients should be aware of the in-home use of these devices and should provide guidance to the patient and family regarding their appropriate application, including regular cleaning and disinfection.[96]

Hazards of aerosol therapy

While aerosol therapy can be a clinically valuable tool when properly applied, certain hazards and considerations are associated with its use. Foremost among these potential hazards is the risk of infection. Other potential risks include the pulmonary and systemic effects of the "bland" solutions aerosolized, reactivity of the airway to particulate aerosols, side effects of medication (including the potential for drug reconcentration), and the omnipresent problem of electrical shock (previously discussed).

Infection. Whereas the potential for humidification devices to spread bacteria has been demonstrated, aerosol generators have long been known to be a primary source of nosocomial infections.[35,97,98] The organisms most commonly associated with contamination of aerosol generators are gram-negative bacilli, particularly *Pseudomonas aeruginosa*. More recently, disturbing case reports of nosocomial infection with *Legionella pneumophila* (the cause of the highly virulent legionnaires' disease) have been disseminated.[99]

That aerosol generators spread bacteria via the airborne route has been clearly demonstrated. In a recent study involving canine models with *P aeruginosa* pneumonia, dogs were divided into three groups: a control group, a group supported by mechanical ventilation with heated humidification, and a group breathing a continuous heated aerosol. Careful air sampling revealed that the control animals did not spread the organism at all. Animals supported by mechanical ventilation exhaled contaminated aerosols, but organisms could not be recovered at distances greater than 2 feet from the source. On the other hand, contaminated aerosols were recovered at distances as great as 15 feet from the animals breathing the heated aerosol.[100]

Various procedures have been recommended for reducing contamination of and infection from respiratory care equipment.[13,98] Recent guidelines promulgated by the Centers for Disease Control recommend that humidification and nebulization reservoir systems should (1) start sterile and (2) be changed or replaced with disinfected or sterile water (not tap or simple distilled water) every 24 hours.[101] More details on procedures for infection control are provided in Chapter 14.

Pulmonary and systemic effects. Given the rapid absorption of fluid that can occur through the lung, even "bland" aerosols present potential risks. Excess water can cause overhydration, and excess normal saline solution has the potential to cause fluid and electrolyte imbalances and hypernatremia.[102] Research on animal models has shown that inhalation of water aerosols for as little as 72 hours results in focal tissue abscesses, localized inflammation, weight gain, increased respiratory rates, and decreased serum osmolarity. Aerosolized normal saline solution (0.9%)

administered over the same period resulted in atelectasis and pulmonary edema.[103] Although not directly generalizable to human beings, such findings suggest that indiscriminate use of continuous aerosol therapy should be avoided. Beyond this, it is clear that careful preassessment of the need for and potential risks of continuous aerosol therapy should be conducted before its implementation, especially among those who are at potential risk from these pulmonary and systemic effects. Patients presumably at risk include all infants, those with preexisting fluid and electrolyte imbalances, those with a high potential for fluid and electrolyte imbalances, and any patient with diagnosed atelectasis or pulmonary edema.

A related problem is that of the patient who has difficulty in evacuating mobilized secretions. Care should always be taken to ensure that patients are capable of clearing secretions, once they are mobilized by aerosol therapy. Proper coughing techniques, controlled deep breathing, and postural drainage and percussion should accompany aerosol therapy to promote evacuation of secretions from the bronchial tree (see Chapter 27). For those patients who are unable to clear secretions adequately, mechanical tracheobronchial aspiration or fiberoptic bronchoscopy may be indicated.

Airway reactivity. It has been shown that high-density bland aerosols produced by ultrasonic nebulization can cause reactive bronchospasm and increased airway resistance, especially in patients with preexisting respiratory disease.[64] Administration of bronchodilators before high-density mist therapy can help prevent this problem. Apparently, heated jet aerosols do not produce the same increase in airway resistance. Less is known about the effect of cool mists on airway reactivity.

It is also well known that common mucolytic agents such as acetylcysteine can produce significant bronchospasm in sensitive persons. Therefore, it is generally recommended that a bronchodilator drug also be used to prevent or minimize this occurrence.[61,69]

In light of this knowledge, the potential for inducing bronchospasm should always be considered when one is giving high-density bland aerosols or nebulized drug agents to which the airway may be sensitive. Monitoring of patients for reactive bronchospasm should include peak flow measurements before and after therapy; auscultation for adventitious breath sounds; observation of the patient's breathing pattern and overall appearance; and, most essentially, communication with the patient during therapy.

Drug reconcentration. During the baffling and recycling of solutions undergoing nebulization, as droplets are continuously returned to the fluid reservoir the potential exists for the solute concentration of the solution to increase. Under such conditions, the patient is subjected to increasingly higher concentrations of the agent during the course of therapy; this poses a risk of drug toxicity. It was at first believed that this phenomenon occurred only in jet nebulizers, but an excellent study has demonstrated that drug reconcentration can occur in both jet and ultrasonic nebulizers.[104]

One of the drugs used was the mucolytic acetylcysteine. When subjected to 30 minutes of ultrasonic nebulization with ambient air as the carrier gas, acetylcysteine concentrations rose from 20.5% to 40.1%. When control of temperature and humidity ensured full water vapor saturation of the carrier gas, reconcentration did not occur. Table 23-4 vividly illustrates these differences. The conclusion drawn was that, under conditions of low humidity in the carrier gas, evaporation of solvent (water) occurs at a faster rate than that of the heavier drug solute, thereby progressively raising the concentration of the residual solution.

Obviously, this problem is of potential significance only when medications are being nebulized over periods in excess of 10 to 15 minutes, and then only if the total dose available for nebulization exceeds that prescribed. Although these conditions seldom pertain with current practices, practitioners should still be wary of the possibility for and consequences of drug reconcentration.

SUMMARY

Humidity therapy and aerosol therapy are among the most common modes of current respiratory care. The appropriate application of humidity and aerosol therapy entails careful understanding of their proven capabilities, limitations, and potential risks. As a guiding principle, indiscriminate use of either approach is contraindicated. Moreover, when indicated by careful assessment of the patient's needs, humidity and aerosol therapy should generally be considered adjuncts to other modes of clinical care, such as good systemic hydration, oral or parenteral drug administration, and rigorous bronchial hygiene. In this regard, the respiratory care practitioner must play a vital role. Rather than simply administering prescribed treatments, the practitioner must actively participate in the

identification and ongoing assessment of those patients best served by application of these methods. Beyond this, all respiratory care practitioners should continue the process of critically assessing the safety and efficacy of both new and existing methods for the provision of humidity and aerosol therapy. Only in this manner can we expect to assure the best possible respiratory care.

REFERENCES

1. Pierce AK and Saltzman HA, chairmen: Conference on the scientific basis for respiratory therapy, Am Rev Resp Dis 110(2):1, 1974.
2. Pierce AK: Scientific basis of in-hospital respiratory therapy, Am Rev Respir Dis 122(2):1, 1980.
3. Brian J: Aerosol and humidity therapy, Am Rev Respir Dis 122(2):17, 1980.
4. Chatburn RL and Primiano FP: A rational basis for humidity therapy (editorial), Resp Care 32:249, 1987.
5. American National Standards Institute: American national standard for humidifiers and nebulizers for medical use (ANSI Z79:9-1979), New York, 1979, American National Standards Institute.
6. McPherson SP: Respiratory therapy equipment, ed 3, St Louis, 1985, The CV Mosby Co.
7. Inglestent S: Studies on the conditioning of air in the respiratory tract, Acta Otolaryngol (Stockh) [Suppl] 131, 1956.
8. Sara C: The management of patients with a tracheostomy, Med J Aust 1:99, 1965.
9. Sykes MK, McNicol MW, and Campbell EJM: Respiratory failure, ed 2, Oxford, England, 1976, Blackwell Scientific Publications.
10. Bendixen HH et al: Respiratory care, St Louis, 1965, The CV Mosby Co.
11. Shapiro BA, Harrison RA, and Trout CA: Clinical applications of respiratory care, ed 3, Chicago, 1985, Year Book Medical Publishers.
12. Petty TL: Intensive and rehabilitative respiratory care, ed 2, Philadelphia, 1974, Lea & Febiger.
13. Burton GG and Hodgkin JE, editors: Respiratory care; a guide to clinical practice, ed 2, Philadelphia, 1984, JB Lippincott Co.
14. Forbes AR: Humidification and mucus flow in the intubated trachea, Br J Anaesth 45:874, 1973.
15. Forbes AR: Temperature, humidity and mucus flow in the intubated trachea Br J Anaesth 46:29, 1974.
16. Chalon Jr, et al: Humidity and the anesthetized patient, Anesthesiology 50:195, 1979.
17. Chalon, J, Loew DAY, and Malebranche J: Effects of dry anesthetic gases on tracheobronchial ciliated epithelium, Anesthesiology 36:338, 1972.
18. Tsuda T et al: Optimum humidification of air administered to a tracheostomy in dogs, Br J Anaesth 49:965, 1977.
19. Chamney AR: Humidification requirements and techniques, Anaesthesia 24:602, 1969.
20. Noguchi H: Studies on proper humidification in tracheostomized dogs, Nagoya Med J 17:159, 1972.
21. Noguchi H, Takumi A, Aochi O: A study of humidification in tracheostomized dogs, Br J Anaesth 45:844,
22. Cushing IE and Miller WF: In Safar P, editor: Respiratory therapy, Philadelphia, 1965, FA Davis Co.
23. Miller WF: Fundamental principles of aerosol therapy, Respir Care 17:295, 1972.
24. Miller WF: Aerosol therapy in acute and chronic respiratory disease, Arch Intern Med 131:148, 1973.
25. Klein EF et al: Performance characteristics of conventional and prototype humidifiers and nebulizers, Chest 64:690, 1973.
26. Dolan GK, and Zawadski JJ: Performance characteristics of low-flow humidifiers, Respir Care 21:393, 1976.

Table 23-4 Drug Reconcentration During Ultrasonic Nebulization

Aerosolization time (minutes)	Percent acetylcysteine	
	Ambient air	Humidified air
0	20.5	20.5
5	21.7	20.4
10	23.0	20.2
15	26.4	20.1
20	29.0	20.2
25	32.8	20.6
30	40.1	20.5

Modified from Glick RV: Drug reconcentration in aerosol generators, Inhal Ther 15:179, 1970.

27. Branson RD and Hurst JM: Laboratory evaluation of moisture output of seven heat and moisture exchangers, Respir Care 32:741, 1987.

28. Hemholz HF and Burton GG: Applied humidity and aerosol therapy. In Burton GG and Hodgkin JE, editors: Respiratory care: a guide to clinical practice, Philadelphia, ed 2, 1984, JB Lippincott Co.

29. Poulton TJ and Downs JB: Humidification of rapidly flowing gas, Crit Care Med 9:59, 1981.

30. Comer PB et al: Airway maintenance in patients with long-term endotracheal intubation, Crit Care Med 4:211, 1976.

31. Emergency Care Research Institute: Heat and moisture exchangers, Health Devices 12:155, 1983.

32. Walker AKY and Bethune DW: A comparative study of condenser humidifiers, Anesthesia 31:1086, 1976.

33. Mebius C: A comparative study of disposable humidifiers, Acta Anaesth Scand 27:403, 1983.

34. Shelly M, Bethune DW, Latimer RD: A comparison of five heat and moisture exchangers, Anesthesia 41:527, 1986.

35. Graff TD: Humidification: indications and hazards in respiratory therapy, Anesth Analg 54:444, 1975.

36. Bancroft ML: Problems with humidifiers, Int Anesthesiol Clin 20:95, 1982.

37. Geevarghese KP, Aldrete JA, and Patel TC: Inspired air temperature with immersion heater humidifiers. Anesth Analg 55:331, 1975.

38. Kirch TJ and Dekornfeld TJ: An unexpected hazard while using the Emerson post-operative ventilator, Anesthesiology 28:1106, 1967.

39. Sladen A, Laver M, and Pontoppidan H: Pulmonary complications of water retention in prolonged mechanical ventilation, N Engl J Med 279:448, 1968.

40. Korones SB: High-risk newborn infants, ed 3, St Louis, 1981, The CV Mosby Co.

41. Klaus MH and Fanaroff AA, editors: Care of the high risk neonate, ed 3, Philadelphia, 1986, WB Saunders Co.

42. Thibeault DW and Gregory GA, editors: Neonatal pulmonary care, ed 2, Menlo Park, Calif, 1986, Addison-Wesley Publishing Co, Inc.

43. Klein EF and Graves SE: Hot pot tracheitis, Chest 65:225, 1974.

44. Schulze T, Edmondson EB, and Pierce AK: Studies of a new humidifying device as a potential source of bacterial aerosols, Am Rev Respir Dis 96:517, 1967.

45. Ahlgren EW, Chapel JF, and Dorn GL: *Pseudomonas aeruginosa* infection potential of oxygen humidifying devices, Respir Care 22:383, 1977.

46. Rhame FS, et al: Bubbling humidifiers produce microaerosols which carry bacteria, Infect Control 7:403, 1986.

47. Stange K and Bygdeman S: Do moisture exchangers prevent contamination of ventilators? Acta Anaesth Scand 24:487, 1980.

48. Saravolatz LD et al: Lack of bacterial aerosols associated with heat and moisture exchangers, Am Rev Respir Dis 134:214-216, 1986.

49. Powner DJ, Sanders CS, and Bailey BJ: Bacteriologic evaluation of the Servo 150 hygroscopic condenser humidifier, Crit Care Med 14:135, 1986.

50. Goularte TA, Manning M, and Craven DE: Bacterial colonization in humidifying cascade reservoirs after 24 and 48 hours of continuous mechanical ventilation, Infect Control 8:200, 1987.

51. Scanlan CL: Electrical safety in respiratory therapy (Part II), Dallas, 1977, American Association for Respiratory Care.

52. Swift DL and Litt M: Physical and physiological properties of aerosol deposition and mucocilary clearance. In Burton GG and Hodgkin JE, editors: Respiratory care; a guide to clinical practice, ed 2, Philadelphia, 1984, JB Lippincott Co.

53. Goetz A: The physicochemical behavior of submicron aerosols, Am Rev Respir Dis 83:410, 1961.

54. Stahlhofen W, Gebhart J, and Heyder J: Experimental determination of the regional deposition of aerosol particles in the human respiratory tract, Am Indust Hyg Assoc J 41:385, 1980.

55. Newman SP: Aerosol deposition considerations in inhalation therapy, Chest 88(Suppl):152S, 1985.

56. Hatch TF and Gross P: Pulmonary deposition and retention of inhaled aerosols, New York, 1964, Academic Press, Inc.

57. Altshuler B, et al: Aerosol deposition in the human respiratory tract, Arch Industr Health 15:293, 1957.

58. Dautrebande L, et al: Lung deposition of fine dust particles, Arch Industr Health 16:179, 1957.

59. Brain JD and Valberg PA: Deposition of aerosol in the respiratory tract: state of the art, Am Rev Respir Dis 120:1325, 1979.

60. Hayek A: Cellular structure and mucus activity in the bronchial tree and alveoli, Ciba Foundation Symposium on Pulmonary Structure and Function, Boston, 1962, Little, Brown & Co.

61. Miller WF and Geumei AM: In Petty TL, editor: Chronic obstructive pulmonary disease, New York, 1978, Marcel Dekker.

62. Miller WF, Johnston FF, and Tarkoff MP: Use of ultrasonic aerosols with ventilatory assistors, J Asthma Res 5:355, 1968.

63. Wanner A, and Rao A: Clinical indications for and effects of bland, mucolytic and antimicrobial aerosols, Am Rev Respir Dis 122:79, 1980.

64. Cheney FW and Butler J: The effects of ultrasonically produced aerosols on airway resistance in man, Anesthesiology 29:1099, 1968.

65. Godwin CR, et al: Induced sputum as a rapid and efficient technique for diagnosing *Pneumocystis carinii* pneumonia in AIDS patients, Respir Care 32:895, 1987 (abstract).

66. Yue WY and Cohen SS: Sputum induction by newer inhalation methods in patients with pulmonary tuberculosis, Dis Chest 51:611, 1967.

67. Hensler N et al: The use of hypertonic aerosol in production of sputum for diagnosis of tuberculosis, Dis Chest 40:639, 1961.

68. Lillehei JP: Sputum induction with heated aerosol inhalations for the diagnosis of tuberculosis, Am Rev Respir Dis 84:276, 1961.

69. Ziment I: Respiratory pharmacology and therapeutics, Philadelphia, 1978, WB Saunders Co.

70. Lehnert BE, and Schachter EN: The pharmacology of respiratory care, 1980, St Louis, The CV Mosby Co.

71. Dautrebande L: Microaerosols, New York, 1962, Academic Press, Inc.

72. Hill TV and Sorbello JG: Humidity outputs of large-reservoir nebulizers, Respir Care 32:255, 1987.

73. Wells RE et al: Humidification of oxygen during inhalation therapy, N Engl J Med 268:644, 1963.

74. Litt M and Swift DF: The Babington nebulizer: a new principle for generation of therapeutic aerosols, Am Rev Respir Dis 105:308, 1972.

75. Swift DL: Generation and respiratory deposition of therapeutic aerosols, Am Rev Respir Dis 122:71, 1980.

76. Mercer TT, Goddard RF, and Flores RL: Effect of auxiliary air flow on the output characteristics of compressed-air nebulizers, Ann Allergy 27:211, 1969.

77. Chiov WL: Aerosol propellants: cardiac toxicity and long biological half-life, JAMA 227:658, 1974.

78. Silverglade A: Aerosol propellants, JAMA 231:135, 1975.

79. Newman SP et al: Effects of various inhalation modes on the deposition of radioactive pressurized aerosols, Eur J Respir Dis 63(Suppl):57, 1982.

80. Epstein SW et al: Survey of the clinical use of pressurized aerosols, Can Med Assoc J 120:813, 1979.

81. Newman SP et al: Deposition of pressurized suspension aerosols inhaled through extension devices, Am Rev Respir Dis 124:317, 1981.

82. Dolovich M, Ruffin R, and Corr D: Clinical evaluation of a simple demand inhalation MDI aerosol delivery device, Chest 84:36, 1984.

83. Barry W et al: Ribavirin aerosol for acute bronchiolitis, Arch Dis Child 61:593, 1986.

84. Craig CP: Product commentary: room humidifiers and hospitals; colonization of water sources, Infect Control 6:129, 1985.

85. Andrews AH Jr: Ultrasonic aerosol generator, Presbyt St Luke Hosp Med Bull 3:155, 1964.

86. Proceedings of the First Conference on Clinical Application of the Ultrasonic Nebulizer, Somerset, Penn, 1966, DeVilbiss Co.

87. Abramson HA, editor: Proceedings of the Second Conference on Clinical Application of the Ultrasonic Nebulizer, J Asthma Res 5:213, 1968.

88. Boucher RMG and Kreuter J: Ultrasonic nebulization, Ann Allergy 26:591, 1968.

89. Gauthier WD: Operational characteristics of the ultrasonic nebulizer, Proceedings of the First Conference on Clinical Application of the Ultrasonic Nebulizer, Somerset, Penn, 1966, DeVilbiss Co.

90. Stevens HR and Albregt HB: Assessment of ultrasonic nebulization, Anesthesiology 27:648, 1966.

91. Modell JH et al: Effect of ultrasonic nebulized suspensions of pulmonary surfactant, Dis Chest 50:627, 1966.

92. Modell JH et al: Effect of chronic exposure to ultrasonic aerosols on the lungs, Anesthesiology 28:680, 1967.

93. Tabachnik E, and Levison H: Clinical application of aerosols in pediatrics, Am Rev Respir Dis 122:97, 1980.

94. Allan D: Artificial humidification, Med Sci 17:41, 1966.

95. Boucher RGM and Kreuter J: Fundamentals of the ultrasonic atomization of medicated solutions, Ann Allergy 26:591, 1968.

96. Spendlove JC and Fannin KF: Source, significance, and control of indoor microbial aerosols: human health aspects, Public Health Rep 98:229, 1983.

97. Reinarz JA, Pierce AK, and Mays BB: The potential role of inhalation therapy equipment in nosocomial pulmonary infections, J Clin Invest 44:831, 1965.

98. Pierce AK and Sanford JP: Bacterial contamination of aerosols, Arch Intern Med 131:156, 1973.

99. Kaan JA, Simoons-Smit AM, and McLaren DM: Another source of aerosol causing nosocomial legionnaires' disease, J Infect 11:145, 1985.

100. Christopher KL et al: The potential role of respiratory therapy equipment in cross infection: a case study using a canine model for pneumonia, Am Rev Respir Dis 128:271, 1983.

101. Simmons BP and Wong ES: Guidelines for the prevention of nosocomial pneumonia, Infect Control 3:327, 1982.

102. Lyons HA: Use of therapeutic aerosols, Am J Cardiol 12:462, 1969.

103. Stehlin CS and Schare BL: Systemic and pulmonary changes in rabbits exposed to long-term nebulization of various therapeutic agents, Heart Lung 9:311, 1980.

104. Glick RV: Drug reconcentration in aerosol generators, Inhal Ther 15:179, 1970.

24

Production, Storage, and Delivery of Medical Gases

F. Robert Thalken

The distribution of therapeutic gases is a major responsibility of the respiratory care practitioner. Although practitioners have assumed many more challenging duties, providing assurances of the safe and uninterrupted supply of medical gases remains a foundation of the practitioner's role and function.

In this chapter, we consider the production and storage of medical gases and the devices used to control their delivery in the clinical setting. We will call on some previously discussed principles as we describe both the gaseous and liquid forms of medical gases. Much of the information in this chapter is drawn from two sources with which all respiratory care practitioners should be familiar: the codes of the National Fire Protection Association[1] and the pamphlets of the Compressed Gas Association.[2] In addition, the reader can find useful information in the many brochures and publications available from gas and equipment manufacturers.

OBJECTIVES

After completion of this chapter, the reader should be able to:

1. Compare and contrast the roles of regulating and recommending agencies as related to the production, storage, and distribution of medical gases.

2. Differentiate the characteristics and principles of operation of gas- and liquid-filled cylinders, including measurement of contents and calculation of duration of flow.

3. Describe the characteristic features of gaseous and liquid bulk oxygen storage and delivery systems.

4. Differentiate the three major safety systems used in medical gas distribution systems.

5. Compare and contrast common high-pressure gas regulators according to their design characteristics, safety features, and appropriate clinical use.

6. Apply the principle of pressure compensation to differentiate among the various flow-metering devices employed in clinical practice.

KEY TERMS

Most terms used in this chapter are defined in context. The following terms are introduced without explicit definition but may be found in the text glossary:

ambient	flange
anode	inadvertent
bore	inert
by-product	pollutant
carbonaceous	protocol
cathode	statutory
combustion	tempered
distillation	transfill
efficacy	vaporizer
fermentation	

AGENCIES

Many agencies are involved in the control of manufacturing and safe use of medical gases and devices employed in respiratory care. With more detailed information available from other sources, we provide only a general description of these various agencies.[3-9]

According to their control authority, the agencies discussed in this chapter can be divided into two general groups: those that recommend standards and procedures and those that actually regulate by statutory authority. The key recommending and regulating agencies associated with respiratory care are listed in the box on p. 585.

Recommending agencies

Recommending agencies are usually made up of individuals or formal organizations involved in some aspect of technology. Through the consensus of their members, they

REGULATING AND RECOMMENDING AGENCIES INVOLVED WITH MEDICAL GASES

RECOMMENDING AGENCIES

Compressed Gas Associations (CGA)

The CGA is made up of individuals involved in the compressed gas industry. It has created standards and safety systems for compressed gas systems.

National Fire Protection Association (NFPA)

The NFPA is an agency involved in improved methods of fire protection and prevention, including creating standards for the storage of flammable and oxidizing gases.

International Standards Organization (ISO)

The ISO is the international agency for standardization covering most areas of technology.

American National Standard Institute (ANSI)

ANSI is a private nonprofit organization that coordinates the voluntary developments of national standards in the US and represents US interests in the area of international standardization.

Z-79 Committee

Z-79 is a committee of ANSI and is the American National Standards Committee on standards for anesthesia and ventilatory devices. These devices include anesthesia machines, reservoir bags, tracheal tubes, humidifiers, nebulizers, and other oxygen-related equipment.

REGULATING AGENCIES

Department of Transportation (DOT)

The department of the federal government given the responsibility in 1970 for compressed gas cylinders, which were previously regulated by the Interstate Commerce Commission (ICC).

Department of Health and Human Services (HHS)

This department of the federal government was formerly called the Department of Health, Education and Welfare (HEW). HHS has created many agencies that are involved in health delivery. As an example, the Food and Drug Administration (FDA) is an agency that requires a certain level of purity for medical gases.

Food and Drug Administration (FDA)

The FDA is an agency of HHS and requires a certain level of purity for medical gases.

Bureau of Medical Devices (BMD)

The BMD is an agency of FDA and was formed in 1976 to classify, provide standards for, and regulate medical devices.

Occupational Safety and Health Agency (OSHA)

OSHA is an agency of the federal Department of Labor and is responsible for occupational safety.

---

establish and encourage voluntary compliance with pertinent standards. A good example of a recommending agency is the Compressed Gas Association (CGA), which is made up of manufacturers and distributors of equipment, containers, and valves as well as others involved in the production of compressed and liquefied gases.[7]

Practitioners involved in respiratory care can and should provide input to recommending bodies. An example of a recommending body to which a clinician can and should provide input is the Z-79 Committee of the American National Standards Institute (ANSI).

Regulating agencies

Regulating agencies are federal, state, and local bodies that have the statutory authority to enforce laws controlling the manufacture and safe use of compressed gases and medically related drugs and devices. A good example of a regulatory agency is the Food and Drug Administration (FDA). Among its many responsibilities, the FDA has the authority to establish standards of purity for medical gases and requirements for demonstrating the safety and efficacy of medical devices.

Regulatory agencies often adopt the voluntary standards developed by recommending agencies as their legal requirements. For example, a local county government might adopt the National Fire Protection Association standards for the storage of bulk oxygen. Under such circumstances, the voluntary standards of a recommending agency become the statutory requirements of a governmental regulating body.

Because both voluntary standards and legal requirements are under constant review and revision, no text can possibly assure complete and up-to-date coverage, particularly in the area of state and local regulations. Health care institutions and their professional staffs share the responsibility to keep abreast of current knowledge in these areas and, where applicable, to assure ongoing compliance.

PRODUCTION OF MEDICAL GASES

Of the many gases that are produced and used commercially, we are interested in the few that are called medical gases (Table 24-1). Of these, we will focus on the therapeutic gases, generally excluding laboratory and anesthetic gases. From a safety standpoint, however, the respiratory care practitioner should be familiar with all gases used in the clinical setting, especially as related to their potential fire risk.

In regard to fire risk, medical compressed gases are classified as either nonflammable (will not burn), nonflammable but will support combustion, or flammable (will burn readily). According to this classification, medical gases are grouped as follows:

Nonflammable: Nitrogen, carbon dioxide, helium
Support combustion: Oxygen, nitrous oxide, air, oxygen-nitrogen, oxygen-carbon dioxide, helium-oxygen
Flammable: Cyclopropane, ethylene

In the remainder of this section, we will address the characteristics and production of the therapeutic gases and gas mixtures commonly used in respiratory care.

Oxygen

Characteristics. Oxygen is a colorless, odorless, transparent, and tasteless gas that occurs in nature as free molecular oxygen and as a component of a host of chemical compounds. It comprises almost 50% by weight of the earth's crust and in combination with hydrogen occurs as water in all living matter. At 0°C and 1 atmosphere pressure, oxygen has a density of 1.429 g/L, being slightly heavier than air (1.30 g/L). Oxygen is only slightly soluble in water; at room temperature and 1 atmosphere pressure, only 3.3 ml of oxygen can dissolve in 100 ml of water. Nonetheless, this small amount is sufficient for all oxygen-dependent aquatic life.

As indicated previously, oxygen is nonflammable. It does, however, greatly accelerate combustion, which is of considerable importance in its widespread use. A match would be consumed in an instant if lighted in an oxygen-rich environment, but the flame would also die with equal speed unless it ignited another combustible material. The relationship between the burning intensity of a combustible substance and the amount of ambient oxygen is direct but not simple. Burning speed increases with an increase in the concentration of oxygen at a fixed total pressure or with an increase in total pressure of a constant gas concentration. Burning speed will also increase if only oxygen concentrations are raised and the partial pressure of the various oxygen percentages is kept constant by lowering the total pressure. These data demonstrate that both oxy-

gen concentration and partial pressure influence the rate of burning.

Production. Oxygen is produced by several methods, including: (1) fractional distillation of atmospheric air, (2) electrolysis of water, (3) chemical decomposition, and (4) physical separation.

Fractional distillation. Fractional distillation is the most common and least expensive method for the commercial production of oxygen. The process involves several related steps. First, atmospheric air is filtered to remove pollutants, water, and carbon dioxide. The purified air is then converted to a liquid by first compressing it to high pressure, and then cooling the mixture by rapid expansion (the Joule-Thompson effect).

The resultant mixture of liquefied oxygen and nitrogen is heated slowly in a distillation tower. Nitrogen, with its boiling point of −195.8°C (−320.5°F), escapes first, followed by the trace gases argon, krypton, and xenon. The remaining liquid oxygen is then transferred to specially insulated cryogenic (low-temperature) storage cylinders or converted to gas for storage under high pressure in metal cylinders.

This method produces oxygen that is approximately 99.5% pure. The remaining 0.5% is mostly nitrogen and trace argon. FDA standards require an oxygen purity of at least 99%.

Electrolysis. Electrolysis is the process of applying an electrical current across an anode and a cathode in water. As a result, molecular hydrogen and oxygen are produced in their gaseous form. Because the current requirements necessary to produce large volumes of oxygen by this method are prohibitively expensive, electrolysis is generally used only as a source of hydrogen gas.

Chemical decomposition. Although many chemical reactions are capable of producing oxygen, only one is of any clinical significance. Controlled heating of solid sodium chlorate ($NaCLO_3$) produces sodium chloride (NaCL) and gaseous oxygen, with carbon dioxide, water, and trace amounts of carbon monoxide being the primary by-products. The method can produce about 99.5% oxygen at flows of up to 4.5 L/min. Small portable devices based on this principle are used as remote emergency sources of low-pressure oxygen. Such devices have been termed solid-state oxygen generators (SSOG).[10]

Physical separation. Physical separation is accomplished by one of two methods.[5] The first method employs molecular "sieves" composed of inorganic sodium aluminum silicate pellets to absorb nitrogen and water vapor from atmospheric air, thereby making available a concentrated mixture of more than 90% gaseous oxygen for patient use. The second method uses a semipermeable plastic membrane to filter nitrogen (but not water vapor) from ambient air and is capable of producing an oxygen mixture of approximately 40%. These devices, called oxygen concentrators, are used primarily to supply oxygen in the home

Table 24-1   Therapy and Anesthetic Gases

Limited therapy, laboratory gases	Therapy gases	Anesthetic gases
Carbon dioxide	Air	Cyclopropane
Helium	Helium-oxygen	Ethylene
Nitrogen	Oxygen	Nitrous oxide
	Oxygen-carbon dioxide	
	Oxygen-nitrogen	

care setting. For this reason, details of their principles of operation and appropriate use will be covered in Chapter 35.

Air

Oxygen and nitrogen may be mixed to produce a gas with an oxygen concentration equivalent to that of air.[5] More commonly, air for medical use is produced simply by filtering and compressing atmospheric air.[2]

A typical large medical air-compressor system is depicted in Fig. 24-1. These systems typically use an electrical motor to power a piston in a compression cylinder. On its downstroke, the piston draws air in through a filter system via an inlet valve. On its upstroke, the piston compresses the air in the cylinder (closing the inlet valve), and delivers it through an outlet valve to a reservoir tank. Air from the reservoir tank is dried and reduced to the desired working pressure by a pressure-reducing valve before being delivered to the piping system.

For medical gas use, it is essential that the air provided be free of oil or particulate contamination. This is usually accomplished by the use of Teflon piston rings, as opposed to the carbon rings or oil lubrication sometimes used in nonmedical air compressors. Moreover, large compressor systems used to provide air to a hospital unit must be capable of maintaining high flows (at least 100 L/min) at the standard working pressure of 50 psig for all equipment in use.

Smaller compressors are available for bedside or home use. Typically, these units employ a diaphragm or turbine to compress the air and generally do not have a reservoir tank. Because of their limited flow and pressure capabilities, the use of these small compressors is restricted to powering equipment that does not require unrestricted flows at 50 psig, such as small-volume medication nebulizers (see Chapter 23).

Carbon dioxide

At normal atmospheric temperatures and pressure, carbon dioxide is a colorless and odorless gas about 1.5 times as heavy as air. Carbon dioxide does not support combustion or maintain animal life. Unrefined carbon dioxide gas may be obtained from the combustion of coal, coke, natural gas, oil, and other carbonaceous fuels; as a by-product of ammonia production from lime kilns, carbide furnaces, or fermentation processes; and from certain natural springs and wells. For medical purposes, carbon dioxide usually is produced by heating limestone in contact with water. The gas is recovered from this process and liquefied by compression and cooling.[2] The FDA purity standard for carbon dioxide is 99.9%.

Helium

Helium is second only to hydrogen as the lightest of all gases, with a density at STPD of 0.1785 g/L. Helium is

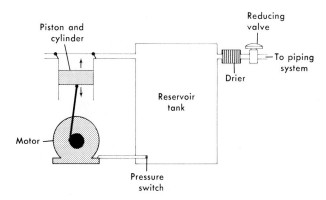

Fig. 24-1 Large air-compressor system for piping system. Compressor sends gas to reservoir at higher than line pressure. When preset pressure level is reached, pressure switch shuts compressor off. Gas leaves reservoir and passes through dryer to remove moisture, and reducing valve reduces gas to desired line pressure. When reservoir pressure has dropped to near line pressure, pressure switch turns compressor back on. (From McPherson SP and Spearman CB: Respiratory therapy equipment, ed 3, St Louis, 1985, The CV Mosby Co.)

odorless and tasteless and is both chemically and physiologically inert (therefore nonflammable). It is a good conductor of heat, sound, and electricity but is poorly soluble in water. Although present in small quantities in the atmosphere, helium is commercially produced from natural gas by liquefication to purity standards of at least 95%.[2] Free helium can also be liberated from uranium ore by heating.

STORAGE OF MEDICAL GASES

Gas cylinders

Compressed or liquid medical gases are stored and shipped in high-pressure cylinders, which are carefully controlled by both industrial standards and federal regulations. Gas cylinders are made of seamless steel, finely tempered and nonreactive with their gaseous or liquid contents, and are classified according to their fabrication method as either type 3A or type 3AA.

Markings and identification. Medical gas cylinders are marked by metal stampings on their shoulders that supply specific information (Fig. 24-2). Although the exact location and order of these markings may vary, the practitioner should be able to identify several key items of information.

The letters ICC (Interstate Commerce Commission) or DOT (Department of Transportation) are followed by the cylinder classification (3A or 3AA) and the maximum working pressure in pounds per square inch. This pressure represents the filling pressure of the cylinder, which can generally be exceeded by 10%. For example, a cylinder marked with a pressure of 2015 psi can be filled to about 2200 psi.

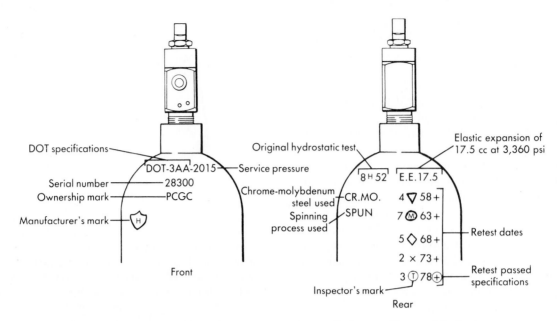

Fig. 24-2   Typical markings for cylinders containing medical gases. Front and back views are for illustration purposes only; exact location and order of markings are variable.

Below this, one normally finds the letter size of the cylinder (E, G, etc), followed by its serial number. A third line provides a mark of ownership, often followed by the manufacturer's stamp or a mark identifying the inspecting authority.

On the opposite surface of the cylinder one normally finds an abbreviation indicating the method by which the cylinder was manufactured, often noted as "Spun Cr-Mo," indicating the use of chrome-molybdenum. Also in this vicinity are a series of symbols that include data on the cylinder's original safety test and dates of all subsequent tests as prescribed by regulation. These tests occur every 5 or 10 years, as specified in DOT regulations. Under high-pressure hydrostatic test conditions, such factors as leaks, cylinder expansion, and wall stress are determined, and the cylinders are inspected internally and cleaned. The notation "E.E." followed by a number indicates the cylinder's elastic expansion, in cubic centimeters, under these test conditions.

In addition to these permanent marks, all cylinders are color coded and labeled to identify their contents. The box opposite lists the color code for therapeutic and anesthetic gases as adopted by the National Institute of Standards and Technology of the US Department of Commerce. Since these codes are not yet standardized internationally (oxygen cylinders are white in many foreign countries), it is strongly emphasized that the color of a cylinder should be used only as a rough guide. As with any medicinal agent, the practitioner must always positively identify the cylinder contents by carefully reading the label.

Cylinder sizes and contents. Cylinders are given a letter designation according to size (Fig. 24-3). Table 24-2 provides a listing of the most common cylinder sizes and

COLOR CODE FOR SIZE E GAS CYLINDERS	
GAS	COLOR
Oxygen	Green
Carbon dioxide	Gray
Nitrous oxide	Light blue
Cyclopropane	Orange
Helium	Brown
Ethylene	Red
Carbon dioxide and oxygen	Gray and green
Helium and oxygen	Brown and green
Air	Yellow

net contents for the gases with which the respiratory care practitioner will have frequent contact.

Sizes AA through E are referred to as "small cylinders" and are used most often for anesthetic gases and portable oxygen supplies. These small cylinders differ from the larger ones in the mechanism by which they attach to the appliances they serve. Small cylinders employ a connector called a yoke, whereas the large cylinders (F to H and K) have a threaded outlet from their valves for attachment of a pressure-regulating device.

Filling (charging) cylinders. We differentiate here between gases that can be stored in cylinders in gaseous or liquid forms at room temperature and those that must be maintained in a cryogenic (low-temperature) state. Cryogenic storage of gases in the liquid form will be discussed in a following section.

Compressed gases. The general rule is that gas cylinders will be filled at a temperature of 70°F to the pressure

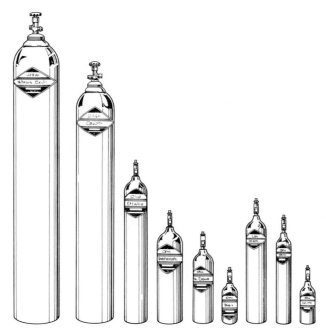

Fig. 24-3   Cylinder sizes by letter code.

specified for a given cylinder, as stamped on its shoulder. However, oxygen, helium-oxygen, and oxygen-carbon dioxide, may be filled to 10% in excess of the stated pressure. Thus a cylinder certified for 2015 psi may be filled to a pressure of 2217 psi and is generally referred to as a 2200-pound cylinder.

Liquefied gases. Medical gases with critical temperatures above room temperature can be stored in cylinders as liquids at room temperature. These gases include carbon dioxide, nitrous oxide, and cyclopropane. Rather than using a filling pressure, cylinders of these gases are filled according to a specified filling density. The filling density is the ratio between the weight of liquid gas put into the cylinder and the weight of water the cylinder could contain if full. For example, the filling density for carbon dioxide (68%) allows the manufacturer to fill a cylinder with liquid CO_2 up to 68% of the weight of water that a full cylinder could hold. The filling densities of cyclopropane and nitrous oxide are 55% and 68%, respectively.

Cylinder pressures for these liquid gases are considerably lower than those for vaporous gases. Because liquid gas does not fill the entire volume of a given cylinder, the space above the liquid surface contains gas vapor in equilibrium with the liquid. The measured pressure in a liquid-filled cylinder is thus equivalent to the pressure of the vapor at any given temperature.

The pressure in a cylinder is therefore a function of the state of matter in which the gas is stored. The pressure in a cylinder filled with a gas in its gaseous form represents the force required to compress its volume into the available space. However, the pressure in a cylinder of gas stored in its liquid form represents the vapor pressure of the gas over its surface.

Measuring cylinder contents. Because of these differences in the physical state of matter, different methods of measuring the contents of compressed and liquid gas cylinders must be employed.

Compressed-gas cylinders. For gas-filled cylinders, the volume of gas in a cylinder is directly proportional to the cylinder pressure at a constant temperature. If a cylinder is full at 2200 psig, it will be half full when the pressure drops to 1100 psig. Therefore the contents of a compressed-gas cylinder are usually monitored by means of a pressure gauge. If greater accuracy is needed, the cylinder may be weighed. However, measurement of the contents of a compressed-gas cylinder by weight requires prior knowledge of the weight of the empty cylinder and the density of the gas it contains.

Liquid-gas cylinders. Because the pressure in a liquid-gas cylinder represents the vapor pressure above the liquid, pressure measurements give no indication of how much liquid remains in the cylinder at any one time. As long as there is some liquid in the cylinder and the temperature remains constant, the vapor pressure—and thus the displayed gauge pressure—will remain unchanged, even though gas is being used up. Only when the liquid is completely gone and the cylinder contains just vapor will the pressure fall in proportion to the reduction in remaining gas volume. Thus gauge pressure is of use in monitoring cylinder contents only after all the liquid vaporizes. If the contents of liquid-filled cylinders must be determined, they must be weighed.

Fig. 24-4 compares the behavior of compressed-gas and liquid-gas cylinders during use. Of course, the vapor pressure of liquid-gas cylinders will vary with the temperature of their contents. Nitrous oxide has a cylinder pressure of

Table 24-2 Typical Medical Gas Cylinders' Volume and Weight of Available Contents* (All Volume at 70°F [21.1°C])

Cylinder style and dimensions	Nominal volume cu in./liter	Contents	Air	Carbon dioxide	Cyclo-propane	Helium	Nitrogen	Nitrous oxide	Oxygen	Mixtures of oxygen — Helium	Mixtures of oxygen — Carbon dioxide
B 3½" od × 13" 8.89 × 33 cm	87/1.43	psig		838	75		1900	745	1900	†	†
		Liters		370	375				200		
		Lbs.-oz.		1-8	1-7¼				—		
		Kilograms		0.68	0.66						
D 4½" od × 17" 10.8 × 43 cm	176/2.88	psig	1900	838	75	1600	1900	745	1900	†	†
		Liters	375	940	870	300	370	940	400	300	400
		Lbs.-oz.		3-13	3-5½	—		3-13	—		
		Kilograms		1.73	1.51			1.73			
E 4¼" od × 26" 10.8 × 66 cm	293/4.80	psig	1900	838		1600	1900	745	1900	†	†
		Liters	625	1590		500	610	1590	660	500	660
		Lbs.-oz.		6-7		—		6-7	—		
		Kilograms		2.92				2.92			
M 7" od × 43" 17.8 × 109 cm	1337/21.9	psig	1900	838		1600	2200	745	2200	†	†
		Liters	2850	7570		2260	3200	7570	3450	2260	3000
		Lbs.-oz.		30-10		—		30-10	122 cu ft		
		Kilograms		13.9				13.9	—		
G 8½" od × 51" 21.6 × 130 cm	2370/38.8	psig	1900	838		1600		745	—	†	†
		Liters	5050	12,300		4000		13,800		4000	5330
		Lbs.-oz.		50-0		—		56-0	—		
		Kilograms		22.7				25.4			
H or K 9¼" od × 0.51" 23.5 × 130 cm	2660/43.6	psig	2200			2200	2200	745	2200‡	†	†
		Liters	6550			6000	6400	15,800	6900		
		Lbs.-oz.				—		64	244 cu ft		
		Kilograms						29.1	—		

*These are computed contents based on nominal cylinder volumes and rounded to no greater variance than ± 1%.

†The pressure and weight of mixed gases will vary according to the composition of the mixture.

‡275 cu ft/7800 liter cylinders at 2490 psig are available on request.

From Standard for Nonflammable Medical Gas Systems (NFPA 56 F), 1990, copyright National Fire Protection Association, Boston, Mass. From the Compressed Gas Association, Inc.

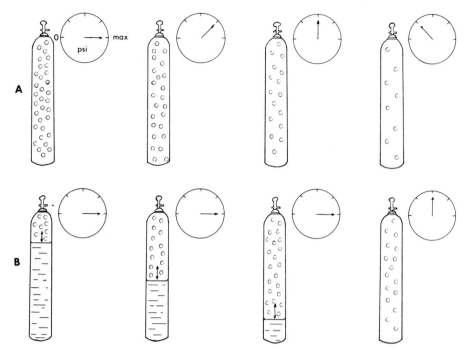

Fig. 24-4   The content of a gas-filled cylinder, **A,** is directly proportional to the gas pressure. As gas is withdrawn, for example, a pressure drop of 50% indicates a loss of 50% of the contained gas. In a liquid-gas cylinder, **B,** gauge pressure measures only the vapor pressure of gas in equilibrium with the liquid phase, and this remains constant at a given temperature as long as liquid is present. Only when all the liquid phase has vaporized, as the cylinder nears depletion, does the gauge pressure drop proportionately to the terminal volume of remaining gas.

745 psig at 70°F; at 60°F, it has a cylinder pressure of only 660 psig. As the temperature rises and approaches the critical point, more liquid will vaporize in the cylinder and pressure will rise. Should a cylinder of nitrous oxide warm to 97.5°F, the entire liquid contents will convert to gas, cylinder pressure will rise to the critical value of 1054 psig, and, if tapped, the cylinder gauge pressure will fall in direct proportion to usage.

Estimating the duration of compressed-gas cylinder flow. When one is initiating a therapeutic procedure that uses a compressed-gas cylinder, it is a matter of both safety and convenience to be able to predict how long its contents will last. An estimate of a cylinder's duration of flow can be made if the following factors are known: (1) the average anticipated gas flow, (2) the cylinder size, and (3) the cylinder pressure at the start of therapy.

The length of time a cylinder will last is simply a function of its gaseous contents divided by the average flow:

$$\text{Duration of flow} = \frac{\text{Contents}}{\text{Flow}}$$

Unfortunately, commercial gas cylinder contents are generally specified in English units of cubic feet or gallons, whereas actual gas flow normally is measured in metric liters. Table 24-3 provides factors by which the

practitioner can quickly convert one unit of measure to another.

Instead of laboriously memorizing contents for each cylinder size and constantly converting between metric and English units of measure, one can quickly calculate the duration of flow with values designed specifically for this purpose. These values, called *cylinder factors,* can be derived for each common gas and cylinder size by the following formula:

$$\text{Cylinder factor (L/psig)} = \frac{\text{Cubic feet in full cylinder} \times 28.3}{\text{Pressure of full cylinder in psig}}$$

The numerator of the equation uses the English-metric conversion factor (28.3) to convert the cylinder contents from cubic feet to liters. Dividing the resulting volume (in liters) by the denominator (the pressure in a full cylinder) yields the cylinder factor. Of course, the cylinder factor is

Table 24-3   Gas Volume Conversion Factors

Liters	Cubic feet	Gallons
28.316	1	7.481
1	0.03531	0.2642
3.785	0.1337	1

simply a ratio of the number of liters of gas that leave the cylinder for every 1 psig drop in pressure.

For example, an oxygen G cylinder contains about 187 cubic feet of gas under a filling pressure of 2200 psig. Therefore, the volume of gas leaving the cylinder for every pound per square inch gauge drop in pressure would be (187 × 28.3)/2200, or 2.41 L/psig. Based on this formula, Table 24-4 provides cylinder factors for the therapeutic medical gases and common cylinder sizes. The factors for O_2, O_2/N_2, and air will be used in the vast majority of situations.

Once the factors for a given gas and cylinder are known, calculation of the duration of flow is a simple matter of applying the following equation:

$$\text{Duration of flow (minutes)} = \frac{\text{Gauge pressure (psig)} \times \text{cylinder factor}}{\text{Flow (L/min)}}$$

As an example, let us estimate the duration of a G cylinder of oxygen with a gauge pressure of 800 psi if we use a flow of 8 L/min. Referring to Table 24-4, we find the oxygen G cylinder factor of 2.41. Applying the prior equation:

$$\text{Duration of flow (minutes)} = \frac{800 \times 2.41}{8}$$

$$= 241 \text{ minutes (about 4 hours)}$$

Given this estimate, the practitioner would plan to exchange this cylinder well in advance of its estimated time of depletion.

Bulk oxygen

Because of the tremendous volume of oxygen used in the average hospital, a separate discussion of special large-bulk storage systems is warranted. Bulk oxygen storage consists of any system capable of accommodating more than 13,000 cubic feet of gas ready for use. Such systems may be located out-of-doors or in a special building set aside for the purpose. Strict regulations for locating and maintaining bulk oxygen systems have been established by the NFPA and are subject to further control by local community fire and building codes.

The supervision and maintenance of bulk oxygen units are not always the responsibility of the respiratory care department. Nevertheless, in order to deal with the potential risk of emergency interruptions in gas supply, practitioners should be thoroughly acquainted with bulk systems in general and, more specifically, with the system used in their own institutions.

Bulk oxygen systems may provide either gaseous or cryogenic liquid oxygen. They are discussed separately below. Bulk oxygen is used as a "central supply," or "piped-in system," in which the gas is carried from a central source to the hospital floors by a system of pipes built into the walls. It is therefore possible to have oxygen outlets conveniently located by each patient's bed and any other area desired. As opposed to cylinder gas supply, a central system is referred to as a "low-pressure system."

The great value of such a centrally located oxygen supply should be obvious. There is less risk of a depletion of oxygen supply, and the inconvenience and hazard of transporting and storing individual cylinders are eliminated. Finally, pressure regulation of oxygen is accomplished at the central station, and the gas piped to the clinical areas is already reduced to the standard working pressure of 50 psig. This eliminates the need for pressure-reducing valves at the patient outlets and requires only the use of flowmeters (to be discussed in a subsequent section).

Gaseous bulk oxygen. There are three general systems that provide large central supplies of gaseous oxygen, including (1) standard cylinder manifolds, (2) fixed cylinders, and (3) trailer units. Although not as common as liquid bulk systems, the practitioner may encounter these in selected clinical settings.

Standard cylinder manifolds. Large (normally H or K size) compressed-oxygen cylinders can be banked together into a manifold system (Fig. 24-5). Manifolds usually include two sides: a "primary bank" and a "reserve bank." When the primary system falls to a set pressure, the control valve automatically switches over to the reserve bank. The manifold mechanism also contains pressure-reduction valves and an alarm system to warn of reserve switch-over, impending depletion, or malfunction. Groups of six or more cylinders may be joined together and replaced as needed with full ones.

Fixed cylinders. In contrast to the cylinders just described, fixed cylinders consist of large banks of up to 75 cylinders permanently fixed at a stationary site. When empty, they are refilled on location from a truck that contains liquid oxygen and converts the liquid to gas for pumping into the cylinders.

Trailer units. Very large cylinders mounted on trailers can be towed to the central area and connected to the distribution circuit. For heavy oxygen consumption, large trailers with up to 30 permanently attached long horizontal tubes are available. Replacement is a simple matter of switching trailers. As in the other cylinder systems, trailer gas is at 2200 psig pressure. Trailer units are useful to provide a replacement supply in the event of primary system failure or needed maintenance.

Table 24-4 Factors to Calculate Duration of Cylinder Flow in Minutes

| Gas | Cylinder size | | | |
	D	E	G	H&K
O_2, O_2/N_2, air	0.16	0.28	2.41	3.14
O_2/CO_2	0.20	0.35	2.94	3.84
He/O_2	0.14	0.23	1.93	2.50

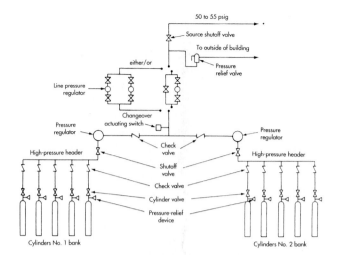

Fig. 24-5 Typical cylinder supply system without reserve supply (schematic). Supply systems with different arrangement of valves and regulators are permissible if they provide equivalent safeguards. (Type I Gas Systems.) For SI Units, 1 psig is equal to 6.895 kPa gauge. (From Standard for Nonflammable Medical Gas Systems [NFPA 56 F], 1990, Copyright National Fire Protection Association, Boston, Mass.)

Liquid bulk oxygen. Because they represent an extremely economical method of both transporting and storing oxygen, liquid gas systems are widely used. Of prime importance is the fact that at its boiling point of $-297.3°F$, 1 cubic foot of liquid oxygen is the equivalent of 860.6 cubic feet of gaseous oxygen at ambient temperature and pressure. Thus a relatively small volume of liquid oxygen can provide a very large amount of the gaseous form.

Although we have already discussed the liquid form of some medical gases packaged in standard cylinders, liquid oxygen deserves special consideration because of its physical characteristics. The major physical difference between oxygen and those liquid gases noted previously is that its critical temperature $(-181.1°F)$ is well below room temperature. For this reason, the mechanisms for producing and maintaining the liquid state of oxygen are much more complex than those used for other liquid medical gases.

Brief reference was made earlier to the method of producing liquid oxygen from the compression and cooling of air. To prevent the cryogenic liquid from reverting back to its gaseous form, the liquid must be kept well below its critical temperature. This is accomplished by keeping it in special containers, under a pressure not to exceed 250 psig. All such containers for liquid oxygen, whether tank trucks or hospital supply stations, are constructed on the principle of a large Thermos bottle. They consist of inner and outer steel shells, separated by a vacuum, which effectively blocks the transfer of heat into the liquid. This evacuated space is filled with a noncombustible insulation, and the inner shell is coated with silver to aid in repelling heat. The containers are vented so that vaporized liquid oxygen

can escape if warming occurs. It should be apparent that when the temperature of liquid oxygen is kept below its boiling point, it can be exposed to atmospheric pressure for short periods of time without immediately vaporizing. Otherwise, transferring liquid between bulk containers would be difficult.

There are two types of container for use with liquid oxygen: the liquid oxygen cylinder and the permanent station or stand tank.

Liquid-oxygen cylinders. Liquid-oxygen cylinders are used as a primary gas supply when gas usage is too large for a gaseous cylinder bank but not great enough to require a permanently installed liquid vessel. Smaller cylinders of this type are also used for oxygen supply in private homes.[11]

Large liquid-oxygen cylinders are 58 inches high and 20 inches in diameter and hold the equivalent of 3000 cubic feet of gas, matching the contents of more than 12 size standard cylinders. These cylinders can be banked into manifold-like gas cylinders, but they must also incorporate a vaporizer to convert the cryogenic liquid to a gas. Such liquid manifold systems may be used for primary oxygen supplies in very small hospitals or in larger nursing homes.

Small liquid-oxygen cylinders are designed primarily for home use. These cylinders come in three different sizes, ranging from 25 to 40 inches high and from 12 to 14 inches in diameter. Depending on their size, they may hold the equivalent of between 600 and 1200 cubic feet of gaseous oxygen. Small liquid-oxygen cylinders are refilled on site by the transfer of liquid oxygen from a large cylinder. Because of their extensive use in home care, details on the design and use of these small liquid oxygen cylinders are provided in Chapter 35.

Fixed stations (stand tanks). Fixed stations are large cylindrical or spherical containers with capacities up to the gaseous equivalent of 130,000 cubic feet (Fig. 24-6). As with small cryogenic cylinders, the liquid oxygen is converted to gas by vaporizers, which may be heated externally or simply draw heat from the surrounding air. Elaborately controlled to ensure a steady, even conversion of liquid to gas according to need, these systems are designed to ensure an uninterrupted gas supply. They are refilled from service tank trucks according to schedules designed for each hospital. All liquid bulk systems also incorporate pressure-reducing valves to lower pressure to 50 psig.

Bulk oxygen safety precautions. As previously described, bulk systems must include reserve or backup gas supplies. The standard established by the NFPA requires that the reserve supply be equal to the average daily gas use in the hospital. Most liquid-oxygen systems use a bank of fixed cylinders for this purpose. However, larger institutions may actually need a second, smaller liquid cylinder to meet this reserve standard.

Although rare, total failure of hospitals' bulk oxygen supply systems has been reported.[12] Obviously, since such a situation presents immediate danger to patients receiving

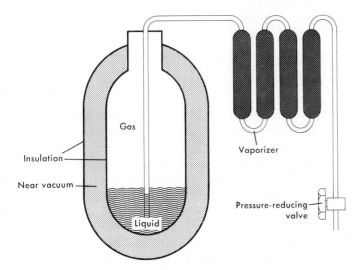

Fig. 24-6 A liquid-oxygen stand tank (fixed station). (From McPherson SP and Spearman CB: Respiratory therapy equipment, ed 3, St Louis, 1985, The CV Mosby Co.)

oxygen or gas-powered ventilatory support, the respiratory care department must be prepared. Established protocols should provide a quick means for identifying affected patients and responding according to a predetermined priority scheme. Each practitioner should be familiar with this departmental protocol and their role in addressing such an emergency.

DISTRIBUTION AND REGULATION OF MEDICAL GASES

Before medical gases can actually be administered to a patient, they must be delivered to the site of use and reduced to a workable range of pressure. This is the primary function of gas-distribution and regulation systems.

Modern hospital gas-distribution systems deliver bulk stored oxygen and compressed air to patients' rooms and specialized care areas via an elaborate piping network. Included in this network may be a vacuum source and—for surgical areas—nitrous oxide. However, whenever patients are transported or gases other than these are required, cylinders must still be employed as the gas source.

Gas pressures are regulated either within the piping network or directly at the cylinder source. In either case, various safety systems are used to minimize the likelihood of administering the wrong gas to a patient.

Patient safety is always the primary consideration in the distribution and regulation of medical gases. However, a system is only as safe as those who use it. For these reasons, practitioners must be proficient in the use of both central gas supply systems and cylinder-stored gas.

Central piping systems

Structural requirements for piping systems are established by the NFPA and are described in more detail else-

where.[1,5,6] An example of a central piped-gas system is shown in Fig. 24-7. Normally, the gas pressure in a central piping system is reduced to the working pressure at the bulk source or storage location. A main alarm provides warning of pressure drops or interruptions in flow from the source. Zone valves throughout the distribution system can be closed for maintenance of the system or in case of fire. Wall outlets at the delivery sites provide connections to the system for various equipment. Normally, oxygen and air are provided to the delivery outlets at the standard working pressure of 50 psig, with unrestricted flow. Since delivery outlets may include not only oxygen but also air, vacuum, and possibly nitrous oxide, special safety connectors are used to prevent inadvertent misconnections.

Safety-indexed connector systems

With the large number of compressed gases in current commercial, medical, and scientific use, one of the greatest risks in medical gas therapy is the inadvertent administration of the wrong gas to a patient. Certainly, care on the part of the practitioner in reading labels or other identifying marks is the most important deterrent to such an accident. However, human error is always a potential risk. For this reason, specially designed connectors, or indexed safety systems, have been developed for gas delivery and regulation equipment.

The purpose of an indexed safety system is to make certain connections between cylinders and delivery systems impossible. When properly used, such a system should prevent, for example, a cylinder of nitrous oxide from being attached to a system for administration of oxygen. We will describe only the key elements of the indexed safety systems in common use; the practitioner is encouraged to become familiar with their details as provided in the applicable CGA publications.[7-9]

There are three basic indexed safety systems involved in the delivery and regulation of medical gases: (1) the American Standard Compressed Gas Cylinder Outlet and Inlet Connections, or American Standard Safety System (ASSS) for short, (2) the Diameter-Index Safety System (DISS), and (3) the Pin-Index Safety System (PISS).

American Standard Safety System (ASSS). Adopted in the US and Canada, the American Standard Safety System provides specifications for threaded high-pressure connections between compressed-gas cylinders and their attachments. Standardized for each gas, these specifications are explained in detail in the applicable CGA publication.[9]

The ASSS standards are limited to large cylinders with threaded valve outlets (sizes F through H/K). They provide specifications for the mating nipples and hexagonal nuts by which an appliance (usually a pressure regulator) is attached to the valve.

Fig. 24-8 illustrates a cutaway of a joined threaded outlet and nipple. The gas channel through the nipple of the regulator is aligned with the channel through the threaded outlet. The two parts are secured by a hexagonal nut that is

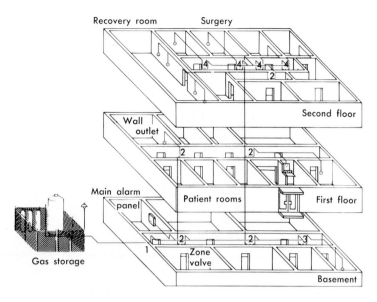

Fig. 24-7 A hospital piping system. Numbers indicate zone values. (From McPherson SP and Spearman CB: Respiratory therapy equipment, ed 3, St Louis, 1985, The CV Mosby Co. Courtesy Puritan-Bennett Corp, Los Angeles, Calif.)

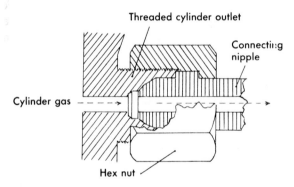

Fig. 24-8 This sketch illustrates the structure of a typical American Standard connection, such as might be used to attach a reducing valve to a large high-pressure cylinder. The hexagonal nut is held onto the nipple of the reducing valve by a circular collar, seen as a cross-sectional projection on the nipple. As the hex nut is tightened on the threaded cylinder outlet, the end of the nipple is snugly seated into the conical outlet. (Modified from CGA Pamphlet V-1, connection no. 540, Compressed Gas Association, Inc, New York.)

attached to the nipple by a shoulder-and-flange mechanism.

By varying the size (or "bore") of the cylinder outlet and nipple for each gas, the ASSS standards should make misconnections impossible. For example, it should not be possible to connect CO_2 cylinders to an oxygen bank.

There are two fundamental divisions of the ASSS: thread position and thread direction. Thread position may be internal or external. Thread direction may be right-handed or left-handed. Each division is further segmented by varying the number, pitch, and diameter (bore) of the threads. In general, left-handed threads are used for fuel gases, and right-handed threads are used for nonfuel (in-

cluding medical) gases. Most of the valve outlets have external threads, and their corresponding nipples have internal threads.

Most threads of the ASSS are usually classified as National Gas Outlet (NGO), but a few are National Gas Taper (NGT). It is important to note that each gas may not have its own specific connection. Indeed, there are only 26 different connections for the 62 listed gases. This means that some gases must share identical connections.

In catalogs of cylinder gas dealers, the practitioner will see the connection specifications listed for each type of cylinder and gas. A typical description is as follows for a large cylinder of oxygen:

$$CGA-540 \times 0.903\text{-}14NGO\text{-}RH\text{-}Ext$$

This tells us that the connection for the threaded outlet of this cylinder is listed by the CGA as connection no. 540, that the outlet has a thread diameter (bore) of 0.903 inch, that there are 14 threads per inch of the NGO type, and that the threads are right-handed (RH) and external (Ext).

Generally, respiratory care practitioners will use but one or two outlet connections, since most of the relatively small number of different gases they employ are grouped within a few connector sizes. However, practitioners should be familiar with the classification scheme in general, since expanding instrumentation and scope of services in the future may bring them into contact with other gases and gas systems.

Pin-Indexed Safety System (PISS). Pin-indexing is incorporated in the specifications of the American Standard listing just described, but as a subsection applicable only to the valve outlets of small cylinders, up to and including

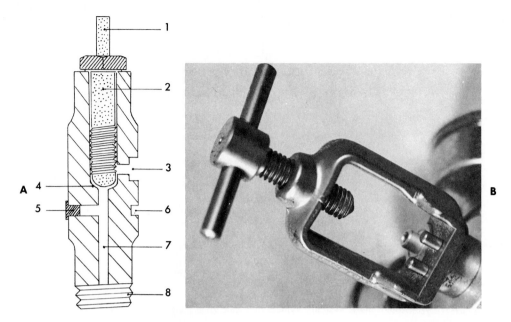

Fig. 24-9   A, Diagrammatic sectional sketch of a small cylinder valve. **B,** Photograph of the yoke connector used with small cylinders. (See text for description.)

size E. These cylinders use a yoke type of connection.

Fig. 24-9 illustrates the general structure of cylinder valves and the yoke used with small cylinders. Fig. 24-9, *A,* presents a cross-sectional view of a small-cylinder valve, similar in principle to cylinder valves in general. The valve stem, *1,* connects to a threaded valve plunger, *2.* The cylinder outlet, *3,* is separated from the gas channel, *7,* by the valve seat, *4.* Turning of the stem by means of a handgrip (not shown) opens and closes the valve seat, permitting or restricting gas outflow.

An emergency pressure release, *5,* allows gas to escape, should pressures within the cylinder rise to dangerous levels. A pair of borings in the valve body of small cylinders, *6,* represents part of the Pin-Index Safely System. Finally, the valve is attached to the body of the cylinder by means of a threaded connection, *8.*

Fig. 24-9, *B,* shows a yoke connector for cylinders of sizes A through E. The handscrew is used to hold the yoke firmly onto the valve. The small receiving nipple (background) fits into the gas outlet, *3,* which is normally sealed with a nylon bushing. The two pins (foreground) are positioned to mate with the borings in the valve stem, *6,* of the Pin-Indexed Safety System.

Like the ASSS, the PISS is designed to prevent the wrong cylinder from being attached to a given appliance. The exact position of the two holes drilled in the face of the valve and the two pins on the yoke varies for each gas. Unless the pins and holes align perfectly, the yoke nipple will not seat in the recess of the valve. The total system comprises six hole/pin positions and, because of overlapping, adjacent holes cannot be used inadvertently. There

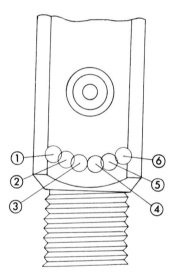

Fig. 24-10   Location of the Pin-Index Safety System holes in the cylinder valve face, various pairs of which constitute indices for different gases. (See text for the complete pairings.) (Modified from CGA Pamphlet V-1, Pin-Index Safety System, Compressed Gas Association, Inc, New York.)

are therefore ten possible combinations, of which nine are now in use.

Fig. 24-10 is a composite illustration of the location of all six possible holes and the numbers by which they are indexed. Table 24-5 lists the gases included in the PISS system, including their index positions.

Diameter-Indexed Safety System (DISS). Whereas the ASSS and PISS deal with high-pressure connections between cylinders and gas-regulating equipment in general, the DISS was established specifically to prevent accidental interchanging among low-pressure (less than 200 psig) connectors used for administration of medical gas. Specifically, the DISS is used in respiratory care to connect flowmeters and other therapy devices, such as nebulizers, ventilators, and anesthesia apparatus, to a low-pressure gas source. This low-pressure gas source may be either that available after pressure reduction from a cylinder or that directly provided at the outlet connection of a central piping system.

As illustrated in Fig. 24-11, the DISS connection consists of an externally threaded body and a mated nipple with a hex nut. The body of the connector has two concentric borings: a primary bore, noted as bore 1, and a counterbore, or bore 2. The accompanying nipple has two shoulders, identified as 1 and 2, and a loose hex nut secured by a flange behind shoulder 2. As the two parts are joined, the corresponding shoulders and bores mate, and the union is held together by the tightened hex nut.

Indexing is achieved by varying the dimensions of the borings and shoulders. Starting with a basic set of dimensions, bore 1 is increased and bore 2 is decreased in increments of 0.012 inch. The nipple shoulders are varied accordingly. The final connection is a smooth-bored body and a nipple of regular diameter.

There are 11 indexed connections, which accommodate 11 gases or gas mixtures. Table 24-6 lists the DISS connection numbers with the gases assigned to each.[9] It should be noted that the standard removable threaded oxygen connector (0.5625 inch in diameter and 18 threads per inch), became commonplace before the DISS gained widespread adoption. Although technically not part of the system, oxygen has been given a DISS number of 1240.

Although the practitioner will generally use oxygen or air from a central outlet, he or she may have occasion to administer helium-oxygen mixtures and oxygen-carbon dioxide mixtures, both of which have DISS connections. To avoid the cumbersome stocking of a large variety of pressure regulators and tubing connectors for special gas use,

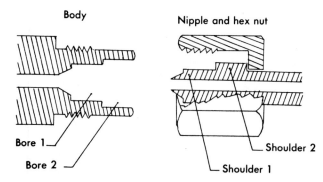

Fig. 24-11 Schematic illustration of components of a representative DISS connection. The two shoulders of the nipple allow the nipple to unite only with a body that has corresponding borings. If the match is incorrect, the hex nut will not engage the body threads. (Modified from CGA Pamphlet V-5, DISS connection no. 1100, Compressed Gas Association, Inc, New York.)

the practitioner can use adapters to convert among various DISS connections. Of course, the use of adapters to circumvent any safety system carries with it the increased risk of misconnection. For this reason, practitioners should exercise extreme caution when adapting equipment connections.

Quick-connect systems. Quick-connect systems represent a variation of the standard DISS connections, designed specifically to provide easy attachment of equipment to the wall-station outlets of built-in piping systems.[5] Various manufacturers have designed specially shaped connectors for each gas (Fig. 24-12). Because the connector for each gas has a distinct shape, it will not fit an outlet for another gas. Unlike the DISS system, however, each manufacturer has independently developed its own system. For this reason, connectors from different manufacturers are totally incompatible with each other. As long as a single quick-connect system is used throughout an institution, this incompatibility is seldom a problem.

Table 24-5   Pin-Indexed Gases

Gas	Index hole position
O_2	2-5
O_2/CO_2 (CO_2 not over 7%)	2-6
He/O_2 (He not over 80%)	2-4
C_2H_4	1-3
N_2O	3-5
$(CH_2)_3$	3-6
He/O_2 (He over 80%)	4-6
O_2/CO_2 (CO_2 over 7%)	1-6
Air	1-5

Table 24-6   DISS Connection Numbers and Assigned Gases

Connection number	Gas	Connection number	Gas
1020	Unassigned	1120	Unassigned
1040	N_2O	1140	C_2H_4
1060	He	1160	Air
	He/O_2 ($O_2 <20\%$)	1180	He/O_2 (He 80% or less)
1080	CO_2	1200	O_2/CO_2 (CO_2 7% or less)
	O_2/CO_2 ($CO_2 >7\%$)	1220	Suction
1100	$(CH_2)_3$	1240	O_2 (standard)

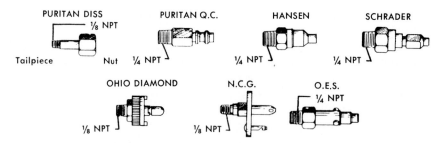

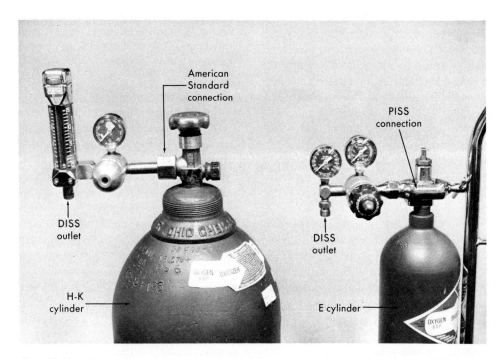

Fig. 24-13   Comparison of safety systems used for compressed gases. Note that the DISS connections are for outlets that have reduced pressures (less than 200 psig), while the American Standard connection is shown for a large cylinder and the PISS connection is shown for a small cylinder.

In summary, various safety systems have been developed to prevent inadvertent misconnections among medical gases. Fig. 24-13 illustrates the use of and relationships among the ASSS, PISS, and DISS systems as applied to cylinder gases. Proficiency in the proper use of these systems is a basic requirement for respiratory care practitioners.

Regulation of gas pressure and flow

Whatever the source of medical gas, a device is needed to regulate its pressure and flow as it is administered to a patient. When the goal is simply to reduce gas pressure, a *reducing valve* is employed. A *flowmeter* is a device that controls the flow of a gas. A device that controls both pressure and flow is called a *regulator*.

For cylinder gases such as oxygen or compressed air, the high pressure leaving the cylinder must first be reduced to a lower "working" pressure. For respiratory care in the US, this working pressure is standardized at 50 psig. For bulk delivery systems with individual station outlets, built-in reducing valves drop the system pressure to 50 psig. This standardized pressure may then be applied directly to power devices such as ventilators (see Chapter 30). However, when the goal is to control the delivery of medical gas to a patient (as described in the next chapter), a flow-metering device must be used in conjunction with pressure reduction.

High-pressure reducing valves. There are three types of high-pressure reducing valves: the preset reducing valve, the adjustable reducing valve, and the multiple-

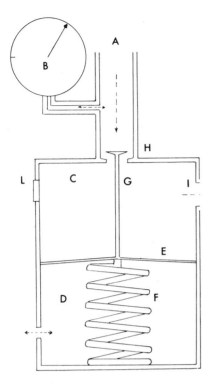

Fig. 24-14 Diagram of preset, high-pressure–reducing valve. (See text for details.)

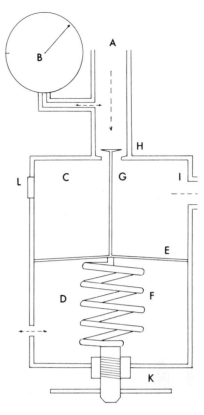

Fig. 24-15 Diagram of an adjustable, high-pressure reducing valve. (See text for details.)

stage reducing valve.[5] Although all of these valves function on the same basic principle, their design characteristics and use are different enough to deserve individual description.

Preset reducing valve. Fig. 24-14 portrays the basic design features of a high-pressure preset reducing valve. High-pressure gas (2200 psig for oxygen) enters the valve through *A,* with the inlet pressure displayed on the pressure gauge, *B.* The body of the valve is divided into a high-pressure chamber, *C,* and an ambient-pressure chamber, *D,* by a flexible diaphragm, *E.* Attached to the diaphragm in the ambient-pressure chamber is a spring, *F,* which is fixed to the other side of the chamber. Also attached to the diaphragm, but in the high-pressure chamber, is a valve stem, *G,* seated on the high-pressure inlet, *H.* Gas flows through the valve seat, *H,* into the high-pressure chamber, and on to the gas outlet, *I.* The pressure chamber is supplied with a safety vent, *L,* that is preset to 200 psig to release pressure in the event of malfunction.

The spring tension is calibrated to "give" when the pressure on the diaphragm exceeds 50 psig. When this happens, the valve stem will be pulled back and close the high-pressure inlet, thereby preventing further entry of gas into the reducing valve. However, as long as gas is allowed to escape from the pressure chamber through the outlet, *I,* the inlet valve will remain open and permit gas flow. Thus a balance between outlet flow and inlet pressure is maintained. Automatic adjustment of the dia-

phragm-spring combination maintains the pressure in the high-pressure chamber at a nearly constant 50 psig; hence the name *preset.* Preset reducing valves are normally used in conjunction with high-pressure gas cylinders to lower the pressure to the standard 50 psig used with most respiratory care equipment.

Adjustable reducing valve. Although most respiratory care equipment is designed to function at the standard 50 psig, some devices require variable pressures in order to operate effectively. Variable outlet pressures from a high-pressure gas source are provided with an adjustable reducing valve. Fig. 24-15 shows the basic design features of a high-pressure adjustable reducing valve. As with the preset reducing valve, the inlet valve, *H,* remains open until the gas pressure exceeds the spring tension, thus displacing the diaphragm and preventing further gas entry. However, whereas the preset reducing valve provides a fixed pressure, the adjustable reducing valve allows the clinician to change outlet pressures. This is accomplished by means of a threaded hand control, *K,* attached to the end of the diaphragm spring. Changing the tension on the valve spring permits pressures to be varied over a wide range, usually between 0 and 100 psig.

The most common application of the adjustable reducing valve is in combination with a Bourdon type of flow

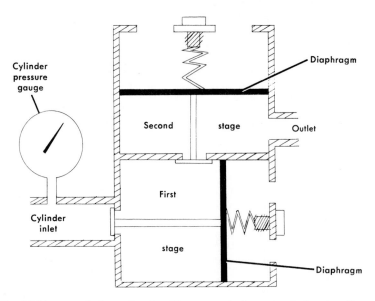

Fig. 24-16   Multistage reducing valve. Double-stage reducing valve is functionally two single-stage reducing valves working in tandem. Gas enters first stage (first reducing valve), and its pressure is lowered. Gas then enters second stage (second reducing valve), and pressure is lowered to desired working pressure (usually 50 psig). A three-stage reducing valve would have one more reducing valve in series. (From McPherson SP and Spearman CB: Respiratory therapy equipment, ed 3, St Louis, 1985, The CV Mosby Co.)

gauge, to be described subsequently. As previously indicated, this combination of a reducing valve and a flow-metering device is called a regulator.

Multiple-stage reducing valve. As the name implies, the multiple-stage reducing valve accomplishes pressure reduction in two or more steps. Multiple-stage reducing valves may be either preset or adjustable, and they can be combined with a flow-metering device as a true regulator. Practitioners may have occasion to use two-stage reducing valves, but rarely three-stage ones.

As shown in Fig. 24-16, which depicts a two-stage pressure-reducing valve, gas from a cylinder inlet initially enters a first-stage pressure-reduction chamber. Usually, the diaphragm spring tension of the first stage is factory preset to an intermediate pressure level between 200 and 700 psig. Then the second stage lowers this intermediate pressure to the working level (in three-stage units, the second stage lowers the pressure to about one half that of the first). Since each pressure chamber will have one safety relief vent, the number of stages in a reducing valve usually can be determined by noting the number of relief vents present.

Because pressure is reduced in multiple steps, these reducing valves are able to effect more precision and smoothness in flow control. However, multiple-stage reducing valve regulators are larger and more costly than single-stage reducing valves. For this reason, they are indicated only when minimal fluctuations in pressure and flow are critical factors, as in research activities. For routine hospital work, the simpler single-stage reducing valves are quite satisfactory.

Low-pressure gas flowmeters. It is not enough that we be able to simply reduce the pressure of gases used in the clinical setting. As with drugs, the administration of medical gases to patients requires some knowledge of the "dosage" being delivered. This is accomplished, in part, by metering the rate of gas flow to the patient through a device appropriately called a flowmeter.

When a high-pressure gas cylinder is used to provide medical gas for patient use, both a reducing valve and a flowmeter are combined into a regulator. However, when gas is provided through a central supply system, the pressure has already been reduced to the desired working pressure (50 psig) by the time it reaches the outlet stations. This eliminates the need for pressure-reducing devices at the bedside and requires only a device for regulating the gas flow.

There are three primary types of flowmeter used in respiratory care: the flow restrictor, the Bourdon gauge, and the Thorpe tube. The Thorpe tube type of flowmeter can be further categorized as being either "pressure compensated" or not pressure compensated (uncompensated). Although the uncompensated Thorpe tube is seen infrequently today, respiratory care practitioners may have occasion to apply all of these flow-metering devices under different clinical circumstances. For this reason, we will compare and contrast the principles underlying all four of these devices.

Flow restrictors. The flow restrictor is the simplest and least expensive type of flow-metering device. As shown in Fig. 24-17, a flow restrictor consists solely of a fixed orifice, calibrated to deliver a specific flow at a constant pressure (50 psig).

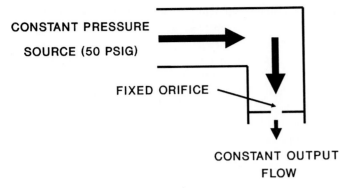

Fig. 24-17 Flow restrictor.

The operation of the flow restrictor is based on the principle of flow resistance, as described in Chapter 4. Specifically, we may quantify the flow of gas through a tube according to the following equation:

$$R = \frac{P_1 - P_2}{\dot{V}}$$

Rearranging the equation to solve for flow ($\dot{V}$) yields the following:

$$\dot{V} = \frac{P_1 - P_2}{R}$$

where $\dot{V}$ is the volumetric flow per unit time, P_1 is the pressure at the upstream point (point 1), P_2 is the pressure at the downstream point (point 2), and R is the total resistance to gas flow.

Because a flow restrictor is always used in conjunction with a source of constant pressure (usually 50 psig), $P_1 - P_2$ normally remains constant. With a constant pressure difference and a fixed orifice, the resistance to gas flow (R) also remains constant. With both the numerator and the denominator of the equation fixed, the resultant flow will also be a constant value for any given orifice size.

Given a constant driving pressure and a constant gas density, the actual flow through an orifice is proportional to the square of the orifice diameter[13]:

$$\dot{V} \propto \text{Diameter}^2$$

Thus, as long as the downstream pressure (P_2) remains negligible, an orifice of a given size attached to a 50 psig gas source will always produce a constant flow of known value. A flow restrictor therefore may be classified as a fixed orifice, constant-pressure flow-metering device.[14]

Commercially produced flow restrictors designed for clinical use are always calibrated at 50 psig. A selection of models is available, each providing a specific preset flow. Typically, these devices are used to provide calibrated low flows of oxygen, in the range of 0.5 to 3 L/min.

In addition to low cost and simplicity, flow restrictors provide an added advantage of safety, especially in patients who require precise low flows of oxygen (see Chapter 25). Since the flow through the device is fixed, it is im-

possible for the patient or the practitioner to inadvertently alter the prescribed liter flow. Moreover, the accuracy of flow restrictors is independent of gravity, meaning that they may be used in any position. As we shall see, this is an important advantage when oxygen is used in transport situations.

However, the advantages of the flow restrictor must be weighed against its limitations. Obviously, the fixed flow provided by these devices limits their utility, and requires that the device be changed whenever a new flow is prescribed. To overcome this limitation, some manufacturers provide flow restrictors that incorporate a number of calibrated orifice sizes, which can be selected by the practitioner with the use of a rotary dial. However, these devices can be as expensive as other flow-metering instruments capable of providing a continuous range of flows. Finally, the accuracy of a flow restrictor is dependent on the maintenance of a constant and specific pressure difference across the orifice. For example, should the upstream pressure drop below 50 psig, or should the downstream pressure rise significantly, the flow provided by these devices will be less than that designated. Although a significant drop in upstream (or source) pressure is uncommon in the hospital setting, rises in pressure downstream, or distal to the restrictor, can readily occur. Downstream pressure will rise whenever a device with high flow resistance is connected in series with the flow restrictor. For this reason, flow restrictors should not be used with any equipment that itself creates high flow resistance. This includes jet-type nebulizers and some types of humidification equipment (described previously in Chapter 23).

Bourdon gauge. A Bourdon gauge is a low-pressure flow-metering device that is always used in conjunction with an adjustable high-pressure–reducing valve. Like the flow restrictor, the Bourdon gauge employs a fixed-size orifice. Unlike the flow restrictor, however, the Bourdon gauge operates under variable pressures, as determined by adjustment of the pressure-reducing valve. The Bourdon gauge therefore may be classified as a fixed-orifice, variable-pressure flow-metering device.[14]

As shown in Fig. 24-18, outflow resistance in a Bourdon gauge is created by a calibrated orifice of fixed size, *A*. The gauge itself is attached to the system proximal to the calibrated orifice by a connector, *B*. Inside the gauge is a curved, hollow, closed tube, *C*, that responds to pressure changes by changing shape. The force of gas pressure tends to straighten the tube, causing its distal end to move. This motion is transmitted to a gear assembly and an indicator needle, *D*. A numbered scale is calibrated to read the needle movement in units of flow (liters per minute).

As in the flow restrictor, the fixed-size orifice used in the Bourdon gauge assures that the output flow will be proportional to the driving pressure. That is, each unit of pressure pushing gases through the orifice will do so at a known rate of flow. Thus, although the gauge is actually sensing pressure, it is calibrated to display flow.

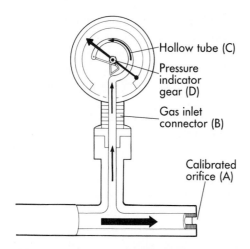

Fig. 24-18 Components of a Bourdon pressure gauge.

When used in conjunction with an adjustable high-pressure–reducing valve (a combination often referred to as a "Bourdon regulator"), a Bourdon gauge provides the clinician with a continuous selection of metered flows over its scale range. Of course, this is accomplished simply by alteration of the spring tension on the attached reducing valve.

Like the flow restrictor, the accuracy of the Bourdon gauge is not affected by gravity. For this reason, the Bourdon gauge is ideal in situations in which the upright positioning of the flow-metering device cannot be assured. This situation is common when patients must be transported with a portable oxygen source, either inside or outside the hospital setting. In these cases, upright positioning of the oxygen supply (usually small cylinders) is seldom convenient, and movement of both the oxygen supply and the patient is common. Also, the continuous range of flows available with a Bourdon regulator provides increased flexibility of use over simple flow restrictors.

However, as with the simple flow restrictor, the accuracy of the Bourdon gauge can be affected by variations in downstream pressures. Since the Bourdon gauge measures only the pressure of gas proximal to its calibrated outflow orifice, any significant increase in pressure distal to this orifice will affect the gauge reading. Specifically, if resistance distal to the calibrated orifice increases, the total pressure difference across it will decrease, resulting in a lower flow. In such a situation, however, the proximal pressure as measured by the Bourdon gauge remains constant. Thus, since the flow reading is based on gas pressure proximal to the orifice, the Bourdon gauge will indicate a flow *higher than that actually delivered* whenever it is faced with significant increases in downstream pressure.[5] Indeed, because the gauge records reducing valve chamber pressure, it will register flow on its printed face, even when the outlet is completely blocked (Fig. 24-19)! For these reasons, when the situation demands accurate

flows in conjunction with the application of any device that creates high downstream flow resistance, the Bourdon gauge should not be used.

Thorpe tube flowmeter. The Thorpe tube flowmeter is always used in conjunction with a low gas pressure source, as provided by either a preset pressure-reducing valve or a 50 psig bulk delivery system station outlet at the bedside. As compared to the flow restrictor and the Bourdon gauge, the Thorpe tube is classified as a variable-orifice, constant-pressure flow-metering device.[14]

The principle of operation of the Thorpe tube flowmeter is depicted in Fig. 24-20. The heart of this type of meter consists of a tapered transparent tube with a float. The diameter of the tube increases from bottom to top (exaggerated here for clarity). While in use, the float is suspended in the tube against the force of gravity by the flow of gas. Its position is noted against an adjacent scale, which is normally calibrated in liters per minute.

Whereas the Bourdon gauge actually measures pressure, the Thorpe tube flow-metering device truly measures flow. The ability of the Thorpe tube flowmeter to measure flow is based on the complex interaction of the forces of fluid dynamics and gravity.[13] Displacement of the float requires that the force of gravity be overcome. When gas from a 50 psig source begins to flow through the tube, a pressure difference ($P_1 - P_2$) is created across the float. As the float rises in the widening tube, the space available for gas to flow around the float (equivalent to the orifice) increases, thereby decreasing the restriction to flow. A decrease in the restriction to flow allows a greater flow for a given pressure difference. Ultimately, the float position is stabilized when the pressure difference across the float (an upward force) equals the opposing downward force of gravity.

An increase in input flow initially disrupts this balance, creating an increase in the pressure difference across the float (the upward force of $P_1 - P_2$ becomes greater than the downward force of gravity). This causes the float to rise. As the float rises, however, the available "orifice" increases in diameter, flow resistance around the float drops, and the difference in pressure once again equilibrates with the force of gravity. The position of the float thus stabilizes at a higher level, proportionate to the greater flow around it.

As previously indicated, Thorpe tube flow-metering devices are of two basic designs: pressure compensated and not pressure compensated (uncompensated). The term *pressure compensation* refers to a design in the Thorpe tube flowmeter that prevents a change in downstream resistance (or "back pressure") from affecting its liter flow calibration. For therapeutic gas administration, all manufacturers now supply only pressure-compensated Thorpe tubes. However, some older equipment that is still in use might not conform to these standards, and some gas-metering devices used in ventilators and anesthesia equipment

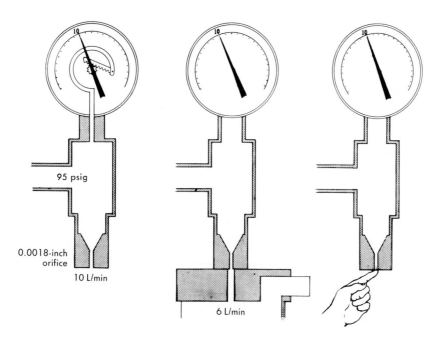

95 psig

0.0018-inch orifice

10 L/min

6 L/min

Fig. 24-19 Bourdon regulator with resistance downstream. If resistance is placed on Bourdon regulator, postrestriction pressure is no longer constant, as it will be somewhat higher than atmospheric pressure. Pressure gradient is then decreased; because only prerestriction pressure and not actual pressure gradient is monitored, the reading will be erroneously high. (From McPherson SP and Spearman CB: Respiratory therapy equipment, ed 3, St Louis, 1985, The CV Mosby Co. Courtesy Puritan-Bennett Corp, Los Angeles, Calif.)

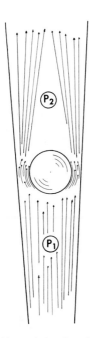

Fig. 24-20 The position of the float in the Thorpe tube-type flowmeter is based on a balance between the force of gravity and the pressure difference ($P_1 - P_2$) across it, as determined by the variable-sized orifice created between the float and tube wall.

are still of the uncompensated design. For these reasons, it is important that the practitioner understand the effect of pressure compensation on the accuracy of these devices.

As we have learned, an increase in downstream resistance is common when a flowmeter is connected to several types of respiratory care equipment. Practically all gas-administration equipment contains some restriction to flow in its circuitry. With some devices, such as jet nebulizers, these restrictions generate very high downstream resistance. Depending on their design, Thorpe tube flowmeters respond to downstream resistance in one of two different ways.

Uncompensated Thorpe tube. The uncompensated Thorpe tube flowmeter is calibrated in liters per minute, but at atmospheric pressure (without restriction).[5] Gas from a 50 psig source flows into the meter at a rate controlled by a needle valve proximal to the flow tube (Fig. 24-21, *A*). When flow-restricting equipment is attached distal to the meter, downstream resistance is generated, raising pressures in the flow tube. As long as this pressure does not exceed the source pressure of 50 psig, gas will continue to flow through the tube. However, the added downstream resistance increases the pressure in the flow tube above atmospheric pressure. At higher operating pressures, a greater amount of gas per unit time will flow through a given restriction than at atmospheric pressure. Thus, with the float at a given height, more gas will be

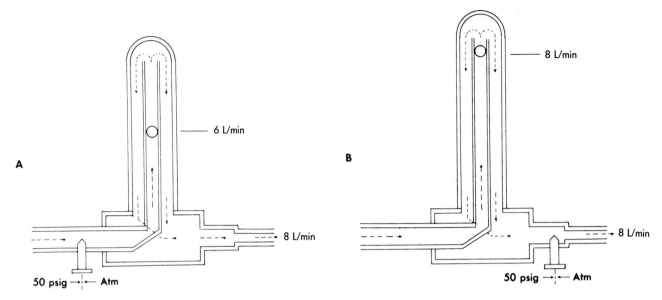

A

6 L/min

8 L/min

50 psig →⊦← Atm

B

8 L/min

8 L/min

50 psig →⊦← Atm

Fig. 24-21   Comparison of, **A,** pressure-uncompensated, and **B,** pressure-compensated flowmeters. In the former, the flow-control valve is proximal to the meter, and the gauge records less than the actual output. In the latter, location of the valve distal to the meter correlates the gauge reading with the output. (See text for detailed explanation.)

flowing between it and the flow tube walls than indicated on the scale. Therefore, when faced with a restriction to outlet flow, an uncompensated Thorpe tube flowmeter displays *less gas flow than the patient actually receives.*[5]

Compensated Thorpe tube. In contrast to the uncompensated Thorpe tube, the scale of the compensated Thorpe tube flowmeter is calibrated against a constant pressure of 50 psig instead of the atmospheric pressure.[5] Its major structural feature, shown in Fig. 24-21, *B,* is placement of the flow control needle valve distal to the flow tube. Thus the entire meter, including the flow tube, is at a constant pressure of 50 psig. With an increase in downstream resistance, pressure will increase only in that portion of the circuit distal to the needle valve. As long as the pressure generated by the downstream resistance does not exceed 50 psig (in which case flow will cease), the position of the float in the tube will accurately reflect actual outlet flow. For this reason, the pressure-compensated Thorpe tube is the preferred instrument in most clinical situations.

The only factor limiting the use of the pressure-compensated Thorpe tube is gravity. With its accuracy dependent on the maintenance of an upright position, clinical applications in which this cannot be assured (for example, during certain types of patient transport) represent a relative contraindication to use. In these situations, the gravity-independent Bourdon gauge can be used as a satisfactory alternative.

In summary, Fig. 24-22 graphically portrays the effects of downstream resistance or "back pressure" on the Bourdon gauge and the pressure-compensated and pressure-uncompensated Thorpe tube type of flow-metering devices.

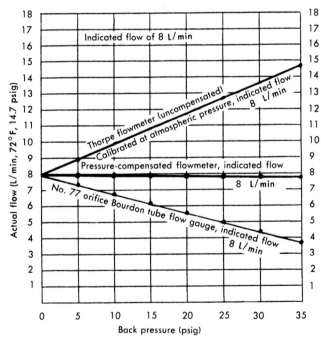

Fig. 24-22   Comparative accuracy of flow-metering devices. (From McPherson SP and Spearman, CB: Respiratory therapy equipment, ed 3, St Louis, 1985, The CV Mosby Co. Modified from Puritan-Bennett Corp, Los Angeles, Calif.)

SUMMARY

Knowledge of how medical gases are produced, stored, and distributed represents a cornerstone in the delivery of quality respiratory care. Although practitioners have assumed many more challenging duties, provision of assurances of the safe and uninterrupted supply of medical gases remains a foundation of the practitioner's role and function.

Beyond ensuring compliance with various regulatory standards, the respiratory care practitioner must assume primary responsibility for selecting and applying appropriate devices to regulate gas pressure and control gas flow. Although safety systems have been established to minimize errors in the delivery of medical gases to patients, such systems are no substitute for the careful application of clinical knowledge. Only in this manner can safety and quality be assured.

REFERENCES

1. National Fire Protection Association, Batterymarch Park, Quincy Mass: Pamphlet nos. 50, 53m, 56F, and 99C.
2. Compressed Gas Association, 1235 Jefferson Davis Highway, Arlington, Va: Pamphlet P-2, Characteristics and safe handling of medical gases.
3. Bancroft ML and Steen JA: Health device legislation: an overview of the law and its impact on respiratory care, Respir Care 23:1179, 1978.
4. Dorsch JA and Dorsch SE: Understanding anesthesia equipment: construction, care, and complications, Baltimore, 1975, Williams & Wilkins Co.
5. McPherson SP: Respiratory therapy equipment, ed 3, St Louis, 1985, The CV Mosby Co.
6. Webb JM: Manufacture, storage, and transport of medical gases. In Burton GG and Hodgkin JE, editors: Respiratory care: a guide to clinical practice, ed 2, Philadelphia, 1984, JB Lippincott Co.
7. Compressed Gas Association, 1235 Jefferson Davis Highway, Arlington, Va: Handbook of compressed gas, ed 2.
8. Compressed Gas Association, 1235 Jefferson Davis Highway, Arlington, Va: Pamphlet P 2.6.
9. Compressed Gas Association, 1235 Jefferson Davis Highway, Arlington, Va: Pamphlet V-5, Diameter Index Safety System.
10. Scott Aviation Products: Aviox Instruction Manual, Lancaster, NY, 1980, A-T-O Corp.
11. Puritan Bennett Corporation: Companion Liquid Oxygen System Training Manual, Lanexa, Kan, Puritan Bennett Corp.
12. Bancroft ML, duMoulin GG, and Headley-Whyte: Hazards of bulk oxygen systems, Anesthesiology 52:504, 1980.
13. Grant WJ: Medical gases: their properties and uses, Chicago, 1978, Year Book Medical Publishers.
14. Ward JJ: Equipment for mixed gas an oxygen therapy. In Barnes TA, editor: Respiratory care practice, Chicago, 1988, Year Book Medical Publishers.

25

Medical Gas Therapy

F. Robert Thalken

The administration of therapeutic gases is the most common mode of respiratory care in both the acute and long-term care settings. Indeed, the early development of respiratory care as a specialized field of health care delivery was closely associated with the introduction of medical gas therapy—in particular oxygen—as a legitimate treatment modality.

Since that time, significant changes have occurred in both our understanding of the physiologic effects of the various therapeutic gases and the technology employed to deliver them. Of particular importance is the growing acceptance of the premise that therapeutic gases must be treated as is any pharmacologic agent. Dosages must be chosen, responses monitored, and changes made according to predetermined therapeutic goals.

Within this context, the respiratory care practitioner must possess more than just technical knowledge of equipment capabilities and operation. In consultation with the physician, the skilled clinician should be able to determine the desired goals of gas therapy, select the appropriate mode of administration, monitor the patient's response to the prescribed regimen, and recommend changes in the approach taken according to individual patient need.

OBJECTIVES

A comprehensive knowledge of therapeutic gas administration, including applicable indications, hazards, methods of delivery, and techniques of assessment, is required before the respiratory care practitioner can apply these skills in clinical practice. This chapter provides an in-depth analysis of medical gas therapy, emphasizing the role of the respiratory care practitioner in selecting, evaluating, and adjusting therapy according to desired patient outcomes. Specifically, after completing this chapter, the reader should be able to:

1. Define the general goals, objectives, and guiding principles in the administration of therapeutic gases;
2. Cite the major hazards associated with therapeutic gas administration, emphasizing the physiologic and morphologic effects of high inspired partial pressures of oxygen;
3. Differentiate the principles underlying low-flow, reservoir, and high-flow gas delivery systems;
4. Describe the design characteristics, operating principles, clinical capabilities, and limitations of current gas therapy modalities;
5. Given relevant clinical data, select the appropriate initial mode of gas therapy and make recommendations regarding changes in the therapeutic regimen according to patient need;
6. Describe the theory of operation, advantages, disadvantages, appropriate clinical use, and limitations of current oxygen analysis systems.

KEY TERMS

Most terms used in this chapter are defined in context. The following terms are introduced without explicit definition but may be found in the text glossary:

actinomycoses	metaphase
actuator	mitochondria
aerobic	mitosis
ambient	obliterate
anode	obtunded
aspiration	ocular
cathode	orifice
chronic obstructive pulmonary disease (COPD)	pallor
	parenteral
debilitating	patency
enzyme	polyps
exacerbate	radionecrosis
extrapolation	retina
exudate	rheostat
flaccid	sclerosis
galvanometer	thrombosis
hyperpnea	titrate
infiltrate	untoward
inspissated	

OXYGEN THERAPY

As the basic "fuel" for all aerobic life, oxygen is the most widely used—and abused—therapeutic gas. Although less common today than in the past, the clinical abuse of oxygen is based mainly on a lack of clarity regarding its capabilities and hazards. As the primary member of the health care team responsible for its rational use, the respiratory care practitioner must be well versed in both the goals and objectives of oxygen therapy and its hazards and limitations.

Goals

The general goal of administering supplemental oxygen is to maintain adequate tissue oxygenation with a minimum amount of energy expenditure by the cardiopulmonary system. Specifically, the clinical objectives for administration of supplemental oxygen are to prevent or correct arterial hypoxemia and tissue hypoxia and to prevent or minimize the increased cardiopulmonary workload associated with compensatory responses to hypoxemia and hypoxia.

Correction of arterial hypoxemia. Simple oxygen therapy can be used to correct hypoxemia caused by hypoventilation, diffusion defects, or moderate ventilation-perfusion ($\dot{V}/\dot{Q}$) imbalances. The hypoxemia caused by a physiologic shunt is generally less responsive to supplemental oxygen therapy. With shunt fractions of 25% or less, and otherwise normal physiologic conditions, moderate to high concentration of oxygen may maintain the Pao_2 above 60 mm Hg. When the shunt fraction rises above 25%, supplemental oxygen administration alone is generally not sufficient to maintain adequate arterial oxygenation.[1] In these situations, special modes of airway pressure therapy, such as positive end-expiratory pressure (PEEP) or continuous positive airway pressure (CPAP), are indicated (see Section VII).

Minimizing cardiopulmonary workload. The compensatory response of the cardiopulmonary system to hypoxemia involves both increased ventilation and cardiac output. The resultant increase in physiologic work associated with hypoxemia can be alleviated by oxygen therapy.

For example, in some patients, acceptable arterial oxygenation breathing room air may be achieved only by a significant increase in alveolar ventilation and thus the work of breathing. When supplemental oxygen is given in appropriate amounts, this high ventilatory demand—and its accompanying high work of breathing—can be reduced.

On the other hand, patients with arterial hypoxemia can maintain normal or near normal oxygen delivery to the tissues only by increasing their cardiac output. If oxygen therapy can adequately relieve the hypoxemia, the workload on the circulatory system can be reduced. Such use is particularly important when the heart is already stressed by disease, as in myocardial infarction, or as a result of cardiac surgery.

Guiding principles

Because oxygen has both beneficial and detrimental effects, it should be treated as a drug. As such, the minimum amount or dose required to obtain the appropriate response should be used. Depending on the device or system employed, oxygen is generally ordered either in liters per minute or as a concentration of oxygen.[2-5] When a concentration is prescribed, it may be either as a percentage, such as 24%, or as a fractional concentration (Fio_2), such as 0.24.

Once the desired amount of oxygen is being administered, the patient's response should be assessed. Depending on the therapeutic objectives, assessment may include observation, inspection, and analysis of arterial and mixed venous blood gases (see Section V). If the response indicates that the clinical objectives are not being met, then the amount of oxygen being administered should be adjusted and the patient reevaluated. This dose-response approach should provide the least amount of oxygen necessary to obtain the desired therapeutic objective, thereby minimizing the likelihood of oxygen's detrimental effects.

Detrimental effects

Ironically, oxygen is both vital for and potentially threatening to life. The detrimental effects of oxygen include alterations in both structure and function and are largely determined by a combination of two key factors: the inspired partial pressure and the length of exposure. Among the most important detrimental effects of supplemental oxygen administration are oxygen-induced hypoventilation, absorption atelectasis, oxygen toxicity, and retrolental fibroplasia.

Oxygen-induced hypoventilation. In our prior discussion of ventilatory control mechanisms and the role of the peripheral chemoreceptors, we made brief reference to oxygen-induced hypoventilation.

The effect of oxygen administration on ventilation is well documented in the literature.[6] When a healthy subject breathes 100% oxygen, the peripheral chemoreceptors remain essentially inactive. However, because of the increased oxygen in the blood, there is less reduced hemoglobin available for carbon dioxide transportation, and $Paco_2$ tends to rise slightly. This increased $Paco_2$ stimulates the medullary respiratory center and typically produces a 5% to 20% increase in ventilation. On the other hand, in the presence of moderate hypoxemia, the peripheral chemoreceptors are stimulated. The resultant augmentation of ventilation also results in a mild hypocapnia, although for obviously different reasons.

In contrast, when hypoxemia exists with chronic hypercapnia, the central response to carbon dioxide is blunted and the primary stimulus to breathing is mediated through

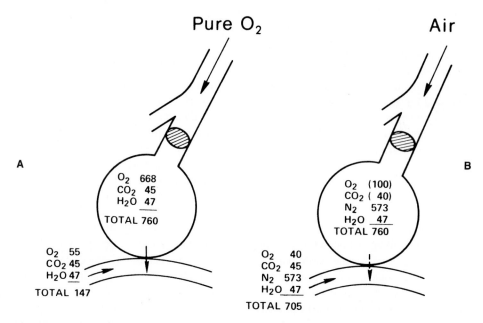

Fig. 25-1 Reasons for atelectasis of alveoli beyond blocked airways when oxygen is breathed, **A,** and when air is breathed, **B.** Note that in both cases, the sum of the gas partial pressures in the mixed venous blood is less than in the alveoli. In **B,** the P_{O_2} and P_{CO_2} are shown in parentheses because these values change with time. However, the total alveolar pressure remains within a few mm Hg of 760. (From West JB: Respiratory physiology: the essentials, ed 3, Baltimore, 1985, Williams & Wilkins.)

hypoxemic stimulation of the peripheral chemoreceptors. In this situation, oxygen administration can suppress the peripheral chemoreceptors. Patients with chronic hypercapnea tested for their response to concentrations of oxygen in the 90% to 100% range tend to hypoventilate. Because the respiratory center in these patients is unresponsive to the elevation in P_{CO_2}, the expected compensatory response does not occur. Although the patient with chronic hypercapnea and its associated hypoxemia presents the greatest hypoventilation risk, patients whose respiratory center has been depressed by sedatives or narcotics are also subject to oxygen-induced hypoventilation. In general, the risk of oxygen-induced hypoventilation increases when Pa_{CO_2} has remained at or above 50 mm Hg long enough for a compensatory acid-base response (see Chapter 10).

This detrimental effect of oxygen should never prevent its use when indicated. The prevention of hypoxia is always the most critical therapeutic need. As a guide for the use of oxygen in patients with chronic hypercapnea, the therapeutic objective should be to maintain Pa_{O_2} between 50 and 60 mm Hg. Generally, this will maintain adequate tissue oxygenation while minimizing the likelihood of inducing hypoventilation.[6-10] Moreover, this level of oxygen will prevent rapid deterioration of the patient until the effect of higher blood oxygen levels can be assessed.[10]

In clinical practice, we usually assume that oxygen can be safely administered to patients with chronic hypercapnea at controlled low concentrations. A 24% to 28% oxy-

gen concentration carries little risk and can be delivered accurately by a variety of methods. The Pa_{CO_2} may rise slightly but, after perhaps 1 hour, will usually plateau at a level still within the bounds of safety.

In these patients, the importance of continuous therapy cannot be overemphasized. If oxygen therapy is stopped, even for short periods such as for meals, the Pa_{O_2} may fall rapidly below pretreatment levels.[7] To ensure adequate oxygenation for these patients, oxygen should be given continuously until the pathophysiologic process that caused the need for oxygen therapy has been alleviated.[8]

Absorption atelectasis. Normally, nitrogen constitutes the majority of the mixed gases in both the alveoli and blood. Breathing pure oxygen depletes both alveolar and blood nitrogen within several minutes. Removal of nitrogen from the blood greatly lowers the total pressure of gases in the venous system. This creates a large pressure gradient for diffusion of gases between the venous blood and any body cavity with total gas pressures at or near atmospheric. Indeed, this concept of nitrogen "washout" was applied in the past to relieve postoperative intestinal distention.

In the lung, the large pressure gradient established between the pulmonary capillary blood and alveoli by breathing 100% oxygen is of no major consequence unless the respiratory zone becomes obstructed. Under these circumstances, as depicted in Fig. 25-1, *A,* a large gradient for oxygen diffusion is established. With no source for repletion, the oxygen will rapidly diffuse into the blood, lower-

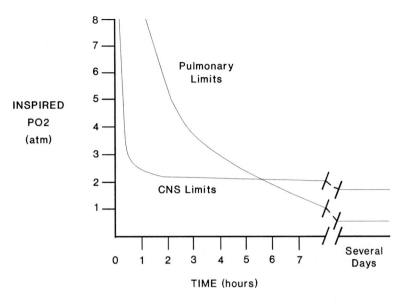

Fig. 25-2   Relationship between P_{O_2} and exposure time responsible for oxygen toxicity. (From Lambertsen CJ: In DiPalma JR, editor: Drill's pharmacology in medicine, New York, 1971, McGraw-Hill. Used by permission of McGraw-Hill.)

ing the total pressure in the alveolus until it collapses. Because collapsed alveoli are perfused but not ventilated, absorption atelectasis will increase the physiologic shunt fraction.[11] Moreover, because surface tension forces make it particularly difficult to reopen collapsed alveoli, special modes of ventilatory support such as CPAP may be needed to restore normal $\dot{V}/\dot{Q}$ relationships in the affected areas (see Chapters 28 and 29).

The risk of absorption atelectasis is compounded when patients breathe at a minimal tidal volume (V_T) as a result of sedation, surgical pain, or central nervous system (CNS) dysfunction. Also, alveoli that are partially obstructed, or those with poor ventilation as a result of a dependent location, may become unstable when the oxygen in the alveoli diffuses into the pulmonary circulation faster than it can be replaced.[11] This can result in a more gradual shrinking of the alveoli and may lead to complete collapse, even when the patient is not breathing supplemental oxygen (Fig. 25-1, *B*). In the alert patient this is not as great a risk, since the natural "sigh" mechanism periodically hyperinflates the lung, ventilating those alveoli that may be considered sluggish in their tidal exchange.

Oxygen toxicity. The classic description of pulmonary oxygen toxicity was written by Lorrain Smith in 1897. He accurately describes the typical congestion, inflammation, and edema that we have come to recognize as the pathologic manifestation of long-term exposure to a high P_{O_2}. As a modern clinical entity, oxygen toxicity represents both an untoward consequence of our advanced technologic abilities and a limiting factor in the treatment of hypoxemia and tissue hypoxia.

Oxygen toxicity is a complex syndrome involving many organ systems. Primary involvement includes the CNS and the lungs. Although the tolerance of these two organ sys-

tems differs, the observance of detrimental effects is related directly to the magnitude of the P_{O_2} and the cumulative time of exposure (Fig. 25-2). CNS manifestations become most apparent when the person is breathing oxygen at hyperbaric pressures and include tremors, twitching, and convulsions (discussed later in this chapter). Of primary importance to the respiratory care practitioner are the pulmonary effects of long-term exposure to a high P_{O_2}.

It is generally accepted that 100% oxygen breathed continuously for more than 24 hours can result in pulmonary damage. Healthy dogs die after about 70 hours exposure to 100% oxygen at ambient pressure.[12] Guinea pigs develop pulmonary edema within 48 hours of exposure to 100% oxygen.[13] A healthy man shows a significant drop in diffusing capacity within hours of breathing 100% oxygen, accompanied by a progressive fall in vital capacity (VC) after 24 to 60 hours.[14]

Breathing oxygen at pressures above atmospheric pressure greatly accelerated the development of oxygen toxicity symptoms.[15-17] Twelve hours of exposure to 100% oxygen in a hyperbaric chamber at 2 atm pressure results in complaints of a cough, substernal chest tightness and burning, and dyspnea, accompanied by decreases in VC, residual volume (RV), and lung compliance (C_L).[18]

Clinical picture. The clinical picture of prolonged exposure to high inspired P_{O_2} is like that of a diffuse bronchopneumonia.[19] On chest x-ray film, patchy infiltrates, usually most prominent in the lower lung fields, are observed. Pathologic examination reveals alveolar wall edema and an intra-alveolar exudate of large cells. Unlike bacterial pneumonia, however, polymorphonuclear leukocytes usually are not prominent, and bacteria are few.

As with any pneumonia, the alveolar exudate and consolidation occurring with oxygen toxicity creates areas with low $\dot{V}/\dot{Q}$ ratios and physiologic shunting. A vicious cycle is established whereby attempts to alleviate the hypoxemia by increasing supplemental oxygen only worsen the toxic effects. However, if patient survival can be maintained while inspired oxygen concentrations are lowered, the pulmonary lesion may resolve.

Exactly how much oxygen is too much is still the subject of debate. In their review of the literature on oxygen toxicity, Winter and Smith suggested that no significant damage occurs to the human lung at F_{IO_2} levels up to 0.50 for extended periods.[18] Contrary to this observation is the report of patients receiving low-flow oxygen therapy at home for 7 to 61 months whose lungs at autopsy showed evidence of oxygen toxicity.[20] However, this study concluded that the pulmonary changes exhibited in these patients did not contribute to an accelerated mortality. The long-term exposure of US astronauts to 100% oxygen at $\frac{1}{3}$ atmospheric pressure without any deleterious effects suggests that a safe upper limit may be in the range of 250 to 280 mm Hg.[13,14]

Biochemical basis. It is believed that oxygen toxicity is mediated through the actions of chemical units known as free radicals. These are extremely reactive atoms or molecules that carry at least one unpaired electron. They exist in the free form only momentarily, quickly combining with other atoms. The hydroxyl, perhydroxyl, and superoxide free radicals all are implicated in oxygen toxicity, with superoxide being the best understood.

In its normal molecular form, oxygen is essentially inactive. However, as oxygen participates in cellular biochemical actions, it takes on electrons and is reduced, while its electron donors are oxidized. This intracellular reduction of oxygen is responsible for producing the superoxide radical. As metabolic reactions continue, superoxide is converted to perhydroxyl, and this in turn reacts with additional superoxide to produce the powerful hydroxyl radical. Finally, this hydroxyl radical is stabilized by combining with a hydrogen atom, producing water. Superoxide is thus an intermediate (as opposed to final) product of oxygen reduction.

Free radicals such as superoxide have been directly implicated in the inhibition of tissue growth and the inactivation of essential cellular enzymes. It is known that 100% oxygen at 1 atm pressure can inhibit growth of living tissue cultures, apparently by interfering with the synthesis of DNA and RNA. It is now believed that free radicals are responsible for this action, possibly by blocking the metaphase stage of cellular mitotic reproduction.

Free radicals are also able to inactivate some enzyme systems that regulate cellular metabolism. Especially vulnerable are those enzymes whose functions depend on sulfhydryl (SH) groups. Mitochondrial activity is highly dependent on sulfhydryl enzymes, which are easily blocked by the products of oxygen reduction.[21] This evidence suggests that one of the major sites of injury caused by oxygen is the mitochondria.

Tolerance. Oxygen-free radicals are normally produced by cellular elements of the lung and detoxified rapidly by superoxide dismutase (SOD). Other naturally occurring detoxifying agents include catalase, glutathione peroxidase, lipid membrane constituent, vitamin E, ascorbate, glutathione, cysteine, and cysteamine. However, SOD attracts the most interest.[22-26]

By definition, a dismutase is an enzyme able to effect simultaneous oxidation-reduction. SOD specifically catalyzes the transformation of superoxide into hydrogen peroxide and molecular oxygen. Hydrogen peroxide, in turn, is metabolized into two harmless by-products, water and molecular oxygen.

The role of SOD in protecting the lung from the effects of high P_{O_2} has been demonstrated in animal models. Most experimental rats exposed to 100% oxygen die within 72 hours. However, if they are first exposed to 85% oxygen for a week, they can then survive 100% oxygen for an extended period. This phenomenon is called *oxygen tolerance.* While it is developing, lung content of SOD increases by about 50%. Apparently SOD production is stimulated by inhalation of moderately elevated oxygen concentrations, and the body subsequently can tolerate a higher P_{O_2} than it could before exposure.

It has been established that while experimental oxygen tolerance is developing and pulmonary SOD levels are rising, alveolar type II pneumocytes increase by up to 300%. This tremendous proliferation of alveolar cells is obviously related to the increasing levels of SOD. It probably represents a high initial dismutase cell content or stimulation of increased SOD production by the granular pneumocytes. Thus, it seems that type II alveolar cells are an important source of superoxide dismutase and may represent the primary defense mechanism of the lung against oxygen toxicity.

Pathologic changes in the alveolar region. The first observable effect of high P_{O_2} on the lung is damage to the capillary endothelium, followed by a thickening of the alveolar-capillary membrane resulting from edema. As previously indicated, the type II alveolar cells begin proliferating at an early stage, but the type I cells may actually decrease in number or be destroyed.[27] Destruction of basement membranes and an exudative phase follows. Capillary beds swell and in some cases may become obliterated.[18] Hyaline membranes and fibrosis are final results of this process.[18] The most useful index for following these changes is the VC, which becomes progressively reduced as the damage progresses.[17] These changes eventually manifest themselves in the clinical picture previously described, that is, a diffuse bronchopneumonia-like syndrome with edema, congestion, atelectasis, and hemorrhage.

Other detrimental effects. Feline experiments have shown that the rate of upward movement of minute particles deposited on the distal tracheal mucosa is markedly slowed in the presence of 100% oxygen.[28] If this action of oxygen in animals can be extrapolated to the human airway, serious clinical implications become obvious. It is also of interest that exposure to low concentrations of oxygen also slows mucus transport time.

Of potential clinical importance is the fact that the retarding action of high oxygen tensions on ciliary function can be prevented or reversed by parenteral or aerosol administration of epinephrine, isoproterenol, and adenosine triphosphate.

Further animal experiments have established that prolonged exposure to high Po_2 can interfere with the production of pulmonary surfactant.[21] The primary mechanism appears to be disruption or inactivation of the methyltransference pathway for lecithin synthesis.

Factors affecting response. The susceptibility of patients to the detrimental effects of high Po_2 varies considerably. Other than the duration and magnitude of prior exposure, several factors are known to alter the development of oxygen toxicity. The box below summarizes the major factors currently known to hasten or impede the development of the pathologic changes characterizing the lung's response to high Po_2.[27] Although the exact mechanisms by which these factors alter the lung's response to high Po_2 are not fully known, alterations in cellular immune responses and free radical production and detoxification are implicated.

Retrolental fibroplasia. The term retrolental means "behind the lens," and retrolental fibroplasia (RLF) refers to an ocular condition of premature infants associated with oxygen administration. The disease was established as a specific entity in the 1950s, when it was observed that some premature infants given oxygen developed damage to the eyes severe enough to produce permanent blindness. The pathologic condition is basically a fibrotic process behind the ocular lenses, which impairs light penetration to the retina. Excessive blood oxygen levels produce retinal vasoconstriction, and if this is severe enough to persist after oxygen therapy ceases, permanent damage is likely.[29-32] This risk poses a serious management problem, since the premature infant often requires supplementary oxygen. The American Academy of Pediatrics has recommended maintaining Pao_2 between 50 and 70 mm Hg to minimize the risk of RLF in premature infants.[33]

Note that oxygen-induced eye damage may not be limited to neonates. Near-total blindness was reported in a 32-year-old man following prolonged exposure to supplemental oxygen that produced a Pao_2 between 250 and 300 mm Hg.[34] The apparent cause of visual loss in this case was retinal arterial constriction.

Guidelines to avoid unnecessary risk. We can summarize our discussion on the dangers of oxygen by emphasizing that when oxygen is needed, it must be given, even though we recognize its potential risk. Because reactions to high oxygen tensions cannot be predicted with any degree of precision, patients may suffer toxic effects. Failure to supply needed oxygen, however, will surely cause irreversible tissue damage or death.

Nevertheless, oxygen, like any potent medicine, should be used with reason and according to indications. If high concentrations of oxygen are necessary, the duration of administration should be kept to a minimum and reduced as soon as possible. In general, the objective of therapy is to administer oxygen sufficient to maintain Pao_2 between 60 and 100 mm Hg. The exceptions are those circumstances in which oxygen delivery to the pulmonary blood is normal but the oxygen-carrying capacity of the hemoglobin is impaired. Anemia and carbon monoxide inhalation are two common clinical conditions needing high blood-gas ten-

---

FACTORS AFFECTING OXYGEN TOXICITY

HASTENED ONSET OR INCREASED SEVERITY	DELAYED ONSET OR DECREASED SEVERITY
Adrenocortical hormones	Acclimatization to hypoxia
Adrenocorticotropic hormone	Adrenergic blocking drugs
Carbon dioxide inhalation	Anesthesia
Convulsions	Antioxidants
Dexamethasone	Chlorpromazine
Destroamphetamine	Gamma-aminobutyric acid
Disulfiram (ATA base)	Ganglionic blocking drugs
Epinephrine	Glutathione
Hyperthermia	Hypothermia
Insulin	Hypothyroidism
Norepinephrine	Immaturity
Paraquat	Intermittent exposure
Thyroid hormones	Reserpine
Vitamin E deficiency	Starvation
X-irradiation	Tris (hydroxymethyl)aminomethane
	Vitamin E

sions to increase dissolved plasma oxygen, compensating for the deficient hemoglobin transport. Frequent arterial blood monitoring is a mandatory safety measure when concentrations above 50% are used.

Oxygen delivery systems

Historically, oxygen delivery systems have evolved sporadically according to both available technology and our changing understanding of physiologic needs. Devices such as the nasal catheter have remained basically unchanged over time, whereas various masks, tents, and whole oxygen rooms have come and gone or have been refined and developed to better meet specific clinical objectives.[35]

Today, the respiratory care practitioner is confronted with a wide array of modalities for the administration of oxygen and other therapeutic gases. Given the practitioner's role in the initial selection of the appropriate therapeutic modality, it is essential that he or she understand the capabilities and limitations of these various devices and be skilled in using them under a variety of clinical conditions.[36]

General performance characteristics. Selection of an oxygen delivery system should be based on matching its performance characteristics to both the clinical objectives of the therapy and the patient's needs.[37] System performance is judged according to two critical factors: (1) the delivered F_{IO_2} and (2) the stability of this F_{IO_2} under varying patient demands. An ideal oxygen system would be capable of delivering any desired F_{IO_2} under all clinical conditions. Generally, this ideal is achieved only with expensive and complex positive-pressure breathing devices and requires establishing an artificial airway. Although falling short of ideal, simpler and less costly methods of oxygen administration are generally satisfactory under all but the most demanding situations.

The F_{IO_2} an oxygen system provides, and whether the provided F_{IO_2} remains stable under varying patient demand, depends primarily on the amount of oxygen available to the patient during inspiration. As long as the device provides all the inspired gas needed by the patient during inspiration, a stable F_{IO_2} is ensured. This inspiratory need can be met either by providing a volume of therapeutic gas equal to the inspired volume or by matching the patient's inspiratory flow with an equivalent flow of the prescribed mixture. Devices that can supply all a patient's inspired gas needs at a given F_{IO_2} are often called *fixed-performance oxygen delivery systems.*[38,39]

On the other hand, should the patient's inspiratory volume or flow needs not be met fully, the therapeutic gas will be mixed with ambient air and its F_{IO_2} diluted proportionately. Moreover, under these circumstances, the F_{IO_2} provided will be unstable, varying according to the patient's ventilatory demands. Devices not capable of meeting all the patient's inspiratory volume or flow needs,

thereby delivering an F_{IO_2} that varies with ventilatory demand, are referred to as *variable-performance oxygen delivery systems.*[38,39]

Categories of oxygen delivery systems. Based on these fundamental considerations, we may categorize oxygen delivery devices into three general groups: (1) low-flow systems, (2) reservoir systems, and (3) high-flow systems.[37-39] Because of their limited application and unique characteristics, a fourth category of oxygen delivery systems, termed enclosures, will be discussed separately.

Low-flow systems provide supplemental oxygen directly to the airway at flows ranging from 0 to 15 L/min. Since the average inspiratory flow rate of an individual with a normal minute ventilation ($\dot{V}_E$) exceeds the high end of this range, the 100% oxygen provided by the low-flow device will be diluted with ambient air. How much dilution occurs is directly proportional to the difference between the flow of oxygen provided by the device and the patient's inspiratory flow rate. All low-flow systems are of the variable performance type.

Reservoir systems generally provide comparable flow rates of oxygen but include a volume reservoir in which the therapeutic gas accumulates during patient expiration. When the patient's inspiratory flow rate exceeds that provided by oxygen inflow to the device, the reservoir volume is tapped. A reservoir device can be characterized as a fixed-performance system only if (1) the volume in the reservoir is sufficient to meet all inspired volume demand and (2) no ambient air can enter the system during inspiration. If these conditions are not met, reservoir system performance will be variable.

High-flow systems are devices that supply a given F_{IO_2} at a flow rate that equals or exceeds that generated by the patient during inspiration, there by ensuring a stable F_{IO_2}. To accommodate variations in patients' inspiratory demands, a high-flow device should provide at least 50-60 L/min total flow; under some conditions 100 L/min or more may be required. Nonetheless, as long as the total flow meets or exceeds that of the patient during inspiration, a high-flow device can be categorized as a fixed-performance system.

To enhance performance, combinations of the above device types may be employed. Both high- and low-flow systems may incorporate reservoirs to enhance or stabilize the delivered F_{IO_2}. Likewise, the flow into a reservoir system may be increased to ensure that the "reserve" volume is not depleted during inspiration.

Low flow systems. Among the most common low-flow devices currently employed in respiratory care are the nasal cannula and nasal catheter. More recently, low-flow oxygen-conserving devices have been developed to minimize oxygen waste in long-term therapy, especially in the home (see Chapter 34).

Nasal cannula. The nasal cannula (Fig. 25-3) is a plastic appliance (formerly made of metal) consisting of two

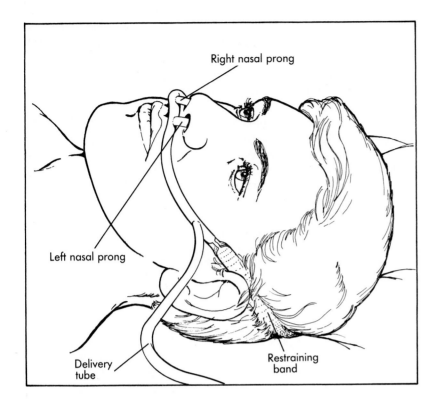

Right nasal prong

Left nasal prong

Delivery tube

Restraining band

Fig. 25-3 Nasal cannula.

tips about ½-inch long arising from an oxygen supply tube that is attached to a pressure-compensated flowmeter and a simple bubble or diffusion humidifier. It is inserted into the vestibule of the nose. The cannula has the advantages of ease of application, lightness of weight, economy, and disposability. It has the disadvantage of instability, being easily dislodged from a restless or unobserved patient. It is also necessary to pay attention to the patient's comfort when instituting treatment, since excessive flows can produce considerable pain in the frontal sinuses. Finally, such nasal conditions as a deviated septum, mucosal edema, excessive mucus drainage, and polyps may interfere with adequate oxygen delivery.

Nasal catheter. The nasal catheter is so named because it is placed through the nasal passage with its tip in the oropharynx (Fig. 25-4). Its function is nearly identical to the nasal cannula. Made of nontoxic plastic, the catheter has several holes at its end. Success in catheter therapy depends on its proper insertion and maintenance, techniques with which every respiratory care practitioner should be familiar.

Before introduction, the distal third to half of the catheter is lubricated. Although use of a water-soluble lubricant precludes ingestion or aspiration of oil-based products, subsequent removal of the catheter may be facilitated by the judicious application of small amounts of petroleum jelly. A low flow of oxygen is started to ensure patency of the tube and is continued during the insertion. The catheter is gently slid along the floor of either naris into the

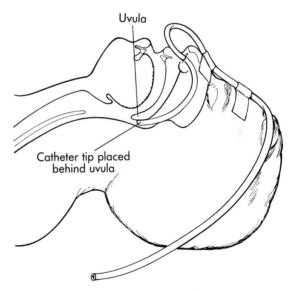

Uvula

Catheter tip placed behind uvula

Fig. 25-4 Placement of nasal catheter in nasopharynx.

oropharynx until direct visualization (with tongue depressor) confirms placement of its tip just below the uvula. It is then retracted about ½ inch or until just out of sight and is fastened to the bridge of the nose with adhesive tape.

If direct visualization is not possible, a "blind" procedure can be used. The catheter can be placed on the side of the patient's face and the distance from tip of the nose to the ear lobe measured. This length of the catheter is then inserted through the nose into the pharynx.

Under no circumstances must force be used to advance the catheter through the nose; if significant resistance is encountered, the opposite naris should be used. The same nasal disorders affecting the use of the nasal cannula (previously described) may block passage of the catheter, and attempts to force it through will only produce mucosal damage and worsen the condition. For patients who cannot tolerate a nasal catheter, the practitioner should recommend an alternative approach.

Although made of nontoxic materials, catheters do increase the production of nasal secretions. Inspissated secretions can cause the catheter to adhere to the nasal mucosa. Frequent changing and the use of small quantities of oil-based lubricants can minimize this problem. Catheters should be removed and fresh ones inserted in the opposite naris at least every 8 hours. Generally, a well-placed catheter is not uncomfortable and allows some mobility for the patient. Most current usage is limited to short-term therapy (less than 1 hour), as might be needed during bronchoscopy or in the recovery room.

Some controversy exists regarding the relative performance characteristics of the nasal cannula and catheter. Compared with the cannula, many assume that the nasal catheter provides a slightly higher F_{IO_2} for a given flow. The reason given to support this assumption is that the catheter, because of its placement, should make more effective use of the upper airway as an "anatomic" reservoir. It has also been suggested that for the mouth-breathing patient a catheter is preferable to a cannula.

Some studies have shown that the eventual delivery of oxygen to the blood does not significantly differ among these devices, nor according to the route of breathing.[40-42] Other studies show tracheal concentration differences under similar conditions.[43] Lacking firm evidence of differences in performance between these devices, the decision on which is best in a given circumstance should be based mainly on consideration of patient comfort and tolerance. Clearly, the cannula should be considered first choice for the cooperative and alert patient who can be depended on to keep the appliance in its proper position.

Oxygen-conserving devices. Oxygen-conserving devices are low-flow delivery systems modified to reduce the waste of oxygen that typically occurs during the expiratory phase of breathing.[44] Because they can lower the cost of oxygen delivery, such devices are finding widespread application in the home care setting. For this reason, details on their principles of operation, performance characteristics, and advantages and disadvantages are covered in the chapter on respiratory home care (see Chapter 34).

Estimating the F_{IO_2} of low-flow devices. Precise measurements of the F_{IO_2} delivered by low-flow oxygen delivery systems are neither practical nor necessary in the clinical setting. Indeed, it is the patient's response to the therapy, as assessed by astute observation and laboratory measurements, that ultimately determines the adequacy of the device's performance. Nonetheless, estimation of the F_{IO_2} being delivered to the patient is useful, particularly when initiating therapy or assessing the underlying cause of the hypoxemia (see Chapter 15).

The oxygen enrichment of inhaled air provided by low-flow delivery systems depends on the balance between the patient's ventilatory need and the oxygen supply during inhalation. The deeper the tidal volume or the greater the inspiratory flow of the patient, the more the oxygen will be diluted by supplementary air. Conversely, the more oxygen supplied during inhalation, the greater will be its alveolar concentration as less room air is inspired.

Clearly, the final fraction or concentration of inspired oxygen must represent a proportionate mixture of the pure oxygen supplied by the device and that provided in the diluting air. This relationship can be represented by a simple estimating equation:

$$F_{IO_2} \text{ (estimated)} \cong \frac{O_2 + 0.21 (\dot{V}_{insp} - O_2)}{(\dot{V}_{insp})}$$

O_2 represents the flow in liters per minute of 100% oxygen provided by the device. The $\dot{V}_{insp}$ is the patient's average inspiratory flow rate. To estimate the average inspiratory flow, simply multiply the patient's $\dot{V}_E$ by the sum of the I:E ratio parts (I:E ratio being observed or estimated).[45] As an example:

> V_T = 600 ml
> Respiratory rate = 15
> $\dot{V}_E$ = 15 × 600 ml = 9.0 L/min
> Observed I:E ratio = 1:2
> Sum of I:E parts 1 + 2 = 3
> Estimated average inspiratory flow:
>   3 × 9.0 L/min = 27 L/min

Returning to the F_{IO_2} estimation equation, assume that a 2 L/min flow is being provided by a nasal cannula to a patient with the above ventilatory parameters. Using these values, the estimated F_{IO_2} would be calculated as follows:

$$F_{IO_2} \text{ (estimated)} \cong \frac{2 \text{ L/min} + .21(27 \text{ L/min} - 2 \text{ L/min})}{(27 \text{ L/min})}$$

$$\cong 7.25/27$$

$$\cong 0.27$$

A faster inspiratory flow, as would occur with an I:E ratio of 1:3, would decrease F_{IO_2} by mixing more room air with the set flow of oxygen. This same effect would occur even with a constant I:E ratio as long as the $\dot{V}_E$ increased. A proportionately higher F_{IO_2} will occur when the inspiratory flow or $\dot{V}_E$ decreases.

Confounding this relationship is the contribution of the "anatomic" reservoir to the performance of low-flow delivery systems.[37] Portions of the upper airway (and trachea with transtracheal catheters) will collect oxygen from the device during the normal pause between a given expiration and the following inspiration. In concept, this collection adds a bolus of oxygen to each breath, causing an increase in F_{IO_2}.

In practice, it is difficult to estimate the effect of the anatomic reservoir. Although it theoretically accumulates 100% oxygen (which is inspired first into the trachea), actual measurements of peak tracheal oxygen fraction with simple nasal devices have demonstrated concentrations of only 24% to 47%.[42,43] The anatomic reservoir may thus add as little as 1% or as much as 20% to the inspired oxygen concentration, depending on the pattern of breathing and oxygen flow rates.

As a rule of thumb, the practitioner may estimate that each liter per minute flow provided through a standard nasal low-flow device increases the inspired oxygen concentration by approximately 3% to 4%. Because flows through standard nasal devices greater than 6 to 8 L/min are generally uncomfortable for most patients, neither the nasal cannula or catheter should be considered when the desired concentration of inspired oxygen exceeds 40% to 45%.[40] Higher concentrations require the use of a reservoir system.

Reservoir systems. Compared with low-flow systems, reservoir devices generally can provide a higher F_{IO_2} for a given oxygen input. In principle, this is accomplished by extension of the anatomic reservoir. When the patient's inspiratory flow rate exceeds that provided by oxygen inflow to the device, the system's reservoir volume is tapped, providing an additional supply of oxygen.

The most common reservoir systems currently in use are facial masks. The performance characteristics of facial masks vary according to three key factors: (1) the flow into the device, (2) the volume of the reservoir, and (3) the amount of air leakage. Variations in these factors among the various mask designs determine whether the device operates as a variable- or fixed-performance system.

Before discussing these critical differences, it is important to note the common characteristic of masks. The practitioner will note variation in the use of masks among the hospitals with which he or she may have contact. In general, we can say that the oxygen mask is used when moderate to high concentrations of oxygen are needed quickly and for relatively short periods. It is the emergency equipment of choice, and some type of mask should be available wherever patients are being treated. A mask may be used for up to several hours, but other techniques are more appropriate for prolonged therapy.

To achieve maximum performance from a mask, a tight seal between the unit and the patient's face is necessary, making these devices somewhat uncomfortable. The head strap or harness necessary to hold it in place adds to the discomfort. Masks are often quite hot, since they confine heat radiating from the face about the nose and mouth. An oxygen mask can be hazardous on a patient who is prone to vomit, since it can block the flow of vomitus, potentially causing aspiration. Because of the risk of aspiration

and the possibility of airway obstruction by a flaccid tongue, a mask generally is contraindicated with unconscious patients. However, in those situations in which oxygen by mask must be delivered to unconscious patients, an oral airway should be inserted to prevent the tongue from retracting into the pharynx, and the mask should be loosely set on the face.

Despite these shortcomings, oxygen masks are among the most versatile gas administration systems. However, the effective use of masks requires a sound understanding of the principles underlying their operation. In this section, we describe the principles of operation and performance characteristics of the following three types of masks: simple, partial rebreathing, and nonrebreathing.

Simple mask. The simple mask, shown in Fig. 25-5, is a disposable nontoxic plastic unit with neither valves nor a reservoir bag. Exhaled air is vented through holes in its body. If oxygen supply is interrupted, air is drawn in

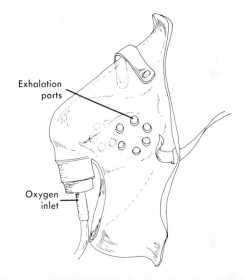

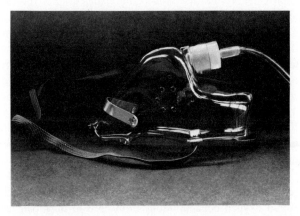

Fig. 25-5 Simple mask. Oxygen is delivered to cone-shaped face piece from which patient both inhales oxygen and draws in room air through exhalation ports. On exhalation, gas exits exhalation ports. (From McPherson SP: Respiratory therapy equipment, ed 3, St Louis, 1985, The CV Mosby Co.)

through the exhalation ports as well around the edge of the mask. A minimal flow of 5 to 6 L/min is necessary to ensure that the mask volume is replenished with oxygen at the end of exhalation. Should the flow rate be less than this amount, the mask volume will act as an extension of the patient's anatomic deadspace and cause rebreathing of expired carbon dioxide.

The F_{IO_2} delivered by a simple mask is a function of the oxygen input flow, the mask (reservoir) volume, and the patient's ventilatory characteristics.[46] Because this reservoir volume is small, and because air readily enters through the numerous vent holes during inspiration, the simple mask functions as a variable-performance delivery system. As with any variable-performance system, the exact F_{IO_2} is impossible to predict with certainty. In general, the delivered concentrations vary from 35% to 55% at gas flows of 6 to 10 L/min.[40,46] As with any oxygen delivery system, these values give no indication of the arterial oxygen levels, which vary from patient to patient.

Because of its convenience and relative comfort, the simple mask has been widely used whenever moderate oxygen concentrations have been desired for short periods. This includes the postoperative recovery state, temporary therapy while awaiting definitive plans, and interim therapy while weaning a patient from continuous oxygen administration.

Partial rebreathing mask. The partial rebreathing mask provides additional reservoir volume through a reservoir bag. The purpose of the partial rebreathing mask is to conserve oxygen by a technique that, as the name implies, permits the patient to rebreathe some exhaled air. Fig. 25-6, *A,* schematically illustrates the basic parts and function of the partial rebreathing mask. Source oxygen flows into the neck of the mask and passes directly into the mask itself during the inspiratory phase. During exhalation oxygen inflow enters the reservoir bag. As the patient exhales, approximately the first third of the exhaled air is returned to fill the reservoir bag and to mix with source oxygen. This fraction of the exhaled volume essentially represents the anatomic deadspace, which contains mostly oxygen and little carbon dioxide. As the bag fills with both source oxygen and exhaled air, rising pressure in the system directs the terminal two thirds of exhaled air (with its carbon dioxide load) out the exhalation ports. If the oxygen inflow is adjusted so that the bag does not collapse during inhalation (usually at least 5 to 6 L/min), the amount of carbon dioxide contaminating the reservoir is negligible.[47]

With a well-fitted partial rebreathing mask, adjusted so that the patient's inhalation does not deflate the bag, inspired oxygen concentrations from 35% to 60% can usually be achieved at delivered flows between 6 and 10 L/min.[41] The fact that higher F_{IO_2} levels are not observed with this system indicates that significant amounts of room air are inspired. This dilution occurs mainly through the exhalation ports, which in most disposable devices consist of simple vents in the face piece. These ports also provide a mechanism for breathing air if source oxygen becomes disconnected. For this reason, partial rebreathing masks with open exhalation ports are best characterized as variable-performance gas delivery systems.

Nonrebreathing mask. Also a mask and reservoir bag device, the name of the nonrebreathing mask indicates that there is no exhaled gas rebreathing. Fig. 25-6, *B,* shows the essential differences between the partial and nonrebreathing mask. The distinguishing features of the nonrebreathing mask are its series of one-way valves. One valve is placed between the bag and the mask. As in the partial rebreather, source oxygen flows either into the bag (during exhalation) or into the mask. The valve separating the bag and mask prevents exhaled air from returning to the bag and diverts it into the atmosphere through one or more one-way exhalation valves in the face piece. A third emergency intake valve permits room air to enter the system should source oxygen fail or the patient's needs suddenly exceed the available oxygen flow. Because a tight-fitting nonrebreathing mask with competent valving that is set at the appropriate flow rate can deliver close to 100% source gas, it approximates the characteristics of a fixed-performance delivery system. For this reason, the well-designed nonrebreather is the system of choice for short-term administration of high concentrations of oxygen as well as other premixed therapeutic gases.

In most disposable units, however, exhalation valves do not preclude air entrainment, and air leaks around the body of the mask are common. Moreover, the safety inlet in these systems is often no more than a series of open vent holes. These holes allow additional ambient air to be inhaled even when oxygen is attached, causing further dilution. Indeed, controlled laboratory studies with healthy volunteers indicate that a typical disposable nonrebreathing mask delivers oxygen concentrations in the 57% to 70% range, with an average of only 63%.[40] Common disposable nonrebreathing masks should therefore be considered variable-performance systems.

High-flow systems. Whereas reservoir devices attempt to meet inspiratory demands by providing reserve volume, high-flow systems aim to provide constant concentrations of oxygen by meeting or exceeding the patient's flow requirements during inspiration. This is accomplished either by (1) entraining air with oxygen at fixed ratios, as with air entrainment devices, or by (2) premixing high-pressure air and oxygen source gases, as with blending systems.

Regardless of approach, as long as the gas flow meets or exceeds the inspiratory flow rate generated by the patient, a constant F_{IO_2} will be provided. However, air entrainment and blending systems do differ in the range of oxygen concentrations available. By definition, entrainment devices dilute the source gas with air, thereby providing oxygen concentrations less than 100%. Moreover, because the oxygen concentrations provided by air entrainment devices

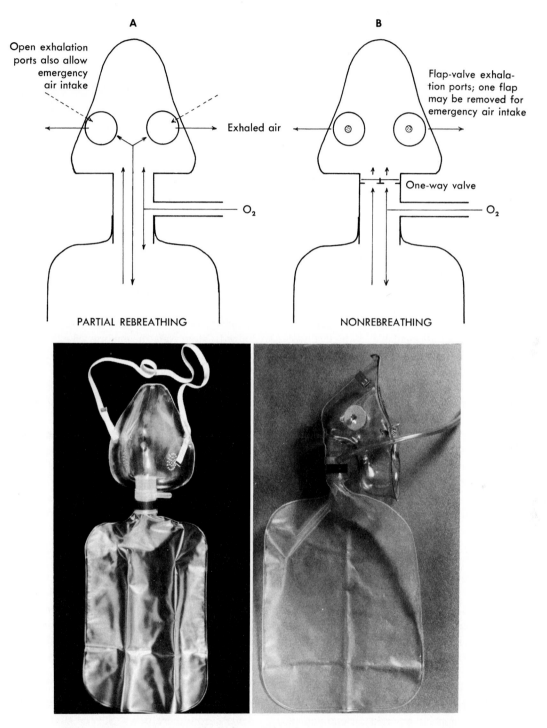

Fig. 25-6   Diagrammatic illustrations of the difference between, **A,** disposable partial rebreathing oxygen mask and, **B,** disposable nonrebreathing mask. In both, oxygen flows directly into the mask during inspiration and into the reservoir bag during exhalation. However, the early portion of exhaled air in **A** returns to the bag to be rebreathed with incoming oxygen in the next breath. Terminal air escapes through exhalation ports. In **B** all exhaled air is vented through a port in the mask, and a one-way valve between the bag and mask prevents rebreathing.

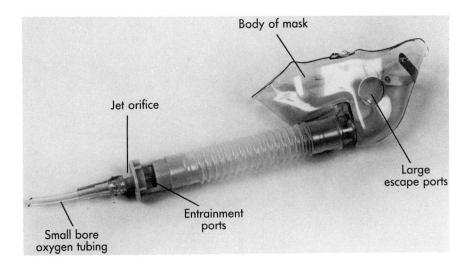

Fig. 25-7 Parts of air entrainment mask.

are inversely proportional to their total output flow, they function as true fixed-performance systems only when delivering low to moderate concentrations of oxygen. On the other hand, because blending devices premix air and oxygen at high source pressures, a full range of oxygen concentrations (21% to 100%) is available at high flows, thereby approaching our earlier definition of an "ideal" gas delivery system. Choosing the appropriate high-flow system requires matching clinical objectives with patient needs and equipment capabilities.

Air entrainment systems. Air entrainment systems are indicated when the clinical objective is to provide stable or controlled F_{IO_2} at low to moderate levels, generally between 0.24 to 0.40. The two most common systems in this category are the air entrainment mask and the "all-purpose" nebulizer. In general, masks are indicated for alert patients with normal humidification mechanisms intact. Air entrainment nebulizers, on the other hand, are employed to deliver oxygen when either the upper airway is bypassed or a humidity deficit is contributing to problems in airway clearance.

The use of an oxygen mask that provided controlled oxygen concentrations was first reported in 1941 by Barach and Eckman.[48,49] Oxygen was mixed by passing it through a jet and entraining specific amounts of room air. This device is often called a "Venturi" or "injector."[1,35] Barach's system provided relatively high concentrations of oxygen (above 40%) and controlled the amount of air mixed with oxygen by adjustable air entrainment ports or orifices. Some 20 years later, Campbell reported an entrainment mask designed to provide a low oxygen concentration with high-flow rates of air over the patient's face, calling it a Venturi or "Venti-mask."[50] Fig. 25-7 provides a diagram of a mask fashioned after Campbell's prototype.

As the name "Venti-mask" suggests, the principle of operation of these devices has often been attributed to the Venturi phenomenon, usually in combination with the Bernoulli effect. This is incorrect.[51,52] Rather than using an actual Venturi tube to entrain air, air entrainment masks

employ a restricted orifice or jet through which oxygen flows at high velocities. Air is entrained at the jet site in direct proportion to the velocity with which oxygen moves through the orifice. The smaller the orifice, the greater will be the velocity of oxygen, and the more air will be entrained. Moreover, the mixing of oxygen and air at this point is caused by the forces of fluid viscosity and not, as the Bernoulli theorem would suggest, by pressure gradients.[52] Air is entrained by shear forces occurring at the boundary of the jet flow, not by low lateral pressures at the jet orifice.

To provide a controlled oxygen concentration at flow rates sufficient to ensure that no further dilution of room air occurs during inspiration, the total flow must exceed that patient's *peak* inspiratory flow.[1,5,52] During normal quiet breathing, peak inspiratory flows seldom exceed 30 L/min, but this can easily double or triple as a result of hyperpnea or hyperventilation. As a general clinical guide, a minimum total flow of 40 L/min should be established; higher flows may be necessary for patients with greater than normal $\dot{V}_E$ or rates of breathing.[5]

The actual oxygen concentration and total flow provided by an air entrainment mask is a function of three variables: (1) the oxygen flow to the jet, (2) the air to oxygen ratio of the device, and (3) the amount of resistance encountered after leaving the jet system.[51,52]

Most manufacturers list a single or narrow range of oxygen flow for the jet on their entrainment device for each concentration desired, and users appear to be reluctant to deviate from these flows. Several studies have shown that oxygen concentrations remain within 1% to 2% of that specified when flows of 2 to 15 L/min are used to drive the jet.[51,53,54] Some individual exceptions do exist, and variations up to 6% oxygen have been measured under changing jet flow.[54] Clinicians using these devices should become familiar with the brand of masks they use by measuring the oxygen concentration coming from the mask at different flows.

The air to oxygen entrainment ratio is a constant mathematical value for each oxygen percentage. Calculation of both the final concentration of a mixture of air and oxygen, and the ratio of air and oxygen needed to obtain a given FIO_2, is based on a modification of the dilution equation for solutions, as discussed in Chapter 5.

In diluting any solution, the initial volume times the initial concentration equals the final volume times the final concentration. This relationship can be expressed in the following formula:

$$V_1 C_1 = V_2 C_2$$

Given that a gas or gas mixture is equivalent to a solution, both air and oxygen may be considered solutions, with oxygen as the "solute." For example, if we dilute 2 L of 100% oxygen with 2 L of nitrogen (0% oxygen), use of the above dilution equation would yield a final oxygen concentration of 50%:

$$V_1 C_1 = V_2 C_2$$
$$(2\text{ L}) \times 100\% = (4\text{ L}) \times C_2$$
$$C_2 = \frac{2\text{ L}}{4\text{ L}} \times 100\%$$
$$= 50\%$$

Of course, in clinical practice we commonly combine two gases of different oxygen concentrations (air and oxygen) to derive a third mixture. Modification of the simple dilution equation to accommodate the mixing of two "solutions" to derive a third is as follows:

$$V_F C_F = V_1 C_1 + V_2 C_2$$

where V_1 and V_2 are the volumes of the two gases being mixed, C_1 and C_2 the respective concentrations of the applicable gas in these volumes (usually oxygen), and V_F and C_F are the final volume and concentration of the resultant mixture. Depending on the values known, various forms of this equation allow us to compute the final concentration of a mixture of air and oxygen, the ratio of air and oxygen needed to obtain a given FIO_2, or the amount of supplemental oxygen that must be added to a quantity of air to obtain a given FIO_2.

For example, let us assume that we wish to know the FIO_2 that would result from mixing 3 vol of air ($FIO_2 = 0.21$) with 1 vol of oxygen ($FIO_2 = 1.0$). First we rearrange the above equation to solve for the final concentration of oxygen (C_F):

$$C_F = \frac{V_1 C_1 + V_2 C_2}{V_F}$$

Then we substitute the values for V_1 and C_1 (the air) and V_2 and C_2 (the oxygen):

$$C_F = \frac{(3 \times 0.21) + (1 \times 1.0)}{4}$$
$$C_F = \frac{1.63}{4} = 0.41$$

Thus the FIO_2 resulting from mixing 3 vol of air with 1 vol of oxygen is approximately 0.40, or 40%.

To compute the ratio of air to oxygen needed to achieve a given FIO_2, a more complex rearrangement of the general mixing equation is required:

$$V_F C_F = V_1 C_1 + V_2 C_2$$

Step 1: Because $V_F = V_1 + V_2$:

$$(V_1 + V_2)C_F = V_1 C_1 + V_2 C_2$$

Step 2: Multiplying $(V_1 + V_2)$ by C_F we derive:

$$V_1 C_F + V_2 C_F = V_1 C_1 + V_2 C_2$$

Step 3: Subtracting $V_2 C_F$ from both sides of the equation:

$$V_1 C_F = V_1 C_1 + V_2 C_2 - V_2 C_F$$

Step 4: Subtracting $V_1 C_1$ from both sides of the equation:

$$V_1 C_F - V_1 C_1 = V_2 C_2 - V_2 C_F$$

Step 5: Combining terms, we derive:

$$V_1(C_F - C_1) = V_2(C_2 - C_F)$$

Step 6: Finally, dividing both sides of the equation by V_2:

$$V_1/V_2 = \frac{(C_2 - C_F)}{(C_F - C_1)}$$

As applied to mixing air and oxygen, V_1 represents the volume of air (with an oxygen concentration of 21% [C_1]); V_2 represents the volume of pure oxygen ($C_2 = 100$); and C_F represents the oxygen percentage desired ($O_2\%$). Therefore:

$$\text{Liters air entrained/liter } O_2 = \frac{(100 - O_2\%)}{(O_2\% - 21)}$$

For example, suppose we wish to generate an oxygen concentration of 70% by mixing air with pure oxygen. The ratio of air to oxygen needed to achieve this concentration would be computed as follows:

$$\text{Liters air entrained/liter } O_2 = \frac{(100 - O_2\%)}{(O_2\% - 21)}$$
$$\text{Liters air entrained/liter } O_2 = \frac{(100 - 70)}{(70 - 21)}$$
$$= \frac{30}{49}$$
$$\cong \frac{0.6}{1.0}$$

Thus, to obtain a final mixture of 70% oxygen, we would have to mix approximately 0.6 L of air with every 1.0 L of oxygen.

To avoid these complex computations, many clinicians employ a simple estimation aid referred to as the "magic box."[55] As shown in Fig. 25-8, the clinician draws a box

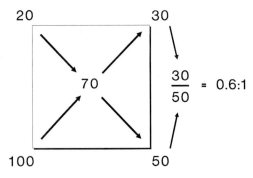

Fig. 25-8 "Magic box."

and places 20 at the top left* and 100 at the bottom left. Then the percentage of oxygen desired is placed in the middle of the box (in this case 70%). Next, the practitioner subtracts diagonally from lower left to upper right (disregarding the sign) and from upper left to lower right (disregarding the sign). The resulting top right number is the value for air (in this case 30 L/min), with the bottom right number being the value for oxygen (in this case 50 L/min). Since these ratios are traditionally expressed in terms of liters of air per liter (1 L) of oxygen, we simply divide 30 by 50 to derive a 0.6:1.0 ratio of air to oxygen (equivalent to that previously computed the long way).

Based on computations using the actual mixing equation, Table 25-1 lists the approximate air-to-oxygen ratios for several common oxygen percentages. To calculate total flow at any given ratio, simply multiply the sum of the ratio parts times the oxygen input flow in liters per minute. For example, with an oxygen concentration of 40%, the approximate air to oxygen ratio is 3:1, for a total of 4 parts. Assuming an input flow of 12 L/min, the total flow would be estimated at 4×12, or 48 L/min.

Crucial in clinical practice is the fact that downstream resistance to flow in air entrainment devices decreases the amount of air entrained, thereby decreasing total flow. Although the delivered oxygen concentration must therefore rise, the actual FIO_2 received by the patient may actually decrease as room air is inhaled around and through the mask parts.[51] A similar effect is produced with partial or complete occlusion of the air intake ports surrounding the jet. Under either circumstance, the system will assume the characteristics of a variable-performance device.

These masks are generally best used for relatively short periods when precise control over inspired oxygen is needed, such as during exacerbations of chronic ventilatory insufficiency. Because of their relative size, comfort, and appearance, they are less well tolerated for long-term therapy than are nasal cannulas. Moreover, unlike cannu-

las, these masks must be removed for eating and drinking. As previously discussed, even a short interruption in oxygen therapy among chronically hypercapneic patients can cause the PaO_2 to fall rapidly.[8] To ensure continuous oxygenation for patients when the mask must be removed, a cannula set at a flow producing an equivalent FIO_2 should be used.

The high air flow produced by these masks can be quite drying. For this reason, attempts should be made to humidify the gases.[56,57] Although simple humidifiers can be used to saturate the oxygen flow to the jet without affecting the FIO_2, very little increase in overall humidification occurs because of the relatively large amounts of room air entrained.[56] This is particularly true when the entrainment ratios are high, that is, with 40% oxygen or less (see Table 25-1). A better method is to add aerosol to the entrained air through a standard 22 mm collar, using either an air-powered jet or ultrasonic nebulizer. This technique should be considered whenever the adequacy of humidification is in question. As an added benefit, aerosol collars help prevent accidental occlusion of the entrainment ports of these devices, such as may occur with bedsheets.

The gas-powered air entrainment nebulizer represents an alternative high-flow oxygen delivery system that additionally generates particulate water for deposition in the respiratory tract. The most significant advantages these systems provide are their humidification and heat control capabilities, especially for intubated patients (see Chapter 23). The oxygen and aerosol can be delivered by an aerosol mask, tracheostomy mask, or an aerosol T-tube connector (Briggs adapter).[45,58]

Unlike entrainment masks, in which mixing ratios usually are determined by variable jet sizes, the gas-powered nebulizer has a fixed orifice. Instead, ratios of air to oxygen are altered by varying the size of the air entrainment

Table 25-1   Approximate Air-to-Oxygen Ratios for Oxygen Concentrations in Common Use

% Oxygen	Approximate air-to-oxygen ratio*	Total ratio parts†
100	0:1	1
80	0.3:1	1.3
70	0.6:1	1.6
60	1:1	2
50	1.7:1	2.7
45	2:1	3
40	3:1	4
35	5:1	6
30	8:1	9
28	10:1	11
24	25:1	26

*Assuming 20.9% oxygen in air.
†Total flow of mixed air and oxygen can be calculated by multiplying the total ratio parts times the oxygen flow rate (L/min).

---

*The number 20 is used for ease of estimation; for accuracy in determining ratios needed for concentration of 30% or below, the clinician must use 21.

port. Permanent nebulizers typically have fixed entrainment settings, such as 100%, 70%, and 40%. Disposable nebulizers usually provide a continuously adjustable air entrainment port that provides oxygen concentrations ranging from approximately 28% to 100%.

In reality, the oxygen concentration delivered by an air entrainment nebulizer to the patient's airway is usually higher than that set. The reason for this discrepancy is the added downstream resistance created by the 4 to 6 feet of tubing used to deliver the gas.[58] In general, this effect is most pronounced at high mixing ratios (lower oxygen concentrations) or when the tubing becomes blocked with water.[58] Even in the latter situation, the lumen of the tube must be decreased by more than 70% before changes in oxygen percentage occur.[59] In some situations, delivery of oxygen concentrations below 28% may require the use of compressed air to drive the jet and the addition of oxygen through a T-tube connector at a point distal to the entrainment site.[60-62] Oxygen is then titrated into the system and measured until the desired percentage is achieved.

Because of the extremely small size of the nebulizer jet orifice, the maximum oxygen inflow is restricted to between 12 and 15 L/min at 50 psig. With a set oxygen concentration of 40%, the total output flow will range from about 48 to 60 L/min. This may be barely adequate for some patients and inadequate for those with increased peak inspiratory flow rates or high $\dot{V}E$.

An air entrainment nebulizer may therefore be treated as a fixed-performance device only when system output meets the patient's inspiratory demands. Generally, this situation exists only when the device is set to delivery 40% oxygen or less. However, even at the 40% setting, some variance in delivered FIO_2 may occur.[40,41,43,47] Certainly, when these devices are set at concentrations above 40%, matching of the patient and device flow rates must be evaluated. Additional flow can be attained by connecting two or more nebulizers together with a Y adapter or by adding supplemental oxygen through a T adapter.[60]

When the oxygen is delivered to a patient with an endotracheal or tracheostomy tube through a T-tube connector, an alternative approach is to add an open-volume reservoir, consisting of 50 to 150 ml of aerosol tubing, to the expiratory side of the T tube. As long as the flows through the system are adequate to flush this reservoir volume with source gas during the pre-inspiratory pause, the effect will be comparable to the use of a reservoir mask.

Should it not be possible to meet the patient's inspiratory demands in this manner, a true nonrebreathing system can also be established. This requires a T tube with one-way inspiratory and expiratory valves and a reservoir bag in the inspiratory limb of the circuit. In such a system, provision must be made for emergency inflow of ambient air should the source gas fail.

Oxygen blender systems. Oxygen blenders or controllers are devices that use 50 psig sources of oxygen and com-

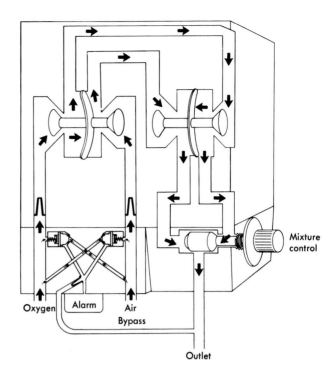

Fig. 25-9 Oxygen blending device. (From McPherson SP: Respiratory therapy equipment, ed 3, St Louis, 1985, The CV Mosby Co.)

pressed air and mix the two gases with a proportioning valve.[60] A typical oxygen blender consists of (1) pressure-regulating valves that equalize the inlet pressures of air and oxygen, (2) a precision metering device or mixture control, and (3) an alarm system that provides an audible alert to drops in source gas pressure (Fig. 25-9). By proportionately varying the size of the air and oxygen inlets, blenders can deliver oxygen concentrations of 21% to 100% at flows ranging from about 2 to 100 L/min (depending on the model). With these performance characteristics, oxygen blenders approach the ideal of a true fixed-performance gas delivery system. As long as the outlet flow exceeds the patient's peak inspiratory flow rate, a stable FIO_2 can be delivered at any level, even with a simple mask.

The major problem with blending systems is the provision of adequate humidification at high-flow rates. If jet nebulizers are used for humidification, flow capabilities are limited by both the restricted orifice and the necessity to set the device at the 100% source gas setting. Simple bubble or diffusion humidifiers also can restrict flow and tend to lose efficiency at higher flow rates.[60] Low-resistance cascade or wick-type heated humidifiers can provide as much as 90% relative humidity at 37°C with continuous flow rates up to 60 L/min.[60] When higher levels of water vapor content are desired or particulate water deposition is indicated, an in-line ultrasonic nebulizer may be required.

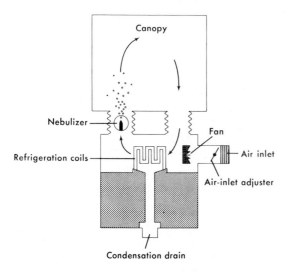

Fig. 25-10 Adult oxygen tent incorporating refrigeration coils for cooling. (From McPherson SP: Respiratory therapy equipment, ed 3, St Louis, 1985, The CV Mosby Co.)

Enclosures. The concept of enclosing a patient in a controlled oxygen atmosphere is among the oldest approaches to the therapeutic use of oxygen. Indeed, whole rooms were once used for this purpose.[35] Today, with simpler and more precise airway modalities available, the use of enclosures for oxygen therapy is generally limited to infants and children. Tents, incubators, and hoods are the primary types of oxygen therapy enclosures in current use.

Tents. Oxygen tents were once popular for use with both adults and children. Their use today is rare in adults, but they are still used with pediatric patients. In general, tents are air conditioned or cooled by ice to provide a relatively comfortable temperature within a plastic sheet enclosure (Fig. 25-10). Of course, frequent opening and closing of this plastic enclosure causes great fluctuations in oxygen concentrations. Moreover, the maximum oxygen concentrations that can be achieved in a tent is limited. In larger tents, input oxygen flows of 12 to 15 L/min produce oxygen concentrations in the 40% to 50% range. Comparable concentrations are achieved in smaller pediatric or "croup" tents with input flows in the 8 to 10 L/min range. Because of these limitations, tents today are used primarily to provide an enclosed environment for pediatric aerosol therapy, which may be desirable for children with croup, epiglottitis, or cystic fibrosis.

Any enclosure such as a tent with an oxygen-enriched atmosphere is at increased risk of fire. All electrical appliances with the potential for sparks, such as call bells and electric toys, should be kept out of an oxygen tent.

Hoods. Oxygen hoods are the most convenient method of providing therapy to infants.[29] As shown in Fig. 25-11, "oxyhoods" cover only the head, leaving the patient's body available for nursing care. Historically, hoods or "head tents" were also used with adults,[35] although this

approach has been supplanted by the other methods of oxygen delivery previously described.

Controlled oxygen therapy through a hood is accomplished with either a heated air entrainment nebulizer or a blending system with heated humidification (see Fig. 25-11). Minimum flows of 4 to 5 L/min are generally required to prevent accumulation of carbon dioxide. Above this level, flows are adjusted to achieve the prescribed F_{IO_2} (which should be continuously monitored) and the desired Pa_{O_2} range of 50 to 60 mm Hg.[33] Depending on the size of hood, flows of 10 to 15 L/min may be needed to maintain stable high oxygen concentrations. Greater flows are generally unnecessary and may produce harmful noise levels.[63] Total flows from nebulizers should also be limited if these are used to supply mixed gas to the hood.

It is especially important for a premature infant that the oxygen be properly warmed and humidified and not directed toward the face or head. Low temperatures or the convection cooling created by high flows over the head can cause substantial heat loss or cold stress. Such cold stress can increase oxygen consumption or cause apnea in preterm infants.[29-31]

For these reasons, the temperature of the gases in the hood should be precisely maintained to provide a neutral thermal environment. The temperature required to maintain these conditions varies according to the infant's age and weight, generally ranging from 35°C for newborns under 1200 g to 30°C for older infants of 2500 g or more.[31,64] More detail on these concepts is provided in Chapter 32.

Incubators. Incubators are Plexiglass enclosures that combine convection heating through an electrical coil and fan, with a mechanism for providing humidification and supplemental oxygen (Fig. 25-12). Humidification is available through a baffled blow-over water reservoir under the patient platform. However, because of the high risk of infection associated with this system, alternative sources of humidification are generally employed. Oxygen can be provided by a simple connection to a compensated flowmeter and is normally monitored continuously by either a polarographic or fuel-cell analyzer (see following section). In most units, a filtered air entrainment device limits concentrations to about 40%. Obviously, leakages and frequent opening of the incubator will dilute the oxygen levels well below 40%. Conversely, blockage of the inlet filter can restrict air entrainment and result in a higher than expected ambient oxygen concentration.

If higher concentrations of oxygen are actually needed, the entrainment port can be manually closed, normally by raising a red visual indicator. Alternatively, precise oxygen levels in incubators can be maintained by a controlling system that combines an oxygen analyzer with a flow-controlling solenoid valve. Desired oxygen levels are set on the controller and are monitored by the analyzer. Should the concentration fall below the preset value, the solenoid

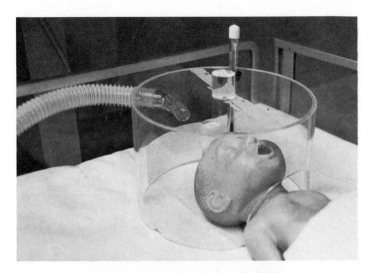

Fig. 25-11   Infant oxygen hood.

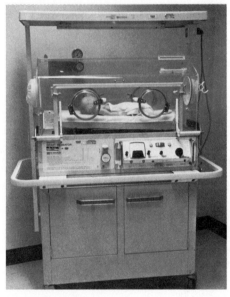

Fig. 25-12   Infant incubator.

is opened and additional oxygen flows into the system until the analyzer value again matches the value chosen. Even with such a device, the relatively large airspace of the incubators makes it difficult to provide true controlled oxygen therapy.

Because hoods provide greater overall oxygen control, and because radiant heating servocontrolled warmers are generally more convenient than incubators, the indications for this type of enclosure increasingly have become limited to providing a neutral thermal environment to more stable infants. Newer incubators incorporate a double-walled construction to help slow radiant heat loss from infants, thereby decreasing oxygen consumption by significant amounts.[65,66]

Oxygen analysis

Whenever possible, the oxygen therapy delivery system should be analyzed to monitor the concentration given. This is especially true for fixed-performance devices and for enclosures. Depending on the clinical objectives of therapy and the patient's status, monitoring may be continuous or intermittent. At a minimum, when oxygen analysis is indicated, monitoring should be conducted at least every 1 to 2 hours, or after any change in prescribed settings.

Common commercially available analyzers for routine bedside use are of three types: physical, electrical, and electrochemical.[60,67,68]

The principle underlying the physical analyzer is oxygen's unique paramagnetic susceptibility. Based on this physical property, oxygen molecules tend to locate themselves in the strongest portion of a magnetic field. Conversely, diamagnetic gases (such as nitrogen) tend to be attracted to the weakest portion of a magnetic field.

The physical analyzer measures the presence of oxygen molecules using a small glass dumbbell that is filled with nitrogen and suspended on a taut quartz fiber in the field of a permanent magnet (Fig. 25-13). In the absence of oxygen, the forces of the torque (rotary force) of the quartz

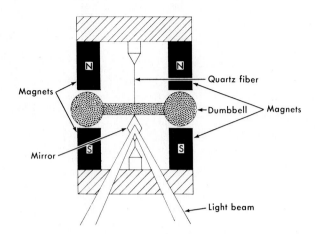

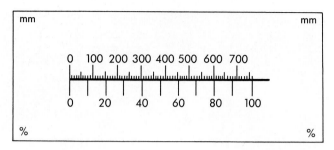

Fig. 25-14   Calibrated scale for physical analyzer showing oxygen percentage and mm Hg.

Fig. 25-13   Physical oxygen analyzer principle of operation. (From McPherson SP: Respiratory therapy equipment, ed 3, St Louis, 1985, The CV Mosby Co.)

fiber and the magnetic field are equal and in balance. Oxygen molecules introduced into the system disrupt the magnetic field in direct proportion to their number. By migrating toward the space between the magnets, the oxygen molecules tend to displace any other gas molecules present. This upsets the magnetic balance, overcomes the torque of the quartz fiber, and rotates the glass dumbbell in response to the alterations in the magnetic force. A small mirror attached to the fiber reflects a beam of battery-powered light onto a translucent scale calibrated in both oxygen percentage and Po_2 (mm Hg).

A major advantage of this analyzer is its ability to detect and measure concentrations of oxygen in any mixture of gases. Since the number of oxygen molecules occupying the space between the magnets in the measuring chamber is determined by the Po_2, the physical analyzer actually measures the Po_2 and not the oxygen concentration. However, the indicator scale for this type analyzer is calibrated in both oxygen percentage and Po_2 (Fig. 25-14). For this reason, the percentage concentration reading will only be accurate at sea level. When used at higher altitudes, the Po_2 is accurately indicated but the percentage concentration will be below the actual value. For this reason, the physical analyzer scale must be recalibrated when used above sea level.

Also, since the instrument is calibrated to measure Po_2 in the dry state, water vapor must be removed before analysis. This is accomplished with a drying chamber filled with blue silica gel crystals that absorb water vapor. Also in the drying chamber is anhydrous cobalt chloride, which turns pink when saturated with water. This color change (from blue to pink) indicates the need to replace the crystals in the drying chamber.

Because the physical analyzer system generates no appreciable heat, it is safe to employ with flammable gases such as cyclopropane and ethylene. However, because gas

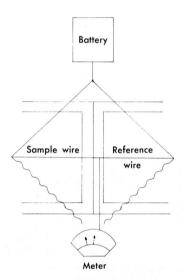

Fig. 25-15   Electrical oxygen analyzer (Wheatstone bridge). (From McPherson SP: Respiratory therapy equipment, ed 3, St Louis, 1985, The CV Mosby Co.)

flow in the chamber would cause the dumbbell to sway vigorously, this type of analyzer can only be used with static gas samples.[68]

The electrical analyzer employs the principle of thermal conductivity in measuring available oxygen. All gases conduct heat, but to varying degrees. The ability of a substance to conduct heat is measured as its coefficient of thermal conductivity (see Chapter 4). Because oxygen has a higher thermal conductivity coefficient than nitrogen, variations in the relative amounts of oxygen and nitrogen in a gas mixture will alter the thermal conductivity of the mixture as a whole in direct proportion to the amount of oxygen present.

The electrical analyzer measures these differences in thermal conductivity using a battery-powered Wheatstone bridge of platinum wires (Fig. 25-15). One limb of the bridge is exposed to the test gas, with the other limb functioning as a variable resistor for calibration. The instrument is calibrated before use by drawing room air into the sample chamber and balancing the bridge by adjusting a

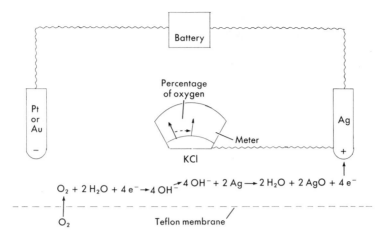

$$O_2 + 2\,H_2O + 4\,e^- \rightarrow 4\,OH^- \quad 4\,OH^- + 2\,Ag \rightarrow 2\,H_2O + 2\,AgO + 4\,e^-$$

Fig. 25-16   Example of diagram for polarographic (Clark-type) electrode for gaseous oxygen measurement. (From McPherson SP: Respiratory therapy equipment, ed 3, St Louis, 1985, The CV Mosby Co.)

rheostat until the scale reads 21%. Because the electrical resistance of a wire varies directly with the temperature, introduction of a nitrogen-oxygen mixture with greater than 21% oxygen will transfer more heat away from the sample wires, lower their resistance, and increase the current flow. This creates an "imbalance" in current across the two limbs of the bridge, registered by a galvanometer calibrated in percentage of oxygen.

Since the comparison is relative to the proportions of oxygen and nitrogen in the mixture, the electrical analyzer measures the concentration of oxygen in nitrogen rather than its partial pressure. For this reason, the introduction of gases other than oxygen and nitrogen, such as carbon dioxide, will alter the accuracy of the device and result in erroneous readings. However, the electrical analyzer can be scaled to measure other gas mixtures. The helium analyzer employed on many pulmonary function devices is a good example of an electrical analyzer calibrated for other gas mixtures.

Because water vapor has a different thermal conductivity coefficient than either oxygen or nitrogen, electrical analyzers must be provided with a constant level of molecular water. This may be accomplished either by ensuring that the sample gas is dry (as with the physical analyzers) or by saturating the sample with water vapor. Electrical analyzers that saturate the gas sample use hydrated silica gel crystals (pink) for this purpose. Last, because of the resistors in their circuits, electrical analyzers generate substantial amounts of heat and can therefore cause flammable gas mixtures to ignite. For this reason, electrical analyzers should not be used to measure oxygen concentrations in a mixture with any flammable gas.

Electrochemical analyzers can be subdivided into two types: the polarographic (Clark) electrode and the galvanic fuel cell. Compared with the physical and electrical ana-

lyzers, electrochemical analyzers offer the advantage of continuous monitoring capabilities.

Both the polarographic electrode and the galvanic fuel cell measure P_{O_2} in proportion to the availability of oxygen molecules for participation in a reduction-oxidation (REDOX) reaction. This reaction takes place in an electrolytic gel across an anode and a cathode separated from the air by a semipermeable membrane such as Teflon. Oxygen diffuses through the membrane at a rate proportional to its partial pressure and is chemically reduced (and therefore consumed) at the cathode. The hydroxyl ions produced in this reduction oxidize a metal (usually lead or silver) at the anode. The REDOX reaction generates a current flow between anode and cathode in direct proportion the number of oxygen molecules reduced. Current is measured on a galvanometer calibrated in percentage oxygen.

The polarographic analyzer probe typically consists of a platinum or gold cathode and a silver anode (Fig. 25-16). A small current, usually provided by a battery, maintains electrode polarity and speeds the reaction, thereby providing a relatively fast response time. This type of electrode is essentially the same design used in blood-gas analyzers.

The galvanic fuel also employs a lead anode but usually incorporates a gold cathode. However, unlike the Clark electrode, polarity and current flow in the galvanic fuel are maintained solely by the chemical reaction itself (Fig. 25-17). Therefore the galvanic fuel cell does not require an external power source unless accessories, such as warning alarms, are incorporated. Against this relative advantage must be weighed the disadvantage of the slower response times characterizing galvanic fuel cells, and the cost of cell replacement.

Table 25-2 summarizes the principles and characteristics of the common types of oxygen analyzers used in respiratory care.[68]

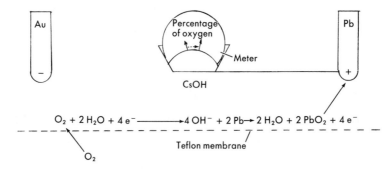

Fig. 25-17 Example of diagram for galvanic fuel cell for gaseous oxygen analysis. (From McPherson SP: Respiratory therapy equipment, ed 3, St Louis, 1985, The CV Mosby Co.)

Selecting an approach

Because of the wide variety of techniques of administering oxygen, it is obvious that there is no one best method. Although a decision to give oxygen to a patient is a medical one, it is not always easy for the physician to know which procedure will be the most effective. For this reason, the respiratory care practitioner should be involved in the initial selection of an appropriate approach and should assume major responsibility for supervision of the prescribed therapy, including recommending necessary changes in the treatment regimen based on sound patient assessment.

In our discussion of various oxygen therapy modalities, we have suggested available ranges of delivered oxygen concentrations for each type. Because the delivered concentration of gas from any appliance is subjected to many modifying influences, these values can only be used as guides to average performance. Indeed, it is generally the pathophysiologic process underlying the disease that best determines the effectiveness of a given approach to oxygen administration. Because of alterations in the lung's ventilatory and gas exchange functions, there may be little correlation between the fractional concentration of inhaled oxygen and the realization of a normal arterial oxygen content. Complete relief of hypoxemia may be easily achieved by low-flow cannula oxygen in one patient and be impossible by mask therapy in another.

For this reason, except for short-term therapy as may occur immediately after surgery with general anesthesia, safe and rational treatment must depend on the actual measurement of blood oxygenation. The initial degree of hypoxemia must therefore be documented by direct measurement and regularly monitored until the desired level of blood oxygenation is reached. After the degree of hypoxemia has been determined, the choice of technique may require some trials and errors, guided by blood oxygen levels, with thought given to patient comfort as well as to avoiding overoxygenation.

Based on these considerations, general goals can be established for several major patient categories. In patients with acute hypoxemia and no preexisting lung disease, the goal should be to restore arterial oxygen contents to normal levels. In patients whose cardiovascular performance is marginal or overtaxed, more liberal usage of oxygen may be indicated over the short term, but only until the underlying problem is resolved. Patients with chronic hypercapnea and an accompanying acute or chronic hypoxemia present a special case. In this group, the goal should be to ensure adequate arterial oxygenation without depressing the hypoxic drive. Adequate arterial oxygenation for these patients generally means achieving an Sao_2 in the 85% to 90% range, with Pao_2 levels between 50 and 60 mm Hg.[2-5,10,19,50] Last, patients in whom chronic hypoxemia has manifested itself in pulmonary vascular hypertension may be considered candidates for long-term continuous low-flow oxygen therapy.[69-71]

Table 25-2 Comparison of Oxygen Analyzers

	Physical (paramagnetic)	Electrical (thermal conduction)	Electrochemical (polarographic)	Electrochemical (galvanic cell)
Parameter measured	Partial pressure	Oxygen concentration	Partial pressure	Partial pressure
Accurate with other gases?	Yes	Oxygen and nitrogen only	Yes	Yes
Sampling technique	Intermittent static sample	Intermittent static sample	Continuous dynamic	Continuous dynamic
Use with flammable gases?	Yes	No	Yes	Yes
Oxygen consumption	No	No	Yes	Yes

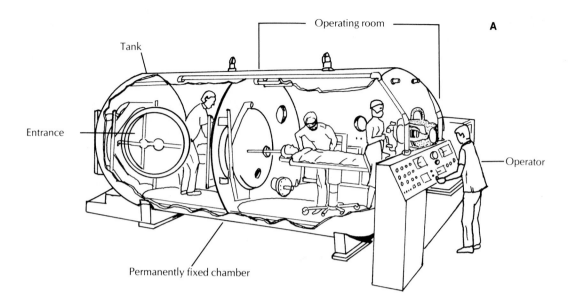

Fig. 25-18 **A,** Fixed hyperbaric chamber. **B,** Monoplace chamber.

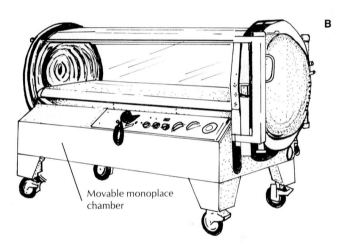

HYPERBARIC OXYGEN THERAPY

Treatment of disorders using increased barometric pressure, with or without increased oxygen concentration, dates back several centuries. Hyperbaric oxygen therapy is presently enjoying a great deal of attention and support after many decades of suspicion, abuse, and condemnation. In the majority of instances over the last 100 years, the suspicion and condemnation were justified. Now, with good scientific research and careful attention to conservative applications, the hyperbaric oxygen chamber is being recognized as an important tool in the primary treatment of certain disorders and as an adjunct treatment modality in other disorders.[72]

Hyperbaric chambers are of two basic designs (Fig. 25-18). The fixed chamber (see Fig. 25-18, *A*) is a walk-in metal-encased room capable of "diving" to many atmospheres below sea level, with many people inside. Whole operating rooms have functioned inside these chambers. The more commonly used chamber is a clear plastic cylinder on wheels designated as a monoplace chamber (see Fig. 25-19, *B*). These chambers are generally limited to 3 atm or 45 psi absolute pressure and can hold only one person at a time. Oxygen concentrations up to 100% are available to achieve high oxygen tissue tensions.

How hyperbaric oxygen works is only partially understood. Oxygen is delivered to the tissues at increased tensions, and Pao_2 levels as high as 1800 to 1900 mm Hg may be achieved at 3 atm pressure while the patient breathes 100% oxygen. Physiologic effects of such increased oxygen tensions include (1) new capillary bed formation (neovascularization), (2) arteriolar constriction, and (3) alteration in the metabolism and growth of both anaerobic and aerobic organisms. The physiologic effects of the increased barometric pressure include reduction in size of nitrogen bubbles dissolved within the blood and other tissue cavities, such as joints.

Over the last 10 years four hyperbaric oxygen therapy treatment categories have evolved. Category I disorders are those best treated by hyperbaric oxygen. Clinical problems in this category include carbon monoxide poisoning, cyanide poisoning, decompression sickness, gas embolism, and gas gangrene.[72]

Category II disorders are those for which hyperbaric oxygen may be used as adjunct to other established modes of therapy. Clinical problems in this category include skin grafts, smoke inhalation, actinomycoses, acute peripheral arterial insufficiency, crush injuries, intestinal obstruction, refractory osteomyelitis, radionecrosis of soft tissue, osteoradionecrosis, and thermal burns.

With category III disorders, data exist that hyperbaric oxygen may be helpful, but no proof exists. Conditions in category III include traumatic head and spinal cord injuries, bone grafts, and sickle cell anemia crises. Last, in category IV are those conditions for which theoretic data suggest some benefit might be realized, but no definitive work has been done to establish this. Examples of category IV conditions are multiple sclerosis, arthritis, and emphysema.

Treatment protocols have been standardized by the hard work of the Undersea Medical Society and have gained wide acceptance by both government agencies and practicing physicians. The protocol for a given disease entity may require 90-minute "dives" to 2 to 3 atm, two to four times a day, sometimes lasting for months. Caring for patients in these circumstances may be taxing and requires skill and compassion.

The harmful effects of hyperbaric oxygen fall into two areas: CNS and pulmonary toxicity (see the previous section on the detrimental effects of oxygen). CNS toxicity is most commonly manifested by convulsions. Early signs of impending CNS complications include twitching, sweating, pallor, and restlessness. Pulmonary toxicity is not noted early in the treatment because the effects are cumulative. Certain drugs are considered helpful in retarding oxygen toxicity to lung tissue. Vitamin E is the most commonly used. Many other drugs, if taken at the same time as the hyperbaric oxygen is being used, can accelerate oxygen toxicity. These substances have been noted previously (see box, p. 611).

The safety aspects of running a hyperbaric chamber are unique and offer many challenges. For this reason, chamber operators should be appropriately qualified according to US Navy protocol or other comparable criteria for personnel in this field. Avoiding fires and sudden decompression (blowouts) are primary safety concerns. Only 100% cotton material can be used so that fire from static electricity is avoided. No products with an alcohol or petroleum base can be used, and the patient must not wear sprays, makeup, or deodorant. Last, pressure- and flow-regulating equipment used in hyperbaric chambers must be specifically designed for operation at chamber pressures or appropriately modified for this use.

OTHER MEDICAL GAS THERAPIES

Although oxygen is the primary medical gas used for therapeutic purposes, helium and carbon dioxide may also be used for therapeutic purposes. Although generally replaced by other approaches, both gases have a rather long history of application in respiratory care and still may find application in carefully delimited clinical situations.

Helium therapy

An earlier chapter mentioned the use of helium in the treatment of obstructive disease, and we now discuss this technique in more detail. It is helium's low-density property that makes the gas a valuable therapeutic tool. Heli-

um's only medical indication is in the management of airway obstruction, specifically that occurring in the larger airways.[73]

For reasons that are not clear, the use of helium (mixed with oxygen) has not been popular in the past 20 years. Barach described the rationale for using helium in 1935 for decreasing work of breathing and was still recommending its use for bronchial asthma in 1976.[74,76] Helium-oxygen therapy has been shown to decrease ventilation, carbon dioxide production, and oxygen consumption in patients with chronic obstructive pulmonary disease (COPD).[76] It has also been shown to decrease resistance to flow in upper airway obstruction.[74,77,78]

Principle. To understand the potential benefits of helium breathing in airway obstruction, we must briefly review the principles of fluid physics applied to the movement of gases into and out of the respiratory tract. In concept, the driving pressure to move gases through the tracheobronchial tree is a function of both the rate of flow and the flow characteristics. For laminar flow, the driving pressure is linearly proportional to the flow ($\dot{V}$) times a constant related to gas viscosity (K_1):

$$P = \dot{V} \times K_1$$

For turbulent flow, the driving pressure is proportional to the square of the flow times a constant related to gas density (K_2):

$$P = \dot{V}^2 \times K_2$$

Normally, the flow pattern in the small airways is mainly laminar, whereas the flow pattern in the large airways is mainly turbulent or mixed. Whether flow is mainly laminar or mainly turbulent is determined by several factors, including gas velocity, tube radius, gas density, and gas viscosity (Reynold's number). According to this formula, with all else being equal, the lower the density of a gas, the greater will be the tendency toward laminar flow. Moreover, low-density gases should be able to maintain laminar flow patterns at higher velocities than heavier gases.

Since the viscosity of helium does not differ substantially from either air or oxygen, breathing helium will have little effect on the pressure gradients associated with the laminar flow occurring in the small airways. However, wherever the flow pattern is turbulent (mainly in the large airways), substituting a low-density helium mixture for higher-density air or oxygen will encourage laminar flow. Because less pressure is required to move a gas at a given velocity under conditions of laminar flow than when the flow pattern is turbulent, breathing a helium mixture will reduce the work of breathing associated with obstruction of the large airways.

Guidelines for use. Currently, helium is the only low-density gas acceptable for medical use, and since it is inert and unable to support life, it must always be mixed with oxygen. All helium-oxygen mixtures must have at least 20% oxygen to supply basic metabolic needs. A popular combination is the so-called 80-20 mixture, with 80% helium and 20% oxygen. For practical purposes such a mixture is comparable with air, with helium substituted for nitrogen. For a more specific comparison, it should be noted that the density of air is 1.293 g/L, whereas that of 80-20 helium is 0.429 g/L. For a comparable flow through obstructed large airways, such a mixture should dramatically lower the work of breathing.[73]

It is possible to mix pure helium and oxygen at the bedside, but the hazards of error and mechanical failure are so great that it is much safer, as well as more convenient, to use commercially prepared cylinders of premixed gases. In addition to the 80-20 combination, another commonly used mixture is 70-30 (density = .554 g/L). This gives an additional quantity of oxygen, which is often helpful in correcting hypoxemia associated with large airway obstruction.

There are six points of practical importance to consider in the therapeutic use of helium-oxygen mixtures:

1. Helium mixtures must always be given in a tightly closed system because their high diffusibilities will allow them to escape from even small leaks. Tents, catheters, and cannulas are not satisfactory. The gases should be given by a well-fitted nonrebreathing mask or through cuffed endotracheal or tracheostomy tubes. It can be administered by inspiratory positive-pressure ventilators.[78]

2. The average hospital gas flow meter is calibrated for oxygen, and since it depends on the kinetic support of a float by the metered gas, gauge readings will not be accurate for the lighter helium-oxygen mixtures. Special meters, calibrated for the helium mixtures, can be used, but they are not necessary because correction can be made for the scales of the oxygen meters. For a 80-20 helium-oxygen mixture a factor of 1.8 is used, whereas 70-30 helium-oxygen requires a factor of 1.6. This means that for every 10 L/min gas flow recorded on the meter, 18 L/min and 16 L/min, respectively, of the above helium mixtures would actually leave the flowmeter. To deliver a desired flow, the flow meter is adjusted to a reading equal to the desired rate divided by either 1.8 or 1.6, depending on the gas mixture being used. Factors for any other combination can be calculated if needed.

3. The low density of the helium mixtures makes them poor vehicles for the transport of aerosols. Humidifiers, of course, must be used with any administered gas, but high therapeutic concentrations of water particles from nebulizers cannot be expected.

4. The low density of helium mixtures make coughing less effective. An expulsive cough depends, in part, on the development of turbulent flow in the large airways. To the extent that helium encourages laminar flow in these airways, clearance of secretions by coughing will be impaired. Assuming the patient can develop an effective cough, this problem can be rectified by washing out the helium before coughing.

5. The only side effect directly attributable to helium is a benign one, but one that should be kept in mind. In the low-density gas the spoken word is badly distorted at a pitch so high as to make it almost unintelligible. This is of importance only to the conscious, nonintubated patient, who should be warned of the phenomenon and reassured that it will disappear within a few seconds after therapy ceases.

6. Because of helium's relatively high cost, systems that conserve the gas during therapy should be used. This cost factor and practical problems in administration have probably limited widespread use of helium-oxygen therapy.

Carbon dioxide therapy

Paradoxical though it may seem, a gas whose removal from the body occupies much of the respiratory care practitioner's attention and efforts is sometimes used therapeutically. The therapeutic inhalation of carbon dioxide is not extensive, but the practitioner may be called on to administer the gas or to apply rebreathing circuits frequently enough to necessitate becoming familiar with physiologic actions.

Respiratory response. Carbon dioxide is basically a respiratory center stimulant, but maximum stimulation is probably attained with the inhalation of a 10% concentration. Higher concentrations depress the respiratory center after initial stimulation.

Circulatory response. Two major effects circulatory effects are recognized. First, carbon dioxide evokes local tissue vasodilation through the metabolic mechanism discussed in Chapter 7. This effect is most profound in the brain, where carbon dioxide is the major factor governing cerebral blood flow.

Second, and more significant, carbon dioxide directly stimulates both the cardiovascular brain centers and the sympathetic nervous system. This results in the following centrally mediated responses:

1. Elevation of the systolic and diastolic blood pressures;
2. Increased heart rate;
3. Increased myocardial contractility; and
4. Constriction of skeletal smooth muscle.

Central nervous system response. Generally, low concentrations of carbon dioxide produce CNS stimulation, whereas high concentrations have a depressant effect. The administration of 5% carbon dioxide may produce mental confusion, and 10% may lead to loss of consciousness within as little as 10 minutes. At 30% or above, carbon dioxide becomes anesthetic. For this reason, 10% carbon dioxide mixtures should never be used for therapeutic purposes. Moreover, carbon dioxide must never be administered unless the patient is definitely known to have a responsive respiratory center. Failure to assure this responsiveness could result in a fatal hypercapnia and respiratory acidosis.

Clinical indications. The clinical indications for carbon dioxide therapy are limited. Most uses for this form of therapy have been replaced by safer and more effective modes of respiratory care. Nevertheless, because it may continue to be used, we briefly describe its therapeutic effects.

Improve cerebral blood flow. The use of carbon dioxide to overcome the cerebral vascular spasm associated with certain forms of cerebral vascular disease has a long history. Results have been less than satisfactory for two reasons. First, in patients with normal respiratory center responses, increases in ventilation minimize the desired elevation of Pco_2. Second, because many of the patients so treated have sclerosis of the cerebral vessels (as opposed to spasm), carbon dioxide has a negligible effect. However, ophthalmologists still use the gas to dilate vessels in the retina of the eye when thromboses have impaired the circulation.

Hyperinflate the lungs. Carbon dioxide has been used to stimulate deep breathing among selected patient categories, including postoperative patients and those who are otherwise unresponsive or obtunded. Like other modes of hyperinflation therapy, the primary goal is to prevent or reverse alveolar collapse and atelectasis. Caution must be employed in such instances to be sure that there is no underlying respiratory dysfunction. Unless the patient can respond to treatment by hyperventilation, not only is the therapy of no value but hypercapnia is a certainty. Modern techniques can usually perform this function better and much more safely than can carbon dioxide.

Abolish singulation (hiccup, hiccough). Although there are other methods of treating singulation, this condition is one of the most specific indications for carbon dioxide therapy. Singulation is an abnormal spasmodic constriction of the diaphragm against a closed glottis, under the stimulation of an irritated phrenic nerve. Such irritation can come from a host of conditions, including gastric distention or irritation, toxins, and metabolic upsets. Often, it plagues postoperative patients as well as those who suffer from debilitating diseases.[79] Prolonged hiccuping can produce severe physical fatigue, interfere with eating, and cause emotional distress.

We all know some of the traditional maneuvers for stopping hiccups, such as forced inspiratory breath holding, taking long drinks of water, and breathing into a paper bag. The efficacy of these maneuvers is based on a common factor: they all elevate alveolar carbon dioxide levels, thereby producing some degree of hypercapnia. This is what stops the hiccups. Subjecting the respiratory center to stimulation of hypercapnia supposedly initiates a rhythmic

discharge of impulses to the diaphragm that overrides the interposed spasmodic contractions and restores a normal breathing cycle. The administration of low concentrations of carbon dioxide usually accomplishes this more quickly and smoothly than the traditional methods described above and in most instances is effective in stopping the hiccups. Sometimes simple mechanical stimulation of the pharynx, with a catheter, will stop the attack through a reflex mediated by the vagus nerve. This technique has been used with success by anesthesiologists on patients suffering from postoperative hiccups. For some patients, combined therapy, including tranquilization, may be necessary to bring relief.

Precautions. Because carbon dioxide, like helium, does not support life, it must be used in combination with oxygen. In addition to its action as an asphyxiant, carbon dioxide produces toxic effects in excess dosage, and it must be given with great care. During its administration the practitioner must remain in constant attendance and watch the patient closely because individuals vary in their responses to the gas. Each department of respiratory care should establish its own procedures governing the use of carbon dioxide. At a minimum, these should ensure that (1) all treatments use mixtures with no more than 5% carbon dioxide and (2) no treatment exceed 10 minutes in duration.

The carbon dioxide mixture should be given with a well-fitted nonrebreathing mask, manually held to the patient's face so that it can be removed as necessary. The potential side effects of carbon dioxide administration include headache, dizziness, dyspnea, nasal irritation, palpitations, dimming of vision, muscle tremors, paresthesia, sensation of cold, and mental depression. These symptoms indicate a potentially adverse response and, if observed, should be grounds for immediate discontinuation of the therapy. Actual toxicity is manifested by severe dyspnea, nausea and vomiting, disorientation, and a dangerous elevation of blood pressure. When systolic blood pressure reaches 200 mm Hg, convulsions and cardiac failure can occur.

Carbon dioxide is contraindicated in patients with significant airway obstruction for two reasons. First, it is this type of patient who is most likely to have a less than normally responsive respiratory center and run the risk of hypercapnia. Second, with an active respiratory center the increased work of breathing under carbon dioxide stimulation against obstruction may more than negate any positive value of therapy.

SUMMARY

Medical gas therapy represents a major responsibility of the respiratory care practitioner. The safe and effective use of medical gases in general, and oxygen in particular, demands careful consideration of the patient's underlying disease process as the basis for determining an appropriate approach. Based on this foundation, the practitioner must be capable of matching a chosen modality to the patient's needs and of monitoring the patient's response according to the therapeutic goals chosen, with due consideration for potential hazards and contraindications.

REFERENCES

1. Nunn JF: Applied respiratory physiology, ed 2, London, 1977, Butterworth Publishers.
2. O'Donohue WJ Jr and Baker JP: Controlled low-flow oxygen for respiratory failure, Chest 63:818, 1973.
3. Petty TL: Intensive and rehabilitative respiratory care, ed 2, Philadelphia, 1974, Lea & Febiger.
4. Bone RC, Pierce AK, and Johnson RL: Controlled oxygen administration in acute respiratory failure in chronic obstructive pulmonary disease: a reappraisal, Am J Med 65:896, 1978.
5. Sykes MK, McNicol MW, and Campbell EJM: Respiratory failure, ed 2, Oxford, England, 1976, Blackwell Scientific Publications.
6. Hodgkin JE, editor: Chronic obstructive pulmonary disease: current concepts in diagnosis and comprehensive care, Park Ridge, Ill, 1979, American College of Chest Physicians.
7. Cullen JH and Kaemmerlen JT: Effect of oxygen administration at low rates of flow in hypercapneic patients, Am Rev Respir Dis 95:116, 1967.
8. Massaro DJ et al: Effect of various modes of oxygen administration on the arterial gas values in patients with respiratory acidosis, Br Med J 2:627, 1962.
9. Mithoefer JC: Indications for oxygen therapy in chronic obstructive pulmonary disease, Am Rev Respir Dis 110 (pt 2):35, 1974.
10. Hutchinson DCS et al: Controlled oxygen therapy in respiratory failure, Br Med J 2:1157, 1964.
11. West JB: Pulmonary pathophysiology—the essentials, Baltimore, 1977, Williams & Wilkins Co.
12. Smith CW, Lehan PH, and Monks JJ: Cardiopulmonary manifestations with high O_2 tensions at atmospheric pressure, J Appl Physiol 18:849, 1963.
13. West JB: Respiratory physiology: the essentials, ed 3, Baltimore, 1985, Williams & Wilkins Co.
14. Bates DV, Macklem PT, and Christie RV: Respiratory function in disease, Baltimore, 1971, WB Saunders Co.
15. Clark JM and Fisher AB: In Davis JC and Hunt TK, editors: Hyperbaric oxygen therapy, Bethesda, Md, 1977, Undersea Medical Society, Inc.
16. Pratt PC: Pathology of oxygen toxicity, Am Rev Respir Dis 110:51, 1974.
17. Clark JM: The toxicity of oxygen, Am Rev Respir Dis 110:40, 1974.
18. Winter PM and Smith G: The toxicity of oxygen, Anesthesiology 37:210, 1972.
19. Hyde RW and Rawson AJ: Unintentional iatrogenic oxygen pneumonitis—response to therapy, Ann Intern Med 71:517, 1969.
20. Petty TL, Stanford RE, and Neff TA: Continuous oxygen therapy in chronic airway obstruction: observations on possible oxygen toxicity and survival, Ann Intern Med 75:362, 1971.
21. Mustafa MG and Tierney DF: Biochemical and metabolic changes in the lung with oxygen, ozone and nitrogen dioxide toxicity: state of the art, Am Rev Respir Dis 118:1061, 1978.
22. Fridovich I: Oxygen: boon and bane, Am Sci 63:54, 1975.
23. Crapo JD: Superoxide dismutase and tolerance to pulmonary oxygen toxicity, Chest 67(suppl):39s, 1975.
24. McCord JM and Fridovich I: Superoxide dismutase, J Biol Chem 244:6049, 1969.
25. Babior BM et al: The production by leukocytes of superoxide: a potential bactericidal agent, J Clin Invest 53:741, 1973.
26. Curvette JT et al: Defect in pyridine nucleotide dependent superoxide production by a particulate fraction from the granulocytes of patients with chronic granulomatous diseases, N Engl J Med 293:628, 1975.
27. Hedley-Whyte, Burgess GE, Feeley TW, Miller MG: Applied physiology of respiratory care, Boston, 1976, Little, Brown & Co.
28. Laurenzi GA et al: Adverse effect of oxygen on tracheal mucus flow, N Engl J Med 279:333, 1978.
29. Klaus MH and Fanaroff AA, editors: Care of the high-risk neonate, ed 3, Philadelphia, 1986, WB Saunders Co.
30. Thibeault DW and Gregory GA, editors: Neonatal pulmonary care, ed 2, Menlo Park, Calif, 1986, Addison-Wesley Publishing Co, Inc.
31. Korones SB: High-risk newborn infants, ed 3, St Louis, 1981, The CV Mosby Co.
32. Kensey V, Jacobus J, and Hemphill F: Retrolental fibroplasia and the use of oxygen, Arch Ophthalmol 56:481, 1956.
33. Standards and Recommendations for Hospital Care of Newborn Infants, ed 6, Evanston, Ill, 1977, American Academy of Pediatrics.
34. Kobayashi and Murakami: Blindness of an adult caused by oxygen, JAMA 219:741, 1972.
35. Leigh JM: The evolution of oxygen therapy apparatus, Anaesthesia 29:462, 1974.
36. Demers RR: Oxygen delivery systems for use in acute respiratory failure, Respir Care 28:553, 1983.
37. Shapiro BA, Harrison RA, and Trout CA: Clinical application of respiratory care, ed 3, Chicago, 1985, Year Book Medical Publishers, Inc.
38. Leigh JM: Variation in performance of oxygen therapy devices, Anaesthesia 25:100, 1970.
39. Leigh JM: Variation in performance of oxygen therapy devices, Ann Royal Coll Surg 52:234, 1973.
40. Redding JS, McAfee DD, and Parham AM: Oxygen concentrations received from commonly used delivery systems, South Med J 71:169, 1978.
41. Kory RC et al: Comparative evaluation of oxygen therapy techniques, JAMA 179:767, 1962.
42. Poulton TJ, Comer PB, and Gibson RL: Tracheal oxygen concentrations with nasal cannula during oral and nasal breathing, Respir Care 25:739, 1980.
43. Gibson RL et al: Actual tracheal oxygen concentrations with commonly used oxygen equipment, Anesthesiology 44:71, 1976.
44. O'Donohue W: Oxygen conserving devices, Respir Care 32:37, 1987.
45. Rarey KP and Youtsey JW: Respiratory patient care, Englewood Cliffs, NJ, 1981, Prentice-Hall, Inc.
46. Collis JM and Berthune DW: Oxygen by face mask and nasal catheter, Lancet 1:787, 1967.
47. Committee on Public Health: A report: effective administration of inhalation therapy with special reference to ambulatory and emergency oxygen treatment, Bull NY Acad Med 38:135, 1962.
48. Barach AL and Eckman M: A mask apparatus which provides high concentrations with accurate control of the percentage of oxygen in the inspired air and without the accumulation of carbon dioxide, J Aviation Med 12:39, 1941.
49. Barach AL and Eckman M: A physiologically controlled oxygen mask apparatus, Anesthesiology 2:421, 1941.
50. Campbell EJM: A method of controlled oxygen administration which reduces the risk of carbon dioxide retention, Lancet 1:12, 1960.
51. McPherson SP: Oxygen percentage accuracy of air-entrainment masks, Respir Care 19:658, 1974.
52. Scacci R: Air entrainment masks; jet mixing is how they work; the Bernoulli and Venturi principles are how they don't, Respir Care 24:928, 1979.
53. Friedman SA et al: Effects of changing jet flows on oxygen concentrations in adjustable entrainment masks Respir Care 25:1266, 1980 (abstract).

54. Spearman CB et al: Effects of changing jet flow on oxygen concentrations in adjustable entrainment masks, Respir Care 15:1266, 1980 (abstract).
55. Riggs JH: Respiratory facts, Philadelphia, 1988, FA Davis Co.
56. Spier WA et al: Oxygen concentration delivered by Venturi masks with in-line humidification, JAMA 216:879, 1971.
57. Cohen JL et al: Air-entrainment masks: a performance evaluation, Respir Care 22:277, 1977.
58. Farney RJ et al: Oxygen therapy: appropriate use of nebulizers, Am Rev Respir Dis 115:567, 1977.
59. Klein EF, Mon BK, and Mon MJ: Oxygen accuracy with Venturi nebulizer systems, Crit Care Med 7:186, 1979 (abstract).
60. McPherson SP: Respiratory therapy equipment, ed 3, St Louis, 1985, The CV Mosby Co.
61. Durham Jr and Miller WF: Controlled oxygen administration with adequate humidification Inhal Ther 14:87, 1969.
62. Pierce AK: In Guenter CA and Welch MH, editors: Pulmonary medicine, Philadelphia, 1977, JB Lippincott Co.
63. Dawes GW and Williams TJ: The oxygen hood as a noise factor in infant care, Respir Care 24:12, 1979 (abstract).
64. Scopes J and Ahmed I: Ranges of critical temperatures in sick and premature newborn babies, Arch Dis Child 41:417, 1966.
65. Yeh TF et al: Oxygen consumption and insensible water loss in premature infants in single- versus double-walled incubators, J Pediatrics 97:967, 1980.
66. Marks KH et al: Oxygen consumption and temperature control of premature infants in a double-wall incubator, Pediatrics 68:93, 1981.
67. Wilson RS and Taver MB: Oxygen analysis: advances in methodology, Anesthesiology 37:112, 1972.
68. Bageant RA: Oxygen analyzers, Respir Care 21:410, 1979.
69. Nocturnal Oxygen Therapy Trial Group: Continuous or nocturnal oxygen therapy in hypoxemic chronic obstructive lung disease, Ann Intern Med 93:391, 1980.
70. Lenfant D: Twelve or 24-hour oxygen therapy: why a clinical trial? JAMA 243:551, 1980.
71. Petty TL et al: Outpatient oxygen therapy in chronic obstructive pulmonary disease: a review of 13 years' experience and an evaluation of modes of therapy, Arch Intern Med 139:28, 1979.
72. Davis JC and Hunt TK: Hyperbaric oxygen therapy, Bethesda, Md, 1977, Undersea Medical Society, Inc.
73. Egan DF: Therapeutic uses of helium, Conn Med 31:355, 1967.
74. Barach AL: The use of helium in the treatment of asthma and obstructive lesions of the larynx and trachea, Ann Intern Med 9:739, 1935.
75. Barach AL and Segal MS: In Weiss EG and Segal MS: Bronchial asthma: mechanisms and therapeutics, Boston, 1976, Little, Brown & Co.
76. Ishikawa and Segal MS: Re-appraisal of helium-oxygen therapy on patients with chronic lung disease, Ann Allergy 31:536, 1973.
77. Lu TS et al: Helium-oxygen in the treatment of upper airway obstruction, Anesthesiology 45:678, 1976.
78. Motley HL: Helium-oxygen therapy, Respir Care 18:668, 1973.
79. Souadjian J and Cain J: Intractable hiccup, Postgrad Med 43:72, 1968.

26

Hyperinflation Therapy

Alan M. Realey

Hyperinflation therapy includes a variety of respiratory care modalities designed to facilitate lung expansion. Historically, intermittent positive pressure breathing (IPPB) was used extensively for this purpose. More recently, incentive spirometry and the intermittent use of continuous positive airway pressure (CPAP) have been introduced as alternative hyperinflation methods.

Ongoing research on these methods continues to demonstrate mixed results. Clearly, certain benefits are derived by some patients, while other individuals or groups exhibit little or no positive outcomes. Current evidence suggest that positive outcomes of hyperinflation therapy should be expected only when patients are carefully selected and the approach chosen is administered and closely monitored by a skilled clinician.

In this context, the respiratory care practitioner must play a vital role. In consultation with the prescribing physician, the practitioner should assist in identifying those candidates most likely to benefit from hyperinflation therapy, recommend and initiate the appropriate therapeutic approach, monitor the patient's response, and alter the treatment regimen according to individual need.

OBJECTIVES

After completing this chapter, the reader should be able to:

1. Describe the physiologic principles underlying hyperinflation therapy;

2. Relate the indications for the various approaches to hyperinflation therapy to their clinical application;

3. Identify the potential detrimental effects and contraindications associated with the various modes of hyperinflation therapy;

4. Compare and contrast the key functional components of hyperinflation therapy equipment;

5. Delineate the primary responsibilities of the practitioner in the planning, implementation, and followup stages of hyperinflation therapy.

KEY TERMS

Most terms used in this chapter are defined in context. The following terms are introduced without explicit definition but may be found in the text glossary:

anecdotal	neurosurgery
cardiogenic	pneumomediastinum
cavitary	pneumonectomy
corroborating	pneumopericardium
diuresis	pneumotachygraph
fistula	prophylactic
hemoptysis	rebreathe
hemostasis	recontamination
impedance	subcutaneous
insufflation	submicronic
intra-alveolar	tracheoesophageal
intracranial	transudation
intrapleural	tourniquet
kyphoscoliosis	Valsalva maneuver
lobectomy	

PHYSIOLOGIC BASIS

All modes of hyperinflation therapy attempt to facilitate lung expansion by increasing the transpulmonary pressure gradient.[1,2] As detailed in Chapter 8, the transpulmonary pressure gradient (P_L) represents the difference between the intra-alveolar pressure, P_{alv}, and the intrapleural pressure, P_{pl}:

$$P_L = P_{alv} - P_{pl}$$

With all else constant, an increase in the transpulmonary pressure gradient will expand the alveoli and dilate the intrathoracic airways in direct proportion to the pressure difference created.

As shown in Fig. 26-1, the P_L can be increased by either (1) decreasing the P_{pl} (see Fig. 26-1, *A*) or (2) increasing the P_{alv} (see Fig. 26-1, *B*). A spontaneous deep inspiration will increase the P_L by decreasing the P_{pl}. On the other hand, positive pressure applied to the airway will increase the P_L by raising the P_{alv}.

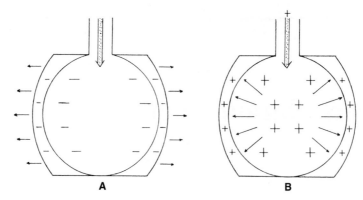

Fig. 26-1   Transpulmonary pressure gradients with spontaneous inspiration, **A,** and positive pressure inspiration, **B.**

Although both approaches are used in hyperinflation therapy, it should be clear that those methods that achieve higher P_L levels by decreasing P_{pl} are physiologically more normal than those that raise P_{alv}. As discussed in Chapter 7, negative intrapleural or intrathoracic pressures play an important role in facilitating venous return to the right heart. On the other hand, positive P_{alv} impedes this normal process and can actually decrease venous return and cardiac output. Moreover, positive P_{alv} may also compress the lung's vascular beds, thereby increasing pulmonary vascular resistance. Other physiologic effects of positive P_{alv}, especially those associated with long-term ventilatory support, are discussed in Chapter 29.

INTERMITTENT POSITIVE PRESSURE BREATHING

Historical overview

IPPB was introduced as a clinical modality by Motley and associates in 1947.[3] Since that time, IPPB has had a volatile history. During the early years after its introduction, IPPB enjoyed widespread use and acclamation. Physicians and respiratory care practitioners alike used IPPB for a broad range of clinical conditions and with various expectations regarding the outcome of therapy. By 1970, despite the fact that little scientific evidence was available to support its use, IPPB became the predominant mode of respiratory care.

Slowly, the pendulum began to shift in the other direction. In 1974, at a conference entitled "The Scientific Basis of Respiratory Therapy," participants concluded that current clinical knowledge provided little support for the widespread use of IPPB.[4] Five years later, at a follow-up conference on in-hospital respiratory therapy, IPPB was again identified as an overused treatment modality.[5]

In the face of growing criticism from within the respiratory care community,[6,7] the Respiratory Care Committee of the American Thoracic Society (ATS) prepared guidelines for the use of IPPB, supporting its rational use in cer-

tain clearly defined clinical situations.[8] More recently, the American Association for Respiratory Care disseminated a statement asserting the effectiveness of IPPB in several, very specific clinical situations.[9]

Apparently, the pendulum has begun to swing back toward a more moderate view on the applicability and effectiveness of IPPB. Clearly, this treatment modality can be effective when appropriately chosen and administered, and it should not be totally condemned or universally applied. Like so many other respiratory care modalities, the effective application of IPPB requires that (1) patients be carefully chosen, (2) indications for therapy be clearly delineated, (3) goals of therapy be clearly understood, and (4) treatment be properly administered by a trained respiratory care practitioner.

Definition and physiologic principle

Although many of the principles involved are similar, IPPB must not be confused with continuous ventilatory support (see Chapters 29 and 30). Continuous ventilatory support involves the long-term application of positive pressure through an artificial airway to patients with acute respiratory failure. IPPB, on the other hand, refers to the application of inspiratory positive pressure, usually with accompanying humidity or aerosol therapy, to a spontaneously breathing patient as a short-term treatment modality, usually for no longer than 15 to 20 minutes. These treatments may be administered several times each day, sometimes as frequently as once every hour.[8,10]

Figs. 26-2 and 26-3 compare P_{alv} and P_{pl} during spontaneous breathing and IPPB administration. During the inspiratory phase of spontaneous breathing, the drop in P_{pl} caused by expansion of the thorax is transmitted to the alveoli, creating a transrespiratory pressure gradient (P_{rs}) equivalent to the difference between the pressure at the airway opening (P_{ao}) and P_{alv}:

$$P_{rs} = P_{ao} (0) - P_{alv} \text{ (negative)}$$

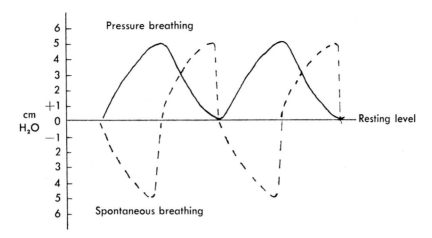

Fig. 26-2 Comparison of intra-alveolar pressure in positive pressure and spontaneous tidal ventilation with driving pressures of 5 cm of water.

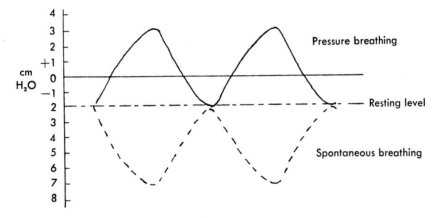

Fig. 26-3 Comparison of intrapleural pressure in positive pressure and spontaneous tidal ventilation with driving pressures of 5 cm of water.

The magnitude of alveolar expansion, and therefore the volume of gas that will flow into the alveoli during a spontaneous inspiration, is proportional to the difference between the P_{alv} and P_{pl} at end inspiration, or to P_L:

$$\text{Alveolar expansion} \cong P_L \text{ (end inspiration)}$$
$$\cong P_{alv} - P_{pl}$$

During spontaneous expiration, as the lungs and chest wall recoil, P_{pl} becomes less negative and P_{alv} rises above atmospheric. This reverses the transrespiratory pressure gradient (P_{alv} becomes greater than P_{ao}), causing gas flow from the alveoli out to the airway opening.

The application of IPPB to the airway reverses the events of inspiration. Rather than being generated by a negative P_{alv} the P_{rs} is created by the application of positive pressure to the airway:

$$P_{rs} = P_{ao} \text{ (positive)} - P_{alv} \text{ (0)}$$

Again, gas flows from the airway opening to the alveoli. However, P_{alv} *rises* during the inspiratory phase of IPPB. This rise also creates a transpulmonary pressure gradient thereby expanding the alveoli. However, compared with spontaneous inspiration, the pressure gradient is reversed. Because P_{alv} is greater than P_{pl} during IPPB, positive pressure is transmitted from the alveoli to the intrapleural space, causing a rise in P_{pl} during inspiration. Depending on the lung's mechanical properties, P_{pl} may actually exceed atmospheric pressure during a portion of inspiration.

As with spontaneous breathing, the recoil force of the lung and chest wall, stored as potential energy during the positive pressure breath, causes a passive exhalation. As gas flows from the alveoli out to the airway opening, P_{alv} drops to atmospheric level, while P_{pl} is restored to its normal subatmospheric range.

Indications for IPPB

In the past, IPPB therapy was administered for a host of reasons, some well substantiated and others without any sound clinical or physiologic basis. Today, this cavalier approach in no longer acceptable. As previously stated, the selection of IPPB as a legitimate treatment modality must be supported by corroborating patient data that clearly indicate a potential benefit. Moreover, IPPB should not be used when a less complex or less expensive modality can be used as effectively. Alternative modes of hyperinflation therapy are discussed later in this chapter.

Indications for IPPB therapy can be divided into three general categories. Category I indications include those clinical situations for which substantiating evidence has demonstrated tangible clinical benefits for IPPB administration. Category II indications include those clinical problems for which IPPB may be useful as an adjunct to other established modes of therapy. Category III indications include situations in which IPPB may be useful but for which no sound substantiating evidence exists. The box below lists these various indications according to these three categories.

Category I indications. Category I indications include the treatment of atelectasis, impending hypercapneic respiratory failure, and the decreased compliance associated with certain restrictive disorders of the thoracic cage.

Atelectasis. IPPB has been successfully employed to treat atelectasis associated with the failure to take deep breaths. Patients who have difficulty in taking deep breaths without assistance include those with neuromuscular disorders, those who are heavily sedated, and those with pain. Frequently, this pain is the result of an abdominal or thoracic surgical procedure. Compounding the effects of the pain itself is the tendency of postoperative patients to contract or "splint" muscles in the incisional area voluntarily,

thereby further decreasing tidal volumes (V_T) and precluding spontaneous deep breaths.

This repetitive, shallow breathing is a major contributing factor in the development of postoperative pulmonary complications. As many as 70% of patients who have undergone upper abdominal surgery exhibit clinical signs of postoperative atelectasis.[11,12]

It is well known that the normal pattern of breathing includes intermittent sighs, occurring as frequently as every 5 to 6 minutes. At times, this sigh volume approaches the inspiratory capacity. This mechanism, along with the ability to cough effectively and clear pulmonary secretions, is vital to maintaining normal lung function. Often the postoperative patient loses the normal sign mechanism, resulting in a progressive decrease in functional residual capacity and the development of atelectasis (Fig. 26-4). Compounding this problem is the inability of many postoperative patients to develop an effective cough, thereby compromising normal clearance mechanisms.

In concept, a correctly administered IPPB treatment should provide these patients with augmented V_T levels, achieved with minimal effort. In fact, an aggressive respiratory therapy regimen that includes IPPB has been shown to be as effective as therapeutic bronchoscopy in treating patients with lobar atelectasis.[11] The optimal breathing pattern to reinflate collapsed lung units with IPPB consists of slow, deep breaths that are sustained or held at end-inspiration. This type of inspiratory maneuver increases the distribution of inspired gas to areas of the lung with low compliance, specifically, the atelectatic areas.

Although the application of IPPB to treat atelectasis is well substantiated, its use prophylactically to prevent the occurrence of this postoperative complication is not well supported.[13] For this reason, the use of IPPB to prevent atelectasis falls under the category III indications.

Impending respiratory failure. IPPB is also indicated as a preliminary measure in the treatment of impending hypercapneic respiratory failure (also called ventilatory failure), specifically that associated with acute exacerbations of chronic obstructive pulmonary disease (COPD). By providing augmented V_T levels, bronchodilation, and improved secretion clearance, IPPB may preclude the necessity for endotracheal intubation and continuous ventilatory support.[9,14] Augmented V_T levels can increase minute ventilation ($\dot{V}_E$), thereby lowering arterial carbon dioxide levels and reversing the worsening respiratory acidosis that characterizes this clinical problem. IPPB may also improve the distribution of ventilation, resulting in better arterial blood oxygenation. The bronchodilatory effect of IPPB can be both mechanical and pharmacologic. The application of positive pressure physically dilates the airways during inspiration, thus helping to distribute inspired gases to areas of the lung previously obstructed with secretions. In addition, bronchodilating agents may be given at appropriate intervals to further decrease airway resistance

---

INDICATIONS FOR IPPB

CATEGORY I (SUBSTANTIATING EVIDENCE SUPPORTS USE)

Treatment of clinically diagnosed atelectasis
Management of impending hypercapneic respiratory failure
Treatment of decreased lung compliance in kyphoscoliosis

CATEGORY II (IPPB MAY BE USEFUL AS ADJUNCTIVE THERAPY)

Enhancement of aerosol drug administration through improved breathing patterns
Treatment of cardiogenic pulmonary edema

CATEGORY III (IPPB MAY BE USEFUL; FURTHER EVIDENCE NEEDED)

Prevention of atelectasis
Management of acute bronchospasm
To decrease the work of breathing

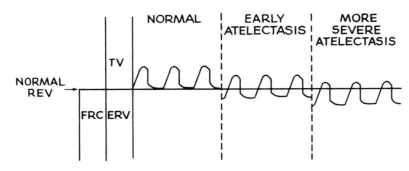

Fig. 26-4 Effect of progressive alveolar collapse on resting expiratory volume (REV). Note that as atelectasis becomes more severe, the tidal volume progressively encroaches on the expiratory reserve volume. Similarly, the level of the resting expiratory volume is displaced downward. (From Sanderson RG: The cardiac patient: a comprehensive approach, ed 2, Philadelphia, 1983, WB Saunders Co.)

(Raw). In combination with aggressive bronchial hygiene measures, increased VT levels and bronchodilation may contribute to improved clearance of pulmonary secretions.[14]

In this manner, the patient suffering from an acute exacerbation of chronic lung disease may be stabilized sufficiently to treat the underlying problem without committing to long-term ventilatory support. Stabilization of such patients may require that treatments be given as frequently as every hour. However, given the poor outcomes and high cost of long-term ventilatory support in these patients, early and aggressive intervention with IPPB during an acute exacerbation of chronic lung disease represents a sound clinical decision.

This approach is not indicated for the hypercapneic patient with full metabolic compensation. Rapid reduction of the Paco₂ in such patients may impose an acute "metabolic" alkalosis on top of their compensated state.[14] IPPB therapy should be directed only toward the patient suffering from impending respiratory failure who is developing an acute-on-chronic respiratory acidosis.

Restrictive disorders. Appropriately applied IPPB has also demonstrated tangible benefits in treating certain restrictive disorders associated with chest wall abnormalities. Specifically, IPPB has been shown to temporarily improve pulmonary mechanics in patients with kyphoscoliosis.

Patients with kyphoscoliosis exhibit both reduced thoracic and pulmonary compliance. Until recently, the decreased lung compliance noted in these patients was believed to be irreversible. However, it recently has been demonstrated that IPPB with high inflation pressures can increase lung compliance (CL) in these patients by an average of 70%.[15] Although temporary, this increase in CL may last up to 3 hours. For the patient with kyphoscoliosis, this effect will decrease the work of breathing during the period of improved CL.

Category II indications. Clinical problems for which IPPB may be useful as an adjunct to other established modes of therapy include its use to facilitate the administration of aerosolized drugs and in the treatment of cardiogenic pulmonary edema.

Aerosol drug administration. The most common current modes of aerosol drug administration are the small-volume pneumatic nebulizer and the metered dose inhaler (MDI). As delineated in Chapter 23, the effectiveness with which these devices deposit aerosolized drugs in the respiratory tract is mainly a function of the patient's breathing pattern. Optimal aerosol deposition occurs only when the patient breathes slowly and deeply, with a breath hold at the end of inspiration.[14] If a patient is unable to maintain this breathing pattern, it is unlikely that the administration of bronchodilators or other medications through these devices will be effective.

The respiratory pattern displayed by pain-stricken postoperative patients or those in acute respiratory distress often results in lower than normal VT levels and higher than normal respiratory rates. Moreover, such patients have difficulty in maintaining a end-inspiratory pause of any significant duration. Under these conditions, aerosol administration through a small-volume pneumatic nebulizer or MDI will result in a larger than normal amount of the aerosolized drugs being deposited in the upper airways or simply wasted on exhalation.

In situations such as these, IPPB may be employed to facilitate restoration and maintenance of a breathing pattern more conducive to aerosol drug administration.[14] Just as with small-volume pneumatic nebulizers, however, the dosage of any pharmacologic agent delivered by nebulization through an IPPB circuit is unpredictable. Indeed, inappropriately applied IPPB may be a less effective vehicle for aerosolized administration of drugs than other simpler methods, even in patients not able to maintain an optimal breathing pattern. For this reason, the decision to use IPPB as an alternative method of aerosol drug administration should be based on clear evidence that the patient is unable to employ effectively a small-volume pneumatic nebulizer or MDI and on the availability of personnel skilled in its use.

Treatment of cardiogenic pulmonary edema. Cardiogenic pulmonary edema is associated with failure of the left ventricle, resulting in increased end-diastolic pressures that are transmitted back to the pulmonary circulation. These increased pulmonary vascular pressures cause fluid transudation across the alveolar-capillary membrane, acutely impairing pulmonary gas exchange. Treatment of cardiogenic pulmonary edema aims at reducing pulmonary vascular pressures by lowering the left ventricular end-diastolic pressure. In addition to the use of potent pharmacologic agents to increase left ventricular performance and enhance diuresis, various techniques have been employed to encourage venous pooling in the capacitance vessels of the circulatory system, thereby effectively reducing circulating blood volume.

Within this context, IPPB was introduced in the 1930s as an adjunctive treatment for cardiogenic pulmonary edema.[16-20] The use of IPPB in acute pulmonary edema is directed toward decreasing the work of breathing, treating the hypoxemia, and retarding venous return. The treatment of hypoxemia is of the highest priority, and very high concentrations of oxygen are often needed to correct the problem. During episodes of acute cardiogenic pulmonary edema, the respiratory care practitioner should immediately administer 100% oxygen while other personnel take other measures.

In attempting to reduce venous return, various measures have been employed. Phlebotomy, or the physical removal of blood from the circulation, is one method of reducing venous return. However, this is a hazardous practice, especially for patients who may already be hypotensive. For this reason, phlebotomy is seldom, if ever, employed to treat acute pulmonary edema. The application of rotating tourniquets applied to the extremities is a more common adjunct approach to decreasing venous return during the acute phase of pulmonary edema.

The application of IPPB in cardiogenic pulmonary edema is based on the retarding effect positive pressure has on venous return to the right heart. IPPB is certainly simpler than other mechanical methods of causing venous pooling, and it can potentially help alleviate the accompanying problems of hypoxemia and high work of breathing associated with acute pulmonary edema.

In employing IPPB for this purpose, the goal is to maximize safely—rather than minimize—intrathoracic pressures. Pressures of 40 cm H_2O or higher may used to enhance the effects of the positive pressure on the capacitance vessels, possibly in conjunction with an inflation hold. In addition, from 5 to 15 ml of 30% to 50% ethyl alcohol can be nebulized simultaneously through the IPPB circuit to destabilize the bubbly edema secretions, reducing them to a liquid state to increase their ease of removal.[21] Although the introduction of rapidly acting diuretics and the improved preventative management of left ventricular failure have reduced the need for this approach, IPPB remains an effective adjunct in the management of

cardiogenic pulmonary edema.[14] Nonetheless, as with any technique designed to reduce venous return artificially, care must be taken to avoid too great a reduction in cardiac output, which ultimately may impair tissue perfusion.

Category III indications. Situations in which IPPB may be useful, but for which no sound substantiating evidence exists, include the prevention of atelectasis, the treatment of acute bronchospasm, and as a method to decrease the work of breathing.

Prevention of atelectasis. As previously discussed, sound evidence supports the use of IPPB in the management of clinically diagnosed atelectasis, but its use as a prophylactic measure to prevent its occurrence is lacking.

Acute bronchospasm. Because of the dilatory effect of positive pressure on the intrathoracic airways, IPPB has been proposed as a useful intervention in the treatment of acute airway obstruction resulting from bronchospasm. In concept, this approach has a sound physiologic basis. However, there is no substantiating clinical evidence to support its use exclusively for this purpose. Part of the problem is the confounding influence of the oxygen and aerosolized bronchodilator therapy typically employed with IPPB in these situations. Moreover, clinical case reports have demonstrated that IPPB alone actually can result in bronchospasm and increased airway resistance in some patients.[14]

Decreased work of breathing. If IPPB is properly administered by a skilled respiratory care practitioner, the positive pressure applied to the airways during inspiration can supply nearly all the work necessary for each breath. Unfortunately, this effect lasts only as long as the treatment itself and thus is of dubious clinical value unless related measures are concurrently applied. Moreover, as with the treatment of bronchospasm, the confounding effects of oxygen and aerosolized bronchodilator therapy on reducing the work of breathing and relieving the accompanying dyspnea have never been addressed. Also, the improper administration of IPPB can actually increase the work of breathing, resulting in further dyspnea, anxiety, and agitation in the patient.[14]

Detrimental effects of IPPB

Consideration of IPPB as a treatment modality for specific patients should go beyond the simple consideration of need. As with any clinical intervention, certain detrimental effects or potential hazards are associated with the application of IPPB. These potential problems should be addressed in the initial stages of planning the treatment regimen and must be considered throughout the course of therapy as part of the process of assessing the patient for unwanted side effects. The box on p. 639 lists the major potential side effects of IPPB therapy. The following discussion highlights these problems and the respiratory care practitioner's related responsibilities.

Decreased cardiac output. As previously discussed, cardiac output may be decreased by applying positive pres-

---

POTENTIAL HAZARDS OF IPPB ADMINISTRATION

Decreased cardiac output
Pulmonary barotrauma
Gastric insufflation
Hyperventilation
Reactive bronchospasm
Infection
Psychologic dependence

---

sure to the thorax. Physiologically, increased intrapleural pressures can impede venous return to the right side of the heart, thereby decreasing its total output. In healthy individuals, some cardiovascular compensation occurs through increased venomotor tone, decreasing the magnitude of this effect. However, if this compensatory response is lacking, or if the patient is already hypotensive, IPPB can dramatically lower cardiac output. For this reason, respiratory care practitioners administering IPPB should conduct a preliminary bedside assessment of the patient's cardiovascular status and monitor high-risk patients throughout the treatment for the signs and symptoms of compromised cardiovascular function.

Pulmonary barotrauma. The high pressures and high volumes associated with some forms of IPPB therapy can cause lung tissue damage, referred to as pulmonary barotrauma. The likelihood of this problem is probably highest in patients with chronic obstructive disorders, especially those with bullous emphysema. In these patients, failure to provide a sufficient expiratory time may result in further gas trapping, greater overinflation, and, in some instances, actual pneumothorax. Air under pressure also may leak into other areas of the body, resulting in subcutaneous emphysema, pneumomediastinum, or pneumopericardium. Again, careful preassessment and ongoing monitoring are vital in preventing pulmonary barotrauma and, if necessary, in responding to its occurrence.

Gastric insufflation. When positive pressure is applied to the pharynx, the esophagus can open and gas can pass directly into the stomach. The exact pressure at which this occurs, called the *esophageal opening pressure,* is not known with precision but is estimated to range from 20 to 25 cm H_2O. Pressures in or above this range may therefore cause gastric insufflation.

Uncommon in the alert and cooperative patient, gastric insufflation with IPPB is a real problem in the neurologically obtunded. Moreover, the problem occurs most frequently during IPPB therapy administered by mask. Gastric insufflation by itself is a minor inconvenience. The most worrisome result of excess air in the stomach is the potential for vomiting and pulmonary aspiration of stomach contents. Proper instruction and supervision of cooperative patients and the avoidance of pressures higher than

necessary to achieve the desired goal should generally minimize the likelihood of this adverse effect. For the obtunded patient receiving IPPB by mask, a functioning nasogastric tube must be in place.

Hyperventilation. Patients tend breathe more rapidly than desired during initial IPPB administration. Since V_T levels are also being augmented, a large increase in $\dot{V}_E$ can result, causing an acute hypocapnia. Moreover, in some chronically hypercapnic patients, abrupt lowering of the Pa_{CO_2} may result in a period of posttreatment hypoventilation and a profound hypoxemia.

In general, keeping the respiratory rate between six to eight breaths per minute will minimize the likelihood of hyperventilation during IPPB. Nonetheless, the practitioner must remain with the patient throughout the treatment and be on guard for the signs and symptoms of hypocapnea. These signs and symptoms include dizziness and numbness or tingling of the extremities (paresthesia).

Bronchospasm. As previously discussed, IPPB without accompanying bronchodilator therapy may result in bronchospasm, especially in those patients with hyperreactive airways. In known asthmatics and others with increased potential for bronchospasm, a bronchodilator must always be administered along with the IPPB treatment. Bland aerosols alone are not recommended, since these may result in bronchospasm in some patients.

Infection. It is well documented that respiratory therapy equipment can be a source of hospital-acquired infection.[22] The use of disposable circuits and proper handwashing technique are vital to prevent infection. To prevent recontamination of the airways, disposable circuits should be changed at least every 24 to 48 hours. The IPPB device itself should be disassembled, when practical, and disinfected on a regular basis. Last, only sterile diluents and medications should be used for aerosolization.

Psychologic dependence. Some patients may come to rely on the psychologic benefits of IPPB even in the absence of proved physiologic effect. Many patients who have been using IPPB for years clearly would receive the same benefits with simpler and less costly approaches. However, habit and psychologic attachment preclude changing the treatment regimen without considerable resistance. Patience and understanding must be displayed in dealing with such patients.

Contraindications for IPPB

In several clinical situations logic dictates that IPPB should not be used (see box on p. 640). Most of these contraindications are derived from anecdotal case reports rather than empirical studies. However, as with all procedures, a sound knowledge of the patient's condition and the indications for and expected outcomes of treatment—tempered with common sense—should guide the practitioner in the decision-making process.

Lack of adequate, skilled supervision. Many of the reported failures associated with IPPB administration are

---

CONTRAINDICATIONS TO IPPB ADMINISTRATION

ABSOLUTE CONTRAINDICATIONS

Lack of adequate, skilled supervision
Availability of simpler, equally effective approach
Tension pneumothorax

RELATIVE CONTRAINDICATIONS

History of pneumothorax
Pulmonary air leak
Recent lobectomy/pneumonectomy
Pulmonary hemorrhage
Cardiovascular insufficiency
Increased intracranial pressure
Air trapping
Active local lung infection (tuberculosis)
Lack of patient cooperation

---

partly a result of the lack of adequate, skilled supervision. As previously noted, the success of this form of therapy depends on careful preliminary planning, effective patient teaching, and skillful application under the watchful eye of a knowledgeable practitioner. IPPB is strictly contraindicated when these most basic conditions cannot be met.

Availability of simpler, equally effective approaches. Equally important as an absolute contraindication to IPPB is the availability of alternative approaches that are simpler, less costly, and at least as effective in achieving the established therapeutic goal. Of course, this decision must be based on careful assessment of the patient's clinical problem and status as related to the overall need for respiratory care.

Tension pneumothorax. The only other absolute contraindication for IPPB is a tension pneumothorax without a functioning chest tube in place. Clearly, this presents a life-threatening situation. Continuation of an IPPB treatment in this circumstance may lead to compression of the heart and great vessels, resulting in complete cardiopulmonary collapse. Common sense dictates that IPPB could serve no purpose but to intensify an already existing medical emergency.

History of pneumothorax. Initiating an IPPB regimen on a patient with a known history of pneumothorax necessitates that great skill and keen observation be employed by the practitioner. Pressures and volumes must be kept within acceptable limits. Inspiratory flows should be kept to a minimum while adequate expiratory time is allowed to prevent gas trapping.

Pulmonary air leak. Patients with subcutaneous emphysema or other forms of pulmonary air leak may not be candidates for IPPB. Careful evaluation of the costs and benefits associated with therapy must be made before initi-

ating treatment on these patients. Any of the several manifestations of pulmonary air leak must be considered a relative contraindication to IPPB therapy.

Recent lobectomy or pneumonectomy. Some practitioners feel that exposing the airways to positive pressure soon after lobectomy or pneumonectomy may damage the excision site and cause air leakage. The latter problem is of minor consequence, since these patients normally have a chest tube in place postoperatively. Of course, spontaneous deep breathing poses the same potential danger for these patients as IPPB and is not normally contraindicated after such surgery. However, depending on the goals of therapy, simpler and less hazardous approaches should be considered first.

Pulmonary hemorrhage. If active bleeding is occurring from pulmonary tissue, positive pressure may further aggravate the situation. If IPPB is indicated in a patient with pulmonary hemorrhage, emphasis first should be placed on identifying the source of bleeding and providing hemostasis. Massive hemoptysis is a medical emergency in which there is no logical rationale for hyperinflation therapy of any kind.

Cardiovascular insufficiency. Patients with preexisting cardiovascular insufficiency are poor candidates for IPPB. Therefore, marked hypotension of any kind, systemic hemorrhage, and myocardial infarction represent relative contraindications to the application of positive pressure to the airway. In these situations, it is essential that the practitioner weigh the benefits of therapy against the potential hazards for each patient.

Increased intracranial pressure. IPPB's effect on venous return is not limited to the thoracic venous system. Positive pressure in the thorax also can retard cerebral venous return. Because the brain is enclosed in a "fixed" container, impedance to the outflow of blood will cause engorgement of the cerebral circulation and potentially increase intracranial pressures. In instances where increased intracranial pressures are problematic, such as after neurosurgery or brain trauma, IPPB generally is contraindicated.

Air trapping. In patients with COPD who also exhibit marked pulmonary distention, the application of IPPB may aggravate preexisting air trapping. Overdistention of the lung tissue resulting from air trapping may result in an increased incidence of barotrauma and cardiovascular embarrassment. Air trapping is most likely to occur when inspiratory flows are incorrectly set and insufficient time is provided for exhalation. Mechanically retarding exhalation—thereby lengthening the expiratory phase and preventing early small airway closure—may help but is not always successful. Moreover, expiratory retarding raises mean pleural pressures, increasing the possibility of detrimental cardiovascular effects and pulmonary barotrauma.

Tracheoesophageal fistula. This rare condition, usually congenital, normally is corrected surgically as soon as it is

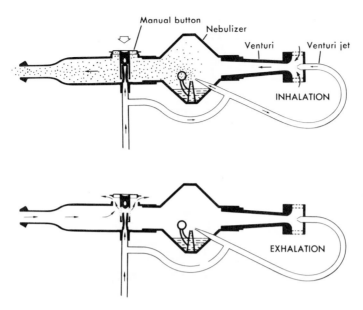

Fig. 26-5 Functional diagram of Bird Asthmastik. (Courtesy Bird Corp, Palm Springs, Calif. From McPherson SP: Respiratory therapy equipment, ed 3, St Louis, 1985, The CV Mosby Co.)

diagnosed. Moreover, the majority of patients with a tracheoesophageal fistula (neonates) are seldom, if ever, candidates for IPPB. However, if positive pressure were applied to the airway of these patients, gas could enter the esophagus, resulting in gastric insufflation. In reality, this problem is associated mainly with the long-term ventilatory support of infants awaiting surgical intervention and normally is addressed by endotracheal intubation.

Active tuberculosis. It has been suggested that IPPB may cause the spread of localized pulmonary infections such as tuberculosis. Although no documentation exists to prove this, the reader should be aware that active tuberculosis may be cited as a relative contraindication in some centers. A more rational reason to delimit the use of IPPB in these cases may be the potential to disrupt the cavitary lesions characterizing the advanced stages of untreated tuberculosis.

Lack of patient cooperation. By now it should be clear that patient understanding and cooperation are vital to the success of IPPB therapy. Patients who cannot or will not cooperate in the treatment are candidates for alternative modes of therapy. Although IPPB can be delivered to these patients with a face mask, the potential hazards of this approach far outweigh any likely benefits of the therapy.

Equipment

IPPB devices are mechanical ventilators and function according to the principles applicable to this category of respiratory care equipment (see Chapters 29 and 30). However, machines designed for the sole purpose of delivering IPPB treatments generally are much simpler in design and function. In this section, we will discuss the gen-

eral characteristics of IPPB devices and look at a few representative examples of devices used for this purpose. More detailed descriptions of the design and functional characteristics of the many IPPB devices in current use are available elsewhere.[23]

General characteristics. IPPB devices are usually powered by either a 50 psig pressure source or an electrical compressor. All function as *assistors,* allowing the patient to determine when inspiration under positive pressure begins. Inspiration may be terminated either manually (as determined by the patient) or when a predetermined pressure is reached at the airway. IPPB devices that end inspiration when a predetermined pressure is reached are termed *pressure-cycled.*

All IPPB devices also incorporate either a true Venturi or air entrainment jet to enhance flow capabilities. The breathing circuit of IPPB devices generally includes a nebulizer (for administration of aerosols) and an exhalation valve that provides a route for expired gases to be vented to the atmosphere.

Manually cycled IPPB devices. Manually cycled IPPB devices include a simple valve mechanism or port that the patient manually closes to begin inhalation and opens to begin exhalation. Typically, an aneroid manometer monitors inspiratory pressure. The peak or end-inspiratory pressure achieved by a manually cycled IPPB device primarily depends on the duration of the inspiratory phase, as determined by the patient.

Examples of manually cycled IPPB devices include the Ohio Hand-E-Vent and the Bird Asthmastick. A functional diagram of the Bird Asthmastick is shown in Fig. 26-5. During inhalation, closure of the manual button by the patient diverts a compressed gas source to a mainstream neb-

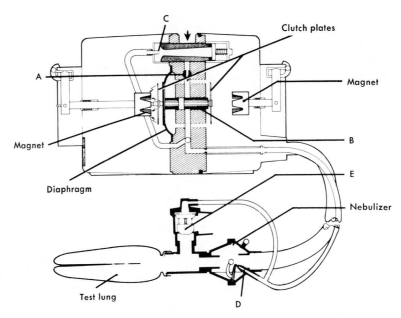

Fig. 26-6   Structure of Bird Mark 7. (Courtesy Bird Corp, Palm Springs, Calif. From McPherson SP: Respiratory therapy equipment, ed 3, St Louis, 1985, The CV Mosby Co.)

ulizer and a Venturi jet. As long as the button is depressed, source gas and entrained air flow through the nebulizer to the patient through a mouthpiece. Exhalation is begun when the patient releases the button, opening an outlet to the atmosphere. With this exhalation valve open, both source gas and the patient's expired gases readily flow out to the atmosphere, until the next inhalation is manually cycled.

Oxygen concentrations available with manually cycled IPPB devices depend on the power source. Obviously, when driven by an air compressor, an F_{IO_2} of 0.21 is provided. Concentrations above this level can only be achieved by providing a supplemental flow of oxygen into the system.

When driven by 100% oxygen, the F_{IO_2} delivered by a manually cycled IPPB devices varies according to the amount of air entrained at the Venturi or jet. Because air entrainment decreases as pressure in the system increases, F_{IO_2} levels are neither stable nor predictable. In general, however, the higher the end-inspiratory pressure and the longer the inspiratory time, the greater the average F_{IO_2}.

Compared with other equipment used to deliver IPPB treatments, manually cycled IPPB devices are simple, dependable, and generally easy for patients to use. On the other hand, they provide limited practitioner control over the parameters of ventilation and can only be used by patients demonstrating a minimum basic level of skill and coordination.

Patient cycled IPPB devices. Whereas manually cycled IPPB equipment requires that a port be activated by hand, patient-cycled devices incorporate a valve that responds directly to pressure differences generated during breathing.

Typically, such valves not only initiate gas flow at the beginning of inhalation but also terminate inhalation once a predetermined pressure is achieved.

Although differing significantly in design characteristics, these valves all function in a similar manner. As a patient begins inspiration, the valve "senses" the drop in pressure and opens to allow gas flow under pressure. As gas continues to flow during inspiration, pressure at the airway and in the system rises. This increase in pressure also is "sensed" by the valve, which closes when the pressure reaches a certain critical level that is preset by the practitioner.

How much negative pressure is required to open the breathing valve and begin inhalation determines the *sensitivity* of the device. Depending on the design of the device, sensitivity may be fixed or adjustable. The amount of pressure required to close the valve, thereby initiating exhalation, is called the pressure limit and is always adjustable, typically up to 30 to 60 cm H_2O. Because ventilators are categorized mainly according to the mechanism ending inspiration (see Chapter 29), these devices are commonly referred to as pressure-cycled ventilators.

The two most common valve designs used in patient-cycled IPPB equipment are the sliding alignment valve and the rotary alignment valve. Bird IPPB devices typify the sliding alignment valve concept. On the other hand, Bennett equipment incorporates the rotary alignment principle. For purposes of comparison, we will provide a brief overview of the functional characteristics of each.

Sliding alignment valve (Bird). A typical Bird ventilator (the Mark 7) is shown in Fig. 26-6. Gas from a 50 psig source flows into the top of the unit (downward arrow), immediately encountering a variable flow control valve, *A*. Distal to the flow control valve is the ceramic sliding alignment valve, *B*. As shown, the valve is shifted to the left, such that its center passage is misaligned with the source gas stream, blocking further flow (the "off" position).

Connected to either end of the valve are metallic plates, called clutch plates, each in proximity to a permanent magnet. The distance between the magnets and the clutch plates can be varied by threaded control levers to either side of the device.

The left and right sides of the device are separated by a flexible diaphragm, which is attached to the alignment valve. Because the left side of the device is open to the atmosphere, it is called the ambient chamber. The right side, or pressure chamber, is continuous with the breathing circuit and patient airway (test lung in this example).

When the patient begins inspiration, negative pressure is transmitted through the breathing circuit back to the pressure chamber, creating a pressure difference across the flexible diaphragm that tends to pull it—and the alignment valve—to the right. However, the attractive force between the left clutch plate and the left magnet opposes movement of the diaphragm, in direct proportion to the distance between the two. If the negative pressure in the pressure chamber is sufficient to overcome this magnetic force, the diaphragm will move to the right, aligning the center passageway of the valve with the main stream of gas and initiating the inspiratory cycle.

Exactly how much negative pressure must be generated by the patient to initiate inspiration (the sensitivity of the device) is determined by the distance between the ambient chamber clutch plate and magnet, as set by the practitioner. The closer the clutch plate and magnet, the greater the negative pressure—and patient effort—necessary to move the diaphragm and open the valve.

Once the sliding alignment valve opens, source gas normally takes two routes. Some goes directly to a Venturi jet, *C*, while the remainder is diverted to the mainstream nebulizer jet, *D*, and exhalation valve chamber, *E*. Pressurization of the exhalation valve forces it closed, preventing gas outflow during inspiration.

As pressure in the pressure chamber rises during inspiration, the flexible diaphragm tends to bow back toward the left. However, its movement is opposed by the attraction between the pressure chamber clutch plate and magnet. Exactly how much positive pressure must be generated to end inspiration (the pressure limit of the device) is determined by the distance between the pressure chamber clutch plate and magnet. As with the sensitivity adjustment, this distance can be adjusted by the practitioner. The closer the pressure chamber clutch plate and magnet, the greater the positive pressure necessary to move the diaphragm back to the left and close the alignment valve.

Once the alignment valve moves back to the left, source gas flow is terminated, allowing the exhalation valve, *E*, to open to the atmosphere and the patient to exhale passively until the next inspiratory cycle is begun.

Unlike the manually cycled IPPB apparatus, this type of device places the control of sensitivity, flow, and end-inspiratory pressure limit in the hands of the clinician. Obviously, this capability allows for more precise adjustment of the parameters of ventilation according to individual patient need. Indeed, other components of the Mark 7 and similar Bird ventilators provide automatic time cycling to inspiration, thereby extending their use to apneic patients.

Limited control over delivered F_{IO_2} levels is provided by a valve that optionally diverts source gas away from the Venturi (the "air-mix" control). Assuming that the device is powered by 100% oxygen, bypassing the Venturi will deliver 100% oxygen to the patient. However, bypassing the Venturi substantially lowers the device's flow capabilities. Moreover, even when the Venturi is in use, oxygen concentrations are extremely variable and generally higher than one might predict. These higher than expected concentrations occur for two reasons: (1) oxygen tends to accumulate in the ambient chamber at high system pressures and (2) nebulizer flow (100% source gas) represents a large component of the total flow provided to the patient. Use of an oxygen blender and reservoir system will provide for exact F_{IO_2} control, but this approach is expensive and complicated and necessitates a source of medical-grade compressed air.

Rotary alignment valve (Bennett). A typical Bennett IPPB device (the AP-5) is shown in Fig. 26-7. Unlike the Bird Mark 7, the Bennett AP-5 has a self-contained power source, consisting of a small-output electrical air pump or compressor (boxed in dotted lines). Compressor output initially passes through a submicronic filter and then follows two pathways. Part of the compressor output goes to a nebulizer control valve, which, if open, allows gas to power the sidestream nebulizer. The remainder of gas flows to a pressure-control device with a built-in Venturi.

The pressure-control device, commonly referred to as a "diluter-regulator," serves two functions. First, it provides air entrainment to enhance the device's flow capabilities. Second, by a simple adjustable spring-loaded pressure-reducing valve, it provides a means for precisely regulating system pressures between 0 and 30 cm H_2O.

Gas at the set pressure then passes to the Bennett rotating alignment valve. The valve consists of a counter-weighted hollow drum and attached vane that can rotate in a special housing (Fig. 26-8). Inspiration is triggered when the patient creates a small pressure difference across the drum vane (about -0.5 cm H_2O). This pressure difference causes the drum to rotate. Rotation aligns two drum windows with the main stream of pressurized gas from the diluter-regulator, allowing gas to flow into the breathing circuit and to the patient. Simultaneously, gas under pressure flows to a balloonlike exhalation diaphragm, which,

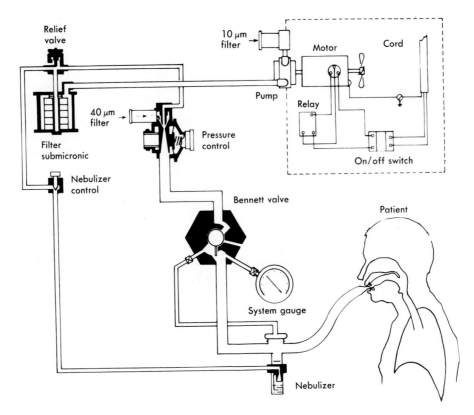

Fig. 26-7   Functional diagram of AP series ventilators. (Courtesy Puritan-Bennett Corp, Los Angeles. From McPherson SP: Respiratory therapy equipment, ed 3, St Louis, 1985, The CV Mosby Co.)

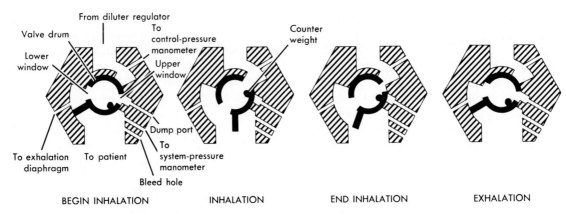

Fig. 26-8   Bennett valve. (From McPherson SP: Respiratory therapy equipment, ed 3, St Louis, 1985, The CV Mosby Co.)

when inflated, occludes the exhalation port in the breathing circuit.

As gas continues to flow through the system during inspiration, pressure distal to the valve increases. Because the pressure proximal to the valve is held constant, the pressure difference across the valve decreases throughout inspiration. As the pressure difference across the valve decreases, the opposing force of the drum counterweight causes the valve to rotate slowly back toward the closed position. Rotation of the drum back toward the closed po-

sition decreases the size of the window openings, thereby decreasing flow throughout inspiration. As the pressures across the valve begin to equalize, flow decreases to a critical minimum value of approximately 1 to 3 L/min. At this point, the force of gravity on the counterweight is sufficient to overcome the small difference in pressure across the valve, closing the valve and terminating flow.

With the Bennett valve closed, pressurized gas in the exhalation diaphragm is dumped to the atmosphere. Deflation of the exhalation diaphragm opens the exhalation port, allowing expired gases to escape into the atmosphere. This cycle is repeated when the patient again initiates an inspiratory effort.

Like the Bird IPPB device, the Bennett design places control of the end-inspiratory pressure limit in the clinician's hands. However, unlike the Bird series, there is no direct control over flow. More advanced models in the Bennett series offer a choice between 100% source gas and air dilution (allowing some variation in total output flow), and the PR-2 line incorporates a simple flow control mechanism. Even so, the flow capabilities of the Bennett-type IPPB devices are determined first by the initial pressure setting. The greater the preset system pressure, the greater the initial flow.

Because of the design of their valves, Bennett IPPB devices also differ from the Bird series in the practitioner's control over sensitivity. Whereas a wide range of negative pressures needed to initiate inspiration are available with Bird ventilators, the sensitivity of the Bennett valve is essentially factory preset. More advanced models in the Bennett series incorporate a mechanism to increase sensitivity, but these devices do not allow sensitivity to be decreased below the level designed into the valve assembly. In the clinical application of IPPB, however, this difference is of minor practical importance.

Like the Bird series, modifications to this basic Bennett design provide for automatic (time) cycling to begin inspiration, thereby allowing its use in long-term ventilatory support. However, pressure-cycled devices such as the Bird and Bennett series have generally been replaced by volume-cycled ventilators designed specifically for long-term support.

Administration of IPPB

Effective use of IPPB as a respiratory care modality requires careful preliminary planning, individualized assessment and implementation, and thoughtful followup. In all three phases of the process, the respiratory care practitioner should work closely with the prescribing physician in determining patient need, selecting the appropriate therapeutic approach, and assessing patient progress toward predefined clinical goals. Only by ensuring that these elements are combined as part of the overall respiratory care plan can the clinician expect tangible and beneficial patient results.

Preliminary planning. Preliminary planning should focus on identifying explicit goals for the IPPB regimen as related to the patient's underlying pathologic disorder and clinical status.

Setting goals. Obviously, the goal or objectives set for a given patient should be based on diagnostic information that supports the potential need for IPPB therapy. Goals that fall outside the indication categories previously delineated are generally inappropriate.

Patient goals for IPPB therapy should be as explicit and measurable as possible. As an example, for a patient exhibiting clinical signs and symptoms of postoperative atelectasis (see Chapter 16), the following therapeutic goals might be established:

1. A spontaneous vital capacity (VC) 70% of predicted;
2. Improvement in the chest x-ray film;
3. Remission of auscultatory signs of atelectasis.

Evaluating alternatives. A critical component in the preliminary planning process must be the consideration of alternative approaches to resolve the problem. Specifically, before implementation of the IPPB regimen, the practitioner and prescribing physician must determine whether simpler and less costly methods might be as effective in achieving the desired objectives.[14] If this is the case, further consideration of IPPB should be postponed until the patient's response to the alternative regimen is assessed.

Baseline assessment. Before initiating therapy, the practitioner should conduct a baseline assessment of the patient. Such information will assist the clinician in individualizing the approach and evaluating the patient's subsequent response to the therapeutic regimen. Used in conjunction with the patient's medical history, this baseline assessment also will alert the practitioner to possible problems or hazards associated with the administration of IPPB to a specific patient.

The baseline assessment should include both a general evaluation of the patient's clinical status and a specific assessment related to the chosen goals of therapy. The general assessment, common to all patients for whom IPPB is ordered, will normally involve the measurement of vital signs, observational assessment of the patient's appearance and sensorium, and chest auscultation. The more focused assessment should be individualized according to the identified clinical goals.

Obviously, different therapeutic goals will require different baseline information. In the situation just cited, the practitioner would obtain a baseline measurement of the patient's VC or IC at bedside. For patients in impending respiratory failure receiving IPPB to forestall intubation and mechanical ventilatory support, arterial blood gas information would be a critical component of the assessment plan. On the other hand, if IPPB is selected to enhance delivery of a bronchodilator aerosol, bedside assessment of forced expiratory flow (FEV%) would be an integral part of the evaluation. Only in this manner can the therapy be individually tailored according to the patient's status and needs.

Implementation. Implementation of the therapeutic regimen involves equipment preparation, patient orientation, and careful adjustment of the treatment parameters according to the patient's response.

Equipment preparation. Although all IPPB equipment should undergo a regular schedule of preventative maintenance and calibration, it is the practitioner's responsibility to ensure that all components are in proper working order before any patient application. Most respiratory care departments have standard protocols for this purpose.

Moreover, because a pressure-cycled IPPB device will not terminate inspiration if leaks in the system occur, it is important to check the patency of the patient's breathing circuit before each use. This can be done by aseptically occluding the patient connector and manually triggering a breath. If the machine rapidly cycles into expiration, the circuit is patent.

Patient orientation. Once chosen, the success with which IPPB therapy will achieve a specified goal depends largely on the effectiveness of initial patient orientation. Before initiating IPPB on a new patient, the practitioner must carefully explain to the patient the purpose of the treatment regimen. This explanation should be tailored to the patient's level of understanding and address, at a minimum, the following points: (1) why the physician ordered the treatment, (2) what the treatment does, (3) how it will feel, and (4) what the expected results are. To confirm patient understanding, minimize anxiety, and set the stage for effective participation, the practitioner should solicit feedback from the patient and attempt to answer all questions thoroughly.

The IPPB device must not be brought to the bedside until the practitioner feels that the patient adequately understands the nature of the procedure and the importance of cooperation in the therapy. Once the practitioner decides to bring the equipment to the bedside, a simple functional description may allay any fear or anxiety associated with the use of such an unfamiliar device.

Particularly useful in this regard is providing a simulated demonstration of the procedure. This may be done effectively with a test lung or, if deemed necessary, by self-application using a separate breathing circuit maintained for this purpose. For some patients, an effective demonstration can make the difference between success and failure in implementing the treatment regimen.

Patient positioning. For best results, the patient should be positioned in as close to an upright posture as possible. Slouching should be discouraged because it will hamper the excursion of the diaphragm, which will, in turn, decrease the volume of gas delivered to the patient's airways. An obese patient should ideally be positioned standing upright next to the bed, but this often is not practical.

Initial application. To eliminate airway leaks in the alert patient, an initial trial of nose clips may be necessary until the technique is understood and the treatment can be accomplished without them. The mouth piece must be inserted well past the lips and a tight seal must be encouraged to prevent gas leakage from the site. A flanged mouth piece may be necessary for some patients. The use of a mask is fraught with hazards and is suggested only for alert and cooperative patients otherwise unable to accomplish the treatment without leakage from the system.

The machine should be set so that a breath can be initiated with minimal patient effort. A sensitivity of -1 to -2 cm H_2O is adequate for most patients. System pressure can be set initially to between 10 to 15 cm H_2O, with resulting volumes to be measured and pressures adjusted accordingly after the treatment has begun. If the IPPB device has a flow control, the practitioner should begin the treatment with low to moderate flows and adjust them according to the patient's breathing pattern. Generally, the goal will be to establish a breathing pattern consisting of six to eight breaths per minute, with an inspiratory to expiratory time (I:E) ratio of between 1:2 and 1:3. Obviously, these parameters may need to be adjusted according to individual needs and patient response. Moreover, careful monitoring of the breathing pattern—and coaching to maintain it—must be conducted throughout the duration of the treatment.

Adjustment of initial parameters. Once the treatment is initiated and the patient's basic ventilatory pattern is established, ventilatory parameters should be individually adjusted and monitored according to the goals of the therapy. Examples of this individualized approach to IPPB administration include the different strategies characterizing the treatment of atelectasis, the management of impending respiratory failure, the administration of aerosolized medications, and the mechanical reduction of respiratory work.

Treatment of atelectasis. When applied to treat atelectasis, IPPB therapy should be volume oriented. In these situations, arbitrary pressure settings are not acceptable, and V_T levels must be monitored. A V_T goal must be set for each individual patient and the therapy delivered on the basis of these goals.

There are various ways of determining these volume goals. The method used in most clinical centers involves measurement of either the patient's vital capacity (VC) or inspiratory capacity (IC) at the bedside. If the VC exceeds 15 ml/kg of body weight, or the IC is greater than ⅓ of the predicted value, IPPB is not given and another treatment regimen, such as incentive spirometry, is considered. If the VC is less than 15 ml/kg, or the IC is less than ⅓ of the predicted value, IPPB is initiated, with the pressure gradually manipulated from the initial setting to deliver a volume equivalent to 15 ml/kg or to exceed ⅓ of the predicted IC. Of course, the delivered pressure can be increased further to deliver an even larger inspiratory volume if tolerated and deemed necessary.

It has been shown that larger inspiratory volumes can be achieved if the patient is encouraged to breathe actively during the administration of the positive pressure breath.[24] However, no definitive studies exist that demonstrate the need to have the patient actively participate in inspiration. Regardless of approach, IPPB is only useful in the treatment of atelectasis if the volumes delivered exceed those volumes achieved by the patient's spontaneous efforts.[25-28]

Treatment of impending respiratory failure. When IPPB is used as a preliminary measure in the management of impending hypercapneic respiratory failure, the goal is to stabilize or prevent further deterioration in lung function, as assessed by astute observation, regular bedside measurements of lung mechanics, and serial blood gas analysis. Absolute volume adjustments in these situations are less important than ensuring that (1) alveolar ventilation is sufficient to meet metabolic needs, (2) adequate oxygenation is maintained, and (3) sufficient mechanical reserves exist to forestall commitment to long-term ventilatory support. Treatment should therefore focus on establishing a ventilatory pattern that minimizes the work of breathing (discussed in more detail below), maintains acceptable levels of arterial carbon dioxide between treatment sessions, and provides oxygen concentrations equivalent to those otherwise being administered.

Administration of aerosolized medications. As with the administration of all aerosolized medications, the best particle deposition occurs when the IPPB device is set to deliver a slow, deep breath and the practitioner encourages a sustained breath hold at end-inspiration, ideally for 5 or more seconds.[22] In certain patients the practitioner may encourage an appropriate breath hold by momentarily occluding the exhalation port of the IPPB circuit. Of course, the limits of comfort and tolerance for the individual patient must not be exceeded.

As previously discussed, when the objective of aerosol drug administration is bronchodilation, it is essential that the practitioner determine the effect of the treatment on relevant pulmonary function measures. Preassessment of forced expiratory flows should therefore be repeated on completion of the therapeutic session, with the results being documented through appropriate followup activities.

Decreasing the work of breathing. If IPPB is used primarily to decrease the work of breathing, volume adjustment during inspiration is less critical. Instead, the clinician should attempt to ensure that the IPPB device provides as much of the inspiratory work as possible. This may be accomplished by combining active patient coaching with careful manipulation of the controls to provide a physiologically beneficial respiratory rate and inspiratory-expiratory ratio.

When applying IPPB to reduce the work of breathing in patients with chronic obstructive disorders involving collapse of the small airways during expiration, an extended expiration time may be required. Since such patients cannot perform pursed-lip breathing with an IPPB mouth piece in place, a similar effect can be achieved by placing a retard cap on the exhalation limb of the IPPB circuit. A typical retard cap has several orifices of various sizes. In principle, exhalation through a restricted orifice increases upstream airway pressure, prolongs exhalation, and prevents air trapping caused by small airway collapse.

Discontinuation. Depending on the goals of therapy and the patient's condition, IPPB treatments typically vary from 10 to 30 minutes. Should the practitioner observe any untoward effects, or should the patient exhibit signs of tiring, the practitioner should immediately discontinue the treatment and stay at the bedside until the patient's condition is stabilized.

Follow up. Follow-up activities include posttreatment assessment of the patient, recordkeeping, and equipment maintenance.

Posttreatment assessment. At the conclusion of a treatment session, the practitioner should repeat the initial assessment of the patient. As with the baseline assessment, this follow-up evaluation has two components. The general follow-up evaluation of the patient's clinical status should focus on determining any pertinent changes in vital signs, sensorium, and breath sounds, with emphasis on identifying possible untoward effects. The more specific follow-up assessment must gather posttreatment information relevant to evaluating progress toward achieving the chosen goals of therapy.

Record keeping. A succinct but complete account of the treatment session, including the results of preassessment and postassessment, must be entered in the appropriate location of the patient's medical record according to approved institution protocol. Any untoward patient responses must also be reported immediately to responsible personnel, including at least the prescribing physician and attending nursing personnel. As noted above, if assessment indicates a deterioration in patient status, the practitioner must remain with the patient until the problem is resolved or deferred to other personnel with direct responsibility for the patient's welfare.

ALTERNATE METHODS OF HYPERINFLATION

Historical perspective

When simple deep breathing is indicated to prevent and treat atelectasis, and the patient can take an adequate breath, maneuvers other than IPPB must be considered. Historically, several techniques other than IPPB have been used for this purpose.[29]

Carbon dioxide inhalation. Having the patient rebreathe exhaled carbon dioxide or a medical gas containing higher than ambient concentrations of this gas induces hyperventilation in healthy subjects. Unfortunately, the first response of the respiratory center is to increase rate of breathing rather than the V_T. Clearly, it is a deeper breath that is the goal of therapy. Moreover, carbon dioxide inhalation is fraught with numerous hazards, especially in patients with chronic hypercapnea or depressed central nervous system (CNS) responses (see Chapter 25). For these reasons, carbon dioxide inhalation is no longer recommended as a hyperinflation technique.

Blow bottles. The use of "blow bottles" to treat or prevent postoperative atelectasis was once popular in many clinical centers. With blow bottles the patient must generate sufficient pressure during expiration to move water from one bottle to another. In principle, this expiratory resistance was thought to stabilize alveoli and prevent their closure. In reality, if blow bottles have any beneficial effect, it is probably better associated with the initial deep inspiration taken and not the forced expiratory maneuver. Indeed, the forced expiratory maneuver may actually worsen atelectasis. If patients are encouraged to exhale into their expiratory reserve volume, small airways may begin to close prematurely. In addition, this maneuver may be quite painful for the postoperative patient.[28]

Current approaches

In addition to IPPB, two alternative approaches to hyperinflation therapy are in current use: incentive spirometry (IS) and the intermittent use of CPAP. Whereas we have well over a decade of experience with IS, the intermittent use of CPAP to treat atelectasis represents a relatively new approach to the problem. Indeed, intermittent CPAP is considered by many to be in the investigational stage of development. Nonetheless, preliminary results appear favorable. For this reason, intermittent CPAP will be included in our discussion of alternative methods of hyperinflation therapy.

Incentive spirometry. IS is a simple technique designed to encourage patients in maximal deep breathing. The incentive for each deep breath is provided by a visual volume or flow indicator. A goal is established by the practitioner for each patient on the basis of preliminary trials or by observation of initial effort and achievement.

Goal. The primary goal of IS is to treat atelectasis, especially in postoperative patients.[29] As previously discussed, pain, narcotic analgesia, and loss of the normal sigh mechanism in postoperative patients all can contribute to a progressive loss of lung volume. Adverse effects of the loss of the normal sigh mechanism become evident clinically in as little as 1 hour.[28]

In areas of the lung that become less compliant, ventilation-perfusion ($\dot{V}/\dot{Q}$) ratios drop, intrapulmonary shunting increases, and arterial oxygen levels fall. Moreover, the decreased compliance associated with atelectasis imposes an acute restrictive condition on the patient that tends to increase respiratory work and promote a rapid, shallow breathing pattern (see Chapter 8).

As with IPPB, the efficacy of incentive spirometry is best documented in the treatment of clinically diagnosed atelectasis. Currently, its role in the prevention of atelectasis is less clear.[30-33]

Physiologic basis. The physiologic basis underlying IS is a breathing maneuver called a sustained maximal inspiration (SMI). The SMI maneuver attempts to mimic the normal physiologic sigh mechanism by having patients inspire from the resting expiratory level up to their inspiratory capacity (IC).

Physiologically, the SMI increases the P_L by decreasing the P_{pl} below that normally achieved by the patient during quiet breathing:

$$P_L = P_{alv} (0) - P_{pl} \text{ (more negative)}$$

With all else being constant, the greater the P_L the greater will be the magnitude of alveolar expansion. Moreover, because the patient is instructed to sustain the effort at end-inspiration, better gas distribution to areas of the lung with abnormal time constants also should occur.

Hazards and contraindications. The major advantage of IS as a mechanism to facilitate lung expansion is its relative safety. Unlike IPPB, which increases P_L by increasing P_{alv} and thus P_{pl}, the SMI maneuver affects lung expansion through a physiologically normal mechanism. For this reason, when IS is properly performed, adverse cardiovascular effects are not a consideration.

The exception to this generalization occurs when the sustained end-inspiratory pause of IS is incorrectly maintained against a closed glottis, with contraction of the expiratory muscles. This Valsalva-like maneuver can increase intrapleural pressures and also result in a vagal reflex that can depress the cardiac rate. This situation is readily preventable by proper patient instruction.

Since airway pressures are maintained at atmospheric during the SMI, the potential problem of gastric insufflation, common with IPPB, is not of concern with IS. Last, IS alone has never been associated with bronchospasm in patients with reactive airways.

On the other hand, IS can potentially result in pulmonary barotrauma. Pulmonary barotrauma is associated with the magnitude of increase in the P_L, not necessarily its direction. Therefore, any intervention that increases the P_L can cause pressure damage to the lung, including subcutaneous emphysema, pneumothorax, pneumomediastinum, and pneumopericardium. Although this hazard is always a potential risk, its probability is extremely low at the volumes and pressures typically achieved in patients with otherwise healthy lungs.

Equipment. Part of the appeal of IS is the relative simplicity and low cost of the equipment used. Although recent advances in technology have made available some very sophisticated approaches, including microprocessor-based IS devices, there is no evidence that these devices produce any better outcomes than their lower cost—often disposable—counterparts.

Indeed, it has never been demonstrated conclusively that equipment of any sort is essential in achieving the goals of IS. Traditional prescriptions for the patient to "deep breath and cough," if aggressively followed, may well be as effective as the use of a given IS device with cooperative patients.[31-33]

However, the introduction of IS equipment as a substitute for this traditional regimen has a sound clinical basis. First, IS equipment facilitates setting and monitoring progress toward measurable goals, thereby providing some degree of patient motivation (the "incentive" of IS). Second, once a patient is properly instructed in the method, the treatment regimen can be conducted without direct supervision, thus making this approach more cost effective than the one-on-one intervention otherwise required.

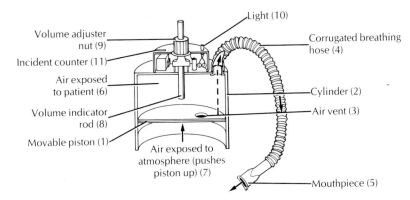

Volume adjuster nut (9)
Incident counter (11)
Air exposed to patient (6)
Volume indicator rod (8)
Movable piston (1)
Light (10)
Corrugated breathing hose (4)
Cylinder (2)
Air vent (3)
Air exposed to atmosphere (pushes piston up) (7)
Mouthpiece (5)

Fig. 26-9   Bartlett-Edwards incentive spirometer. (From Eubanks DH and Bone RC: Comprehensive respiratory care, St Louis, 1985, The CV Mosby Co.)

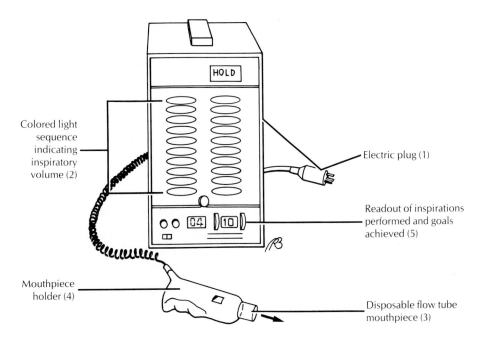

HOLD

Colored light sequence indicating inspiratory volume (2)
Electric plug (1)
Readout of inspirations performed and goals achieved (5)
Mouthpiece holder (4)
Disposable flow tube mouthpiece (3)

Fig. 26-10   Spirocare incentive breathing exerciser. (From Eubanks DH and Bone RC: Comprehensive respiratory care, St Louis, 1985, The CV Mosby Co.)

IS devices can generally be categorized as volume or flow oriented. Volume-oriented devices actually measure and visually indicate the volume achieved during the SMI. Flow-oriented devices, on the other hand, measure and visually indicate inspiratory flow. This flow is equated with volume by assessing the duration of inspiration or time (flow × time = volume).

Volume-oriented devices. The prototype volume-oriented IS device, the Bartlett-Edwards incentive spirometer, is shown in Fig. 26-9. This device is a true volume-displacement IS. Inspired volume displaces a piston, *1,* that moves within a cylinder, *2.* An air vent, *3,* allows air intake should the piston be fully displaced. A corrugated large-bore breathing hose, *4,* and mouth piece, *5,* connect the patient to the air in the piston cylinder, *6.* During inspiration, the negative pressure generated by the patient in the cylinder causes atmospheric pressure to displace the

piston upward, in proportion to the inhaled volume. Piston displacement is measured by an indicator rod, *8.* When the rod rises to a level preset by a volume adjuster nut, *9,* an electrical contact is established, lighting a visual indicator, *10.* Repetitions of the maneuver are recorded by a mechanical accumulator or incident counter, *11.* After completion of the maneuver, the patient removes the mouth piece, allowing gravity to return the piston to its initial starting position. To minimize the likelihood of cross-contamination, the piston-cylinder component is disposable. Only the volume indicator assembly is permanent.

Rather than actually measuring volume by displacement, some volume-oriented IS devices employ a modified pneumotachometer to convert inspired flow into a volume measurement. The Spirocare Incentive Breathing Exerciser is a good example of this approach (Fig. 26-10).

The Spirocare Incentive Breathing Exerciser is electri-

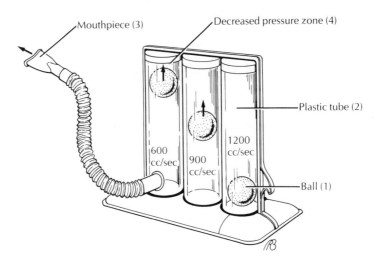

Fig. 26-11 TriFlo II incentive deep breathing exerciser. (From Eubanks DH and Bone RC: Comprehensive respiratory care, St Louis, 1985, The CV Mosby Co.)

cally powered by standard line current, *1*. The main component of the device provides a colored light sequence by which the volume goal is set and patient achievement monitored, *2*. Flow is translated into volume through a rotating turbine housed within a disposable flow tube, *3*. Light transmitted from the mouth piece holder, *4*, is alternately "cut" by the rotating turbine in direct proportion to the mass movement of gas through the flow tube. These alternating light impulses are counted by a sensor, also in the mouth piece holder, and translated into volume by a processor in the main unit of the spirometer. A light-emitting diode display at the bottom of the unit, *5*, counts the number of successful attempts at the prescribed volume goal compared with a number preset by the practitioner. A breath-hold indicator at the top of the unit encourages the patient to sustain the inspired volume once it is achieved.

Flow-oriented devices. Whereas volume-oriented IS devices actually measure and display volume, flow-oriented devices provide only an indirect indicator of the patient's inspired volume. Typically, this is achieved with calibrated flow indicators that function on the same principle as the Thorpe-tube flowmeter.

Fig. 26-11 shows a representative example of a flow-oriented incentive spirometer. Ping-pong-like balls, *1*, are enclosed in three interconnected plastic flow tubes, *2*. As the patient inhales through the mouth piece, *3*, a drop in proximal pressure, *4*, causes the ball in the first tube to rise to a level proportionate to the flow around it. Each tube is calibrated such that full displacement of its ball is equivalent to a specific flow, as indicated on the wall of the tube (600, 900, and 1200 cc/s in the device shown in Fig. 26-11). As flow exceeds the maximum for the first tube, the ball in the second tube rises, followed by that in the third tube. Motivation to maintain an end-inspiratory hold in this type of flow-oriented incentive spirometer is provided by instructions to keep the indicator balls elevated to full displacement for as long as possible.

Inspired volume is estimated as the product of inspired flow times time:

$$V \text{ (liters)} = \frac{\dot{V} \text{ (cc/s)} \times \text{time (s)}}{100}$$

For example, if a patient were to maintain displacement of the balls in the first and second chamber of this device for 3 seconds, the estimated inspired volume would be calculated as 900 cc/s × 3 s/100 = 2.7 L. Obviously, given the relative lack of precision of such devices and the errors inherent in the bedside measurement of these short time intervals, volume measurements derived from flow-oriented incentive spirometers should be treated only as rough estimates of actual inspired volume.

Because there are no definitive studies comparing the relative efficacy of volume and flow-oriented incentive spirometers, the decision regarding which type of equipment is best currently must be based on empirical assessment of patient acceptance, ease of use, and cost.

Technique. As with IPPB, the successful application of IS involves three phases: planning, implementation, and follow up. Since many of the components of this process are similar to those previously described, we will highlight only the key points and differences in approach.

Planning. As with IPPB, preliminary planning for IS should focus on identifying explicit goals related to the patient's underlying pathologic disorder and clinical status. The most critical component of planning for IS is the baseline assessment. Ideally, patients scheduled for upper abdominal or thoracic surgery should have been screened before undergoing the procedure. Assessment conducted at this point will help identify patients at high risk for postoperative complications and provide an opportunity to determine their baseline lung volumes and capacities. Moreover, this approach provides an opportunity to orient high-risk patients to the procedure before they undergo surgery, thereby increasing the likelihood of success when and if IS is implemented postoperatively.

If hyperinflation therapy is clearly indicated, preliminary planning also should help determine the most effective approach. In general, if the patient's postoperative VC is less than 12 to 15 ml/kg of body weight, or the IC is less than $\frac{1}{3}$ of predicted, then IPPB should be considered as the initial approach. Values above this range indicate that SMI is feasible and should be the first choice. Obviously, changes in a patient's ventilatory parameters and clinical status are grounds for altering the approach taken.

Implementation. Successful implementation of IS depends first on effective patient teaching. When instructing a patient in the use of an incentive spirometer, it is important that the practitioner set a goal that is attainable but that requires some moderate effort. Setting an initial goal that the patient can achieve easily results in little incentive and an ineffective maneuver, at least initially. The patient should be instructed to inspire slowly and deeply to maximize the distribution of ventilation.

A common problem in initial instruction is that the patient may tend to inspire rapidly, using the accessory muscles of ventilation to aid the work of the diaphragm. Correct technique will emphasize diaphragmatic breathing at a slow to moderately inspiratory flow. As with IPPB, demonstration is probably the most effective way to ensure patient understanding and cooperation. By using oneself as an example, both the operation of the device and the proper breathing technique can be easily explained and much trial and error avoided.

On maximal inspiration, the patient should be instructed to sustain the breath for at least 5 seconds. A normal exhalation should follow the breath-hold, and the patient should be given the opportunity to rest as long as necessary before the next SMI maneuver. A rest period of 30 seconds to 1 minute may be necessary for some patients in the early postoperative stage. This rest period helps avoid a common tendency among some patients to perform repetitively the maneuver at rapid rates, thereby causing respiratory alkalosis. The goal is not rapid, partial lung inflation but intermittent, maximal inspiration.

The exact number of sustained maximal inspirations needed to accomplish the therapeutic goal is not known and surely varies according to the patient's clinical status. However, because healthy individuals average about six sighs per hour, an IS regimen should probably aim to ensure a minimum of 8 to 10 SMI maneuvers each hour.[34]

Follow up. After initial implementation, follow-up activities should focus on assessing patient progress toward the prespecified goal of therapy. Because the degree of supervision necessary to ensure ongoing compliance and document progress varies significantly among patients, the practitioner must assume primary responsibility for determining the frequency and intensity of follow-up activities. Some patients will require regular visits by the practitioner to verify correct technique and appropriate effort, whereas others can progress with minimal supervision. In either case, records of progress, as related to the patient's clinical status, must be maintained throughout the course of treatment. Such records provide the only sound basis for considering alternative approaches to therapy and terminating the regimen once its goals are achieved.

Intermittent CPAP. CPAP has been used for well over a decade in the management of patients with respiratory failure and accompanying refractory hypoxemia. In these situations, CPAP is used as a continuous mode of therapy and is normally applied to the patient through an artificial airway (see Chapters 29 and 30). More recently, CPAP has been identified as a possible alternative to other hyperinflation techniques in the treatment and prevention of postoperative atelectasis.[16,35-38] For this purpose, CPAP generally has been applied by mask on an intermittent basis.

Physiologic basis. Unlike IPPB, which provides positive pressure during inspiration only, CPAP maintains an increased PL throughout the breathing cycle. Moreover, with CPAP, the transrespiratory pressure gradient necessary to move gases from the airway opening to the alveoli must be provided by the patient. In essence, the patient spontaneously provides the work necessary to ventilate the lungs; the CPAP simply maintains the alveoli and lungs as a whole, at a greater resting volume (FRC) than otherwise attainable.

This concept is illustrated in Fig. 26-12. By maintaining airway pressures above atmospheric while the patient breathes spontaneously, CPAP keeps the patient's FRC at an elevated level. With all else constant, this elevation in FRC is directly proportional to the pressure applied.

The exact mechanism by which CPAP aids in the treatment of atelectasis is unknown. However, the following factors probably contribute to its beneficial effects: (1) the recruitment of collapsed or partially collapsed alveoli through the increase in the FRC, (2) a decrease in the work of breathing associated with increased pulmonary compliance, (3) an improved distribution of ventilation through collateral channels, such as the pores of Kohn and canals of Lambert, and (4) a potential increase in the efficiency of secretion removal.[28,35,36]

Effectiveness. Recent investigations have shown that CPAP may be superior to a regimen of incentive spirometry, coughing, and deep breathing in preventing atelectasis and in its ability to increase a patient's FRC.[39,40] In one study, CPAP pressures up to 15 cm H_2O for 15 to 30 continuous breaths hourly facilitated lung reexpansion and improved PaO_2s within 12 hours.[32] Similar results obtained by others indicate that CPAP treatment must exceed 10 minutes in duration if it is to have beneficial effects.[41] Other investigators have demonstrated the resolution of lobar atelectasis in patients treated with mask CPAP, but only when administered continuously for 6 to 10 hours.[42]

Even though evidence exists to support the use of CPAP

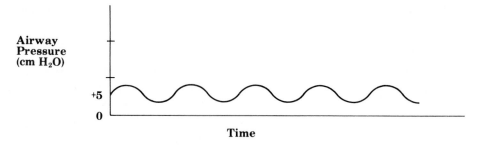

Fig. 26-12   During CPAP the airway pressure remains above ambient at all times as the patient breathes spontaneously. (From Pilbeam SP: Mechanical ventilation: physiological and clinical applications, Denver, 1986, Multimedia Publishing Inc.)

therapy in the treatment of postoperative atelectasis, the duration of beneficial effects appears limited. Indeed, the corresponding increase in FRC may be lost within 10 minutes after the end of the treatment.[41,43] For this reason, it has been suggested that CPAP should be used on a continuous, not intermittent, basis.[38]

Moreover, some recent studies show no significant difference between the use of CPAP and other methods of hyperinflation in preventing atelectasis, as measured by changes in arterial blood gas values and pulmonary function parameters.[43,44] Because the evidence on the effectiveness of CPAP is still contradictory, its current application should be limited to the treatment of atelectasis in those situations where alternative approaches have been tried without success.

Hazards and complications. Although there are documented incidences of complications with continuous CPAP, no documented complications have yet been reported for intermittent CPAP.[45] However, the potential complications of intermittent CPAP are threefold.[42] First, because CPAP represents the application of positive pressure to the airway, complications common to any positive pressure therapy may apply. Second, potential complications arising because of the mask delivery system may also occur. Last, since CPAP alone provides no enhancement to ventilation, patients with an accompanying ventilatory insufficiency may hypoventilate during application.

The possible hazard of barotrauma always exists when positive pressure is applied to the airways. However, CPAP is most often applied at lower levels than the peak inspiratory pressures associated with mechanical ventilation and IPPB. Decreased venous return and decreased cardiac output are also potential hazards, but, for the same reason, it would seem that the likelihood of this occurring would be less than that associated with machine-delivered positive pressure breaths. Although intermittent CPAP at pressures as high as +15 cm H_2O has been used effectively, the appropriate level for a given patient must be determined on an individual basis.[36]

When CPAP is applied by mask, a tight seal must be maintained to keep pressure levels above atmospheric. Any significant leaks in the system will result in the loss of

positive airway pressure. Because a tight seal requires a tight-fitting mask, some patients may experience pain and irritation. More serious is the possibility of gastric insufflation and the potential for aspiration of stomach contents. As with IPPB by mask, this potential hazard can be eliminated by use of a nasogastric tube.

Whereas hyperventilation is a major hazard of IPPB, CPAP poses a real danger of hypoventilation. Experience with long-term CPAP clearly demonstrates that patients must be able to maintain adequate excretion of carbon dioxide on their own if the therapy is to be successful.

For these reasons, patients receiving CPAP must be closely and continuously monitored for untoward effects. In addition, it is vital that the CPAP device be equipped with means to monitor the level of pressure delivered to the airways and with alarms to indicate the loss of pressure caused by system disconnect or mechanical failure. These are essential components of any CPAP device.

Equipment. Equipment currently used to deliver CPAP varies substantially in design and complexity. More detail on this approach, as applied in the management of respiratory failure, is provided in Chapter 30.

For purposes of illustration, the key elements of a simple CPAP circuit employing a continuous-flow principle is shown in Fig. 26-13. A breathing gas mixture from an oxygen blender, *A,* flows continuously through a humidifier, *B,* into the inspiratory limb of a breathing circuit, *C.* A reservoir bag, *D,* provides reserve volume if the patient's inspiratory flow exceeds that of the system.

The patient connection, *E,* includes four key components. One-way inspiratory and expiratory valves (*F* and *G,* respectively) minimize the likelihood of rebreathing expired gases. An emergency inlet valve, *H,* ensures that atmospheric air could be available to the patient should a failure occur in source gas delivery. A manometer, *I,* monitors CPAP pressure at the patient's airway.

The expiratory limb of the circuit, *J,* is immersed in a water column, *K.* With gas flowing continuously through the circuit, the pressure in the system will be proportional to the length (in centimeters) of the immersed tubing, *L.* Airway pressure can be varied by changing the depth of the water column in the expiratory circuit.

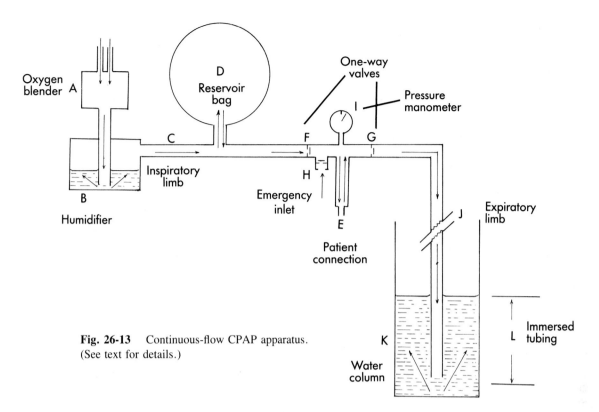

Fig. 26-13   Continuous-flow CPAP apparatus. (See text for details.)

Technique. Whether intermittent or continuous, CPAP represents a complex and potentially hazardous approach to patient management. Initial application and monitoring require a broader range of knowledge and skill than that required for simpler modes of hyperinflation therapy. For this reason, discussion on the techniques of administering CPAP and managing patients receiving this form of therapy will be deferred to Section VII.

SUMMARY

Hyperinflation therapy includes a variety of modalities designed to facilitate or maintain lung expansion. When applied to achieve rationally selected goals among carefully chosen patients, hyperinflation therapy represents an important tool in the provision of comprehensive respiratory care.

In the past, IPPB was applied to patients without much attention to careful planning, implementation, or followup. Later, this modality was nearly abandoned, with little consideration for its possible benefits with carefully chosen patients. Over time, other approaches to hyperinflation therapy have developed, including IS and intermittent CPAP. With these developments has come a more scientific approach to their use. Continuing investigation into the safety and efficacy of these modalities is providing the framework within which practitioners can rationally deliver hyperinflation therapy.

As our understanding of these approaches grows, it is apparent that positive outcomes can be achieved only with careful planning, implementation, and followup. In this context, the respiratory care practitioner will continue to play a primary role.

REFERENCES

1. Ingram RH Jr: Mechanical aids to lung expansion, Am Rev Respir Dis 122:23, 1980.
2. Martin RJ, Roger RM, and Grant BA: The physiologic basis for the use of mechanical aids to lung expansion, Am Rev Respir Dis 122:105, 1980.
3. Motley HL, Werko L, Cournand A, and Richardo DW: Observations on the clinical use of intermittent positive pressure, J Aviat Med 18:417, 1947.
4. Pierce AK and Saltzman HA, chairmen: Conference on the scientific basis for respiratory therapy, Am Rev Respir Dis 110:1, 1974.
5. Pierce AK: Scientific basis of in-hospital respiratory therapy, Am Rev Respir Dis 122:1, 1980.
6. O'Donohue WJ: IPPB past and present, Respir Care 27:588, 1982.
7. Demers RR: IPPB treatments: indications and alternatives, Respir Care 23:758, 1978.
8. The Respiratory Care Committee Of The American Thoracic Society: Guidelines for the use of intermittent positive pressure breathing, Respir Care 25:365, 1980.
9. American Association For Respiratory Care: The pros and cons of IPPB: AARC provides an assessment of its effectiveness, AARC Times, 10:48, 1986.
10. Kittredge P: What is not an IPPB treatment? Respir Care 23:262, 1978.
11. Hughes RL: Improving postoperative tidal volumes, Respir Care 26:985, 1981.
12. Indihar RJ, Forsberg DP, and Adams AB: A prospective comparison of three procedures used in attempts to prevent postoperative pulmonary complications, Respir Care 27:564, 1982.
13. Pontoppidan H: Mechanical aids to lung expansion in nonintubated surgical patients, Am Rev Respir Dis 122:109, 1980.

14. Ziment I: Intermittent positive pressure breathing. In Burton GG and Hodgkin JE, editors: Respiratory care: a guide to clinical practice, ed 2, Philadelphia, 1984, JB Lippincott Co.

15. Sinha R and Bergofsky EH: Prolonged alteration of lung mechanics in kyphoscoliosis by positive-pressure hyperinflation, Am Rev Respir Dis 106:47, 1972.

16. Barach AL, Bickerman HA, and Petty TL: Perspective in pressure breathing, Respir Care 20:627, 1975.

17. Barach AL, Martin S, and Eckman M: Positive pressure respiration and its application to the treatment of acute pulmonary edema and respiratory obstruction, Proc Am Soc Clin Invest 16:664, 1937.

18. Barach AL, Martin S, and Eckman M: Positive pressure respiration and its application to the treatment of acute pulmonary edema, Ann Intern Med 12:754, 1938.

19. Poulton EP: Left-sided heart failure with pulmonary edema treated with the pulmonary plus machine, Lancet 2:93, 1936.

20. Miller WF and Sproule BJ: Studies on the role of intermittent inspiratory positive pressure oxygen breathing in the treatment of edema, Dis Chest 35:5, 1959.

21. Rau JL: Respiratory therapy pharmacology, Chicago, 1984, Year Book Medical Publishers, Inc.

22. Shapiro BA et al: Clinical application of respiratory care, Chicago, 1985, Year Book Medical Publishers.

23. McPherson SP: Respiratory therapy equipment, ed 3, St Louis, 1985, The CV Mosby Co.

24. Welsh MZ et al: Methods of intermittent positive pressure breathing, Chest 78:463, 1980.

25. Morrison J: A proposal for the more rational use of IPPB, Respir Care 24:318, 1976.

26. O'Donohue WJ: Maximum volume IPPB for the management of pulmonary atelectasis, Chest 76:683, 1979.

27. Powers WE and Morrison J: Evaluation of inspired volumes in postoperative patients receiving volume-oriented IPPB, Respir Care 23:39, 1978.

28. O'Donohue WJ: Measures for lung expansion in postoperative patients, Respir Care 26:987, 1981.

29. Bartlett RH, Gazzaniga AB, and Geraghty T: Respiratory maneuvers to prevent postoperative complications: a critical review, JAMA 224:1017, 1973.

30. Celli BR, Rodriguez KS, and Snider GL: A controlled trial of intermittent positive pressure breathing, incentive spirometry, and deep breathing exercises in preventing pulmonary complications after abdominal surgery, Am Rev Respir Dis 130:12, 1984.

31. O'Connor M, Tattersall MP, and Carter JA: An evaluation of the incentive spirometer to improve lung function after cholecystectomy, Anaesthesia 43:785, 1988.

32. Schwieger I, Gamulin Z, and Forster A: Absence of benefit of incentive spirometry in low-risk patients undergoing elective cholecystectomy: a controlled randomized study, Chest 89:652, 1986.

33. Stock MC, Downs JB, and Gauer PK: Prevention of postoperative pulmonary complications with CPAP, incentive spirometry, and conservative therapy, Chest 87:151, 1985.

34. Pilbeam SP: Mechanical ventilation: physiological and clinical applications, St Louis, 1986, The CV Mosby Co.

35. Anderson JB, Qvist J, and Kann T: Recruiting collapsed lung through collateral channels with positive end expiratory pressure, Respir Dis 260, 1979.

36. Anderson JB, Oleson KP, Eikard B et al: Periodic continuous positive airway pressure, CPAP, by mask in the treatment of atelectasis: a sequential analysis, J Dis 61:20, 1980.

37. Covelli HD, Weled BJ, and Beekman JF: Efficacy of continuous positive airway pressure administered by face mask, Chest 81:147, 1982.

38. Williamson DC and Modell JH: Intermittent continuous positive airway pressure by mask, Arch Surg 117:170, 1982.

39. Freid JL, Downs JB, Davis JEP, and Heenan TJ: A new Venturi device for administering continuous positive airway pressure (CPAP), Respir Care 26:133, 1981.

40. Stock CM, Downs JB, Gauer PK, and Cooper RB: Prevention of atelectasis after upper abdominal operation, Crit Care Med 11:220, 1983 (abstract).

41. Paul WL and Downs JB: Postoperative atelectasis: intermittent positive breathing, incentive spirometry and face mask positive end-expiratory pressure, Arch Surg 116:861, 1981.

42. Branson RD, Hurst JM, and DeHaven CB: Mask CPAP: state of the art, Respir Care 30:846, 1985.

43. Stock CM et al: Comparison of continuous positive airway pressure, incentive spirometry and conservative therapy after cardiac operations, Crit Care Med 12:969, 1984.

44. Carlson C, Sondem B, and Tyhler V: Can post-operative continuous positive airway pressure prevent pulmonary complications after abdominal surgery? Intensive Care Med 7:225, 1981.

45. Shapiro BA, Peterson J, and Cane RD: Complications of mechanical aids to intermittent lung inflation, Respir Care 27:467, 1982.

27

Chest Physical Therapy

Craig L. Scanlan

Chest physical therapy (CPT) represents a collection of diverse techniques designed to facilitate clearance of airway secretion, improve the distribution of ventilation, and enhance the efficiency and conditioning of the muscles of respiration.[1,2] These methods include positioning techniques, chest percussion and vibration, directed coughing, and various breathing and conditioning exercises.[3,4]

As with many of the methods of respiratory care, the various components of CPT were often introduced without scientific assessment for one specific medical indication and then applied to other, sometimes dissimilar conditions in the hope that they would help.[5] This approach resulted in the widespread and indiscriminate application of CPT to patients with many different cardiopulmonary disorders. For example, in the late 1970s, more than 55% of the patients admitted to a single critical care recovery unit received some form of this therapy.[6] With the decrease in popularity of other respiratory care methods (eg, intermittent positive pressure breathing) during the early 1980s, the use of CPT continued to grow at a rapid pace.[7]

Seldom during this period was the efficacy of chest physical therapy questioned. Indeed, it was not until recently that rigorous scientific methods have been applied to study the effectiveness of CPT in groups of patients with similar conditions.[8] Results of these studies indicate that selected methods of CPT are effective with certain patients under specific clinical circumstances.

Thus chest physical therapy can be a valuable component of comprehensive respiratory care, but only if it is used in a discriminating manner. Successful outcomes require careful evaluation and selection of patients, a clear definition of therapeutic goals, rigorous application of the appropriate methods, and ongoing assessment and follow-up.

OBJECTIVES

This chapter focuses on the rational application of chest physical therapy in patients with disorders that affect the respiratory system. Specifically, after completion of this chapter, the reader will be able to:

1. Cite the general goals and specific indications for chest physical therapy;

2. Describe the importance of initial and ongoing patient assessment in the planning and implementation of chest physical therapy;

3. Differentiate among the underlying principles, relative efficacy, and methods of application of the following modes of chest physical therapy:
   a. Therapeutic positioning;
   b. Chest percussion and vibration;
   c. Cough and related expulsion techniques;
   d. Breathing retraining;
   e. Conditioning exercises;

4. Identify the major complications and adverse effects of chest physical therapy, including their treatment implications.

KEY TERMS

Most terms used in this chapter are defined in context. The following terms are introduced without explicit definition but may be found in the text glossary:

airway conductance (G)	lateral decubitus
bronchopleural fistula	MSVC
efficacy	P_{Imax}
epigastric	radioaerosol
hyperreactivity	Trendelenburg
ICP	

GOALS OF CHEST PHYSICAL THERAPY

The box on p. 656 summarizes the five primary goals of chest physical therapy.[1-3] Preventing the accumulation of secretions is a prophylactic goal, which is most often applied to high-risk surgical patients or those with neurologic

---

GOALS OF CHEST PHYSICAL THERAPY

To prevent the accumulation of secretions
To improve the mobilization of secretions
To promote more efficient breathing patterns
To improve the distribution of ventilation
To improve cardiopulmonary exercise tolerance

---

conditions that can potentially impair respiratory tract clearance. Improving the mobilization of secretions applies mainly to patients with preexisting disorders that cause an abnormal increase in the volume or viscosity of respiratory tract secretions, such as cystic fibrosis. The promotion of more efficient breathing patterns is an appropriate goal when structural or functional abnormalities result in the inefficient use of the respiratory muscles. Improving the distribution of ventilation is a legitimate goal of chest physical therapy when ventilation-perfusion abnormalities impair pulmonary gas exchange. Finally, improving cardiopulmonary exercise tolerance represents a long-term goal associated with comprehensive programs for patient rehabilitation as discussed in depth in Chapter 34.

The importance of identifying a specific goal or goals for a given patient cannot be overemphasized. Without a clear goal in mind, it is difficult to justify the application of CPT. Moreover, only by identifying the goal of therapy can one choose the appropriate mode of CPT and assess its effects. Rational selection of the goals of chest physical therapy therefore must be based on knowledge of its indications as related to patient assessment and selection.

INDICATIONS FOR CHEST PHYSICAL THERAPY

Recent studies on the effectiveness of CPT in groups of patients with similar conditions have refined our understanding of the indications for this mode of respiratory care.[8] In general, these conditions may be grouped into those representing acute clinical disorders and those of a more chronic nature.[8,9] A separate category—the preventive use of CPT—also warrants examination.[1,3] Current indications for CPT are summarized in Table 27-1.

Chest physical therapy for acute conditions

Among the acute conditions for which scientific evidence currently supports the application of chest physical therapy are (1) acute illness with copious secretions,[10] (2) acute respiratory failure with clinical signs of retained secretions (audible abnormal breath sounds, deteriorating ABGs, chest radiographic changes),[11] (3) acute lobar atelectasis[12-14] and $\dot{V}/\dot{Q}$ abnormalities caused by lung infiltrates or consolidation.[15-17]

Acute conditions for which research has shown that chest physical therapy is not beneficial include (1) acute exacerbations of COPD,[18-20] (2) pneumonia without clinically significant sputum production,[21] and (3) status asthmaticus.[4,8]

Chest physical therapy for chronic conditions

There are two broad categories of chronic conditions for which scientific evidence currently supports the application of selected chest physical therapy techniques. These include (1) conditions characterized by chronic production of large volumes of sputum and (2) chronic obstructive pulmonary disease accompanied by inefficient breathing patterns and/or decreased exercise tolerance.

Chronic production of large volumes of sputum. Chest physical therapy has been shown effective in facilitating the clearance of both central and peripheral airway secretions in chronic conditions associated with copious sputum production, as occurs in cystic fibrosis,[22-25] bronchiectasis,[26-27] and certain cases of chronic bronchitis.[28-30] In general, sputum production must exceed 30 ml per day for CPT to significantly improve clearance of secretions from the respiratory tract.[31]

Chronic obstructive pulmonary disease. The theoretical objectives of chest physical therapy in these patients are reduction of dyspnea and respiratory disability and improvement of exercise tolerance and the activities of daily living.[32]

To acquire a new, more efficient breathing pattern, simple physical conditioning methods (walking, climbing stairs, etc) are combined with breathing retraining and ventilatory muscle exercise, with the use of a variety of manual or mechanical techniques.[32-34] With a few exceptions, most studies indicate that these methods have an immediate objective benefit on blood gases and alveolar ventilation because of a reduction in respiratory rate and an in-

Table 27-1   Indications for Chest Physical Therapy

Category	Indications
Acute conditions	Copious secretions
	Acute respiratory failure with retained secretions
	Acute lobar atelectasis
	V/Q abnormalities caused by unilateral lung disease
Chronic conditions	Copious secretions
	COPD with inefficient breathing patterns or decreased exercise tolerance
Preventative use	Postoperative respiratory complications
	Neuromuscular disorders?
	Exacerbations of COPD?

? indicates unproven benefit.

crease in tidal volume.[32] Maximum exercise capacity, maximum work rate, and respiratory muscle endurance may also be improved over the short term.[35]

However, long-term results are contradictory and more difficult to interpret.[32,36] Whereas some studies have noted both clinical and functional improvements with fewer relapses and hospital admissions, other studies have not been able to show any benefit to the patient. Unfortunately, such long-term studies often lack control groups or suffer from imprecise definition of the clinical state being managed. Clearly, more research is needed before the appropriate indications for CPT in long-term rehabilitation are clearly delineated.[32,36]

Preventive use of chest physical therapy

Chest physical therapy has been suggested as a preventive or prophylactic mode of respiratory care in patients with a variety of disorders.[1,3] These include patients at high risk of postoperative respiratory complications, patients with neurologic disorders that compromise respiratory tract clearance, and patients with chronic lung disease who are likely to have acute exacerbations of their disorder. Current evidence presents a mixed picture regarding the benefits of prophylactic CPT.

Preventing postoperative respiratory complications. The three most common respiratory complications associated with surgery are atelectasis, pulmonary aspiration, and postoperative pneumonia.[37] Among those at highest risk of having these complications are patients with chronic obstructive pulmonary disease.[38] Chest physical therapy, when used in combination with other respiratory care modalities designed to promote hyperinflation of the lungs, has been shown effective in decreasing the incidence of postoperative respiratory complications in these and other selected high-risk patients.[39-41] CPT immediately after surgery also lowers the risk of postoperative pulmonary complications in elderly patients, and a regimen of preoperative therapy further decreases the incidence of postoperative atelectasis in these patients.[42] However, the benefits of CPT alone in reducing complications in other surgical patients are questionable.[43]

Preventing respiratory problems in neuromuscular dysfunction. Patients with neuromuscular dysfunction are at increased risk of secretion retention.[44] Typically, the underlying disease process compromises the ability to cough effectively. Although lung function may remain normal, neuromuscular disease also predisposes to breathing at low lung volumes, a pattern that increases the likelihood of alveolar collapse. As ventilatory reserve decreases, the risk of progressive atelectasis and secretion retention is increased. In concept, prompt recognition and treatment of abnormal respiratory function in neuromuscular disorders should help prevent problems related to ineffective airway clearance. Although this is a logical assumption supported by numerous case reports, there currently are no comparative studies that demonstrate the benefits of prophylactic CPT in these patients.

Preventing exacerbations of chronic lung disease. Although CPT is still used extensively to prevent acute exacerbations of chronic lung disease, firm evidence to support this application in scanty. Only in the long-term management of cystic fibrosis have comparative studies shown the potential effect of CPT in preventing acute deterioration in patient status. Specifically, when CPT is administered on a regular basis to patients with cystic fibrosis, little or no functional improvement is realized. However, periods without CPT tend to result in a progressive worsening of the patients' functional status, which can be reversed with renewal of regular CPT.[45]

PATIENT ASSESSMENT

The appropriate use of chest physical therapy depends, first and foremost, on proper initial and ongoing assessment of the patient. Obviously, all the key elements involved in establishing the need for respiratory care apply, as detailed in Section V of the text. Formulation of the respiratory care plan thus depends on the results of initial physical assessment, laboratory testing (including pulmonary function tests), and radiologic evaluation.

As an essential element of treatment implementation, initial and follow-up assessment enables the practitioner to[3]:

1. Understand the underlying medical or surgical condition as it relates to the patient's altered respiratory status.
2. Select and plan an appropriate treatment regimen.
3. Evaluate the effectiveness of the selected treatment regimen.
4. Recommend changes in the treatment regimen.
5. Identify the appropriate point at which to discontinue treatment.
6. Formulate a discharge and home care plan for those in need of continued care outside the institutional setting.

Special considerations in initial and ongoing assessment of the patient for chest physical therapy include evaluation of the patient's posture, muscle tone, ability to cough, sputum production (or lack thereof), breathing pattern, state of relaxation, and general physical fitness.[3] For surgical patients, particular attention must also be paid to the nature of the operative procedure, its duration, and the immediate postanesthesia response. Emphasis must be placed on the relative cardiovascular stability of the patient, as determined by blood pressure, heart rate, and rhythm.

In combination, comprehensive review and evaluation of these various factors will determine the likelihood of successful outcomes. Such assessment, when incorporated into the respiratory care planning process, clearly distinguishes the "bang, breathe, and cough" approach from an effective and individually tailored treatment plan.[3]

CHEST PHYSICAL THERAPY METHODS

Five primary methods are employed in chest physical therapy. Used alone or in combination, these methods include therapeutic positioning, chest percussion and vibration, coughing and related expulsion techniques, breathing retraining, and conditioning exercises. Appropriate application of these techniques requires an understanding of their underlying principles, relative efficacy, and methods of application.

Therapeutic positioning

Therapeutic positioning involves the simple application of gravity to achieve specific clinical objectives. The three primary objectives of therapeutic positioning are (1) to facilitate the mobilization of secretions (postural drainage), (2) to improve the distribution of ventilation (dependent positioning), and (3) to relieve dyspnea (relaxation positioning).

Postural drainage. The purpose of postural drainage is to facilitate the mobilization of respiratory tract secretions by positioning of the patient and the use of gravity to aid in their removal.[3] This is accomplished by simply placing the segmental bronchus to be drained in a vertical position relative to the force of gravity.[46,47]

Efficacy of postural drainage. Assessing the efficacy of postural drainage alone is difficult, since most studies combine this method with one or more other modes of chest physical therapy.[48] Moreover, several different criteria have been used to judge its effectiveness, including the volume and consistency of sputum produced, the clearance of radioactive albumin particles, and various measures of pulmonary function.

Despite these limitations, the current literature supports the following conclusions:

1. Postural drainage does not facilitate mucociliary clearance in normal subjects.[49]
2. Postural drainage does not improve pulmonary function in patients with stable chronic lung disease who produce scanty amounts of secretions.[50,51]
3. Postural drainage is most effective in patients with conditions characterized by excessive sputum production (30 ml or more per day).[8,31,52]
4. To be effective, postural drainage probably requires head-down positions in excess of 25 degrees.[8,28,49]
5. Adequate systemic and airway hydration is a prerequisite for effective mucociliary clearance in general and postural drainage in particular.[53]

Technique. On the basis of a preliminary assessment of the patient and a substantiation of the need for postural drainage, the respiratory care practitioner, in consultation with the ordering physician, identifies the appropriate lobe(s) and segments for drainage. Also on the basis of the preliminary assessment, the practitioner determines the potential need for modification of the position(s) chosen. Modification of head-down positions may be required for

patients with unstable cardiovascular status, hypertension, cerebrovascular disorders, and orthopnea.[46]

Treatment times should be scheduled either before or at least 1-½ to 2 hours after meals or tube feedings.[3] If the patient assessment indicates that pain may hinder implementation of treatment, consideration also should be given to coordinating the treatment regimen with prescribed pain medication.

Before positioning, the procedure (including adjunctive techniques) is explained to the patient. As necessary, clothing around the waist and neck should be loosened.[3] Also, any monitoring leads, intravenous tubing, and oxygen therapy equipment connected to the patient should be inspected and adjusted to ensure continued function during the procedure. Vital signs, including pulse, respiration rate, and blood pressure, should be taken before initiation of the procedure. Auscultation should also be conducted before the initiation of drainage. These simple assessments will serve as baseline measures for monitoring the patient's response during the procedure and can assist in determining its effect after completion.[46]

Figs. 27-1 through 27-9 show the primary positions used for drainage of the various lung lobes and segments.[46] For head-down positions in general, the foot of the bed must be elevated above the head by at least 16 to 18 inches to achieve the desired 25-degree angle. In the ambulatory care setting, a tilt table may be used in lieu of a hospital bed. A tilt table allows precise positioning at head-down angles of up to 45 degrees. When angles this large are used, shoulder supports must be provided to prevent the patient from sliding off the table. Modifications of these positions for infants and children are discussed in Chapter 32.

Once the patient is in position, the practitioner should confirm his or her comfort and ensure proper support of all joints and bony areas with pillows or towels. Stippled areas in Figs. 27-1 through 27-9 indicate the anatomic locations for percussion and vibration, if the latter are to accompany the procedure.

The indicated position should be maintained for a minimum of 5 to 10 minutes, if tolerated, and longer if good sputum production results.[1] During the procedure, the practitioner should continually observe the patient for signs of ill effects and monitor the pulse rate and blood pressure as needed. The practitioner's presence also ensures appropriate coughing technique, both during and after positioning. When the patient is in the head-down positions, strenuous coughing should be avoided, since this will markedly raise intracranial pressure. Rather, the patient should use the forced-expiration technique (described later). In general, total treatment time should not exceed 30 to 40 minutes.

Both the patient and the practitioner should understand that postural drainage does not always result in the immediate production of secretions. More often, secretions are

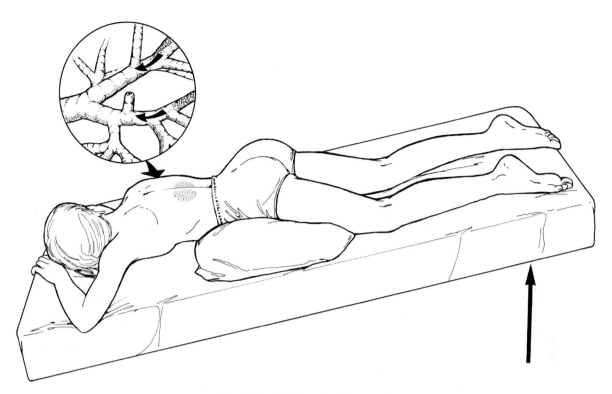

Fig. 27-1   Position for drainage of posterior basal segment of lower side.

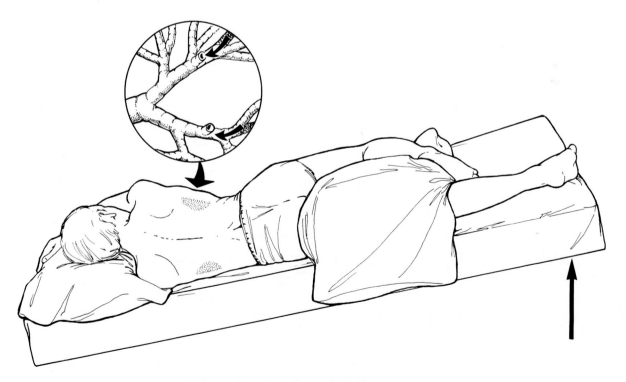

Fig. 27-2   Position for drainage of lateral basal segment of lower lobe.

Fig. 27-3 Position for drainage of anterior basal segment of lower lobe.

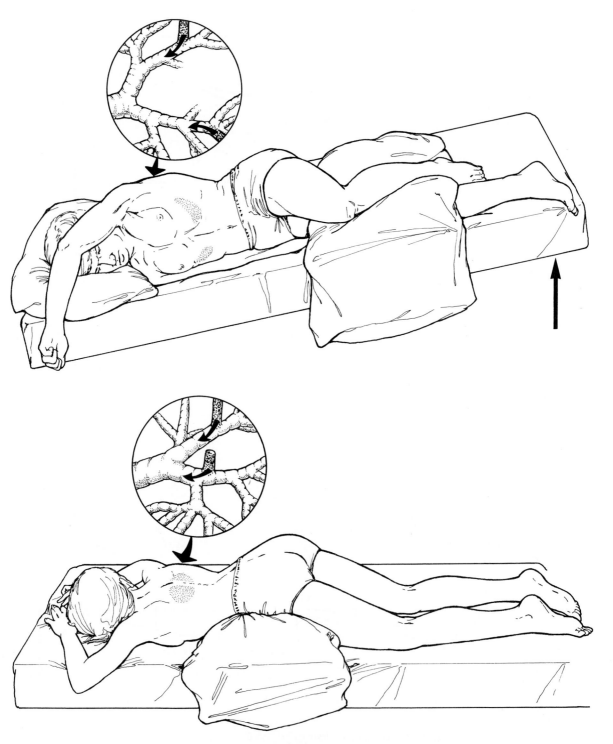

Fig. 27-4 Position for drainage of superior segment of lower lobe.

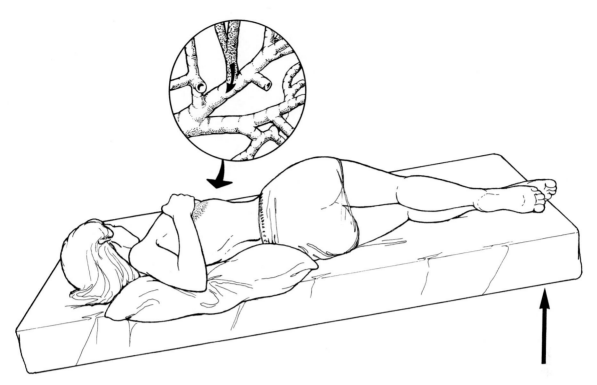

Fig. 27-5   Position for drainage of lateral and medial segments of middle lobe.

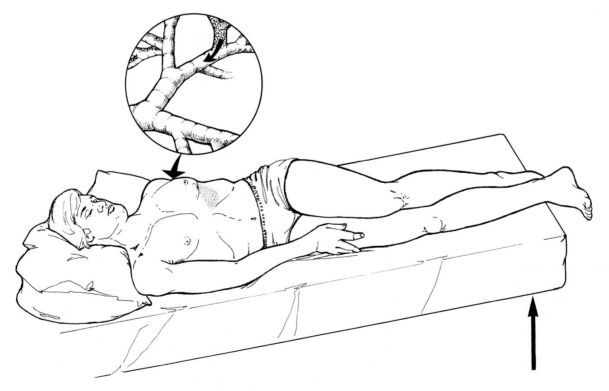

Fig. 27-6   Position for drainage of superior and inferior lingular segment.

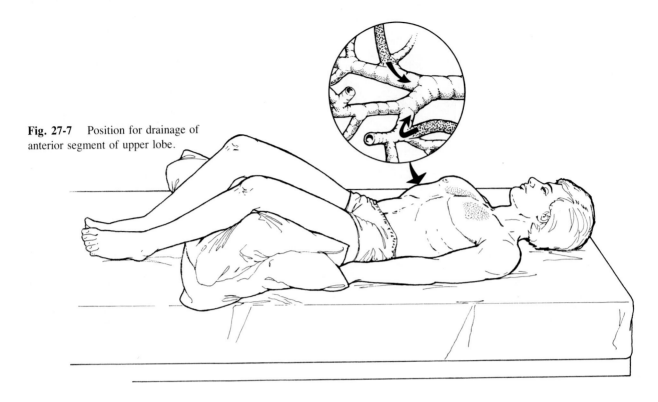

Fig. 27-7   Position for drainage of anterior segment of upper lobe.

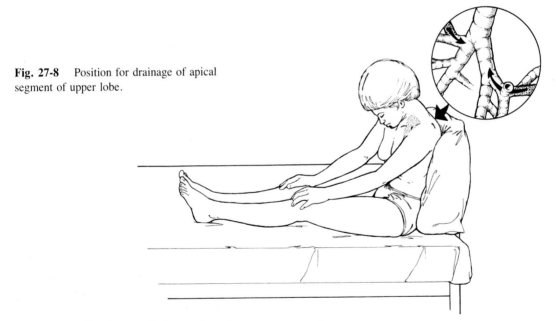

Fig. 27-8   Position for drainage of apical segment of upper lobe.

simply mobilized toward the trachea for easier removal with a less effortful cough after the procedure. If the drainage should be effective at once, so much the better, and if it precipitates vigorous coughing, the patient should sit up until the cough subsides.

On completion of the procedure, the practitioner should restore the patient to the pretreatment position and ensure his or her stability and comfort. Immediate posttreatment assessment should include repeat vital signs, chest auscultation, and questioning of the patient regarding his or her subjective response to the procedure. Charting should in-

clude specification of position(s) used, time in the position, the patient's tolerance, subjective and objective indicators of treatment effectiveness (including the amount and consistency of sputum produced), and any untoward effects observed. Since the effects of the procedure may not be immediately evident, the practitioner should make a return visit within 1 to 2 hours after treatment or obtain follow up information from the patient's nurse.

sure change and hence better ventilation.[55,56] Thus, as when the patient is in the upright position, the "down" portion of the lung always receives the best ventilation and also the best blood flow.

Unilateral lung disease. The effects of the side-lying position on $\dot{V}/\dot{Q}$ ratios in patients with unilateral lung disease clearly support the application of dependent positioning to improve oxygenation in these patients. In patients with unilateral chest infiltrates, the Pa_{O_2} tends to fall significantly when the "bad" lung is in the dependent or down position.[57,58] This fall in Pa_{O_2} is attributable to an increase in intrapulmonary shunting caused by a gravity-enhanced increase in perfusion through collapsed lung units. Because these units are in the collapsed state, most of the ventilation would tend to go to the upper lung, further worsening the $\dot{V}/\dot{Q}$ relationship.

Logically, the opposite of this effect—that is, placement of the good lung in the dependent or down position—may be employed for therapeutic purposes to enhance oxygenation in patients with unilateral lung disease.[16,17,59] Coincidentally, placement of the patient with the good lung down is also the position of choice for most postural drainage. In certain conditions, however, such as lung contusions resulting in internal pulmonary bleeding, it may at times be necessary to place the nonaffected lung in the up position to prevent blood that has accumulated in the diseased lobes or segments from entering the good lung.[6] Placement of the diseased lung in a down position is also indicated in the presence of a completely or partially filled lung abscess and in unilateral pulmonary interstitial emphysema (PIE).[59]

Generalized decreases in lung volume. The therapeutic benefits of positioning in patients with a generalized decrease in lung volume associated with the adult respiratory distress syndrome (ARDS) also have been reported.[15] In this study, patients receiving mechanical ventilation were turned from the supine to the prone position. In addition, support was provided to the upper thorax and pelvis, thereby allowing the abdomen to protrude. Once placed in this position, patients exhibited a mean increase in arterial oxygen tension of 69 mm Hg (range, 2 to 178 mm Hg), without a change in tidal volume, inspired oxygen concentration, or level of positive end-expiratory pressure (PEEP). No significant change in mean arterial carbon dioxide tension, respiratory frequency, or effective compliance was observed after positioning.

This maneuver alone made it possible to reduce the inspired oxygen concentration in four of the five patients who required mechanical ventilation of the lungs and to defer intubation in the one patient who was breathing spontaneously. Arterial P_{O_2} decreased in 12 of 14 instances after patients were turned from the prone to the supine position.

The physiologic basis for this positioning effect is less clear than in patients with unilateral lung disease. Im-

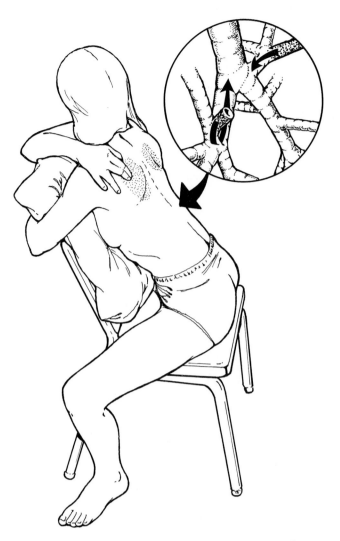

Fig. 27-9 Position for drainage of posterior segment of upper lobe.

Dependent positioning. A less frequent application of positioning, but one that is gaining acceptance as a clinically useful maneuver, is to enhance the distribution of ventilation in patients with $\dot{V}/\dot{Q}$ imbalances that significantly impair gas exchange.[7] Problems that are amenable to this simple approach include acute localized conditions, such as unilateral pneumonias, and conditions resulting in a more generalized decrease in lung volume, such as the adult respiratory distress syndrome (ARDS).

In concept, dependent positioning at first seems illogical. In normal subjects, both the side-lying (lateral decubitus) and head-down positions result in a decrease in functional residual capacity, of about 18% and 27%, respectively.[54] This is caused by displacement of the dome of the dependent diaphragm farther up into the thorax than in the sitting or standing position.

However, this diaphragmatic displacement and lower functional residual capacity place the dependent zones of the lung on a steeper portion of the pressure-volume curve, resulting in a greater change in volume for a given pres-

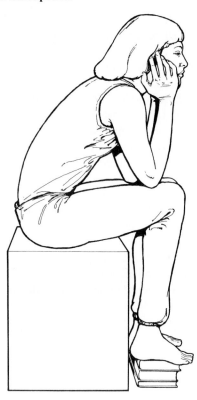

Fig. 27-10   Resting position 3, patient seated while leaning on hands.

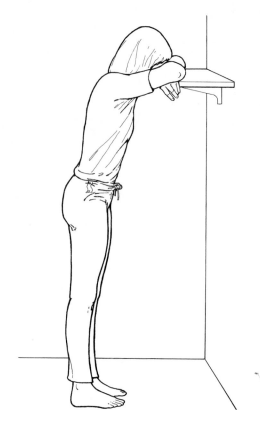

Fig. 27-11   Resting position 2, patient standing while leaning on elbows that have been placed on wall or chest-high object.

proved arterial oxygenation caused by a reduction in abdominal restriction to the movement of the diaphragm is unlikely, since no change in effective compliance of the lungs and thorax was observed. Clearly, the switch to the prone position somehow improves the $\dot{V}/\dot{Q}$ relationship, but it is not known exactly how this occurs. Studies of prone positioning in infants suggest that a decrease in asynchronous chest wall movement may be partly responsible for improvements in the distribution of ventilation,[60] although these findings cannot necessarily be generalized to adults.

Relaxation positioning. Relaxation positioning is a simple technique designed to help relieve dyspnea occurring in patients with COPD or those with acute shortness of breath caused by an attack of asthma. Figs. 27-10 and 27-11 portray the relaxation positions useful when patients are sitting and standing, respectively.

In both positions, the patient leans the body forward, while placing the elbows and upper arms against a support (the thighs or a wall). This position has two major effects. First, the forward flexion about the waist relaxes the abdominal muscles, thereby facilitating descent of the diaphragm. Second, fixing the upper arms allows the patient to make more efficient use of the accessory muscles of inspiration, especially the pectoralis groups (refer to Chapter 6). In combination with a purposefully slower breathing pattern, this posture can help reduce the work of breathing, increase tidal volumes, and decrease the subjective sensation of dyspnea.[61]

In reality, many patients with COPD have already "learned" to assume this relaxation position when they experience shortness of breath. When properly reinforced by the practitioner and combined with other maneuvers designed to improve diaphragmatic activity and slow the breathing pattern, the full benefits of this positional technique can be realized.

Percussion and vibration

Percussion and vibration involve the application of mechanical energy to the chest wall by means of either the hands or various electrical or pneumatic devices. Both methods are designed to augment the clearance of secretions.[62] In theory, percussion should help jar retained secretions loose from the tracheobronchial tree, making them easier to remove by coughing or suctioning. Vibration, on the other hand, is designed to facilitate movement of secretions toward the central airways during the expiratory phase of breathing.

Efficacy of percussion and vibration. As with postural drainage, assessment of the efficacy of percussion and vibration is difficult, since most studies combine this method with one or more other modes of chest physical therapy.[8] Moreover, the patients studied often have substantially different underlying disorders. For example, in a study of ten patients with a variety of disorders (including atelectasis,

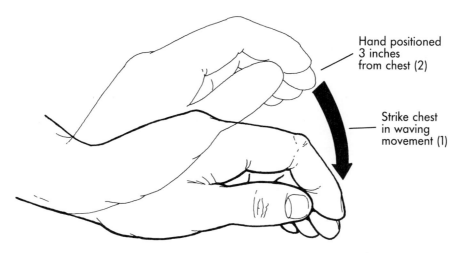

Hand positioned
3 inches
from chest (2)

Strike chest
in waving
movement (1)

Fig. 27-12 Movement of cupped hand at wrist to percuss chest.

pleural effusion, and pneumonia), mechanical vibration, when combined with positional changes and suctioning, resulted in significant improvements in Sao_2 measured at 30 and 60 minutes after therapy.[63] Of course, it could not be determined whether the vibration alone caused these improvements. In a more specific study, patients with cystic fibrosis treated with mechanical percussion and postural drainage did produce significantly more sputum than those treated with postural drainage alone.[64] More recent studies involving inhaled radioaerosol techniques confirm that percussion and vibration may increase the volume of sputum production but have consistently failed to demonstrate any independent beneficial effect on mucociliary clearance.[65-67]

Interpretation of these findings is made difficult by the fact that there is no general consensus as to what represents the appropriate force or frequency for percussion or vibration.[3,43,66] For this reason, and in light of current knowledge, the indiscriminate application of these methods cannot be justified.[8] However, since percussion and vibration methods may increase the volume of sputum production in selected patients, their application on a delimited basis is appropriate. Specifically, percussion and vibration should be considered only when other more proven methods are unsuccessful in mobilizing secretions. Good examples include patients who are unable to cough or who cannot assume the appropriate position for postural drainage.[68]

Percussion technique. Percussion, when indicated, is applied over the surface landmarks of the area being drained (Figs. 27-1 to 27-9). Manual percussion is accomplished with the hands in a cupped position, with fingers and thumb closed. In this manner, a cushion of air is trapped between the hand and the chest wall. The striking force may be against the bare skin, although a thin layer of cloth, such as a hospital gown or a bed sheet, does not significantly impair transmission of the energy wave.

The practitioner, holding his or her arm with the elbow partially flexed and the wrist loose, rhythmically strikes the chest wall in a waving motion, using both hands alternately in sequence (Fig. 27-12). Slower, more relaxing rates are better tolerated by patient and practitioner alike.[1] This is not a difficult technique to master, but skill and experience are needed to determine the appropriate force and to maintain a rhythmic pattern.

Ideally, the percussion should proceed back and forth in a circular pattern over the localized area for a period of 3 to 5 minutes. Naturally, care must be exercised by the practitioner to avoid tender areas or sites of trauma or surgery, and percussion must never be performed directly over bony prominences, such as the clavicles or vertebrae.

Vibration technique. When indicated, chest vibration is often used in conjunction with percussion but its application is limited to the expiratory phase of breathing. Typically, the practitioner lays one hand over the involved area of the patient's chest and places the other hand on top of the first (Fig. 27-13). Alternatively, the hands may be placed on either side of the chest. After the patient takes a deep breath, the practitioner exerts slight to moderate pressure on the chest wall and initiates a rapid vibratory motion of the hands throughout expiration.

Adjunctive devices. Various electrical and pneumatic devices have been developed to generate and apply the energy waves used during percussion and vibration. Although they are no substitute for a skilled practitioner, these devices do not tire the patient and can deliver consistent rates, rhythms, and impact forces.[69] However, there is currently no firm evidence to indicate that these devices are any more effective than manual techniques.

Coughing and related procedures

Although generally taken for granted, the cough is one of our most important protective reflexes.[70] By ridding the

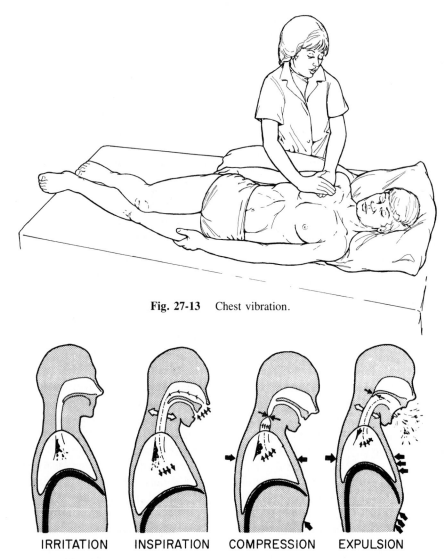

Fig. 27-13   Chest vibration.

IRRITATION   INSPIRATION   COMPRESSION   EXPULSION

Fig. 27-14   The cough reflex. (From Cherniack RM and Cherniack L: Respiration in health and disease, ed 3, Philadelphia, 1983, WB Saunders Co.)

larger airways of excessive mucus and particulate matter, the cough complements the mucociliary clearance mechanism, thereby ensuring airway patency.

Mechanism. Normally, a cough is induced either by irritation of the sensory endings of the vagus nerve in the larynx, trachea, or larger bronchi or by afferent fibers of the glossopharyngeal nerve in the pharynx. A cough may also be induced by stimulation of nerve endings in the mucous membranes of the esophagus, pleural surface, and auditory canal. Whatever the source, these impulses are transmitted to the cough center in the medulla, which reflexly stimulates the muscles of the chest and larynx to initiate the cough sequence.[71,72]

Fig. 27-14 shows the sequence of events characterizing a normal cough reflex. Four distinct phases are evident. In the initial irritation phase, an abnormal stimulus provokes sensory fibers to send afferent impulses to the cough center. This stimulus normally is either inflammatory, me-

chanical, chemical, or thermal. Infection is a good example of cough stimulation caused by an inflammatory process. Foreign bodies can provoke a cough through mechanical stimulation. Chemical stimulation can occur when irritating gases are inhaled. Finally, cold air may cause thermal stimulation of sensory nerves and produce a cough.

Once these afferent impulses are received and processed, the cough center stimulates the respiratory muscles to initiate a deep inspiration (the second phase). In normal adults, this inspiration ranges in volume from 1 to 2 L.

During the third or compression phase, efferent nerve impulses cause glottic closure and a forceful contraction of the expiratory muscles. Lasting about 0.2 second, this compression phase results in a rapid rise in intrapleural and alveolar pressures, often in excess of 100 mm Hg.

At this point, the glottis opens, initiating the expulsion phase. With the glottis open, a large pressure gradient is established between the lower and upper portions of the respiratory tract. In combination with the continued contraction of the expiratory muscles, this pressure gradient causes a violent, expulsive flow of air from the lungs, with a velocity often approaching 500 miles per hour! Because the nasopharynx is closed off when the glottis opens, foreign material expelled from the respiratory tract enters the mouth, where it can be expectorated or swallowed.

In terms of therapeutic application, it is important to realize that a cough also may be initiated voluntarily, without the presence of irritating stimuli. This is in distinct contrast to a similar reflex, the sneeze, which generally cannot be induced without local irritation. It is also important to understand that a cough generally is an effective clearance mechanism only down to about the sixth or seventh branching of the tracheobronchial tree.[1] Thus, retained secretions beyond this level must first be mobilized into the larger airways by other methods if they are to be effectively cleared. Finally, and of utmost concern in the clinical setting, is the fact that interference with any one of its four phases can result in an ineffective cough, thereby impairing the patient's ability to clear respiratory tract secretions. Table 27-2 provides examples of factors that can impair the normal cough reflex, according to the phase affected.

Efficacy. How important is an effective cough in facilitating the clearance of respiratory tract secretions and achieving the goals of chest physical therapy? The answer is simple. In patients with copious secretions, properly directed coughing is at least as effective in clearing the respiratory tract as more complicated methods.[8,28] Vigorous directed coughing alone has been shown to provide radio-aerosol clearance as good as that resulting from a combination of postural drainage, percussion, and vibration administered by a skilled therapist, although the more comprehensive treatments did produce a greater volume of sputum.[23]

However, current knowledge suggests that coughing and other modes of chest physical therapy may differ in regard to the location of their action. Apparently, directed coughing is at least as effective in clearing secretions in the central airways as other methods of chest physical therapy but not as effective in clearing secretions arising from the peripheral airways.[29] This difference is consistent with our understanding of the physiology of the normal cough mechanism, as previously discussed.

Cough technique. Although the cough is a normal reflex, the appropriate voluntary use of this mechanism to facilitate respiratory tract clearance depends on effective teaching of the patient by the practitioner, combined with individually tailored supervision and reinforcement.

The three most important aspects involved in teaching the patient to develop an effective cough regimen are (1) instruction in proper positioning, (2) instruction in breathing control, and (3) exercises to strengthen the expiratory muscles.[70] These activities are modified according to the patient's underlying clinical problem.

Positioning. Proper positioning is an essential prerequisite for an effective cough. Patients must be taught to assume a position that facilitates exhalation and compression of the thorax.[1,70] Because of the tension on the abdominal muscles, it is difficult, if not impossible, to generate an effective cough in the supine position.[70] Rather, the patient ideally should be placed in a sitting position, with shoulders rotated inward, the head and spine slightly flexed, and the forearms relaxed or supported. To provide abdominal and thoracic support, the feet should be supported. If the patient is unable to sit up, the head of the bed can be raised, the patient's knees slightly flexed, and the feet braced on the mattress.

Breathing control. Breathing control measures help ensure that the inspiration, compression, and expulsion phases of the cough are maximally effective and coordinated. For effective inspiration, the patient should be taught to inspire slowly and deeply through the nose, using the diaphragmatic method (discussed later). In patients with copious amounts of sputum, such breaths alone may stimulate coughing by loosening secretions in the larger airways.

After the patient is able to achieve a satisfactory deep inspiration, he or she is told to bear down against the glottis, in much the same manner as during straining at stool. In patients with pain, or those subject to bronchiolar collapse, it is probably best that they be shown how to "stage" their expiratory effort into two or three short bursts. For these patients, this method is generally less fatiguing and more effective in producing sputum than a single violent expulsion.[1,70]

Effective breathing control is best achieved when instruction is supplemented with demonstration. In this manner, the practitioner can show the patient exactly what is expected by going through the various phases of the cough sequence, such as simple throat clearing, and pointing out both the correct technique and common errors.

Table 27-2   Mechanisms Impairing the Cough Reflex

Phase	Examples of impairments
Irritation	Anesthesia
	CNS depression
	Narcotics-analgesics
Inspiration	Pain
	Neuromuscular dysfunction
	Pulmonary restriction
	Abdominal restriction
Compression	Laryngeal nerve damage
	Artificial airway
	Abdominal muscle weakness
	Abdominal surgery
Expulsion	Airway compression
	Airway obstruction
	Abdominal muscle weakness

Strengthening the expiratory muscles. At times, proper positioning and appropriate breathing control alone may not result in the development of an effective cough. More often than not, this limitation results from a significant weakness in the muscles of expiration. Expiratory muscle weakness is common in patients with chronic obstructive pulmonary disease who suffer from a general lack of muscle conditioning and in patients who have undergone long-term ventilatory support, during which muscles may have atrophied from lack of use. In either case, an effective cough cannot be developed until these muscles are reconditioned. Details on expiratory muscle exercises are provided in the next section of this chapter.

Modifications in method. Several modifications of this coughing technique are warranted in special circumstances. Among these special circumstances are those involving the surgical patient, the patient with COPD, and the patient with a neuromuscular disorder that precludes a sufficiently deep inspiration.

Surgical patients. Preoperative training in breathing control can help prepare patients for the postoperative regimen, thereby minimizing the anxiety over pain that commonly impairs an effective cough in these patients. The postoperative regimen can be enhanced by coordination of the coughing sessions with prescribed pain medication, and assisting the patient in "splinting" the operative site. This may be accomplished initially by the practitioner, using his or her own hands to support the area of incision. Later, the patient can be taught to use a pillow to splint the site. The forced-expiration technique (to be discussed later) may also be of value in these patients.

COPD patients prone to bronchiolar collapse. In patients prone to bronchiolar collapse, high intrapleural pressures during a forced cough may compress the smaller airways and limit the cough's effectiveness. In this case, the patient should be placed in the sitting relaxation positioned described previously (Fig. 27-10).[70] The practitioner then instructs the patient to inhale slowly through the nose while concurrently moving to a full upright position. The goal is a moderate, as opposed to full, inspiration. This reduces the volume of air to be removed by the patient and results in less increase in intrapleural pressure.

To compensate for characteristic loss of expulsive force, the patient is told to exhale with moderate force through pursed lips, while bending forward.[70] This forward flexion of the thorax enhances expiratory flow by upward displacement of the abdominal contents. After three or four repetitions of this maneuver, the patient is encouraged to bend forward and initiate short staccato-like bursts of air. This technique relieves the weak patient of the strain of a prolonged hard cough, and the staccato rhythm at a relatively low velocity minimizes airway collapse. This technique has a modification called "huffing" whereby the patient is instructed to make the sound of "huff, huff, huff" rapidly with the mouth open, the sound audibly coming from the throat.[73]

Patients with neuromuscular conditions. Patients with neuromuscular conditions present the practitioner with a special challenge in cough management. Depending on the nature of the neuromuscular disorder, the normal reflex reaction to irritation may be impaired or absent, deep inspiration may be impossible, glottic closure may be incomplete, or expiratory muscles may not be able to contract. In cases in which one or more of these factors cause significant retention of secretions, an artificial airway normally is indicated (refer to Chapter 21). This allows direct access to the central airways for removal of secretions by suctioning.

Regardless of whether an artificial airway is present, these patients typically are unable to generate the forceful expulsion necessary to move secretions toward the trachea. In such cases, chest compression may be a useful adjunct to other modes of chest physical therapy. In this technique, the patient takes as deep an inspiration as possible, assisted as necessary by the application of positive pressure with a self-inflating bag or an IPPB device. At the end of the patient's inspiration, the practitioner begins exerting pressure on the lateral costal margin with both hands, increasing the force of compression throughout the expiration. This mimics the normal cough mechanism by generating an increase in the velocity of the expired air and may be helpful in moving secretions toward the trachea, where they can be removed by either nasotracheal or tracheobronchial suctioning.

Acute chest compression. Acute chest compression is similar in concept to the procedure just described for cough control, but it is specifically indicated in the patient with severe emphysema and air trapping.

Not only may the mechanism of air trapping interfere with effective cough, as already noted, but it may place the patient's life in jeopardy. The emphysematous patient with chronic bronchial secretions may suddenly be stimulated by the need to cough, take a deep breath, start the cough, and suddenly find the airflow shut off before end-expiration. At this point the patient may be unable either to exhale or to inhale, and the chest becomes "frozen" and immobile. The patient continues to strain in an attempt to move air, the neck veins distend from the increased intrapleural pressure, the face becomes plethoric or cyanotic, and the patient is suddenly in acute danger of suffocation.

Fortunately, most such episodes are self-limiting, as perhaps weakness causes enough reduction in intrapleural pressure to permit air to move. Nonetheless, the experience is frightening to patient and family alike and, in the worst cases, can severely compromise cardiac output and cerebral blood flow.

The respiratory care practitioner should be prepared to manage this event, since coughing and certain breathing exercises may precipitate an attack of acute air trapping. Should this happen or should the patient give a history of its occurrence at home, family members also should be taught how to treat it.

The technique is simple but effective and is applied as soon as the patient's distress becomes apparent. If the patient is relatively slight in stature, the practitioner, standing behind the patient, places both hands over the lateral costal margins and the lower chest and exerts a series of short, strong compressions, releasing the pressure completely after each. This develops short bursts of pressure sufficient in most cases to open the small airways and allow completion of exhalation. If the patient is large, with a heavy chest wall, the practitioner can exert greater expulsive force by standing to the patient's side and, grasping him or her in a bear hug around the lower thorax, sharply squeezing the patient laterally against his or her own body. Regardless of method, forceful compression of the costal margins is not without its hazards; rib fracture, lung puncture, and injury to liver are all possible but infrequent complications.

Forced-expiration technique. The forced-expiration technique (FET) represents a modification of the normal cough sequence. The FET consists of one or two forced expirations from mid to low lung volume *without* closure of the glottis, followed by a period of diaphragmatic breathing and relaxation. The goal of this method is to facilitate clearance of bronchial secretions with less change in intrapleural pressure and with less likelihood of bronchiolar collapse.[8]

Maintenance of an open glottis may be facilitated by having the patient phonate or "huff" during expiration. The period of diaphragmatic breathing and relaxation following the forced expiration is essential for restoring lung volume and minimizing fatigue.

Comparative clinical studies on the effectiveness of this method have demonstrated favorable results. In general, when self-applied by patients with copious secretions, the forced expiration technique results in better sputum production in less time than traditional therapist-supervised intervention.[24] Moreover, the FET has been shown to provide better radioaerosol clearance than directed coughing, especially when combined with postural drainage.[27] This evidence suggests that the ideal chest physical therapy regimen in patients with copious secretions may well be postural drainage combined with the forced expiration technique.

Breathing exercises

Breathing exercises represent a broad category of activities designed to achieve a variety of purposes, including the following[74]:

1. To promote greater use of the diaphragm and decreased use of the upper rib cage and other accessory muscles of inspiration.
2. To increase awareness of the muscles of respiration and to suppress the tendency for hurried and gasping respiration.
3. To provide patients with the tools necessary to better handle the distressful symptom of dyspnea.

4. To identify and provide a means by which inefficient and inappropriate muscle use can be diminished or eliminated.
5. To improve the efficiency of alveolar ventilation by increasing tidal volume, slowing the rate of breathing, prolonging the expiratory time, and promoting better distribution of ventilation to perfusion.
6. To improve the strength and endurance of the respiratory muscles.
7. To improve the effectiveness of the cough.
8. To improve the delivery of therapeutic aerosols.
9. To teach patients to coordinate their breathing with body motions and the activities of daily living.
10. To relieve exertional dyspnea so that patients can improve their overall cardiopulmonary fitness and general exercise tolerance.

Our analysis will focus first on the application of specific inspiratory and expiratory breathing exercises, followed by a discussion of more general conditioning activities. Integration of these exercises and conditioning activities into a comprehensive rehabilitation program are discussed in Chapter 34.

Although emphasis is placed on the application of these techniques in patients with COPD, where appropriate, mention will be made of their potential use among other patient groups, including those with chronic neuromuscular disorders and those with acute problems (eg, postsurgical patients).

Inspiratory breathing exercises. There are three primary types of inspiratory breathing exercise: diaphragmatic (abdominal) breathing, lateral costal breathing, and inspiratory resistive breathing.

Diaphragmatic (abdominal) breathing exercises. As discussed in previous chapters, COPD, especially those forms characterized by loss of elastic tissue, pulmonary distention, and air trapping, result in grossly inefficient use of the diaphragm and excessive dependence on the accessory muscles of inspiration.[75] The primary purpose of diaphragmatic or "abdominal" breathing exercises is to promote greater use of the diaphragm and decreased use of the accessory muscles of inspiration. Initially, this is accomplished by developing in the patient an increased awareness of diaphragmatic activity, followed by exercises designed to increase the strength of this primary muscle of inspiration. Long-term benefits to the patient may include an increased efficiency of alveolar ventilation, achieved by virtue of an increased V_T, a slower rate of breathing, and increased exercise tolerance.

Efficacy. Three questions are critical in addressing the effectiveness of diaphragmatic breathing exercise. First, we must ask whether it is possible to voluntarily alter one's breathing pattern from mainly accessory to mainly diaphragmatic breathing. Second, if it is possible to voluntarily change the nature of inspiratory muscle use, we must know whether or not this change affects the pattern of ventilation or its distribution. Finally, we must know whether such exercises can improve overall muscle strength and endurance.

With regard to the ability of diaphragmatic breathing exercises to alter the pattern of breathing, the evidence is clear.[76] In patients with COPD, diaphragmatic breathing exercises have been shown to increase the relative contribution of this muscle to ventilation from about 40% (during uncoached spontaneous breathing) to about 67%.[76]

The effect of diaphragmatic breathing exercises on the pattern of ventilation and its distribution is more controversial. There is a general consensus that diaphragmatic breathing exercises can result in increased V_T and slower rates of breathing.[74] However, studies of the effect of diaphragmatic breathing exercises on the distribution of ventilation provide mixed results. In normal subjects, breathing mainly with the intercostal and accessory muscles results in a greater distribution of the inspired air to the upper lung regions as compared with either normal or diaphragmatic breathing. At low inspiratory flows, the distribution of ventilation with diaphragmatic breathing does not differ significantly from normal spontaneous breathing; at higher inspiratory flows, however, a normal breathing pattern causes a maldistribution of ventilation to the upper lung regions, not unlike that occurring during use of intercostal and accessory muscles.[77] Unfortunately, similar studies in patients with COLD have shown no systematic difference in the overall distribution of ventilation between spontaneous and augmented diaphragmatic breathing.[76]

Research results also provide a mixed picture regarding the effect of diaphragmatic breathing exercises on muscle strength and endurance. In one study of patients with chronic obstructive bronchitis with moderate disability, 3 weeks of controlled diaphragmatic breathing had no beneficial effects on exercise performance (walking) or the perceived strain of exercise, as compared with a placebo treatment.[78] However, several other studies have demonstrated positive results in the application of inspiratory breathing retraining, most often when included as a component of general conditioning exercise activity.[35,79-81] Although the outcome measures in these studies vary, the following general benefits of retraining in inspiratory muscle breathing were realized: a decrease in respiratory rate and an increase in V_T, Pao_2, and oxygen consumption during exercise; an increased maximum sustainable ventilatory capacity; and an increased maximum 12-minute walking distance.

Technique. Changing the breathing pattern is a slow and difficult process, which requires the utmost patience on the part of the practitioner. This is because it is often difficult for a patient who has come to rely extensively on the thoracic accessory muscles to revert back to diaphragmatic breathing. Indeed, many patients may never be able to fully accomplish this changeover.

Before starting a breathing exercise, the practitioner should make sure that the patient is relaxed, both mentally and physically. Before teaching any new breathing exercise, the practitioner also should demonstrate it on himself or herself, explaining both the purpose of each maneuver and how the patient can best accomplish it.

The best position for initiation of diaphragmatic breathing exercises is similar to that used for cough training, that is, a 45-degree sitting position, with shoulders rotated inward, the head and spine slightly flexed, the forearms relaxed or supported, and the knees bent. To minimize use of the upper thoracic respiratory muscles, a modification of the Jacobeson relaxation exercise may be employed.[1] In this technique, the patient is asked to shrug the shoulders and hold them up for a short period. Alternatively, the practitioner asks the patient to tighten the muscles of the arms and chest and then relax.

Once the patient is properly prepared, the practitioner places a hand on the patient's upper abdomen in the epigastric region below the xiphoid process (Fig. 27-15). The patient is then encouraged to inhale slowly through the nose, "taking air into the abdomen" with an effort forceful enough to lift the practitioner's hand. As the patient initiates the effort, the practitioner provides progressive resistance to the outward movement of the epigastric region, releasing the pressure at the end of inspiration.

The patient's awareness of the effort should be confirmed, and the exercise should be repeated (with rest as necessary) until satisfactory movement is achieved. Because of the physical work involved, the initial time tolerated by the patient may be short, but as performance improves the exercise may be extended to 30 minutes three to four times daily. Ideally, the patient can be taught to perform the exercise on himself or herself, using progressive epigastric pressure in the same manner as the practitioner.

During this early learning phase, the practitioner must be on guard for common errors, including arching of the patient's back or simple protrusion of the abdomen.[74] Both these maneuvers mimic true diaphragmatic breathing but are readily recognized. If a patient persists in these ineffective actions despite appropriate instruction and feedback, the practitioner should consider use of the lateral costal breathing exercises (discussed next) as an alternative.

In patients who can tolerate head-down positions, it may be possible to enhance this exercise with the patient in a Trendelenburg position in bed or on a tilt table. In this variation the patient is positioned in a 20-degree head-down tilt. As with the standard procedure, diaphragmatic action is taught and confirmed with progressive hand pressure. In subsequent treatment sessions, resistance to inspiration is provided by a weight placed over the epigastric region. Initially, this weight may be as little as 5 lb, but with strengthening of the diaphragm, the load may be progressively increased in 5 lb increments up to 20 to 30 lb, as tolerated.

Once the patient masters diaphragmatic breathing in the

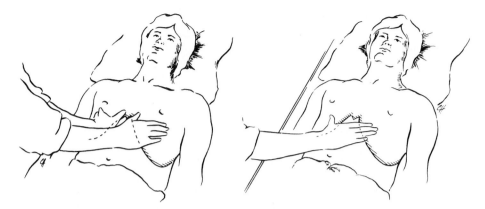

Fig. 27-15   Placement of therapist's hand for diaphragmatic breathing. (From Frownfelter D: Chest physical therapy and pulmonary rehabilitation: an interdisciplinary approach, ed 2, Chicago, 1987, Year Book Medical Publishers.)

sitting position, the practitioner should assist the ambulatory patient in application of this technique while standing, and, subsequently, as a component of the walking regimen.

Lateral costal breathing exercises. Lateral costal breathing exercises are intended to augment abdominal breathing. This modification of the diaphragmatic technique consists of expansion and contraction of the costal margin, which increases mobility of the diaphragm and, in theory, increases ventilation to the lung bases. Lateral costal breathing exercises are a viable alternative to the diaphragmatic method, especially in patients who have undergone abdominal surgery. As such, lateral costal breathing exercises have an effect comparable to that of the diaphragmatic technique on alveolar ventilation, muscle strength and endurance, and the patterns of breathing.

Technique. The patient will best understand the purpose of the exercise if introduced to it in the relaxed supine position. The practitioner places his or her hands over the costal margins so that they almost cup the lower rib edges (Fig. 27-16). At the end of exhalation, the practitioner begins application of pressure. The patient is instructed to "breathe around the waist and push the hands away" to direct attention to this area. As inhalation begins, the practitioner gradually increases the manual pressure to the expanding ribs while encouraging a slow, deep breath. Finally, the patient is taught to use his or her own hands to mobilize the lower ribs.

Inspiratory resistive breathing. Research conducted in the mid-1970s clearly demonstrated that both respiratory muscle strength and endurance in healthy subjects could be increased by a 6-week training program that involved resistive breathing exercises.[82] Subsequently, this technique was introduced and successfully applied as a simple alternative to traditional breathing exercises in patients with pulmonary disease.[83-88]

In concept, inspiratory resistive breathing represents the simple imposition of an additional work load on the in-

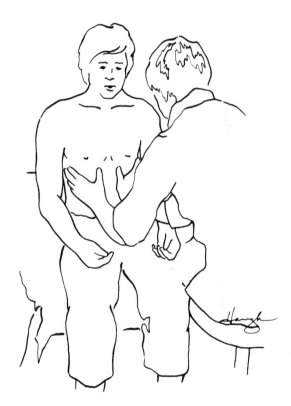

Fig. 27-16   Lateral costal breathing exercises. (From Frownfelter D: Chest physical therapy and pulmonary rehabilitation: an interdisciplinary approach, ed 2, Chicago, 1987, Year Book Medical Publishers.)

spiratory muscles (mainly the diaphragm) during breathing. Over time, this increased work load should increase both the strength and the endurance of these muscles. In turn, the increased strength and endurance of the inspiratory muscles should improve the patient's exercise tolerance.

The first device designed for this purpose was a simple adjustable flow resistor combined with a one-way valve

(Fig. 27-17). During inspiration, the patient breathes through a restricted orifice of variable size. Flow resistance across this orifice creates a pressure difference between the atmosphere and the mouth, thereby increasing the load placed on the inspiratory muscles. During expiration, gas flows unimpeded out the exhalation valve. Because the pressure difference during inspiration varies directly with the rate of flow, the load placed on the inspiratory muscles with this type of device is greater when the patient breathes fast and less when the patient breathes more slowly.

More recently, a threshold resistor has become commercially available for this purpose (Fig. 27-18). Instead of using a restricted orifice to increase the pressure differential, the threshold resistive breathing device uses an adjustable spring-loaded valve. This assures a relatively constant load, regardless of how fast or how slowly the patient breathes.[89] With this device, it is possible to set a specific load in terms of the negative inspiratory pressure (cm H_2O) necessary to open the valve.

Efficacy. In clinical trials with comparison groups, various researchers have shown that an inspiratory resistive breathing exercise training program can result in significant patient benefits. Among the positive outcomes generally reported are: decreased dyspnea and respiratory frequency, increased inspiratory muscle strength, and increased respiratory muscle endurance.[83-88] However, these benefits tend to occur without a change in either resting pulmonary function or overall exercise performance, as assessed by cycle ergometer exercise, stair climbing, walking distance, or treadmill walking.[90] Moreover, some studies have failed to show any significant benefit at all.[90,91]

Recently, it has been suggested that variations in the breathing strategy used during inspiratory resistive exercise may have a profound effect on its outcomes. Specifically, analysis of the breathing patterns used by patients has shown that a reduction in the peak mouth pressure, breathing frequency, and external resistive work, combined with a longer inspiratory time, is the most beneficial approach.[91]

Related to the general concern over variations in patients' breathing strategies has been a lack of validated clinical guidelines for prescribing inspiratory resistive exercises.[92] With the availability of the threshold resistive device, however, this situation is changing. A recent clinical study has shown that a resistive load of 30% of the maximum inspiratory pressure, or P_{Imax}, represents the minimum load necessary to effect an increase in inspiratory muscle strength and endurance.[93] Moreover, the use of this minimum load over a 2-month training program resulted in an increase in general exercise tolerance, as measured by the maximum 12-minute walking distance.

Technique. From these findings, it is evident that the success of this method depends on proper patient evaluation, training, and follow up, as conducted by a knowledgeable practitioner.

In terms of evaluation, in addition to the general assessment of the patient (previously described), the practitioner initially should measure the patient's maximum inspiratory

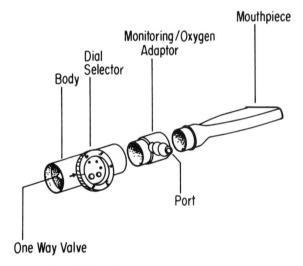

Fig. 27-17   Flow-resistive breathing device.

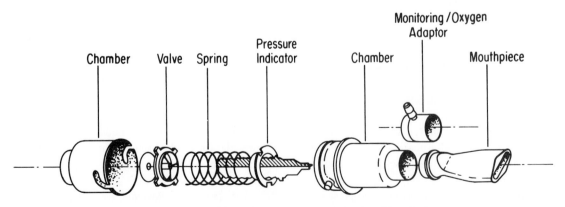

Fig. 27-18   Threshold (spring-loaded) resistive breathing device.

pressure with the use of a calibrated pressure manometer like that shown in Fig. 27-19. Once the P_{Imax} is obtained, the practitioner can compare the patient's value with established norms, as shown in Table 27-3.[94] This preliminary measure of inspiratory muscle strength thus helps in establishment of initial loads and provides the basis for the subsequent monitoring of the patient's progress.

In preparation for exercise training, the patient should be instructed to assume a position that relaxes the abdominal muscles, such as that used for cough training. Instruction in diaphragmatic breathing should ideally precede application of the inspiratory resistive exercises, thereby assuring appropriate emphasis on the use of this muscle of respiration.

If using a flow-resistive device, the practitioner initiates instruction at the maximum orifice setting, while measuring the inspiratory pressure generated through a monitoring/oxygen adapter (a second adapter may be necessary if the patient is receiving supplemental oxygen). The practitioner encourages the patient to inhale and exhale slowly through the device, at a rate of no more than 12 to 15 breaths per minute. If the generated inspiratory pressure is less than 30% of the measured P_{Imax}, the next smaller orifice is selected, with this procedure repeated until the 30% effort is consistently achieved.

Once the appropriate effort is achieved, the patient is instructed to begin exercise with the device in one or two regular daily sessions of 10 to 15 minutes' duration. As the level of resistance becomes more tolerable over time, the patient progressively increases the duration of the sessions to 30 minutes. A self-maintained log of treatment times can help motivate the patient and assist the practitioner in subsequent progress monitoring.

At this point the patient should be reevaluated by the practitioner, and this evaluation should include measurement of the P_{Imax}. If the patient exhibits an increase in the P_{Imax}, the level of resistance should be increased (by decreasing the size of the orifice) to the new 30% level, with session time restored to 10 to 15 minutes and the exercise progression and follow up should be repeated. If, on the other hand, the P_{Imax} is not increased, the practitioner should attempt to determine the cause by questioning the patient and inspecting the log. In many cases, a failure to demonstrate an improvement in P_{Imax} can be attributed to simple noncompliance with the exercise regimen.

When a threshold resistive device is used, the technique is essentially the same, except that loads can be set directly on the device. As with the flow-resistive device, once the initial load is determined, the patient progressively increases the duration of the session. On reevaluation by the physician or the practitioner, the load may be increased, with the patient then repeating the cycle of increasing session time.

Expiratory breathing exercises. There are two primary types of expiratory breathing exercise: pursed-lip breathing and forced-exhalation abdominal breathing. The former technique is used exclusively in patients with COPD who are prone to early airway collapse. The latter method has been used in these patients but may also be useful as an adjunct to cough training in other groups with expiratory muscle dysfunction.

Pursed-lip breathing. Pursed-lip breathing is a simple maneuver that many patients with COPD adopt without instruction. The purpose of pursed-lip breathing is to prevent the air trapping caused by bronchiolar collapse, especially that associated with pulmonary emphysema.[95]

By increasing expiratory flow resistance, pursed-lip breathing has two primary effects. First, pursed-lip breathing increases upstream pressures in the tracheobronchial tree during exhalation.[96] This causes the equal pressure point (EPP) to move farther up toward the larger airways, thereby decreasing the likelihood of bronchiolar collapse.[97] Second, pursed-lip breathing decreases expiratory flow

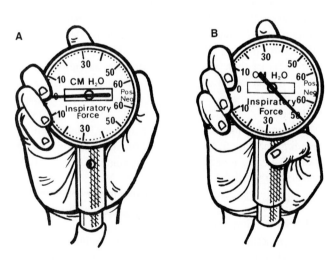

Fig. 27-19 An inspiratory force measurement. The gauge is attached to the patient's airway, **A.** The patient is instructed to take a deep breath while the clinician obstructs the airway by closing the open port on the gauge, **B.** The negative pressure detection, measured here as −50 cm of water, is the patient's maximum inspiratory force. (From Pilbeam SP: Mechanical ventilation: physiological and clinical applications, ed 1, St Louis, 1986, Multimedia Publishing, Inc.)

Table 27-3 Normal Maximum Inspiratory Pressure (cm H_2O) By Age and Sex

Age group	Mean (± SD) P_{Imax} from residual volume	
	Male	Female
9-18	−96 ± 35	−90 ± 25
19-50	−127 ± 28	−91 ± 25
51-70	−112 ± 20	−77 ± 18
>70	−76 ± 27	−66 ± 18

From Rochester DF and Hyatt RE: Respiratory muscle failure, Med Clin North Am 67:573-579, 1983.

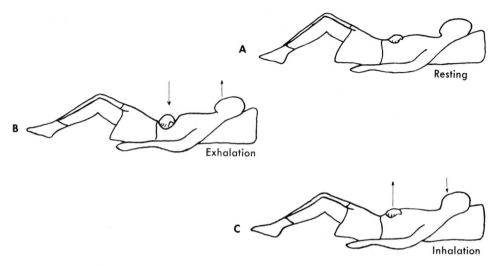

Fig. 27-20   Forced-exhalation abdominal breathing. (See text for description.)

rates. This decreases the frequency of breathing and prolongs the expiratory time.[95,98]

Efficacy. Patients with chronic obstructive pulmonary disease who breathe through pursed lips tend to exhibit both an increase in alveolar ventilation and an improvement in $\dot{V}/\dot{Q}$ distribution, as indicated by a decrease in the $P(A-a)O_2$.[99] Whether these beneficial effects are caused mainly by the movement of the EPP or to the decrease in respiratory rates is not known. The fact that simple deep breathing at slow rates alone may have similar effects in these patients suggests that it is the pattern of breathing that is of primary importance.[98] However, the changes in airway pressure generated during pursed-lip breathing may help diminish feelings of dyspnea by altering tension relationships of the respiratory muscles.[100]

Technique. In preparation for training in pursed-lip breathing, the patient should be placed in a comfortable position. The practitioner instructs the patient to inhale slowly through the mouth. During exhalation, the patient is taught to purse the lips as if whistling, controlling the velocity of exhaled air to the slowest that is consistent with comfortable ventilation. Ideally, this should lower the rate of breathing and increase the expiratory time so that it is at least twice as long as inspiration. Efforts should be made to avoid strenuous expiratory efforts, since this may simply increase the tendency toward bronchiolar collapse. The technique should be reinforced as needed, and the patient should be encouraged to apply this method whenever dyspnea is sensed.

Forced-exhalation abdominal breathing. Forced-exhalation abdominal breathing exercises are designed to strengthen the contractile force of the abdominal wall muscles. This technique is useful in patients with poor muscle conditioning that limits exercise capacity or in those who have an ineffective cough because of a specific weakness of the expiratory muscles. Forced-exhalation abdominal

breathing exercises are best taught with the patient in the supine position, with a pillow under the patient's head and the knees drawn up comfortably to relax the anterior abdominal wall. The principles of the technique are illustrated in Fig. 27-20. The patient's hand is placed on the epigastrium to focus attention to this area, *A*. Much of the success of therapy will depend on the degree to which the practitioner can keep the patient's mind on this epigastric movement. Exercise is always started in the same manner, by exhaling from the resting level. At the same time, the patient is instructed to pull in the upper abdomen gradually, with conscious force, prolonging exhalation as long as possible, *B*. At end-exhalation the patient is told to inhale easily through the nose, letting the upper abdomen balloon out, *C,* and the cycle is repeated. The patient is advised to think of all breathing as taking place in the abdomen rather than in the chest; therefore, as the patient inhales, the abdomen should swell, lifting up the hand, and as he or she exhales, the hand should fall with the receding abdomen.

During the maneuver, the practitioner must keep reminding the patient to concentrate on all respiratory movement as taking place in the area in contact with the hand and to disregard the chest completely. Many patients, trying hard to cooperate, will suddenly forget the sequence they were taught, contracting the epigastric wall during inhalation and attempting to relax it during exhalation.

The practitioner who encounters this problem will find two techniques useful in correction of the breathing pattern. The first is the steady repetition over several breathing cycles of "inhale, abdomen out, exhale, abdomen in" to help fix the rhythm in the patient's mind. The second is the placement of a hand over the patient's hand on the abdominal wall to exert gentle but firm pressure, depressing the epigastrium during the prolongation of exhalation. Much practice may be required for this seemingly simple

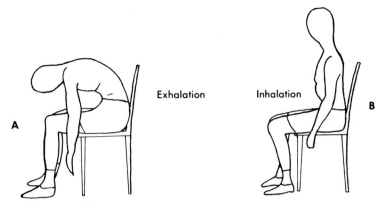

Fig. 27-21   Forced-exhalation abdominal breathing, seated. (See text for description.)

procedure, but as proficiency is acquired, the patient is encouraged to make a positive effort to use the diaphragm and the abdominal muscles rather than the upper thoracic accessory muscles.

To vary the forced-exhalation exercise, the patient may be taught to do it in the seated position, employing the added techniques of forward bending as shown in Fig. 27-21. The patient relaxes in a straight-backed chair, sitting upright to commence the maneuver. With the arms hanging loosely by the side to promote relaxation of the thoracic skeletal muscles, he or she slowly exhales through pursed lips while slowly bending forward and retracting the upper abdomen (Fig. 27-21, *A*). When properly timed, flexion of the trunk should be complete at the moment of end-expiration. The body is then raised while the patient inhales through the nose, letting the abdomen distend as the lungs fill. When inhalation is completed, the patient should be back in the upright position. To aid exhalation, the forward bending uses the flexion of the trunk to compress the abdomen and elevate the diaphragm. This exercise is especially helpful to the patient who has difficulty clearing secretions, because it tends to stimulate their mobility and facilitate their removal by cough.

Coordinating breathing with walking. The ultimate objective of all breathing exercises is to increase the patient's tolerance for physical activity. Of all the major complaints expressed by patients with COPD, none is more important than the inability to walk comfortably. This may manifest itself as difficulty in walking from room to room within the home or as a hesitancy to leave the home at all. In the hospital, the respiratory care practitioner will observe that many patients breathe with ease while resting in bed or on a chair but revert to severe thoracic or paradoxical ventilation as soon as they start to walk. Improvement of walking tolerance generally does more to increase the patient's morale than any other therapeutic intervention.

The primary purpose of walking exercises is to help minimize dyspnea during exertion, thereby increasing the patient's tolerance for increased activity. Ideally, this is achieved by coordinating physical exertion with the rhythm of breathing, with the prolonged phase of exhalation as the period of maximum effort. This implies that the patient has mastered the act of diaphragmatic breathing and fully understands its purpose.

To prepare for walking exercise, the patient must first practice diaphragmatic breathing in the standing relaxation position, as previously described (Fig. 27-11). The patient is then instructed to begin movement while breathing slowly, taking two steps during inhalation and three steps during exhalation. This rhythm helps the patient to maintain a ventilatory ratio in which exhalation time exceeds that devoted to inhalation. Moreover, it lets the patient perform the most exertion when it is easier, during the relatively passive expiratory phase. Because this exercise is developed so that it can be done smoothly, the patient will find that walking will consume much less energy than when his or her breathing was haphazard.

Patients who master this coordinated walking technique will find it applicable to many other activities. For example, it will greatly help the patient in climbing stairs, which ordinarily is one of the most difficult chores for those with severe COPD. In this adaptation of the method, the patient learns to manage two or three steps during exhalation and to rest during inhalation.

Graded exercises. As the culmination, or end objective, of the breathing exercises just described, a system of graded exercises is used to increase the patient's overall physical conditioning. Graded exercises are designed to gradually increase the patient's overall physical conditioning over an extended period of time. This progressive approach minimizes the likelihood of ill effects and allows careful monitoring of progress by the practitioner.

A patient is ready for this aspect of physical therapy only after any acute exacerbation of the disease process is under control and he or she has mastered the basic breath-control techniques previously discussed.

Whereas techniques in performing progressive exercises may vary, the general principles are the same. Assessments of pulmonary and cardiac function, including blood gas analysis, are made before the program is started and are repeated according to the needs of each treatment schedule. Whether a treadmill or an exercise bicycle is used is less important than the ability to vary the patient's work load in a quantitative fashion. We will limit our discussion here to the use of the treadmill.

The first exposure of the patient to exercise is tentative, to judge response and tolerance, and to teach the proper technique. Supplemental oxygen is normally given to the patient as needed, usually through a nasal cannula. Initially, the treadmill is adjusted to 0% grade and a rate not to exceed 1 mph. The practitioner must give encouragement to those patients who initially are apprehensive and assure them that they can step off the moving surface at any time. During the first trial the practitioner must see that the patient is using the diaphragm to breathe, since it is under such conditions of stress that he or she is likely to revert to thoracic or paradoxical breathing, and this cannot be permitted if the exercise regimen is to be successful.

Graded exercises are scheduled on a regular basis, usually daily, over a period of weeks to months. The pitch of the walking surface, its speed, and the duration of exercise are increased in increments tailored to each patient, and these are good criteria for evaluation of progress. For example, if a patient walks 10 minutes at 0% grade and 1 mph initially and later walks 15 minutes at 2% grade and 1.5 mph, this represents significant improvement.

Even more important is the gradual reduction in the need for supplemental oxygen as the intensity of the exercise increases. It may seem paradoxical that increasing exercise of a patient with respiratory insufficiency should lower the oxygen requirement, but the physiologic reason is the foundation for this aspect of rehabilitation. We must remember that patients with COPD often become sedentary, which results in a progressive deterioration of the skeletal muscles. Since poorly conditioned skeletal muscle consumes more oxygen per minute for a given work load than does properly conditioned muscle, this progressive deterioration places disproportionately high energy demands on the patient—demands that cannot always be met.

The clinical improvement from a graded exercise program is attributed to two factors.[101,102] First, although pulmonary function tests may show little functional change, exercise improves the patient's respiratory muscle strength and endurance, thereby increasing maximum ventilatory capacity. Second, physical conditioning will lower the maximum oxygen consumption for a given work load, thereby increasing the dyspnea threshold. Together, both factors greatly increase the patient's exercise tolerance.

Although the program just described would have to be conducted under the constant supervision of trained personnel in a rehabilitation facility, there may be instances in which such supervision is not practical or possible.[103,104] With proper selection, many patients can profit from a well-planned program of graded exercise at home. One of

the many valuable services of the respiratory care practitioner is the training and follow-up supervision of patients for such programs.

Graded exercises with oxygen also can be done at home but should be attempted only if both the patient's attending physician and the respiratory care practitioner consider the patient responsible and intelligent enough to follow directions accurately.[105] Home exercise can be provided by an exercise cycle or by level walking, if space permits. Supportive oxygen, supplied in small liquid or compressed-gas cylinders, can be carried in a shoulder sling by the walking patient. According to the patient's capabilities, an individualized schedule of graded walking can be developed. However, such a schedule must be reviewed frequently to assess results, and it should be modified as necessary. More details on the proper use and integration of graded exercise activity within an organized rehabilitation program are provided in Chapter 34.

COMPLICATIONS AND ADVERSE EFFECTS OF CHEST PHYSICAL THERAPY

When they occur, the complications and adverse effects of CPT can be significant and severe. However, either these problems are infrequent or they are significantly under reported.[7] Among the major complications of CPT, pulmonary hemorrhage and rib fractures are potentially the most severe. Lesser adverse effects include increased intracranial pressure, hypoxemia, decreased cardiac output, and increased airway resistance.

Hemorrhage

Massive pulmonary hemorrhage leading to death has been cited as a major complication of chest physical therapy.[7,106] In case reports of this fatal complication, the underlying cause was attributed to either a pulmonary abscess or a bronchopleural fistula. Moreover, hemoptysis or bleeding of bright red blood was always observed before the incident. On the basis of these reports, one should logically avoid CPT when there is active hemoptysis.

Rib fractures

Rib fractures are often identified as a complication of CPT, most often attributed to percussion and vibration. However, only one report of this potential problem appears in the medical literature, and then only in association with the management of an infant with hyaline membrane disease, a condition in which rib fractures are common anyway.[7,107] For this reason, the likelihood of properly performed chest physical therapy causing rib fractures should be considered small, and the presence of rib fractures should not be considered an absolute contraindication to percussion and vibration. If, as the literature suggests, percussion and vibration should not be used extensively, the possibility of this complication is even more remote.

Increased intracranial pressure

Obviously, both coughing and the use of any head-down position in CPT pose the risk of increased intracranial pressure (ICP). Increases in ICP averaging as high as 23 mm Hg have been reported when patients with head injuries were placed in the Trendelenburg position.[108] Although this effect is blunted by certain anesthetic agents and high oxygen concentrations, any form of CPT that could raise ICP must be applied with extreme caution to high-risk patients. In the absence of ICP monitoring, CPT should be attempted in these patients only when the benefits clearly outweigh the risks.[7]

Hypoxemia

The fact that CPT can decrease arterial PaO_2 was clearly demonstrated some 20 years ago.[109] Subsequent studies have shown that this decrease in arterial oxygenation is most likely in patients with cardiovascular instability or those with profuse bronchial secretions.[110,111]

As previously discussed, arterial hypoxemia also is worsened in patients with unilateral lung disease when they are positioned with the bad lung down.[16,17,57] Tyler and associates[112] have found PaO_2 differences as great as 100 mm Hg between right and left side-lying positions in such patients, although the average decrease was less than 17 mm Hg. The factor most associated with the effect of CPT on oxygenation appears to be the baseline PaO_2.[7] In general, the higher the PaO_2 before chest physical therapy, the greater will be the drop in this measure during treatment.

In patients with chronic obstructive pulmonary disease (COPD), measurements of arterial oxygen saturation (SaO_2) during CPT indicate only a small risk of hypoxemia in this group. In a series of patients being treated for acute exacerbations of COPD, none exhibited a significant change in SaO_2 during CPT.[113] In stable patients with COPD being managed on an outpatient basis, only one of 15 exhibited a clinically significant fall in SaO_2 (from 94% to 67%).[114] Moreover, this decrease occurred only after bronchodilator administration but not during CPT alone.

Thus the potential risk of hypoxemia during CPT is real, but it is generally predictable and small. This risk can be minimized by provision of supplemental oxygen or an increase in the delivered FIO_2 during chest physical therapy.

Impaired cardiac output

Decreases in cardiac output of as much as 50% have been reported in some patients receiving a CPT regimen that included an artificial cough with positive pressure hyperinflation.[115] These changes occurred only in those who were unconscious or too ill to resist the treatment procedure. Impaired venous return resulting from increased intrathoracic pressure was the probable cause of this effect, along with failure of the normal cardiovascular compensatory mechanisms.[7]

In a group of patients recovering from mitral valve surgery, CPT (consisting of percussion, vibration, and costal breathing, followed by coughing) caused a mean drop in cardiac output of 14% and an average decrease in mixed venous PO_2 of 9 mm Hg (from 41 to 32 mm Hg).[116] Although the fall in mixed venous PO_2 observed in this study suggests that tissue oxygenation can be compromised during CPT procedures, contrary results have been reported.[7]

As with arterial oxygenation, the likelihood that CPT will adversely affect cardiac output and oxygen delivery is probably related to the relative cardiovascular stability of the patient. The probability of an adverse cardiovascular effect is therefore greatest when CPT is applied to those with hypovolemia, those in shock from any cause, or those who have lost the compensatory mechanisms normally responsible for regulation of blood pressure and flow.

Increased airway resistance

It is logical to assume that CPT should improve airway caliber and lower airway resistance. Indeed, application of chest physical therapy to patients with either chronic bronchitis or cystic fibrosis has been shown to increase expiratory flow rates after therapy.[117,118] However, this improvement appears to be substantially less among those patients who exhibited signs of bronchospasm, such as wheezing, during therapy.

That CPT may actually increase airway resistance in some patients has also been demonstrated. In a study of patients with chronic bronchitis during an acute exacerbation of their illness, nearly half exhibited a decrease in FEV_1 immediately after CPT, with restoration of baseline values within 30 minutes after therapy.[19] Significantly, subjects with the greatest fall in FEV_1 tended to have the most reactive airways, as judged by their response to bronchodilators. Moreover, administration of a bronchodilator before CPT abolished this adverse response in all patients.

Likewise, although chest physical therapy has been shown to result in an overall improvement in the specific airway conductance (the inverse of airway resistance) among a group of patients, about one in five exhibited a decrease in this measure of airway caliber.[119] Why airway resistance increased in these patients remains unclear, since neither a failure to clear sputum nor hyperreactivity of the airways was considered a contributing factor.

Apparently, CPT can cause an increase in airway resistance in some patients. The primary mechanism responsible for this adverse effect is probably reversible bronchospasm in patients with hyperreactive airways. Ideally, these patients can be identified in advance by virtue of a positive response to bronchodilator agents. For these persons, the administration of a bronchodilator before therapy may minimize or abolish this adverse response.

SUMMARY

Chest physical therapy represents a collection of physical techniques designed to facilitate clearance of airway secretion, improve the distribution of ventilation, and enhance the efficiency and conditioning of the muscle of respiration. It was not until recently that rigorous scientific methods have been applied to study the effectiveness of these methods in groups of patients with similar conditions. Results of these studies indicate that selected methods of CPT are effective for certain patients under specific clinical circumstances.

Among those for whom scientific evidence currently supports the application of chest physical therapy are (1) acutely ill patients with copious secretions, (2) patients in acute respiratory failure with clinical signs of retained secretions, (3) patients with acute lobar atelectasis, (4) patients with $\dot{V}/\dot{Q}$ abnormalities caused by lung infiltrates or consolidation, (5) patients with chronic conditions characterized by production of large volumes of sputum, and (6) patients with COPD who exhibit inefficient breathing patterns and/or decreased exercise tolerance.

Five primary methods are employed in chest physical therapy. Used alone or in combination, these methods include therapeutic positioning, chest percussion and vibration, coughing and related expulsion techniques, breathing retraining, and conditioning exercises. Each method differs according to its underlying principle, relative efficacy, and method(s) of application. The appropriate selection and application of these techniques depends, first and foremost on proper initial and ongoing assessment of the patient. This should include the results of the initial physical assessment, laboratory testing (including pulmonary function tests), and radiologic evaluation.

The complications and adverse effects of CPT can be significant and severe. However, either these problems are infrequent or they are significantly underreported. Among the major complications of CPT, pulmonary hemorrhage and rib fractures are potentially the most severe. Lesser adverse effects include increased intracranial pressure, hypoxemia, decreased cardiac output, and increased airway resistance. Recognition of the potential for these problems and careful preliminary respiratory care planning can minimize their likelihood and ensure the safe and effective provision of chest physical therapy.

REFERENCES

1. Frownfelter D: Chest physical therapy and pulmonary rehabilitation: an interdisciplinary approach, ed 2, Chicago, 1987, Year Book Medical Publishers.
2. American Physical Therapy Association, Cardiopulmonary Section: Definition of chest physical therapy, American Physical Therapy Association, 1982.
3. Frownfelter D: Chest physical therapy and airway care. In Barnes TA: Respiratory care practice, Chicago, 1988, Year Book Medical Publishers.
4. Rochester D and Goldberg S: Techniques of respiratory physical therapy, Am Rev Respir Dis 122(suppl):133-146, 1980.
5. Murray J: The ketchup-bottle method, N Engl J Med 300:1155-1157, 1979.
6. MacKenzie CF, Ciesla N, Imle PC, and Klemic N, editors: Chest physiotherapy in the intensive care unit, Baltimore, 1981, Williams & Wilkins Co.
7. Tyler ML: Complications of positioning and chest physiotherapy, Respir Care 27:458-466, 1982.
8. Kirilloff LH, Owens GR, Rogers RM, and Mazzocco MC: Does chest physical therapy work? Chest 88:436-444, 1985.
9. Sutton P, Pavia D, Bateman J, and Clarke S: Chest physiotherapy: a review, Eur J Respir Dis 63:188-201, 1982.
10. Connors AF Jr et al: Chest physical therapy: the immediate effect on oxygenation in acutely ill patients, Chest 78:559-564, 1980.
11. MacKenzie CF, Shin B, McAslan TC: Chest physiotherapy: the effect on arterial oxygenation, Anesth Analg 57:28-30, 1978.
12. Marini JJ, Pierson DJ, and Hudsson LD: A prospective comparison of fiberoptic bronchoscopy and respiratory therapy, Am Rev Respir Dis 119:971-978, 1979.
13. Marini JJ: Postoperative atelectasis: pathophysiology, clinical importance, and principles of management, Respir Care 29:515-522, 1984.
14. Hammond WE and Martin FJ: Chest physical therapy for acute atelectasis, Phys Ther 61:217-220, 1981.
15. Douglas WW et al: Improved oxygenation in patients with acute respiratory failure: the prone position, Am Rev Respir Dis 115:559-566, 1977.
16. Dhainaut JF, Bons J, Bricard C, and Monsallier JF: Improved oxygenation in patients with extensive unilateral pneumonia using the lateral decubitus position, Thorax 35:792-793, 1980.
17. Syracuse DC, Hyman AI, and King TC: Postural influences on arterial blood gases in patients with unilateral pulmonary consolidation, Surg Forum 30:173-174, 1979.
18. Anthonisen P, Riis P, and Sogaard-Anderson T: The value of lung physiotherapy in the treatment of acute exacerbations in chronic bronchitis, Acta Med Scand 175:715-719, 1964.
19. Campbell AH, O'Connell JM, and Wilson F: The effect of chest physiotherapy upon the FEV_1 in chronic bronchitis, Med J Aust 1:33-35, 1975.
20. Newton D and Stephenson A: Effects of physiotherapy on pulmonary function, Lancet 2:228-230, 1978.
21. Graham W and Bradley D: Efficacy of chest physiotherapy and intermittent positive pressure breathing in the resolution of pneumonia, N Engl J Med 299:624-627, 1978.
22. De Boeck C and Zinman R: Cough versus chest physiotherapy, Am Rev Respir Dis 129, 182-184, 1984.
23. Rossman CM et al: Effect of chest physiotherapy on the removal of mucus in patients with cystic fibrosis, Am Rev Respir Dis 126:131-135, 1982.
24. Pryor S, Webber B, Hosdon M, and Batten J: Evaluation of the forced expiration technique as an adjunct to postural drainage in treatment of cystic fibrosis, Br Med J 2:417-418, 1979.
25. Zach MS and Oberwaldner B: Chest physiotherapy—the mechanical approach to antiinfective therapy in cystic fibrosis, Infection 15:381-384, 1987.
26. Mazzocco MC, Owens GR, Kirilloff LH, and Rogers RM: Chest percussion and postural drainage in patients with bronchiectasis, Chest 88:360-363, 1985.
27. Sutton P et al: Assessment of the forced expiration technique, postural drainage, and directed coughing in chest physiotherapy, Eur J Respir Dis 64:62-68, 1983.
28. Oldenburg FA et al: Effects of postural drainage, exercise, and cough on mucus clearance in chronic bronchitis, Am Rev Respir Dis 120:739-745, 1979.
29. Bateman JR et al: Is cough as effective as chest physical therapy in the removal of excessive bronchial secretions? Thorax 36:683-687, 1981.
30. Bateman JR et al: Regional lung clearance of excessive bronchial

secretions during chest physiotherapy in patients with stable chronic airways obstruction, Lancet 1:294-279, 1979.

31. Sergysels R: Can respiratory kinesitherapy palliate the functional sequelae of chronic obstructive bronchopathies? Rev Fr Mal Respir 11:605-608, 1983.

32. Gimenez M: Technics and results in respiratory kinesitherapy of chronic obstructive bronchopneumopathies, Rev Fr Mal Respir 11:525-43, 1983.

33. Faling LJ: Pulmonary rehabilitation—physical modalities, Clin Chest Med 7:599-618, 1986.

34. Make BJ: Pulmonary rehabilitation: myth or reality? Clin Chest Med 7:519-540, 1986.

35. Casciari RJ et al: Effects of breathing retraining in patients with chronic obstructive pulmonary disease, Chest 79:393-398, 1981.

36. Housset B, Tetard C, and Derenne JP: Respiratory physiotherapy and respiratory mechanics of chronic respiratory insufficiency, Rev Fr Mal Respir 11:915-921, 1983.

37. Bartlett RH et al: Studies on the pathogenesis and prevention of postoperative pulmonary complications, Surg Gynecol Obstet 137:925, 1973.

38. Tarhan S et al: Risk of anesthesia and surgery in patients with chronic bronchitis and chronic obstructive pulmonary disease, Surgery 74:720, 1973.

39. Bartlett RH: Respiratory therapy to prevent pulmonary complications of surgery, Respir Care 29:667-679, 1984.

40. Kigin CM: Chest physical therapy for the postoperative or traumatic injury patient, Phys Ther 61:1724, 1981.

41. Vraciu J and Vraciu R: Effectiveness of breathing exercises in preventing pulmonary complications following open heart surgery, Phys Ther 57:1367-1370, 1977.

42. Castillo R and Haas A: Chest physical therapy: comparative efficacy of preoperative and postoperative in the elderly, Arch Phys Med Rehabil 66:376-379, 1985.

43. Torrington KG, Sorenson DE, and Sherwood LM: Postoperative chest percussion with postural drainage in obese patients following gastric stapling, Chest 86:891-895, 1984.

44. Hoffman LA: Ineffective airway clearance related to neuromuscular dysfunction, Nurs Clin North Am 22:151-166, 1987.

45. Desmond KJ et al: Immediate and long-term effects of chest physiotherapy in patients with cystic fibrosis, J Pediatr 103:538-542, 1983.

46. Harris JA and Jerry BA: Indications and procedures for segmental bronchial drainage, Respir Care 20:456, 1975.

47. Tecklin JS: Positioning, percussing, and vibrating patients for effective bronchial drainage, Nursing 79 9:64-71, 1979.

48. Zausmer E: Bronchial drainage: evidence supporting the procedures, Phys Ther 48:586-591, 1968.

49. Wong JW et al: Effects of gravity on tracheal transport rates in normal subjects and in patients with cystic fibrosis, Pediatrics 60:146-152, 1977.

50. March H: Appraisal of postural drainage for chronic obstructive pulmonary disease, Arch Phys Med Rehabil 52:528-530, 1971.

51. May D and Munt P: Physiologic effects of chest percussion and postural drainage in patients with stable chronic bronchitis, Chest 79:29-32, 1979.

52. Loring M and Denning C: Evaluation of postural drainage by measurement of sputum volume and consistency, Am J Phys Med 50:215-219, 1971.

53. Chopra SK et al: Effects of hydration and physical therapy on tracheal transport velocity, Am Rev Respir Dis 115:1009-1014, 1974.

54. Marini JJ et al: Influence of head-dependent positions on lung volume and oxygen saturation in chronic airflow obstruction, Am Rev Respir Dis 129:101-105, 1984.

55. Clauss RH et al: Effects of changing body position upon improved ventilation-perfusion relationships, Circulation 37(suppl):214-217, 1968.

56. Kaneko K, Mille-Emili J, and Dolowich MB: Regional distribution of ventilation and perfusion as a function of body position, J Appl Physiol 21:767-777, 1966.

57. Zack MB, Pontoppidan H, and Kazemi H: The effect of lateral positions on gas exchange in pulmonary disease: a prospective evaluation. Am Rev Respir Dis 110:49-55, 1974.

58. Remolina C et al: Positional hypoxemia in unilateral lung disease, N Engl J Med 304:523-525, 1981.

59. Demers RR: Down with the good lung—(usually) Respir Care 32:849-850, 1987 (editorial).

60. Martin RJ et al: Effect of supine and prone positions on arterial oxygen tension in the preterm infant, Pediatrics 63:528-531, 1979.

61. Barach AL: Chronic obstructive lung disease: postural relief of dyspnea, Arch Phys Med Rehabil 55:494, 1974.

62. Radford R et al: A rational basis for percussion-augmented mucociliary clearance, Respir Care 27:556-563, 1982.

63. Holody B and Goldberg H: The effect of mechanical vibration physiotherapy on arterial saturation in acutely ill patients with atelectasis or pneumonia, Am Rev Respir Dis 124:372-375, 1981.

64. Denton R: Bronchial secretions in cystic fibrosis: the effects of treatment with mechanical percussion vibration, Am Rev Respir Dis 86:41-46, 1962.

65. Pavia D, Thompson M, and Phillipakos D: A preliminary study of the effects of a vibrating pad on bronchial clearance, Am Rev Respir Dis 113:92-96, 1976.

66. Sutton PP et al: Assessment of percussion, vibratory-shaking and breathing exercises in chest physiotherapy, Eur J Respir Dis 66:147-152, 1985.

67. Wollmer P et al: Inefficiency of chest percussion in the physical therapy of chronic bronchitis, Eur J Respir Dis 66:233-239, 1985.

68. van der Schans CP, Piers DA, and Postma DS: Effect of manual percussion on tracheobronchial clearance in patients with chronic airflow obstruction and excessive tracheobronchial secretion, Thorax 41:448-452, 1986.

69. Eubanks DH and Bone RC: Comprehensive respiratory care, St Louis, 1985, The CV Mosby Co.

70. Langerson J: The cough: its effectiveness depends on you, Respir Care 24:142-149, 1979.

71. Leith DL: Cough. In Brain JD, Proctor DF, and Reid LM, editors: Respiratory defense mechanisms, New York, 1977, Marcel Dekker.

72. Irwin RS et al: Cough: a comprehensive review, Arch Intern Med 137:1189, 1977.

73. Petty TL: Chronic obstructive pulmonary disease, New York, 1978, Marcel Dekker.

74. Barrascout AR: Chest physical therapy and related procedures. In Burton GG and Hodgkin JE, editors: Respiratory care: a guide to clinical practice, ed 2, Philadelphia, 1984, JB Lippincott Co.

75. Grassino A, Bellemare F, and LaPorta D: Diaphragm fatigue and the strategy of breathing in COPD, Chest 85(suppl 6):515-545, 1984.

76. Grimby G, Oxhoj H, and Bake B: Effects of abdominal breathing on distribution of ventilation in obstructive lung disease, Clin Sci Mol Med 48:193-199, 1975.

77. Fixley MS et al: Flow dependence of gas distribution and the pattern of inspiratory muscle contraction, J Appl Physiol 45:733-741, 1978.

78. Williams IP, Smith CM, and McGavin CR: Diaphragmatic breathing training and walking performance in chronic airways obstruction, Br J Dis Chest 76:164-166, 1982.

79. Levine S, Weiser P, and Gillen J: Evaluation of a ventilatory muscle endurance training program in the rehabilitation of patients with chronic obstructive pulmonary disease, Am Rev Respir Dis 133:400-406, 1986.

80. Belman M and Mittman C: Ventilatory muscle training improves

exercise capacity in chronic obstructive pulmonary disease patients, Am Rev Respir Dis 121:273-280, 1980.

81. Pardy RL et al: Inspiratory muscle training compared with physiotherapy in patients with chronic airflow limitation, Am Rev Respir Dis 123:421-425, 1981.

82. Leith DE and Bradley M: Ventilatory muscle strength and endurance training, J Appl Physiol 41:508-516, 1976.

83. Anderson JB et al: Resistive breathing training in severe chronic obstructive lung disease: a pilot study, Scand J Respir Dis 60:151-156, 1979.

84. Sonne LJ and Davis JA: Increased exercise performances in patients with severe COPD following inspiratory resistive training, Chest 81:436-439, 1982.

85. Asher MI et al: The effects of inspiratory muscle training in patients with cystic fibrosis, Am Rev Respir Dis 126:855-859, 1982.

86. Keens TG et al: Ventilatory muscle endurance training in normal subjects and patients with cystic fibrosis, Am Rev Respir Dis 116:853-860, 1977.

87. Falk P et al: Relieving dyspnea with an inexpensive and simple method in patients with severe chronic airflow limitation, Eur J Respir Dis 66:181-186, 1985.

88. Chen H, Dukes R and Martin BJ: Inspiratory muscle training in patients with chronic obstructive pulmonary disease, Am Rev Respir Dis 131:251-255, 1985.

89. Clanton TL et al: Inspiratory muscle conditioning using a threshold loading device, Chest 87:62-66, 1985.

90. McKeon JL et al: The effect of inspiratory resistive training on exercise capacity in optimally treated patients with severe chronic airflow limitation, Aust NZ J Med 16:648-662, 1986.

91. Belman MJ, Thomas SG, and Lewis MI: Resistive breathing training in patients with chronic obstructive pulmonary disease, Chest 90:662-669, 1986.

92. Sobush DC and Dunning M: Providing resistive breathing exercise to the inspiratory muscles using the PFLEX device: suggestion from the field, Phys Ther 66:542-544, 1986.

93. Larson JL, Kim MJ, and Sharp JT: Inspiratory muscle training with a threshold resistive breathing device in patients with chronic obstructive pulmonary disease, Am Rev Respir Dis 133:A100, 1986.

94. Rochester DF and Hyatt RE: Respiratory muscle failure, Med Clin North Am 67:573-579, 1983.

95. Evans TW and Howard P: Whistle for your wind, Br Med J 289:449-450, 1984.

96. Ingram RH and Schilder DP: Effect of pursed lips expiration on the pulmonary pressure-flow relationship in obstructive lung disease, Am Rev Respir Dis 95:381-388, 1967.

97. Martin L: Pulmonary physiology in clinical practice; the essentials for patient care and evaluation, St Louis, 1987, The CV Mosby Co.

98. Thoman RL, Stoker GL, and Ross JC: The efficacy of pursed lips breathing in patients with chronic obstructive pulmonary disease, Am Rev Respir Dis 3:100-106, 1966.

99. Mueller RE, Petty TL, and Filley GF: Ventilation and arterial blood gas changes induced by pursed-lip breathing, J Appl Physiol 28:784, 1970.

100. Howell JBL: Breathlessness in pulmonary disease. In Howell JBL and Campbell EJM, editors: Breathlessness, Oxford, England, 1966, Blackwell Scientific.

101. Pierce AK et al: Responses to exercise training in patients with emphysema, Arch Intern Med 113:28, 1964.

102. Barach AL and Petty TL: Is chronic obstructive lung disease improved by physical exercise? JAMA 234:854, 1975.

103. Haas A et al: Pulmonary therapy and rehabilitation: principles and practices, Baltimore, 1979, Williams & Wilkins Co.

104. Lertzman MM and Cherniack RM: Rehabilitation of patients with chronic obstructive pulmonary disease, Am Rev Respir Dis 114:1145, 1976.

105. Pierce AK, Paez PN, and Miller WF: Exercise therapy with the aid of a portable oxygen supply in patients with emphysema, Am Rev Respir Dis 91:653, 1965.

106. Hammon WE and Martin RJ: Fatal pulmonary hemorrhage associated with chest physical therapy, Phys Ther 59:1247-1248, 1979.

107. Puorhit DM, Caldwell C, and Lerkoff AH: Multiple rib fractures due to physiotherapy in a neonate with hyaline membrane disease, Am J Dis Child 129:1103-1104, 1975.

108. Moss E, Gibson JS, and Mcdowall GD: The effects of nitrous oxide, Althesin and thiopentane on intracranial pressure during chest physiotherapy in patients with severe head injuries. In Shulman K et al, editors: Intracranial pressure IV, New York, 1980, Springer-Verlag.

109. Halloway R et al: Effect of chest physiotherapy on blood gases of neonates treated with intermittent positive pressure respiration, Thorax 24:421-426, 1969.

110. Gormenzano J and Branthwait MA: Effects of physiotherapy during intermittent positive pressure ventilation: changes in arterial blood gas tensions, Anaesthesia 27:258-263, 1972.

111. Gormenzano J and Branthwaite MA: Pulmonary physiotherapy with associated ventilation: arterial blood gas tension changes following pulmonary physiotherapy with IPPB, Anaesthesia 27:249-257, 1972.

112. Tyler ML et al: Prediction of oxygenation during chest physiotherapy in critically ill patients, Am Rev Respir Dis 121(part 2):218, 1980 (abstract).

113. Buscaglia A and St Marie M: Oxygen saturation during chest physiotherapy for acute exacerbation of severe chronic obstructive pulmonary disease, Respir Care 28:1009-1013, 1983.

114. Moody LE and Martindale CL: Effect of pulmonary hygiene measures on levels of arterial oxygen saturation in adults with chronic lung disease, Heart Lung 7:315-319, 1978.

115. Laws AK and McIntyre RW: Chest physiotherapy: a physiologic assessment during intermittent positive pressure ventilation in respiratory failure, Can Anaesth Soc J 16:487-493, 1969.

116. Barrell SE and Abbas HM: Monitoring during physiotherapy after open heart surgery, Physiotherapy 64:272-273, 1978.

117. Feldman J, Traver GA, and Taussig LM: Maximal expiratory flows after postural drainage, Am Rev Respir Dis 119:239-245, 1979.

118. Tecklin JS and Holsclaw DS: Evaluation of bronchial drainage in patients with cystic fibrosis, Phys Ther 55:1081-1084, 1975.

119. Cochrane GM, Webber BA, and Clarke SW: Effects of sputum on pulmonary function, Br Med J 2:1181-1183, 1977.

SECTION VII

Care of the Critically Ill

28

Respiratory Failure and the Need for Ventilatory Support

Craig L. Scanlan

Before 1960 the term *respiratory failure* was essentially absent from the medical literature.[1] Advances in life support and monitoring techniques over the last two decades have refined our ability to define and manage this now commonly recognized problem.

In simple terms, respiratory failure represents the inability of the lung to fulfill its primary function of gas exchange. Specifically, this means that the process of external respiration, or the exchange of oxygen and/or carbon dioxide between the alveoli and the pulmonary capillaries is inadequate.[2] Despite this simple definition, abnormalities of pulmonary gas exchange can occur in a wide diversity of clinical disorders, ranging from an uncomplicated drug overdose to the complex pathophysiologic processes characterizing the adult respiratory distress syndrome (ARDS).

As with the failure of other organ systems, such as the kidneys or the heart, respiratory failure is a potentially life-threatening event that demands clinical intervention. Given the diversity of clinical disorders that can cause respiratory failure, it is not surprising that clinical intervention strategies for respiratory failure are also numerous. Depending on the underlying problem, clinical management strategies for respiratory failure may range from the aggressive use of traditional therapeutic modalities, such as oxygen therapy and drugs, to advanced life support techniques, such as mechanical ventilation and other forms of ventilatory support.

Thus, as suggested by its diverse causes and multiple management approaches, respiratory failure is really a complex clinical concept. Of course, respiratory failure cannot be effectively managed without an in-depth understanding of its causes and clinical manifestations. Toward that end, this chapter will focus on the etiologic, pathophysiologic, and clinical features of respiratory failure, with special emphasis on identifying the need for ventilatory support.

OBJECTIVES

After completion of this chapter, the reader will be able to:

1. Define respiratory failure and differentiate its two primary physiologic types.

2. Compare and contrast the concepts of acute and chronic respiratory failure.

3. Identify the common causes of respiratory failure according to their affect on the respiratory apparatus.

4. Differentiate the six primary pathophysiologic processes underlying respiratory failure and the mode(s) of ventilatory support indicated in each.

5. Compare and contrast the justification for ventilatory support in selected special circumstances.

6. Recognize the limitations of quantitative approaches in assessment of patients' needs for ventilatory support.

KEY TERMS

Most terms used in this chapter are defined in context. The following terms are introduced without explicit definition but may be found in the text glossary:

bradykinin
hypersomnolence
micrognathia
myxedema
normocapnia
Ondine's curse

pancreatitis
serotonin
syringomyelia
uvulopalatopharyngo-
    plasty

Section on Indications for Ventilatory Support adapted with permission from Pierson DJ: Indications for mechanical ventilation in acute respiratory failure, Respir Care 28:570-577, 1983.

BASIC CONCEPTS IN RESPIRATORY FAILURE

If respiratory failure is defined as the inadequate exchange of carbon dioxide or oxygen between alveoli and pulmonary capillaries, then it should manifest itself in terms of altered arterial blood gases. The first objective criteria for the diagnosis of respiratory failure were based on the results of blood gas analysis. In 1965 Campbell[3] defined respiratory failure as a condition in which the Pao_2 is below 60 mm Hg or the $Paco_2$ is above 50 mm Hg in a resting subject breathing air at sea level.

This simple definition provided by Campbell is still used extensively today. However, we now realize that the absolute arterial levels of both oxygen and carbon dioxide signaling respiratory failure may be above or below these values, depending on the specific clinical circumstances. For example, whether a Pao_2 of 60 mm Hg indicates respiratory failure depends, in part, on the patient's age, the Fio_2 being breathed, and the barometric pressure.[4] Likewise, as discussed later, an arterial Pco_2 above 50 mm Hg may or may not signal "failure" in the clinical sense of the term. Moreover, for respiratory failure to exist, these abnormal changes in arterial blood gases must be associated with a pulmonary or respiration-related abnormality. For example, hypoxemia caused by intracardiac shunting and hypercapnea resulting from metabolic alkalosis are not indicative of respiratory failure.[5]

Problems of oxygenation versus problems of ventilation

Implicit in Campbell's early definition of respiratory failure is the fact that oxygenation and ventilation are two separate but interrelated physiologic processes. Thus abnormalities of oxygen exchange can occur separately from inadequacies in ventilation or CO_2 excretion.

On the basis of this knowledge, the concept of respiratory failure can be further refined to include two broad physiologic types: that associated with abnormalities of oxygenation and that resulting from inadequacies in ventilation.[1,6-9] Respiratory failure caused by abnormalities of oxygenation is also called type I respiratory failure or, better, *hypoxemic respiratory failure*. Synonyms for respiratory failure resulting from inadequate ventilation are type II respiratory failure, ventilatory failure, and *hypercapnic respiratory failure*.[2]

As indicated in Table 28-1, the primary manifestation of hypoxemic respiratory failure is a lower than predicted Pao_2 and a higher than predicted $P(A-a)o_2$. Moreover, by definition, hypoxemic respiratory failure occurs in the presence of a normal or low $Paco_2$. Thus the underlying physiologic processes leading to hypoxemic respiratory failure include all the causes of arterial hypoxemia except hypoventilation and a low Fio_2. Specifically, hypoxemic respiratory failure may be caused by a diffusion impairment (rare), a low $\dot{V}/\dot{Q}$ ratio, or intrapulmonary shunting.

On the other hand, the hallmark of hypercapnic respiratory failure is an elevated $Paco_2$. As with hypoxemic respiratory failure, the Pao_2 in pure hypercapnic respiratory failure is less than would be expected for a given Fio_2, but this is because of the simple displacement of oxygen in the alveoli by carbon dioxide (refer to Chapter 9). Indeed, the alveolar-to-arterial oxygen tension gradient in hypercapnic respiratory failure is usually normal, indicating normal oxygen exchange across the lungs. Thus the underlying physiologic process leading to pure hypercapnic respiratory failure is alveolar hypoventilation.

Of course, as Table 28-1 indicates, hypoxemic and hypercapnic respiratory failure can occur together, in which case the Pao_2 would be decreased, and both the $Paco_2$ and the alveolar-to-arterial oxygen tension gradient would be increased.[8] The problem underlying this combined form of respiratory failure is therefore some combination of alveolar hypoventilation with a $\dot{V}/\dot{Q}$ inequality.[1]

Acute versus chronic respiratory failure

Further refinement of the concept of respiratory failure can be made according to the duration of the underlying abnormality as related to the body's compensatory abilities. Thus the term *acute respiratory failure* refers to situations in which hypoxemia, hypercapnea, or both develop too rapidly to allow physiologic compensation. According to this definition, acute respiratory failure may be considered a life-threatening event that necessitates drastic clinical intervention, including some form of ventilatory support.[1,9,10]

On the other hand, *chronic respiratory failure* develops over a period of weeks to months, thus providing time for the body to partially compensate for the underlying pathophysiologic disturbance.[1] Compensatory responses to chronic hypoxemia include various mechanisms to improve oxygen transport, as discussed in Chapter 15. The primary compensatory response to chronic hypercapnea is renal buffering of hydrogen ions, as described in Chapter 10.

Acute respiratory failure may be superimposed on chronic respiratory failure. This so-called "acute-on-

Table 28-1   Hypoxemic and Hypercapnic Respiratory Failure

Type of respiratory failure	Blood gas changes		
	Pao_2*	$Paco_2$	$P(A-a)o_2$
Hypoxemic	Low	Normal to low	High
Hypercapnic	Low	High	Normal
Combined	Low	High	High

*In each case, Pao_2 is lower than predicted for the Fio_2. When breathing high Fio_2, Pao_2 can be adequate, eg, 90 to 100 mm Hg, in the face of severe oxygenation failure.

From Martin L: Pulmonary physiology in clinical practice, ed 1, St Louis, 1987, The CV Mosby Co.

chronic" form of respiratory failure generally involves patients with a preexisting chronic pulmonary disorder, such as COPD.[11] Typically, these patients have developed partial compensation for both the hypoxemia and the hypercapnea that characterize their disease process. Because this compensation does not correct the underlying problem, any acute worsening or exacerbation of the disorder, such as might occur with a severe bacterial pneumonia, can cause a rapid deterioration in respiratory status. In these cases, the deterioration in respiratory status usually involves both a rise in the $Paco_2$ level and an abnormal drop in the Pao_2 level, signalling a combined form of respiratory failure.

Respiratory failure versus respiratory insufficiency

Although the terms respiratory failure and respiratory insufficiency are often used interchangeably, it is clinically useful to draw a distinction between their meanings. Whereas respiratory failure is always manifested by alterations in arterial blood gases, this is not necessarily so with respiratory insufficiency. Indeed, respiratory insufficiency is best defined as a condition in which breathing is accompanied by abnormal signs or symptoms, such as dyspnea or paradoxical breathing. Signs and symptoms like these usually signal an abnormal increase in the work of breathing. Thus a patient with respiratory insufficiency may maintain normal or near normal blood gas levels, but at the expense of an increased work of breathing.[12]

Because respiratory insufficiency generally foreshadows respiratory failure, the importance of the clinical (as opposed to the laboratory) picture of the patient cannot be overemphasized. Early recognition of the signs and symptoms of respiratory insufficiency, before the development of overt respiratory failure, may forestall the need to institute hazardous ventilatory support measures. This is particularly true in patients with chronic hypercapnic respiratory failure who are suffering from an acute exacerbation of their disease process.[11]

ETIOLOGY OF RESPIRATORY FAILURE

As previously discussed, a diversity of clinical disorders can result in abnormalities of gas exchange and therefore cause respiratory failure.[1,5,8] The classification of respiratory failure according to cause enhances our ability to compare similar groups of patients, thus facilitating therapeutic decision making and aiding in the determination of clinical outcomes.[1]

Major categories of respiratory failure

The causes of respiratory failure can be logically categorized according to the manner in which they impair breathing or gas exchange. Fig. 28-1 shows the key functional divisions of the respiratory system, including its central and peripheral nervous system components, the chest wall

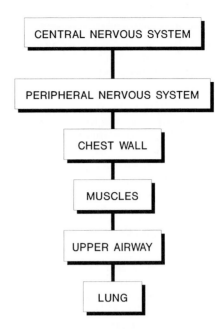

Fig. 28-1   In addition to its pulmonary element (the lung), the respiratory system incorporates several extrapulmonary elements. (Redrawn from Respir Care 24:4, April 1979.)

and muscles, the major conducting airways, and the lung itself.

According to this scheme of the respiratory apparatus, an abnormality affecting any one of these divisions can result in inadequate gas exchange. The box on p. 686 lists several specific clinical disorders that can impair gas exchange and that are associated with each of these key functional divisions of the respiratory system.

In general, most disorders of the central and peripheral nervous system or the muscles of respiration result in a reduction in alveolar ventilation and thus a primary hypercapnic respiratory failure. Disorders of the chest wall and pleura have variable effects on respiration. As restrictive disorders, these abnormalities typically result in a reduction in lung volumes, including V_T. However, as long as the patient compensates for this reduced V_T with an increase in the frequency of breathing, it may be possible to maintain adequate alveolar ventilation, although at the expense of an increased work of breathing. Some patients with restrictive disorders of the chest wall or pleura actually tend to hyperventilate.

Nonetheless, the reduced V_T values common to most restrictive disorders may result in progressive atelectasis. Moreover, disorders of the chest wall and pleura can cause direct compression of lung tissue (as in kyphoscoliosis) or a maldistribution of ventilation (as in flail chest) and also result in atelectasis or areas of low $\dot{V}/\dot{Q}$. Thus restrictive disorders also can result in hypoxemic respiratory failure.

Disorders of the upper airway associated with impaired gas exchange typically cause either partial or complete air-

---

CAUSES OF RESPIRATORY FAILURE

CENTRAL NERVOUS SYSTEM

Drug overdose (eg, opiates, barbiturates, tranquilizers, alcohol)

Obesity-related hypoventilation (pickwickian syndrome)

Primary alveolar hypoventilation syndrome ("Ondine's curse")

Central sleep apnea syndrome

Stroke

Tumors

Brain, brainstem, or spinal cord trauma

Multiple sclerosis

Syringomyelia

Myxedema

Metabolic imbalances (hyperglycemia, hyponatremia, etc)

Infections (meningitis, encephalitis, etc)

PERIPHERAL NERVOUS SYSTEM

Poliomyelitis (also acts centrally)

Amyotrophic lateral sclerosis

Guillain-Barré syndrome

Botulism poisoning

Tetanus

Drugs (curare, succinylcholine)

CHEST WALL (INCLUDING PLEURA)

Kyphoscoliosis

Ankylosing spondylitis

Morbid obesity

Flail chest

Restrictive pleural diseases

MUSCLES

Muscular dystrophy

Polymyositis

Myasthenia gravis

Muscle fatigue or atrophy

UPPER AIRWAY

Epiglottis

Laryngotracheitis

Trauma

Tracheal stenosis

Internal or external (compressing) tumors

Foreign body

Micrognathia

INTRINSIC LUNG DISEASES

COPD

Asthma

Cystic fibrosis

Pneumonia

Pulmonary emboli (thromboemboli, fat emboli, etc)

Interstitial/parenchynal lung diseases (including fibrosis)

Oxygen toxicity

Pulmonary edema

ARDS

---

way obstruction, resulting in both a hypoxemic and a hypercapnic respiratory failure.

Finally, severe intrinsic lung disease most commonly results in either a combined hypoxemic and hypercapnic respiratory failure (as in COPD) or a purely hypoxemic respiratory failure (as in pneumonia, pulmonary edema, and ARDS).

Differences in etiology according to age

The most common causes of respiratory failure vary according to the patient's age group.[1] In neonates, the most common cause of respiratory failure is an intrinsic lung disorder called hyaline membrane disease, or newborn respiratory distress syndrome. Common causes of respiratory failure in infants between the ages of 1 and 24 months are immature immune defenses (causing infection) and small airway obstruction (resulting from infection). In older children, respiratory failure is most often caused by status asthmaticus, cystic fibrosis, or aspiration of a foreign body. More detail on the conditions associated with respiratory failure in infants and children is provided in Chapter 32. The remainder of this chapter will focus on respiratory failure in the adult patient.

Interrelationship among problems

Of course, two or more of these problems may coexist at the same time or be complicated by related conditions. Motor vehicle trauma resulting in both brain injury and flail chest and heroin drug overdose resulting in pulmonary edema are good examples of situations in which two problems—both capable of leading to respiratory failure—coexist.

An excellent example of complications caused by related conditions is the interrelation between heart disease and respiratory failure. Respiratory failure may complicate an acute myocardial infarction directly, as in pulmonary edema, or indirectly as a result of decreased cerebral perfusion. On the other hand, a myocardial infarction may complicate respiratory failure by decreasing oxygen transport to the tissues and increasing the metabolic demands on the heart.[13]

Finally, the presence of a critical illness in general in-

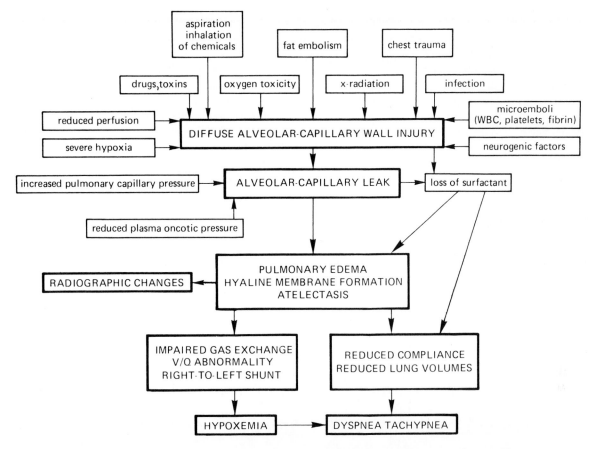

Fig. 28-2 Pathogenesis and pathophysiology of adult respiratory distress syndrome. (From Farzan S: A concise handbook of respiratory diseases, ed 2, East Norwalk, Conn, 1985, Appleton & Lange.)

creases the risk of other complications and causes of respiratory failure, such as pulmonary infection, pulmonary embolization, hyponatremia, and renal failure.[1]

The adult respiratory distress syndrome (ARDS)

Nowhere is the interrelationship among the various causes and complicating factors in respiratory failure more apparent than in the large number of disorders grouped together under the general term *adult respiratory distress syndrome* (ARDS).

As the term suggests, ARDS is not a disease itself but, rather, a remarkably uniform pattern of clinical, physiologic, and pathologic features characterizing the lung's response to a variety of both pulmonary and extrapulmonary injuries.[14] The box on p. 688 lists the broad range of disorders that have been associated with ARDS.

As shown in Fig. 28-2, the pathophysiologic "common denominator" in all these conditions is diffuse damage to the alveolar-capillary membrane, specifically the type I pneumocytes. Regardless of cause, such damage results in an increase in the permeability of this membrane and the leakage of fluid high in protein content from the capillaries into the interstitial space and alveoli (Fig. 28-3).[15-18]

In conjunction with necrosis of the type I pneumocytes, the collection of this proteinaceous exudate in the alveoli results in the formation of hyaline membranes and the loss of surfactant (Fig. 28-3).[19] Alveoli not filled with exudate thus become unstable and collapse, causing progressive atelectasis and the characteristic changes seen in radiographs of the chest over time (Fig. 28-4).

ARDS is also associated with a marked increase in the concentration of certain hormones and other blood-borne chemical mediators.[14,20] These substances include histamine, bradykinin, serotonin, and certain prostaglandins. Such substances have potent vasoactive properties, including the ability to cause constriction of the pulmonary venous circulation and the tendency to increase capillary endothelial permeability. Whether these substances represent a primary contributing factor in the cause of ARDS or simply an effect of the initial injury is not yet known.

In combination, the noncardiac pulmonary edema, hyaline membrane formation, and atelectasis severely impair gas exchange, resulting in a hypoxemia that does not respond well to oxygen therapy. This so-called "refractory" hypoxemia is one of the primary clinical hallmarks of ARDS.[14-18]

CONDITIONS ASSOCIATED WITH THE ADULT RESPIRATORY DISTRESS SYNDROME

PULMONARY-RELATED CONDITIONS

Infections (viral, bacterial, fungal)

Aspiration

Gastric contents
Near-drowning
Hydrocarbon fluids

Inhaled toxins

Oxygen
Smoke inhalation
Chemicals (NO_2, Cl_2, NH_3, phosgene)

Trauma

Lung contusion
Chest trauma

Other

Radiation pneumonitis
Postperfusion (cardiopulmonary bypass)
High-altitude pulmonary edema

NONPULMONARY CONDITIONS

Shock of any cause
Drug overdose
Disseminated intravascular coagulation
Massive blood transfusion
Sepsis
Fat embolism
Hemorrhagic pancreatitis
Uremia
Anaphylaxis
Nonthoracic trauma
Neurogenic pulmonary edema
Eclampsia

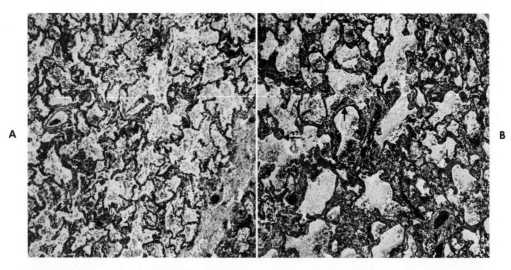

A   **B**

Fig. 28-3   Characteristic early light microscopic abnormalities in ARDS caused by viral pneumonia. **A,** Alveolar filling with proteinaceous and cellular debris. **B,** Abnormalities after 48 to 72 hours, showing hyaline membranes *(arrows)* in addition to alveolar filling. (From Moser KM and Spragg RG: Respiratory emergencies, ed 2, St Louis, 1982, The CV Mosby Co.)

Pulmonary edema, atelectasis, and surfactant loss also combine to reduce lung volumes and compliance. As shown in Fig. 28-5, this decrease in lung volumes and compliance increases the pressure differences necessary to produce the same tidal volume, thereby progressively increasing the patient's work of breathing. Clinically, this increased work of breathing manifests itself in dyspnea, tachypnea, and signs of respiratory muscle fatigue, such as paradoxical breathing.

In summary, the causes of respiratory failure are extremely diverse and often interrelated. For these reasons, key elements in the management of respiratory failure, including selection of the mode of ventilatory support, tend to emphasize common pathophysiologic abnormalities as opposed to specific disease processes. These common pathophysiologic abnormalities and their clinical manifestations are discussed in the next section.

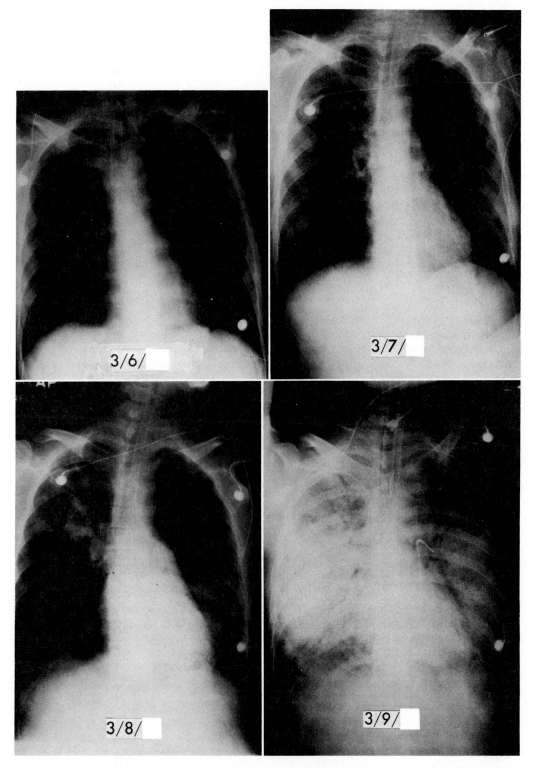

Fig. 28-4   Characteristic roentgenographic changes as ARDS develops. (From Moser KM and Spragg RG: Respiratory emergencies, ed 2, St Louis, 1982, The CV Mosby Co.)

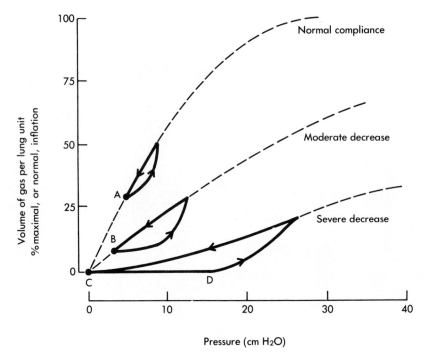

Fig. 28-5 Conceptualization, based on data from several sources, of the relationship of unit lung volume to transpulmonary pressure. *Solid lines* represent inflation and deflation curves during constant tidal volume; *dashed lines* represent deflation curves over full range of transpulmonary pressures. As ARDS increases in severity and compliance progressively decreases, functional residual capacity decreases from point A to B to C. At C the unit is collapsed. Before it can be reinflated, a critical opening pressure (D) must be exceeded. Thus, with ARDS of increasing severity, the pressure required to produce the same tidal volume progressively increases. (From Moser KM and Spragg RG: Respiratory emergencies, ed 2, St Louis, 1982, The CV Mosby Co.)

INDICATIONS FOR VENTILATORY SUPPORT

By definition, acute respiratory failure is the primary indication for institution of ventilatory support. However, despite three decades and millions of patient hours of experience, no absolute consensus has emerged on the appropriate use of the various modes of ventilatory support or on when they should be initiated in patients with acute respiratory failure.

Modes of ventilatory support

All modes of ventilatory support facilitate lung expansion by increasing the transpulmonary pressure gradient. With all else constant, an increase in the transpulmonary pressure gradient will expand the alveoli in direct proportion to the pressure difference created.

As defined in the box on p. 691,[21] the primary modes of ventilatory support in current use are (1) continuous mandatory ventilation (CMV), in either the control or the assist/control mode; (2) intermittent mandatory ventilation (IMV); (3) pressure support ventilation (PSV)[22]; and (4) continuous positive airway pressure (CPAP). Continuous positive airway pressure may be used alone or in combination with any of the other three modes. When it is combined with either CMV, IMV, or PSV, the term positive

end-expiratory pressure (PEEP) is used. Thus, for example, CMV with PEEP represents the application of pressure greater than atmospheric at the airway opening during every inspiration, with pressure maintained above atmospheric during expiration. More details on the selection and application of these various modes of ventilatory support are provided in Chapters 30 and 31.

Parameters indicating the need for ventilatory support

An implicit assumption in clinical practice is that patient management will inevitably become more precise and effective, once the definitive studies are performed and the right quantitative measures become available. Over the last three decades, numerous quantitative measures have been suggested as indicating the need to institute ventilatory support. Table 28-2 provides a summary of these indicators, as synthesized from various sources.[5,23-29] These measurements vary from simple bedside observations to complex determinations that require sophisticated research equipment. Moreover, the specific measurements most widely relied on in practice are used differently by some authorities.

Confounding the use of these measures as criteria for instituting ventilatory support is the fact that some patients

PRIMARY MODES OF VENTILATORY SUPPORT

CONTINUOUS MANDATORY VENTILATION (CMV)

The application of pressure greater than atmospheric at the airway opening during every inspiration, used to support ventilation. During expiration, pressure returns to atmospheric. The older term intermittent positive pressure ventilation (IPPV) is synonymous with CMV. CMV may be applied in either the control or the assist/control mode:

Control mode CMV

Continuous mandatory ventilation in which the frequency of breathing is determined by the ventilator according to a preset cycling pattern without initiation by the patient

Assist/control mode CMV

Continuous mandatory ventilation in which the minimum frequency of breathing is predetermined by the ventilator controls but the patient can initiate ventilation at a faster rate

INTERMITTENT MANDATORY VENTILATION (IMV)

Periodic ventilation with positive pressure, with the patient breathing spontaneously between breaths. These periodic breaths may be controlled (control mode IMV) or assisted, as with synchronous intermittent mandatory ventilation (SIMV).

PRESSURE SUPPORT VENTILATION (PSV)

Pressure limited assisted ventilation designed to augment a spontaneously generated breath. The patient has primary control over the frequency of breathing, the inspiratory time, and the inspiratory flow.

CONTINUOUS POSITIVE AIRWAY PRESSURE (CPAP)

The maintenance of a pressure above atmospheric at the airway opening throughout a spontaneous breathing cycle.

Table 28-2   Some Measurements Used in Determining the Need for Ventilatory Support*

Measurement	Values	
	Normal	Ventilatory support indicated†
Tidal volume (V_T) (ml/kg)	5-8	<5
Vital capacity (VC) (ml/kg)	65-75	<10; <15
Forced expiratory volume in one second (FEV_1) (ml/kg)	50-60	<10
Functional residual capacity (FRC) (% of predicted value)	80-100	<50
Respiratory rate (f) (breaths/min)	12-20	>35
Maximum inspiratory force (MIF) (cm H_2O)	80-100	<20; <25; <30
Minute ventilation ($\dot{V}_E$), (L/min)	5-6	>10
Maximum voluntary ventilation (MVV) (L/min)	120-180	<20; <(2 × $\dot{V}_E$)
Dead space fraction (V_D/V_T) (%)	0.25-0.40	>0.60
Pa_{CO_2} (mm Hg)	35-45	>50; >55
Pa_{O_2} (mm Hg)	75-100 (breathing air)	<50 (air); < 70 (mask O_2)
Alveolar-to-arterial P_{O_2} gradient.[$P(A-a)_{O_2}$], breathing 100% O_2 (mm Hg)	25-65	>350; >450
Arterial/alveolar P_{O_2} ratio (Pa_{O_2}/PA_{O_2})	0.75	<0.15
Arterial P_{O_2}/inspired O_2 fraction ratio (Pa_{O_2}/FI_{O_2}) (mm Hg)	350-450	<200
Intrapulmonary right-to-left shunt fraction ($\dot{Q}s/\dot{Q}_T$) (%)	≤5	>20; >25; >30

Adapted from Pierson DJ: Indications for mechanical ventilation in acute respiratory failure, Respiratory Care 28:5, May 1983.
*Adapted in part from references 5, 23-29.
†Multiple cut-off values indicate different recommendations by different sources.

with severe chronic obstructive or restrictive lung disease exhibit marked abnormal values on some indicators and yet are ambulatory and stable. In these cases, common sense would dictate that ventilatory support is not necessary. This example illustrates both the difficulty and the limitations of applying strict numerical criteria in determining when to initiate ventilatory support.

Nonetheless, an analysis of the physiologic bases underlying these numerous indicators provides a useful perspective on the need for ventilatory support. In Table 28-3 these measurements are rearranged according to the six main physiologic processes they assess. Each of these processes will be reviewed, after which the application of ventilatory support in several special clinical situations, including its prophylactic use, will be discussed.

Inadequate alveolar ventilation. Arterial P_{CO_2} reflects alveolar ventilation and, by definition, when the Pa_{CO_2} is elevated there is hypoventilation. When alveolar hypoventilation occurs rapidly enough to produce life-threatening respiratory acidosis, acute hypercapnic respiratory failure (or ventilatory failure) is present.[30] On the other hand, long-standing or slowly developing hypoventilation that is adequately compensated by metabolic alkalosis poses no immediate threat to life and can be tolerated for months or years. For example, two patients might have the following arterial blood values:

	Patient A	Patient B
Pa_{CO_2}	60	60
HCO_3^-	25	36
pH	7.25	7.38

Although both patients have hypercapnia of the same severity, only one of them (patient A) exhibits acute respiratory failure. Patient B, on the other hand, exhibits a compensated respiratory acidosis, and thus is suffering from chronic hypercapnic respiratory failure. The distinction between these two states is of fundamental importance in respiratory care, and on it rests the use of Pa_{CO_2} and pH as indications for ventilatory support.

From the foregoing, it is clear that Pa_{CO_2} values alone are not adequate criteria for initiating ventilatory support. The threshold values shown in Table 28-2 are valid only when they represent a sudden change from a patient's usual state, something that can be detected only by examination of the pH as well.

When CO_2 retention develops acutely, how far must the arterial pH fall before life is threatened? No clear answer to this question is available, although most clinicians do not regard pH values above 7.30 as necessarily constituting an emergency. In one study of complications occurring during mechanical ventilation, mortality and morbidity were increased in patients whose pH values fell below 7.30,[31] and this value is often used as a cutoff point at which intubation and ventilatory support are indicated. No clinical comparisons of 7.30 with 7.25 or lower values have been made, however, and some clinicians prefer to use values lower than 7.30 as the criterion.

Although arterial pH is a more appropriate indicator of acute hypercapnic respiratory failure than is Pa_{CO_2}, trends in these values are more important still. Worsening acute respiratory acidosis over minutes or hours, particularly in the face of vigorous therapy, is an indication for ventilatory support, regardless of the specific pH value used as a threshold.

Since an elevated Pa_{CO_2} increases ventilatory drive in normal subjects, the very existence of hypercapnic respiratory failure suggests the presence of one or more other abnormalities of the respiratory apparatus. Specifically, the presence of acute hypercapnic respiratory failure indicates that either (1) the patient is not responding in a normal manner to the elevated Pa_{CO_2}, (2) the patient is responding normally, but the "signal" is not getting through to the respiratory muscles, or (3) despite normal afferent and efferent response mechanisms, the lungs and chest bellows are simply incapable of providing adequate ventilation, because of parenchymal disease or muscular weakness.[32]

In pure hypercapnic respiratory failure, the most appropriate mode of ventilatory support depends, in part, on the underlying cause of the alveolar hypoventilation. When the problem is solely caused by a decrease in ventilatory drive, as in an uncomplicated drug overdose, simple CMV in either the control or the assist/control mode is usually sufficient. However, when the problem is a result of a restrictive disorder of the lungs or chest bellows and the patient is responding normally to the elevated Pa_{CO_2}, the application of control-mode CMV may result in the patient's "fighting" the ventilator.[33] Moreover, the high frequencies of spontaneous breathing typically exhibited by these patients may cause a rapid swing to respiratory alkalosis, once they are placed in the assist/control mode of CMV. For this reason, some authorities suggest that IMV is the mode best able to normalize alveolar ventilation in these cases.[33]

Table 28-3 Indications for Ventilatory Support, Classified by Physiologic Mechanism

Mechanism	Best available indicator
Inadequate alveolar ventilation	Pa_{CO_2} and pH
Inadequate lung expansion	V_T; VC; f
Inadequate respiratory muscle strength	MIF; MVV; VC
Excessive work of breathing	$\dot{V}_E$ required to keep P_{CO_2} normal; V_D/V_T; f
Unstable ventilatory drive	Breathing pattern, clinical setting
Severe hypoxemia	$P_{(A-a)O_2}$; Pa_{O_2}/PA_{O_2}; Pa_{O_2}/F_{IO_2}; Q_S/Q_T

Adapted from Pierson DJ: Indications for mechanical ventilation in acute respiratory failure, Respiratory Care 28:5, May 1983.

Inadequate lung expansion. Even when alveolar ventilation is adequate, the patient may be unable to maintain normal lung expansion. Inadequate lung expansion may occur during general anesthesia, after upper abdominal surgery, after cervical spinal cord injuries, and in acute restrictive lung disease, such as ARDS. The inability to maintain normal lung expansion may lead to atelectasis and pneumonia.

Measurements used to gauge the need for ventilatory support in these and other conditions characterized by inadequate lung expansion include tidal volume (V_T), vital capacity (VC), respiratory rate (f), and functional residual capacity (FRC). Of these, the FRC is simple to measure in the pulmonary function laboratory but is prohibitively difficult to measure in the intensive care unit on an acutely ill, often uncooperative patient. Although useful in research, FRC assessed at the bedside cannot be considered a readily available measurement to routinely indicate or monitor ventilatory support.

Spontaneous V_T is the most direct measure of lung expansion. Most authorities consider a value of 5 ml/kg or less in an acutely ill patient as indicating the need for ventilatory assistance. Experimental support for this belief comes from studies of patients with otherwise normal lungs who are undergoing general anesthesia. Bendixen and associates[34,35] showed that anesthetized, spontaneously breathing patients had progressive hypoxemia and loss of lung compliance, both of which could be reversed by intermittent deep breaths. This group of investigators demonstrated the same ill effects with the use of controlled ventilation with physiologically normal V_T levels.[36] These studies were largely responsible for the introduction in the late 1960s of the automatic "sigh" mechanisms now found on most mechanical ventilators.

Subsequent studies showed that CMV with "supernormal" V_T levels (in the range of 10 to 15 ml/kg) without intermittent sighs effectively prevented both hypoxemia and loss of lung compliance.[37,38] These observations are the basis for the current practice of routinely using "supernormal" V_T settings in both the CMV and the IMV modes in acutely ill patients with inadequate lung expansion.

Indirect data on the value of augmented lung inflation in acute lung injury come from animal studies of near-drowning. Ruiz and associates[39] induced fresh-water drowning in dogs under general anesthesia and compared the effects of four different modes of therapy on the Pao_2.[39] CMV with a V_T of 15 ml/kg and combined with 10 cm H_2O of PEEP produced significantly better oxygenation than did spontaneous ventilation, CPAP, or simple CMV. In a similar study that involved salt-water drowning, the same group of investigators found that either CPAP or CMV with PEEP was more effective in reversing hypoxemia in the early postinjury period than was CMV alone; results achieved with the latter were indistinguishable from those with simple spontaneous ventilation.[40] In these studies the continuous positive airway pressure maintained at the airway by either PEEP or CPAP, rather than the intermittent positive pressure breaths, appears to have been the important therapeutic modality.

Thus the best modes of ventilatory support in situations in which the primary cause of acute respiratory failure is inadequate lung expansion are those that maintain positive pressure at the patient's airway throughout the ventilatory cycle. If alveolar ventilation is adequate, simple CPAP should suffice. On the other hand, if inadequate lung expansion coexists with inadequate alveolar ventilation, then CMV with PEEP or IMV with PEEP is indicated.

Inadequate respiratory muscle strength. Effective ventilation requires that the respiratory muscles be capable of bearing the work load associated with overcoming the elastic and frictional forces opposing lung inflation (refer to Chapter 8). As indicated in Fig. 28-6, there exists a range of work loads within which the respiratory muscles can maintain the conditioning necessary to fulfil this function. Subnormal work loads can lead to muscle atrophy or an actual loss of muscle mass and contractile force. A good example of respiratory muscle atrophy occurs in patients with spinal cord trauma (for example, quadriplegics). On the other hand, work loads in excess of a muscle's energy-utilization capabilities can lead to muscle fatigue or a reversible decrease in the force developed during sustained or repeated contractions. Muscle fatigue may occur whenever the elastic or frictional work load imposed on the respiratory muscles is excessive, as in pulmonary fibrosis (excessive elastic work) or asthma (excessive frictional work).[41]

In either case, the strength of the respiratory muscles may be inadequate to support normal levels of ventilation. Thus respiratory muscle weakness can lead to inadequate lung expansion, loss of lung compliance, hypoventilation, atelectasis, and pneumonia. As shown in Table 28-3, the measurements used most commonly to assess respiratory muscle strength are the maximum inspiratory force (MIF),[42] maximum voluntary ventilation (MVV), and VC.

Although the threshold value used by different authorities varies, the MIF is a readily available measurement that can be made in any patient who is intubated or who can achieve a seal with the use of a mouthpiece. Patients who can generate an inspiratory pressure of -30 cm H_2O probably have sufficient muscle strength for continued spontaneous ventilation; a value less than this is compatible with adequate lung inflation in some persons with chronic neuromuscular conditions, but in acutely ill patients it implies little reserve and the threat of progressive ventilatory insufficiency. The MVV maneuver can be performed at the bedside with a hand-held spirometer such as the Wright respirometer. The MVV is useful in assessment of ventilatory reserve, but it requires cooperation and cannot be performed by many patients.

As with most of the parameters listed in the tables, these traditional measurements have not been investigated prospectively as criteria for initiation of ventilatory support.

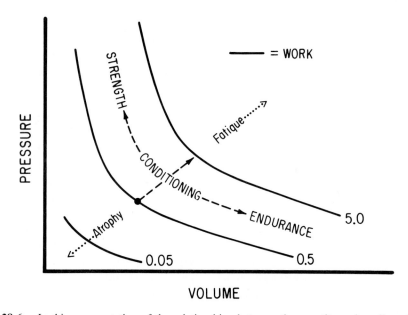

Fig. 28-6 In this representation of the relationships between the quantity and quality of work loads placed on ventilatory muscles, the isopleths represent three rates of work. A subnormal work rate (0.05 kg·m·mm^{-1}) can result in atrophy, whereas a supranormal work rate (5 kg·m·mm^{-1}) can condition or, if high enough, fatigue muscles. Note that the quality of a constant work load can be characterized by the relationship between the muscle pressure generation *(pressure)* and the muscle contraction distance *(volume change)*. A high-pressure low-volume change work load emphasizes isometric conditioning and improves strength; low-pressure high-volume change work load emphasizes isobaric conditioning and improves endurance. (Redrawn from Problems in pulmonary disease, Winter 1986.)

Data justifying their use come mainly from studies of ventilator weaning.[43,44] Supplementing these methods of assessing the strength of the respiratory muscles are a variety of new quantitative research methods, some of which may soon be available at the bedside. These new methods are discussed in Chapter 31.

The most appropriate mode of ventilatory support for the patient with inadequate respiratory muscle strength is a matter of considerable controversy. In general, if the cause of respiratory muscle weakness is fatigue, it seems logical to have a mechanical ventilator assume all the work of breathing, as occurs with CMV in the control mode.[45] How long this may be necessary varies with the degree of fatigue. Typically, however, it takes fatigued respiratory muscles anywhere from 24 to 48 hours to fully recover. During this period, the continuing need for ventilatory support should be carefully monitored with both observational assessment and quantitative measurements. Since the respiratory muscles are not used during this period, care must be taken to ensure that, once recovered, they do not proceed to a state of atrophy.

On the other hand, if the cause of respiratory muscle weakness is atrophy, it seems reasonable to allow their progressive "loading" by providing opportunities for the patient to breath spontaneously, as occurs during IMV.[33] The problem with this approach is the significant additional work of breathing imposed on the patient by artificial airways, ventilator circuits, and demand valve systems.

Pressure support ventilation (PSV) recently has been proposed as an alternative approach to ventilatory support in patients with respiratory muscle weakness.[22,46,47] Besides counteracting the imposed work of breathing created by artificial airways, ventilator circuits, and demand systems, PSV may help recondition the respiratory muscles, thus aiding in the discontinuation of ventilatory support.[48-51] At the time of this writing, however, more research is needed to confirm these proposed benefits of PSV.

Excessive work of breathing. Respiratory muscle weakness may be a primary cause of respiratory failure, as with atrophy. However, most respiratory muscle weakness is due to fatigue, which, in turn, is attributable to an excessive work of breathing. Clinically, a rapid and increasing respiratory rate is a cardinal sign of an excessive work of breathing. Sustained breathing frequencies of 35 breaths per minute or higher in the adult usually indicate a need for some form of ventilatory support.

Whether because of an increase in elastic or frictional opposition to ventilation, patients whose work of breathing is excessive may develop acute respiratory acidosis, as well as $\dot{V}/\dot{Q}$ imbalances as a result of inadequate lung expansion. The overall demand placed on the ventilatory apparatus is reflected in the minute ventilation ($\dot{V}_E$) required to maintain adequate alveolar ventilation, as indicated by a normal Pa_{CO_2} (Table 28-3). Although, as in the foregoing discussion, available data have come from studies of ventilatory weaning,[43] a $\dot{V}_E$ of 10 L/min or less can be considered an acceptable ventilatory demand for most adult patients. $\dot{V}_E$ requirements in excess of 10 L/min are difficult for most adults to sustain, particularly if the process causing the acute episode continues for a period of days.

The $\dot{V}_E$ necessary to maintain normocapnia is determined by two factors: CO_2 production ($\dot{V}_{CO_2}$), which reflects metabolic needs, and the dead space fraction (V_D/V_T), which indicates the efficiency of ventilation. An increase in either or both of these components can produce excessive ventilatory demand for a given patient. A V_D/V_T of 0.6 or greater is sometimes offered as an indication for ventilatory support. This criterion was first given by Pontoppidan and associates [5] and was applied in patients with severe hypoxemic respiratory failure compatible with ARDS. ARDS is characterized not only by increased V_D/V_T but also by severe hypoxemia, tachypnea, and poor lung expansion, and it is not known for certain whether V_D/V_T measurements provide a more accurate gauge for instituting mechanical ventilation than do these other signs. Some COPD patients have baseline V_D/V_T values in excess of 0.6. Thus, once again, this criterion should be used in conjunction with clinical judgment in deciding when to initiate ventilatory support in persons with underlying lung disease.

In situations in which the increased work of breathing is caused by poor lung expansion and decreased compliance, modes of ventilatory support that increase the FRC by the application of positive pressure throughout the respiratory cycle, such as CMV or IMV with PEEP, are generally the methods of choice. On the other hand, when the excessive work of breathing is a result of increased resistance to airflow in either upper or lower airways, as in status asthmaticus, the pure CMV mode is normally indicated. In either case, it is important to remember that a too narrow endotracheal tube can impose an additional burden on the ventilatory apparatus.[30,52] Especially in the presence of a high $\dot{V}_E$, patients who can breathe comfortably through an 8 mm tube may be unable to do so through a 6 or 7 mm tube without ventilatory assistance.

Unstable ventilatory drive. As indicated in Table 28-3, at present there are no objective measurements that will identify the patient whose ventilatory drive may become insufficient. In patients whose spontaneous ventilation is initially adequate, there is a risk of sudden apnea or life-threatening hypoventilation in the early hours after closed head injury, drug overdose, or cerebrovascular accident.

At the present time, it is reasonable to apply CMV to patients with severe acute brain injury whose neurologic status is unstable or deteriorating, whose measured intracranial pressure is increasing, or who have apneic episodes or irregular respiratory patterns. These indications are not applicable in patients who have stabilized after the first 24 hours and have no other reasons for mechanical ventilation or in those with stable patterns of irregular breathing, such as Cheyne-Stokes respiration. Deliberate hyperventilation to diminish brain swelling is a separate indication that will be discussed later.

Severe hypoxemia. The sixth physiologic abnormality that may be considered in determining the need for ventilatory support is impaired oxygenation of the arterial blood. Severe hypoxemia is a finding common to many patients who require ventilatory support, but it is difficult to prove that this is an indication in and of itself. As we have seen, hypoxemic respiratory failure is defined in terms of degree of hypoxemia[8,9,53]; yet the relationship between ventilatory support and oxygenation is unclear in many patients.[30] CMV with PEEP is the mainstay of therapy to correct hypoxemia in patients with significant intrapulmonary shunting. However, the treatment of severe hypoxemia need not involve mechanical ventilation, as when continuous positive airway pressure (CPAP) is used by itself.[33] Although many authorities still cite hypoxemia of a certain severity as an indication for CMV, such citations antedate the current widespread use of CPAP in these situations.

Severity of hypoxemia is a good indicator of the critical nature of a patient's illness, even if the specific need for ventilatory assistance is unclear. Table 28-2 presents five different measures of hypoxemia that have been stated as indications for instituting ventilatory support. Most of these attempt to quantify the degree of arterial hypoxemia against either the F_{IO_2} or Pa_{O_2}.

The most commonly used and accepted measure of the severity of hypoxemia is the alveolar-to-arterial oxygen tension gradient, or $P_{(A-a)O_2}$. As described in Chapter 9, the alveolar P_{O_2} in the alveolar-to-arterial oxygen tension gradient is calculated according to the alveolar air equation:

$$P_{AO_2} = F_{IO_2}(P_B - P_{H_2O}) - \frac{Pa_{CO_2}}{R}$$

Because the respiratory exchange ratio, R, cannot readily be measured at the bedside, R is assumed to be either 0.8 or 1.0 for the purpose of this calculation. A $P_{(A-a)O_2}$ of 350 mm Hg or greater during breathing of 100% O_2 indicates severe hypoxemia, and patients with this finding usually (but not always) require some form of ventilatory support.

Ways of quantifying severe hypoxemia other than with the A-a gradient include the arterial-to-alveolar P_{O_2} ratio (also known as the a/A ratio) and the less exact but easier to calculate arterial P_{O_2}-to-F_{IO_2} (P/F) ratio. Using the latter, one finds that a patient with a Pa_{O_2} of 80 mm Hg breathing 40% O_2 would have a Pa_{O_2}/F_{IO_2} ratio of 200, a threshold value used by some clinicians to indicate the need for ventilatory support with PEEP or CPAP. Calculation of the shunt fraction, or $\dot{Q}s/\dot{Q}t$, also is used by some clinicians to indicate the severity of hypoxemia in acute respiratory failure, although whether a value of 0.20, 0.25, or 0.30 should be used has not been decided. More details on these measures of the adequacy and efficiency of oxygenation are provided in Chapter 31.

Since hypoxemia causing shunts as large as these can occur only in the presence of significant airway closure and atelectasis, the mode of ventilatory support chosen in these cases must be capable of recruiting collapsed alveoli and maintaining their patency throughout the breathing cycle. In the presence of adequate alveolar ventilation, the application of CPAP alone is usually sufficient to achieve this end.[33] However, patients with severe hypoxemia often have other problems, such as alveolar hypoventilation or respiratory muscle fatigue. In these situations, CMV with PEEP is the preferred mode of ventilatory support.

Prophylactic ventilatory support. In addition to the six general indications listed in Table 28-3, some clinicians suggest that ventilatory support should be considered whenever there is a high probability that one or more of these problems will develop, even though none are currently present. This recommendation is based on the premise that institution of ventilatory support before the development of respiratory acidosis, poor lung expansion, or respiratory muscle fatigue could prevent the deleterious effects of these processes. From the preceding discussion, it is evident that "hard data" are scanty for each of the six mechanisms under consideration; there is even less substantiating information with respect to prophylactic ventilatory support.

The most obvious potential application of prophylactic mechanical ventilation is for surgical patients in the early postoperative phase. We know that in the initial hours after some types of surgery, particularly upper abdominal procedures, VC may fall to one third or less of its preoperative value. We also know that hypoxemia, atelectasis, and pneumonia are frequent complications in the postoperative period. Together these factors suggest that mechanical ventilation could be applied to maintain adequate alveolar expansion and thus prevent these problems from occurring.

Nonetheless, a controlled study of prophylactic mechanical ventilation in this setting failed to show any differences in gas exchange, morbidity, or mortality between patient groups.[54] Thus, the theoretical value of prophylactic mechanical ventilation is yet to be confirmed in practice. Because of the numerous disadvantages and complications associated with ventilatory support,[55-58] clinicians should be cautious about applying these methods to patients without sound justification.

Special uses for ventilatory support. The literature is replete with descriptions of various modes of ventilatory support in specific or delimited clinical situations. Among those most often cited are closed head injuries, flail chest, obstructive lung disease, and sleep apnea.

Closed head injury. An indication separate from all of the foregoing is deliberate hyperventilation with CMV to reduce brain swelling and intracranial pressure in patients with severe closed head trauma. Hypocapnia and alkalosis have additive effects in reducing cerebral blood flow, and two groups of investigators report better survival rates with intensive regimens that include mechanical hyperventilation to $Paco_2$ values of 25 to 30 mm Hg.[59,60] However, the clinical benefits associated with hyperventilation are diminished after 24 to 48 hours as the brain's acid-base balance is restored (despite peripheral alkalosis). For this reason, mechanical ventilation in cases of closed head trauma is limited to the initial day or two following the injury. Perhaps because of the older age of the patients and the focal nature of the disease process, mechanical hyperventilation does not improve survival or neurologic outcome after cerebrovascular accidents.[61]

Flail chest. Traumatic flail chest is another condition that in the past has been considered a separate indication for mechanical ventilation, often for prolonged periods.[62]

In the last 15 years, however, an increasing body of evidence suggests that the majority of patients with flail chest do not require mechanical ventilation. Three retrospective studies[63-65] and one prospective investigation[66] of flail chest cases have found that such patients can be managed in much the same way as trauma patients in general. The results of these studies are consistent with the concept that it is not the flail segment but the associated lung contusion, aspiration of gastric contents, and other injuries that determine the course of illness. In the absence of other indications, only rarely is the disruption of thoracic integrity itself severe enough to require ventilatory support.[67-68]

Obstructive lung disease. For status asthmaticus and acute exacerbations of chronic obstructive pulmonary disease, most clinicians consider the indications for mechanical ventilation to be somewhat different from those discussed up to this point. There are two main reasons for this. First, patients with severe obstructive lung disease are especially prone to complications of mechanical ventilation and to difficult weaning, once the acute episode is resolved. Second, and more important, early and aggressive intervention with more conservative management approaches can make mechanical ventilation unnecessary in most of these patients.

While mild to moderate acute respiratory alkalosis is the rule in acute asthma attacks, a $Paco_2$ value rising to or above normal despite treatment is regarded as an ominous sign,[69] even if usual criteria for hypercapnic respiratory failure (eg, $Pco_2 > 50$, pH 7.30) have not yet been met. In the past, mechanical ventilation has often been initiated in such cases, with the idea that progression to life-threatening respiratory acidosis was predictable, once the $Paco_2$ began to climb. This assumption is refuted by the observations of Bondi and Williams,[70] who found that although hypercapnia is an indicator of severity in status asthmaticus, intubation and mechanical ventilation can be avoided in many patients despite $Paco_2$ values of 60 mm Hg or higher. The authors of recent guides to the management of severe acute asthma agree that intubation can be deferred, even in the face of moderate hypercapnia, as long as the patient remains alert and cooperative during therapy. However, when consciousness becomes impaired, mechanical ventilation usually becomes necessary.[71-73]

Acute respiratory failure that occurs during an exacerbation of COPD is usually reversible through aggressive application of the same modes of therapy used in long-term management.[30,74,75] A combination of judicious oxygen therapy, administration of bronchodilators, corticosteroids, respiratory stimulants, and appropriate antibiotics, and vigorous bronchial hygiene measures can enable the clinician to avoid mechanical ventilation in most instances.[75,76] As in status asthmaticus, the main indications for intubation are uncontrollable, progressive respiratory acidosis, despite vigorous therapy, and an altered mental status. The latter may consist either of stupor or of uncontrollable agitation that makes sedation mandatory and renders adequate nursing and respiratory care impossible.

Sleep apnea. Sleep apnea is a general term for episodic cessation of respiration during sleep. Since brief periods of apnea are normal during sleep, the sleep apnea syndrome is strictly defined as the occurrence of five or more apneic periods per hour, each lasting at least 10 seconds. Moreover, these episodes must manifest themselves in clinically discernible signs or symptoms, such as polycythemia or daytime hypersomnolence.[8]

Currently, there are two recognized forms of the sleep apnea syndrome: central sleep apnea and obstructive sleep apnea. As the name implies, central sleep apnea is most likely caused by a defect in the respiratory control mechanism of the central nervous system. Typically, patients with central sleep apnea do not make efforts to breathe during the apneic periods. Patients with the central sleep apnea syndrome may be of any age, weight, or sex. The central sleep apnea syndrome is relatively rare.

FACTORS THAT INCREASE RISK FOR OBSTRUCTIVE SLEEP APNEA

Obesity (particularly in men)
Alcohol (only in men and when consumed before bedtime)
Irregular work shift (eg, night shift)
COPD
Large tonsils
Craniofacial deformities (eg, acromegaly)
Enlarged tongue
Hypothyroidism
Chest wall deformities
Tranquilizers (particularly when added to any other risk factor)

From Martin L: Pulmonary physiology in clinical practice, ed 1, St Louis, 1987, The CV Mosby Co.

Obstructive sleep apnea, on the other hand, is characterized by occlusion of the oropharyngeal airway, accompanied by continuing efforts to breathe. Moreover, the occurrence of obstructive sleep apnea is associated with a number of well-defined factors, with obesity in men being the most common finding (refer to box below, left).

Until recently, treatment of moderately severe sleep apnea syndrome was limited to weight reduction for obesity, the use of respiratory stimulants, or mechanical devices, such as a tongue retainer. Sleep apnea that was not responsive to these methods was sometimes treated surgically with either tracheostomy or uvulopalatopharyngoplasty, a procedure involving shortening of the soft palate and removal of the uvula and tonsils.

Over the last decade, continuous positive airway pressure (CPAP) has emerged as an alternative treatment for obstructive sleep apnea. As depicted in Fig. 28-7, the continuous positive airway pressure, usually administered through a nasal device, distends the oropharynx, thereby preventing occlusion by the tongue and soft palate.[77] Comparative studies indicate that, among all sleep apnea treatment modalities, CPAP is generally the most successful, the least hazardous, and the best tolerated.[78]

More recently, CPAP also has been used with success in central sleep apnea disorders.[79,80] Exactly why CPAP should be effective in this type of sleep apnea is not en-

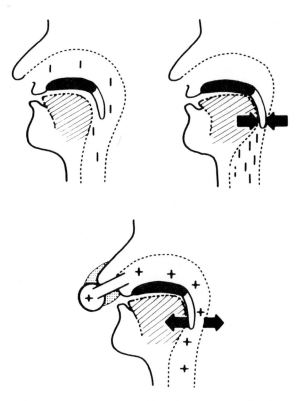

Fig. 28-7   Nasal constant positive airway pressure for obstructive sleep apnea. The positive airway pressure can prevent pharyngeal collapse *(arrows).*

tirely clear. However, recent research suggests that upper airway collapse may also play a role in the induction of central sleep apnea. Specifically, central sleep apnea may be due in part to a reflex inhibition of respiration caused by activation of the supraglottic mucosal receptors during upper airway closure.[80]

SUMMARY

Although simple in concept, respiratory failure represents a complex clinical phenomenon that is best understood in terms of the underlying pathophysiologic disturbance(s). Numerous objective measures exist to help quantify the nature and severity of the underlying disturbance. In the final analysis, however, these criteria cannot substitute for the more subjective judgment and perspective that come with clinical experience.

In addition to objective criteria, several subjective aspects of a patient's acute episode must be considered. These include the individual patient's "baseline status," the severity of preexisting lung disease, the presence of related chronic cardiovascular problems, and the nature of the acute episode. In view of these considerations, efforts to avoid ventilatory support during an acute asthma attack in a patient who could be expected to improve within hours might be appropriate. However, in the face of severe lung trauma or progressive neuromuscular disease, the need to commit to ventilatory support is more apparent. In any case, the hazards of endotracheal intubation and mechanical ventilation must be weighed against the expected benefits for each person.

Clinical judgment should never be translated completely into a list of numeric thresholds for which every patient is treated in the same manner. Some authors avoid strict use of numeric criteria, emphasizing instead the importance of serial observations and the individual patient's medical history in the decision as to when to commit to ventilatory support.[12,81] Nonetheless, the use of objective measurements that assess the mechanisms underlying respiratory failure can provide a physiologic framework for the application of sound clinical judgment to this fundamental aspect of respiratory care.

REFERENCES

1. Bryan CL: Classification of respiratory failure. In Kirby RR, Smith RA, and Desautels DD, editors: Mechanical ventilation, New York, 1985, Churchill Livingstone.
2. Shapiro BA, Harrison RA, and Walton JR: Clinical application of blood gases, ed 3, Chicago, 1982, Year Book Medical Publishers.
3. Campbell EJM: Respiratory failure, Br Med J 1:1451, 1965.
4. Petty TL: Acute respiratory failure. In Petty TL, editor: Intensive and rehabilitative respiratory care, Philadelphia, 1982, Lea & Febiger.
5. Pontoppidan H, Geffin B, and Lowenstein E: Acute respiratory failure in the adult, Boston, 1973, Little, Brown & Co.
6. Martin L: Respiratory failure, Med Clin North Am 61:1369, 1977.
7. Balk R and Bone RC: Classification of acute respiratory failure, Med Clin North Am 67:551, 1983.
8. Martin L: Pulmonary physiology in clinical practice: the essentials for patient care and evaluation, St Louis, 1987, The CV Mosby Co.
9. Bone RC: Acute respiratory failure: classification, differential diagnosis, and introduction to management. In Burton GG, and Hodgkin JE, editors: Respiratory care: a guide to clinical practice, ed 2, Philadelphia, 1984, JB Lippincott Co.
10. Demling RH and Nerlich M: Acute respiratory failure, Surg Clin North Am 63:337, 1983.
11. Demers RR and Irwin RS: Management of hypercapnic respiratory failure: a systemic approach, Respir Care 24:328-335, 1979.
12. Shapiro BA, Harrison RA, and Trout CA: Clinical applications of respiratory care, ed 3, Chicago, 1985, Year Book Medical Publishers.
13. Suter PM: Cardiopulmonary interactions in acute respiratory failure: update in intensive care and emergency medicine series, vol 2, New York, 1987, Springer-Verlag.
14. Lake KB: Adult respiratory distress syndrome (high permeability pulmonary edema). In Burton GG and Hodgkin JE, editors: Respiratory care; a guide to clinical practice, ed 2, Philadelphia, 1984, JB Lippincott Co.
15. Shale DJ: The adult respiratory distress syndrome—20 years on, Thorax 42:641-645, 1987.
16. Biondi JW et al: The adult respiratory distress syndrome, Yale J Biol Med 59:575-597, 1986.
17. Brandstetter RD: The adult respiratory distress syndrome—1986, Heart Lung, 15:155-164, 1986.
18. Bernard GR and Brigham KL: The adult respiratory distress syndrome, Annu Rev Med 36:195-205, 1985.
19. Mason RJ: Surfactant in adult respiratory distress syndrome, Eur J Respir Dis 153(suppl):229-236, 1987.
20. Hechtman HB, Valeri CR, Shepro D: Role of humoral mediators in adult respiratory distress syndrome, Chest 86:623-627, 1984.
21. Pulmonary terms and symbols: a report of the ACCP-ATS Joint Committee on Pulmonary Nomenclature, Chest 67:583, 1975.
22. Kacmarek RM: The role of pressure support ventilation in reducing the work of breathing, Respir Care 33:99-120, 1988.
23. Pierce AK: Acute respiratory failure. In Guenter CA and Welch MH, editors: Pulmonary medicine, Philadelphia, 1982, JB Lippincott Co.
24. Mclees BD: Critical care medicine. In Wyngaarden and Smith LH Jr, editors: Cecil's textbook of medicine, ed 16, Philadelphia, 1982, WB Saunders Co.
25. Geer RT: Mechanical ventilation. In Fishman AP, editor: Pulmonary diseases and disorders, New York, 1980, McGraw-Hill Book Co.
26. Jay SJ: Acute respiratory failure. In Stein JH, editor: Internal medicine, Boston, 1983, Little, Brown & Co.
27. Caprio GS and Riley MA: The mechanically ventilated patient. In Morrison ML, editor: Respiratory intensive care nursing, ed 2, Boston, 1979, Little, Brown & Co.
28. Stauffer JL: Establishment and care of the airway. In Petty TL, editor: Intensive and rehabilitative respiratory care, ed 2, Philadelphia, 1982, Lea & Febiger.
29. Peters RM: Work of breathing and abnormal mechanics, Surg Clin North Am 54:955-966, 1974.
30. Pierson DJ: Acute respiratory failure. In Sahn SA, editor: Pulmonary emergencies, New York, 1982, Churchill-Livingstone.
31. Zwillich CW et al: Complications of assisted ventilation, Am J Med 57:161-169, 1974.
32. West JB: Causes of carbon dioxide retention in lung disease, N Engl J Med 284:1232, 1971.
33. Downs JB: Ventilatory patterns and modes of ventilation in acute respiratory failure, Respir Care 28:586-591, 1983.
34. Bendixen HH et al: Atelectasis and shunting during spontaneous ventilation in anesthetized patients, Anesthesiology 25:297-301, 1964.
35. Egbert LD, Laver MB, and Bendixen HH: Intermittent deep breaths and compliance during anesthesia in man, Anesthesiology 24:57-60, 1963.

36. Bendixen HH, Hedley-White J, and Laver MB: Impaired oxygenation in surgical patients during general anesthesia with controlled ventilation: a concept of atelectasis, N Engl J Med 269:991-996, 1963.

37. Sykes MK, Young WE, and Robinson BE: Oxygenation during anesthesia with controlled ventilation, Br J Anaesth 37:314-325, 1965.

38. Visick WD, Fairley HB, and Hickey RF: The effects of tidal volume and end-expiratory pressure on pulmonary gas exchange during anesthesia, Anesthesiology 39:285-290, 1973.

39. Ruiz BC et al: Effect of ventilatory patterns on arterial oxygenation after near-drowning with fresh water: a comparative study in dogs, Anesth Analg 52:570-576, 1973.

40. Modell JH et al: Effects of ventilatory patterns on arterial oxygenation after near-drowning in sea water, Anesthesiology 40:376-384, 1974.

41. Macklem PT: Respiratory muscle dysfunction, Hosp Pract 21(3):83-90, 95-96, 1986.

42. Black LF and Hyatt RE: Maximal static respiratory pressures in generalized neuromuscular disease, Am Rev Respir Dis 103:641-647, 1971.

43. Sahn SA and Lakshminarayan S: Bedside criteria for discontinuation of mechanical ventilation, Chest 63:1002-1005, 1973.

44. Pierson DJ: Weaning from mechanical ventilation in acute respiratory failure: concepts, indications, and techniques, Respir Care 28:646-660, 1983.

45. Grassino A and Macklem PT: Respiratory muscle fatigue and ventilatory failure, Annu Rev Med 35:625-647, 1984.

46. Brochard L, Pluskwa F, and Lemaire F: Improved efficacy of spontaneous breathing with inspiratory pressure support, Am Rev Respir Dis 136:411-415, 1987.

47. MacIntyre NR: Respiratory function during pressure support ventilation, Chest 89:677-683, 1986.

48. Marini JJ, Capps JS, and Culver BH: The inspiratory work of breathing during assisted mechanical ventilation, Chest 87:612-618, 1985.

49. Fiastry JF, Quan BF, and Habib MP: Pressure support compensation for inspiratory work due to endotracheal tubes and demand CPAP, Chest 89:441S, 1986 (abstract).

50. MacIntyre NR: Weaning from mechanical ventilatory support: volume assisting intermittent breaths versus pressure assisting every breath, Respir Care 33:121-125, 1988.

51. Brochard L, Pluskwa F, and Lemaire F: Pressure support (PS) of spontaneous breathing (SB) assists weaning from mechanical ventilation, Am Rev Respir Dis 134:A122, 1986 (abstract).

52. Sahn SA, Lakshminarayan S, and Petty TL: Weaning from mechanical ventilation, JAMA 235:2208-2212, 1976.

53. Murray JF: Pathophysiology of acute respiratory failure, Respir Care 28:531-540, 1983.

54. Shackford SR, Virgilio RW, and Peters RM: Early extubation versus prophylactic ventilation in the high risk patient: a comparison of postoperative management in the prevention of respiratory complications, Anesth Analg 60:76-80, 1981.

55. Zwillich CW et al: Complications of assisted ventilation: a prospective study of 354 consecutive episodes, Am J Med 57:161-169, 1974.

56. Stauffer JL, Olson DE, and Petty TL: Complications and consequences of endotracheal intubation and tracheotomy: a prospective study of 150 critically ill adult patients, Am J Med 70:65-76, 1981.

57. Johanson WG: Infectious complications of respiratory therapy, Respir Care 27:445, 1982.

58. Bone RC: Complications of mechanical ventilation and positive-end expiratory pressure, Respir Care 27:402-407, 1982.

59. Crockard HA, Coppel DL, and Morrow WFK: Evaluation of hyperventilation in treatment of head injuries, Br Med J 4:634-640, 1973.

60. Becker DP et al: The outcome from severe head injury with early diagnosis and intensive management, J Neurosurg 47:491-502, 1977.

61. Christensen MS et al: Cerebral apoplexy (stroke) treated with and without artificial hyperventilation. Pt I. Cerebral circulation, clinical course, and cause of death, Stroke 4:568-619, 1973.

62. Avery EE, Morch ET, and Benson DW: Critically crushed chests: a new method of treatment with continuous mechanical hyperventilation to produce alkalotic apnea and internal pneumatic stabilization, J Thorac Surg 32:291-311, 1956.

63. Cullen P et al: Treatment of flail chest: use of intermittent mandatory pressure and positive end-expiratory pressure, Arch Surg 110:1099-1103, 1975.

64. Trinkle JK et al: Management of flail chest without mechanical ventilation, Ann Thorac Surg 19:355-363, 1975.

65. Shackford SR et al: The management of flail chest: a comparison of ventilatory and nonventilatory treatment, Am J Surg 132:759-762, 1976.

66. Shackford SR, Virgilio RW, and Peters RM: Selective use of ventilator therapy in flail chest injury, J Thorac Cardiovasc Surg 81:194-201, 1981.

67. Parham AM, Yarbrough DR III, and Redding JS: Flail chest syndrome and pulmonary contusion, Arch Surg 113:900-903, 1978.

68. Lead article: Management of the stove-in chest with paradoxical movement, Br Med J 2:1242, 1977.

69. Rebuck AS and Read J: Assessment and management of severe asthma, Am J Med 51:788-798, 1971.

70. Bondi E and Williams MH Jr: Severe asthma: course and treatment in the hospital, NY State J Med 77:350-353, 1977.

71. Williams MH Jr: Life-threatening asthma, Arch Intern Med 140:1604, 1980.

72. Fish JE and Summer WR: Acute lower airway obstruction: asthma. In Moser KM and Spragg RG, editors: Respiratory emergencies, ed 2, St Louis, 1982, The CV Mosby Co.

73. Scoggin CH: Acute asthma and status asthmaticus. In Sahn SA, editor: Pulmonary emergencies, New York, 1982, Churchill-Livingstone.

74. Hudson LD and Pierson DJ: Comprehensive respiratory care for patients with chronic obstructive pulmonary disease, Med Clin North Am 65:629-645, 1981.

75. Light RW: Conservative treatment of hypercapnic acute respiratory failure, Respir Care 28:561-566, 1983.

76. Martin TR, Lewis SW, and Albert RK: The prognosis of patients with chronic obstructive pulmonary disease after hospitalization for acute respiratory failure, Chest 82:310-314, 1982.

77. Sullivan CE et al: Reversal of obstructive sleep apnea by continuous positive airway pressure applied through the nares, Lancet 1:862, 1981.

78. Katsantonis GP et al: Management of obstructive sleep apnea: comparison of various treatment modalities, Laryngoscope 98:304-309, 1988.

79. Hoffstein V and Slutsky AS: Central sleep apnea reversed by continuous positive airway pressure, Am Rev Respir Dis 135:1210-1212, 1987.

80. Issa FG and Sullivan CE: Reversal of central sleep apnea using nasal CPAP, Chest 90:165-171, 1986.

81. Moser KM: Management of acute respiratory failure. In Isselbacker KJ, Adams RD, and Braunwald E, editors: Harrison's principles of internal medicine, New York, 1980, McGraw-Hill Book Co.

29

Physics and Physiology of Ventilatory Support

Craig L. Scanlan

No aspect of respiratory care is as challenging, or as potentially rewarding, as the successful application of modern methods of ventilatory support to the patient with a critical but reversible failure of the cardiopulmonary system. As with all respiratory care interventions, the success with which ventilatory support is applied depends first and foremost on the practitioner's understanding of both its underlying principles and physiologic effects.

OBJECTIVES

Toward that end, this chapter will focus on the physical principle and physiologic effects—both helpful and harmful—that characterize modern modes of ventilatory support. Specifically, after completing this chapter, the reader will be able to:

1. Differentiate the physiologic concepts of positive and negative pressure ventilation and continuous positive airway pressure (CPAP);

2. Describe the major mechanisms by which the inspiratory phase of positive pressure ventilation can be initiated;

3. Identify the various mechanisms by which positive pressure is generated and applied during inspiration and how alterations in the inspiratory phase affect the parameters of respiration.

4. Differentiate the four primary parameters that are used to cycle a positive pressure ventilator from the inspiratory into the expiratory phase and their clinical significance;

5. Explain the mechanisms by which the expiratory phase of positive pressure ventilation may be manipulated to achieve specific ends;

6. Differentiate the physiologic effects of positive pressure ventilation on the respiratory, cardiovascular, renal, hepatic, and gastrointestinal systems;

7. Describe the physical and physiologic principles underlying alternative and experimental approaches to ventilatory support, including negative pressure ventilation and ventilation at high frequencies.

TERMS

Most terms used in this chapter are defined in context. The following terms are introduced without explicit definition but may be found in the text glossary:

angiotensin	pendelluft
autoregulation	peribronchial
bilirubin	poliomyelitis
biphasic	sinusoidal
convective	splanchnic
Hz	tetany
juxtamedullary	vasopressin

PHYSIOLOGIC BASIS OF VENTILATORY SUPPORT

All modes of ventilatory support attempt to facilitate lung expansion by increasing the transpulmonary pressure gradient (P_L). As detailed in Chapter 8, the P_L represents the difference between the intra-alveolar pressure, P_{alv}, and the intrapleural pressure, P_{pl}:

$$P_L = P_{alv} - P_{pl}$$

With all else constant, an increase in P_L will expand the alveoli in direct proportion to the pressure difference created.

As shown in Fig. 29-1, the P_L can be increased by either (1) decreasing the P_{pl} (see Fig. 29-1, *A*) or (2) increasing the P_{alv} (see Fig. 29-1, *B*). A spontaneous inspiration increases the P_L by decreasing the P_{pl}. Negative pressure ventilation exerts a similar effect by decreasing the pressure at the body surface or chest wall during inspiration.

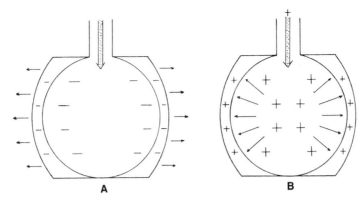

Fig. 29-1   Diagrammatic illustration of the difference between inspiratory forces of, **A,** negative pressure and, **B,** positive pressure ventilation.

On the other hand, positive pressure ventilation increases the P_L by raising the P_{alv} during inspiration.

A third mode of ventilatory support, CPAP, maintains an increased P_{alv} throughout both inspiration and expiration. Since CPAP maintains airway pressure at a constant level throughout the breathing cycle, gas flow into and out of the lung depends on spontaneously generated changes in pleural pressure, as with normal breathing.

Negative pressure ventilation

In concept, negative pressure ventilation is similar to spontaneous breathing. During the inspiratory phase of spontaneous breathing, muscle contraction causes expansion of the thorax, which, in turn, causes a drop in P_{pl}. This drop is transmitted to the alveoli, creating a transrespiratory pressure gradient (P_{rs}) equivalent to the difference between the pressure at the airway opening (P_{ao}) and the P_{alv}:

$$P_{rs} = P_{ao}\ (0)\ -\ P_{alv}\ (negative)$$

The amount of alveolar expansion, and therefore the volume of gas that will flow into the alveoli during a spontaneous inspiration, is proportional to the magnitude of P_L:

$$\text{Alveolar expansion} \cong P_L\ (end\ inspiration)$$
$$\cong P_{alv} - P_{pl}$$

Whereas in spontaneous ventilation the decreases in alveoli pressures during inspiration are a result of active muscle contraction, negative pressure ventilation creates these pressure drops by decreasing the pressure at the body surface (P_{bs}) to negative or subatmospheric levels. This negative P_{bs} is transmitted first to the pleural space and then to the alveoli:

$$\downarrow P_{bs} \rightarrow\ \downarrow P_{pl} \rightarrow\ \downarrow P_{alv}$$

Since the airway during negative pressure ventilation remains exposed to atmospheric pressure ($P_{ao} = 0$), a P_{rs} comparable to that generated during a spontaneous inspira-

tion is created. Therefore, gas will flow from the area of relatively high pressure (the airway opening) to the area of relatively low pressure (the alveoli). As with spontaneous breathing, the amount of gas that will expand the alveoli during negative pressure ventilation is determined by the magnitude of P_L.

During expiration in both spontaneous breathing and negative pressure ventilation, the lungs and chest wall are allowed to recoil passively back to their resting end-expiratory levels. As this occurs, P_{pl} values become less negative, and alveolar pressures rise above atmospheric. This reverses the P_{rs} (P_{alv} becomes greater than P_{ao}), causing gas to flow from the alveoli out to the airway opening.

Positive pressure ventilation

As depicted in Figs. 29-2 and 29-3 , positive pressure ventilation reverses the pressure gradients that occur during normal spontaneous breathing (or negative pressure ventilation). Rather than being generated by a negative P_{alv}, the P_{rs} is created by applying positive pressure to the airway:

$$P_{rs} = P_{ao}\ (positive)\ -\ P_{alv}\ (0)$$

Again, gas flows from the airway opening to the alveoli. However, alveolar pressures rise during the inspiratory phase of positive pressure ventilation. This rise in alveolar pressure also creates a transpulmonary pressure gradient thereby expanding the alveoli. However, compared with spontaneous inspiration or negative pressure ventilation, the pressure gradient is reversed. Because P_{alv} is greater than P_{pl} during intermittent positive pressure ventilation (IPPV), positive pressure is transmitted from the alveoli to the intrapleural space, causing a rise in P_{pl} values during inspiration. Depending on the lung's mechanical properties, P_{pl} may actually exceed atmospheric pressure during a portion of inspiration.

As with spontaneous breathing, the recoil force of the lung and chest wall, stored as potential energy during the positive pressure breath, causes a passive exhalation. As

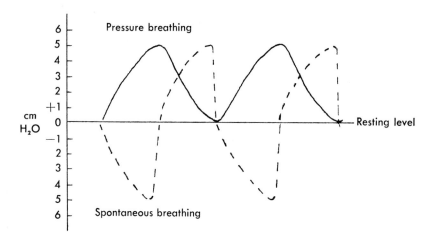

Fig. 29-2 Comparison of P_{alv} in positive pressure and spontaneous ventilation with driving pressures of 5 cm H_2O.

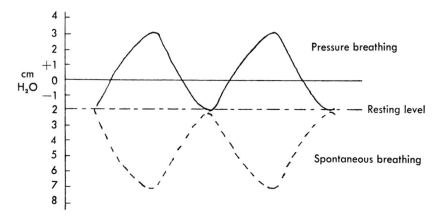

Fig. 29-3 Comparison of P_{pl} in positive pressure and spontaneous ventilation with driving pressures of 5 cm H_2O.

gas flows from the alveoli out to the airway opening, P_{alv} drops to atmospheric level, while P_{pl} is restored to its normal subatmospheric range.

Continuous positive airway pressure

Like negative and positive pressure ventilation, application of CPAP increases the transpulmonary pressure gradient, thereby causing alveolar expansion. However, unlike both negative and positive pressure ventilation, airway pressure with CPAP remains essentially constant throughout the breathing cycle (Fig. 29-4). Thus the difference between the pressure at the airway opening (P_{ao}) and the alveolar pressure (P_{alv}) with CPAP remains relatively constant. In other words, the transrespiratory pressure gradient created with CPAP is zero. Since a transrespiratory pressure gradient is necessary for gas to flow from the airway opening to the alveoli, CPAP alone does not provide ventilation.

If gas is to move into the lungs during CPAP administration, the patient must spontaneously create a transrespi-

ratory pressure gradient by expanding the thorax, thereby lowering P_{pl} and P_{alv}. Thus, whereas negative and positive pressure ventilation create the pressure gradients necessary for gas flow into the lungs, CPAP serves only to maintain alveoli at greater inflation volumes.

Continuous positive pressure ventilation can be combined with positive pressure ventilation. In this mode of ventilatory support, airway pressure is maintained above atmospheric levels throughout both inspiration and expiration, as with CPAP. However, during inspiration, a positive transrespiratory pressure gradient is created by applying additional positive pressure to the airway, above and beyond the CPAP level (Fig. 29-5).

During the expiratory phase, airway pressure is allowed to return to the CPAP level. Because the positive airway pressure is maintained during expiration, this mode of ventilation is commonly referred to as CMV with positive end-expiratory pressure breathing, or CMV with PEEP (some texts still use the older term IPPV with PEEP).

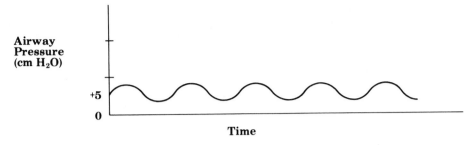

Fig. 29-4   CPAP. (From Pilbeam SP: Mechanical ventilation: physiological and clinical applications, St Louis, 1986, The CV Mosby Co.)

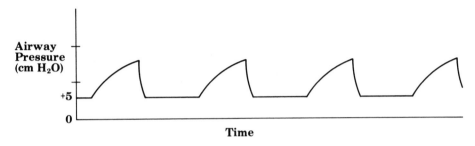

Fig. 29-5   CPAP combined with CMV (CMV with PEEP). (From Pilbeam SP: Mechanical ventilation: physiological and clinical applications, St Louis, 1986, The CV Mosby Co.)

Because the predominant mode of ventilatory support in current use is positive pressure ventilation (with or without PEEP), we will emphasize the physical principles and physiologic effects underlying this approach first. Following our discussion of positive pressure ventilation will be an analysis of alternative methods of ventilatory support, including negative pressure ventilation and ventilation at high frequencies.

PHYSICAL AND MECHANICAL PRINCIPLES OF POSITIVE PRESSURE VENTILATION

The physical and mechanical principles underlying positive pressure ventilation are best understood within the context of an orderly framework of analysis. The framework most commonly employed divides the events of mechanical ventilation into four related components[1]:

1. The mechanism by which inspiration is initiated;
2. The nature of the inspiratory phase;
3. The mechanism by which inspiration is terminated;
4. The nature of the expiratory phase.

Initiating inspiration

A positive pressure ventilator can initiate the inspiratory phase of the breathing cycle in various ways. These mechanisms are commonly referred to as cycling or triggering modes. The three major cycling modes are the assist mode, the control mode, and the assist-control mode. Manual cycling is also available on many ventilators.

Assist mode—patient cycled or triggered. In the assist mode of ventilation, the patient initiates inspiration and determines the frequency of breathing.[2,3] In assist mode ventilation, the patient's inspiratory effort causes a drop in pressure within the ventilator circuit. This pressure drop is "sensed" by the ventilator and initiates the inspiratory phase of the breathing cycle.

The clinician can usually adjust the amount of negative pressure needed to initiate the mechanical breath. This adjustable mechanism is called the *sensitivity* or patient-effort control.[4] Ideally, the amount of negative pressure needed to cycle the ventilator into the inspiratory phase should be as little as possible. Requiring a large amount of negative pressure to initiate inspiration can significantly increase the patient's work of breathing.

How fast the ventilator mechanism responds to the patient's inspiratory effort is called the *response time*. Unlike sensitivity, the response time of a ventilator is an inherent characteristic of its design and is therefore not normally adjustable. Generally, the response time of a ventilator is critical only at high ventilatory frequencies, such as may be used in infants and small children.

As described in Chapter 26, the assist mode is commonly used with intermittent positive pressure breathing (IPPB) therapy. The primary advantage of the assist mode of ventilation is that it gives the patient total control over the rate of breathing. However, the pure assist mode provides no mechanism to ventilate a patient who stops breathing. For this reason, the pure assist mode is con-

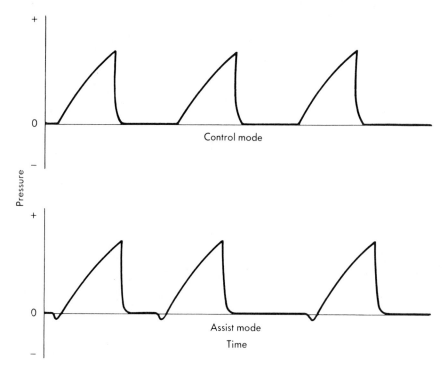

Fig. 29-6   Pressure waveforms for CMV during control mode (top) and assist mode (bottom). Note regular time intervals for control mode while time intervals for assist mode are more variable. Slight negative pressure "triggers" assist breaths.

traindicated in the continuous ventilatory support of critically ill patients.

Control mode—time cycled or triggered. In the control mode of ventilation, the frequency of cycling to inspiration is established by the ventilator according to a predetermined time interval, independent of the patient's efforts or breathing pattern.[2,3] In this mode of mechanical support, the parameters of ventilation are entirely in the clinician's hands. For this reason, controlled ventilation is the only mode of cycling to inspiration that can provide precise and consistently predictable physiologic results. However, controlled ventilation is poorly tolerated by many conscious patients, often requiring sedation or induced neuromuscular paralysis to be successful. More specific considerations for control mode ventilation are presented in Chapters 30 and 31.

Specific systems for establishing a controlled breathing rate can vary from one ventilator to another.[1,4] Rate can be set as an individual control that divides each minute in equal time segments, allotting one time segment for each full ventilatory cycle. With this method, inspiration and expiration are adjusted by using other controls such as flow and volume while the rate remains separate. Separate timers for inspiration and expiration can also set a control rate on some ventilators. Changing either or both of these timers can affect the control rate the patient receives. Alternatively, the expiratory time may be set by the clinician, with the inspiratory time determined by other parameters, such as flow and volume.

Assist-control (guarantor) mode. The assist-control mode of cycling to inspiration represents a combination of the two mechanisms just described. In the assist-control mode of ventilation, the minimum frequency of cycling to inspiration is established by the ventilator according to a predetermined time interval. However, the patient can override this minimum frequency by initiating inspiration at a faster rate.[2,3]

In the assist-control mode, the patient is normally allowed to establish an acceptable breathing rate, with the control rate set somewhat below that of the patient. In this case the control rate serves as a guarantor should the patient's breathing pattern slow or stop completely.

The assist-control mode of cycling to inspiration, available on modern devices since the 1960s, is used mainly to ventilate patients who are conscious and spontaneously breathing. Because patients can establish their own rate of breathing and therefore influence their own Pco_2 levels, acceptance is generally good. However, the practitioner will encounter some patients in whom the assist-control mode results in hypocapnea. The resulting respiratory alkalosis produced in these circumstances can lead to significant problems, considered in more detail later in this chapter and subsequently in Chapter 31.

Fig. 29-6 diagrams typical pressure waveforms created during controlled and assisted ventilation. Pressure is graphed on the vertical axis, with time being plotted on the horizontal axis. Note in the assist mode that each positive-pressure breath begins with a slight drop in pressure, indi-

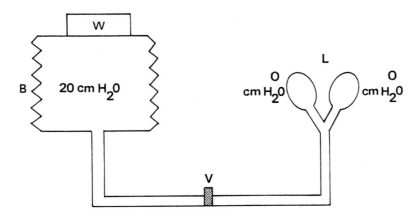

Fig. 29-7   Mechanical properties of constant pressure generator.

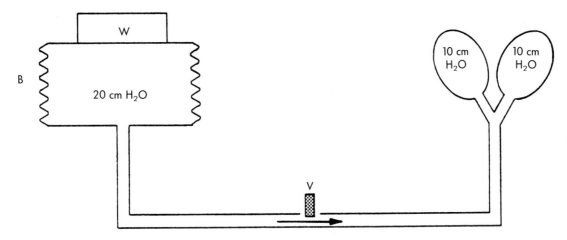

Fig. 29-8   Constant pressure generator (mid-inspiration).

cating patient cycling to inspiration. Moreover, the time between breaths in the assist mode is somewhat variable. In the control mode, on the other hand, the time between breaths is constant. Patient inspiratory effort, even if it were to occur, would not influence the predetermined rate.

Nature of the inspiratory phase

It is during the inspiratory phase of mechanical ventilation that the ventilator generates and delivers a volume of gas under pressure to the patient. We will analyze two major aspects of the inspiratory phase: (1) how the positive pressure is generated and applied and (2) how alterations in the inspiratory phase affect the parameters of respiration.

Generation and application of positive pressure. There are two major ways in which positive pressure can be generated and applied to the airway: pressure generation and flow generation.[1,5-7] Within each of these two major categories we will explore two subcategories.

Pressure generation. A pressure generator is a ventilator that develops a pressure pattern not influenced by the mechanical characteristics of the patient's respiratory system. Although the pressure pattern exhibited by a pressure

generator remains unaffected by changes in the mechanical properties of a patient's lungs, the flow pattern will vary with alterations in lung compliance (C_L) and airway resistance (Raw).[1,5-7] There are two subcategories of pressure generators: the constant pressure generator and the nonconstant pressure generator.

Constant pressure generator. The mechanical principles underlying a constant pressure generator are depicted in Fig. 29-7. A bellows, B is connect to a pair of elastic lungs, L. The bellows and lungs are separated by a closed valve, V. A weight, W, on top of the bellows creates a constant force per unit area, or pressure, equivalent to 20 cm H_2O. The lungs are at atmospheric pressure (0 cm H_2O).

Opening the valve, V, will immediately creates an initial difference in pressure between the bellows and lungs of 20 cm H_2O − 0 cm H_2O, or 20 cm H_2O. Gas will therefore flow from the area of higher pressure (the bellows) to the area of relatively lower pressure (the lungs).

As gas flows into the lungs, their pressure rises (Fig. 29-8). However, the pressure in the bellows remains constant at 20 cm H_2O. Thus the pressure difference between the bellows and lungs progressively decreases throughout inspiration. During mid-inspiration, as shown in Fig. 29-8, the pressure difference between the bellows and lungs has decreased to 20 cm H_2O − 10 cm H_2O, or 10 cm H_2O.

Of course, flow into the airway will vary directly with the difference in pressure between the bellows and lungs. Since the pressure difference across this system decreases throughout inspiration, we would expect the flow also to decrease. However, the pressure applied by the bellows system should remain constant. These pressure and flow events, characteristic of a constant pressure generator, are graphically portrayed in Fig. 29-9, *A*.

As is evident in Fig. 29-9, *A,* airway pressure remains constant throughout inspiration. This pressure pattern, typical of a constant pressure generator, is often called a *square wave* pressure pattern. Because of the large initial pressure gradient, flow, on the other hand, starts out high. However, as the pressure gradient drops, the flow progressively decreases throughout inspiration. This flow pattern, also typical of a constant pressure generator, is often referred to as a *decelerating or tapering flow wave.*

Although the pressure pattern exhibited by a constant pressure generator is unaffected by changes in the mechanical properties of a patient's lungs, the flow pattern does vary with alterations in patient compliance and resistance. Fig. 29-9, *B* and *C,* demonstrates these effects.

In Fig. 29-9, *B,* a reduction in C_L causes more rapid filling of the lung units, due to a decreased time constant (see Chapter 8). Under these circumstances, the pressure difference between ventilator and lung drops more rapidly than normal, resulting in a steeper and more rapid drop in flow. On the other hand, when the Raw increases (see Fig. 29-9, *C*), the flow created by the constant pressure starts out lower and tapers more slowly throughout inspiration.

In addition to devices using a weighted bellows as the pressure-generating mechanism, several other ventilator designs produce a constant pressure pattern. Ventilators that generate their driving pressure using an air injector or Venturi device, a second-stage reducing valve or low-pressure regulator, or a blower or turbine are also considered

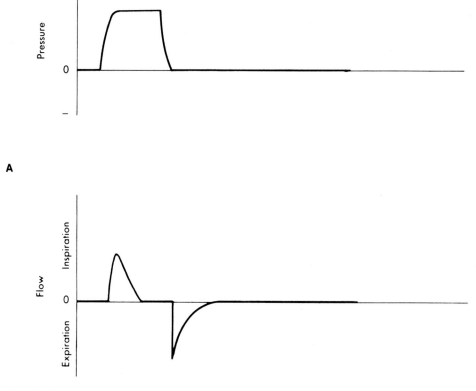

Fig. 29-9   Pressure and flow waveforms for a constant pressure generator. **A** represents "normal" conditions while **B** illustrates a decrease in C_L and **C** shows an increase in Raw.

constant pressure generators.[1,7] Examples include the Chemtron Gill-1 (weighted piston), Bird Mark 7 and 8 in the air-mix modes (air injector/Venturi), and the Bennett PR-1 and PR-2 (second-stage reducing valves). The box opposite summarizes the characteristics of a constant pressure generator.

Nonconstant pressure generator. Like the constant pressure generator, the nonconstant pressure generator develops a pressure pattern that is not influenced by the mechanical characteristics of the patient's respiratory system. However, rather than producing a square wave or constant pressure pattern, the nonconstant pressure generator produces a pattern of either decreasing or increasing force throughout inspiration.

An example of a decreasing force nonconstant pressure generator would be a bellows system compressed by a weak spring.[1] As the bellows empties, the spring relaxes, and progressively less force (pressure) is applied throughout inspiration. However, with such a device, the pattern

---

CHARACTERISTICS OF A CONSTANT PRESSURE GENERATOR

The pressure pattern throughout inspiration is constant (a square wave).

The pressure pattern is not influenced by the patient's lung characteristics.

The flow delivered varies with respect to both time and the patient's lung characteristics.

Flow starts out high during the initial phase of inspiration and progressively decreases toward the end of inspiration.

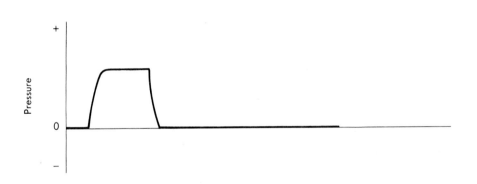

B

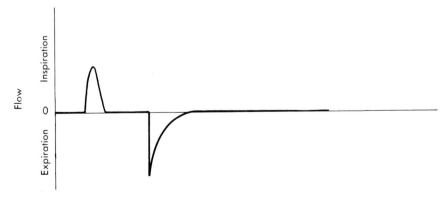

Fig. 29-9, cont'd   For legend see opposite page.

Continued.

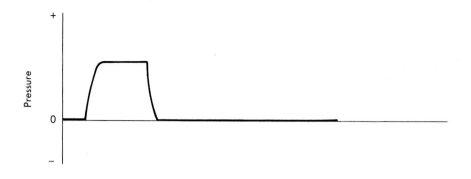

c

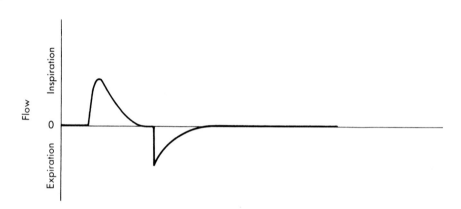

Fig. 29-9, cont'd   For legend see page 706.

of applied pressure remains the same, regardless of changes in the mechanical properties of the lungs or thorax. The Servo 900 series ventilators, when set at low driving pressures, behave as decreasing force nonconstant pressure generators.

Increasing force nonconstant pressure generators are less common in clinical practice. However, a nonconstant flow generator with a built-in internal leak would exhibit the characteristics of a increasing force nonconstant pressure generator. The early Engstrom ventilators (ER 150 and 300) combined nonconstant flow generation with an internal leak in their piston chambers and would thus be characterized as increasing force nonconstant pressure generators. More recently, microprocessor-controlled ventilators that provide accelerating flow patterns (Siemens Servo 900C, Bear 5, Hamilton Veolar) will function as increasing force nonconstant pressure generators at high airway pressures. The box opposite summarizes the characteristics of nonconstant pressure generators.

Flow generation. A flow generator is a ventilator that develops a flow pattern not influenced by the mechanical

---

CHARACTERISTICS OF A NONCONSTANT PRESSURE GENERATOR

The pressure pattern throughout inspiration is not constant; it may increase or decrease.

The pressure pattern is not influenced by the patient's lung characteristics.

The flow delivered varies with respect to time, the patient's lung characteristics, and the nature of the pressure pattern (increasing or decreasing force).

With an increasing force nonconstant pressure generator, flow starts out low during the initial phase of inspiration and progressively increases toward the end of inspiration.

With a decreasing force nonconstant pressure generator, flow starts out high during the initial phase of inspiration and progressively decreases toward the end of inspiration.

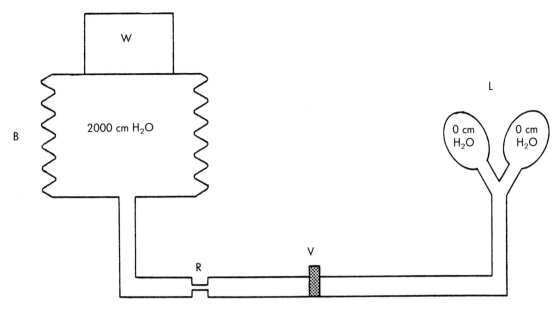

Fig. 29-10   Mechanical principles underlying constant flow generator.

characteristics of the patient's respiratory system. Although the flow pattern exhibited by a flow generator remains unaffected by changes in the mechanical properties of a patient's lungs, the pressure pattern will vary with alterations in compliance and airway resistance.[1,5-7] As with pressure generators, there are two subcategories of flow generators: the constant flow generator and the nonconstant flow generator.

Constant flow generator. The mechanical principles underlying a constant flow generator are depicted in Fig. 29-10. As is evident, all components are the same as with the constant pressure generator, with two critical exceptions.

First, the small weight on top of the bellows has been replaced with one having 100 times the mass. Now the generated pressure in the bellows is 100 times that previously generated, or about 2000 cm H_2O. Second, a high resistance element, *R*, has been placed between the bellows and lungs. Were it not for the presence of this small orifice, opening of the valve, *V*, would expose the lungs to unacceptably high pressures and flows.

The initial pressure difference between the bellows and lung is tremendous (2000 cm H_2O). However, when the valve, *V*, is opened to initiate inspiration, a large drop in pressure occurs across the restricted orifice. This orifice limits both the absolute rate of flow and the rate with which pressure in the system rises.

Unlike that developed by a constant pressure generator, the pressure gradient established between the bellow and lungs with a constant flow generator remains extremely large at end-inspiration (2000 − 20 = 1980 cm H_2O).

Thus, for all intents and purposes, the pressure difference across the system remains constant throughout inspiration.

Of course, flow into the airway will vary directly with the difference in pressure between the bellow and lungs. Since the pressure difference across this system is essentially constant throughout inspiration, we would expect the flow also to remain constant. Moreover, with a constant flow occurring between the bellows and lungs throughout inspiration, we would expect the pressure at the airway and in the lungs to rise progressively.

The pressure and flow events typical of a constant flow generator applied to a lung with normal mechanical properties are graphically portrayed in Fig. 29-11, *A*. As is evident, flow throughout inspiration assumes a constant or square wave pattern. Pressure, on the other hand, increases progressively throughout inspiration.

Fig. 29-11, *B*, demonstrates the effect of a decrease in C_L on the pressure and flow characteristics exhibited by a constant flow generator. As expected, the flow pattern remains unaffected by this mechanical change in lung characteristics. However, the pressure pattern is altered. The pressure rises faster and (if the delivered volume is constant) to a higher level than that observed in Fig. 29-11, *A*. Higher than normal resistance would also result in a greater pressure for a given volume, but the slope of the pressure curve would be less steep than normal.

In addition to a weighted bellows generating high working pressures, several other ventilator mechanisms can produce a constant flow pattern. Ventilators that generate their driving pressure from a first-stage reducing valve (50

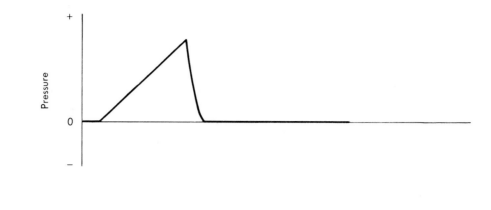

A

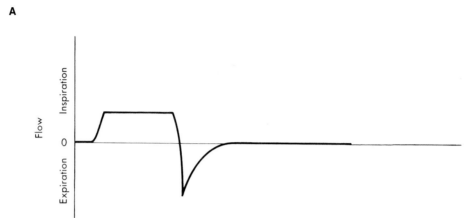

Fig. 29-11   Pressure and flow waveforms for a constant flow generator under different patient conditions. **A** shows typical wave forms for "normal" conditions. **B** illustrates a decrease in C_L. Note that in **B** the inspiratory flow pattern remains unchanged while inspiratory pressure increases and expiratory flow increases.

psig) with high resistance are considered constant flow generators. The Bird Mark 7 and 8 in the pure source gas mode, the Bear 2 and 5 in the square wave flow mode, the Foregger 210, and the Veriflow CV 2000 are examples of this type of driving mechanism. Positive displacement pumps or compressors that generate driving pressures well in excess of the actual pressure necessary to inflate the lungs (five to ten times greater) are also considered constant flow generators. The compressor driven Bennett MA-1, when operating against low to moderate airway pressures, functions as a constant flow generator. Last, ventilators that use a gear-driven piston mechanism, in which the rate of piston displacement is constant over time, also produce a constant flow pattern.[1,7] The Bourns LS104-150 is an example of a ventilator that uses a linearly driven piston to generate a constant flow. The box opposite summarizes the characteristics of a constant flow generator.

Nonconstant flow generator. The mechanical principles underlying a nonconstant flow generator are depicted in

Fig. 29-12, *A*. A piston in a cylinder is being driven by a connecting rod attached to a rotating wheel. The wheel is driven by an electric motor (not shown). During the forward stroke of the piston, gas is displaced out of the cylinder and directed to the patient. On the return stroke, the

---

CHARACTERISTICS OF A CONSTANT FLOW GENERATOR

The flow throughout inspiration is constant (a square wave).

The flow pattern is not influenced by the patient's lung characteristics.

The pressure delivered varies with respect to both time and the patient's lung characteristics.

Pressure progressively increases in a linear manner throughout inspiration.

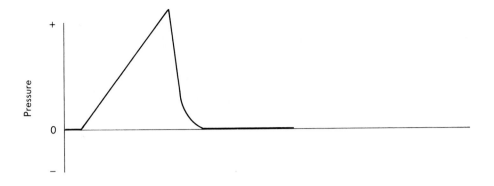

B

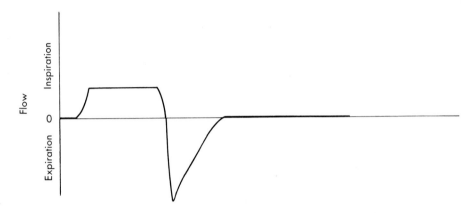

Fig. 29-11, cont'd   For legend see opposite page.

piston moves back, and a fresh volume of gas is drawn into the cylinder. Unidirectional flow of gas is maintained by one-way valves.

In this system, the angular motion of the wheel is translated into the linear motion of the piston. Thus the linear motion of the piston is greatest when the connecting rod is moving parallel to the piston and least when the connecting rod is moving perpendicular to the piston.

The piston's movement through the cylinder, and therefore the flow of gas to the patient during inspiration, occurs in an accelerating, then decelerating, fashion (Fig. 29-12, *B*). This pattern, typical of a nonconstant flow generator, is often termed a *sine wave flow pattern,* after the sinusoidal motion of the piston.[1,7,8]

The pressure and flow waveforms generated by this type of nonconstant flow generator reflects the change in flow over time (see Fig. 29-12, *B*). Initially, because flow is slow, pressure rises slowly. As the middle portion of inspiration is reached, flows rise rapidly. This rapid rise in

flow results in a rapid upswing in pressure during mid-inspiration. However, as flows taper off toward the end of inspiration, the rise in pressure slows. The pressure pattern characterizing this type of nonconstant flow generator thus resembles the S-shaped oxyhemoglobin dissociation curve.

Some newer-generation microprocessor-controlled ventilators can mimic the sinusoidal flow pattern produced by a eccentrically driven pistons. Examples include the Bennett 7200, the Bear 5, and the Hamilton Veolar ventilators. The box on p. 712 summarizes the characteristics of a nonconstant flow generator.

Alterations to the inspiratory phase. Besides the differences in inspiratory flow and pressure waveforms created by various types of ventilators, it is also possible to create a pause at the end of inspiration. This pause, referred to as an end-inspiratory pause (EIP), inflation hold, or inspiratory hold, follows active inspiration and precedes the expiratory phase (Fig. 29-13). The option to provide

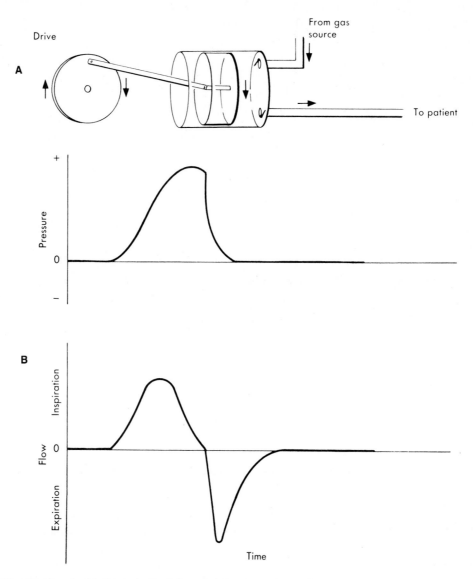

Fig. 29-12   **A,** Mechanical principle underlying nonconstant flow generator. **B,** Pressure and flow waveforms of nonconstant flow generator.

CHARACTERISTICS OF A NONCONSTANT FLOW GENERATOR

The flow pattern throughout inspiration remains the same from breath to breath but is not constant.

The flow pattern is not influenced by the patient's lung characteristics.

The pressure delivered varies with respect to time, the patient's lung characteristics, and the nature of the flow pattern.

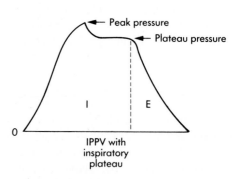

Fig. 29-13   End-inspiratory pause (see text for details). (From Martin L: Pulmonary physiology in clinical practice, St Louis, 1987, The CV Mosby Co.)

an EIP is found on most ventilators used in critical care. Indeed, some ventilator waveforms, such as that created by the Engstrom 300 series, automatically incorporate an EIP as part of the inspiratory phase.

With most ventilators, however, EIP is invoked *after* delivery of a preset inspiratory pressure or volume. EIP is typically determined either in direct time increments or as a percentage of total ventilatory cycle time. In this case, adding an EIP effectively increases the total inspiratory time, thereby shortening the time available for exhalation (see the following section on inspiratory-expiratory time ratios). The Bennett MA-1, MA-2, and 7200; the Bear 1, 2, and 5; and the Siemens Servo 900 series ventilators are examples of ventilators with adjustable EIP mechanisms.

When an EIP is established, rather than allowing immediate exhalation, the ventilator exhalation valve remains closed for a predetermined time interval.[4] During this time interval, the inspired volume is held in the patient's lungs, with no gas flow allowed into or out of the system (for this reason some authors refer to the EIP as a "volume hold"). With no gas flow, pressure in the ventilator and tubing system attempts to equilibrate with the P_{alv}. This equilibration between the system and alveolar pressures manifests itself as a pressure drop at the airway, as recorded on the ventilator's pressure manometer. When pressure equilibration is complete, a pressure "plateau" can be observed (see Fig. 29-13).

The EIP is used for both therapeutic and diagnostic purposes. Its role as a therapeutic modality, discussed in the next section, remains controversial. However, the role of the EIP maneuver in the bedside monitoring of pulmonary mechanics is well established.[9,10]

As a bedside monitoring tool, the EIP allows the clinician to separate out the elastic and frictional resistive components opposing inspiration during mechanical ventilation. Whereas the peak pressure during positive pressure ventilation represents the total pressure necessary to overcome both elastic and flow-resistive opposition to gas movement, the EIP plateau pressure (taken during conditions of no flow) provides a rough estimate of the pressure needed to overcome elastic forces only, that is, lung-thorax compliance. Moreover, the difference between the peak and plateau pressure can be used as a rough estimate of flow-resistive opposition to ventilation, that is, Raw. More detail on the use of the EIP in monitoring the ventilator patient is provided in Chapter 31.

Clinical importance of the inspiratory phase. Most modern positive pressure ventilators provide the clinician with a choice of various inspiratory flow and pressure patterns. Interestingly, years of research using mechanical analogs, animal models, and human subjects has generally failed to provide conclusive evidence that any one of these pressure or flow waveforms is clinically superior to the others. The sole exception to this generalization is the physiologic effect of the EIP.

In mechanical models, the decelerating flow pattern characteristic of constant pressure or some nonconstant flow generators does result in better distribution of volume to lung units with high time constants.[11,12] However, nitrogen washout curve analysis of laboratory lung models has failed to demonstrate a significant difference in the efficiency of gas distribution among these various flow patterns.[13] Similar analysis in humans using argon washout curves tend to confirm that no one inspiratory flow pattern is clinical superior to another.[14]

However, studies have demonstrated that an EIP can and does affect physiologic parameters. By momentarily maintaining airway pressure under conditions of zero flow, an EIP provides additional time for redistribution of gas between lung units with short and long time constants. This movement of gas from "fast" to "slow" filling spaces during EIP is called *pendelluft* and has been demonstrated in both laboratory and computer simulations.[12,13]

In concept, pendelluft should improve the distribution of ventilation, thereby improving oxygenation. As applied clinically, however, EIP tends to affect mainly the efficiency of ventilation, not oxygenation.[15] In both animal and human studies, increasing EIP time intervals are associated with a decrease in the V_D/V_T ratio, $Paco_2$, and inert gas washout times.[14-16]

Changes in inspiratory waveform or EIP notwithstanding, the rate of positive pressure ventilation tends to exert the greatest effect on gas distribution in lungs with uneven time constants.[11,12] High rates (with high flows) tend to worsen gas distribution, while low rates (with low flows and long inspiratory times) tend to enhance the distribution of gases within the lung. Unfortunately, both long inspiratory times and the use of an EIP increase mean airway and intrapleural pressures and can negatively affect cardiovascular performance (as described subsequently).

Just as alterations in the inspiratory phase can affect the patient, so too can the patient affect the inspiratory phase. As we have seen, flow patterns delivered by pressure generators can change with changes in the mechanical properties of the patient's lungs. Perhaps more important clinically is the fact that alterations in the mechanical properties of the patient's lungs can actually cause some flow generators to behave more like pressure generators.

As noted previously, the primary difference between a flow generator and a pressure generator is the amount of driving pressure used. In clinical practice, only a few ventilators produce the very high driving pressures necessary to be categorized as true flow generators. Examples of true flow generators are the Monaghan 225 Volume Ventilator, the Bourns Bear 2 and 5 (set to deliver a "square wave" flow pattern), the Puritan-Bennett 7200, the Hamilton Veolar, and the Ohio CPU 1.

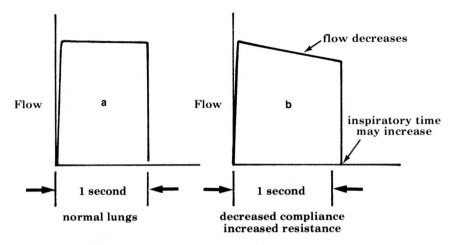

Fig. 29-14   The above inspiratory curves represent the changes in flow that can occur using a constant pressure generator with moderate generating pressures. Under normal conditions, flow is nearly constant (curve on left, *a*). As C_L decreases or Raw increases, the flow decreases slightly (curve on right, *b*). If the ventilator is volume limited, the volume will be delivered from the ventilator but inspiratory (*I*) time may increase (*b*), and this can affect the I:E ratio. (From Pilbeam SP: Mechanical ventilation: physiological and clinical applications, St Louis, 1986, The CV Mosby Co.)

From a practical viewpoint, however, many ventilators categorized as flow generators develop only moderate driving pressures. Such devices can and do maintain the same flow rate or flow pattern against low to moderate airway pressures. However, when these ventilators encounter high airway pressures, such as might occur with markedly decreased lung compliance or increased airway resistance, the difference between the generated and applied pressure drops substantially, causing a decrease in flow throughout inspiration. Under these conditions, flow generators that develop only moderate driving pressures behave more like pressure generators. As depicted in Fig. 29-14, this change in flow characteristics can increase the inspiratory time and thereby alter other time-dependent parameters of ventilation.[4,6]

Examples of ventilators that are characterized as flow generators, but whose flows can decrease at high airway pressures, are the Bennett MA-1 and MA-2, the Bourns Bear 1, and the Siemens 900 Series (at low working pressures).

Terminating inspiration

Various methods can be used to end the inspiratory phase, thereby starting expiration. The literature refers to these methods as either "cycling" or "limiting" mechanisms.[1,3,4,17] For consistency, we will use the term *cycle* to indicate the changeover from inspiration to expiration. A *limit,* on the other hand, will be applied here to indicate the maximum available value of a parameter, such as pressure or volume.

In general, one of four parameters can be used to cycle a positive pressure ventilator from the inspiratory into the expiratory phase: pressure, volume, flow, or time. Manual cycling is also available on the majority of modern ventilators. Although most ventilators end inspiration according to a single cycling mechanism, others combine two parameters simultaneously, such as flow and pressure.

Pressure cycling. A pressure-cycled device delivers gas under positive pressure during inspiration until an adjustable, preselected pressure has been reached.[1-3] When the preselected pressure is achieved, inspiration is ended, the machine cycles "off," and the expiratory phase begins. The volume and flow delivered by a pressure-cycled ventilator vary according to other ventilator and patient characteristics. Although pressure-cycled ventilators are most commonly used to administer IPPB therapy, they may also be applied for continuous ventilatory support under selected conditions.

Volume cycling. A volume-cycled ventilator provides gas under positive pressure during inspiration until an adjustable, preselected volume has been expelled from the device.[1-3] When the preselected volume is delivered out of the system, inspiration is ended, the machine cycles "off," and the expiratory phase begins. The pressure and flow delivered by a volume-cycled ventilator vary according to other ventilator and patient characteristics. Common examples of volume-cycled ventilators include the Bennett MA-1, MA-2, and 7200; the Bear 1, 2, and 5; and the Hamilton Veolar.

Time cycling. A time-cycled ventilator provides gas under positive pressure during inspiration for a preselected time interval.[1-3] When the preselected time interval elapses, inspiration ends, the machine cycles "off," and the expiratory phase begins. With time-cycled ventilators, inspiratory time is constant breath to breath. The pressure, volume, and flow delivered by a time-cycled ventilator may vary according to other ventilator and patient characteristics. Common examples of adult ventilators that are primarily time cycled are the Foregger 210 and the Veriflow CV 2000. Except for the Bourns LS104-150, essentially all infant ventilators in current use cycle to expiration by time.

Flow cycling. A flow-cycled ventilator provides gas under positive pressure during inspiration until flow drops down to a specified terminal level. When this specified low "terminal" flow time is reached, inspiration ends, the machine cycles "off," and the expiratory phase begins.

Flow cycling is the least common means used by positive pressure ventilators to end inspiration. Because of the unique design of their valve mechanism (see Chapter 26), the Bennett PR and AP series ventilators all cycle off when a low "terminal" flow rate is reached. However, the terminal or cycling flow is reached simultaneously with a preset pressure. Thus the pressure used to ventilate the patient is also the same each breath, and these ventilators are often considered to end inspiration using a combination of pressure and flow cycling.

More recently, flow cycling has been incorporated as the mechanism to end inspiration in some modes of pressure support ventilation (PSV).[18] PSV is a form of positive pressure ventilation similar to IPPB but applied during continuous ventilatory support. During the PSV mode, positive pressure is applied and maintained until the patient's inspiratory flow decreases to some minimal level. At this point, inspiration is terminated by opening of the exhalation valve. More detail on the application of PSV is provided in the following chapter.

Manual cycling. Some ventilators end the inspiratory phase only by a manually operated control. This method is commonly employed with some hand-held IPPB devices, such as the Ohio Hand-E-Vent and the Bird Asthmastik (see Chapter 26).[4]

Many positive pressure ventilators used for continuous ventilatory support also incorporate a manual cycling mechanism. This control, usually a simple button, allows the clinician to end inspiration at any time.

Combined cycling. Many ventilators end inspiration when two parameters are reached simultaneously. As just discussed, the Bennett PR and AP Series ventilators are combined pressure- and flow-cycling devices. The Emerson 3PV delivers a specified volume simultaneously with the end of a preset time interval and is therefore considered a combined volume- and time-cycling device. Such combined cycling mechanisms should not be confused with the application of an inspiratory limit.

The concept of inspiratory limits. As described earlier, we take limit to mean a parameter that has a maximum setting but does not necessarily end inspiration. As an example, some ventilators use a pressure relief valve, which opens and vents gases when a preset pressure is reached. Under such circumstances, inspiration may continue with the pressure held at the preset level until some cycling mechanism actually ends inspiration. This maneuver is often referred to as a "pressure hold" to distinguish it from the EIP "volume hold" previously described. In this case, the pressure is limited by the relief valve, but inspiration ends only when a volume- or time-cycling mechanism is activated. The Bourns LS104-150 infant ventilator is an example of a volume-cycled ventilator that incorporates a pressure-limiting relief valve. The Sechrist IV-100B and Bird Babybird are time-cycled ventilators using a pressure-limiting relief system.

An inspiratory limit may alternatively serve to actually end inspiration, but only as a backup or safety mechanism to normal cycling modes. For example, all modern volume-cycled ventilators incorporate a pressure-limiting mechanism. Normally, the pressure limit is set to a level above that required to deliver the preset volume. Should the pressure required to deliver the volume rise to the preselected limit, as might occur with a decrease in patient lung-thorax compliance or an increase in airway resistance, the ventilator would automatically cycle to end inspiration. Some ventilators, such as the Bear series, also can place an upper limit on the inspiratory time or inspiratory-expiratory time ratio. Such a safety mechanism serves to override volume cycling when the inspiratory time interval become dangerously long, as might occur at high airway pressures or with failure of a ventilator component.

In clinical practice, when an inspiratory limiting control is used to override a primary cycling mechanism, the parameters of ventilation that are normally in effect no longer apply. For example, if the primary cycling mechanism is volume, but a preset pressure limit is reached first, the selected volume will not be delivered. Likewise, the selected volume will not be delivered if a preset time limit is reached before volume cycling occurs.

Clinical importance of the cycling mechanism. The parameter used to cycle a positive pressure ventilator from the inspiratory into the expiratory phase is the primary basis for its categorization. The use of the cycling mechanism as the primary distinguishing feature among positive pressure ventilators is based on the critical importance of this characteristic in clinical practice. In this section we discuss some of the technical and clinical differences among the three primary cycling mechanisms, that is, volume cycling, pressure cycling, and time cycling to end inspiration.

Volume-cycled ventilation. Volume-cycled ventilation is the most commonly employed cycling mechanism for continuous ventilatory support of the critically ill. Many critically ill patients have rapidly changing compliance or airway resistance, and it has long been believed that volume ventilators can maintain more adequate ventilation despite these changes, especially when compared with pressure-cycled ventilators.[8,19-22]

Modern volume-cycled ventilators generally have substantial pressure available with which to deliver the set volumes, often exceeding 80 cm of water. With a volume-cycled ventilator, the volume delivered by the ventilator remains relatively constant, while the airway pressure varies according to the mechanical characteristics of the patient's lungs. For example, should compliance decrease or airway resistance increase, the pressure required to deliver the preset volume will increase. Only if the pressure developed exceeds an established limit will inspiration end or some of the volume be vented out of the circuit and lost.

It is critical to note that the cycling of a volume ventilator is based on the volume of gas expelled from the device itself and not necessarily that actually delivered to the patient. In reality, the volume of gas delivered into the patient's lung by a volume-cycled ventilator (and, for that matter, any positive pressure ventilator) is always less than that expelled from the machine.[4] This "loss" of volume is attributable to two factors. First, gases are compressed when delivered under positive pressure. Thus, the expelled volume (at atmospheric pressure) occupies less space when delivered at the airway under positive pressure. Second, the circuitry of most ventilators is somewhat flexible. Expansion of this flexible tubing during inspiratory positive pressure "robs" some of the volume that would otherwise go to the patient. In combination, these factors contribute to the compressed volume of the ventilator.

In general, compressed volume loss is critical only when delivered volumes are small, as in pediatric and high-frequency applications. Compressed volume loss must also be accounted for in certain monitoring functions, such as when performing bedside estimation of compliance and airway resistance. More detail on the calculation of compressed volume and its application in bedside monitoring is provided in Chapters 30 and 31.

An additional factor contributing to the difference between the volume delivered by a volume-cycled ventilator and that actually received by the patient is the presence of leaks in the patient-ventilator system. Because volume ventilators cycle off when a set volume has been expelled from the machine, the presence of a leak in the system will result in less of the expelled volume's actually reaching the patient's lungs. For this reason, volume-cycled ventilators are said to compensate poorly for leaks in the sys-

tem.[8] Because volume-cycled ventilators compensate poorly for system leaks, either low-exhaled-volume or low-inspiratory-pressure alarm systems should be incorporated into their design.[4]

From these examples we can see that a "volume ventilator" may not provide an absolute constant volume under all conditions. The physiologic changes that necessitate different pressures may also cause changes in gas distribution within the lung, as manifested by alterations in the $\dot{V}_A/\dot{Q}_C$ ratio. Because of these changes, even if a volume-cycled ventilator provided nearly the same overall ventilation against different pressure requirements, the resulting arterial blood gases could still vary. All these factors make it important to monitor exhaled volumes as well as physiologic parameters and to make ventilator adjustments accordingly, regardless of cycling mode.

Pressure-cycled ventilation. In contrast with volume-cycled ventilators, pressure-cycled ventilators terminate inspiration whenever their set pressure is reached, regardless of the volume delivered. Although the peak pressure remains relatively constant, the volume delivered by a pressure-cycled ventilator fluctuates with changes in the mechanical properties of the patient's lungs or thorax. Thus pressure-cycled ventilators are very susceptible to compliance and airway resistance changes.[8,21,22] Indeed, even if the patient simply begins to exhale actively or to become tense, the pressure will build abruptly and cycle inspiration prematurely.

However, when adequate supervision is provided by a qualified, knowledgeable practitioner, pressure-cycled ventilation can be successfully used with selected patients. Patients with normal lungs who require ventilatory support, such as those with a neurologic impairment to breathing or those being ventilated postoperatively for brief periods, can be successfully managed with pressure-cycled ventilation.

Most pressure-cycled ventilators, such as the Bird Mark 7 and Mark 8 and the Bennett PR-1 and PR-2, have both limited pressure (50 to 60 cm H_2O) and flow capabilities (80 to 100 L/min). Moreover, these devices typically do not include mechanisms to apply PEEP or CPAP.[4] Also, without special adaptation, oxygen concentrations with most pressure-cycled ventilators are variable and difficult to control. For these reasons, pressure-cycled ventilators are generally unsuitable for long-term use on patient with severe lung disease.

However, pressure-cycled ventilators generally are better able to compensate for leaks than are volume ventilators.[8] Of course, this situation pertains only when the leak is not large enough to prevent cycling altogether. Some models, such as the Bennett PR-2, have leak-compensating controls that add gas flow to compensate specifically for the presence of a leak.

Because these ventilators are compact and lightweight, they are sometimes used with transport systems, both in hospital as well as in ground or air transport. Since most pressure-cycled ventilators are also pneumatically powered (see Chapter 30), they may also be used to back up electrically powered volume ventilators in case of electrical failure. For these reasons, it is vital that the practitioners responsible for ventilatory support be thoroughly familiar with the function and application of pressure-cycled ventilators.

Time-cycled ventilation. Depending on the nature of the application, time-cycled ventilation can effectively mimic either volume or pressure cycling. Flow generators that are time cycled function essentially the same as a volume-cycled ventilator. This is because the product of a constant flow and a constant time yields a constant volume:

$$\dot{V} \ (L/s) \times time \ (s) = V \ (L)$$

If, on the other hand, a pressure limit that does not end inspiration is established during the timed inspiration, then both the flow and volume received by the patient may vary according to changes in patient compliance and airway resistance, as with true pressure-cycled ventilation. This ventilatory mode, called time-cycled, pressure-limited ventilation, is common in many pediatric applications.[4,23,24] More recently, this mode has been incorporated as an option on many newer-generation adult ventilators. In this configuration, the option is referred to as PSV.[18]

As applied in pediatric and neonatal ventilatory support, time-cycled, pressure-limited ventilation is commonly used with continuous flow-type ventilators. These devices deliver a set flow rate continuously through the patient's tubing circuit, allowing spontaneous breathing between controlled positive pressure breaths (intermittent mandatory ventilation [IMV]). Periodically, at preset time intervals, an exhalation valve is closed, and the continuous flow is diverted into the patient's airways. If the pressure limit is reached before the inspiratory time cycle is completed, then some or all of the flow vents to the atmosphere, and the pressure is maintained at the preset limit.

Under these circumstances, the volume the patient receives depends primarily on two factors: (1) the pressure applied and (2) the patient's lung-thorax compliance. As an example, if an infant has a compliance of 2 ml/cm of water and the pressure limit used is 20 cm of water, then the tidal volume (V_T) reaching the lung (assuming pressure equilibration occurs) will be 40 ml (2 × 20). If the same infant's compliance drops to 1 ml/cm of water, then the volume received from the same 20 cm of water of lung pressure will be only 20 ml. Because these small volumes are so difficult to measure, especially in a continuous flow system, this change in volume delivered

would not be indicated by the ventilator itself. Measurements such as arterial blood gases would have to be used instead.

The effect of time-cycled, pressure-limited ventilation on a patient with increased airway resistance depends on the time available for pressure equilibration. Delivered volume will not change if there is sufficient inspiratory time for the lung pressure to equilibrate with the pressure generated at the airway (pressure limit). However, if insufficient time is available for pressure equilibration, delivered volume will decrease with increased airway resistance. The length of time needed for pressure equilibration is longer if airway resistance is increased and shorter if it is decreased. Fig. 29-15 illustrates the fundamental features of time-cycled, pressure-limited ventilation under different patient conditions.

PSV incorporates the same basic concept, although the pressure limit is maintained by microprocessor control of system flow and not by a mechanical relief valve.[18] Moreover, some PSV systems, in addition to cycling by time, may also provide a means to cycle off when a low or terminal flow is reached. This type of PSV may be termed time- or flow-cycled, pressure-limited ventilation.

Regardless of whether applied to children or adults, V_T values provided by time-cycled, pressure-limited ventilation may be increased or decreased by changing the pressure limit. As with pressure-cycled ventilation, monitoring of arterial blood gases and clinical parameters is of utmost importance in this type of ventilation. Details on the application of pediatric ventilatory support and PSV are provided in subsequent chapters.

The nature of the expiratory phase

Regardless of the mechanism by which gas is delivered to the lungs during positive pressure ventilation, it must leave before the next inspiratory cycle begins. Exhalation normally occurs through the stored potential energy in the expanded lungs and thorax. In simple positive pressure ventilation, exhalation begins when the machine cycles to end inspiration. As the expiratory valve of the ventilator opens, P_{alv} becomes greater than airway pressure, gas moves unimpeded from alveoli to the atmosphere, and the lungs and thorax passively recoil down to their resting volume (FRC).

The expiratory phase of positive pressure ventilation need not be entirely passive. Modern mechanical ventilators allow the clinician to purposefully manipulate expiratory flow or pressure waveforms to achieve specific ends. The three most common alterations to the expiratory phase of positive pressure ventilation are (1) expiratory resistance or retard, (2) PEEP, and (3) negative end-expiratory pressure (NEEP).

Moreover, the clinician can also determine whether the

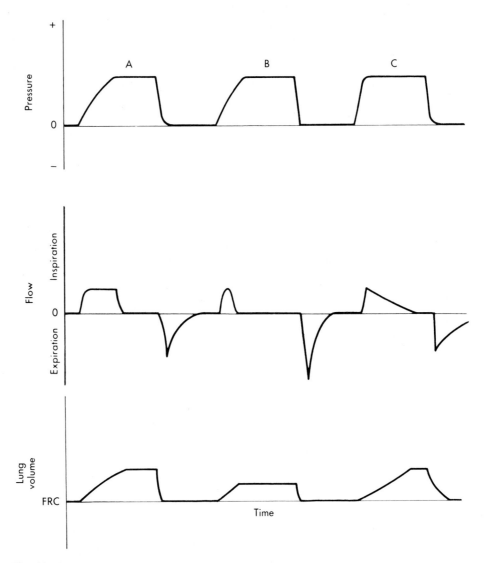

Fig. 29-15 Comparison of pressure, flow, and volume waveforms for time-cycled, pressure-limited ventilation with different patient conditions. *A* shows normal conditions while in *B* there is a decrease in C_L and *C* illustrates an increase in Raw. Inspiratory time is equal in *A, B,* and *C*. Note that *B* shows a decrease in volume due to a decrease in C_L. *C* shows the same volume as *A*, but more time is required during inspiration to reach that volume in the lung because of the increased Raw.

patient can breath spontaneously between mechanically provided breaths. Modes that allow the patient to breath spontaneously between positive pressure breaths are called intermittent mandatory ventilation (IMV).

As shown in Fig. 29-16, these combined capabilities provide four major alternatives for the clinician regarding control over the expiratory phase of positive pressure ventilation. Option 1, in which expiration is passive and spontaneous breathing is not allowed between mechanical breaths, is synonymous with simple continuous mechanical ventilation (CMV). Option 2 adds expiratory resistance, PEEP, or NEEP to CMV. Option 3, in which spontaneous

breathing is allowed between mechanical breaths, but expiration remains passive, represents simple IMV. Option 4 combines IMV with an alteration in expiratory waveform, most commonly PEEP.[25]

Allowing spontaneous breathing (IMV and synchronized intermittent mandatory ventilation [SIMV]). Intermittent mandatory ventilation allows the patient to breath spontaneously between controlled positive pressure breaths.[2,3,26,27] During IMV, some systems provide fresh gas by which spontaneous breathing can occur at a rate and volume that is patient determined. Fig. 29-17, *A*, depicts the airway pressure events occurring during IMV.

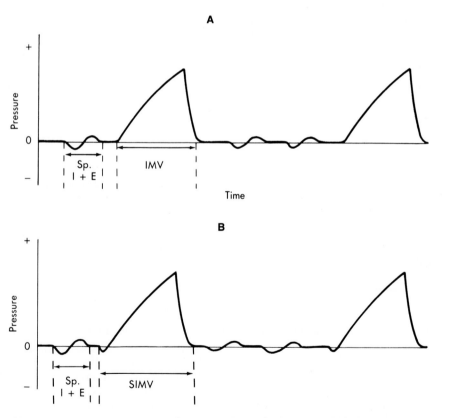

Spontaneous Breathing Allowed?

	No	Yes
No	*Option 1* <u>Example:</u> Simple CMV	*Option 3* <u>Example:</u> Simple IMV
Yes	*Option 2* <u>Example:</u> CMV with PEEP	*Option 4* <u>Example:</u> IMV with PEEP IMV with CPAP

Expiratory Waveform Altered?

Fig. 29-16   Options in manipulating the expiratory phase of positive pressure ventilation.

A

Pressure

Time

Sp. I + E   IMV

B

Pressure

Sp. I + E   SIMV

Fig. 29-17   Pressure waveforms for IMV and SIMV. Spontaneous inspiration and expiration *(Sp. I + E)* are shown combined with pressurized (IMV) breaths. **A** shows the IMV breaths occurring like control mode breaths while **B** shows IMV breaths triggered by patient (SIMV).

Table 29-1 compares the physiologic effects of IMV with traditional CMV.

IMV has been used both as a weaning methods and as a primary mode for ventilatory support in infants and adults for the past decade.[26] Not all patients are candidates for IMV, and although it has become a useful adjunct in ventilatory support, many of its purported advantages are yet to be studied in a controlled fashion.[28,29]

IMV allows (or requires) the patient to provide some of the work of breathing during ventilatory support. When the patient can provide more work, the ventilator's control rate is decreased accordingly. This allows for smooth transitions during ventilatory support and may also decrease the mean P_{pl} compared with simple CMV.[26,27,29] IMV is also useful when it is combined with expiratory pressure maneuvers, which are described subsequently. Most newer-generation ventilators incorporate a system for application of the IMV mode[4]; for ventilators not equipped with an IMV mechanism, special circuits can be added.[26]

SIMV represents a technical adaptation of IMV. Compared with true IMV, in which the periodic mechanical breaths are purely time cycled (control mode), SIMV can synchronize the machine-provided breaths to coincide with the patient's inspiratory effort, as with assisted ventilation (Fig. 29-17, B). Other terms used by manufacturers and authors to describe this same mode are intermittent demand ventilation (IDV) and intermittent assisted ventilation (IAV).[2,4,30,31]

The real role of SIMV compared with IMV is yet to be determined, although theoretically it should prevent the "stacking" of a controlled breath on top of a spontaneous breath. With SIMV, there is some amount of delay time when a mandatory breath is to occur until the patient begins the next inspiratory effort. One study comparing IMV and SIMV failed to show any significant difference between the two modes when various hemodynamic parameters, blood gases, and the incidence of pulmonary barotrauma were compared.[32]

Manipulation of the expiratory phase. Manipulation of the expiratory phase of positive pressure ventilation may involve application of expiratory resistance, PEEP, or NEEP. The use of NEEP is primarily of historical interest and is included here for completeness only.

Expiratory resistance or retard. Resistance to expiration can be applied during positive pressure ventilation to slow the flow of exhaled gases from the patient. Expiratory resistance can be created in a mechanical ventilator circuit by adding a restricted orifice to the exhalation limb of the system. Such a device is often referred to as a *flow resistor.*[4]

Fig. 29-18 illustrates the effect of expiratory resistance on airway pressure during positive pressure ventilation. In concept, by creating high resistance to expiratory flow, this maneuver mimics the effect of pursed-lip breathing commonly observed in patients with chronic obstructive pulmonary disease (COPD), particularly emphysema. *Spontaneous* pursed-lip breathing has been shown to decrease expiratory flows, prolong exhalation, decrease ventilatory rates, increase V_T values, improve arterial oxygen and carbon dioxide tensions at rest, and reduce the oxygen ventilation equivalent.[33] Presumably, these effects are caused by pressure stabilization of the small airways, which prevents their collapse on exhalation (see Chapter 8).

In theory, the application of mechanical flow resistance during the expiratory phase of positive pressure ventilation should have a similar effect when applied to patients with small airways disease. However, the beneficial effects of mechanically applied expiratory resistance during CMV have never been conclusively demonstrated.[25] Moreover, the detrimental effects of expiratory resistance more than outweigh any potential benefits attributable to this maneuver.[25] Table 29-2 compares the beneficial and detrimental effects of expiratory resistance.

Unfortunately, some mechanical ventilation circuits create significant expiratory flow resistance. This phenome-

Table 29-1   Physiologic Effects of Continuous Mechanical Ventilation Versus Intermittent Mandatory Ventilation

Continuous mechanical ventilation	Intermittent mandatory ventilation
Spontaneous breathing prohibited	Spontaneous breathing allowed
Patient may (assist-control mode) or may not (control mode) determine rate of breathing	Above IMV rate patient controls rate and depth of breathing
Ventilator responsible for minute ventilation	Patient contributes to $\dot{V}_E$
Respiratory muscle use minimal	Patient must use respiratory muscles
Higher mean P_{pl} for given minute ventilation ($\dot{V}_E$)	Lower mean P_{pl} for given $\dot{V}_E$

Table 29-2   Physiologic Effects of Expiratory Resistance

Beneficial	Detrimental
Decreased expiratory flows	Increased mean P_{pl}
Prolonged expiratory times	Potential decrease in venous return
Prevention of airway closure?*	Potential decrease in cardiac output
Improved gas distribution?*	Increased likelihood of pulmonary barotrauma

*? indicates a questionable effect.

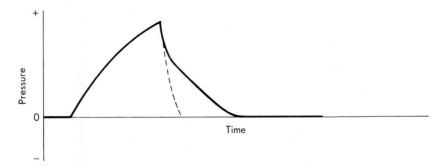

Fig. 29-18   Pressure waveform during CMV with expiratory resistance (retard) applied. (The dotted line represents the normal slope of the pressure drop from peak to baseline during expiration for comparison.)

non is a result of the sizes of various tubings and ports through which expiratory gases must flow. Since unnecessary expiratory flow resistance can increase the work of breathing, especially in IMV modes, efforts must be made to ensure that ventilatory circuits pose the least amount of resistance possible.

Positive end-expiratory pressure. The term PEEP is broadly used to denote the application and maintenance of pressure above atmospheric at the airway throughout the expiratory phase.[2] When combined with mechanically provided inspiratory positive pressure breaths, the terms CMV with PEEP, IPPV with PEEP, or continuous positive pressure ventilation (CPPV) are applied.[34,35] PEEP can also be added to the IMV mode of mechanical ventilation. This approach is referred to as either IMV with PEEP or IMV with CPAP.[26,27]

When pressure above atmospheric is maintained at the airway during both the inspiratory and expiratory phases of spontaneous breathing, the terms continuous positive-pressure breathing (CPPB)[36] or CPAP[37] are used. When positive pressure is applied only during the expiratory phase of spontaneous breathing, with inspiration occurring at or near atmospheric pressure, the terms spontaneous PEEP (sPEEP) or expiratory positive airway pressure (EPAP) have been used.[38-42]

Fig. 29-19 illustrates the various airway pressure waveforms created by a PEEP mechanism. In contrast to expiratory resistance, which employs a flow resistor to limit expiratory flows, true PEEP mechanisms are characterized as *threshold resistors.*[4,43] As shown in Fig. 29-20, a true threshold resistor maintains a given pressure level independent of flow. The box opposite lists the most common types of devices that provide threshold resistance. Most newer-generation positive pressure ventilators incorporate one of these approaches to provide PEEP or CPAP.[4] More detail on the design and use of these PEEP mechanisms is provided in Chapter 30.

PEEP is primarily used to increase FRC, decrease physiologic shunting, and increase the efficiency of oxygenation, thereby allowing for lower inspired oxygen concen-

trations (F_{IO_2}).[36,37,44-48] Other parameters such as the C_L and $\dot{V}_D/\dot{V}_T$ ratio may also be improved by using PEEP in some patients.[48] However, PEEP also can have detrimental effects on the patient. Table 29-3 summarizes the beneficial and detrimental effects of PEEP. More detail on these effects is provided in the subsequent section on the physiologic effects of positive pressure ventilation.

Up to 15 cm H_2O PEEP is commonly used, although some patients may require end expiratory pressures as high as 40 cm H_2O to maintain adequate oxygenation.[34,44-49] When infants are receiving PEEP or CPAP, 15 cm H_2O pressure or less is normally applied, although, as with adults, higher pressures have been used.[50] The clinical application of PEEP is discussed further in Chapters 30 and 31.

DEVICES USED TO GENERATE PEEP

Underwater columns
Spring-loaded diaphragms or disks
Balloon valves with preset internal pressures
Reverse Venturi devices
Electromechanical valves

Table 29-3   Physiologic Effects of Positive End-Expiratory Pressure

Beneficial	Detrimental
Increased FRC	Increased mean P_{pl}
Decreases CC/FRC ratio	Potential decrease in venous return
Decreased shunt fraction	Potential decrease in cardiac output
Increased C_L	Increased likelihood of pulmonary barotrauma
Increase Pa_{O_2} for given F_{IO_2}	Increased pulmonary vascular resistance

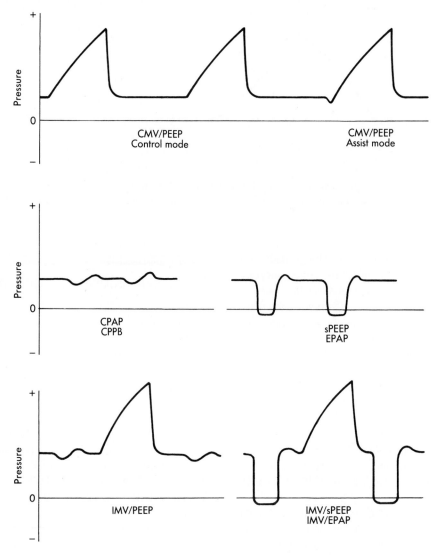

Fig. 29-19   Pressure waveforms for various forms of ventilatory support with end-expiratory pressure at a positive level. See text for description.

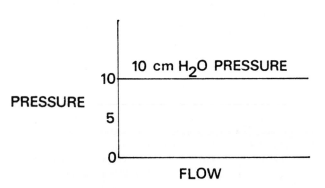

Fig. 29-20   Characteristics of a true threshold resistor.

Negative end-expiratory pressure. NEEP applies a sub-atmospheric pressure to the airway during the expiratory phase of positive pressure ventilation (Fig. 29-21). NEEP has also been referred to as "positive/negative pressure ventilation." In concept, NEEP was developed to overcome the detrimental cardiovascular effects of positive pressure ventilation. The assumption underlying NEEP was that the application of negative pressure during exhalation would counterbalance the impedance to venous return created by the positive pressure during inspiration.

Compared with positive pressure alone, application of NEEP does lower mean airway and pleural pressures and enhance venous return.[1] However, NEEP can also cause airway closure, decrease the FRC, and worsen $\dot{V}/\dot{Q}$ relationships.[1,25] Because other, safer approaches to minimizing the cardiovascular effects of positive pressure ventilation are available to the clinician, there is presently no in-

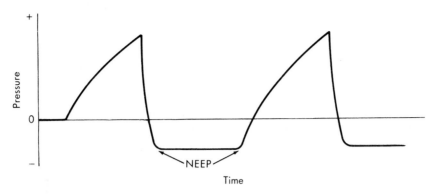

Fig. 29-21 Pressure waveform during CMV with NEEP added.

dication for the use of NEEP in the management of patients requiring continuous ventilatory support.

The application of negative pressure in a ventilator circuit during exhalation has been used in some pediatric ventilators, but not to lower airway pressure below zero. In these devices, the combination of high frequencies of breathing with small, high-resistance tubing often makes it impossible for airway pressure to return to zero during exhalation. The negative pressure mechanism is incorporated simply to assist in the evacuation of gases from the ventilator circuit and restore expiratory pressures to zero. In these cases, there is no intent to apply negative airway pressure to the airway.[25]

Inspiratory-expiratory time ratios

The relationship between the inspiratory and expiratory time provided during positive pressure ventilation is called the inspiratory-expiratory (I:E) time ratio. Although the increased use of IMV has diminished the importance of time variables in ventilatory support, the practitioner will still encounter situations in which adjustments in the time allocated for inspiration and expiration are critical.

In general, I:E time ratios are most important in the control and assist-control modes of CMV.[25] In these modes, the I:E ratio, combined with the frequency of positive pressure breaths, determines the net effect of positive pressure ventilation on both the efficiency of ventilation and the cardiovascular system. When inspiration is ended by volume or time cycling, both the inspiratory and expiratory time can and sometimes must be manipulated to achieve an acceptable balance between efficient ventilation and the least cardiovascular effect.

Table 29-4 summarizes the major terms, symbols, and formulas used in calculating the time variables that may be manipulated during the control and assist-control modes of mechanical ventilation. As previously noted, the frequency of positive pressure breaths exerts a substantial effect on gas distribution in lungs, especially under conditions of uneven time constants.[12] High rates, short inspiratory times, and low I:E ratios (such as 1:4 or 1:5) tend to

worsen gas distribution, while low rates, long inspiratory times, and high I:E ratios (such as 1:2 or 1:1) tend to enhance the distribution of gases within the lung. Unfortunately, those time patterns that enhance gas distribution and the efficiency of ventilation are most likely to exert a detrimental effect on the cardiovascular system. How one can achieve an acceptable balance between efficient ventilation and the least cardiovascular effect is discussed in the next section.

PHYSIOLOGIC EFFECTS OF POSITIVE PRESSURE VENTILATION

Positive pressure ventilatory support cannot be used either safely or effectively unless those responsible for it are proficient in its mechanics and knowledgeable of both its beneficial and detrimental physiologic effects. When artificially ventilating a patient, we deliberately attempt to change a physiologic condition, ideally from a poor to an

Table 29-4 Time Variables in Mechanical Ventilation

Term	Symbol	Formula for Calculation
Frequency (rate)	f	Count breaths/minute or $\dfrac{60}{t_I + t_E}$
Cycle time	$t_I + t_E$	Add $t_I + t_E$ or $\dfrac{60}{f}$
Inspiratory time	$t_I(I)$	$t_I = \dfrac{60}{f} - t_E$ or $t_I = \%t_I \times (t_I + t_E)$
Expiratory time	$t_E(E)$	$t_E = \dfrac{60}{f} - t_I$
Inspiratory-expiratory time ratio	I:E or $t_I{:}t_E$	$I{:}E = \dfrac{t_I}{t_E}$, usually numerator (t_I) expressed as 1
Percentage inspiratory time	$\%t_I$	$\%t_I = \dfrac{t_I}{t_I + t_E} \times 100$

improved status. Nonetheless, we are interfering with a level of function, even if that function is pathologic. It is therefore vital that respiratory care practitioners be fully knowledgeable of not only the objectives of treatment, but also the effect of intervention on the body as a whole, including its unwanted to adverse consequences.

Generally, the effects of positive pressure ventilation are most apparent as they apply to the lung itself and to the circulatory and renal systems. Effects of positive pressure ventilation on other elements of physiologic function are evident, although less pronounced.

Pulmonary effects of positive pressure ventilation

The beneficial effects of positive pressure ventilation on the lungs provide the basis for its clinical use. Detrimental effects, on the other hand, represent the potentially harmful consequences of applying this mode of support to a critically ill patient. Obviously, when positive pressure ventilation is indicated, it must never be withheld from a patient. However, knowledge of the detrimental effects of positive pressure ventilation must be incorporated into the clinical decision-making process. Moreover, once positive pressure ventilation is instituted, the clinician must continuously be on guard for the many potentially harmful consequences of this mode of ventilatory support.

Beneficial effects. Properly applied positive pressure ventilation can maintain or improve alveolar ventilation, help restore normal acid-base balance, and reduce a patient's work of breathing. Further, when used in conjunction with oxygen and supplementary manipulation of expiratory pressures, positive pressure ventilation can assist the clinician in normalizing or improving oxygenation. Of course, these beneficial effects can be realized only when consideration is given to establishing appropriate parameters of ventilation, as described in detail in the following chapter.

The relationship between improved alveolar ventilation and the correction of abnormal acid-base balance is apparent, and in these areas positive pressure ventilation performs some of its most important functions. More effective alveolar ventilation is evidenced by a decrease in arterial blood carbon dioxide tension and an elevation of arterial blood pH.

Positive pressure ventilation can also significantly reduce the work energy expended by patients with actual or impending respiratory muscle fatigue.[51] The respiratory care practitioner will frequently see the gratifying physical relaxation enjoyed by patients as a mechanical ventilator assumes a major portion of their work of breathing.

Obviously, to lessen the work of breathing, ventilation must be sufficient to meet the patient's needs. Otherwise, the spontaneously breathing patient will tend to "fight" the ventilator. Early studies demonstrated that inappropriately applied positive pressure ventilation actually resulted in alveolar hypoventilation and, as a result of patient struggling, an increase in the work of breathing of as much as 250%.[52]

In terms of improving oxygenation, early studies on the effects of simple positive pressure breathing demonstrated an elevation in arterial blood oxygen tension, even with ambient air as the source gas.[53,54] Although these findings were taken as evidence of an increased uniformity of alveolar ventilation and an improved $\dot{V}A/\dot{Q}c$ ratio, more recent analysis suggests that this is not the case. More likely, the improved oxygenation observed in these early studies was probably the result of increased alveolar ventilation or decreased work of breathing. Indeed, as discussed in the next section, positive pressure ventilation can actually worsen the $\dot{V}A/\dot{Q}c$ ratio!

On the other hand, when PEEP (with CMV or IMV or as simple CPAP) is applied to patients with refractory hypoxemia due to a decreased FRC and physiologic shunting, dramatic improvements in oxygenation can occur. This is attributable to the recruitment of collapsed alveoli and their associated capillary beds, resulting in a decrease in the portion of pulmonary blood flow perfusing unventilated alveoli, that is, a decrease in alveolar shunting.

Detrimental effects. Positive pressure ventilation represents an abnormal means of moving gas into and out of the lungs. As such, we should expect application of this mode of support to have detrimental effects on the respiratory system. The potentially harmful pulmonary consequences of positive pressure ventilation include alteration in $\dot{V}/\dot{Q}$ ratios, hyperventilation and respiratory alkalosis, pulmonary barotrauma, atelectasis, air trapping, and an increased work of breathing.[6] Other pulmonary problems not directly associated with positive pressure ventilation per se include airway complications (see Chapter 21), the detrimental effects of oxygen (see Chapter 25), and nosocomial pulmonary infections (see Chapter 14).

Ventilation-perfusion imbalances. Early studies with COPD patients reported increases in the alveolar-arterial oxygen tension gradient $P(A-a)O_2$ during positive pressure breathing.[51] These findings suggested that the inspired gas was not being normally distributed throughout the lung.

The early notion that positive pressure ventilation might alter the distribution of gases in the lungs has subsequently been confirmed with healthy subjects. The reasons for this alteration in gas distribution are apparent when one compares spontaneous ventilation with positive pressure breathing.

As discussed in Chapter 8, spontaneous ventilation results in gas distribution mainly to the dependent and peripheral zones of the lungs. Application of positive pressure ventilation, on the other hand, tends to reverse this normal pattern of gas distribution, directing the majority of delivered volume to nondependent and central or peribronchial lung zones.[6] This phenomenon is partly a result of the inactivity of the diaphragm and chest wall. Whereas in spontaneous breathing these structures actively facilitate gas movement, their inactivity during positive pressure ventilation impedes ventilation to the dependent and peripheral lung zones.[55,56]

An increase in ventilation to the nondependent zones of the lung, where there is proportionately less perfusion, will tend to increase the $\dot{V}_A/\dot{Q}_C$ ratio, effectively increasing the physiologic deadspace and V_D/V_T. Indeed, positive pressure ventilation can increase the physiologic deadspace by this mechanism.[57] However, the increase in $P(A-a)_{O_2}$ gradient that is sometimes observed with positive pressure ventilation must be caused by a lower than normal $\dot{V}_A/\dot{Q}_C$ ratio in some portions of the lung.

Positive pressure ventilation lowers the $\dot{V}_A/\dot{Q}_C$ ratio in portions of the lung mainly by its effect on the pulmonary circulation. Positive pressure ventilation can compress the capillaries in the respiratory zones of the lung, thereby increasing pulmonary vascular resistance and decreasing perfusion volume.[58] Since this effect is in proportion to the pressure applied, the least blood flow will go to the areas with the greatest positive pressure, contributing to a further increase in physiologic dead space. Conversely, blood from these areas will be diverted to regions with lower vascular resistance, that is, those receiving the least pressure and ventilation. Thus the majority of pulmonary blood flow during positive pressure ventilation tends to perfuse the least well-ventilated lung regions, thereby lowering the $\dot{V}_A/\dot{Q}_C$ ratio in these areas and increasing the $P(A-a)_{O_2}$ gradient.[59]

A good clinical example of the effect of positive pressure ventilation on $\dot{V}/\dot{Q}$ relationships are the changes that can occur in oxygenation of patients with a unilateral lung disease as their positions are shifted. In most cases, oxygenation is significantly better when the affected lung is maintained in the superior position.[6] This phenomenon is explained in part by the fact that ventilation under positive pressure is preferentially distributed to the nondependent areas, in this case, the superior lung.

Hyperventilation and respiratory alkalosis. As with IPPB therapy (see Chapter 26), positive pressure ventilation, particularly in the assist-control mode, can result in hyperventilation, a decreased Pa_{CO_2} and respiratory alkalosis.[56,60,61] As described in Chapter 9, a high pH (alkalosis) impairs oxygen unloading at the tissue level. Moreover, a high pH can cause hypokalemia. Hypokalemia can disturb electrical conduction in both the heart and skeletal muscles, resulting in cardiac arrhythmias or tetany. Low Pa_{CO_2} levels also cause cerebral vasoconstriction, which, if severe, can impair perfusion of the brain.

For these reasons, mechanical hyperventilation generally should be avoided. Exceptions to this rule are conditions in which the physician desires to decrease cerebral perfusion pressures, such as may occur with cerebral trauma, or when temporary depression of the respiratory drive is indicated, as when a patient is "fighting" the ventilator. In the latter case, pharmacologic intervention is preferable, and hyperventilation should be applied only until appropriate pharmacologic intervention can be initiated (see Chapter 30).

Pulmonary barotrauma. Pulmonary barotrauma is the rupture of lung tissue by excessive positive pressure. Rupture of lung tissue manifests itself clinically in a variety of conditions, including pneumothorax, pneumomediastinum, pneumoperitoneum, and subcutaneous emphysema (Fig. 29-22).[61,62]

Generally, the incidence of pulmonary barotrauma in patients with normal lungs being ventilated with positive pressure is low. Studies in animals indicate that frank damage to lung tissue is unlikely at pressures below 80 cm H_2O.[6] However, patients with unstable lung tissue, such as occurs with bullous emphysema, are more prone to pulmonary barotrauma than those with normal lungs. Moreover, high levels of PEEP increase the incidence of pulmonary barotrauma.[63]

Atelectasis. As shown in Fig. 29-23, prolonged positive pressure ventilation with unvarying V_T values less than 10 ml/kg can result in a gradual and progressive atelectasis.[64] This progressive atelectasis manifests itself in an increase in the proportion of pulmonary blood flow perfusing unventilated alveoli (alveolar shunting) and an increase in the $P(A-a)_{O_2}$ gradient. This detrimental effect of positive pressure ventilation is easily addressed by the use of periodic sighs or V_T values in the range of 12 to 15 ml/kg.

Air trapping. Air trapping represents the incomplete emptying of lung units. As described in Chapter 8, lung units prone to trapping air are those with long time constants, that is, high airway resistance or high compliance. Since both of these conditions apply in patients with pulmonary emphysema, the possibility of air trapping with positive pressure ventilation is highest in this group. Air trapping can increase P_{alv}, thereby impeding pulmonary blood flow and increasing the possibility of pulmonary barotrauma.[6]

Air trapping during positive pressure ventilation tends to occur only when insufficient time is allowed for exhalation.[65] Although an I:E ratio of 1:2 is generally sufficient to ensure complete exhalation in patients with normal lungs, ratios of 1:4 or less may be required in some patients with severe COPD. Unfortunately, achieving these low ratios can require very short inspiratory times. As we have seen, short inspiratory times with high inspiratory flows tend to promote further maldistribution of inspired gas in lungs with uneven time constants.

Increased work of breathing. As just described under beneficial effects, properly applied positive pressure ventilation can decrease the work of breathing in patients with disorders characterized by low compliance of the lungs or thorax or high airway resistance. This beneficial effect, however, is limited to modes of support in which the ventilator does essentially all the work, as in the control or assist-control modes. When the patient is allowed to

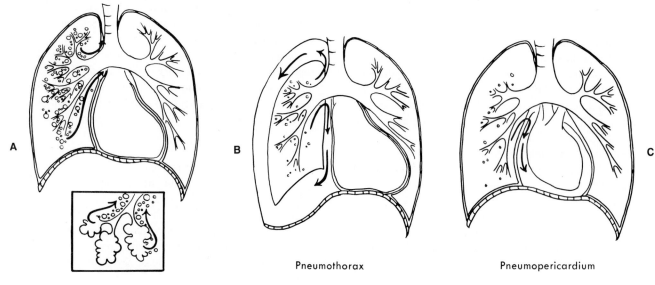

Interstitial emphysema

Pneumothorax

Pneumopericardium

Fig. 29-22 **A,** Pulmonary barotrauma. Ruptured alveoli are indicated in framed alveoli at bottom. Air dissects from alveoli along vascular sheaths to hilus and thence to pleural space. **B,** Pneumothorax, indicating origin of air in lung tissue and its pathway to inflate pleural space. Heart shifts to left because of high pressure created in right chest. **C,** Course of air from lung to pericardial space. Distended pericardial space causes cardiac tamponade, small heart. (From Korones SB: High-risk newborn infants, ed 4, St Louis, 1986, The CV Mosby Co.)

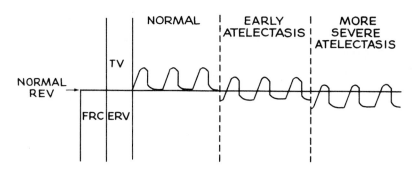

Fig. 29-23 Effect of progressive alveolar collapse on FRC due to ventilation at constant, small volumes. (From Sanderson RG: The cardiac patient: a comprehensive approach, ed 2, Philadelphia, 1983, WB Saunders Co.)

breathe spontaneously, as with IMV or CPAP, it is possible to increase the patient's work of breathing.[56]

This seeming paradoxical effect is due mainly to shortcomings in existing equipment function. Increased inspiratory work is necessary in many IMV or CPAP circuits due to the high resistance to gas flow through some humidifiers and the slow response time of some demand valve systems.[66-68] Increased expiratory work is attributed mainly to high-resistance expiratory valves.[69] The problem of adding to the patient's work of breathing by applying a IMV or CPAP system can be avoided by using a continuous high flow of gas through a circuit with minimal flow resistance.[56] More recently, some clinicians recommend applying PSV to "unload" the respiratory muscles from the

work of breathing during IMV or CPAP.[18] More detail on the theory and application of PSV is provided in Chapters 30 and 31.

Cardiovascular effects of positive pressure ventilation

With the close functional relationship between the respiratory and circulatory systems, it is not surprising that interference with the performance of one will affect the other. The great potential hazard of a detrimental circulatory response to positive pressure ventilation makes it mandatory for the practitioner to understand fully what does and can happen to cardiovascular function when a patient is artificially ventilated.

Early studies on the effect of positive pressure ventila-

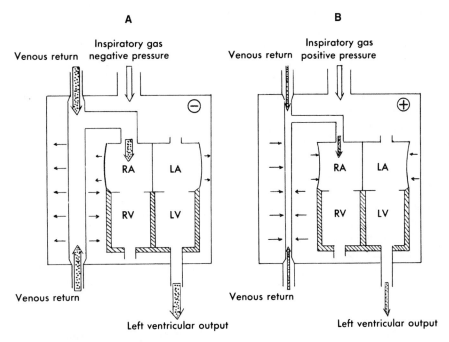

Fig. 29-24   Relationship between P_{pl} and cardiac output in, **A**, spontaneous and, **B**, positive pressure breathing. (Details are explained in the text.)

tion on the cardiovascular system all demonstrated an early, small, and transient increase in cardiac output, followed almost immediately by a significant reduction in left ventricular outflow.[70-73] In general, the reduction in cardiac output observed in these cases was directly related to the magnitude of the pressure applied, more specifically, the rise in P_{pl} that occurred with application of pressure to the airway.[74-76]

Spontaneous versus positive pressure ventilation. Fig. 29-24 graphically compares the effects of a spontaneous (negative pressure) inspiration with that observed during positive pressure ventilation. Normally (see Fig. 29-24, *A*), increasingly negative P_{pl} values during inspiration enhance venous return, increase right atrial filling, and improve pulmonary blood flow. Combined, these factors enhance left atrial and left ventricular filling, thereby increasing left ventricular stroke volume.

When the lung is ventilated under positive pressure, P_{pl} can become positive (Fig. 29-24, *B*). Positive P_{pl} compresses the intrathoracic veins, thereby raising the central venous and right atrial filling pressures. As these pressures rise, venous flow back to the heart is impeded, and right ventricular preload and stroke volume decrease, as does the pulmonary blood flow. Initially, blood already in the pulmonary circulation is displaced into the left heart, causing a transient increase in its filling pressure and output. However, this initial effect lasts for but a few heart strokes, and, if the positive pressure is continued, flow both to and from the left heart falls.

Moreover, the high impedance encountered by blood returning to the right heart causes venous pooling, mainly in

the capacitance vessels of abdominal viscera.[73] This effect effectively removes from the circulation a volume of blood large enough to further reduce the left ventricular output and constitutes a serious potential danger to the patient.

The venous impedance caused by positive pressure ventilation is not limited to return flow coming from the abdomen. An increase in the central venous pressure can also restrict return flow from the brain. Impedance to venous return from the brain can increase the intracranial pressure (ICP), thereby potentially reducing cranial perfusion pressures. Combined with a fall in left ventricular output, an increase in ICP during positive pressure ventilation can significantly impair cerebral perfusion and potentially cause cerebral ischemia and tissue hypoxia.

In healthy subjects, the effects of positive pressure ventilation on cerebral blood flow are minimized by autoregulatory mechanisms that maintain cranial perfusion pressures within a narrow range. However, patients with preexisting cerebrovascular problems, and those already exhibiting an elevation in ICP, may be at risk for decreased cerebral perfusion with CMV, CMV with PEEP, and CPAP. Examples include neurosurgical patients and those with head injuries, intracranial tumors, or cerebral edema of any cause. In these patients, ICP monitoring may be necessary.[6]

Factors affecting the cardiovascular impact. The magnitude of the deleterious effect of positive pressure ventilation on the circulatory system depends on two major factors: (1) the subject's cardiovascular status and (2) the resulting mean P_{pl}.

Cardiovascular status. In terms of cardiovascular status, the effects of moderate elevations in P_{pl} on cardiac output in healthy subjects are minimal. In healthy subjects, as left ventricular stroke volume decreases, compensatory responses increase both the cardiac rate and the tone of the capacitance vessels of the venous system (see Chapter 7). These normal responses ensure maintenance of blood flow and perfusion pressures sufficient to meet body needs.

However, should the subject have compromised cardiac function, already be hypovolemic, or have lost peripheral venomotor tone, cardiovascular compensation may be impossible. In these cases, even a small rise in P_{pl} may result in a precipitous fall in cardiac output.

Mean intrapleural and airway pressures. For a given cardiovascular status, the effects of positive pressure ventilation are also directly related to the mean or average P_{pl}. Since in clinical practice the direct measurement of P_{pl} is difficult, we commonly use the mean airway pressure as our gauge of the potential cardiovascular impact of positive pressure ventilation. Although the airway pressure is not quantitatively the same as the P_{pl}, the mean values of both are linearly related and thus can be used interchangeably to monitor qualitative changes.

The concept of a mean or average pressure is essential to understanding the cardiovascular impact of positive pressure ventilation. As an example of this concept, Fig. 29-25 plots a biphasic positive and negative pressure curve against arbitrary time units. Initially, pressure rises from its starting point to a peak pressure of 20, dropping back to zero during the first five time units. For the last five time units, a negative pressure of the same magnitude—but opposite direction—is applied.

The mean of any parameter plotted on a curve is proportional to the area "under" the curve. In this case, the area under the curve is described by the product of pressure (y-axis) times time (x-axis):

$$\text{Mean pressure} \cong \text{Pressure} \times \text{time}$$

If the pressure pattern in Fig. 29-25 was a true square or constant pressure wave, calculation of the mean pressure would be simply a matter of multiplying the height of the curve (pressure) times its width (time). However, since the pressure waveform in Fig. 29-25 is variable, the area under the curve must be calculated by summing an infinite number of points along the curve (a, b, c, d, etc, in Fig. 29-25). In theory, the calculation of the area under a variable curve is accomplished using integral calculus. In practice, these calculations are performed by a microprocessor incorporated into the electronic circuitry of the device used to monitor the applied pressure.

Even without using calculus, it is obvious in our illustration that the mean pressure of the terminal half of the curve is the same as that of the first but with the opposite sign. Common sense tells us that these two opposing pressures curves will counterbalance each other, yielding an average or mean pressure of zero.

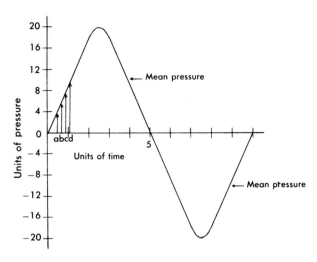

Fig. 29-25   Illustrations of the concept of mean pressure and the relationship between pressure and time.

Factors affecting mean intrapleural pressure. The mean P_{pl} is affected by many variables, the most important of which are summarized in the box below.[25] We will discuss each of the key variables in terms of their potential impact on a patient's cardiovascular status.

In regard to the magnitude of pressure applied, Fig. 29-26 portrays five inspiratory pressure waveforms of equal time, all generated by a constant flow ventilator. With all else being equal, the one with the greatest area will exert the greatest cardiovascular effect. Clearly, waveform E in Fig. 29-26 has the greatest area and would comparatively exert the greatest cardiovascular effect.

Obviously, the nature of the inspiratory waveform will also affect the mean airway and intrapleural pressures. The three curves in Fig. 29-27 illustrate this point. All three curves are applied for the same time interval. Curve A, characteristic of a constant pressure generator (or time-cycled, pressure-limited ventilation), clearly has the greatest area and would therefore tend to exert the greatest cardiovascular effect. On the other hand, curves B and C depict the pressure waveforms of a nonconstant and constant flow generator, respectively. Both have less area than curve A

**FACTORS AFFECTING MEAN
INTRAPLEURAL PRESSURE**

Magnitude of applied positive pressure
Nature of inspiratory waveform
Duration of positive pressure
Duration of expiratory phase
Nature of expiratory phase
Mechanical properties of lungs and thorax

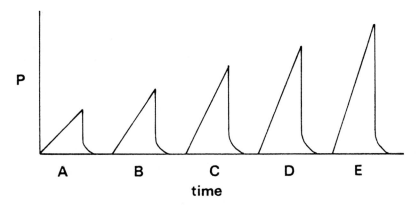

Fig. 29-26   Effect of changes in peak pressure on mean airway pressure.

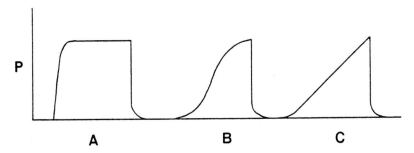

Fig. 29-27   Effect of inspiratory waveform on mean airway pressure.

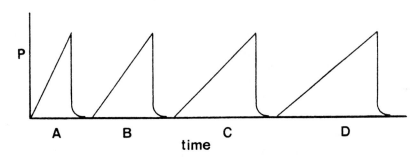

Fig. 29-28   Effect of inspiratory time on mean airway pressure.

and would consequently tend to exert less cardiovascular effect.

Without varying the peak pressure or inspiratory waveform, changes in the duration of inspiration will affect mean P_{pl} and thus the magnitude of cardiovascular effect. In Fig. 29-28, four inspiratory pressure curves are shown, all with the same peak pressure, but with progressively increasing inspiratory times. Clearly, curve D has the greatest area and therefore the greatest potential to affect cardiac output negatively. Moreover, to the extent that a longer inspiration shortens the time available for expiration, less time will be available for P_{pl} to return toward normal, further aggravating the cardiovascular effect.

Conversely, the greater the duration of expiration, the

more time will be available for P_{pl} to return toward normal. Thus, for a constant rate of breathing, longer expiratory times are associated with a lesser cardiovascular effect. In general, the detrimental cardiovascular effects of positive pressure ventilation are most likely when the time available for expiration is less than twice that provided for inspiration, that is, when the I:E ratio is greater than 1:2.[70]

Of course, this relationship applies only when ventilation is provided in the assist-control or control mode and the expiratory phase is passive. Purposeful manipulation of the expiratory phase can be expected to affect cardiovascular performance. In general, IMV modes minimize the cardiovascular effects of positive pressure ventilation,

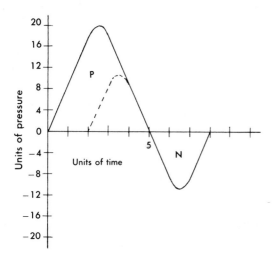

Fig. 29-29 Effect of spontaneous breathing (IMV) on mean airway pressure.

whereas PEEP increases the potential for a deleterious circulatory effect.

When the patient is allowed to breath spontaneously during the expiratory phase, as with IMV, the negative P_{pl} developed during inspiration offset some or all of the positive pressure generated during the mechanical phase of breathing.[26,27]

This phenomenon is illustrated in Fig. 29-29. The positive pressure segment P represents the inspiratory airway pressure curve generated by a positive pressure ventilator over a five-unit time period. The mean inspiratory pressure is thus equivalent to the area under curve P. The negative pressure segment N represents the subatmospheric pressure generated by a spontaneous inspiration, as during IMV. The net circulatory effect of the pressure over the entire cycle will be proportional to the difference between the areas P and N, graphically shown by superimposing N on P, with the dotted outline. Thus the mean airway pressure for the whole ventilatory cycle has been lowered by adding a subatmospheric component, in this case due to a spontaneous breath.

Of course, PEEP will have exactly the opposite effect.[77,78] Since PEEP elevates the expiratory pressure baseline above atmospheric, the beneficial effects that would otherwise occur with passive expiration at atmospheric pressure are lost. However, since PEEP is generally applied to patients with pathologic conditions characterized by low lung compliance, less of the positive airway pressure is transmitted to the pleural space than would be the case with normal lungs. This is because of the relationship between P_{pl} and the mechanical properties of the patient's lungs and thorax.

Positive pressure generated by a ventilator eventually reaches the alveoli, where it is transmitted across alveolar walls to the pleural space and thoracic cavity. How much of this alveolar pressure is actually transmitted to the pleu-

ral space depends on the mechanical properties of the patient's lungs and thorax.

In general, for a given alveolar pressure, the more compliant the lung, the greater will be the increase in P_{pl}. Thus, a patient with a disease process causing a loss of elastic tissue, such as occurs in pulmonary emphysema, will be more subject to the cardiovascular effects of a given level of positive pressure than an individual with healthy lungs.

In contrast, a lung with low compliance will transmit less of the alveolar pressure to the pleural space. This explains, in part, why high levels of PEEP may often be used with minimal cardiovascular effects on patients with pathologic conditions characterized by low lung compliance (the cardiovascular effect of high PEEP levels can also be minimized by combining PEEP with IMV).

On the other hand, when the compliance of the chest wall (rather than the lung) is reduced, expansion of the thorax is limited, and more of the alveolar pressure will be transmitted to the pleural space. Therefore, patients who have healthy lungs but suffer from conditions restricting thoracic expansion (such as kyphoscoliosis and spondylitis) will be more subject to the cardiovascular effects of a given level of positive pressure than will individuals with normal thoracic compliance. However, a similar effect can occur in patients with normal thoracic compliance who actively oppose a positive pressure inspiration by contracting their expiratory muscles (as might occur when a patient "fights" a ventilator). Contraction of the expiratory muscles effectively lowers the thoracic cage compliance, also causing more of the alveolar pressure to be transmitted to the pleural space.

Finally, if airway resistance is high, less of the pressure generated at the airway will actually reach the alveoli. Thus the high airway pressures common in patients with obstructive disorders are not necessarily reflected in high pleural pressures.

Renal effects of positive pressure ventilation

It has long been known that many patients receiving long-term positive pressure ventilatory support exhibit significant salt and water retention, as manifested by either a weight gain or failure to lose weight as anticipated. In addition, such patients typically show a reduction in hematocrit, consistent with hypervolemia caused by water retention.[79,80] These early observations are now attributed to both the direct and indirect effect of positive pressure ventilation on renal function.

In terms of its direct effect, positive pressure ventilation can reduce urinary output by as much as 50%.[80,81] This phenomenon has been attributed to a reduction in renal blood flow and glomerular filtration rates, caused by a decrease in cardiac output. Reductions in mean arterial blood pressure below 75 mm Hg reduce renal blood flow, glomerular filtration rates, and urinary output. However, mean arterial pressures this low are seldom caused by positive pressure ventilation alone, and autoregulatory mechanisms within the kidney are generally able to maintain renal perfusion pressures within normal limits over a wide range of mean arterial pressures. Moreover, since restoring cardiac output to normal does not entirely restore urinary output compromised by positive pressure ventilation, other mechanisms must be involved.[6]

Recent evidence suggests that the decreased urinary output common with positive pressure ventilation is not caused by a reduction in renal blood flow per se but rather to a redistribution of blood flow within the kidney.[82] During positive pressure ventilation (especially with PEEP), blood flow to juxtamedullary nephrons increases, while flow to the cortical nephrons decreases.[83] Because the juxtamedullary nephrons are more efficient at sodium reabsorption than their cortical counterparts, this shift in the distribution of blood flow increases both sodium and water reabsorption. Exactly why positive pressure ventilation causes a redistribution of blood flow within the kidney is unknown; however, an increase in renal sympathetic tone or the release of humoral agents such as catecholamines, vasopressin, or angiotensin are possible explanations.[6]

The indirect impact of positive pressure ventilation on renal function is believed to occur through humoral mechanisms, specifically by an increase in the release of antidiuretic hormone (ADH), also called vasopressin. ADH is a hormone secreted by the posterior pituitary gland that inhibits urine excretion, thereby increasing water retention.

Experimental evidence indicates that a decrease in blood pressure increases ADH secretion by stimulating the left atrial stretch receptors, which innervate the posterior pituitary. Since an increase in the pressure surrounding the atria is comparable to the decrease in internal pressure that occurs with hypotension, positive pressure ventilation causes a similar stimulation of these stretch receptors and a similar increase in ADH secretion.[80,83-85] As might be assumed, negative pressure ventilation has exactly the opposite effect, causing diuresis rather than water retention.[86]

For these reasons, it is clear that the management of the patient receiving long-term positive pressure ventilatory support must include close attention to maintaining a safe balance between fluid intake and output.

Other effects of positive pressure ventilation

Related to its effects on the cardiovascular system is the effect of positive pressure ventilation on the liver and gastrointestinal system. Hepatic dysfunction with positive pressure ventilation can occur in patients with otherwise normal livers and is manifested by an increase in serum bilirubin levels.[83] This may be a result of a decrease in portal venous flow associated with mechanical compression of the liver, a direct increase in resistance to splanchnic blood flow, or simple vascular engorgement. Regardless of cause, these effects are aggravated by PEEP.

An increase in splanchnic resistance may also contribute to gastric mucosal ischemia and help explain the high incidence of gastrointestinal bleeding and stress ulceration in patients receiving long-term positive pressure ventilation.[83]

ALTERNATIVES TO TRADITIONAL POSITIVE PRESSURE VENTILATION

Given the number and potential seriousness of problems associated with positive pressure ventilation, it is not surprising that clinicians have sought to develop and apply alternative approaches to ventilatory support. Negative pressure ventilation actually preceded ventilation by positive pressure as a method of managing respiratory failure. More recently, experimentation with positive pressure ventilation at high frequencies has led some to suggest this mode as a viable alternative to traditional CMV.

Negative pressure ventilation

Classically, negative pressure ventilation was provided by the body tank ventilator, commonly known as the "iron lung." First described in 1929, the tank ventilator saw widespread, lifesaving use through many poliomyelitis epidemics.[87] The body tank ventilator is an airtight cylinder that accommodates the patient up to the neck, leaving the head exposed to atmosphere. At the opposite end, or underneath the tank, is a large electrically powered bellows or diaphragm, equipped with a handle for manual operation in the event of electric failure. Expansion of the bellows creates a negative pressure within the cylinder proportional to its displacement.

This negative pressure is applied to the body surface and transmitted first to the pleural space and then to the alveoli. Since the airway during negative pressure ventilation remains exposed to atmospheric pressure ($P_{ao} = 0$), a transrespiratory pressure gradient comparable to that generated during a spontaneous inspiration is created. Therefore, gas will flow from the area of relatively high pressure (the airway opening) to the area of relatively low pressure (the alveoli).

Unlike spontaneous breathing, in which negative pressure is transmitted only to the pleural space, the negative pressure generated in the cylinder is transmitted to the whole body (except for the head and neck). Since the abdomen tends to be more compliant than the chest wall, a disproportionate amount of negative pressure is transmitted to the abdominal viscera and blood vessels. This drop in intra-abdominal pressure eliminates the normal venous pressure gradient that facilitates return flow from the abdomen into the thorax. Consequently, blood tends to pool in the abdominal capacitance vessels of the venous system.

As with positive pressure ventilation, the pooling effect that occurs with whole body negative pressure ventilation effectively removes a volume of blood from the circulation. This "relative" hypovolemia can potentially cause a reduction in CVP, right atrial filling pressures, and cardiac output. During the years of the poliomyelitis epidemics, when body respirators were extensively used, the circulatory depression caused by this venous pooling was called "tank shock."

In an attempt to retain the benefits of negative pressure ventilation while minimizing the disadvantages of the whole-body tank respirator, the cuirass ventilator was developed. Basically, the cuirass consists of a rigid turtlelike shell, with its edges designed to conform to the lateral surfaces of the thorax, base of the neck, and hip-pubic area. From the top of the shell a flexible hose leads to an electric pump.

Like the full body respirator, the cuirass employs negative pressure at the body surface to generate the necessary pressure gradient. However, since the negative pressure is confined mostly to the thorax, abdomen venous pooling is minimized.

Although use of the cuirass, along with that of the whole-body ventilator, has declined, negative pressure ventilation remains a viable alternative to the positive pressure approach with certain patient categories. Specifically, patients with permanent neuromuscular impairments who retain adequate upper airway protective and clearance reflexes (thereby not needing an artificial airway) are ideally suited to ventilatory support with negative pressure ventilation.[88] In particular, improvement in the design of the cuirass, including an assist-sensing mechanism and new, lightweight construction, have made this approach more acceptable to patients, especially for use in the home setting (see Chapter 35).

Ventilation at high frequencies

Recently there has been substantial interest in ventilation systems that use frequencies above 60 per minute.[89-94] Investigations began to appear in the literature with regularity in the early 1970s, primarily in Scandinavian journals.[89,94,95] A tremendous interest has developed, exemplified by numerous reviews, reports, and editorials.[89,94-103]

However, hard knowledge regarding these nontraditional methods remains limited.[99,100,103] Ongoing research efforts are attempting to establish whether these modes of ventilatory support can assume a proper role in respiratory care.

Modes of high-frequency ventilation. Although often referred to simply as high-frequency ventilation (HFV), there are really three distinct types of high-frequency ventilatory support.[94,103] According to the rates, volumes, and systems used, these modes are designated as high-frequency positive pressure ventilation (HFPPV), high-frequency jet ventilation (HFJV), or high-frequency oscillation (HFO). Table 29-5 compares the current modes of high-frequency ventilation.

High-frequency positive pressure ventilation. HFPPV was originally developed in the late 1960s as a research tool designed to eliminate blood pressure fluctuations caused by traditional ventilation during cardiovascular studies on animals.[94,95] HFPPV was found ideal for this purpose. As applied to animals, pleural pressures remained negative, and spontaneous breathing efforts ceased (cessation of spontaneous respiration with HFV subsequently has been attributed to stimulation of the lung's stretch receptors). Yet ventilatory and oxygenation parameters with HFPPV remained comparable to those observed with spontaneous breathing. For these reasons, the technique was tested and successfully applied on humans as an alternative clinical mode of ventilatory support.

Today, HFPPV is characterized by (1) ventilatory rates between 60 and 100/min, (2) I:E ratios of 1:3 or less, (3) constant pressure generation (decelerating inspiratory flow), (4) small V_T values, often approaching the anatomic dead space, and (5) the maintenance of positive airway pressure but subatmospheric P_{pl} throughout the breathing cycle.[89,103]

Gas delivery during HFPPV is accomplished with specially designed time-cycled, pressure-limited devices developed specifically for this purpose.[6] Gas is routed through an insufflation catheter that is passed through an endotracheal tube, laryngoscope, or bronchoscope. As

Table 29-5   Modes of High-Frequency Ventilation

Mode	Respiratory rate per minute	Tidal volume	Peak inspiratory pressure	Comment
High-frequency positive pressure ventilation	60 to 100	3 to 5 ml/kg body weight	Low	Similar to conventional IPPV
High-frequency jet ventilation	100 to 200	3 to 5 ml/kg body weight	Low	Short bursts delivered into upper airways; requires a special "jet" ventilator
High-frequency oscillation	60 to 3600	Less than 3 ml/kg body weight	Low	Uses piston, or audio loud-speaker, or flow interrupter to oscillate column of gases in airway

shown in Fig. 29-30, the rapid closing and opening of a pneumatically or electrically controlled exhalation valve determines gas movement into and out of the lungs. Some HFPPV systems have no valve at all, using fluidic principles to control the direction of gas flow. Since the volumes delivered are typically small compared with traditional modes of mechanical ventilation, the ventilator circuitry must have a small internal volume and low gas compression factor.

In clinical practice, HFPPV tidal volumes are only 20% to 30% as large as those used during traditional CMV, or about 3 to 5 ml/kg. Rates are generally varied between 60 and 100/min, with I:E ratios kept at 1:3 or less.[6] Carbon dioxide levels respond best to changes in rate, whereas adjustments in oxygenation are made mainly by altering the F_{IO_2} or applied pressure. As with traditional CMV, oxygenation with HFPPV can be further enhanced by applying PEEP where indicated.

High-frequency jet ventilation. HFJV was first described in 1977.[104] Originally, this method was designed to deliver gas from a variable-pressure regulator through a 14- to 18-gauge percutaneous transtracheal catheter. Because of the high velocity of gas exiting the tip of the catheter, air or mixed gases are entrained at this site, yielding a volume somewhat larger than that delivered by the system alone. These pulses of pressurized gas are provided in short bursts at rates between 100 and 200/min, as controlled by a pneumatic, electric, or mechanical valve assembly.[90,91,104]

Because the position of the jet outlet relative to the carina determines, in part, the effectiveness of both oxygenation and ventilation, a special endotracheal tube, which incorporates both the jet catheter and a pressure monitor line, has been developed (Fig. 29-31). This approach elim-

inates the need to establish a percutaneous route, provides better control over jet position, and maintains a constant and optimum ratio of jet to lumen size for gas entrainment. Alternatively, a special adapter is available that allows HFPPV to be provided through a standard endotracheal tube.[105]

In clinical practice, HFJV rates are generally varied between 100 and 200/min, with I:E ratios kept at 1:1 or less.[6] Peak airway pressures are usually only 8 to 10 cm H_2O above the baseline pressure, with mean airway pressures comparable to those occurring with traditional CMV (Fig. 29-32). Pco_2 levels with HFJV respond best to relative changes in airway pressure, whereas Po_2 changes correspond mainly to the mean airway pressure.[6] As with HFPPV, oxygenation with HFJV can be further enhanced by applying PEEP where indicated.

Interestingly, percutaneous HFJV prevents oropharyngeal fluid from entering the trachea and can therefore prevent aspiration.[106] Moreover, HFJV allows airway access without interrupting ventilatory support, an important con-

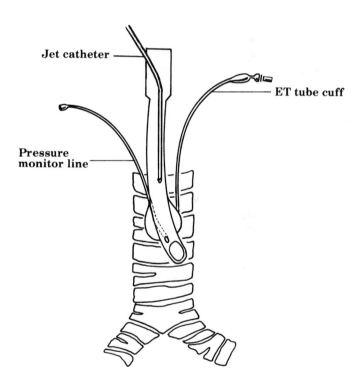

Fig. 29-31   A special HFJV airway tube (endotracheal tube) has been developed. In addition to the standard endotracheal tube with its cuff and standard connector, two additional lines have been added. A special line is connected to a pressure manometer. The line is fused to the main catheter and opens just above the end of the endotracheal tube. This opening is exposed to the inside of the endotracheal tube. A second additional line is the jet catheter that is also fused to the endotracheal tube. Its opening inside the endotracheal tube at the distal end is about 5 cm above the opening for the pressure manometer. (From Pilbeam SP: Mechanical ventilation: physiological and clinical applications, St Louis, 1986, The CV Mosby Co.)

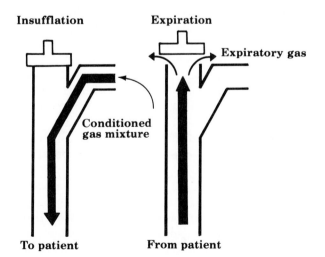

Fig. 29-30   HFPPV value system. (From Pilbeam SP: Mechanical ventilation: physiological and clinical applications, St Louis, 1986, The CV Mosby Co.)

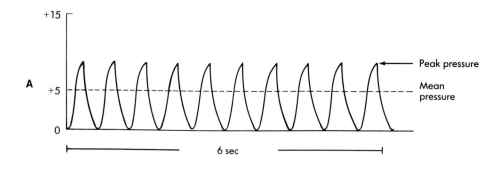

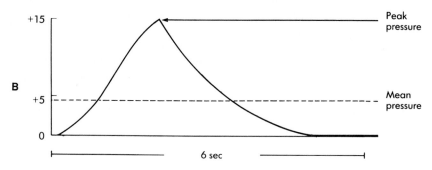

Fig. 29-32 Airway pressure during high-frequency jet ventilation (HFJV). **A,** HFJV. **B,** Conventional IPPV. In the time it takes to deliver one IPPV breath, HFJV delivers approximately ten breaths. In this example, HFJV delivers each breath at a lower peak pressure than is reached with IPPV, but the mean airway pressure is approximately the same. Pressures are in cm H_2O. (From Martin L: Pulmonary physiology in clinical practice, St Louis, 1987, The CV Mosby Co.)

sideration during bronchoscopy and tracheobronchial aspiration. On the other hand, HFJV can lead to air trapping, especially in patients with lung units characterized by long time constants.[6]

High-frequency oscillation. Of the three modes of high-frequency ventilation in current use, HFO is the most radical approach. HFO rates may range from 60 to 3600/min, or 1 to 60 Hz. V_T values with HFO are probably in the 1.5 to 3.0 ml/kg range.[6,92-94]

Three different systems are currently employed to provide HFO: an eccentric wheel-driven piston, an audio loudspeaker, and a rotating flow interrupter.[6] The basic design of a piston-driven HFO system is depicted in Fig. 29-33. Fresh gas is provided by a continual biased flow at the airway connection. Resistance to the outflow of the source gas can create PEEP and aid in regulating airway pressures during oscillation.

Physical principles and physiologic effects. Currently, the mechanisms by which these high-frequency modes of ventilatory support maintain adequate gas exchange are not well understood.[99,100] This theoretical shortcoming is compounded by substantial differences in the technical apparatus used and its application. Nonetheless, a few generalizations can be made.

First, it appears that HFV, particularly at higher frequency ranges, results in a larger mean lung volume than

traditional CMV, even at the same mean airway pressure.[107] This phenomenon explains, in part, the relative effectiveness of HFV in the management of conditions associated with alveolar collapse, such as the infant and adult respiratory distress syndromes.

Although increased mean lung volumes can improve oxygenation, this effect does not explain how HFV provides adequate alveolar ventilation. At lower rates, and volumes in excess of the anatomic dead space, HFV probably provides alveolar ventilation by convective gas transport, much as with traditional CMV.[94] However, as the volumes drop below the anatomic dead space, other gas exchange mechanisms must be involved. Other mechanisms that may explain the effectiveness of HFV at volumes below the anatomic dead space include proximal alveolar ventilation, parabolic flow, coaxial streaming, pendelluft, and molecular diffusion.[6,108,109]

The concept of proximal alveolar ventilation is based on the fact that the distance between the airway opening and alveoli varies. Even if the volume delivered by HFV is less than the anatomic dead space, those alveoli closest to the airway opening will receive some fresh tidal exchange.

The principle of parabolic flow recognizes that gas movement into and out of the airways is characterized by a conical as opposed to square wave pattern, with gas mixing occurring rapidly on cessation of flow (Fig. 29-34).[110]

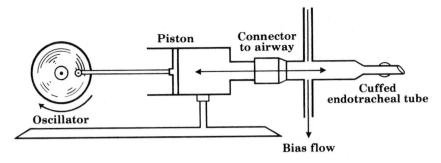

Fig. 29-33   This high-frequency oscillator operates by using a piston connected to an eccentric wheel. As the piston moves forward it forces a small volume to the patient. As it moves back the same volume of gas is withdrawn. A bias flow of gas brings in fresh air and oxygen and helps to remove the carbon dioxide. Gas exchange occurs at the top of the endotracheal tube. (From Pilbeam SP: Mechanical ventilation: physiological and clinical applications, St Louis, 1986, The CV Mosby Co.)

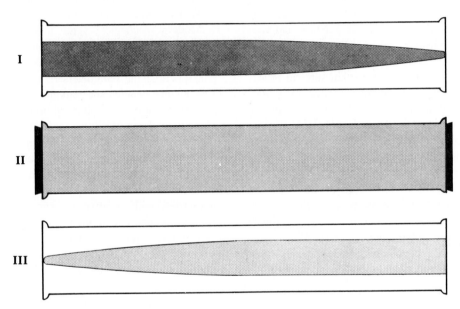

Fig. 29-34   Example of parabolic flow. *I* represents inspiration. *II* shows rapid mixing when flow ceases. *III* demonstrates return to parabolic flow on exhalation. (From Pilbeam SP: Mechanical ventilation: physiological and clinical applications, St Louis, 1986, The CV Mosby Co.)

Again, with parabolic flow, some of the volume of fresh gas will reach the alveoli, even if the total volume is less than the anatomic dead space.

The theory of coaxial streaming is based on the assumption that inspiratory and expiratory gases coexist in the conducting airways at the same time but follow different pathways because of different velocity profiles. Inspiratory gases, with higher incoming velocity, would tend to travel down the center of the airway, whereas expiratory gases (traveling at lower velocity) would tend to exit around the periphery.

The concept of pendelluft has already been discussed as related to the inspiratory phase of traditional CMV. As applied to HFV, convective mixing between lung units with different time constants could result in adequate gas ex-

change, even with volumes smaller than the anatomic dead space.

Experience with apneic diffusion oxygenation suggests that molecular diffusion may also play a role in HFV, especially in the high-frequency oscillation mode.[92,93,108] Supporting this assumption is the observation that the rhythmic action of cardiac contractions facilitates gaseous diffusion in the lungs of patients not spontaneously breathing.[6]

Of course, these various mode of gas movement are not mutually exclusive and probably interact to effect gas exchange during HFV.[109] However, as with traditional CMV, high-frequency systems control carbon dioxide elimination mainly by varying the rate and relative airway pressure and regulate oxygenation mainly by altering F_{IO_2}

values and mean airway pressures (including PEEP).[89-94] Because of these similarities, it is likely that convective transport of some type plays an important in both approaches.

Many potential physiologic advantages of high-frequency ventilation over traditional CMV have been cited (see the box below). Most of these cited advantages are cardiovascular and are attributed to the lower peak airway pressures that characterize HPV. However, recent animal studies have failed to show a significant difference in cerebral, cardiac, pulmonary, or renal blood between HFV and traditional CMV modes of ventilation.[109] Moreover, it now appears that the cardiovascular effects of PEEP during HFV (once thought to be less than with traditional CMV) are essentially the same as those observed during traditional positive pressure ventilation.[112]

Currently, the best documented indication for HFV over traditional CMV is bronchopleural fistula.[113,114] In this situation, HFV tends to maintain better oxygenation and ventilation than that provided by traditional positive pressure ventilation. Ventilation at high frequencies also appears to hold promise as an adjunct tool in certain surgical procedures impeded by either gross lung motion or CMV-caused blood pressure fluctuations, such as those involving the thorax, the larynx, and the brain. Lastly, HFV appears to be of value in preventing major disturbances in gas exchange during bronchoscopy, laryngoscopy, and tracheobronchial aspiration.

Despite its promise, then, the widespread use of HFV in the management of patients with respiratory failure is currently not indicated. Further research is necessary to determine the best and most appropriate use of HFV.[103]

SUMMARY

Modern modes of ventilatory support cannot be used either safely or effectively unless those responsible for these applications understand both the underlying physical principles and physiologic effects.

As we have seen, all modes of ventilatory support facilitate lung expansion by increasing the transpulmonary pressure gradient. Negative pressure ventilation decreases the pressure at the body surface or chest wall during inspiration. Positive pressure ventilation increases the transpulmonary pressure gradient by raising the P_{alv} during inspiration, thereby reversing the normal pressure gradients that occur during spontaneous breathing.

Likewise, CPAP increases the P_L airway pressure, but solely by maintaining a constant airway pressure throughout the breathing cycle. Therefore, gas flow into and out of the lung during CPAP depends on spontaneously generated changes in pleural pressure, as with normal breathing.

To understand the physical and physiologic principles underlying ventilatory support, we divided the events of mechanical ventilation into four related components:

1. The mechanism by which inspiration is initiated;
2. The nature of the inspiratory phase;
3. The mechanism by which inspiration is terminated;
4. The nature of the expiratory phase.

Modern mechanical ventilators allow the clinician to manipulate purposefully the various parameters underlying these components to achieve specific clinical objectives. Manipulating the parameters of positive pressure ventilation ideally benefits the patient. However, positive pressure ventilation is not a normal process and is therefore accompanied by a variety of unwanted or adverse consequences. These potentially detrimental effects include interference with gas exchange itself and cardiovascular, renal, and gastrointestinal complications.

Given the number and potential seriousness of problems associated with positive pressure ventilation, clinicians have developed and applied various alternative approaches to ventilatory support. Although negative pressure ventilation actually preceded positive pressure ventilation as a method of managing respiratory failure, it still maintains a role in the support of certain critically ill patients. More recently, experimentation with positive pressure ventilation at high frequencies shows promise, also in specific applications.

Perhaps most important, our experience with positive pressure ventilation at high frequencies is providing new insights on the physical and physiologic principles of ventilatory support. Continued research on innovative approaches to ventilatory support can only enhance our ability to provide safe and effective management to patients in respiratory failure.

PROPOSED ADVANTAGES OF VENTILATION AT HIGH FREQUENCIES

Reduced peak airway pressures
Reduced pleural pressures
Potential improvement in cardiac output
Decreased incidence of pulmonary barotrauma
Less fluctuation in ICP
Increased mucociliary clearance
Less air leakage with bronchopleural fistulas

REFERENCES

1. Mushin WW, Rendell-Baker L, Thompson PW, and Mapleson WW: Automatic ventilation of the lungs, ed 3, Oxford, England, 1980, Blackwell Scientific Publications.
2. Report of the ACCP-ATS Joint Committee on Pulmonary Nomenclature, Chest 67:583, 1975.
3. Eros B, Powner D, and Grenvik A: Common ventilatory modes: terminology, Int Anesthesiol Clin 18:11-23, 1980.
4. McPherson SP: Respiratory therapy equipment, ed 3, St Louis, 1985, The CV Mosby Co.

5. Eros B, Powner D, and Grenvik A: Mechanical ventilators: principles of operation, Int Anesthesiol Clin 18:23-37, 1980.

6. Pilbeam SP: Mechanical ventilation: physiological and clinical applications, St Louis, 1986, The CV Mosby Co.

7. Scanlan CL: Classification of mechanical ventilators. V. Clinical application—inspiratory phase (individual independent study package), Dallas, 1978, American Association for Respiratory Therapy.

8. Rattenborg CC and Via-Reque E, editors: Clinical use of mechanical ventilation, Chicago, 1981, Year Book Medical Publishers.

9. Bone RC: Monitoring respiratory function in the patient with adult respiratory distress syndrome, Semin Respir Med 2:140, 1981.

10. Bone RC: Diagnosis of causes for acute respiratory distress by pressure-volume curves, Chest 70:740, 1976.

11. Boysen PG, Banner MJ, and Jaeger MJ: Inspiratory times and flow wave patterns in relation to distribution of ventilation, Anesthesiology 63:A560, 1985.

12. Sullivan M, Saklad M, and Demers RR: Relationship between ventilator waveform and tidal-volume distribution, Respir Care 22:386-393, 1977.

13. Dammann JF and McAslan TC: Optimal flow pattern for mechanical ventilation of the lungs—evaluation with a model lung, Crit Care Med 5:128-136, 1977.

14. Dammann JF, McAslan TC, and Maffeo CJ: Optimal flow pattern for mechanical ventilation of the lungs. II. The effect of a sine versus square wave flow pattern with and without an end-inspiratory pause on patients, Crit Care Med 6:293-310, 1978.

15. Lindahl S: Influence of an end inspiratory pause of pulmonary ventilation, gas distribution, and lung perfusion during artificial ventilation, Crit Care Med 7:540, 1979.

16. Fulheihan SF et al: Effect of mechanical ventilation with end-expiratory pause on blood gas exchange, Anesth Analg 55:122, 1976.

17. Shapiro BA, Harrison RA, and Trout C: Clinical applications of respiratory care, ed 3, Chicago, 1985, Year Book Medical Publishers.

18. Kacmarek RM: The role of pressure support ventilation in reducing the work of breathing, Respir Care 33:99-120, 1988.

19. Mapleson WW: The effects of changes of lung characteristics on the functioning of automatic ventilators, Anaesthesia 17:300, 1962.

20. Bendixen HH et al: Respiratory care, St Louis, 1965, The CV Mosby Co.

21. Elam JO, Kerr JH, and Janney CD: Performance of ventilators: effects of changes in lung-thorax compliance, Anesthesiology 19:56, 1958.

22. Fleming WH and Bowen JC: A comparative evaluation of pressure-limited and volume-limited respirators for prolonged post-operative ventilatory support in combat casualties, Ann Surg 176:49, 1972.

23. Lough MD, Williams TJ, and Rawson JE: Newborn respiratory care, Chicago, 1979, Year Book Medical Publishers.

24. Reynolds EOR: In Thibeault DW and Gregory GA, editors: Newborn pulmonary care, Menlo Park, Calif, 1979, Addison-Wesley Publishing Co, Inc.

25. Scanlan CL: Classification of mechanical ventilators. VI. Clinical application—expiratory phase (individual independent study package), Dallas, 1978, American Association for Respiratory Therapy.

26. Kirby RR and Graybar GB, editors: Intermittent mandatory ventilation, Int Anesthesiol Clin 18:1, 1980.

27. Weisman JM, Rinaldo JE, Rogers RM, and Sanders MH: Intermittent mandatory ventilation, Am Rev Respir Dis 127:641-647, 1983.

28. Fairley HB: In Kirby RR and Graybar GB, editors: Intermittent mandatory ventilation, Int Anesthesiol Clin 18:179, 1980.

29. Luce JM, Pierson DJ, and Hudson LD: Critical review: intermittent mandatory ventilation, Chest 79:678, 1981.

30. Shapiro BA et al: Intermittent demand ventilation (IDV): a new technique for supporting ventilation in critically ill patients, Respir Care 21:521, 1976.

31. Harboe S: Weaning from mechanical by means of intermittent assisted ventilation (IAV): case reports, Acta Anesth Scand 21:252, 1977.

32. Hasten RW, Downs JB, and Hesman TJ: A comparison of synchronized and nonsynchronized intermittent mandatory ventilation, Respir Care 25:554, 1980.

33. Mueller Petty TL, and Filley GF: Ventilation and arterial blood gas changes induced by pursed lip breathing, J Appl Physiol 28:784-789, 1970.

34. Ashbaugh DG and Petty TL: Positive end-expiratory pressure: physiology, indications and contraindications, J Thorac Cardiovasc Surg 65:165, 1973.

35. Kumar A et al: Continuous positive-pressure ventilation in acute respiratory failure, N Engl J Med 283:1430, 1970.

36. Barach AL, Bickerman HA, and Petty TL: Perspective in pressure breathing, Respir Care 20:627, 1975.

37. Gregory GA, et al: Treatment of the idiopathic respiratory distress syndrome with continuous positive airway pressure, N Engl J Med 284:1333, 1971.

38. Gillick JS: Spontaneous positive end-expiratory pressure (sPEEP), Anesth Analg 56:627, 1977.

39. Sturgeon CL et al: PEEP and CPAP: cardiopulmonary effects during spontaneous ventilation, Anesth Analg 56:633, 1977.

40. Schmidt GB et al: EPAP without intubation, Crit Care Med 5:297, 1977.

41. Greenbaum DM et al: Continuous positive airway pressure without tracheal intubation in spontaneously breathing patients, Chest 69:615, 1976.

42. Eros B, Powner D, and Grenvik A: In Kirby RR and Graybar GB, editors: Intermittent mandatory ventilation, Int Anesthesiol Clin 18:11, 1980.

43. Kacmarek RM, Dimas S, Reynolds J, and Shapiro BA: Technical aspects of positive end-expiratory pressure (PEEP). Pt I, II, and III, Respir Care 27:1478-1517, 1982.

44. Tyler DC: Positive end-expiratory pressure: a review, Crit Care Med 11:300-307, 1983.

45. Sugerman HJ, Rogers RM, and Miller LD: Positive end-expiratory pressure (PEEP): indications and physiologic considerations, Chest 62 (pt 2):86s, 1972.

46. Gallagher TJ and Civetta JM: Goal-directed therapy of acute respiratory failure, Anesth Analg 59:831, 1980.

47. Ralph D and Robertson HT: Respiratory gas exchange in adult respiratory distress syndrome, Semin Respir Med 2:114, 1981.

48. Suter PM, Fairley HB, and Isenberg MD: Optimal end-expiratory pressure in patients with acute pulmonary failure, N Engl J Med 292:284, 1975.

49. Kirby RR et al: High-level positive end-expiratory pressure (PEEP) in acute respiratory insufficiency, Chest 67:156, 1975.

50. Gregory GA: In Thibeault DW and Gregory GA, editors: Neonatal pulmonary care, ed 2, Menlo Park, Calif, 1986, Addison-Wesley Publishing Co, Inc.

51. Ayres SM and Giannelli S Jr: Oxygen consumption and alveolar ventilation during intermittent positive pressure breathing, Dis Chest 50:409, 1966.

52. Sheldon GP: Pressure breathing in chronic obstructive lung disease, Medicine 42:197, 1963.

53. Gray FD Jr and MacIver S: The use of inspiratory positive breathing in cardiopulmonary disease, Br J Tuberc 52:2, 1958.

54. Motley HL: Intermittent positive pressure breathing therapy, Inhal Ther 7:1, 1962.

55. Froese AB and Bryan AC: Effects of anesthesia and paralysis on diaphragmatic mechanics in man, Anesthesiology 41:242, 1974.

56. Downs JB: Ventilatory patterns and modes of ventilation in acute respiratory failure, Respir Care 28:586-591, 1983.

57. Hedenstierna G: The anatomic and alveolar deadspaces during res-

piratory treatment: influence of respiratory frequency, minute volume, and tracheal pressure, Br J Anesthesiol 47:993, 1975.

58. Hedenstierna G, White FE, and Wagner PD: Spatial distribution of pulmonary blood flow in the dog with PEEP ventilation, J Appl Physiol 47:938-946, 1979.

59. Campbell EJM, Nunn JF, and Peckett BW: A comparison of artificial ventilation and spontaneous respiration with particular reference to ventilation-blood flow relationships, Br J Anesthesiol 30:166-172, 1958.

60. Downs JB, Douglas ME, Ruiz BC, and Miller NL: Comparison of assisted and controlled mechanical ventilation in anesthetized swine, Crit Care Med 7:5-8, 1979.

61. Bone RC: Complications of mechanical ventilation and positive end expiratory pressure, Respir Care 27:402-407, 1982.

62. Bone RC: Mechanical trauma in acute respiratory failure, Respir Care 28:618-623, 1983.

63. Bone RC: Pulmonary barotrauma complicating positive end expiratory pressure, Am Rev Respir Dis 113:921A, 1976.

64. Bendixen HH et al: Imparied oxygenation in surgical patients during general anesthesia with controlled ventilation, N Engl J Med 269:991, 1963.

65. Bergman NA: Intrapulmonary gas trapping during mechanical ventilation at rapid frequencies, Anesthesiology 37:626-633, 1972.

66. Poulton TJ and Downs JB: Humidification of rapidly flowing gas, Crit Care Med 9:59-63, 1981.

67. Op't Holt TB, Hall MW, Bass JB, and Allison RC: Comparison of changes in airway pressure during continuous positive airway pressure (CPAP) between demand valve and continuous flow devices, Respir Care 27:1200-1209, 1982.

68. Gibney RTN, Wilson RS, and Pontoppidan H: Comparison of work of breathing on high gas flow and demand valve continuous positive airway pressure systems, Chest 82:692-695, 1982.

69. Hall JR, Rendelman RC, and Downs JB: PEEP devices: flow dependent increases in airway pressure, Crit Care Med 6:100, 1978.

70. Cournand A, Motley HL, and Werko L: Physiologic studies of the effects of intermittent positive pressure breathing on cardiac output in man, Am J Physiol, 152:162, 1948.

71. Kilburn KH and Sicker HO: Hemodynamic effects of continuous positive and negative pressure breathing in normal man, Circ Res 8:660, 1960.

72. Opie LH et al: Intrathoracic pressure during intermittent positive-pressure respiration, Lancet 1:911, 1961.

73. Bashour FA et al: Effect of intermittent positive pressure breathing on the cardiac output and the splanchnic blood flow, Inhal Ther 13:47, 1968.

74. Coonse GK and Aufrance OE: The relation of the intrapleural pressure to the mechanics of the circulation, Am Heart J 9:347, 1934.

75. Printzmetal M and Kounts WB: Intrapleural pressure in health and disease and its influence on body function, Medicine 14:457, 1935.

76. Christie RV and McIntosh CA: The measurement of intrapleural pressure in man and its significance, J Clin Invest 13:279, 1934.

77. Pick RA, Handler JB, and Friedman AS: The cardiovascular effects of positive end expiratory pressure, Chest 82:345-350, 1982.

78. Marini JJ, Culver BH, and Butler J: Mechanical effects of lung distention with positive pressure on ventricular function, Am Rev Respir Dis 124:382-386, 1981.

79. Drury DR et al: The effects of continuous pressure breathing on kidney function, J Clin Invest 26:945, 1947.

80. Sladen A et al: Pulmonary complications and water retention in prolonged mechanical ventilation, N Engl J Med 279:448, 1968.

81. Murdaugh HV et al: Effect of altered intrathoracic pressure on renal hemodynamics, electrolyte excretion, and water clearance, J Clin Invest 39:834, 1959.

82. Marquez JM et al: Renal function and cardiovascular responses during positive airway pressure, Anesthesiology 50:393, 1979.

83. Hedley-Whyte J, Burgess GE, Feeley TW, and Miller MG: Applied physiology of respiratory care, Boston, 1976, Little, Brown and Co.

84. Henry JP and Pierce JW: Possible role of cardiac atrial stretch receptors in induction of changes in urine flow, J Physiol 131:572, 1956.

85. Davis JT: The influence of intrathoracic pressure on fluid and electrolyte balance, Chest 62 (suppl):118S-125S, 1972.

86. Boyd AD and Antkowiak DE: Mechanisms of diuresis during negative pressure breathing, J Appl Physiol 14:116-120, 1959.

87. Drinker P and McKhann C: The use of a new apparatus for prolonged administration of artificial respiration, JAMA 92:1658, 1929.

88. Holtakers TR, Loosborck LM, and Gracey DR: The use of the chest cuirass in respiratory failure of neurologic origin, Respir Care 27:271-275, 1982.

89. Sjostrand U: High frequency positive pressure ventilation (HFPPV): a review, Crit Care Med 8:345, 1980.

90. Carlon GC et al: Clinical experience with high frequency jet ventilation, Crit Care Med 9:1, 1981.

91. Carlon GC et al: Technical aspects and clinical implications of high frequency jet ventilation with a solenoid valve, Crit Care Med 9:47, 1981.

92. Butler WJ et al: Ventilation by high frequency oscillation in humans, Anesth Analg 59:577, 1980.

93. Marchak BE et al: Treatment of RDS by high-frequency oscillation ventilation: a preliminary report, J Pediatr 99:287, 1981.

94. Sjostrand U and Eriksson IA: High rates and low volumes in mechanical ventilation—not just a matter of ventilatory frequency, Anesth Analg 59:567, 1980.

95. Jonzon A et al: High-frequency positive-pressure ventilation by endotracheal insufflation, Acta Anaesth Scand 43(suppl), 1971.

96. Heebrink DM: Reports: the high frequency ventilation saga, Respir Care 26:991, 1981.

97. Chatburn RL: High frequency ventilation: a report on a state of the art symposium, Respir Care 19:839-849, 1984.

98. Smith RB and Sjostrand UH: High frequency ventilation, Int Anesthesiol Clin 21, 1983.

99. Kirby RR: High-frequency positive-pressure ventilation (HFPPV): what role in ventilatory insufficiency? Anesthesiology 52:109, 1980 (editorial).

100. Froese AB and Bryan AC: High frequency ventilation, Am Rev Respir Dis 123:249, 1981 (editorial).

101. Gallagher RJ, Klain MM, and Carlon GC: Present status of high frequency ventilation, Crit Care Med 10:613-617, 1982.

102. Bland RD et al: High frequency ventilation in severe hyaline membrane disease: an alternative treatment? Crit Care Med 8:275, 1980.

103. Bone RC: High frequency ventilation: exciting, but still a research tool, Respir Care 28:1007-1008, 1983.

104. Klain M and Smith RB: High frequency percutaneous jet ventilation, Crit Care Med 5:280-287, 1977.

105. Chatburn RL, McClellan LD, and Lough MD: A new patient circuit adapter for use with high frequency jet ventilation, Respir Care 28:1291-1293, 1983.

106. Keszler H and Klain M: Tracheobronchial toilet without cardiorespiratory impairment, Crit Care Med 8:298, 1980.

107. Kolton M, Cattran CB, Kent G, et al: Oxygenation during high-frequency ventilation compared to conventional mechanical ventilation in two models of lung injury, Anesth Analg 61:323-332, 1982.

108. Fredberg JJ: Augmented diffusion in the airways can support pulmonary gas exchange, J Appl Physiol 49:232, 1980.

109. Chang HK: Mechanisms of gas transport during ventilation by high-frequency oscillation, J Appl Physiol 56:553-563, 1984.

110. Henderson Y, Chillingsworth FP, and Whitney JL: The respiratory deadspace, Am J Physiol 38:1-19, 1915.

111. Bunegin L, Smith RB, Sjostrand UH et al: Regional organ blood flow during high-frequency positive pressure ventilation (HFPPV) and intermittent positive pressure ventilation, Anesthesiology 61:416-419, 1984.

112. Mikhail MS, Banner MJ, and Gallagher TJ: Hemodynamic effects of positive end-expiratory pressure during high-frequency ventilation, Crit Care Med 13:733-737, 1985.

113. Hoff BH, Wilson E, Smith RB et al: Intermittent positive pressure ventilation and high-frequency ventilation in dogs with experimental bronchopleural fistulae, Crit Care Med 11:598-602, 1983.

114. Sjostrand UH, Smith RB, Hoff BH et al: Conventional and high-frequency ventilation in dogs with bronchopleural fistula, Crit Care Med 13:191-193, 1985.

30

Selection and Application of Ventilatory Support Devices

Craig L. Scanlan

The provision of respiratory care to patients in need of ventilatory support has become increasingly dependent on a variety of complex and sophisticated equipment. The burden of responsibility for the selection and application of these devices to patients in respiratory failure ultimately falls on the respiratory care practitioner. The practitioner involved in critical care must have an in-depth knowledge of both the mechanical and physiologic principles underlying ventilatory support equipment.

Changes in this technology are so rapid that no text can hope to provide complete and up-to-date technical information on each new device that is put on the market. For this reason, we have chosen to focus on the general principles common to these devices. With this foundation, the reader can apply these principles to specific devices using standard reference works, in combination with the technical manuals provided by the manufacturers.

OBJECTIVES

After completion of this chapter, the reader will be able to:

1. Apply a systematic classification scheme to describe and categorize selected mechanical ventilators;

2. Identify the common elements of a patient circuit for continuous mechanical ventilation;

3. Describe the significance and calculate the compressed volume of a ventilator circuit;

4. Describe the major mechanical and physiologic principles involved in the application of selected modes of ventilatory support, to include the following:
   a. Controlled ventilation;
   b. IMV and SIMV;
   c. PEEP and CPAP;
   d. Pressure support ventilation (PSV);
   e. Mandatory minute ventilation (MMV);

5. Delineate the minimum essential characteristics of a ventilatory support device;

6. Specify the most appropriate type of ventilatory support mode for a given clinical situation.

TERMS

Most terms used in this chapter are defined in context. The following terms are introduced without explicit definition, but may be found in the text glossary:

agonist	hypnotic
anxiolytic	hypopneic
barbiturate	msec (millisecond)
Coanda effect	rebreathed volume
fasciculation	sinusoidal
FDA	vagolytic
HEPA	

CLASSIFICATION OF VENTILATORY SUPPORT DEVICES

Many available references describe the origin and development of mechanical ventilators and ventilatory support devices, classifying them according to both structural and functional criteria.[1-3] Unfortunately, the increasing diversity and complexity of these devices is making application of a strict classification scheme difficult.

However, classification of ventilatory support equipment provides an orderly approach to its selection and use. The following box indicates the classification approach most commonly applied to such equipment.[1-5] Using this system, we will review the major mechanical characteristics underlying ventilatory support devices in general. Since there are ample descriptions of individual devices in other texts, we will use specific ventilators only as examples of the principles discussed. However, each person responsible for applying ventilatory support must become

CLASSIFICATION OF VENTILATORY SUPPORT DEVICES

POWER VARIABLES	VENTILATORY SUPPORT DEVICE	PHASE VARIABLES	VENTILATORY SUPPORT DEVICE
Pressure differential	Intermittent positive pressure	Initiating inspiration	Controller
	Intermittent negative pressure		Assistor
			Assistor/controller
	Continuous pressure differential	Inspiratory phase	Constant flow generator
			Nonconstant flow generator
Power source	Pneumatic		Constant pressure generator
	Electrical		Nonconstant pressure generator
	Combined		
Circuitry	Single circuit	Ending inspiration	Pressure-cycled
	Double circuit		Volume-cycled
Power application	Pneumatic drive systems:		Time-cycled
(Drive mechanism)	High pressure/high resistance		Flow-cycled
	Low pressure	Expiratory phase	Spontaneous breathing?
	Piston drive systems:		Yes—IMV/SIMV/MMV
	Rotary		No—simple CMV
	Linear		Alterations:
	Spring driven		PEEP
	Weighted drive systems		Expiratory retard
CONTROL MECHANISM	Mechanical		
	Pneumatic		
	Fluidic		
	Electronic		

thoroughly familiar with each device used, including its principles of operation, capabilities, and limitations.

Three major categories constitute our classification system: (1) ventilator power variables, (2) ventilator control mechanisms, and (3) ventilator phase variables.

Ventilator power variables

The first major category used in classifying ventilatory support devices is based on differentiating their power variables.[6] Power variables useful in distinguishing these devices include the pressure differential used, the power source, the power circuitry, and the way in which the power is applied (drive mechanism).

Pressure differential. Ventilatory support devices may first be categorized as operating via an intermittent negative, intermittent positive, or a continuous-pressure differential (see Chapter 29). Devices using either an intermittent-negative or intermittent-positive pressure differential are true ventilators; they provide the power necessary to move gas into the lung during inspiration. Although ventilators using a negative-pressure differential have been largely replaced by the positive-pressure type, there remain specific clinical indications for negative-pressure ventilation.

Devices employing a continuous-pressure differential are not ventilators per se, since they do not provide the power necessary to move gas into the lung during inspiration. Instead, a continuous-pressure differential, usually positive, is created at the airway to maintain or restore the patient's FRC. In this case, the patient is responsible for generating the change in transpulmonary pressure necessary to move gas into and out of the lungs. Continuous-positive airway pressure (CPAP) devices are the best example of this category of ventilatory support equipment.

Intermittent negative pressure ventilators. The classic negative-pressure ventilation method is the time-honored body tank ventilator, known as the "iron lung" (Fig. 30-1). This ventilator has the advantages of ruggedness and durability, combined with a relative ease of operation. However, because of its many disadvantages, the tank ventilator has been largely replaced with devices using positive, as opposed to negative, pressure.

The body tank ventilator is large and cumbersome, requiring considerable space for its physical size and its operational noise. From both nursing and medical viewpoints, it makes patient care difficult and awkward. Patients ill enough to require ventilator care generally need much personal attention, and yet they are isolated from their surroundings, accessible only through arm ports in the wall of the tank or by being removed from the machine

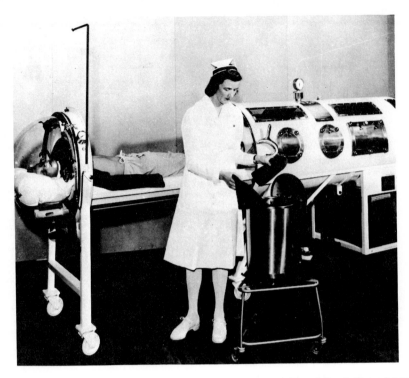

Fig. 30-1   Emerson iron lung. (Courtesy JH Emerson Co, Cambridge, Mass.) (From McPherson SP: Respiratory therapy equipment, ed 4, St Louis, 1989, The CV Mosby Co.)

for hurried care. Monitoring of physiologic functions and the administration of intravenous infusions are also impaired.

Even more important than these inconveniences is the inflexibility of the tank ventilator's function. The classic body tank ventilator is a controller with an adjustable negative-pressure that moves the thorax at set, predetermined intervals, with no provisions for patients to breathe spontaneously. Moreover, there is no way of controlling or regulating flows, a feature that is less important in ventilating patients with normal lungs, than it is in ventilating the larger number of patients with abnormal lungs. Finally, the negative pressure by which the tank ventilator functions can, itself, be a hazard to the patient. The negative pressure is applied not only to the semirigid thorax but also the much more pliant abdomen and is, accordingly, transmitted to the abdominal cavity. Here it tends to cause the venous blood to pool in the large vascular abdominal reservoirs, with a resulting decrease in venous return and cardiac output. This "tank shock" was not an uncommon complication when negative-pressure body ventilators were in widespread use.

Still, negative-pressure ventilation represents an appropriate approach in selected patients, especially those who have both normal lungs and adequate upper airway protective reflexes. To meet this small but continuing demand for negative-pressure ventilation, various types of cuirass (shield-like appliances) have been developed (Fig. 30-2).

The cuirass consists of a shell (available in a number of sizes) with its edges designed to conform to the lateral surfaces of the thorax, base of the neck, and hip-pubic area. Whereas early models were characterized by a heavy, rigid, and uncomfortable chest piece, new models use a lightweight, fenestrated, plastic shell that sits loosely over the patient's trunk with no close skin contact. An airtight seal is achieved by a plastic wrapping that encloses the shell and the patient's back and is snugly applied around the legs. The device is powered by an electrical pump connected to the shell via a flexible hose. In this manner, negative pressure is intermittently applied mostly to the thorax, avoiding the undesirable effect on the abdomen as described above. Early cuirass units were strictly controllers; newer modes employ an electronic flow sensor to synchronize the negative-pressure application to the patient's inspiratory efforts.

The major advantage of negative-pressure ventilators is their ability to ventilate a patient without the need for an artificial airway. However, this advantage must be viewed with some reservation. First, patients with chronic bronchopulmonary disease in respiratory failure need frequent aspiration of secretions, done most effectively through an artificial airway. Second, even patients in respiratory failure with normal lungs may have obtunded upper airway reflexes, and normal oral secretions may pool in the mouth or hypopharynx. In such instances, the inspiratory phase of a negative-pressure ventilator may actually draw these

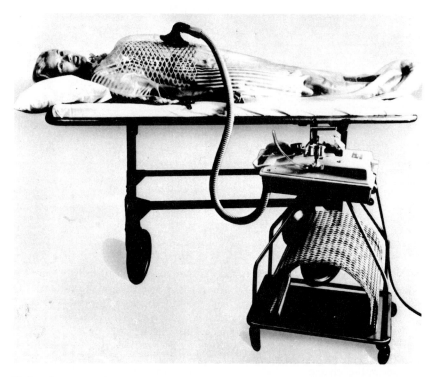

Fig. 30-2   Emerson cuirass. (Courtesy JH Emerson Co, Cambridge, MA) (From McPherson SP: Respiratory therapy equipment, ed 4, St Louis, 1989, The CV Mosby Co.)

fluids into the bronchial tree, causing aspiration, pneumonitis, and atelectasis. Intubation is usually necessary to prevent such complications.

In addition to the problems of size and patient isolation posed by the negative-pressure machines, the much greater versatility of the positive-pressure generators has placed these machines in the therapy foreground of respiratory failure. However, because there are some patients who can benefit from the use of negative-pressure ventilation (especially in the home setting), this category of ventilator should be available on an "as needed" basis.

Intermittent positive-pressure ventilators. Most ventilatory support today is provided by ventilators operating under an intermittent positive-pressure differential. Intermittent positive-pressure ventilators function by applying positive pressure to the airway, thereby raising the intraalveolar pressure and increasing the transpulmonary pressure gradient during inspiration. Although more versatile than negative-pressure ventilators, these devices generally can provide long-term support only when an artificial airway is in place. Modern intermittent positive-pressure ventilators tend to be more complex than their negative-pressure counterparts. Given the complexity and widespread use of these positive-pressure ventilators, most of the remainder of this chapter will be devoted to their use.

Continuous-pressure differential devices. Since continuous-pressure differential devices need only produce a constant distending pressure, they are generally much sim-

pler than true ventilators. The use of a continuous-pressure differential was first described over 50 years ago for the treatment of pulmonary edema.[7,8] However, the first modern application of this concept was described in 1971 for use with infants suffering from Respiratory Distress Syndrome.[9]

As shown in Fig. 30-3, this simple device was assembled from existing materials. A pressurized gas source, *A*, provides continuous flow through a tubing system, from which the patient can spontaneously inhale. Exhalation occurs through a separate outflow or expiratory limb of the circuit, *B*. The continuous-pressure differential was created by varying a restriction to the gas outflow, *E*. A pressure monitor line, *C*, provides the connection for both a monitoring gauge and a simple underwater pressure relief valve, *D*.

Based on their success in treating infant respiratory distress syndrome, continuous positive airway pressure (CPAP) devices subsequently were tested and applied on adults with similar pathologic problems causing an increase in physiologic shunting and a reduction in FRC. Over time, CPAP devices have become more complex and now include commercially available designs that have more sophisticated control and monitoring systems. Most new generation mechanical ventilators also incorporate a CPAP mode capable of providing a continuous-pressure differential to the spontaneously breathing patient. More details on the mechanics of continuous-pressure differen-

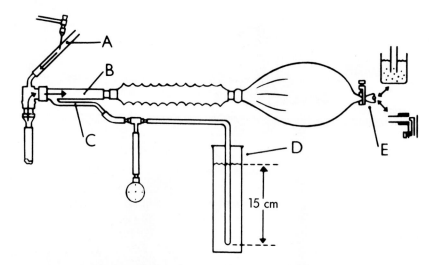

Fig. 30-3   Continuous-flow CPAP system using orificial resistor as originally described by Gergory. *A,* Premixed and humidified source gas to patient connector inlet; *B,* expiratory line; *C,* attachment to pressure manometer and to, *D,* underwater seal pressure pop-off system; *E,* screw clamp on tail of anesthesia bag used to vary size of orifice and adjust PEEP level. (From Blodgett D: Manual of pediatric respiratory care procedures, Philadelphia, 1982, JB Lippincott.)

tial devices are provided later in this chapter.

Power source. Some source of power is required for all ventilatory support devices. Typically, these devices are powered either pneumatically or electrically. Some devices require a combination of these power sources to deliver anything more than room air.

Pneumatically powered ventilators. Pneumatically powered ventilators require only a pressurized gas source to operate, typically oxygen at 50 psig. These ventilators can vary in complexity from hand-operated units, such as the Hand-E-Vent from Ohio Medical Products, to the sophisticated Monaghan 225/SIMV volume ventilator.[1] In units such as the Monaghan 225/SIMV, fluidic principles (discussed separately under the section on Ventilator Control Mechanisms) are applied for controlling various functions.

The obvious advantage of pneumatically powered ventilators is their ability to function without electricity. They are ideal in situations where electrical power is unavailable, (eg, during certain types of patient transport) or as a backup to electrically powered ventilators during power failures.

Pneumatically powered ventilators are also being applied to support patients during sophisticated magnetic resonance imaging procedures, where electrically powered devices simply cannot be used.

However, some pneumatically powered ventilators are electrically controlled (see section on control mechanisms). These devices will not function properly without both a pneumatic power source and an electrical supply to the control mechanism.

Examples of pneumatically powered adult ventilators that can function without an electrical supply are the Bird Mark 7 and 8 and the Bennett PR-I and PR-II. Pneu-

matically powered adult ventilators that require an electrical supply include the Siemens Servo 900 Series, the Engstrom Erica ventilator, the BEAR Series ventilators (when supplied with both compressed air and oxygen), and the Hamilton Veolar. Infant ventilators using a pure pneumatic power source that can function without an electrical supply include the original BabyBird and the Bio-Med MVP-10. The BEAR BP-200 and BEAR Cub (BP-2001) ventilators, the BabyBird 2, the Healthdyne Model 105, the Infrasonic Infant Star ventilator, and the Sechrist IV-100B are examples of pneumatically powered infant ventilators that require an electrical supply.

Electrically powered ventilators. Electricity is a common source of power for many of the ventilators in use today.[1] When a ventilator requires only electric current to function, it should be assumed that only room air is being used to ventilate the patient. If concentrations of oxygen above 21% are to be used, then a source of compressed oxygen must also be available. However, if the oxygen source were to fail or be depleted, a ventilator that is truly electrically powered would not stop ventilating the patient. In other words, the oxygen source is used to control the inspired oxygen percent but not to drive the ventilator. Often electric motors that drive compressors or pistons are used to produce the positive pressure needed. Examples of ventilators needing only electrical current to operate on room air are the Emerson 3-PV and 3MV (IMV) ventilators, the Engstrom ER 300, the Bennett MA-1 and MA-2 ventilators, and the BEAR Series ventilators (when external compressed air is unavailable).

Combined power ventilators. All mechanical ventilators need a source of compressed oxygen to provide F_{IO_2} values above 21%. Therefore, electrically powered ventilators

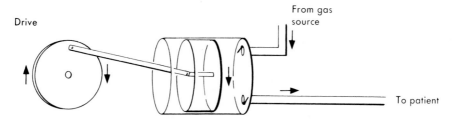

Fig. 30-4   Example of single-circuit ventilator system.

used to deliver anything other than room air require both a compressed oxygen and an electric power source. In this case, the pneumatic source is used to provide the oxygen concentration needed, while the electric power is used to compress the gas for delivery under positive pressure into the lungs. All the electrically powered ventilators previously described fall into this category when delivering gas with an oxygen concentration above 21%.

It is important not to confuse the power source with the control mechanism used by a mechanical ventilator. The control mechanism represents how the various parameters of ventilation are determined, and can include some combination of mechanical, pneumatic, fluidic, or electronic circuitry (see section on control mechanisms). Thus a ventilatory support device may be pneumatically powered but electrically controlled. In this case, a failure of *either* the power source or control mechanism will cause the device to become inoperable.

Examples of pneumatically powered ventilators that will fail to operate if either the power source or control mechanism is lost are the Siemens Servo 900 Series, the Engstrom Erica ventilator, the Hamilton Veolar, the BEAR BP-200 and BEAR Cub (BP-2001), the BabyBird 2, and the Infrasonic Infant Star ventilator. With the BEAR Series ventilators, failure of the pneumatic power supply causes an internal air compressor to take over as the primary power source.

Internal circuitry. Regardless of how the positive pressure is generated, one of two internal drive systems may be used to apply this pressure to the patient's lungs. These two types of internal drives are the single and the double-circuit systems.

Single circuit ventilators. A ventilator with a single circuit is one that provides gas flow directly to the patient from the power source. For example, if a piston is used to provide the necessary driving force and the gases in the piston's cylinder go directly to the patient circuit, as in Fig. 30-4, the system constitutes a single circuit. Most pneumatic and some electrically powered ventilators are of the single-circuit design. Examples of adult ventilators using a single circuit include the Bird Mark 7 and 8, the Bennett PR Series ventilators, the Bennett 7200 Series ventilators, the Siemens Servo 900 Series ventilators, the Emerson 3-PV and 3MV (IMV) ventilators, the Engstrom

Erica ventilator, the BEAR Series ventilators, and the Hamilton Veolar. All infant ventilators in current use employ a single internal circuit.[1,2]

Double circuit ventilators. A double-circuit ventilator has two circuits: the power circuit and the patient circuit. The power circuit drives the patient circuit. Fig. 30-5 diagrams a piston use again, but instead of the piston force being directly transmitted to the patient, it is used to compress a bag, which in turn sends its contents into the patient. In this case, the piston is used as the *drive* circuit, and the bag and tubing are considered the *patient* circuit. Commonly used ventilators employing the double-circuit principle include the Engstrom ER-300 series, the Bennett MA-1 and MA-2, the Monaghan 225/SIMV volume ventilator, and the Ohio CCV-2.[1,2,10]

There are three potential advantages inherent in the double-circuit design. First, double-circuit devices protect the patient from direct exposure to the power source, which may generate pressures as high as 50 psig. Second, some double-circuit devices, such as the Engstrom ER 300, can provide specific flow, pressure, and inspiratory maneuvers that, until recently, were not possible with single-circuit designs. Lastly, should contamination of the internal circuitry occur, only the patient circuit of a double-circuit ventilator need be decontaminated.

Today, however, these advantages are no longer critical. Most single-circuit ventilators employ safety systems that preclude exposure of the patient to dangerously high pressures. Moreover, new microprocessor control mechanisms on many of today's single-circuit ventilators can provide all the flow, pressure, and inspiratory maneuvers previously available only on some double-circuit devices. Finally, in regard to contamination of the internal circuitry of the ventilator, high efficiency particulate air (HEPA) filters now protect this component of single-circuit ventilators from retrograde spread of infectious agents. Moreover, some single-circuit ventilators, such as the Siemens 900 Series, provide easy access to the internal circuit for purposes of cleaning and disinfection. Thus, the functional differences between modern single- and double-circuit ventilators are now much less important than they once were.

Power application (drive mechanisms). The drive mechanism of a positive-pressure ventilator represents the

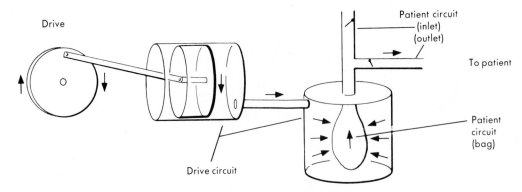

Fig. 30-5 Example of double-circuit ventilator system.

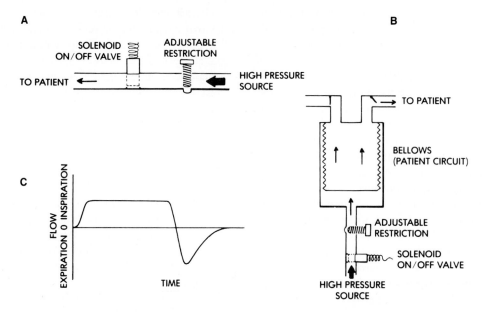

Fig. 30-6 High-pressure pneumatic drive systems with high internal flow resistance. **A,** Single-circuit system. **B,** Double-circuit system. Adjustable restrictions control flow from high-pressure source gas. Electrical solenoids open (solid line drawings) and closed (dashed line drawings), creating inspiration and expiration, respectively. **C,** Constant inspiratory flow pattern typical of these systems. (From Kirby RR, Smith RA, and Desautels DD, editors: Mechanical ventilation, New York, 1985, Churchill Livingstone.)

way in which the generated power is applied to ventilate the patient. There are four major categories of power application systems used by modern ventilators to effect gas flow during inspiration: pneumatic, piston, spring-loaded, and weight driven. Since these various drive mechanisms give a ventilator some of its operational characteristics, a familiarity with their principles is important to the respiratory care practitioner.

Pneumatic drive systems. There are two types of pneumatic drive systems: (1) high pressure (with high internal resistance) and (2) low pressure. Both types of pneumatic drive mechanisms may be incorporated into either a single- or double-circuit design.[10]

High-pressure pneumatic drive systems. Fig. 30-6 shows the high-pressure, high internal resistance power

application, as used in both a single and double-circuit system. In both cases, a valve (pneumatic, mechanical, or electromechanical) controls when power is applied to the system. In the single-circuit design (Fig. 30-6, *A*), the ventilator is driven by a blended gas source under relatively high pressure (3 to 50 psig). A high internal resistance, such as a needle valve, controls the flow of gas into the patient circuit. Examples of single-circuit ventilators using a high-pressure, high internal resistance pneumatic-power application are the Bird Mark 7 and Mark 8 set on "100%," the Bennett 7200 Series ventilators, the latter BEAR Series ventilators (BEAR 2 and 5), and the Hamilton Veolar ventilator.

Fig. 30-6, *B* illustrates the high-pressure, high internal resistance power application in a double-circuit system. In

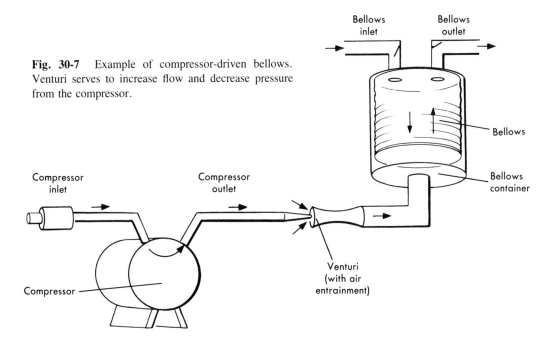

Fig. 30-7 Example of compressor-driven bellows. Venturi serves to increase flow and decrease pressure from the compressor.

this modification, the pressure source is applied to a patient circuit consisting of a bellows in a canister. Like the single-circuit application, a needle valve controls the flow of gas. In this case, however, the needle valve determines the rate of bellows compression, thereby indirectly controlling flow into the patient's lungs. The Monaghan 225/SIMV ventilator is a good example of a high-pressure, high internal resistance power application in a double-circuit system.

Because the driving pressure is relatively high in both these applications, ventilators employing a high-pressure, high internal resistance power application are generally categorized as flow generators and typically produce a constant flow pattern, as shown in Fig. 30-6, C.

Low-pressure pneumatic drive systems. There are three subcategories of low-pressure pneumatic drive systems: (1) pressure reducing valves, (3) venturi/injector systems, and (3) turbine/compressor systems.[10]

A pressure-reducing-valve power application uses an adjustable pressure regulator to reduce a high source pressure to a workable range, usually between 0 to 100 cm H_2O. Typically, ventilators using a pressure-reducing-valve power application are of single-circuit design. The Bennett PR-I and PR-II are good examples of ventilators using this drive mechanism.

A venturi/injector system employs a high-pressure gas source to drive an entrainment device, either of the true venturi or modified injector design. The amount of pressure generated by the venturi/injector system is proportional to, but substantially less than, the driving pressure applied to the jet.[10] Good examples of ventilators using a venturi/injector system are the Bird Mark 7 and Mark 8 set on the "Air Mix" mode.

All low-pressure reducing valves and venturi systems

are susceptible to the effects of downstream pressure and will exhibit a decrease in total flow when significant resistance is applied to them. Devices using either of these low-pressure drive mechanisms are generally characterized as constant-pressure generators, which have a decreasing flow pattern during inspiration.

A turbine or compressor system can also be used to produce positive pressure. Commonly, these compressors are of two general types: those producing relatively low pressures with high flow rates, such as the rotary turbine of the Ohio CCV-2, or those producing relatively high pressures but at low flow rates, such as the compressor pump used on the Bennett MA-1 and MA-2.

Fig. 30-7 portrays the latter type applied in a double-circuit system, such as used in the Bennett MA-1. As indicated, the compressor supplies the pressure necessary to push the bellow upward during inspiration. Outflow from the compressor is enhanced via air entrainment through a venturi. As compared with the compressor alone, the use of this venturi limits the driving pressure so that flow can taper as pressure increases within the patient circuit.[1] This tapering of flow at high working pressure is a characteristic of a constant-pressure generator.

Piston drive systems. Pistons moving back and forth in a cylinder have been used in mechanical ventilators for many years.[10,11] When powered by an electric motor, they provide a convenient mechanism for driving air into a patient's lungs. There are two major types of piston drive systems: rotary and linear.

Rotary–drive pistons. A rotary-drive piston is connected to an electrically driven wheel (Fig. 30-8). If the ventilator is a single-circuit device, then the tidal volume to be delivered can be pulled into the piston during the backward stroke. One-way valves are used to separate the

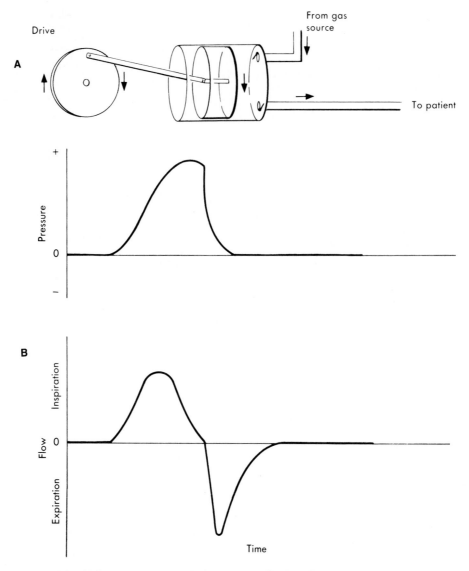

Fig. 30-8 Rotary-driven piston power application. See text for description.

patient's exhaled gases from fresh gases during this phase. On the forward stroke of the piston, gases are pushed into the patient's circuit. A piston drive may also be used in a double-circuit ventilator (see Fig. 30-5).

A unique flow pattern is established by a ventilator with a rotary-driven piston. Because the piston is connected eccentrically to the wheel (Fig. 30-8, *A*) the piston's movement through the cylinder, and the flow of gas out of the cylinder, occurs in an accelerating, then decelerating, fashion. This pattern is typical of a nonconstant flow generator.

As the wheel turns, the piston's movements at the beginning of inspiration are slow because much of the movement of the piston's rod is upward and very little is forward (Fig. 30-8, *B*). During the middle of the piston's movement through the cylinder, much of the movement is forward, creating an accelerating flow out of the cylinder.

The last part of the piston's movement provides a slowing of flow or a deceleration as the piston's movement is less forward again. This type of movement by the piston is termed *sinusoidal,* or producing a sine wave. Thus we often call the inspiratory flow pattern produced by such a device a *sine-wave flow pattern,* although it is more precisely one half of a sine wave.

Since rotary-driven piston ventilators, such as the Emerson 3-PV and 3-MV, are powered by electric motors, they are capable of providing very high airway pressures and are considered flow generators. These devices are very simple, reliable, and have proved themselves over the years. The sine-wave flow pattern produced does mimic the normal flow pattern generated by spontaneously breathing people, and, in concept, may offer some advantage over other flow patterns.[12-14]

Linear-drive pistons. If a piston is used for the driving

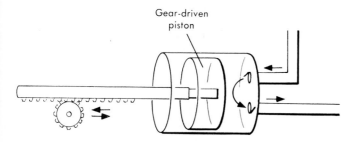

Fig. 30-9   Linear drive (gear-driven) piston.

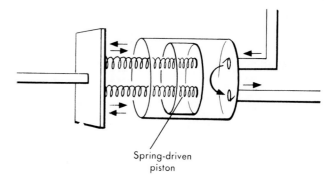

Fig. 30-10   Example of spring-driven ventilator system.

mechanism but is pushed through its cylinder at the same speed rather than in an accelerating-decelerating fashion, then it is considered to have a linear drive (Fig. 30-9). Since the piston's rate of movement is constant throughout its stroke, then the flow of air being pushed into the patient is also constant. Thus a ventilator powered by a linear-drive piston is considered a constant flow generator. The Bourns LS104-150 Infant ventilator, which employs a constant speed gear-driven piston, is a good example of a device using a linear-drive piston power application.[1]

Spring-driven power applications. Although they are a less common power application, springs can be used as the drive mechanism for ventilating the lungs. In Fig. 30-10, springs are used to power a piston in a cylinder. Although no longer in production, the Searle Volume Ventilator Adult (VVA) was a good example of a spring-driven piston power application. Of course, springs may also be used to compress a bag or bellows system.[3]

Regardless of circuit design, the pressure and flow wave-forms produced by a ventilator using a spring-driven power application will depend on the spring tension. Spring tensions that generate working pressures at least three times greater than the airway pressure will generally perform as flow generators, whereas those with less tension will assume the characteristics of a pressure generator.

Weighted-drive mechanisms. A simple device used for a driving mechanism in some ventilators is a weight, such as weighted bellows or piston.[1,3] The weight provides the necessary force to overcome the resistance to airflow during inspiration. This system has also been referred to as "gravity driven." The Chemtron Gill 1 respirator (also out of production) was the sole American example of a ventilator using a weighted-drive mechanism.[1] As with the spring-loaded power application, the pressure and flow waveforms produced by a ventilator using a weighted-drive mechanism depend on the magnitude of the force applied (see Chapter 29).

Ventilator control mechanisms

To allow the operator to regulate the various parameters of ventilatory support, including pressure, volume, flow, and time, a ventilator must have a control mechanism. These mechanisms can be based on mechanical, pneu-

matic, fluidic, or electrical principles, although most modern ventilators combine two or more of these methods to provide user control.

Mechanical control mechanisms. Mechanical control mechanisms are a common component of most ventilators, used mainly to regulate pressure or flow. The simple adjustable pressure reducing valve found on the Bennett PR-I and II is a good example of a mechanical control mechanism (Fig. 30-11). Adjustment of the pressure-reducing valve determines the peak pressure delivery by the system during inspiration.

The adjustable orifice, or needle valve, (Fig. 30-12) is also a good example of a mechanical control mechanism used mainly to control flow from a high-pressure source. A needle valve may also be used to create a constant rate of leakage from a pressurized canister, thereby giving control over time parameters. Both applications of this simple control mechanism are used in the Bird Mark 7 and 8 ventilators.

Simple mechanical devices are also commonly applied to create positive end-expiratory and continuous positive airway pressure (PEEP and CPAP). Such devices, including spring-loaded or gravity-weighted expiratory valves, will be discussed in detail later in this chapter.

Despite the widespread use of mechanical control devices, few ventilators would be considered predominantly controlled by mechanical means. More commonly, modern ventilators are controlled by either pneumatic, fluidic, or electrical means.

Pneumatic control mechanisms. Pneumatic control is provided by using pressurized gas to regulate most or all of the parameters of ventilation. In addition to mechanical pressure regulators and needle valves, pneumatically controlled ventilators rely heavily on pressurized gas cartridges or balloon/valve systems to control the various time parameters of ventilation. Among the ventilators that depend primarily on pneumatic control are the Bennett PR-II, the BabyBird infant ventilator, and the IMV Bird ventilator.[1,2]

Fluidic control mechanisms. Like pneumatically controlled ventilators, fluidically controlled devices use pressurized gas to regulate most or all of the parameters of

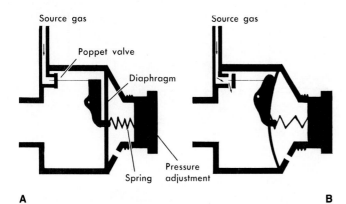

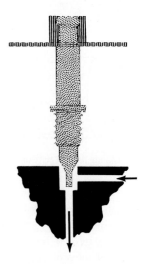

Fig. 30-11   Bennett diluter regulator. **A,** Pressure equals spring tension. **B,** Pressure is below spring tension. (From McPherson SP: Respiratory therapy equipment, ed 4, St Louis, 1989, The CV Mosby Co.)

Fig. 30-12   Needle valve adjusts opening through which gas may pass as a result of pressure gradient across it. (From McPherson SP: Respiratory therapy equipment, ed 4, St Louis, 1989, The CV Mosby Co.)

ventilation. However, instead of simple pressurized valves and timers, fluidically controlled devices employ specialized fluidic "switches" or gates.[15]

All fluidic switches function according to the Coanda effect, as described in Chapter 4.[1] The simplest type of a fluidic switch, called the flip-flop valve, is shown in Fig. 30-13. As illustrated in Fig. 30-12, *A,* once gas flow is established at outflow port 2 (O_2), the low pressure along the outflow wall will cause it to remain there unless disturbed. In Fig. 30-13, *B,* a small pressure pulse is directed through input port 1 (C_1). This pressure pulse is sufficient to disrupt the wall adherence of the gas stream, diverting it to output port 1 (O_1). Diversion of the stream back to output port 2 can now be accomplished by pressurizing input port 2 (C_2).

Fig. 30-14 diagrammatically portrays several other common types of fluidic switches. For the OR/NOR gate, the back-pressure switch, and the AND/NAND gate, output flow will always be at O_2 unless a pressure signal is received from an input port. With the OR/NOR gate, a pressure signal at C_1 will cause the gate to switch its output to O_1. With the back-pressure switch, some source pressure (Ps) is normally allowed to escape out C_1. If, on the other hand, C_1 is occluded, a portion of the source gas will flow through C_1, causing a switch to output port 2. With the AND/NAND gate, both input ports (C_1 and C_2) must be activated for the switch to O_1 to occur.

The proportional amplifier diverts gas out two output ports (O_1 and O_2) equally unless there is an input signal. With an input signal, the relative amount of gas exiting at

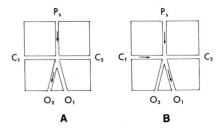

Fig. 30-13   Example of fluidic flip-flop component. Outflow remains at O_2, **A,** until input signal (pressure) is applied at C_1, **B,** which causes outflow to flip to O_1. (From McPherson SP: Respiratory therapy equipment, ed 4, St Louis, 1989, The CV Mosby Co.)

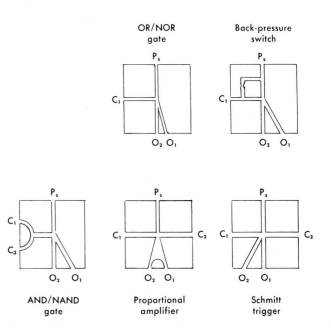

Fig. 30-14   Symbols for some common fluidic elements. (From McPherson SP: Respiratory therapy equipment, ed 4, St Louis, 1989, The CV Mosby Co.)

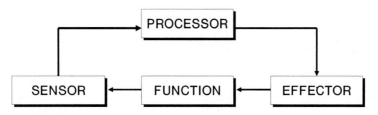

Fig. 30-15   Components of an electronic control mechanism.

O_1 and O_2 will be proportional to the difference in pressure between C_1 and C_2. The Schmitt trigger, as the name implies, is actually a sensing device capable of detecting small changes between the input signals C_1 and C_2, thereby "triggering" a change in the direction of output flow. Thus, the Schmitt trigger can be used as a mechanism to cycle a ventilator to inspiration based on patient effort (an assist mechanism).

Typically, these and similar fluidic switches are combined into an integrated fluidic logic circuit, which functions like an electronic circuit board. This fluidic logic circuit can provide overall control of most ventilator parameters, including pressure, volume, flow, and time. The best example of this approach is incorporated into the Monaghan 225/SIMV ventilator, which is entirely controlled by fluidic logic. Other ventilators using fluidic components to control ventilator parameters include the Bio-Med MVP-10 Pediatric/Neonatal ventilator, the Bio-Med IC-2 ventilator, the Ohio 550, and the Sechrist IV-100B Infant ventilator.[2]

The advantage of fluidic control is simple: there are no moving parts to wear out. On the other hand, fluidic logic circuits waste a portion of the source gas in controlling the ventilator functions. This source gas "consumption" can be substantial, amounting to as much as 8 to 10 L/min. Although not a key consideration when a bulk gas storage and delivery system is available, such gas loss can be a critical factor in certain transport situations.

Electronic control mechanisms. Electronic control, especially that incorporating preprogrammed microprocessors, has quickly become the predominant means of controlling ventilator function. There are two primary reasons for this growth in the use of electronic control mechanisms. First, like fluidic control, electronic control of ventilator parameters can be accomplished with a minimum of moving parts. This increases reliability. Second, electronic control using microprocessors provides functions heretofore unavailable on mechanical ventilators. This increases versatility.

Although there has been a significant evolution in electrical components, the basic concept underlying this type of control mechanism has remained essentially the same over the years. As shown in Fig. 30-15, an electronic control mechanism consists of three key components: a sen-

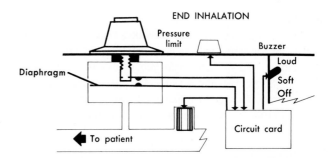

Fig. 30-16   Functional diagram of pressure limit mechanism for MA-1 ventilator. (Courtesy Puritan-Bennett Corp, Los Angeles.) (From McPherson SP: Respiratory therapy equipment, ed 4, St Louis, 1989, The CV Mosby Co.)

sor, a processor, and an effector. The sensor, using either electrical or electromechanical means, "measures" a given parameter, such as pressure or flow. The processor receives this signal and interprets it according to either preprogrammed instructions or those provided by operator input. By comparing the sensor signal to the internal or operator provided instructions, the processor determines if an alteration is needed in the effector device, usually an electromechanical valve, alarm, or indicator system. If an alteration is needed, the processor sends the appropriate signal to the effector, while continuing to monitor the effect of this change via the sensory loop.

A simple example of this type of electronic control is the pressure-limit mechanism on the MA-1 ventilator, as illustrated in Fig. 30-16. The sensor, in this case an electromechanical diaphragm, continually "monitors" airway pressure. The "instructions" for setting the pressure limit are provided by the operator via a manual adjustment of the diaphragm tension. When the pressure exceeds this diaphragm tension, an electrical circuit is closed and a signal is sent to the "processor," in this case a simple circuit card. Once this input signal is received, the processor immediately sends output signals to several "effectors", namely the audible and visual alarm indicators and the main solenoid switch. The main solenoid switch closes, immediately ending the inspiratory phase.

In this example, the processor is simply serving as a "dumb" relay, transferring the input signal from the sensor to the effector. More recently, "smart" processors have been incorporated into mechanical ventilator control systems. Using preprogrammed computer chips, these microprocessors can not only receive and forward signals, but may also interpret and independently act on this information, sometimes making thousands of minute adjustments in the effector system per second!

This latter type of sophisticated microprocessor control is characteristic of the so-called "new generation" of ventilatory support devices, including the Siemens Servo 900C, the Puritan-Bennett 7200 Series, the BEAR 5, and the Hamilton Veolar ventilators.[16] Microprocessor control systems in these devices now provide a clinician with techniques previously unavailable, such as pressure support ventilation (PSV) and mandatory minute ventilation (MMV). Moreover, the sensory data that is used by these processors to alter the parameters of ventilation can also be stored, retrieved, and manipulated for purposes of monitoring and bedside diagnostics.

Ventilator phase variables

As discussed in Chapter 29, the events of mechanical ventilation can be divided into four related components:
1. The mechanism by which inspiration is initiated,
2. The nature of the inspiratory phase,
3. The mechanism by which inspiration is terminated, and
4. The nature of the expiratory phase.

Relevance of phase variables. In classifying a ventilator, phase variables describe how an individual device functions in each of these components of the breathing cycle. For example, the simplest and most widely used approach to ventilator classification focuses solely on the mechanism by which inspiration is terminated. Thus, in this simple scheme, a "volume ventilator" is one that ends inspiration after a preset volume is delivered from the device, whereas a "pressure ventilator" ends inspiration when a preset system pressure is achieved.

By adding the mechanism used to initiate inspiration to our categorization scheme, we can refine our understanding of the device. For example, use of the term "volume-cycled assistor/controller" not only tells us that the device ends inspiration after a preset volume is delivered, but also that the patient can initiate ventilation at a faster rate than the minimum value set by the operator.

Further elaboration on classification using phase variables would include a description of the ventilator's in-

spiratory phase. For example, use of the term "time-cycled, constant flow, assistor/controller" conveys additional information essential in understanding the clinical application of a ventilator. In this case, knowledge of the nature of the inspiratory phase (constant flow generator) in combination with a description of the means by which inspiration is terminated (time-cycled) informs us that this device is functionally equivalent to a volume-cycled ventilator. Specifically, by setting the flow and inspiratory time, a time-cycled, constant flow generator will yield a consistent breath-by-breath volume.

Finally, by including a description of the ventilator's expiratory phase, we can better understand the clinical options available to support the patient in respiratory failure. For example, it is important to know if the device allows the patient to breathe spontaneously between mechanically provided breaths (IMV mode) and, if available, the nature and type of PEEP control.

Clinical interaction of phase variables. The major importance of phase variables in ventilator classification is more than just descriptive. Understanding how phase variables interact under conditions of changing lung characteristics represents an essential skill for the respiratory care practitioner.[17]

Because of the large number of possible combinations, we will limit our discussion of phase variable interaction to that occurring between the end-inspiratory cycling mechanism (volume, pressure, time, or flow cycling) and the nature of the inspiratory phase (flow or pressure generator). For simplicity, we will assume in each case that continuous mandatory ventilation (CMV) in the control mode is being used, with a constant expiratory time.

Flow generators. As described in Chapter 29, if a ventilator is a flow generator (either constant or nonconstant), then changes in compliance or resistance will affect the pressure waveform delivered to the patient. The nature and magnitude of this effect depends on how the ventilator cycles to end inspiration. Table 30-1 demonstrates the effect of increased impedance (decreased compliance and/or increased resistance) on a flow generator that cycles to end inspiration by volume, pressure, or time. For completeness, the time-cycled/pressure-limited mode is also included.

As can be seen, both the volume and time-cycled flow generators behave in a similar fashion when faced with an increased impedance. Specifically, when faced with a decrease in compliance and/or an increase in resistance,

Table 30-1 Flow Generator–Increased Impedance

Cycling mechanism	Effect on volume	Effect on pressure	Effect on inspiratory time	Effect on rate (exp. time constant)
Volume	—	Increased	—	—
Pressure	Decreased	—	Decreased	Increased
Time	—	Increased	—	—
Time/pressure limited	Decreased	—	—	—

these devices continue to deliver a constant volume, but at a higher system pressure. Delivered volume will decrease only if a preset pressure limit causes the ventilator to prematurely end inspiration. This type of interaction would be typical of most piston and high-pressure, pneumatic-driven ventilators that cycle to end inspiration by volume or time, such as the Emerson models 3-PV and 3-MV, the Bennett 7200 Series, the Siemens Servo 900 Series, the BEAR Series, the Monaghan 225/SIMV, and the Hamilton Veolar ventilator.

On the other hand, when a flow generator that cycles to end inspiration by pressure encounters increased impedance, less volume is delivered, the inspiratory time decreases, and (assuming a constant expiratory time) the rate or frequency of breathing increases. A classic example of this type of interaction would occur with the Bird Mark 7 and 8 ventilators in the pure source gas mode.

Finally, when a flow generator that is time cycled and pressure limited encounters increased impedance, the only change in the parameters of ventilation will be a decrease in the delivered volume. This condition would be common in neonatal ventilatory support, where the time-cycled/pressure-limited mode is the predominant approach currently used (see Chapter 32).

Pressure generators. With constant pressure generators, the interaction among phase variables is a little more complex. This is because the flow delivered by a pressure generator varies with changes in the mechanical characteristics of the patient's lungs and thorax. For this reason, it is necessary to separately discuss the effects of increased resistance and decreased compliance.

Increased resistance. Table 30-2 summarizes the effect of increased resistance on pressure generators that cycle to expiration by either volume, pressure, time, or flow. As is evident, when the volume-cycled constant-pressure generator is faced with increased resistance, the preset volume is still delivered (as long as the pressure limit is not reached), but at a higher working pressure. However, because inspiratory flow decreases, it takes longer to deliver this preset volume. Thus, with the expiratory time held constant, the frequency of mechanical breaths must decrease. This lower rate will result in a decrease in minute ventilation.

How a pressure-cycled constant-pressure generator responds to increased resistance depends on the degree of

obstruction present. When faced with high resistance, a pressure-cycled constant pressure generator will cycle off prematurely. As a result, inspiratory time will decrease and the rate of ventilation will increase. A similar response is noted with constant pressure generators that end inspiration when a low terminal flow is reached (flow-cycled ventilators).

However, when the increase in resistance is moderate, these devices will typically respond with a decrease in flow. Under these circumstances, the delivered volume is still decreased, but the inspiratory time may actually increase, resulting in a decreased rate (with expiratory time constant). These responses are typical of pressure-cycled ventilators using a low-pressure, pneumatic-drive system, such as the Bennett PR-II (pressure reducing valve) and the Bird Mark 7 and 8 in the air mix mode (venturi).

Finally, a time-cycled constant-pressure generator typically responds to an increase in resistance with a decrease in delivered volume. Under such circumstances, system pressure is usually increased.

Decreased compliance. Table 30-3 summarizes the impact of decreased compliance on pressure generators that cycle to expiration by either volume, pressure, time, or flow. As evident, the response is generally the same as that which occurs with increased resistance, except for the pressure-cycled category. In this case, the response is most similar to conditions of high airway resistance: a decrease in delivered volume and inspiratory time and an increase in the rate of ventilation.

In all cases above, if the ventilator maintains a constant rate (as opposed to a constant expiratory time), the major time variable affected would be the I:E ratio. Thus, if the rate was constant and the inspiratory time increased, the I:E ratio would rise. However, if the rate was constant and the inspiratory time decreased, the I:E ratio would fall. The interaction of time variables in these examples, particularly the rate and I:E ratio, assumes control mode ventilation.

It should also be noted that several new generation ventilators provide a variety of inspiratory phase options. Typically, a constant flow option represents the primary mode, with either decelerating flow (mimicking the constant pressure generator) or accelerating/decelerating flow (mimicking the nonconstant flow generator) available.

Table 30-2 Constant Pressure Generator–Increased Resistance

Cycling mechanisms	Effect on volume	Effect on pressure	Effect on inspiratory time	Effect on rate (exp. time constant)
Volume	—	Increased	Increased	Decreased
Pressure	Decreased	—	Increased (mod. R)	Decreased (mod. R)
			Decreased (high R)	Increased (high R)
Time	Decreased	May be increased	—	—
Flow	Decreased	—	Decreased	Increased

Classification examples

Table 30-4 applies the power, control, and phase variables to the classification of selected modern intermittent positive-pressure differential ventilators used in respiratory care. It is suggested that the reader apply the principles of classification to these and other specific devices, ideally by first working with the applicable apparatus in a controlled laboratory setting that allows simulated experimentation.

VENTILATOR CIRCUITRY

All ventilators employ an external tubing circuit that delivers fresh gas to the patient and provides a means for exhaled gases to be diverted out to the atmosphere. Understanding this external ventilator circuitry is important for two reasons. First, the ventilator circuitry provides the primary means for many monitoring and therapeutic functions associated with ventilatory support. Second, the external ventilator circuitry plays a major role in the compressed volume loss that characterizes positive pressure ventilation.

Components of a ventilator circuit

Fig. 30-17 shows the major components common to positive pressure breathing circuits. As shown in Figure 30-17, *A,* five essential elements constitute this patient circuit[18]:

1. A main inspiratory line to deliver fresh gas from the ventilator to the patient connector;
2. A connector to the patient's airway;
3. An expiratory line to divert exhaled gases out to the atmosphere;
4. An expiratory valve that blocks gas outflow during the inspiratory phase of mechanical ventilation; and
5. An expiratory valve line that powers the expiratory valve.

Together, these basic components are often referred to as a "Y" circuit, with the inspiratory and expiratory limbs forming the forks of the Y and the patient connector the tail.

Functionally, when a ventilator cycles to begin inspiration, two events occur simultaneously. As fresh gas begins to flow through the main inspiratory line, the expiratory valve is pressurized, closing the patient circuit to the atmosphere. Once the expiratory valve is closed, gas can flow only into the patient's lungs. At end-inspiration, the ventilator cycles off, and the expiratory valve opens to atmosphere. Exhaled gases from the patient now follow the path of least resistance, out the open expiratory port and into the atmosphere.

With fresh gas entering via one line and exhaled gas exiting through a separate limb, the dead space of the Y circuit is limited to the small volume of two-way gas flow in the patient connector (usually 5 to 10 ml). This design minimizes rebreathing of expired gases. However, any addition of tubing *between* the patient connector and the patient airway will increase mechanical dead space and rebreathed volume, thereby increasing the inspired P_{CO_2} and potentially raising the P_{ACO_2}.

Variations from this simple configuration are common, particularly as related to the design of the expiratory valve. Many ventilators, such as the Siemens Servo 900 Series and the BEAR BP-200 Infant ventilator, use an electromechanical, as opposed to pneumatic, expiratory valve.[10] The expiratory valve can also provide additional functions, including the generation and maintenance of positive airway pressure.

Beyond these five essential components, external ventilator circuits typically include other functional enhancements (Fig. 30-17, *B*). A pressure manometer, *1,* provides continuous monitoring of working pressures, ideally through a direct line to the patient connector, *2*. This configuration allows accurate monitoring of proximal airway pressure, as opposed to pressures elsewhere in the system.

Another important consideration in a patient circuit is the incorporation of a device to monitor the patient's expired volume, *6*. Typically such devices operate either by accumulating expired gases (such as the Bennett Monitoring Spirometer shown in Fig. 30-18) or by measuring exhaled flow and electronically converting it to volume (such as the ultrasonic flow transducer shown in Fig. 30-19). Depending on the circuit design, an expired volume monitor may be placed at or near the patient connector, or distal to the circuit's expiratory valve, *4*.

A humidification device, *9,* is also a standard consideration in a patient ventilator circuit. Although a heat and moisture exchanger may serve this purpose, such devices typically operate via the cascade or wick principle, incorporating both a heating element, and thermostat, *10* (see Chapter 23). Whenever inspired gases are heated to

Table 30-3   Constant Pressure Generator–Decreased Compliance

Cycling mechanism	Effect on volume	Effect on pressure	Effect on inspiratory time	Effect on rate (exp. time constant)
Volume	—	Increased	Increased	Decreased
Pressure	Decreased	—	Decreased	Increased
Time	Decreased	Increased	—	—
Flow	Decreased	—	Decreased	Increased

Table 30-4   Ventilator Classification Examples

Ventilator	Power source	Circuitry	Power application	Control mechanism	Phase variables				
					Initiating inspiration	Inspiratory phase	Ending inspiration	Expiratory phase	
BEAR LS104-150	Combined	Single	Linear drive piston	Electronic	Assist/control	Constant flow	Volume-cycled	PEEP	
BEAR BP-200	Pneumatic	Single	Pneumatic (high)	Electronic	Control	Constant flow	Time-cycled#	IMV/PEEP/CPAP	
BEAR Cub (BP-2001)	Pneumatic	Single	Pneumatic (high)	Electronic	Control	Constant flow	Time-cycled#	IMV/PEEP/CPAP	
BEAR-1	Pneumatic	Single	Pneumatic (variable)	Electronic	Assist/control	Constant flow*	Volume-cycled	SIMV/PEEP/CPAP	
BEAR-2	Pneumatic	Single	Pneumatic (variable)	Electronic	Assist/control	Constant flow	Volume-cycled	SIMV/PEEP/CPAP	
BEAR-5	Pneumatic	Single	Pneumatic (high)	Electronic	Assist/control	Constant flow	Volume-cycled	SIMV/PEEP/CPAP/MMV	
Bennett MA-1	Combined	Double	Pneumatic (low)	Electronic	Assist/control	Constant pressure	Volume-cycled	Simple CMV+	
Bennett MA-2	Combined	Double	Pneumatic (low)	Electronic	Assist/control	Constant pressure	Volume-cycled	SIMV/PEEP/CPAP	
Bennett 7200	Pneumatic	Single	Pneumatic (high)	Electronic	Assist/control	Constant flow	Volume-cycled	SIMV/PEEP/CPAP	
Bio-Med MVP-10	Pneumatic	Single	Pneumatic (high)	Fluidic	Control	Constant flow	Time-cycled#	IMV/PEEP/CPAP	
Bio-Med IC-5	Pneumatic	Single	Pneumatic (high)	Electronic	Assist/control	Constant flow	Volume-cycled	SIMV/PEEP/CPAP	
Bird Mark 7/8	Pneumatic	Single	Pneumatic (variable)	Pneumatic	Assist/control	Constant pressure	Pressure-cycled	Simple CMV+	
BabyBird	Pneumatic	Single	Pneumatic (high)	Pneumatic	Control	Constant flow	Time-cycled#	IMV/PEEP/CPAP	
BabyBird 2	Pneumatic	Single	Pneumatic (high)	Electronic	Control	Constant flow	Time-cycled#	IMV/PEEP/CPAP	
Hamilton Veolar	Pneumatic	Single	Pneumatic (high)	Electronic	Assist/control	Constant flow	Volume-cycled	SIMV/PEEP/CPAP/MMV	
IMV Bird	Pneumatic	Single	Pneumatic (high)	Pneumatic	Control	Constant pressure	Time-cycled	IMV/PEEP/CPAP	
Emerson 3PV	Combined	Single	Rotary drive piston	Electronic	Control+	Nonconstant flow	Time/volume-cycled	Simple CMV+	
Emerson IMV	Combined	Single	Rotary drive piston	Electronic	Control+	Nonconstant flow	Time/volume-cycled	IMV/PEEP/CPAP	
Engstrom ER300	Combined	Double	Rotary drive piston	Electronic	Control	Nonconstant flow	Time/volume-cycled	PEEP	
Engstrom Erica	Pneumatic	Single	Pneumatic (high)	Electronic	Assist/control	Constant flow*	Volume-cycled	SIMV/PEEP/CPAP/MMV	
Healthdyne 102/105	Pneumatic	Single	Pneumatic (high)	Electronic	Control	Constant flow	Time-cycled#	IMV/PEEP/CPAP	
Monaghan 225	Pneumatic	Double	Pneumatic (high)	Fluidic	Assist/control	Constant flow	Volume-cycled	SIMV/PEEP/CPAP	
Ohmeda CPU-1	Pneumatic	Single	Pneumatic (high)	Electronic	Assist/control	Constant flow	Time-cycled	SIMV/PEEP/CPAP/MMV	
Searle VVA	Pneumatic	Single	Pneumatic/spring	Electronic	Assist/control	Constant flow*	Volume-cycled	SIMV/PEEP	
Sechrist IV-100B	Pneumatic	Single	Pneumatic (high)	Fluidic/Elec	Control	Constant flow	Time-cycled#	IMV/PEEP/CPAP	
Servo 900 B & C	Pneumatic	Single	Pneumatic (variable)	Electronic	Assist/control	Constant flow*	Volume-cycled	SIMV/PEEP/CPAP	

Notes: + indicates a standard function; may be modified by optional equipment
  * constant flow (square wave) is primary mode; may be modified by user
  # usually combined with a pressure limit (time-cycled, pressure-limited ventilation)

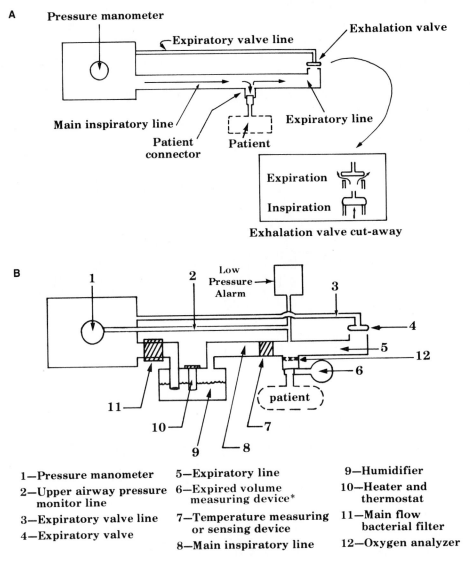

A Pressure manometer

Expiratory valve line

Exhalation valve

Main inspiratory line

Patient connector

Patient

Expiratory line

Expiration

Inspiration

Exhalation valve cut-away

B

1   2   Low Pressure Alarm   3   4   5   12   6

11   10   9   8   7   patient

1—Pressure manometer
2—Upper airway pressure monitor line
3—Expiratory valve line
4—Expiratory valve

5—Expiratory line
6—Expired volume measuring device*
7—Temperature measuring or sensing device
8—Main inspiratory line

9—Humidifier
10—Heater and thermostat
11—Main flow bacterial filter
12—Oxygen analyzer

Fig. 30-17   **A,** Basic components of a patient circuit required to provide a positive-pressure breath. During inspiration the expiratory valve closes and air is forced into the patient's lungs. **B,** A patient circuit containing additional components required for optimum functioning during continuous mechanical ventilation. (From Pilbeam SP: Mechanical ventilation: physiological and clinical applications, St Louis, 1986, The CV Mosby Co.)

help achieve saturation, a temperature measuring, or sensing, device also must be included in the patient circuit, 7.

In order to protect the patient from infectious agents that may be present in the inspired gas, most patient circuits incorporate a bacterial filter, 11, in the main inspiratory line. Typically, these filters are of the high-efficiency particulate air (HEPA) design, using inertial impaction to trap particulate matter as small as 0.3 μm in the gas stream. Finally, a patient circuit may incorporate an in-line oxygen analyzer to provide continuous monitoring of the FIO_2, 12.

Compressed volume

A key consideration related to the patient circuit is the fact that not all the volume delivered by a positive-

pressure ventilator reaches the patient. There are two reasons for this apparent loss of delivered volume. First, gases under pressure are compressed within both the internal and external (patient) ventilator circuit. Second, depending on its compliance, the tubing in the circuit will expand during inspiration. In combination, these factors effectively remove a portion of the delivered volume from participation in ventilation of the patient. When expiration begins, this "trapped" gas will flow out the exhalation valve, but will never have entered the patient's airways. This part of the tidal volume never reaching the patient is commonly referred to as the *compressed volume*.

The volume of trapped gases during inspiration is a function of (1) the internal volume of the ventilator circuit,

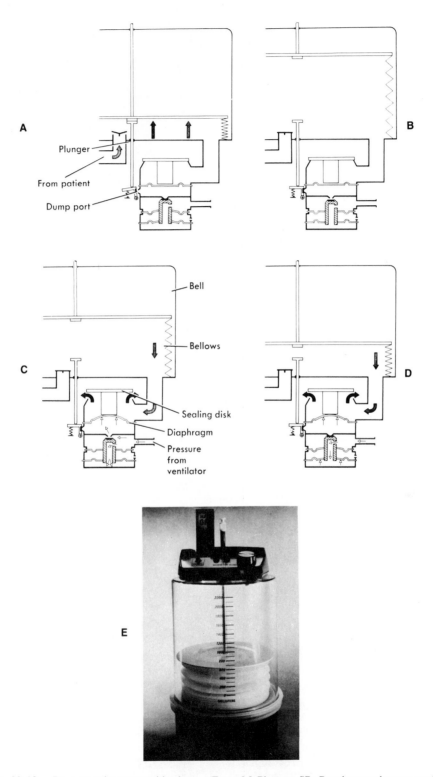

Fig. 30-18   Bennett spirometer with alarm. (From McPherson SP: Respiratory therapy equipment, ed 4, St Louis, 1989, The CV Mosby Co.)

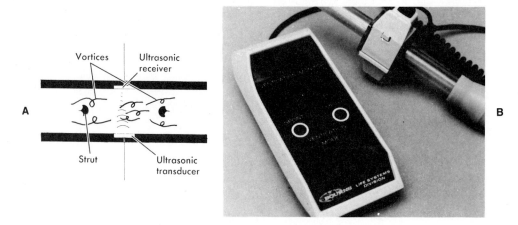

Fig. 30-19   **A,** Functional diagram of vortex shedding-ultrasonic flow transducer. **B,** Bourns LS-75. (**A** modified from Bourns Medical Systems, Inc, Riverside, Calif; from McPherson SP: Respiratory therapy equipment, ed 4, St Louis, 1989, The CV Mosby Co.)

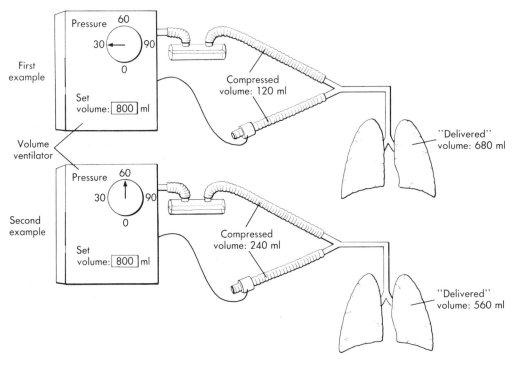

Fig. 30-20   Comparison of volumes delivered to a patient under different end-inspiratory pressures with a volume-cycled ventilator. See text for description of this example.

(2) the compliance of the ventilator system, and (3) the pressure applied. If all the volume used to compress gas is rigid, such as a piston cylinder and stiff, noncompliant tubing, then the amount of compressed volume is about 1 ml/cm H_2O/L of internal ventilator volume.[1] As an example, a ventilator and tubing system having a 4 L noncompliant circuit at end-inspiration would compress about 4 ml of gas/cm H_2O pressure applied. For this example, this system has a "compression factor" of 4 ml/cm H_2O. If the tubing could stretch under pressure, then more volume per

unit of pressure could be trapped, such as 5 ml/cm H_2O. This factor is also referred to as the *compliance factor,* a term generally interchangeable with compression factor.

Fig. 30-20 illustrates the clinical significance of the compression factor for a volume ventilator. In the first example, the tidal volume is set for 800 ml, and the pressure generated at end-inspiration is 30 cm H_2O. In this example, a 4 ml/cm H_2O compression factor is used. To find out how much of the tidal volume is compressed in the system, the airway pressure is multiplied by the factor: 30

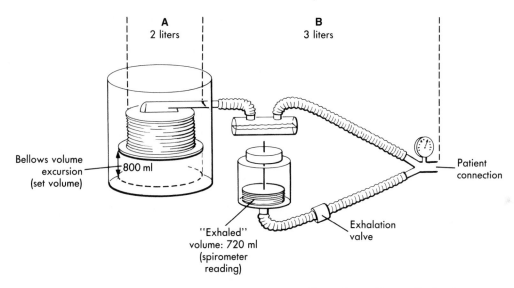

Fig. 30-21 Comparison of internal volume, **A,** and tubing volume, **B,** contributing to compressed volume with a volume-cycled ventilator. See text for description of this example.

$\times$ 4 = 120. Thus, only 680 ml of the set 800 ml actually reaches the patient's airways, while the remaining 120 ml is "trapped" in the system.

Assume that the patient's compliance decreases and, for the second example of Fig. 30-20, is now requiring 60 cm H_2O pressure at end-inspiration. Using the same factor of 4 ml/cm H_2O we multiply the pressure by the factor again: 60 $\times$ 4 = 240. Now only 560 ml of the set 800 reaches the patient, while 240 is compressed in the system. This is a significant drop in patient ventilation, although the majority of the set volume is still delivered.

It should also be appreciated that if the tidal volume were initially 400 ml, and the factor the same, a similar change in ventilating pressures would result in a larger relative change in patient ventilation. Generally, the smaller the tidal volume desired, the smaller the compression factor desired. This is primarily accomplished by using smaller diameter tubing circuits and by using ventilators that have minimal internal volumes, which contribute to the compressed volume.

One practical point about compressed volume is when exhaled volumes are measured from the exhalation valve of a ventilator circuit, the compressed volume of the tubing circuit is also collected. Therefore, an estimation of the patient's exhaled volume can be made by subtracting the amount of calculated compressed volume from the total collected at the exhalation valve. If the ventilator has a large amount of internal volume besides the volume of the external tubing circuit, there can be a discrepancy between the tidal volume set and the amount collected at the exhalation valve. Fig. 30-21 illustrates this point. In this example, the internal volume is 2 L, yielding a factor of 2 ml/cm H_2O, and the tubing circuit volume is 3 L, yielding a factor of 3 ml/cm H_2O. These two factors together mean 5 ml/cm H_2O pressure will be compressed and "lost" to the

patient each breath. However, only the amount compressed in the external tubing (3 ml/cm H_2O) will be collected with the patient's exhaled gases because the internal system returns to atmospheric pressure while the bellows falls and refills. The one-way valve shown at the bellows outlet closes, and any compressed gases within simply expand. Thus, if end-inspiratory pressure is 40 cm H_2O, the set volume is 800 ml; then 80 ml is compressed internally (40 $\times$ 2), 120 ml is compressed externally (40 $\times$ 3), and the patient receives the remaining 600 ml. Only the patient's 600 ml and the tubing's 120 ml are collected during exhalation, while 80 ml remain in the bellows. The set volume of 800 ml differs then from the 720 ml collected because of the internal compressed gas. To determine what the patient received in this example from the exhaled gases, only the 3 ml/cm H_2O factor is subtracted from the collected amount on the spirometer.

MODES OF VENTILATORY SUPPORT

The selection and use of ventilatory support devices depends, in part, on the primary mode of ventilation chosen. Chapters 28 and 29 provided details on the nature of these various modes and their appropriate application to selected groups of patients. In this section, we will focus on how these modes are applied clinically. Specifically, we will analyze the mechanical and physiologic techniques involved in applying controlled ventilation, IMV, PEEP, CPAP, pressure support ventilation (PSV), and mandatory minute ventilation (MMV) to patients using a variety of ventilatory support devices.

Controlled ventilation

As described in Chapter 29, controlled ventilation is in force when the frequency of cycling to inspiration is established by the ventilator according to a predetermined time interval, independent of the patient's efforts or breathing pattern. With the parameters of ventilation entirely in the hands of the clinician, controlled ventilation is the only mode of ventilatory support that can provide precise and consistently predictable physiologic results.

Indications. For this reason, controlled ventilation is the preferred mode of ventilatory support when the desire is to maintain a precise minute ventilation or Pa_{CO_2}, such as in patients with an unstable or changing ventilatory drive. Moreover, controlled ventilation is often useful when the patient's spontaneous breathing efforts in the assist/control or IMV modes would cause either undue work (as with muscle fatigue) or create an undesirable acid-base imbalance (as with hyperventilation syndrome or severe anxiety).

Clinical application. Technically, controlled ventilation is among the simplest modes of ventilatory support to apply, requiring only a ventilator that can be set to prevent patient cycling. Thus, the challenge of controlled ventilation lies not so much in the design of the apparatus as in the management of the patient.

Controlled ventilation is poorly tolerated by many patients, often resulting in asynchronous breathing efforts against the mechanically controlled breaths, or strenuous, but futile attempts to breathe spontaneously. Both conditions can dramatically increase the work of breathing, and with it, the oxygen consumption of the respiratory muscles. Clearly, these adverse effects can negate any advantages to the use of this mode of ventilatory support and have been cited by some as a reason for abandoning this approach altogether.[19] However, most clinicians would argue that controlled ventilation still has a proper, although limited, place in the support of selected patients in respiratory failure.

Suppression of ventilation. Suppression of ventilation by simply "locking the patient out" (placing the ventilator in the control mode) is not acceptable. To be successful, controlled ventilation generally will require some physiologic suppression of the patient's ventilatory efforts. This may be accomplished using several methods. These methods include oxygen suppression of breathing and the use of either tranquilizing agents, sedative-hypnotics, narcotic-analgesics, or neuromuscular blocking agents.[20]

Oxygen suppression of breathing. Oxygen suppression of breathing is especially effective for the patient with long-standing chronic hypercapnia, whose ventilation is mainly dependent on a hypoxic stimulus. We have previously discussed the role played by the peripheral chemoreceptors in chronic hypercapnia accompanying chronic pulmonary disease. We stressed the hazards involved in the indiscriminate use of supplemental oxygen to such patients for fear of inactivating the hypoxic chemoreceptor drive and rendering the patient apneic. Now we do exactly that, inactivate the hypoxic chemoreceptor drive, so that we can

eliminate the patient's own breathing and provide controlled ventilation.

The patient is given an increased F_{IO_2} (usually 70% is sufficient) through the ventilator or by means of a tracheostomy T-tube or mask, for a period not to exceed 10 minutes; results should be realized in that length of time if at all. As the patient becomes hypopneic and ventilatory activity decreases, he or she is placed in the control mode at an appropriate tidal volume and rate. Once the patient is stabilized, the oxygen concentration can be reduced to a safe level. Close observation must be maintained to ensure that the patient remains under adequate control and does not return to the previous pattern. If this procedure is unsuccessful, a tranquilizing agent, sedative-hypnotic, narcotic-analgesic, or neuromuscular blocking agent may be administered.

Tranquilizing agents. The major agents in this category of drugs useful in supporting controlled ventilation are the benzodiazepines, including diazepam (Valium), chlordiazepoxide HCL (Librium), lorazepam (Ativan), and midazolam (Versed). These tranquilizing or anxiolytic agents are all characterized by a high therapeutic dose ratio, low incidence of respiratory depression and excessive sedation, and minimal cardiovascular side effects. Since respiratory depression is minimal at therapeutic dose levels, the benzodiazepines are used mainly to calm the anxious or agitated patient being supported by controlled ventilation. Generally, other more powerful agents will be required to actually suppress breathing.

The exception to this generalization is midazolam. Midazolam doses of 0.15 mg/kg significantly reduce the ventilatory response to CO_2.[21] For this reason, and because of its physical stability, short duration of action, rapid clearance, and minimal activity of its metabolite products, midazolam is the benzodiazepine of choice for IV infusion in patients requiring controlled ventilation.[20]

Sedative-hypnotics. Among the sedative-hypnotics most useful in supporting controlled ventilation are agents commonly used in the induction of anesthesia, such as sodium thiopental (Pentothal) and etomidate (Amidate).

Sodium thiopental is an ultra short-acting barbiturate that has been used successfully as a continuous infusion to sedate patients receiving controlled ventilation.[22] Because of its high pH, sodium thiopental is not compatible with certain acidic agents, and care must be taken to prevent extravasation into the tissues. Myocardial depression is usually limited to a decrease in heart rate during infusion. However, motor responses may take as long as 48 hours to return after cessation of administration.[20]

Etomidate is a nonbarbiturate sedative-hypnotic typically used for the induction and maintenance of anesthesia. It is characterized by a rapid onset of action and recovery. Etomidate has no direct cardiovascular effects and does not cause the release of histamine. However, etomidate may cause suppression of adrenocortical function, thereby abolishing the stress response and indirectly affecting the cardiovascular system.[20] As an agent to support controlled ventilation, etomidate is commonly used in conjunction with a narcotic-analgesic, such as fentanyl.[23]

Narcotic-analgesics. Among the narcotic-analgesics used to support controlled ventilation, morphine sulfate is the best known. Morphine is a potent addictive narcotic with the ability to relieve pain, produce lethargy, and induce a deep-to-stuporous sleep. One of its most specific activities, however, is its depression of ventilation by direct suppression of the medullary respiratory center. Like high concentrations of oxygen, morphine is contraindicated in general medical use in any patient with a compromised ventilatory drive; many deaths have been attributed to its use in patients with asthma, chronic bronchopulmonary disease, and cerebral injury. The respiratory depressant effect of morphine is directly related to its dosage. The respiratory response is a decrease in both frequency and tidal volume.

When used to abolish spontaneous breathing, morphine can be best controlled if given by intravenous injection. By this route, maximum respiratory depression for a given dose occurs within 10 minutes, compared with one hour or more if given intramuscularly. There are no hard-and-fast rules for its administration, but 5 mg given intravenously, repeated every 10 minutes (to a maximum of 20 mg for the series) until the desired effect is realized, represents a common approach. In most patients, if morphine is to be effective, its impact will occur before this amount of the drug has been used. For maintenance, 2 to 3 mg can be given as needed to keep the patient well sedated.

The duration of morphine therapy is usually too short to warrant concern over addiction, but there are occasional side effects that can prove troublesome. Among the most common are nausea and vomiting, which sometimes preclude further use of the drug. Peristalsis is also retarded or stopped by morphine. This can lead to gaseous distention of the bowel severe enough to impair diaphragmatic motion and interfere with ventilation.

The major problem with morphine, however, is its tendency to cause histamine release, and a resultant vasodilation and hypotension.[20] In general, these potential side effects limit the use of morphine in patients with abnormal vasomotor tone or minimal cardiovascular reserve. Because they do not cause histamine release, artificial opiate agonists such as fentanyl (Sublimaze) and its derivatives have been suggested as a substitute for morphine in the application of controlled ventilation. However, at high doses, patients can develop tolerance to these agents. Moreover, these synthetic opiate agonists can have other side effects, such as causing chest wall rigidity, seizures, and respiratory arrest.[20] For this reason, unless pain is contributing to the difficulty in applying controlled ventilation, agents other than the narcotic-analgesics should be considered first.

Neuromuscular blocking agents. A neuromuscular blocking agent is a drug that blocks the transmission of motor nerve impulses to skeletal muscles, effectively paralyzing those muscles. These agents have no CNS activity and do not by themselves alter the patient's level of consciousness, memory, or pain threshold.

There are two major categories of neuromuscular blocking agents: competitive (nondepolarizing) and depolarizing. Competitive neuromuscular blocking agents, such as d-tubocurarine, bind to the acetylcholine receptor sites on the postjunctional membrane, competitively inhibiting acetylcholine from contacting these receptors. This prevents depolarization and muscle contraction. Depolarizing agents, such as succinylcholine (Anectine), also induce paralysis by blocking the acetylcholine receptors of the postjunctional membrane. However, the initial effect is to depolarize the membrane, resulting in a brief period of fine muscle contractions (fasciculations), followed by paralysis.

d-Tubocurarine. d-Tubocurarine is a plant alkaloid whose paralyzing action has been known for centuries and that has been widely used in anesthesiology for many years. When given intravenously (the route of choice), its action is evident in 3 to 5 minutes, lasting about 40 minutes; a dose of 15 mg may be used almost as needed until the desired effect is reached. Since it is a competitive blocking agent, its action can be reversed by administration of an acetylcholinesterase inhibitor, such as neostigmine methylsulfate (Prostigmin).

d-Tubocurarine has many potential side effects. Because of its blocking effect on the sympathetic ganglia, large doses may precipitate hypotension, already a threat to a mechanically ventilated patient. Perhaps even more relevant to patients in respiratory failure is the severe bronchospasm that may follow curarine's use. This bronchospasm is caused both by curarine's effect on the sympathetic ganglia and by the release of histamine.[24]

Pancuronium bromide (Pavulon). Pancuronium bromide is a synthetic competitive blocking agent with a potency some five times that of d-tubocurarine. Unlike d-tubocurarine, pancuronium bromide has little histamine releasing effect and does not block sympathetic ganglia. For this reason, pancuronium bromide does not cause bronchospasm or hypotension. Indeed, pancuronium bromide exhibits vagolytic activity, causing a rise in both pulse rate and systolic blood pressure by as much as 20%.[25] Tachyarrhythmias have also been reported with pancuronium bromide.[26]

Dosage varies with the duration of effect intended. For maintenance of paralysis during controlled ventilation, 4 to 5 mg of pancuronium bromide can be given at intervals of 1 to 3 hours, depending on response. Alternatively, a continuous infusion, at rates between 0.35 to 1.0 μg/kg/min may be used.[20] As with d-tubocurarine, the action of pancuronium bromide can be reversed by administration of an acetylcholinesterase inhibitor.

Succinylcholine (Anectine). Unlike d-tubocurarine and pancuronium bromide, succinylcholine is a depolarizing neuromuscular blocking agent. Also given intravenously, succinylcholine has both a rapid onset and short duration of action, reaching its maximum effect in about two minutes and disappearing within 5 minutes. For this reason, its main use has been in general surgery to provide rapid relaxation for short procedures such as instrumentation. For respiratory suppression, a single dose of 20 mg may be given to test the patient's response or to initiate ventilation and may be repeated as needed until a good ventilatory pattern is established. A smoother response will accompany its prolonged administration in an intravenous infusion, as a 0.1% solution, run at a rate of 2 to 3 mg/min. Because the action is so short, close control over the depth of paralysis can be maintained merely by adjusting the infusion flow. Intravenous succinylcholine administration has been associated with acute cardiovascular collapse. It is believed this is caused by a sudden rise in serum potassium concentration (hyperkalemia) with resulting myocardial depression and ventricular arrhythmias.[27]

Neuromuscular blocking agents must be used under the closest supervision, and patients must never be left unattended. If patients are alert before the administration of blocking agents, they should first be tranquilized or sedated, since the completely helpless feeling of paralysis to patients aware of their condition can be one of the most frightening of experiences.

Intermittent mandatory ventilation (IMV)

As described in Chapter 29, intermittent mandatory ventilation is a mode of ventilation that allows the patient to breathe spontaneously between periodic positive pressure breaths.[28,29] These periodic breaths may be controlled (simple IMV) or assisted (synchronous intermittent mandatory ventilation, or SIMV). IMV may also be combined with PEEP or pressure support ventilation (PSV), both discussed later.

Indications. Considerable controversy still exists regarding the appropriate indications for IMV. Many advocate its use mainly as a method to facilitate weaning,[30] while others claim that IMV should be used as the primary mode of ventilatory support.[19,28] The fact is that many of the purported advantages of IMV have yet to be studied in a controlled fashion.[31]

Clearly, IMV encourages activity of the ventilatory muscles, thereby helping to prevent ventilator dependence. However, there are two additional physiologic benefits of great significance. First, in contrast to the control or assist/control modes, during which the parameters of ventilation are imposed on the patient, the true spontaneous breathing characterizing IMV allows the patient's respiratory center to respond normally to real gas exchange needs. During IMV, the patient's own respiratory drive sets the ventilatory pattern, maintaining a blood carbon dioxide level po-

tentially more suitable to the patient's needs. Second, under the influence of positive-pressure ventilation, intrapleural pressure rises abnormally during each tidal volume, elevating the mean pleural pressure. The major risk of such pressure is its retarding effect on venous return and cardiac output. On the other hand, the spontaneous breaths of IMV cause a drop in intrapleural pressure. The mean intrapleural pressure is thus a function of the ratio of machine to spontaneous breaths, decreasing as patients take over more of their own breathing. For patients in overt, or potential, cardiac failure this may be the most important benefit of IMV.

Despite these proven advantages, IMV must not be viewed as an indispensable ingredient in all ventilator management or as a solution to all management problems.[31,32] We must be careful not to burden some patients too early or too frequently with their own breathing. They may have an adequate central drive to breathe spontaneously, but because of their disease, may not possess adequate musculoskeletal power to convert the drive into significant tidal volumes. For such patients, the assist/control mode may be safer and more effective than IMV until resolution of the underlying disease process can be achieved.[31,33]

Technique. During IMV, some system must provide fresh gas by which spontaneous breathing can occur at a rate and volume that is patient determined. Currently there are two major categories of IMV systems: continuous flow and demand flow.[1,10,34,35] In general, continuous-flow IMV systems are special circuits added to ventilators not equipped with their own IMV mechanism. Demand-flow IMV systems are incorporated into most newer generation ventilators.

Continuous-flow IMV. As the name implies, continuous-flow IMV systems employ a constant flow of fresh gas from which the patient can spontaneously breathe. There are two primary variations of the continuous-flow IMV system: (1) ambient reservoir IMV (also called the parallel flow or "H" system) and (2) pressure reservoir IMV.

Ambient reservoir IMV. Ambient reservoir IMV is the simplest type of equipment adaptation for providing a constant flow of fresh gas to the patient. As shown in Fig. 30-22, a separate blended gas source provides continuous flow through a heated humidifier to a T connector with an open (ambient pressure) reservoir. The T connector attaches this spontaneous breathing circuit to the inspiratory limb of the ventilator circuit. A one-way valve separates the two circuits. During positive-pressure breaths provided by the machine, this one-way valve closes, and gas under pressure goes to the patient as usual.

Should the patient attempt to breathe spontaneously between mechanical breaths, the drop in airway and system pressure will open the one-way valve, allowing the blended gas to be drawn in through the spontaneous breathing circuit. In this respect, the spontaneous breathing circuit functions much like a high-flow oxygen deliv-

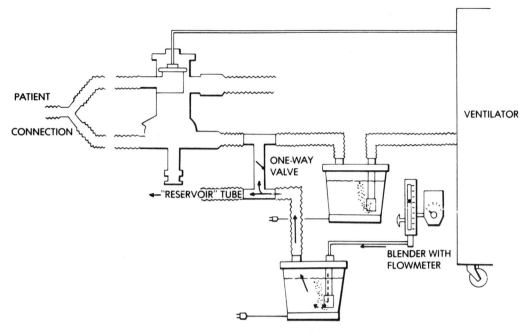

Fig. 30-22   Ambient reservoir IMV system. Gas from the blender passes through a separate humidifier, past a one-way valve, and out the reservoir tube. See text for description. (From Kirby RR, Smith RA, and Desautels DD, editors: Mechanical ventilation, New York, 1985, Churchill Livingstone.)

ery system, requiring sufficient flow to meet the inspiratory demands of the patient (see Chapter 25). Although the added reservoir tube provides some margin of safety in order to prevent dilution with room air, flows through this type of system should generally equal or exceed three times the patient's minute ventilation.

During spontaneous exhalation, the slight rise in system pressure will close the one-way valve, allowing the patient's expired gases to escape out through the open expiratory port of the ventilator circuit. During this phase, gas continues to flow uninterrupted through the spontaneous breathing circuit out to the atmosphere, while replenishing the open reservoir. Since the spontaneous breathing circuit is parallel to (as opposed to in-line with) the ventilator circuit, its continuous flow never enters the ventilator circuit. This allows the patient's exhaled gases to be separated from the continuous flow of the IMV system. Thus, expired gas monitoring, such as volume collection in a spirometer, occurs as usual.

Despite its simplicity, there are two major limitations to the ambient reservoir IMV system. First, the system can only be used effectively when the ventilator is set in the control mode. Otherwise, the negative pressure generated by the patient during spontaneous efforts will tend to cycle the ventilator rather than open the one-way valve. Thus ambient reservoir IMV cannot normally provide synchronization with machine breaths (SIMV). This limitation also means that breath stacking can occur using this system.

The second major limitation of the ambient-reservoir IMV system is related to the use of PEEP. Should the clinician desire to add PEEP to this system, the patient will have to generate a negative inspiratory pressure in excess of the PEEP level to draw a spontaneous breath. This is because the spontaneous breathing circuit operates at ambient pressure (zero relative to atmospheric). PEEP in the ventilator circuit creates a pressure differential across the valve which must be overcome before it will open. The net effect of such a system during spontaneous breathing is called expiratory positive airway pressure (EPAP). As discussed later, EPAP may contribute to lower intrapleural pressure, but can dramatically increase the patient's work of breathing. For these reasons, the application of ambient reservoir IMV is generally limited to situations in which neither synchronous IMV nor PEEP is indicated.

Pressure reservoir IMV. Like ambient reservoir IMV, pressure reservoir IMV employs a continuous flow of fresh gas from which the patient can spontaneously breathe. However, pressure-reservoir IMV differs from ambient reservoir IMV in two major respects. First, the continuous flow of gas occurs in-line with (as opposed to parallel to) the main ventilator circuit. Second, instead of using a reservoir open to the atmosphere, pressure reservoir IMV employs a closed reservoir system, thereby allowing pressures to equilibrate with those in the ventilator circuit.

Fig. 30-23 illustrates a typical pressure reservoir IMV system. As with ambient reservoir IMV, a separate blended gas source provides the necessary continuous

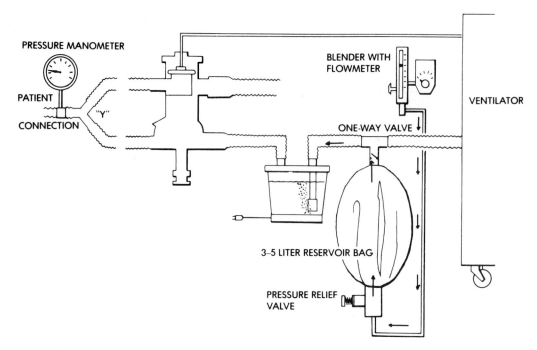

Fig. 30-23   Pressure reservoir IMV system. Continuous gas flow from the blender fills the bag and flows through the circuit to allow spontaneous breathing. The pressure relief valve on the bag is used to vent excess flow during a mechanical breath. See text for description. (From Kirby RR, Smith RA, and Desautels DD, editors: Mechanical ventilation, New York, 1985, Churchill Livingstone.)

flow. However, this flow is diverted into a 3 to 5 L reservoir bag, connected to the inspiratory limb of the ventilator circuit by a T connector at a point proximal to the mainstream humidifier. Although a one-way valve separates the reservoir bag from the ventilator circuit, distension of the bag by continuous gas flow creates a slight pressure differential that normally keeps this valve open, except during machine provided positive pressure breaths.

During positive pressure breaths provided by the machine, this one-way valve closes, and gas under pressure goes to the patient as usual. Simultaneously, the continuous flow fills and distends the reservoir bag, with distention limited by a pressure relief valve.

Between mechanical breaths, the valve opens, and gas flows from the bag into the ventilator circuit. The patient may then draw a spontaneous breath from this flow. During spontaneous exhalation, the patient's expired gases mix with and are flushed out the expiratory port of the ventilator circuit by the continuous flow within the ventilator circuit. In this respect, during spontaneous breathing the pressure reservoir IMV system functions much like a CPAP system, as introduced in Chapter 26 and detailed subsequently in this chapter.

The primary advantage of the pressure reservoir system is the ability to easily incorporate PEEP with IMV. This is because the reservoir bag operates at pressures equivalent to those in the ventilator circuit. Since there normally is

little or no pressure differential across the valve, minimal patient effort is required to draw gas from the circuit and reservoir bag. However, to ensure minimal patient effort, flows through the system generally must be sufficient to meet the peak inspiratory demands of the patient.[10] Alternatively, the use of larger (12 to 18 L) and/or low compliance (highly elastic) reservoir bags may help minimize patient effort during spontaneous breathing.[36-38]

As with the ambient reservoir system, pressure reservoir IMV can be applied only in the control mode. Additional disadvantages of pressure reservoir IMV relate to the in-line nature of the system, which allows continuous flow through the ventilator circuit.

First, since the patient's expired gases mix with the continuous flow within the ventilator circuit, expired volume monitoring is difficult. This problem can be overcome, in part, by using a specialized continuous flow circuit, as shown in Fig. 30-24.[39,40] Such a circuit makes expired volume monitoring possible by diverting the excess flow out the exhalation valve, without passing through the monitoring device.

The second major problem with the pressure reservoir continuous flow system is the potential for increased pressure in the circuit during exhalation. Not only must the patient's expired gases escape through the expiratory port, but also the excess flow from the reservoir bag.[10] This increase in downstream pressure during exhalation is equiv-

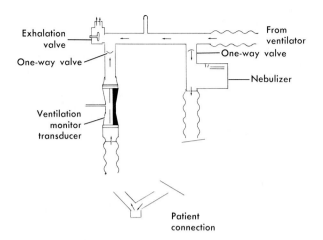

Fig. 30-24   Circuit used for continuous-flow ventilation (CFV). (From McPherson SP: Respiratory therapy equipment, ed 4, St Louis, 1989, The CV Mosby Co.)

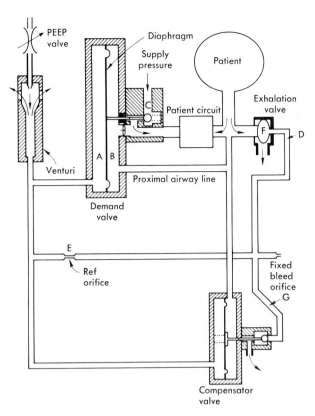

Fig. 30-25   Functional diagram for BEAR-1 and BEAR-2 demand valve, PEEP, and compensator valve systems. (Courtesy Bear Medical Systems, Inc. Riverside, Calif; from McPherson SP: Respiratory therapy equipment, ed 4, St Louis, 1989, The CV Mosby Co.)

alent to the imposition of expiratory resistance, or retard, and can increase the patient's work of breathing.[19]

Pressure reservoir IMV systems may also increase the work of breathing during inspiration, especially if the patient must "pull" gas through a cascade or bubble type humidifier.[10] At inspiratory flows of 120 L/min (mimicking a tachypneic patient), pressure drops as much as 11 cm H_2O have been recorded across some humidifiers.[41] Although higher inspiratory flows through the system can help overcome the increased inspiratory impedance, this effect is negated, in part, by the increase in downstream pressure during exhalation. The use of low-resistance, wick-type humidifiers can help minimize this problem.[10]

Demand flow IMV. In lieu of providing fresh gas for spontaneous breathing by continuous flow, most newer generation ventilators, such as the Siemens Servo 900 Series, the Puritan-Bennett 7200, the BEAR Series, and the Hamilton Veolar, incorporate a demand valve system.

In concept, a demand valve provides flow to the patient in proportion to inspiratory needs. Early versions of this demand valve were simple pneumatic devices, not unlike the gas-powered resuscitator described in Chapter 22. Fig. 30-25 provides a functional diagram of the pneumatic demand valve system incorporated into the BEAR-1 and BEAR-2. Typically, the demand valve consists of a diaphragm in a chamber. One side of the diaphragm, *A*, is exposed to a reference pressure, with the other side exposed to the patient circuit, *B*. Attached to the diaphragm is a valve, *C*, which controls flow from a high-pressure gas source.

During spontaneous breathing, a small drop in pressure (about -1 cm H_2O) on the patient side of the valve, *B* causes the valve to open. Because the valve attempts to maintain a constant pressure differential across the diaphragm, blended gas will enter the system through C at a rate proportional to the patient's inspiratory effort. To accommodate PEEP or CPAP, the reference pressure side of

the diaphragm, *A*, is exposed to this additional pressure. In this manner the pressure drop required to activate the valve will still be about -1 cm H_2O, relative to the PEEP or CPAP pressure. Typically, such valves can provide flows between 0 and 180 L/min.[1] More recently, these simple pneumatic systems have given way to microprocessor-controlled electromechanical valves.[16] These sophisticated valves allow more precise control over both sensitivity and the nature and magnitude of the flow pattern.

Unfortunately, many of these demand valves do not necessarily perform according to specifications. First, ventilator manometers measuring internal or machine (as opposed to airway) pressure tend to significantly underestimate the amount of negative pressure required to open such demand valves.[42] Second, tests of such devices under short inspiratory time conditions have indicated that pressure drops as much as -23 cm H_2O may be necessary to initiate gas flow, with 4 to 10 cm H_2O differentials being the rule.[42,43] As expected, such pressure drops can result in an increase in both the mechanical work and oxygen costs of breathing.[44-46]

Although some of this imposed work of breathing may

be associated with pressure drops across high-resistance humidifiers, most is probably caused by limitations inherent in the design of these valve systems.[47] Of particular concern is the substantial delay time between the initiation of patient inspiratory effort and demand valve opening, ranging between 180 and 250 msec.[46] A continuous-flow pressure reservoir system, however, can "respond" in as little as one-eighth this time, or about 33 msec.[46]

Recent adaptations to ventilator circuitry and microprocessor control mechanisms may overcome these limitations. For example, a new spontaneous breathing update for the Puritan-Bennett 7200A employs a *flow* trigger in the expiratory limb of the circuit to sense changes in ventilatory effort. In combination with new microprocessor instructions, this flow (as opposed to pressure) sensing mechanism should enhance both the sensitivity and response time of the ventilator to spontaneous breathing efforts, thereby minimizing the imposed work of breathing.

However, until such refinements are widely available, demand valve IMV systems should be avoided in patients already breathing under high imposed workloads (such as those with small artificial airways in place), or those with pre-existing respiratory muscle fatigue or significant neuromuscular impairments.[47] Alternatively, pressure support ventilation (PSV), discussed later, may be used to overcome a portion of the workload imposed by these demand valve systems.

Details on the management and monitoring of patients receiving IMV, particularly as they relate to the process of weaning, are provided in Chapter 31. IMV will also be considered in conjunction with positive end-expiratory pressure in the next section.

Positive end-expiratory pressure (PEEP)

One of the most difficult management problems in respiratory care is the patient with persistent hypoxemia, despite the administration of oxygen concentrations of up to 100%. Such a patient may have no significant carbon dioxide retention and may be frankly hypocapnic from hypoxia-induced overbreathing.

Indications. The primary functional defect in patients with hypoxemia that is unresponsive to an increased F_{IO_2} is widespread physiologic shunting. As a rule of thumb, widespread physiologic shunting exists when the arterial oxygen tension of a patient cannot be maintained above 50 mm Hg with an oxygen concentration greater than 50%. Although shunting occurs in a number of diseases, its most serious manifestation is as a component of the infant and adult respiratory distress syndromes. The clinical problem in these cases is correction of a progressive hypoxemia, resulting from airway and alveolar collapse and decreased compliance and FRC.

PEEP is a maneuver that maintains pressure above atmospheric in the patient's lungs at the end of expiration. This combats the collapsing tendency of small airways and alveoli, thereby increasing the FRC. The increased FRC improves compliance, reduces bronchiolar and alveolar collapse, and reduces shunting.[48-51]

Contraindications. The most obvious contraindications to PEEP are known pulmonary hyperinflation and a normal or high compliance. The direct effect of PEEP increases both FRC and compliance, and if they are already elevated, little benefit can be expected. Areas of the lung already hyperinflated will be further distended, and excessive intraalveolar pressure may divert pulmonary capillary flow to poorly ventilated alveoli, increasing venous admixture and worsening the hypoxemia. The same effect may result from the application of PEEP in patients with localized regions of alveolar collapse, such as lobar pneumonia. In this case, normal lung units will be over-distended, causing a diversion of pulmonary blood flow to the poorly ventilated alveoli.

The decision to use or withhold PEEP requires careful scrutiny of clinical and laboratory data, including the establishment of patient risk. PEEP should never be employed as a routine procedure, but only when it has been determined that the hazards of an increased FRC and elevated intrapleural pressure are less than the risks of continued hypoxemia or oxygen toxicity.

Terminology. The mechanics of increasing FRC by retaining gas pressure in alveoli at end-expiration seem fundamentally simple, but safe clinical application requires sound understanding of the desired objective. Unfortunately, it is not enough that practitioners learn the principles and use of PEEP; they must also cope with the confusion of nonuniform terminology relating to the subject.[52,53]

The problem of definition stems from a difference in the use of PEEP on patients who are (1) on controlled, assist/control or IMV mechanical ventilation or (2) breathing spontaneously without mechanical assistance. For consistency, the term positive end-expiratory pressure, or PEEP, will be used in reference to the maintenance of a residual pressure above atmospheric at the airway opening at the end of expiration during *mechanical ventilation,* that is CMV with PEEP or IMV with PEEP. The term constant positive airway pressure, or CPAP, will be used to mean a pressure above atmospheric maintained at the airway opening throughout the respiratory cycle during *spontaneous* breathing.

Technique. There are several methods of applying positive end-expiratory pressure during mechanical ventilation.[10,54] We will look first at the mechanisms by which this additional pressure can be generated, followed by an analysis of differences in the application of PEEP among the control, assist/control, and IMV modes of ventilatory support. Most of the methods used to generate PEEP in a ventilator circuit also apply to the application of CPAP during spontaneous breathing.

Generating PEEP. Ideally, a true PEEP mechanism should be capable of maintaining a given pressure level in a ventilator circuit independent of flow, thereby function-

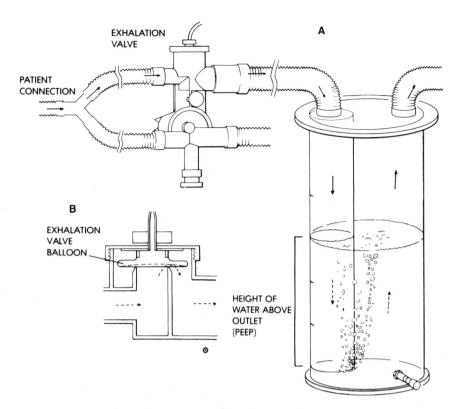

Fig. 30-26 Water-column PEEP device. (From Kirby RR, Smith RA, and Desautels DD, editors: Mechanical ventilation, New York, 1985, Churchill Livingstone.)

ing as a threshold resistor.[54,55] As described in Chapter 29, common PEEP mechanisms include underwater columns, spring-loaded diaphragms or disks, balloon valves with preset internal pressures, reverse venturi devices, and electromechanical valves.

Underwater columns. Fig. 30-26 shows a simple water column PEEP device connected to the expiratory port of a ventilator circuit. By immersing the expiratory line under water, further exhalation of gas below a certain pressure level is impossible. In this case, the PEEP level is adjusted simply by varying either the immersion depth of the expiratory line or the height of the water column. As long as the inlet and outlet of the water column container are not restricted, such a device exhibits the characteristics of a true threshold resistor. However, the resistance to expiration can never be less than the smallest orifice in the system, in this case the space around the exhalation valve balloon.

The water column PEEP device can be noisy (because of the constant bubbling), and evaporation of water can alter the PEEP level unless closely monitored. By diverting exhaled gases to a diaphragm placed *under* a water column, as shown in Fig. 30-27, these problems can be avoided. This is the mechanism used to generate PEEP in the Emerson 3-PV and 3MV (IMV) ventilators.

Spring-loaded diaphragms or disks. Fig. 30-28 illustrates a simple spring-loaded disk PEEP device, also con-

nected to the expiratory port of a ventilator circuit. With this device, the PEEP level is adjusted by altering the tension on the disk, which seats against the expiratory port of the ventilator circuit. When the gas pressure is greater than the spring tension, the disk is displaced, and exhaled air is vented out to the atmosphere. This is the mechanism for generating PEEP in the early Siemens Servo 900 ventilators (models A and B).

Unlike water column PEEP devices, some spring-loaded disks can offer significant resistance to expiratory flow. Whether such a mechanism functions mainly as a flow or threshold resistor depends on both the elastic properties of the spring and the area of the disk seat.[1] A device characterized by a highly elastic ("stiff") spring and a seat with a small cross-sectional area will act as a flow resistor, thereby creating expiratory retard in addition to PEEP.

Pressurized balloon valves. The most common mechanism used to generate PEEP in a ventilator circuit is by pressurization of the expiratory balloon valve. As shown in Fig. 30-29, this may be accomplished in several ways. In Fig. 30-29, *A*, the outlet pressure of a small venturi is used to pressurize the expiratory balloon valve. In this case, the PEEP level is adjusted by altering the flow powering the venturi. This is the mechanism used to generate PEEP in the MA-2 and BEAR-2 ventilators.[10]

The same end can be achieved by pressurizing the expiratory balloon valve with either an adjustable pressure reg-

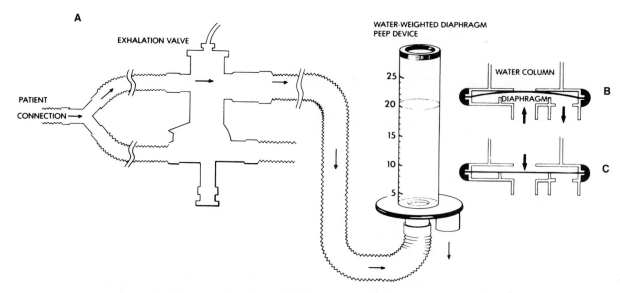

Fig. 30-27   Water-weighted diaphragm PEEP device. **A,** Typical ventilator circuit. **B,** Detail of diaphragm mechanism. When airway pressure is higher than that of the water column, the diaphragm is displaced upward and exhaled gas passes out of the circuit. **C,** When pressures equalize, the diaphragm "seats" and expiratory flow ceases. (From Kirby RR, Smith RA, and Desautels DD, editors: Mechanical ventilation, New York, 1989, Churchill Livingstone.)

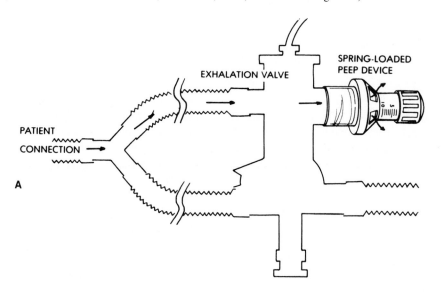

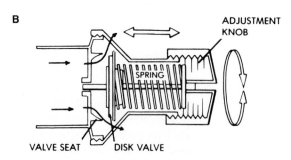

Fig. 30-28   Spring-loaded disk valve. **A,** Typical ventilator circuit. Arrows show direction of expiratory flow. **B,** Detail of spring-loaded valve. See text for description. (From Kirby RR, Smith RA, and Desautels DD, editors: Mechanical ventilation, New York, 1985, Churchill Livingstone.)

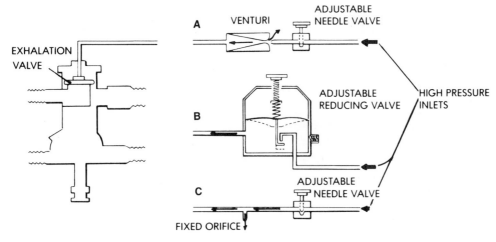

Fig. 30-29   "Trapped" pressure in exhalation valve balloon can be used to generate PEEP in the patient circuit. **A** to **C,** Three ways gas pressure within the balloon is controlled. See text for descriptions. (From Kirby RR, Smith RA, and Desautels DD, editors: Mechanical ventilation, New York, 1985, Churchill livingstone.)

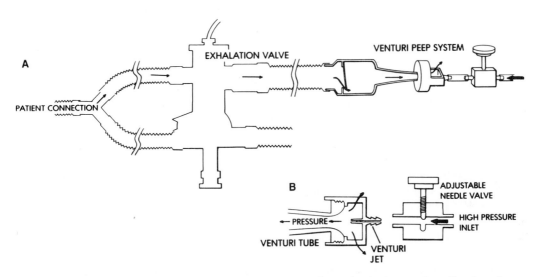

Fig. 30-30   Venturi PEEP system. **A,** Connected to ventilator circuit. Arrows show direction of expiratory flow. **B,** Detail of adjustable needle valve and venturi. (From Kirby RR, Smith RA, and Desautels DD, editors: Mechanical ventilation, New York, 1985, Churchill Livingstone.)

ulator (Fig. 30-29, *B*) or by varying flow through a fixed orifice (Fig. 30-29, *C*). The MA-1 ventilator uses the adjustable pressure regulator/balloon valve system for PEEP, while the Monaghan 225 employs the fixed orifice approach to pressurize its exhalation valve.[1,10]

Like some spring-loaded disks, pressurized balloon valves can offer significant resistance to expiratory flow. A balloon valve's PEEP mechanism will tend to exhibit undesirable flow resistive properties if the balloon cannot empty readily or if the cross-sectional area under the valve is small.[10]

Reverse venturi PEEP devices. Rather than using a venturi indirectly to pressurize a balloon valve, PEEP also may be generated by the direct application of the venturi outlet pressure to a one-way valve in the exhalation port of the ventilator circuit. As illustrated in Fig. 30-30, instead of helping augment inspiratory flow (the usual application), the venturi is used to prevent exhalation below a certain pressure, creating PEEP (thus the use of the term "reverse" venturi). This is the mechanism for generating PEEP in the Bourns LS104-150 and BP-200 infant ventilators. As long as the resistance to flow through the one-way valve and venturi tube is small, this type of PEEP mechanism tends to behave as a true threshold resistor.

Electromechanical valves. More recently, ventilators have begun using electromechanical valves as the PEEP generating mechanisms. In this application, a electromechanical valve (the effector) is used in conjunction with a pressure transducer (to sense pressure fluctuations) and an electronic processing circuit. Once a PEEP pressure is set

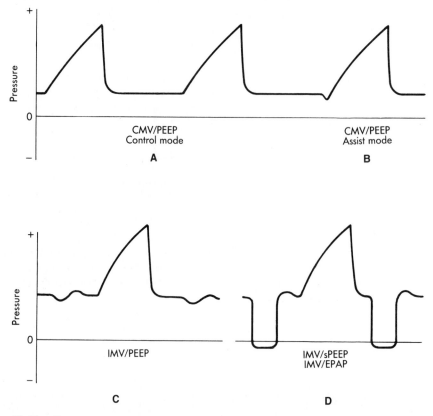

Fig. 30-31   Pressure wave forms for various forms of ventilatory support with end-expiratory pressure at a positive level. See text for description.

by the operator, the processor uses input from the pressure transducer to maintain the desired pressure level, either by closing or opening the electromechanical valve.

In the Hamilton Veolar and Siemens Servo 900C, the electromechanical valve used to control PEEP also serves as the expiratory valve, thereby directly controlling outlet pressures. In the Bennett 7200 and BEAR Cub (BP-2001) ventilators, the electromechanical valve is used to control pressure levels going to a separate pneumatic expiratory valve, thereby controlling PEEP levels indirectly.

PEEP applications in different ventilatory support modes. PEEP may be applied in the control, assist/control, and IMV modes of ventilatory support. PEEP also may be used in conjunction with pressure support ventilation (PSV). Some of the key technical differences in these applications and their clinical significance, will be highlighted subsequently.

PEEP with controlled ventilation. When originally introduced, PEEP was generally limited in application to the control mode of ventilatory support. This limitation was based on the fact that most early ventilator sensitivity mechanisms operated relative to atmospheric pressure, so that an assist breath could be cycled only if the system pressure dropped below zero (relative to atmospheric). Most newer generation ventilators have overcome this problem by providing a sensitivity control that is relative

to system pressure, as opposed to atmospheric pressure.

Nonetheless, there are situations in which controlled ventilation with PEEP may be desirable. On most ventilators, this is accomplished simply by "locking" out the sensitivity control, so that patient effort will not cycle the machine to inspiration. The resulting pressure waveform (Fig. 30-31, *A*) is comparable to control mode CMV, but with an elevated end-expiratory pressure baseline. As with controlled ventilation in general, this approach normally will require some suppression of the patient's ventilatory efforts.

PEEP with assist/control ventilation. The capacity to reliably provide PEEP in the assist/control mode of ventilatory support was developed in the mid-1970s.[56] Technically, this was the result of refinements in sensitivity control mechanisms that gauged patient effort relative to the system pressure, as opposed to atmospheric pressure.

In general, there are two approaches to this application. Either the sensitivity mechanism automatically compensates for PEEP, as in the BEAR-1, BEAR-2, and Puritan-Bennett 7200, or an absolute "trigger" level just below the desired PEEP pressure is set directly, as in the Siemens Servo Series ventilators. In either case, the patient need only cause a small pressure drop below the PEEP baseline to activate the ventilator (see Fig. 30-31, *B*).

Clinically, the major problem with PEEP used in the assist/control mode is the potential for ventilator self-cycling with system leaks. This problem is of particular concern in ventilators using an absolute trigger level. In these cases, any drop in system pressure, whether because of patient effort or system leak, can cycle the ventilator to begin inspiration. If the leak is large, the ventilator will tend to cycle to inspiration as soon as exhalation is completed, resulting in an undesirably fast rate and potential hyperventilation of the patient. Systems incorporating PEEP compensated demand valves overcome this problem, in part, by providing additional flow to the system to "feed" the leak, thereby maintaining PEEP pressure. However, this approach only compensates for, but does not correct, the leak. Obviously, once identified, such a problem should be corrected.

Although IMV has replaced the assist/control mode of ventilatory support in many clinical centers, there are still situations where it is advisable to encourage an inspiratory effort, even if the patient is unable to effect an adequate follow-up tidal volume. Here, assist/control ventilation is helpful, and if PEEP is indicated, it can and should be used. It has even been suggested that PEEP in the assist/control mode administered by face mask might occasionally be useful as a means to avoid tracheal intubation in selected patients.[57] Assisted PEEP simply puts at our disposal another valuable tool in the management of patients in respiratory failure.

PEEP with IMV. In general, the use of PEEP and IMV together is technically possible only when a pressure reservoir or PEEP compensated demand flow system is employed (see Figs. 30-24 and 30-25). Otherwise, the patient must generate an inspiratory force exceeding that of the PEEP level to take a spontaneous breath. Moreover, assist-PEEP with IMV (SIMV with PEEP) is limited to systems using a pneumatic or electromechanical demand flow valve.

The pressure waveform characterizing IMV with PEEP is comparable to simple IMV, but with an elevated end-expiratory pressure baseline (Fig. 30-31, *C*).[58] Normally, only a slight drop in pressure (1 to 3 cm of water) should occur during spontaneous breathing, thus ensuring a minimal work of breathing on the part of the patient.[28]

Using IMV with PEEP results in a lower mean intrapleural pressure than could be achieved in the control or assist/control modes. This approach has allowed application of higher levels of PEEP than would otherwise be used, sometimes as high as 50 to 60 cm H_2O.[59,60] However, regardless of the mode of ventilatory support used, whenever end-expiratory pressures in excess of 20 cm H_2O are needed, more specific cardiovascular monitoring is necessary (see Chapter 31). Moreover, pharmacologic agents may be necessary to support circulation and protect the cardiovascular system from the effects of PEEP.[61]

An alternative approach, as shown in Fig. 30-31, *D,* is requiring the patient to generate an inspiratory force exceeding that of the PEEP level in order to take a spontane-

ous breath. This technique has been referred to as "spontaneous PEEP" (sPEEP) or expiratory positive airway pressure (EPAP).[62,63] The fact that inspiratory pressure dips into the negative range in no way interferes with or negates the function or purpose of PEEP. End-expiration still falls at the desired positive pressure of an elevated resting level, and the FRC is correspondingly enlarged.

Although clearly demanding a greater inspiratory work of breathing than simple IMV with PEEP, this approach is tolerated well by selected patients and offers potential cardiovascular benefits. By having the pressure fall during a spontaneous breath, the mean intrapleural pressure also falls; this may be helpful in reducing the circulatory effects of the positive pressure during expiration in some patients.[64] However, this potential advantage is not consistently observed.[65] Clearly, the real benefits of spontaneous PEEP and the question of which patients would be best served by this approach need further investigation.[32]

Details on the management and monitoring of patients receiving PEEP, including how to establish appropriate PEEP levels, are provided in Chapter 31.

Continuous positive airway pressure (CPAP)

As used here, CPAP represents a method of ventilatory support whereby the patient breathes spontaneously without mechanical assistance against threshold resistance to exhalation for the purpose of increasing the FRC.

Indications. In general, CPAP is the appropriate mode of ventilatory support for patients with adequate spontaneous ventilation, but who continue to exhibit persistent hypoxemia caused by physiologic shunting. However, great care must be taken in judging a patient's adequacy of ventilation. Of and by itself, a normal or low arterial P_{CO_2} is not sufficient evidence that a patient can adequately maintain the spontaneous ventilation necessary for CPAP to be successful.

First, there must be evidence that the patient's ventilation is being achieved efficiently, without unnecessary wasted effort. In general, ventilation is being achieved with satisfactory efficiency if an adult patient is able to maintain a normal or low arterial P_{CO_2} with a minute ventilation less than 10 L/min. Second, there should be no clinical signs or symptoms of respiratory muscle fatigue present. Such signs and symptoms, including dyspnea, tachypnea, asynchronous or paradoxical breathing, and respiratory alternans, are discussed more fully in Chapter 31.

In the presence of refractory hypoxemia, if either or both of these conditions are not met, CMV or IMV with PEEP should be considered the ventilatory support mode of choice. The exception to these rules is the use of CPAP in infants, as discussed in Chapter 32.

Technique. The methods used to generate CPAP are essentially the same as those previously described for PEEP. Since application of CPAP does not require a ventilator, a CPAP system may simply consist of a Y tubing circuit

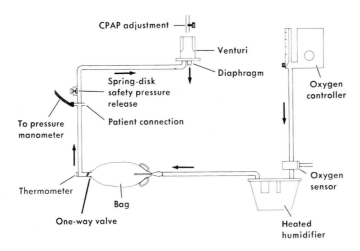

Fig. 30-32   Example of circuit used for CPAP showing essential components. Blended oxygen from controller flows continuously past oxygen sensor, through heated humidifier, into reservoir bag, and past thermometer and patient connection. Pressure near patient is monitored. Expiratory and continuous gases flow past safety pop-off and PEEP device; example shows pressure from venturi opposing flow past diaphragm to establish PEEP/CPAP level. (From McPherson SP: Respiratory therapy equipment, ed 4, St Louis, 1989, The CV Mosby Co.)

powered by a blended source gas, with a threshold resistor on the expiratory limb (see Fig. 30-32).[66,67] Humidification should be provided by a device with low flow resistance, such as a heated wick humidifier. Valving in such a system is unnecessary as long as the breathing gas supply is adequate and adjusted to flow steadily through the threshold resistor.

However, since the work of breathing increases as system pressure decreases from baseline, an ideal CPAP system should be capable of maintaining a near constant ($+/-$ 2 cm H_2O) baseline pressure.[68,69] To minimize pressure fluctuations, flows through the system generally will need to be in the 60 to 90 L/min range.[70] Moreover, to accommodate inspiratory flow demands in excess of this range, a reservoir system, preferably one that is elastically loaded, should be incorporated into the system.[47] Alternatively, lower flows, in the 20 to 30 L/min range, may be used, but only if a reservoir of 12 to 18 L capacity is employed.[36-38] Finally, the device used to develop the CPAP pressure must behave as a true threshold resistor, ideally generating no flow resistance whatsoever over the full range of available flows.[19]

Many newer generation ventilators incorporate a demand flow CPAP mode. However, all of the reservations previously cited regarding demand flow IMV apply to their use with CPAP.[42-47] Indeed, the application of these complex devices may be responsible for many of the reported failures of IMV or CPAP.[19,45] Although the capability to provide pressure support ventilation (PSV) may overcome some of these inherent shortcomings, this approach merely compensates for the problem, rather than solving it. Thus, until substantial improvements are made in the perfor-

mance characteristics of these ventilators, their use exclusively to deliver CPAP should be avoided. Technical considerations notwithstanding, it makes little sense to use a $25,000 ventilator to deliver a mode of ventilatory support that can be provided using a simpler, less expensive apparatus. Even with the addition of appropriate monitoring and alarm functions, an ideal CPAP system (as described above) can be assembled for one tenth of this cost.

Although the application of CPAP to adults was originally based on the presence of an endotracheal tube, recent clinical reports have demonstrated its short-term effectiveness with a tightly fitted face mask.[71-73] Problems with administering CPAP by mask include pressure necrosis on the face, increased dead space in the mask, and gastric rupture. Aspiration of gastric contents can occur if the patient vomits when the mask is strapped to the face, but the use of a nasogastric tube and careful selection of patients can help avoid this problem. In one study, 44 awake, cooperative, spontaneously breathing adult patients with evidence of increased physiologic shunting and a normal or low $Paco_2$ were treated with CPAP by mask, with tracheal intubation avoided in all but one.[73] In this series, no problems with gastric distention or vomiting were reported.

Pressure support ventilation (PSV)

Pressure support ventilation (PSV) is a mode of ventilatory support whereby spontaneous breathing is augmented with a set amount of positive airway pressure.[47] At low support levels, such as 5 cm H_2O, PSV can help unload the respiratory muscles from the imposed work of breathing caused by artificial airways and/or ventilator circuitry.[74-77] At higher levels, pressure support progressively unloads the respiratory muscles from ventilatory work.[78] At pressure support levels resulting in tidal volumes of 10 to 12 ml/kg, essentially all the work of breathing is being assumed by the ventilator.[79]

Regardless of the pressure support level provided, the patient has primary control over the frequency of breathing and the inspiratory time and flow.[47] Thus, the tidal volume resulting from a PSV breath depends on pressure level set, the patient effort, and mechanical forces opposing ventilation.

As compared to spontaneous breathing (including that occurring during IMV), clinical studies have shown that PSV can result in a decreased respiratory rate, increased V_T, reduced respiratory muscle activity, and decreased oxygen consumption.[80-84] Moreover, heart rate, blood pressure, hemoglobin saturation, and end-tidal CO_2 levels achieved with PSV are comparable to those realized with SIMV.[81] PSV may also change the nature of patient work during ventilatory support, improving the endurance conditioning of the respiratory muscles, and thereby facilitating weaning.[79] Finally, PSV apparently is preferred by patients over more traditional modes of ventilatory support.[79,85]

Indications. Although research on PSV is still in progress, there are several specific clinical situations in which this mode of ventilatory support may be indicated. These include the following[47]:
- Spontaneously breathing patients who require ventilatory support and have smaller than optimal artificial airways, especially when breathing at frequencies greater than 20/min and with minute ventilations ($\dot{V}_E$) in excess of 10 L/min;
- Spontaneously breathing patients with a history of COPD or evidence of muscle weakness who require long-term mechanical ventilation (greater than 24 to 48 hours) and are being supported on demand flow systems in the SIMV or CPAP mode; and
- Spontaneously breathing patients who exhibit clinical evidence of muscle weakness or COPD patients who experience difficulty on continuous-flow IMV systems at low frequencies or CPAP.

Technique. PSV is a form of pressure-limited mechanical ventilation, similar in concept to IPPB.[47] Fig. 30-33 portrays the pressure, flow, and volume changes occurring during two different levels of PSV, as compared with those occurring during spontaneous breathing.

As illustrated in Fig. 30-33, when the patient activates a ventilator in the PSV mode, a ventilatory assist is provided at a preset pressure limit. Normally, a pressure plateau or pressure limit is achieved and maintained until the patient's inspiratory flow decreases to some minimal level. At this point, inspiration is terminated by opening of the ventilator's exhalation valve. Thus, when set to deliver pressure support ventilation, a ventilator is providing pressure-limited, flow-cycled, assisted ventilation. PSV

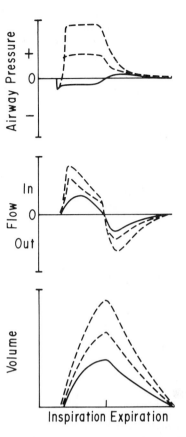

Fig. 30-33 Schema of airway pressure in the distal endotracheal tube (top panel), airflow (middle panel), and lung-volume changes (lower panel), in a spontaneously breathing patient on a mechanical ventilator. Solid lines depict an unassisted breath. Dashed lines depict two levels of pressure-assisted breaths with PSV. Note patient's continued negative-pressure effort when unassisted, compared with the brief period of such patient effort when PSV is used. (From MacIntyre NR: Respir Care 32(6):448, 1987.)

may be used as the sole mode of ventilatory support or incorporated with either IMV, IMV with PEEP, or CPAP.

Although similar in concept to IPPB, PSV is technically more complex, requiring sophisticated, microprocessor-based electromechanical control mechanisms. Only in this manner can the flow be instantaneously adjusted according to both the preset pressure support level and the patient's changing inspiratory demands.

The appropriate level of pressure support depends on both the nature of the patient situation and the goals of ventilatory support. If the goal is simply to overcome the work of breathing imposed by a small artificial airway and/or the patient breathing circuit, then the necessary pressure support level may be estimated by multiplying the total flow resistance of the patient-ventilator system times the patient's peak inspiratory flow.[86,87] Mathematically, this calculation employs the following formula:

$$P_{psv} = \frac{P_{peak} - P_{plateau}}{\dot{V}_{mech}} \times \dot{V}_{Imax}$$

where P_{psv} is the necessary pressure support level in centimeters of water (cm H_2O), P_{peak} is the peak airway pressure in centimeters of water (cm H_2O) during a mechanically provided volume-cycled breath, $P_{plateau}$ is the plateau pressure in centimeters of water (cm H_2O) achieved during an inspiratory hold of the mechanically provided breath, $\dot{V}_{mech}$ is the flow in L/sec provided during the mechanically provided breath, and $\dot{V}_{Imax}$ is the patient's spontaneous peak inspiratory flow in L/sec.

For example, given respective values of 50 and 40 cm H_2O for the peak and plateau pressure during a mechanically provided volume-cycled breath delivered at 60 L/min (1.0 L/sec), and a patient peak inspiratory flow of 30 L/min (0.5 L/sec), we would estimate the appropriate pressure support level as follows:

$$P_{psv} = \frac{50 \text{ cm } H_2O - 40 \text{ cm } H_2O}{1.0 \text{ L/sec}} \times 0.5 \text{ L/sec}$$

$$= 5 \text{ cm } H_2O$$

Alternatively, in patients exhibiting clinical signs and symptoms of respiratory muscle fatigue, such as dyspnea, tachypnea, asynchronous or paradoxical breathing, and respiratory alternans, we would adjust the pressure support level empirically until a reasonable ventilatory pattern can be obtained. In the majority of patients, PSV levels between 5 and 15 cm H_2O are sufficient to achieve this goal.[47]

If the goal is to facilitate weaning from mechanical ventilation, a different protocol has been suggested (see box). In this case, the initial PSV setting is that required to achieve a tidal volume of 10 to 12 ml/kg, referred to as PSV_{max}. Then, the pressure support level is progressively reduced, with an increased frequency of breathing being the primary indicator of patient intolerance. Extubation is indicated when the PSV level can be maintained at 5 cm H_2O with an acceptable ventilatory pattern.[88]

Mandatory minute ventilation (MMV)

The technique called mandatory minute ventilation (MMV) first appeared in the medical literature in 1977.[89] As originally described, MMV was conceived as a ventilatory support technique designed to facilitate patient weaning. According to its originators, the MMV mode ensures delivery of a preset minimum minute volume, with the patient allowed to breathe spontaneously. Should the patient meet this preset $\dot{V}_E$ entirely by spontaneous effort, a ventilator in the MMV mode will remain passive, delivering no positive-pressure breaths. On the other hand, should the patient's spontaneous $\dot{V}_E$ fall below the preset MMV minimum, a ventilator operating in this mode will provide the mechanical support necessary to ensure that the minimum minute ventilation goal is achieved.[90-92]

Currently, MMV represents the only commercially available example of a true "closed-loop" ventilatory support system.[93] This support system incorporates a comput-

---

PRESSURE SUPPORT PROTOCOL

Patient selection: Resolving pulmonary process, reliable respiratory drive (similar to point at which traditional IMV weaning begins)

    Initial settings: Start at PSV_{max} ($V_T = 10$ to 12 ml/kg, work $\simeq 0$)

    Reduce PSV as tolerated (breathing frequency reflects tolerance)

    Extubate at 5 cm H_2O PSV

Consideration: PSV_{max} pressure > 50 cm H_2O is rarely needed. Higher pressures indicate an unstable patient.

Consideration: Backup controlled ventilation can be used as "safety net."

From MacIntyre NR: Weaning from mechanical ventilatory support: volume-assisting intermittent breaths versus pressure-assisting every breath, Respir Care 33(2):124. Modified from Duke University protocol.

---

erized control process that constantly monitors a given parameter (in this case the $\dot{V}_E$) and a means to automatically adjust that parameter to the value previously established by the user. For this reason, only the newer generation microprocessor-based ventilators have the capacity to operate in the MMV mode. Currently, MMV is available as a ventilatory mode option on the Engstrom Erica, Ohmeda CPU-1, BEAR 5, and Hamilton Veolar ventilators.

Two different approaches are presently used to implement MMV. On the Engstrom Erica, Ohmeda CPU-1, and BEAR 5, the practitioner presets both an SIMV frequency and tidal volume, and the minimum MMV level desired. Should the total $\dot{V}_E$ (patient plus IMV breaths) fall below the MMV minimum, then these ventilators will increase the SIMV frequency to maintain the preset $\dot{V}_E$. However, if the patient's $\dot{V}_E$ meets or exceeds the minimum MMV level, the Engstrom Erica and Ohmeda CPU-1 will not deliver any mechanical breaths. The BEAR 5, however, allows the practitioner to set a minimum SIMV frequency that is provided regardless of the total minute ventilation, thereby assuring the delivery of a preset number of periodic positive pressure breaths.

The Hamilton Veolar ventilator employs a slightly different approach. When using this device in the MMV mode, the practitioner sets a minimum minute ventilation and an initial level of pressure support. In turn, the ventilator varies the level of pressure support (P_{psv}) to maintain the desired $\dot{V}_E$. A backup SIMV mode is available should the patient become apneic.

In principle, then, the application of the MMV mode ensures that a constant minute volume of fresh gas is breathed by a patient, despite minute-to-minute changes in his or her ability to breathe spontaneously. Moreover, MMV should allow simpler and more direct control over a patient's Paco$_2$ than that provided by comparable weaning methods.[89] However, there currently is no firm evidence to support the use of MMV as a mode of ventilatory support for patient weaning. Successful use of this mode has been described in the perioperative management of a patient with myasthenia gravis,[94] but as of this writing, no clinical trials comparing MMV with other more traditional modes of ventilatory support or weaning have been conducted.

Moreover, most currently available MMV systems lack a means to ensure *efficient* patterns of ventilation. For example, on current ventilators employing this mode, an MMV setting of 8.0 L/min (8000 ml) could be met by either of the following patterns:

Pattern	Frequency	Tidal Volume	Minute ventilation
A	20	400 ml	8000 ml
B	40	200 ml	8000 ml

Assuming equivalent physiologic dead space, pattern A clearly represents a more efficient combination of frequency and tidal volume, resulting in both less dead space ventilation and a greater alveolar ventilation per minute. Pattern B, on the other hand, is a grossly inefficient combination of frequency and tidal volume, with a large proportion of dead space ventilation per minute. Yet, with current MMV-capable ventilators, both patterns achieve the desired goal of 8.0 L/min and would therefore be acceptable to the machine.

Ideally, this problem would be avoided by allowing the practitioner to set both a minimum $\dot{V}E$ and a maximum allowable spontaneous breathing frequency. In this case, if the spontaneous breathing frequency exceeds the preset maximum, either a ventilator alarm will activate (signaling the practitioner to respond), or the ventilator would automatically increase the tidal volume (or pressure support level) until the spontaneous breathing frequency returned to the desired range.

Because of the current lack of firm evidence to support its use and its present technical limitations, the application of MMV as a primary mode of ventilatory support should be done with extreme caution. Moreover, contrary to those who claim this mode allows patients to "wean themselves," MMV, like any mode of ventilatory support, is no substitute for careful and continuous bedside monitoring by astute respiratory care practitioners.

CHOICE OF VENTILATORY SUPPORT DEVICES AND MODES

The large number of ventilatory support devices on the market testifies to the fact that currently there is no single apparatus capable of meeting all clinical needs or individual practitioner expectations. Each of these devices has its champions, and we are accustomed to hearing debates extolling the virtues of one over another.

The personal preferences among physicians and respiratory care practitioners alike are based on many factors, among which are experience with one type of device, confidence in one over the others, admiration for a particular mechanical principle, and economy. Although all of these are important considerations, most depend more on whim than on the specific objectives sought in each individual patient requiring ventilatory support.

Minimum essential characteristics

Ultimately, the skill and experience of the operating practitioner are probably more important than the specific type of apparatus used. Nonetheless, it is possible to identify some of the essential general characteristics that every ventilatory support device should possess. These include the following:

1. The device should be reliable, that is able to operate for long periods with a minimum of servicing or down-time;
2. The device should be cost-effective, ideally balancing functional versatility against the most common patient needs;
3. The device should be readily upgradeable and not easily subject to obsolescence;
4. The device should be simple to operate and require a minimum amount of training for new users;
5. The device should incorporate a backup mode that ensures essential support of life-sustaining functions in the event of a failure in the primary power or control mechanism;
6. The device should provide mechanisms to warn clinicians of both mechanical failures and changes in critical patient parameters; and
7. The device should meet all applicable regulatory standards, including FDA certification.

Specific performance characteristics that any ventilatory support device should meet include (but need not be limited to) the following:

1. The device should be capable of providing accurate Fio$_2$ values between 0.21 and 1.0 at flows sufficient to meet most patients' peak inspiratory demands (at least 100 L/min);
2. There should be dependable control over, or a safe limit to, the generated or applied pressure;
3. There should be some means of monitoring airway pressure, preferable as close to the patient airway as possible;
4. There must be provisions for adequate humidification of inspired gas, at any available flow; and
5. The patient circuit, including the humidification device and expiratory pressure generator, should exhibit minimal flow resistance in all modes of operation.

This is not an exhaustive list, and practitioners can probably add several more criteria they would like to see met before they would have full confidence in any ventilatory support device. Realistically, the choice of a ventilatory support device will often depend on which of those available in a given hospital is felt to be the safest and most effective for a given patient with due regard for both the clinical circumstances necessitating its use and the number, skill, and experience of those who will be responsible for its operation.

Selection of ventilatory support modes

Given the fact that most newer generation ventilators provide a vast array of ventilatory support options, the key question facing practitioners today is not so much which ventilator to use, but which of the available modes of ventilatory support is most appropriate in a given situation. As previously discussed in Chapter 28, no absolute consensus has yet emerged on the appropriate use of the various modes of ventilatory support; many of the newest approaches are still undergoing clinical investigations. However, current knowledge does allow us to draw some broad generalizations according to the major underlying pathophysiologic process present.

Inadequate alveolar ventilation. The most appropriate mode of ventilatory support for patients with alveolar ventilation varies according to the underlying cause of the problem. If the patient has normal lungs and suffers simply from a decrease in ventilatory drive, as may occur in CNS depression resulting from a narcotic or anesthetic overdose, control or assist/control CMV using either a pressure- or volume-cycled ventilator is usually sufficient. If, on the other hand, the problem is a chronic neuromuscular disorder, and the removal of bronchial secretions or the risk of aspiration is not a clinical consideration, intubation may be avoided and the patient ventilated by a negative-pressure differential ventilator, preferably of the cuirass type.

However, if the problem is caused by a restrictive disorder that decreases the compliance of the lungs or chest bellows, and the patient has a normal ventilatory drive, it is unlikely that either positive- or negative-pressure controlled ventilation will be readily accepted. Moreover, use of CMV in the assist/control mode in these patients may result in respiratory alkalosis. For these reasons, IMV or SIMV should be considered. In any case, because of the decrease in compliance of the lungs or chest wall, a ventilator capable of high driving pressures normally will be required to deliver adequate tidal volumes. Furthermore, if changes in the impedance to ventilation are expected, a volume-cycled ventilator is preferred over one that cycles to end-inspiration by pressure.

Inadequate lung expansion. If the primary cause of acute respiratory failure is inadequate lung expansion, as indicated by a decreased FRC, and the problem is not localized to a particular region of the lung, the application of a continuous distending pressure to the patient's airway is indicated. However, if alveolar ventilation is adequate and

efficient, and there are no overt clinical signs or symptoms of respiratory muscle fatigue, simple CPAP should suffice. If inadequate lung expansion coexists with inadequate alveolar ventilation, then CMV with PEEP or IMV with PEEP is indicated. Pressure support ventilation should be considered as a supplement to these primary modes of ventilatory support if respiratory muscle fatigue is apparent.

Refractory hypoxemia. Usually, refractory hypoxemia is associated with inadequate lung expansion, particularly when caused by widespread airway closure and atelectasis. For this reason, the modes of ventilatory support indicated for refractory hypoxemia are essentially the same as those specified for inadequate lung expansion, that is, CPAP or PEEP. Coexisting alveolar hypoventilation or respiratory muscle fatigue in these patients may necessitate CMV with PEEP or IMV with PEEP and pressure support ventilation.

Inadequate respiratory muscle strength. As discussed in Chapter 28, the "best" mode of ventilatory support for patients with inadequate respiratory muscle strength is still controversial. Logically, if the cause of respiratory muscle weakness is fatigue, the mechanical ventilator should probably assume all or most of the work of breathing. Although this is traditionally accomplished using CMV in the control mode, PSV producing tidal volumes in the 10 to 12 ml/kg range (PSV_{max}) should be considered an alternative, especially in patients with small artificial airways or in those in whom pharmacologic suppression of ventilation is undesirable or not feasible.

On the other hand, if the cause of respiratory muscle weakness is atrophy, IMV is probably the best choice between current ventilatory support modalities. As an alternative approach, one may employ pressure support ventilation, progressively decreasing the support level from PSV_{max} to the minimum necessary to support spontaneous ventilation. This latter alternative may be particularly appealing when there are factors present imposing an additional work of breathing on the patient, such as small artificial airways, high resistance ventilator circuits, or imperfect demand valve systems. As previously discussed, mandatory minute ventilation (MMV) may also be useful in weaning patients with respiratory muscle weakness, but firm evidence in support of its clinical application currently is not available.

Excessive work of breathing. In situations where the increased work of breathing is caused by decreased compliance, without a concomitant reduction in FRC, the mechanical ventilator should probably assume all or most of the work of breathing. As in respiratory failure caused by inadequate respiratory muscle strength, this may be accomplished with either CMV in the control mode or the PSV_{max} approach.

However, if the increased work of breathing is associated with a reduction in FRC and hypoxemia, the application of positive pressure throughout the respiratory cycle in combination with mechanically provided breaths, as with CMV or IMV with PEEP, is generally the strategy of choice.

If the excessive work of breathing is caused by airflow obstruction, mechanical ventilation in the pure CMV mode is normally indicated. In these cases, the ventilator should also give independent control over pressure, flow, and I:E ratio.

Unstable ventilatory drive. In the presence of an unstable ventilatory drive, the ventilatory support mode chosen must assure that the patient's minimum minute ventilation is sufficient enough to prevent respiratory acidosis, while guarding against hyperventilation caused by tachypnea. In general, only CMV in the control mode currently provides this capability. As previously discussed, successfully controlled ventilation generally requires some suppression of the patient's ventilatory efforts.

SUMMARY

The respiratory care practitioner assumes primary responsibility for the selection and application of a variety of complex and sophisticated equipment designed to support patients in respiratory failure. Only by having in-depth knowledge of both the mechanical and physiologic principles underlying this equipment can the practitioner expect to apply it in a safe and effective manner.

Systematic classification provides an orderly approach to the selection and use of ventilatory support equipment that can assist the practitioner. As applied to mechanical ventilators, there are three major classification categories: power variables, control mechanisms, and phase variables.

Power variables distinguish between devices according to the pressure differential used, the power source, the power circuitry, and the way in which the power is applied, or drive mechanism. Control mechanisms include mechanical, pneumatic, fluidic, or electrical principles. Phase variables describe how an individual device functions in each of the four components of the mechanical breathing cycle and help explain the effect of changing lung characteristics on the parameters of ventilation.

Based on this understanding, the key question facing practitioners today is not so much which ventilator to use, but which of the available modes of ventilatory support available is most appropriate in a given situation. Although no absolute consensus has yet emerged, respiratory care practitioners must be well versed in the techniques involved in applying these various modes, including controlled ventilation, IMV, PEEP, CPAP, pressure support ventilation (PSV), and mandatory minute ventilation (MMV). Ultimately, the skill and experience of the operating practitioner with these applications is more important than the specific type of apparatus used.

REFERENCES

1. McPherson SP: Respiratory therapy equipment, ed 3, St Louis, 1985, The CV Mosby Co.
2. Smith RA, Desautels DA, and Kirby RR: Mechanical ventilators. In Kirby RR, Smith RA, and Desautels DD, editors: Mechanical ventilation, New York, 1985, Churchill Livingstone.
3. Mushin WW et al: Automatic ventilation of the lungs, ed 3, Oxford, 1980, Blackwell Scientific Publications.
4. Desautels D: Ventilator classification: a new look at an old subject, Curr Rev Respir Ther 1:82, 1979.
5. Hunter AR: The classification of respirators, Anaesthesia 16:231, 1961.
6. Desautels DA: Ventilator performance evaluation. In Kirby RR, Smith RA, and Desautels DD, editors: Mechanical ventilation, New York, 1985, Churchill Livingstone.
7. Barach AL, Martin S, and Eckman M: Positive pressure respiration and its application to the treatment of acute pulmonary edema and respiratory obstruction, Proc Am Soc Clin Invest 16:664, 1937.
8. Poulton EP: Left-sided heart failure with pulmonary edema treated with the pulmonary plus pressure machine, Lancet 2:983, 1936.
9. Gregory GA, Kitterman JA, Phibbs RH et al: Treatment of idiopathic respiratory distress syndrome with continuous positive airway pressure, N Engl J Med 284:1333, 1971.
10. Spearman CB and Sanders HG Jr: Physical principles and functional design of ventilators. In Kirby RR, Smith RA, and Desautels DD, editors: Mechanical ventilation, New York, 1985, Churchill Livingstone.
11. Morch ET: History of mechanical ventilation. In Kirby RR, Smith RA, and Desautels DD, editors: Mechanical ventilation, New York, 1985, Churchill Livingstone.
12. Dammann JF and McAslan TC: Optimal flow pattern for mechanical ventilation of the lungs—evaluation with a model lung, Crit Care Med 5:128-136, 1977.
13. Dammann JF, McAslan TC, and Maffeo CJ: Optimal flow pattern for mechanical ventilation of the lungs. 2. The effect of a sine versus square wave flow pattern with and without an end-inspiratory pause on patients, Crit Care Med 6(5):293-310, 1978.
14. Boysen PG, Banner MJ, and Jaeger MJ: Inspiratory times and flow wave patterns in relation to distribution of ventilation, Anesthesiology 63:A560, 1985.
15. Smith RK: Respiratory care applications for fluidics, Respir Ther 3:29, 1973.
16. Spearman CB and Sanders SG Jr: The new generation mechanical ventilators, Respir Care 32:403-414, 1987.
17. Scanlan CL: Classification of mechanical ventilators. V. Clinical application—inspiratory phase (individual independent study package), Dallas, 1978, American Association for Respiratory Therapy.
18. Pilbeam SP: Mechanical ventilation: physiological and clinical applications, St Louis, 1986, The CV Mosby Co.
19. Downs JB: Ventilatory patterns and modes of ventilation in acute respiratory failure, Respir Care 28:586-591, 1983.
20. Miyagawa CI: Sedation of the mechanically ventilated patient in the intensive care unit, Respir Care 32:792-805, 1987.
21. Forster A et al: Respiratory depression by midazolam and diazepam, Anesthesiology 53:494-497, 1980.
22. Carlon GC et al: Long-term infusion of sodium thiopental: hemodynamic and respiratory effects, Crit Care Med 6:311-316, 1978.
23. Edbrooke DL et al: Safer sedation for ventilated patients: a new application for etomidate, Anaesthesia 37:765-771, 1982.
24. Greenhouse BB: Muscle relaxants and some problems with their use, Conn Med 34:723, 1970.
25. Clayton BD: Mosby's handbook of pharmacology, ed 4, St Louis, 1987, The CV Mosby Co.
26. Anderson EF and Rosenthal MH: Pancuronium bromide and tachyarrhythmias, Crit Care Med 3:13, 1975.

27. Thomas ET: Circulatory collapse following succinylcholine, Anesth Analg 48:33, 1969.
28. Kirby RR and Graybar GB, editors: Intermittent mandatory ventilation, Int Anesthesiol Clin 18:1-189, 1980.
29. Weisman JM et al: Intermittent mandatory ventilation, Am Rev Respir Dis 127:641-647, 1983.
30. Harboe S: Weaning from mechanical by means of intermittent assisted ventilation (IAV): case reports, Acta Anesth Scand 21:252, 1977.
31. Luce JM, Pierson DJ, and Hudson LD: Critical review: intermittent mandatory ventilation, Chest 79:678, 1981.
32. Fairley HB: In Kirby RR and Graybar GB, editors: Intermittent mandatory ventilation, Int Anesthesiol Clin 18:179, 1980.
33. Hudson LD: Ventilatory management of patients with adult respiratory distress syndrome, Sem Respir Med 2:128, 1981.
34. DeSautels DA and Bartlett JL: Methods of administering intermittent mandatory ventilation, Respir Care 19:187, 1974.
35. Scanlan CL: Classification of mechanical ventilators. V. Clinical application—expiratory phase (individual independent study package), Dallas, 1978, American Association for Respiratory Therapy.
36. Braschi A et al: Functional evaluation of a CPAP circuit with a high compliance reservoir bag, Intens Care Med 11:85-89, 1985.
37. Bishouty ZH, Roeseler J, and Reynaert MS: The importance of the balloon reservoir volume of a CPAP system in reducing the work of breathing, Intens Care Med 12:153-156, 1986.
38. Roeseler J, Bishouty ZH, and Reynaert MS: The importance of the circuit capacity in the administration of CPAP, Intens Care Med 10:305-308, 1984.
39. McPherson SP et al: A circuit that combines ventilator weaning methods using continuous flow ventilation, Respir Care 20:261, 1975.
40. Weled BJ, Winfrey D, and Downs JB: Measuring exhaled volume with continuous positive airway pressure and intermittent mandatory ventilation: techniques and rationale, Chest 76:166, 1979.
41. Poulton TJ and Downs JB: Humidification of rapidly flowing gas, Crit Care Med 9:59-63, 1981.
42. Christopher KL et al: Demand and continuous flow intermittent mandatory ventilation systems, Chest 87:625-630, 1985.
43. Op't Holt TB et al: Comparison of changes in airway pressure during continuous positive airway pressure (CPAP) between demand valve and continuous flow devices, Respir Care 27:1200-1209, 1982.
44. Henry WC, West GA, and Wilson RS: A comparison of the oxygen cost of breathing between a continuous-flow CPAP system and a demand-flow CPAP system, Respir Care 28:1273-1281, 1983.
45. Gibney RTN, Wilson RS, and Pontoppidan H: Comparison of work of breathing on high gas flow and demand valve continuous positive airway pressure systems, Chest 82:692-695, 1982.
46. Viale JP, Annat G, and Bertrand O: Additional inspiratory work in intubated patients breathing with continuous positive airway pressure systems, Anesthesiology 63:536-539, 1985.
47. Kacmarek RM: The role of pressure support ventilation in reducing the work of breathing, Respir Care 33:99-120, 1988.
48. Ashbaugh DG and Petty TL: Positive end-expiratory pressure: physiology, indications, and contraindications, J Thorac Cardiovasc Surg 65:165, 1973.
49. Kumar A et al: Continuous positive-pressure ventilation in acute respiratory failure, N Engl J Med 283:1430, 1970.
50. Tyler DC: Positive end-expiratory pressure: a review, Crit Care Med 11:300-307, 1983.
51. Sugerman HJ, Rogers RM, and Miller LD: Positive end-expiratory pressure (PEEP): indications and physiologic considerations, Chest 62 (pt2):86s, 1972.
52. ACCP-ATS Joint Committee on Pulmonary Nomenclature: Pulmonary terms and symbols, Chest 57:583, 1975.
53. Kittredge P: The difference between PEEP, CPPB, and CPAP, Respir Care 19:14, 1974.
54. Kacmarek RM et al: Technical aspects of positive end-expiratory pressure (PEEP)—parts I, II and III, Respir Care 27:1478-1517, 1982.
55. Banner MJ: Expiratory positive-pressure valves: flow resistance and the work of breathing, Respir Care 323:431-436, 1987.
56. Demers RR and Saklad M: "Assisted PEEP"—assisted mechanical ventilation with positive end-expiratory pressure, Respir Care 19:435, 1974.
57. Ayres SM: Assisted PEEP: helpful or disastrous? Respir Care 19:410, 1974.
58. Gjerde GE: IMV with PEEP versus MV with PEEP, Respir Care 20:894, 1975.
59. Kirby RR et al: High-level positive end-expiratory pressure (PEEP) in acute respiratory insufficiency, Chest 67:156, 1975.
60. Civetta JM et al: "Optimal PEEP" and intermittent mandatory ventilation in the treatment of acute respiratory failure, Respir Care 20:551, 1975.
61. Gallagher TJ and Civetta JM: Goal directed therapy of acute respiratory failure, Anesth Analg 59:831, 1980.
62. Gillick JS: Spontaneous positive end-expiratory pressure (sPEEP), Anesth Analg 56:627, 1977.
63. Eros B, Powner D, and Grenvik A: In Kirby RR and Graybar GB, editors: Intermittent mandatory ventilation, Int Anesthesiology Clin 18:11, 1980.
64. Sturgeon CL et al: PEEP and CPAP: cardiopulmonary effects during spontaneous ventilation, Anesth Analg 56:633, 1977.
65. Weinstein ME et al: Hemodynamic and respiratory response to varying gradients between end-expiratory and end-inspiratory pressure in patients breathing on continuous positive airway pressure, J Trauma 18:231, 1978.
66. Hamilton FN and Singer MM: A breathing circuit for continuous positive airway pressure (CPAP), Crit Care Med 2:86, 1974.
67. Gjerde GE: A method for spontaneous breathing with expiratory positive pressure, Respir Care 20:839, 1975.
68. Kacmarek RM and Goulet RL: PEEP devices, Anesth Clin North Am 5:757-775, 1987.
69. Gherini S, Peters R, and Virgilio RW: Mechanical work on the lungs and the work of breathing with positive endexpiratory pressure and continuous positive airway pressure, Chest 76:251-256, 1979.
70. Civetta JM et al: A simple and effective method of employing spontaneous positive pressure ventilation, J Thorac Cardiovasc Surg 63:312, 1972.
71. Greenbaum DM et al: Continuous positive airway pressure without tracheal intubation in spontaneously breathing patients, Chest 69:615, 1976.
72. Schmidt GB et al: EPAP without intubation, Crit Care Med 5:207, 1977.
73. Smith RA et al: Continuous positive airway pressure (CPAP) by face mask, Crit Care Med 8:483, 1980.
74. Fiastry JF, Quan BF, and Habib MP: Pressure support compensation for inspiratory work due to endotracheal tubes and demand CPAP (abstract), Chest 89:441S, 1986.
75. Forrette TL, Cook EW, and Jones LE: Determining the efficacy of inspiratory assist during mechanical ventilation (abstract), Respir Care 30:864, 1985.
76. Nagy RS and MacIntyre NR: Patient work during pressure support ventilation (abstract), Respir Care 30:860-861, 1985.
77. Linn CR, Gish GB, and Mathewson HS: The effect of pressure support on work of breathing (abstract), Respir Care 30:861-862, 1985.
78. Brochard L et al: Pressure support (PS) decreases work of breathing and oxygen consumption during weaning from mechanical ventilation (abstract), Am Rev Respir Dis 135:A51, 1987.
79. MacIntyre NR: Pressure support ventilation: effects on ventilatory reflexes and ventilatory muscle workload, Respir Care 32:447-457, 1987.

80. Grande CM and Kahn RC: The effect of pressure support ventilation on ventilatory variables and work of breathing (abstract), Anesthesiology 65:A84, 1986.

81. MacIntyre NR: Respiratory function during pressure support ventilation, Chest 89:677-683, 1986.

82. Ershowsky P, Citres D, and Krieger B: Changes in breathing pattern during pressure support ventilation in difficult to wean patients (abstract), Respir Care 31:946, 1986.

83. Thalman TA, Holter JF, and Chitwood WR: Effects of different types of ventilatory support on total body oxygen consumption (abstract), Respir Care 30:859, 1985.

84. Brochard L, Pluskwa F, and Lemaire F: Improved efficacy of spontaneous breathing with inspiratory pressure support, Am Rev Resp Dis 136:411-415, 1987.

85. Prakash O and Meij S: Cardiopulmonary response to inspiratory pressure support during spontaneous ventilation vs. conventional ventilation, Chest 88:403-408, 1985.

86. Chatburn RL: Estimating appropriate pressure support levels (letter); and Mita JF: Response, Respir Care 30:925-926, 1985.

87. Kacmarek RM: Pressure support, another approach to mechanical ventilation, Respir Times 1:1,6, 1986.

88. MacIntyre NR: Weaning from mechanical ventilatory support: volume-assisting intermittent breaths versus pressure-assisting every breath, Respir Care 33:121-125, 1988.

89. Hewlett AM, Platt AS, and Terry VG: Mandatory minute volume: a new technique in weaning from mechanical ventilation, Anaesthesia 32:163-169, 1977.

90. Norlander O: New concepts of ventilation, Acta Anaesthesiol Belg 33:221-234, 1982.

91. Cameron PD and Oh TE: Newer modes of mechanical ventilatory support, Anaesth Intens Care 14(3):258-266, 1986.

92. Shelledy DC and Mikles SP: Newer modes of mechanical ventilation: mandatory minute volume ventilation—part 2, Respir Manage 18(4):21-22, 24, 26-28, 1988.

93. Thompson JD: Computerized control of mechanical ventilation: closing the loop, Respir Care 32:440-446, 1987.

94. Higgs BD and Bevan JC: Use of mandatory minute volume ventilation in the perioperative management of a patient with myasthenia, Br J Anaesth 51:1181-1184, 1979.

31

Management and Monitoring of the Patient in Respiratory Failure

Sharon Williams-Colon
F. Robert Thalken

Management of the patient in respiratory failure involves the integration of many skills. First, the respiratory care practitioner must possess substantial technical expertise in the use of the broad range of sophisticated equipment now commonplace in critical care. Second, the practitioner must possess astute observation and assessment skills, including the ability to evaluate and interpret the patient's clinical presentation and laboratory data. Last, and most important, the practitioner must be able to integrate technical knowledge with assessment skills in order to draw conclusions, make recommendations, and, where appropriate, take action. With sufficient time, effort, and experience, the practitioner can refine these abilities and develop the sound clinical judgment and decision-making skills necessary to provide competent and effective critical care.

Respiratory failure is frequently associated with other organ system dysfunctions. Therefore, successful management must also involve a multisystems approach. Careful attention must be given to the other systems of the body, including assessment of the patient's cardiovascular, renal, neurological, nutritional, and emotional status. While the practitioner may not be an expert in these areas, it is important that significant findings be recognized and related to their potential impact on the patient's cardiopulmonary status. In doing so, it is essential to acknowledge and utilize the expertise of other members of the health care team. The knowledge and skills of the physician, respiratory care practitioner, nurse, and other pertinent health professionals must all be utilized to maximally benefit the patient.

OBJECTIVES

Toward this end, we will present an overview of important components of patient management and cardiopulmo-nary monitoring techniques. Many of the theoretical principles which provide a sound background for patient management have been discussed in detail in previous chapters. We will build onto these principles and relate them to practical applications in the evaluation and management of patients in respiratory failure.

Specifically, after completion of this chapter, the reader will be able to:

1. Outline the general principles of critical care management as applied to care of the patient in respiratory failure;

2. Differentiate the major goals of ventilatory support;

3. Identify the means by which initial ventilatory support parameters are determined and applied;

3. Outline the major components of ongoing monitoring and assessment, including the use of general patient information in respiratory care;

4. Differentiate the specific methods used to obtain pertinent physiologic data on the patient's status and their significance;

5. Given appropriate clinical "clues" involving the patient-ventilator system, state the possible problem and potential solution;

6. Describe the elements of a routine ventilator check, including the importance of appropriate and sequential documentation;

7. Given relevant patient data, recommend appropriate adjustments in the parameters of ventilatory support;

8. Differentiate between the advantages, disadvantages, and appropriate use of current methods for discontinuing ventilatory support.

TERMS

Most terms used in this chapter are defined in context. The following terms are introduced without explicit definition, but may be found in the text glossary:

basilic vein	prothrombin
BUN	PT
capnography	PTT
hematology	pulsus paradoxus
I/O	radiopaque
LC circuit	respirometer
myxoma	spectrophotometry
oximeter	thermistor
percutaneous	thromboplastin

GENERAL PRINCIPLES OF PATIENT MANAGEMENT

The management of critically ill patients is among the most complex and demanding aspects of respiratory care. Patient management is an ongoing process involving three major components: data collection, data analysis and interpretation, and decision-making.

Data collection involves gathering information via repeated or continuous observations. Pertinent information is obtained via traditional physical assessment procedures, in conjunction with standard diagnostic testing, including laboratory and radiologic evaluation. Supplementing this data in the critical care setting are observations made available through physiologic monitoring of the patient's cardiopulmonary status.

The supplementary information provided by physiologic monitoring serves two major purposes. First, physiologic monitoring provides information useful in defining the nature of the problem, its progression, and (ideally) its resolution. Such information provides valuable assistance to health care practitioners in choosing appropriate management strategies and evaluating the patient's response to them, thereby increasing the likelihood of successful outcomes.

Physiologic monitoring also increases our ability to detect complications of management, preferably before they become life-threatening. Given the inherent instability of critically ill patients and the high risk associated with their management, it should come as no surprise that complications are commonplace in the critical care setting. As an example, Table 31-1 summarizes the major complications found over a five-year period in the management of some 350 patients receiving continuous ventilatory support. As many as half of such incidents can result in actual harm to the patient.

Data collection alone is of little value unless it is used to affect patient management. Indeed, health care practitioners today are often inundated with information about the patient, some of which is of questionable utility in patient care. As a general rule of thumb, only information that can and will be used in clinical decision-making should be gathered. Such a rule will minimize the cost and potential patient hazards associated with needless information gathering.

Once needed data has been gathered, it must be analyzed and interpreted. Interpretation of patient data requires extensive knowledge of both normal and abnormal parameters, including their significance in various disease states. In this regard, the respiratory care practitioner should be proficient in gathering and interpreting physiologic data pertinent to assessing patient oxygenation, ventilation, and respiratory mechanics. Moreover, the respiratory care practitioner must possess general knowledge of other elements of patient assessment that are relevant to the care of the patient in respiratory failure, especially hemodynamic monitoring.

Sound clinical decision making follows data collection and interpretation. Decision-making involves assessing the potential benefits and risks associated with available man-

Table 31-1 Potential Complications of Mechanical Ventilation

	No. of cases	Percent incidence
COMPLICATION ATTRIBUTED TO INTUBATION, EXTUBATION OR TUBE MALFUNCTION		
Prolonged intubation attempts	46	30
Intubation of the right mainstem bronchus	34	10
Premature extubation	21	7
Self extubation	30	9
Tube malfunction	21	6
Nasal necrosis	6	2
COMPLICATION ATTRIBUTED TO THE OPERATION OF THE VENTILATOR		
Machine failure	6	2
Alarm failure	13	4
Alarm found off	32	9
Inadequate nebulization of humidification	45	13
Overheating of inspired air	7	2
MEDICAL COMPLICATIONS OCCURRING WITH MECHANICAL VENTILATION		
Alveolar hypoventilation	35	10
Alveolar hyperventilation	39	11
Massive gastric distention	5	2
Pneumothorax	15	4
Atelectasis	16	5
Pneumonia	13	4
Hypotension	16	5

A comprehensive study by Zwillich and associates. From Pilbeam SP: Mechanical ventilation: physiological and clinical applications, Denver, 1986, Multi-Media Publishing, Inc.

agement options and choosing that approach most likely to help and least likely to harm the patient.

Of course, the management process does not end with the initial selection and implementation of a course of action. Patient management is a cyclical and ongoing process. Interventions, once taken, are assessed for their effect. New data is analyzed and interpreted, and refinements or changes are made in the approach used. This process continues until the goals of intervention are achieved, or, as is too often the case in the care of the critically ill, the patient succumbs to the disease process.

As applied to the care of patients receiving ventilatory support, this management process involves the following key elements:

1. Establishment of ventilator settings based on the patient's size and clinical condition. Settings are entered and proper function of the ventilator is verified before connection to the patient.

2. Thorough preliminary assessment of both the patient and ventilator system to assure that all parameters are well tolerated and the patient is stabilized, including assurance of a patent airway, followed by initial data gathering; sampling and analysis of arterial blood gases are to be done within 20 to 30 minutes after stabilization.

3. Setting clinical goals for ventilatory support, in conjunction with the physician and based on the patient's history, physical assessment, and pulmonary status. These goals, along with the length of time the patient is expected to need support, will depend upon the severity of disease and the events leading to initiation of ventilatory support.

4. Adjustment of support parameters, as indicated by arterial blood gas results and the patient's clinical condition. Several adjustments may be necessary before satisfactory results are achieved. However, in order to evaluate the effect of a parameter change on the patient, it is generally wise to make only a single change at a time. Simultaneous changes in support parameters should be reserved for emergency situations.

5. Ongoing monitoring and assessment of the patient and ventilatory system, as often as indicated. The patient's spontaneous ventilatory effort and capabilities also should be assessed regularly, ideally no less than once per shift. Overall cardiopulmonary function and the relative status of other major body systems should be reviewed and discussed with the patient's nurse and attending physician, as appropriate.

6. Additional therapeutic intervention to treat the cause(s) and complications of respiratory failure, keeping in mind that ventilatory support is an interim measure and does not in itself reverse the initial cause of respiratory failure.

7. Weaning from the ventilator once the problems resulting in respiratory failure have been corrected. The

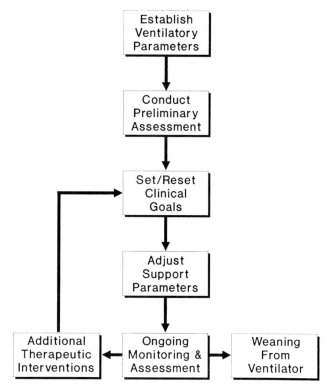

Fig. 31-1   Systematic approach to managing patients in respiratory failure.

physiologic and clinical data collected during the course of ventilation are used by the physician, respiratory care practitioner, and nurse to determine patient readiness for weaning.

As shown in Fig. 31-1, this process, like patient management in general, is cyclical and ongoing. As with any interim life-sustaining strategy, the desired end point of ventilatory support is resolution of the underlying cause of organ failure, with eventual removal of the support measure.

In order to achieve this goal, the patient suffering from respiratory failure requires close attention by skilled respiratory care practitioners who are knowledgeable in the clinical aspects of ventilatory support and patient observation. These patients should be placed in a specialized critical care unit which is staffed on a 24-hour basis by appropriately trained personnel. In addition, such a unit should be equipped to provide a full range of standard and emergency life support measures, including the ability to continuously monitor key physiologic parameters. Only in such a context can a successful outcome be realized.

INITIAL ESTABLISHMENT OF VENTILATORY SUPPORT SETTINGS

In establishing the initial ventilatory support settings, the primary aim is to stabilize the patient by the provision of adequate oxygenation and ventilation. This is accomplished mainly by careful selection of the ventilatory support mode, F_{IO_2}, and parameters of minute ventilation. Additional considerations include the use of periodic sigh breaths, adjustments of inspiratory flow and I:E ratios, provision of adequate humidification, and setting of applicable alarms and indicators.

Mode of ventilatory support

The mode of ventilatory support initially chosen depends mainly upon the patient's underlying pathophysiologic problem. In general, if the patient's respiratory failure is associated with hypercapnea due to inadequate alveolar ventilation, either the CMV or IMV modes may be employed. On the other hand, if the problem is purely a hypoxemia unreponsive to standard oxygen therapy (hypoxemic respiratory failure), then CPAP is indicated. Patients with both inadequate alveolar ventilation and refractory hypoxemia are candidates for CMV or IMV with PEEP. When respiratory failure is associated with respiratory muscle fatigue, a newer mode of ventilatory support, called pressure support ventilation (PSV) may be indicated.

Selection of inspired oxygen concentration (F_{IO_2})

Initial setting of the F_{IO_2} should guarantee an adequate Pa_{O_2} with a wide margin of safety. Since there is no known risk of oxygen toxicity at high concentrations when used for short time periods, an initial F_{IO_2} of 1.0 should be provided whenever a patient's state of oxygenation is in doubt. Moreover, the initial administration of 100% oxygen allows subsequent estimation of the degree of physiologic shunting, as will be discussed in following sections. Although absorption atelectasis is a potential hazard with 100% oxygen administration, its likelihood is diminished by the provision of the large tidal volumes characterizing mechanical ventilatory support.

Even patients whose ventilatory stimulus is mainly oxygen lack should be started on high F_{IO_2} values with ventilatory support, especially when clinical signs indicating a cardiovascular response to hypoxemia are present. If, on the other hand, blood gas data is available prior to initiating ventilatory support and the adequacy of oxygenation is not in question, it may be possible to initiate ventilatory support at an F_{IO_2} equal to or slightly higher than that previously used.

Minute ventilation

In the assist/control, control and IMV modes of ventilatory support, the clinician has control over all or part of the patient's minute ventilation. In the pure CPAP mode, the patient is fully responsible for generating and maintaining an adequate minute ventilation. In either case, the goal is to assure adequate removal of CO_2, as judged by the normalization of the arterial pH. In

Depending upon the ventilator, minute ventilation may be set in one of two ways. Commonly, the ventilator provides separate tidal volume and frequency settings. Minute ventilation is therefore the product of frequency times tidal volume:

$$\dot{V}_E = f \times V_T$$

Alternatively, some ventilators allow the clinician to set the minute ventilation and frequency, with the tidal volume being a derived value:

$$V_T = \frac{\dot{V}_E}{f}$$

Regardless of approach, the total minute ventilation will determine the patient's Pa_{CO_2}. Changes in any variable that alters the total minute ventilation will effect the Pa_{CO_2}.

Nomograms. Prior to 1970, the selection of tidal volumes, rates, and minute ventilations was based, in part, on the Radford nomogram (Fig. 31-2). To use the nomogram, align the parameters of estimated body weight and desired breathing frequency, thereby deriving a predicted tidal volume.

Although correction factors are provided for various conditions, extensive clinical experience with this nomogram has consistently shown that it tends to underestimate the requirements of most patients in need of ventilatory support. This is because the nomogram was developed using data obtained from healthy subjects under basal metabolic requirements. Moreover, even when the application of the nomogram results in an adequate minute ventilation, the predicted tidal volumes generally are insufficient to prevent the progressive atelectasis that can occur in patients receiving ventilatory support (see Chapter 29). For this reason, the Radford nomogram has been replaced with estimating formulas that provide substantially higher tidal volumes.

Estimating formulas. Today, tidal volumes and frequencies of breathing are generally established by estimating formulae, and thereafter adjusted according to the patient's physiologic response to the ventilatory support. These estimates are based on the patient's age, breathing frequency and clinical condition, and the mode of ventilation chosen (see Table 31-2).

With regard to the patient's age, adults are generally started at tidal volumes within the range of 10 to 15 ml/kg, at frequencies between 8 and 20 per minute. For adolescents in the 8- to 16-year-old age range, 8 to 10 ml/kg, at frequencies between 20 to 30 per minute is usually sufficient. Infants and children (birth to 8 years old) normally are managed with tidal volumes in the range of 6 to 8 ml/kg and rates of between 30 to 40 per minute.

Adjustments to these estimates are based, in part, on the mechanical properties of the patient's lungs and thorax. In

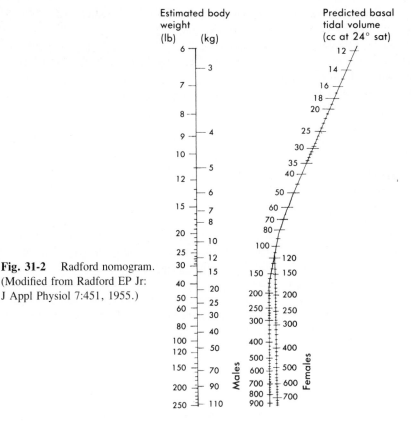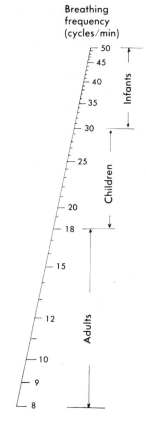

Estimated body weight (lb) (kg)

Predicted basal tidal volume (cc at 24° sat)

Breathing frequency (cycles/min)

Fig. 31-2 Radford nomogram. (Modified from Radford EP Jr: J Appl Physiol 7:451, 1955.)

Corrections of predicted basal tidal volumes.
   For patients not in coma: add 10%
     Fever: add 5% for each °F above 99 (rectal)
         add 9% for each °C above 37 (rectal)
   Altitude: add 5% for each 2000 feet above sea level
         add 8% for each 1000 meters above sea level
   Intubation: subtract volume equal to one-half body weight in pounds
         subtract 1 cc/kg of body weight
   Dead space: add equipment dead space

adult patients with normal lungs and pulmonary mechanics, tidal volumes in the range of 12 to 15 ml/kg of body weight are used, with frequencies in the range of 8 to 12 per minute. Patients with chronic obstructive pulmonary disease tend to do better at lower breathing frequencies, because of the high expiratory resistance to gas flow. Initial frequencies in the range of 8 to 10 per minute are frequently recommended for these patients, with tidal volumes initially set at 10 to 12 ml/kg, and adjusted to maintain an appropriate $Paco_2$. On the other hand, patients with restrictive pulmonary disease may require rates in the 12 to 20 per minute range, sometimes with tidal volumes less than 10 ml/kg.

In terms of the mode of ventilation, the lower ranges of volume and higher ranges of rate generally are used in the assist/control mode, while the higher ranges of volume and lower ranges of rate are more commonly used in the IMV

mode. In the control or assist/control modes, the rate is chosen based on the selected tidal volume, so that the resulting minute volume will achieve a satisfactory $Paco_2$ and pH. In the assist/control mode, the backup rate should depend on the patient's assist rate. In the presence of a respiratory acidosis, it should be high enough to increase the minute ventilation. If the patient has an adequate spontaneous rate, the backup rate should be set at two to four breaths below this value in order to prevent hypoventilation should the patient rate diminish significantly. In the IMV mode, it is best to set the initial frequency close to that of the patient's own spontaneous breathing rate, at the preselected tidal volume. The IMV frequency can then be manipulated based on subsequent blood gas studies.

Obviously, in the pure CPAP mode, the minute ventilation is determined entirely by the patient. However, estimation of the minute ventilation requirements for patients receiving this mode of ventilatory support is useful in establishing monitoring and alarm parameters and in estimating the efficiency of their ventilation (see subsequent sections).

Periodic sighs

The use of periodic sigh breaths is generally limited to the control or assist/control modes, or when tidal volumes are set below the minimum of the specified range. When used, sigh volumes normally are set at one and one-half to two times the tidal volume, at a rate of at least 5 per minute. It is generally unnecessary to use sighs in the IMV mode, since the mandatory breaths are typically set at the high end of the recommended ranges for tidal volumes. Sighs are also considered unnecessary when high tidal volumes and PEEP are being used together.

Inspiratory flows and I:E ratios

In the CMV mode of ventilatory support, inspiratory flows are adjusted to provide the desired inspiratory time, I:E ratio, and breathing pattern. The inspiratory flow necessary to achieve appropriate time parameters in adults generally falls within the 40 to 80 L/min range. However, flows above and below this range may be necessary in some patients to achieve the desired inspiratory time and I:E ratio. As previously discussed, excessively high flows may worsen the distribution of ventilation, whereas low flows lengthen inspiratory times, thereby tending to increase mean intrapleural pressures and potentially resulting in insufficient time for exhalation.

In the control or assist/control modes, the inspiratory flow should be set to provide an I:E ratio of about 1:2 or less. In most patients, this will provide sufficient time for

a full exhalation and a perceptible pause before the next breath, without compromising cardiovascular function.

Patients with chronic obstructive pulmonary disease pose unique problems in setting inspiratory flows. In many of these patients, I:E ratios of 1:4 or lower are necessary in order to provide sufficient time for exhalation and prevent air trapping. However, these I:E ratios generally require short inspiratory times and high inspiratory flows, which tend to worsen gas distribution in these patients. Generally, the solution lies in using low respiratory rates, which can provide for both longer inspiratory and expiratory times. Obviously, use of the IMV mode in these patients can help insure sufficient time for exhalation.

In the CPAP mode, time parameters of breathing are determined by the patient. However, available inspiratory flows are critically important. In order to maintain airway pressure and minimize the work of breathing, available inspiratory flows should be at least three times the patient's minute ventilation.

Humidification and airway temperature

Maintenance of appropriate humidification and airway temperature may be provided by either a hygroscopic condenser humidifier (heat and moisture exchanger) or heated humidifier. If ventilatory support is to be provided on a short-term basis (two days or less), and the patient is normothermic, adequately hydrated, and has no problem with retained secretions, the use of a hygroscopic condenser humidifier is clinically acceptable. Should these conditions not be met, a heated humidifier (preferably servocontrolled) should be employed.

When using a heated humidifier, the proximal airway temperature should be set near normal body temperature, and the humidifier checked for adequate water levels. Caution must be taken against overfilling the humidifier as this may significantly increase circuit resistance and interfere with spontaneous breathing.

Limits and alarms

The high pressure limit on the support system should generally be set at 10 cm H_2O above the peak airway pressure in CMV or IMV modes and 5 cm H_2O above the baseline pressure in the CPAP mode. When sighs are employed, provision must be made to ensure that the pressure limit does not prevent delivery of the full sigh volume.

A low pressure or disconnect alarm should also be incorporated into all systems. In systems used to deliver PEEP or CPAP, the low pressure alarm should be adjustable and set to trigger if baseline pressures fall either 5 cm H_2O or 20% below the set pressure level.

A low exhaled volume alarm is mandatory and should be set to trigger when either the tidal volume or minute ventilation falls 20% below established values. A high tidal volume or minute ventilation alarm, if available,

Table 31-2 Recommended Tidal Volumes and Frequencies*

Patient type	Frequency	Tidal volume
ADULTS		
Normal lungs	8-12	12-15 ml/kg
Chronic obstructive disease	8-10 or less	10-12 ml/kg
Chronic restrictive disease	12-20 or more	10 ml/kg or less
Acute lung injury (ARDS)	12-20 or more	10 ml/kg or less
CHILDREN		
Age 8-16	20-30	8-10 ml/kg
Age 0-8	30-40	6-8 ml/kg

*For control and assist/control modes; for IMV mode, rates below these minimums are common, with volumes set at the high end of the prescribed ranges.
From Kacmarek RM and Venegar JV: Mechanical ventilatory rates and tidal volumes, Respir Care 32:466-474, 1987.

should be set to warn of rises in minute ventilation above 20% of the value established.

If available in the assist/control or control modes, an I:E limit should be set to 1:1, with an alarm indicator to warn of changes in this parameter. Ideally, an airway temperature alarm should be set to warn of unexpected rises in the temperature of inspired gas. Finally, system alarms designed to warn of electrical or gas power failure should be verified for their proper function.

PRELIMINARY ASSESSMENT AND DATA GATHERING

Once the initial ventilatory parameters are established, the clinician should conduct a preliminary assessment of the patient and patient-ventilator system to assure that all parameters are well tolerated and the patient is stable and as comfortable as possible. Also during this phase, the practitioner must assure that all necessary supplementary equipment necessary to provide patient support is available.

After the patient is stabilized and the patient-ventilator system is verified in proper working order, initial arterial blood gases are obtained for analysis.

Initial patient assessment and support

Initial evaluation of the patient should include assessment of the patient's appearance and level of consciousness; measurement of vital signs, including heart rate and blood pressure; simple auscultation to verify bilateral ventilation; measurements of key ventilatory parameters (as provided by the support system); and a preliminary assessment of the airway. Other significant observations, such as cardiac arrhythmias, should also be noted. If the patient is conscious during this period of initial assessment, every effort must be made to attend to his or her psychological needs (see Chapter 13).

Details about the patient's airway should include verification of its position, patency, and cuff pressure. Endotracheal tube placement should be confirmed by either a chest radiograph or fiberoptic laryngoscopy. The initial cuff pressure should be set using either the minimal leak (MLT) or minimal occluding volume (MOV) technique. In either case, cuff pressure at peak airway pressure should ideally be maintained below 25 mm Hg. An extra endotracheal or tracheotomy tube should be kept at the bedside in case of accidental extubation or rupture of the cuff. The necessary equipment for changing each type of airway must be available and easily accessible (see Chapter 21).

A clean, functioning manual resuscitator, connected to oxygen and ready for use, must be available at the bedside in the event of mechanical or electrical failure. A suction source, supply of catheters, and sterile water or saline for instillation must also be available, as frequent suctioning may be required; all patients are at risk of airway occlusion by secretions at any time.

Arterial blood gas analysis

Early arterial blood gas analysis is a critical component of initial patient assessment. However, sampling of the arterial blood should be undertaken only after sufficient time has passed to ensure equilibration between the alveolar and arterial gas tensions.

The amount of time necessary for this equilibration depends upon the underlying disease process. In patients with normal lung function, equilibration can be expected in less than 5 minutes, and arterial blood gases evaluated accordingly. As alveolar ventilation increases and FRC decreases, less time is needed for equilibration of gas tensions. However, in patients with lower than normal alveolar ventilation and larger than normal FRCs, such as those with COPD, equilibration times may be significantly longer than normal. In such patients, it is advisable to wait for 30 minutes after initiation of ventilatory support (or changing support parameters) before sampling the arterial blood.

GOAL SETTING

The effective application of ventilatory support techniques should be founded on tangible clinical goals. Applied as an interim measure only, the primary goal of ventilatory support is to discontinue its use as soon as the underlying problem is resolved.

However, in consultation with the patient's physician, the respiratory care practitioner should establish measurable patient management objectives to guide the course of ventilatory support toward discontinuation. Such objectives should provide clear and consistent direction to those involved in the patient's management, yet allow for tailoring the plan according to the patient's condition and individual needs.

The following box outlines the three primary clinical goals toward which ventilatory support is directed. Associated with each goal should be tangible interim and end-stage indicators used to determine goal achievement. For example, if the primary goal is to ensure adequate patient oxygenation, the interim indicator might be adequate arterial oxygenation (a Pa_{O_2} above 60 mm Hg) at a safe $F_{I_{O_2}}$

GOALS OF VENTILATORY SUPPORT

GOAL	EXAMPLE
To improve alveolar ventilation	pH normalized with Pa_{CO_2} between 35 to 45 mm Hg
To correct hypoxemia	Pa_{O_2} greater than 60 mm Hg with $F_{I_{O_2}}$ less than 0.40
To decrease the work of breathing	Elimination of breathing patterns indicating fatigue (eg, asynchrony or paradox)

(0.40 or less) with minimum cardiovascular depression. On the other hand, the end-stage indicator, associated with discontinuance of the support modality, might be the ability of the patient to maintain a Po_2 above 60 mm Hg on an Fio_2 of less than 0.40 without PEEP or CPAP. Clearly, multiple goals may need to be established for some patients.

ONGOING MONITORING AND ASSESSMENT

Because of the complexities of ventilatory support and its use as a life sustaining measure, meticulous ongoing monitoring of the patient and patient-ventilator system is essential. Both the patient and patient-ventilator system should be thoroughly assessed at least every two hours or whenever changes in parameters are made. With unstable patients, continuous monitoring and assessment may be indicated.

For convenience, we divide the process of ongoing monitoring and assessment into three major components: general patient assessment, physiologic data gathering and interpretation, and patient-ventilator system troubleshooting. In addition, we will discuss the importance of meticulous sequential record keeping.

General patient assessment

General patient information can be obtained through observation and assessment techniques. Some of these procedures will be performed by the respiratory care practitioner; information on others will be gained by chart review or direct communication with the attending physician or nurse. Communication of patient status should also occur through participation in bedside rounds and shift reports. The following assessments are particularly appropriate in monitoring the patient receiving ventilatory support.

Vital signs. Vital signs give the practitioner an indication of the overall status of the patient. The most basic determinations include temperature, pulse, blood pressure, and respiratory rate. Details on the measurement of vital signs are provided in Chapter 13. Table 31-3 provides guidance regarding the interpretation of changes in vital signs as related to the care of patients receiving ventilatory support.

Temperature is usually measured by nursing personnel and found on the nursing flow sheet. An elevated temperature might indicate infection and may warrant further investigation, such as culture and sensitivity tests on sputum, blood, or urine. Elevation of the patient's temperature may also occur when the airway temperature is set too high or the humidifier control mechanism fails.

The pulse rate can and should be obtained and recorded by the respiratory care practitioner. The strength of the pulse in various parts of the respiratory cycle must also be noted. Weakening of the pulse during inspiration may indicate variations in output resulting from positive-pressure cardiac tamponade. The pulse can also yield information on adequacy of circulation (necessary for arterial blood sampling) and blood pressure (weak or thready pulse in hypotension).

A patient heart rate can normally be observed continuously using the electrocardiographic monitor. This index is particularly important during suctioning, which can precipitate arrhythmias. Abnormal rhythms may also indicate ischemic heart disease, an acute cardiopulmonary process such as pulmonary embolism, or the development of congestive heart failure. The practitioner should have a basic understanding of ECG interpretation and should be able to recognize changes from the patient's baseline heart rate and rhythm, including the immediate recognition of life threatening arrhythmias such as complete heart block, ventricular tachycardia, and ventricular fibrillation (see Chapter 22).

Physical assessment. As covered in Chapter 16, physical assessment includes inspection, palpation, percussion, and auscultation. Although it may be more difficult to perform a thorough physical exam on a critically ill patient, the basic principles still apply, but may need to be modified. Astute observation can often spot a potential problem before diagnostic test results are available. Moreover, simple physical assessment, in combination with the measurement of vital signs, can help determine the severity of respiratory failure and the potential outcomes of patient management.

Six simple physical assessment signs have been shown to correlate highly with both the need for continuing ventilatory support and the likelihood of successful outcomes of such care. These simple physical indicators include: (1) a pulse rate over 120 or under 70 beats per minute, (2) a respiratory rate of over 30 per minute, (3) the presence of palpable scalene muscle recruitment during inspiration, (4) the presence of palpable abdominal tensing during expiration, (5) the presence of irregularities of respiratory rhythm with apneic pauses of varying duration, and (6) any condition preventing a patient from responding to commands aimed at producing ventilatory movements (like those needed for vital capacity testing). The chances of a favorable outcome in patients exhibiting none of these six signs is about 90%. Generally, most patients exhibiting one or two of these signs will require further ventilatory support and may not recover at all. When three or more of the signs are present at the same time, the patient's prognosis is extremely poor.

Chest roentgenography. In the critical care setting, roentgenography is used most commonly by the respiratory care practitioner to evaluate endotracheal tube placement. In consultation with the attending physician and/or consulting radiologist, the respiratory care practitioner can also use the chest film to help determine if the lungs are being properly aerated and to detect major pathological changes such as hyperinflation, atelectasis, consolidation, pneumothorax, pleural effusion, and congestion from pneumonia or heart failure (see Chapter 18). A chest film should be obtained immediately after intubation and daily during the critical period of the patient's illness.

Medications. To make informed judgments regarding the patient's stability, need for supplemental therapies, and readiness for weaning, the practitioner should be familiar with all drugs being administered to the patient. Drugs most likely to affect the patient's respiratory status include those given for pain, sedation, muscle relaxation, arrhythmia, and blood pressure control.

Clinical laboratory studies. The major clinical laboratory studies of use in monitoring the patient in respiratory failure are summarized in Table 31-4. Hematology data are useful in assessing the oxygen carrying capacity of the blood, the response to infection, and the potential for bleeding. Clinical chemistry data help in the interpretation of acid-base imbalances, particularly those of metabolic or renal origin. For these reasons, respiratory care practitioners must be familiar with the use, application, and interpretation of these major clinical laboratory studies.

Fluid balance. In most critical care units, nursing personnel assume primary responsibility for monitoring the patient's fluid balance. This is accomplished by evaluating fluid intake and output (I/O), often in conjunction with patient weight. Central venous and pulmonary arterial pressures are also utilized to assess and guide maintenance of fluid balance.

Fluid balance is particularly relevant to the practitioner as it relates to the role of the kidneys in maintaining acid-

Table 31-3   Vital Signs

Clue	Possible problem	Advice
Hypotension	Decreased venous return (caused by changes in intrathoracic pressure)	Evaluate fluid balance and possible need for filling of vascular bed
Hypertension	Anxiety	Reassure, alleviate fears
	Early response to decreased Pa_{O_2}, decreased Pa_{CO_2}	Check patient-ventilator system; if not easily correctable, obtain and evaluate ABG values
Respiratory swing of blood pressure	Decreased venous return (caused by changes in intrathoracic pressure)	If systolic and diastolic pressures below levels for adequate perfusion, evaluate fluid balance and consider filling vascular bed
New arrhythmias, tachycardia, bradycardia	Anxiety	Reassure, alleviate fears
	Decreased Pa_{O_2}, decreased Pa_{CO_2}, increased Pa_{CO_2}	Check patient-ventilator system; if not quickly correctable, obtain and evaluate ABG values
	Decreased venous return	Check other hemodynamic parameters for adequacy of perfusion
Large swings in CVP or PAWP	Decreased venous return	Evaluate other hemodynamic parameters for adequacy of perfusion
Decreased urinary output	Decreased cardiac output owing to decreased venous return	Evaluate other hemodynamic parameters for adequacy of perfusion
Fever	Increased metabolic rate caused by increased inspiratory effort or patient-ventilator asynchrony	Check sensitivity and patient triggering effort settings
	Infection	Treat infection; review preventive measures
	Atelectasis	Check patient-ventilator system for secretions, plugs, slippage of tube into right mainstem bronchus
	Overheated humidifier	Check temperature setting of humidifier heater
Weight gain	Fluid retention caused by decreased venous return	Evaluate other hemodynamic parameters for adequacy of perfusion; consider diuresis
Changes in respiratory rate	Altered settings	Check patient-ventilator settings
	Change in metabolic needs	Evaluate patient metabolic rate
	Anxiety	Reassure, alleviate fears
	Sleep	Normal—metabolic rate is decreased

From Martz KV, Joiner JW, and Shepherd RM: Management of the patient-ventilator system: a team approach, ed 2, St Louis, 1984, The CV Mosby Co.

base balance. In addition. fluid balance management is fundamental to the care of congestive heart failure (CHF). pulmonary edema. and shock of any origin. Moreover. given the sensitivity of the kidneys to changes in oxygen delivery. renal function may be an indicator of disturbances in overall oxygen transport.

Most ventilatory support systems eliminate insensible water loss through the lungs via the provision of saturated gas at body temperature. In essence. this elimination of water loss is equivalent to water gain and should be taken into account. especially in patients whose intake of fluids are restricted. Moreover. any significant water delivery above body humidity levels. such as might occur with supplementary aerosol therapy. should be estimated and reported as fluid intake.

Nutrition. The ability to discontinue ventilatory support can be impacted by a patient's nutritional status. Oxygen consumption and carbon dioxide production are affected by the relative balance among the intake and metabolism of carbohydrates. proteins. and fats. Malnutrition may occur in the critically ill patient as a consequence of decreased nutrient intake and the increased metabolic de-

mands of the body. Careful evaluation should be done by a clinical dietician for all patients receiving long-term ventilatory support. This topic will be discussed later as it relates to patients' ventilatory requirements.

Physiologic data gathering and interpretation

Physiologic data useful in the management of the patient receiving ventilatory support includes information on the patient's state of oxygenation. adequacy and efficiency of ventilation. ventilatory mechanics. and hemodynamics. Table 31-5 provides a summary of the key respiratory parameters according to the function they assess. including the threshold values associated with minimally acceptable physiologic performance (similar guidelines on hemodynamic parameters are provided later in Table 31-10).

Not all such physiologic data need be gathered on all patients. In selecting appropriate parameters for physiologic monitoring of the patient. the clinician should be guided by the nature of the underlying cause of respiratory failure. as balanced against the potential risks and benefits associated with the data gathering procedure.

Generally. invasive procedures. those requiring inser-

Table 31-4   Useful Clinical Laboratory Data

Test	Normal value	Significance
HEMATOLOGY TESTS		
Red blood cells	M 4.6 to 6.2 $\times$ 10^6/mm^3	Oxygen transport
	F 4.2 to 5.4 $\times$ 10^6/mm^3	Response to hypoxemia
		Degree of cyanosis
Hemoglobin	M 16.5 to 16.5 g/dL	Oxygen transport
	F 12.0 to 15.0 g/dL	Response to hypoxemia
		Degree of cyanosis
Hematocrit	M 40% to 50%	Hemoconcentration (high)
	F 38% to 47%	Hemodilution (low)
White blood cells	4500 to 10.000/mm^3	Infection (high)
		Decreased immunity (low)
Platelets	150.000 to 400.000/mm^3	Slow bloodclotting (low)
		Check before ABG
Prothrombin time (PT)	12 to 14 seconds	Slow clotting (high)
		Check before ABG
Partial thromboplastin time (PTT)	25 to 37 seconds	Slow clotting (high)
		Check before ABG
CLINICAL CHEMISTRY TESTS		
Sodium	137 to 147 mEq/L	Acid-base/fluid balance
Potassium	3.5 to 8.4 mEq/L	Metabolic acidosis (high)
		Metabolic alkalosis (low)
		Cardiac arrhythmias (low)
Chloride	98 to 105 mEq/L	Metabolic alkalosis (low)
CO_2 content	25 to 33 mEq/L	Equivalent to HCO_3 + H_2CO_3
Blood urea	7 to 20 mg/dL	Renal failure (high)
Nitrogen (BUN)		Nonvolatile acid
Creatinine	0.7 to 1.3 mg/dL	Renal disease (high)
Glucose	70 to 105 mg/dL	Ketoacidosis (high)

tion of a probe, sensor, or collection device into the body, are associated with greater risk to the patient than noninvasive procedures. However, invasive procedures typically provide more accurate data on physiologic parameters than noninvasive methods. When both approaches are available, the choice of an invasive or noninvasive approach should depend on the relative need for measurement precision. On the other hand, it is often useful to combine the two approaches, using the invasive approach to establish accurate baseline information, while applying the noninvasive method on an ongoing basis to monitor patient status.

Physiologic data may also be gathered intermittently or continuously. Generally, the less stable the patient, the greater the need for continuous data gathering. Continuous

Table 31-5   Key Physiologic Monitoring Data (Respiratory System Parameters)

Function	Parameter	Symbol or formula	Acceptable value(s)
OXYGENATION			
Lung exchange (external)			
Adequacy	Arterial oxygen partial pressure	Pao_2	60 to 100 mm Hg
	Arterial oxygen saturation	Sao_2	>80%
	Trancutaneous oxygen partial pressure	$Ptco_2$	60 to 100 mm Hg
Efficiency	Alveolar to arterial oxygen tension gradient	$P(A-a)o_2$	<350 mm Hg (100% O_2)
	Percent shunt	$\dot{Q}s/\dot{Q}T$	<20%
	a/A ratio	Pao_2/Pao_2	>0.6
	Respiratory index (RI)	$P(A-a)o_2/Pao_2$	<5.0
	P/F ratio	Pao_2/Fio_2	>200
Tissue exchange (internal)	Mixed venous oxygen content	$C\bar{v}o_2$	>10.0 ml/dL
	Mixed venous oxygen partial pressure	$P\bar{v}o_2$	>30 mm Hg
	Mixed venous oxygen saturation	$S\bar{v}o_2$	>65%
	Arterial-venous oxygen content difference	$C(a-\bar{v})o_2$	<7.0 ml/dL
VENTILATION			
Adequacy	Minute ventilation	$\dot{V}E$	>5.0 and <10.0 L/min
	Arterial carbon dioxide partial pressure	$Paco_2$	35 to 45 mm Hg (with normal pH)
	Trancutaneous carbon dioxide partial pressure	$Ptcco_2$	35 to 45 mm Hg (with normal pH)
	End-tidal carbon dioxide partial pressure (percent)	$Petco_2$	35 to 43 mm Hg (4.6 to 5.6%)
Efficiency	Physiologic dead space	V_{Dphy}	see V_D/V_T below
	Deadspace to tidal volume ratio	V_D/V_T	<0.6
	Minute ventilation vs carbon dioxide partial pressure	$\dot{V}E$ vs $Paco_2$	$\dot{V}E$ < 10 L/min with $Paco_2 \leq 40$ mm Hg
	Ventilation quotient	Vq	<3.0
MECHANICS OF VENTILATION			
Work of breathing (direct)	Work kg-m/L or j/L	Work = $P \times V$	<0.20 kg-m/L or 2.0 j/L
Work of breathing (indirect-on ventilator	Dynamic characteristic	$(V_T - Vc)/(P_{peak} - PEEP)$	35 to 50 ml/cm H_2O
	Effective compliance (C_{eff})	$(V_T - Vc)/(P_{stat} - PEEP)$	60 to 100 ml/cm H_2O
Respiratory muscle function (load ability)	Vital capacity	VC	>15 ml/kg
	Maximum voluntary ventilation	MVV	>20 L/min
	Maximum inspiratory force	MIF	>-30 cm H_2O
	Effort index	EI	<0.55
Respiratory muscle fatigue (experimental)	Average asynchrony index	—	Not established
	Percent abdominal paradox	—	Not established
	EMG H-to-L ratio	—	>80% control
	Tension-time index	TT_{di}	<0.15

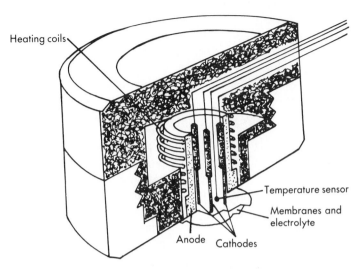

Fig. 31-3   Transcutaneous P_{O_2} electrode. A cross-sectional diagram of the components of the tcP_{O_2} electrode shows a circular anode around a series of cathodes and a temperature sensor. A heating coil causes local hyperemia so that surface P_{O_2} more closely resembles Pa_{O_2}. A double membrane separates the electrode proper from the skin. (From Ruppel G: Manual of pulmonary function testing, ed 3, St Louis, 1982, The CV Mosby Co; in McPherson SP: Respiratory therapy equipment, ed 4, St Louis, 1989, The CV Mosby Co.)

data gathering, which provides indicators of significant changes in physiologic parameters via alarm systems, is equivalent to ongoing patient monitoring.

For each major category of data collection discussed, we will emphasize, where applicable, the variety of options currently available to the practitioner. The final decision on which approach or combination of approaches to physiologic data collection is taken should be made by the care team as a whole, as guided by the above considerations.

Assessment of oxygenation. Oxygenation may be assessed in terms of either oxygen movement between the atmosphere and the blood via the alveolar-capillary membrane (external respiration) or between the blood and the tissue cells (internal respiration). A full evaluation must obviously consider each in careful detail. As the respiratory care practitioner is most directly responsible for external respiratory exchange, we will discuss this aspect first, followed by an analysis of the techniques used to determine oxygen transfer between the blood and the tissue cells.

External (lung) oxygen exchange. Oxygen exchange at the lung should be assessed in terms of both its adequacy and efficiency. The adequacy of oxygen exchange at the lung is generally assessed by measurement of the arterial P_{O_2}. Alternatively or in combination with the Pa_{O_2}, hemoglobin saturation may also be used as an indicator of the adequacy of oxygen exchange at the lung. Both invasive and noninvasive and continuous and intermittent approaches may be used to measure or estimate the adequacy of oxygen exchange occurring at the lungs.

Unfortunately, neither the Pa_{O_2} or Sa_{O_2} individually gives any indication as to the efficiency of oxygen ex-

change at the lung. In order to assess the efficiency of pulmonary oxygen exchange, one must compare the amount of oxygen being delivered to the alveoli with that actually entering the arterial blood. This may be accomplished by the alveolar-arterial oxygen tension gradient $(P(A-a)O_2)$, various ratios that combine arterial and alveolar oxygen tensions, and the estimation, or actual measurement of the degree of physiologic shunting occurring in the lungs $(\dot{Q}s/\dot{Q}_T)$.

Adequacy of oxygen exchange at the lung. The arterial partial pressure of oxygen or Pa_{O_2}, is the most frequently obtained measure of the adequacy of oxygen exchange at the lung. In general, oxygen exchange at the lung is adequate if the arterial P_{O_2} can be maintained in the 60 to 100 mm Hg range.

Usually, the arterial P_{O_2} is obtained intermittently by invasive sampling of arterial blood, either percutaneously or via an indwelling arterial line (see subsequent section). Indwelling intravascular P_{O_2} probes, utilizing a modified Clark electrode, have been developed to provide direct and continuous monitoring of arterial oxygen tensions. However, technical difficulties with these devices, including blood clotting, arterial wall trauma, and motion artifacts, have generally precluded their widespread use.

Alternative noninvasive methods of estimating the Pa_{O_2} include transcutaneous and transconjunctival monitoring. Both methods provide continuous, as opposed to intermittent data.

Transcutaneous P_{O_2} monitoring (Ptc_{O_2}) provides a reasonable estimate of oxygen tension, particularly in infants. A modified Clark electrode, which incorporates heating coils, is utilized (Fig. 31-3). Skin temperatures between $43°$ and $45°C$ cause dilation of capillary beds under the

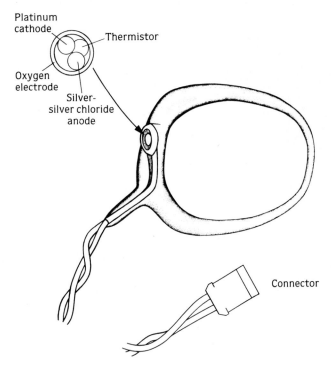

Platinum
cathode

Thermistor

Oxygen
electrode

Silver-
silver chloride
anode

Connector

Fig. 31-4   Diagram of conjunctival Po$_2$ sensor with Clark-type oxygen electrode. (From Wilkins RL, Sheldon RL, and Krider SJ: Clinical assessment in respiratory care, St Louis, 1985, The CV Mosby Co.)

probe and arterialization of the capillary blood. Oxygen diffuses from the cutaneous capillaries, across the dermal and epidermal cell layers, and into the electrode. This diffusion cascade may reduce the Po$_2$ measured at the electrode, particularly as skin thickness increases with patient age. In neonates, the Po$_2$ diffusion gradient between the capillaries and epidermis is largely offset by the heating effect.

In the stable patient with good cardiac output and fluid balance, the Pao$_2$ and Ptco$_2$ are highly correlated, with a relatively constant difference between the two values. In such patients, the Pao$_2$ can be "calibrated" against the Ptco$_2$, thereby minimizing the need for repeated arterial samples. However, the peripheral vasoconstriction that occurs in shock or low flow states dramatically affects cutaneous blood flow, thereby making accurate estimations of Pao$_2$ difficult, if not impossible. For this reason, transcutaneous Po$_2$ monitoring should generally be limited to patients having a stable hemodynamic profile.

Like the transcutaneous monitor, the transconjunctival Po$_2$ monitor incorporates a Clark-type electrode, in this case small enough to be placed against the eye's conjunctiva (Fig. 31-4). The transconjunctival electrode measures the Po$_2$ of the underlying tissue bed, the conjunctival capillaries. Generally, the transconjunctival Po$_2$ electrode is not well tolerated by patients. For this reason, its use has been restricted primarily to surgery. Like the transcutane-

ous Po$_2$ monitor, its accuracy is dependent on the patient's state of tissue perfusion.

The arterial hemoglobin saturation, or Sao$_2$, may also be used as an indicator of the adequacy of oxygen exchange at the lung. As with measurement of the Pao$_2$, both invasive and noninvasive and continuous and intermittent approaches may be used to measure arterial hemoglobin saturation.

Estimation of arterial hemoglobin saturation is normally provided in conjunction with the analysis of arterial blood gas tensions. Using the obtained Pao$_2$, temperature, and pH, the Sao$_2$ is derived by nomogram or computer algorithm. Of course, this derivation assumes that all other parameters are normal, including the type of hemoglobin present.

Actual measurement of the arterial hemoglobin saturation is obtained by spectrophotometric analysis of an arterial blood sample, a procedure called oximetry. Spectrophotometric analysis determines the concentration of a chemical compound in a sample by measuring the amount of light transmitted or absorbed at various wavelengths. Typically, a laboratory oximeter transmits three different wavelengths of light through the blood sample (Fig. 31-5). By comparing the differences in light absorbance at these different wavelengths, the oximeter is able to measure the relative proportion of Hb, Hbo$_2$, and Hbco.

The principle of laboratory oximetry has been adapted for continuous noninvasive monitoring of hemoglobin saturations at the bedside. This method employs transcutaneous Sao$_2$ probes. Transcutaneous oximeter probes transmit two wavelengths of light (red and infrared) from a light emitting diode to a photodetector through a capillary bed, such as those in the finger, toe, or ear lobe (Fig. 31-6). The red light passes easily through red blood (oxyhemoglobin) and is easily absorbed by blue blood (deoxygenated hemoglobin), whereas infrared light passes easily through deoxygenated hemoglobin and is easily absorbed by oxyhemoglobin. Differences in absorption and transmission are proportional to the concentration and type of hemoglobin present, as quantified by a microprocessor.

Oximeters have the advantage of being relatively easy to apply and maintain. However, oximeters have technical limitations and can display inaccurate or misleading data. An underlying assumption of this measurement is that reduced hemoglobin and oxyhemoglobin are the only types of hemoglobin present. Since the analysis is limited to two wavelengths of light, the presence of other hemoglobins, such as carboxyhemoglobin and methemoglobin, can result in an overestimation of the So$_2$. Also, external bright lights can cause optical interference; this can be minimized by covering the sensor with an opaque material. Moreover, optical "shunting" can occur when light from the light-emitting diode reaches the photodetector without passing through the tissue. Correct alignment of the emitter and photodetector flush to the skin helps to eliminate

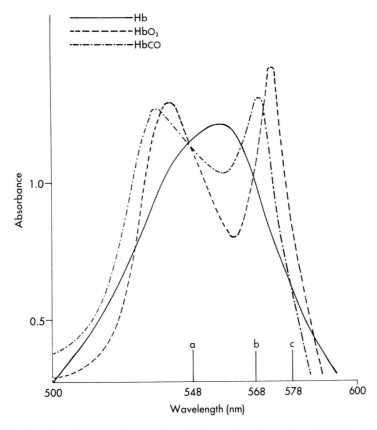

Fig. 31-5 Principle of spectrophotometric oximetry. Absorbance measurements are made at three distinct wavelengths (548, 568, and 578 nm) as light passes through a blood sample. At 548 nm all three forms of Hb (Hb, Hbo$_2$, and Hbco) have identical absorbances. At 568 nm only Hb and Hbo$_2$ coincide, whereas at 578 nm Hb and Hbco coincide. The solution of three simultaneous equations provides the relative proportions of each species as well as the total Hb. (From Ruppel G: Manual of pulmonary function testing, ed 3, St Louis, 1982, The CV Mosby Co; in McPherson SP: Respiratory therapy equipment, ed 4, St Louis, 1989, The CV Mosby Co.)

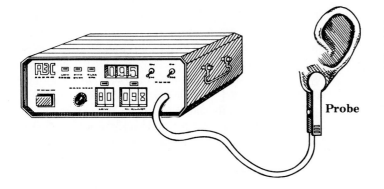

Fig. 31-6 The ear oximeter probe is placed on the ear lobe. (From Pilbeam SP: Mechanical ventilation: physiological and clinical applications, St Louis, 1986, The CV Mosby Co.)

optical shunting. Choosing the proper size sensor for the patient also decreases the risk of optical interference.

The relationship between Pao$_2$ and So$_2$ is described by the oxyhemoglobin dissociation curve. On the middle portion of the curve, where the slope is steep and changes in Pao$_2$ result in larger changes in saturation, oximetry provides a sensitive indication of changes in oxygenation status. However, when operating on the flat upper portion of the curve, where large changes in Pao$_2$ can occur with minor alterations in saturation, oximetry becomes less useful. For this reason, an understanding of the oxyhemoglobin dissociation curve is essential for appropriate interpretation of oximetry data.

Efficiency of oxygen exchange at the lung. The efficiency of oxygen exchange at the lung is commonly assessed by calculation of the alveolar-arterial oxygen tension gradient ($P(A-a)O_2$). Because of the inherent limitations of this measure, calculation of various ratios that combine arterial and alveolar oxygen tensions are often used. One also may estimate or actually measure the degree of physiologic shunting occurring in the lungs ($\dot{Q}s/\dot{Q}T$).

A normal alveolar-arterial oxygen tension gradient breathing 100% oxygen (between 25 and 65 mm Hg) indicates efficient pulmonary oxygen exchange. This small normal difference in oxygen partial pressure is due mainly to anatomic shunting within the lungs and heart. Elevation of the $P(A-a)O_2$ above this level indicates abnormal inefficiencies in oxygen exchange, due mainly to the presence of physiologic shunting.

As a rule of thumb, when breathing 100% oxygen, every 100 mm Hg $P(A-a)O_2$ is equivalent to approximately a five percent physiologic shunt. Unfortunately, when the PaO_2 is below 100 mm Hg, this estimating formula becomes grossly inaccurate. Alternatively, assuming a normal $C(a-\bar{v})O_2$, one may estimate the percent shunt of a patient breathing 100% oxygen as follows:

$$\dot{Q}s/\dot{Q}T \cong \frac{P(A-a)O_2 \times 0.003}{(P(A-a)O_2 \times 0.003) + 5}$$

where 5 represents the normal $C(a-\bar{v})O_2$ in ml/dL.

As long as the inspired oxygen concentration is kept constant, changes in the $P(A-a)O_2$ provide a valuable index of changes in the efficiency of gas exchange over time. However, the $P(A-a)O_2$ does not change linearly with changes in inspired oxygen concentrations. For this reason, various ratios that combine arterial and alveolar oxygen tensions have been proposed and used to assess the efficiency of oxygenation under conditions of changing FIO_2 values.

Unlike the $P(A-a)O_2$, these ratios yield a constant value for a given degree of shunting, regardless of FIO_2. Three such ratios of oxygenation "efficiency" are common in clinical practice settings. These include the ratio of arterial to alveolar oxygen partial pressures (PaO_2/PAO_2), or *a/A ratio*; the ratio of the alveolar-arterial oxygen tension gradient to the arterial partial pressure of oxygen ($P(A-a)O_2/PaO_2$), or *respiratory index* (RI); and the ratio of the arterial partial pressure of oxygen to the inspired fractional concentration of oxygen (PaO_2/FIO_2), or *P/F ratio*.

Normally, the PaO_2/PAO_2 ranges from 0.74 in the elderly to 0.9 in healthy young subjects; a/A values below 0.6 indicate inefficiencies in oxygenation requiring oxygen therapy; values below 0.15 indicate refractory hypoxemia secondary to significant intrapulmonary shunting.

With the PaO_2 as its denominator, interpretation of the respiratory index is opposite to that of the a/A. A low RI (less than 1.0) indicates normal oxygen exchange, whereas higher values indicate increasing inefficiency in pulmonary oxygen transfer. For example, RI values between 1.0 and 5.0 suggest $\dot{V}A/\dot{Q}c$ imbalances amenable to oxygen therapy, while an RI above 5.0 indicates the presence of refractory hypoxemia caused by physiologic shunting.

Unlike the a/A and the RI, the P/F ratio (PaO_2/FIO_2) does not require the calculation of the alveolar oxygen partial pressure and is simpler to compute. In normal subjects, the P/F ratio should exceed 200, regardless of FIO_2. A P/F ratio below 200 indicates a hypoxemia resulting from significant $\dot{V}/\dot{Q}$ inequalities, whereas a P/F ratio less than 150 signifies the presence of a physiologic shunt substantial enough to require ventilatory support.

All three ratios represent useful indices for estimating the severity of impairment of oxygenation across the lung. However, the most accurate and reliable measure of the efficiency of oxygen transfer between the lung and pulmonary circulation is the direct measurement of the physiologic shunt, or $\dot{Q}s/\dot{Q}T$.

The physiologic shunt occurring in the lungs is calculated according to the following equation:

$$\dot{Q}s/\dot{Q}T = \frac{Cc'O_2 - CaO_2}{Cc'O_2 - C\bar{v}O_2}$$

where $\dot{Q}s$ equals the volume of blood effectively bypassing ventilated alveoli, $\dot{Q}T$ equals the total cardiac output, $Cc'O_2$ equals the "ideal" pulmonary end-capillary oxygen content, CaO_2 equals the arterial oxygen content, and $C\bar{v}O_2$ equals the oxygen content of the mixed venous blood.

In order to measure the physiologic shunt, an arterial and a mixed venous blood sample must be obtained and analyzed. Arterial blood is obtained for analysis in the usual manner, with its total oxygen content calculated according to the formulas provided in Chapter 9. A true mixed venous blood sample can be obtained only via the distal sample port of an indwelling pulmonary artery catheter. The total oxygen content of the mixed venous blood is calculated in the same manner as the arterial sample.

True end-capillary pulmonary blood cannot be sampled. However, the oxygen content of "ideal" end-capillary pulmonary blood is assumed to equal that which would be obtained if the end-capillary PO_2 were equal to the alveolar PO_2. To determine the "ideal" end-capillary pulmonary blood content, simply substitute the PAO_2 into the formula for calculating total O_2 content.

If the PAO_2 is sufficient to ensure 100% hemoglobin saturated with oxygen (usually 150 mm Hg or more), the following modified version of the shunt equation may be used:

$$\dot{Q}s/\dot{Q}T = \frac{P(A-a)O_2 \times 0.003}{(P(A-a)O_2 \times 0.003) + C(a-\bar{v})O_2}$$

This modified shunt formula is essentially the same as that used previously to estimate the percent shunt; the only difference is the use of the *actual* arterial-mixed venous oxygen content difference, instead of an estimated normal value.

Although direct measurement of the physiologic shunt is the most accurate and reliable measure of the efficiency of oxygen transfer between the lung and pulmonary circulation, the insertion of a pulmonary artery catheter is warranted only if additional data on the state of hemodynamics and fluid balance are deemed critical in managing the patient. In otherwise stable patients, estimates of the shunt fraction, or the use of indices like the a/A, RI, or P/F ratios are generally sufficient for assessing the efficiency of oxygenation across the lung. More detail on the use of the pulmonary artery catheter in the assessment of a patient's hemodynamic status is provided in a subsequent section.

Internal oxygen exchange (oxygen delivery and uptake). Oxygen delivery to the tissues is a function of both the total arterial oxygen content and the cardiac output:

$$\text{Oxygen delivery (ml/min)} = \dot{Q}_T \text{ (dL/min)} \times Ca_{O_2} \text{ (ml/dL)}$$

Assuring an adequate arterial oxygen content satisfies only half of our concern in providing oxygen to the tissues. To continually meet the cellular needs for oxygen, a sufficient volume of arterialized blood must perfuse the tissues each minute.

Classically, whole body perfusion per minute, or cardiac output, can be measured according to the Fick equation:

$$\dot{Q}_T \text{ (L/min)} = \frac{\dot{V}_{O_2}}{C(a-\bar{v})_{O_2} \times 10}$$

where $\dot{Q}_T$ is the cardiac output in liters per minute, $\dot{V}_{O_2}$ is the whole body oxygen consumption (uptake) in ml/min, and $C(a-\bar{v})_{O_2}$ is the arterial-mixed venous oxygen content difference in ml/dL.

Rearranging the equation to solve for oxygen uptake, we derive:

$$\dot{V}_{O_2} \cong \dot{Q}_T \times C(a-\bar{v})_{O_2}$$

According to this formula, to assess the adequacy of tissue oxygenation, we must not only know how much oxygen is delivered ($\dot{Q}_T \times Ca_{O_2}$), but also how much oxygen is left after its exchange with the tissues. The amount of oxygen left after tissue exchange is expressed by the mixed venous oxygen content, or $C\bar{v}_{O_2}$. Rearranging the equation once again to solve for mixed venous oxygen content, we obtain the following formula:

$$C\bar{v}_{O_2} \cong Ca_{O_2} - \frac{\dot{V}_{O_2}}{\dot{Q}_T}$$

As indicated in this formula, the mixed venous oxygen content will fall if either: (1) the arterial oxygen content (Ca_{O_2}) falls, (2) tissue oxygen uptake ($\dot{V}_{O_2}$) increases, or (3) cardiac output ($\dot{Q}_T$) decreases. Thus the mixed venous oxygen content represents a key indicator of the adequacy of both oxygen delivery and uptake at the tissue level.

In clinical practice, either the mixed venous P_{O_2} or hemoglobin saturation ($S\bar{v}_{O_2}$) are used in lieu of the actual content measure. Normally, blood samples are obtained intermittently from the distal port of a pulmonary artery catheter. The blood sample must be withdrawn slowly and with the balloon deflated. Incorrect technique could cause oxygenated blood to be drawn from the pulmonary capillaries to the catheter, thereby contaminating the sample and increasing its measured oxygen values.

Alternatively, $S\bar{v}_{O_2}$ may be measured continuously by a technique called venous oximetry. Venous oximetry is of potential value in certain conditions of decreased O_2 transport, especially in low cardiac output states. Continuous venous oximetry employs the same general principles of oximetry previously discussed, with two major differences (Fig. 31-7). The first difference is that light transmission occurs through a special fiberoptic pulmonary artery catheter. The second difference is that the device measures the magnitude of reflected, as opposed to absorbed light.

This relatively new assessment technique is of potential value with highly unstable patients for whom continuous knowledge of tissue oxygenation is essential. However, as with indwelling continuous P_{O_2} catheters, the successful use of continuous venous oximetry still presents major technical problems. For this reason, its widespread use cannot be justified at this time.

Regardless of whether an intermittent or continuous sampling method is used, oxygen delivery and tissue uptake are considered adequate if the $P\bar{v}_{O_2}$ is in the normal range of 33 to 53 mm Hg, or the $S\bar{v}_{O_2}$ is between 67% to 88%. Of course, the normal range for $S\bar{v}_{O_2}$ assumes a normal P_{50} of 26.5 mm Hg.

Patient values below these normals indicate a general inadequacy in oxygen delivery to the tissues. $P\bar{v}_{O_2}$ values less than 20 mm Hg indicate severe and potentially life-threatening tissue hypoxia. However, in evaluating the $P\bar{v}_{O_2}$ or $S\bar{v}_{O_2}$, the clinician must take into account the fact that different organ systems have different oxygen requirements. For example, whereas the total body $C(a-\bar{v})_{O_2}$ ranges from 4 to 6 ml/dL, the difference between the arterial and venous oxygen content of the heart is about 11 to 12 ml/dL. Thus a normal mixed venous oxygen content (representing an average for the body as a whole) does not necessarily indicate that tissue oxygenation is adequate for all body systems.

In addition to these considerations, there are two clinical circumstances in which the use of mixed venous oxygen values to assess tissue oxygen may be misleading. First, when oxygen uptake by the tissues is impaired, the $C\bar{v}_{O_2}$ may be higher than normal, because of the failure of the cells to extract the oxygen delivered to them. A failure or inability of the cells to extract the oxygen delivered to them is called dysoxia (see Chapter 15). Dysoxia occurs in septic shock and is also evident in "histotoxic" hypoxia associated with cyanide poisoning. In both cases, disruption of intracellular enzyme systems prevent appropriate oxygen utilization.

The second condition in which mixed venous oxygen values may not be useful indicators of the extent of tissue

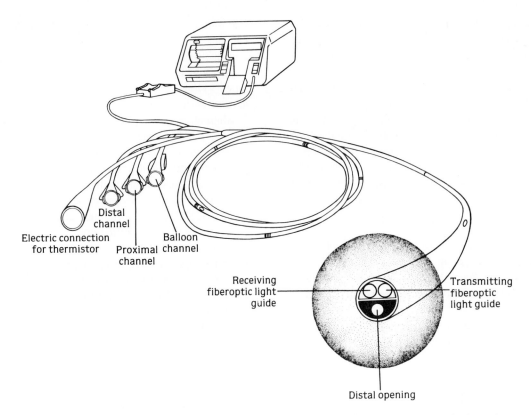

Fig. 31-7   Fiberoptic pulmonary artery catheter system used for continuous monitoring of venous oxygen saturation. (Courtesy Oximetrix, Inc, Mountain View, Calif; from Wilkins RL, Sheldon RL, and Krider SJ: Clinical assessment in respiratory care, St Louis, 1985, The CV Mosby Co.)

hypoxia is ARDS. In some patients with ARDS, the rate of oxygen utilization by the tissues ($\dot{V}O_2$) appears limited by the rate of oxygen delivery. In these cases, as the cardiac output decreases (decreased oxygen delivery), the tissue $\dot{V}O_2$ may decrease. According to the Fick principle, if both the cardiac output ($\dot{Q}T$) and tissue $\dot{V}O_2$ decrease, the $C\bar{v}O_2$ and $S\bar{v}O_2$ may remain unchanged, even in the presence of tissue hypoxia. For this reason, some investigators have suggested using mixed venous levels of lactate and pyruvate (by-products of anaerobic metabolism) as the basis for assessing the state of tissue oxygenation in patients with compromised oxygen delivery.

Assessment of ventilation. To properly assess ventilation, it must be understood that a patient's ventilatory demand is based on the interaction of several factors, including the following:

- Metabolic rate (carbon dioxide production),
- Acid-base status,
- Central respiratory drive,
- Physiologic dead space, and
- Lung and thoracic mechanics.

The following box differentiates between the primary causes of increased and decreased ventilatory demand.

The overall metabolic rate of the body and the type of nutrients being metabolized determines the rate of carbon

---

FACTORS ALTERING VENTILATORY DEMAND

FACTORS INCREASING VENTILATORY DEMAND

Arterial hypoxemia
Increased metabolic rate
Increased physiologic dead space
Metabolic acidosis
J-receptor stimulation (eg, pulmonary edema)
Increased work of breathing
Singultus (hiccup)
Confusion/irritation
CNS stimulation
Early salicylate poisoning

FACTORS DECREASING VENTILATORY DEMAND

Severe metabolic alkalosis
Decreased metabolic rate
Hyperoxia in chronic respiratory acidosis
Narcotic CNS depression
Neurologic disease
Neuromuscular disease

dioxide production. Carbohydrates produce the most CO_2 relative to oxygen consumption, one CO_2 for each O_2. As compared to carbohydrate metabolism, proteins produce 20% less carbon dioxide, with fats generating 30% less. Patients who receive only dextrose IV's may have a comparably higher CO_2 production than those metabolizing only proteins or fats and may exhibit a greater ventilatory demand. Moreover, as indicated in the box below, certain disease states, particularly those resulting from traumatic injury or burns, or those associated with fever, may increase metabolic rates by as much as three or four times.

As described in Chapter 8, the relationship between carbon dioxide production and ventilation is defined by the following relationship:

$$P_{ACO_2} \propto \frac{\dot{V}_{CO_2}}{\dot{V}_A}$$

This formula states that the arterial carbon dioxide tension is directly proportional to the carbon dioxide production and inversely proportional to the alveolar ventilation per minute. Therefore, given a normally functioning lung, CO_2 partial pressures will rise if the metabolic rate rises and the alveolar ventilation remains unchanged. This situation might occur if a patient on ventilatory support with no spontaneous breathing developed an infection, became febrile, and no increase in the ventilator rate or tidal volume were made. The opposite would occur if metabolism were to slow.

In terms of acid-base status, ventilation must always be judged according to its effect on pH. For example, increased ventilatory demands will occur during compensation for metabolic acidosis, yet low levels of alveolar ventilation may be "normal" in compensated respiratory acidosis.

Associated with acid base balance is the patient's central respiratory drive. However, respiratory drive may be increased or decreased independent of alteration in acid-base balance.

The physiologic dead space will also affect the ventilatory demands of a patient. An increase in wasted ventilation is always associated with an increase in ventilatory demand in patients with normal CO_2 response mechanisms.

ALTERATIONS IN METABOLIC RATE

CONDITION	METABOLIC RATE
Basal	25 kcal/kg/day
Fever	Basal + 3.0 kcal/kg/day/°C
Injury	50 to 60 kcal/kg/day
Burns	40 kcal/kg × percent body surface area burned

Finally, the mechanics of the lungs and thorax will affect ventilatory demand, both directly and indirectly. Changes in compliance and resistance directly affect ventilatory demand via their influence on the rate and depth of breathing (see Chapter 8). Decreased compliance or increased resistance indirectly affect ventilatory demand by increasing the work of breathing, thereby increasing metabolic rate and CO_2 production.

In combination then, the assessment of ventilation must take into account the relationship among multiple factors. As with oxygenation, ventilation may be assessed in terms of both its adequacy and efficiency.

Adequacy of ventilation. Although fraught with limitations, measurement of a patient's minute ventilation can be used as a rough approximation of a patient's adequacy of ventilation. More commonly, the adequacy of ventilation is assessed by measurement of the arterial or alveolar P_{CO_2}, as related to the patient's pH.

Before the availability of reliable blood gas analysis, the adequacy of ventilation was judged mainly by observational assessment and the measurement of the minute ventilation, as compared with established norms (such as the Radford nomogram). Although this approach has given way to more precise indices of the adequacy of ventilation, it still has a place in bedside assessment of the patient with respiratory insufficiency or failure.

The minute ventilation is normally measured with a mechanical (vane-type) or electronic respirometer attached to the endotracheal tube or to a mask that is tightly fitted to the patient's face (Fig. 31-8). The patient exhales into the device while the practitioner simultaneously counts the respiratory rate for exactly one minute. With this information, minute ventilation ($\dot{V}_E$), respiratory rate (f), and average tidal volume ($V_T = \dot{V}_E/f$) can be documented. If the respirometer is placed after the exhalation valve in a ventilator circuit, volume added to patient ventilation because of tubing compression must be subtracted if the exact patient value is to be reported.

A normal adult minute ventilation ranges between 5 to 7 L per minute. Of and by itself, a normal minute ventilation does not necessarily indicate that ventilation is adequate. However, the use of the minute ventilation in conjunction with other measures can be helpful in assessing the efficiency of ventilation and certain elements of respiratory mechanics. The use of minute ventilation for these purposes will be discussed subsequently.

The arterial partial pressure of carbon dioxide, or P_{ACO_2}, is the most frequently obtained measure of the adequacy of ventilation. The P_{ACO_2} is usually obtained invasively by arterial puncture or, alternatively, through an indwelling arterial line. In general, ventilation is adequate if the arterial P_{CO_2} is associated with a normal arterial pH. For patients with an otherwise normal acid-base balance, ventilation is considered adequate if the P_{ACO_2} is in the 35 to 45 mm Hg range.

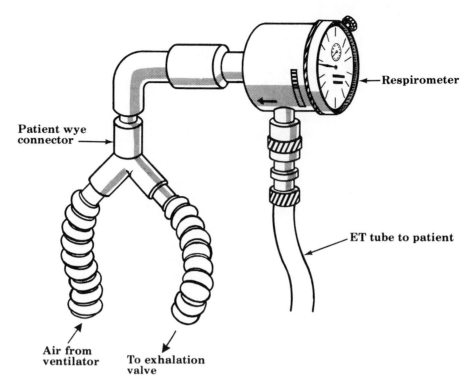

Fig. 31-8   Minute volume measurement at the endotracheal tube. The respirometer is attached to the endotracheal tube so that the patient's actual exhaled air can be measured. The respirometer can also be attached at the exhalation valve. Some respirometers read both inspiration and expiration by measuring flow in both directions. (From Pilbeam SP: Mechanical ventilation: physiological and clinical applications, St Louis, 1986, The CV Mosby Co.)

Continuous, noninvasive monitoring of the adequacy of ventilation can be a useful addition to this standard practice: this may be accomplished by a transcutaneous CO_2 electrode or capnography.

Transcutaneous CO_2 monitoring ($Ptcco_2$) is similar to $Ptco_2$ monitoring. Many devices combine O_2 and CO_2 electrodes into a single sensor. A transcutaneous CO_2 probe is a miniaturized Severinghaus pH electrode, combined with a heating element for warming the skin which attaches to the skin surface. The heating from the probe causes a localized increase in CO_2 production which causes the probe to overestimate $Paco_2$. This error is accounted for by comparing the $Ptcco_2$ to a baseline $Paco_2$. As with measurement of $Ptco_2$, transcutaneous CO_2 monitoring is affected by low perfusion states. However, transcutaneous CO_2 monitoring can be a useful technique for analyzing changes in ventilation, especially when used in conjunction with intermittent arterial Pco_2 analysis and minute ventilation measurements.

Capnography is a measurement technique by which exhaled gas is analyzed for its CO_2 content. Capnographs generally withdraw a sample of gas from an adaptor placed between the endotracheal tube and the ventilator tubing and analyze the sample using either infrared or mass spectrophotometric methods. An example of a capnograph sys-

tem using a mass spectrometer designed for multiple patient sampling is shown in Fig. 31-9.

Fig. 31-10 shows a typical normal single breath capnographic tracing. During the first portion of exhalation (Phase I), the expired partial pressure of carbon dioxide, or $Peco_2$ is near 0, indicating exhalation of deadspace gas. In Phase II, alveolar gas begins mixing with deadspace gas causing an increase in the $Peco_2$. In Phase III, as pure alveolar gas enters the capnograph, the peak, or end-tidal carbon dioxide, partial pressure ($Petco_2$) is achieved.

$Petco_2$ levels can be displayed and reported as either a partial pressure or as a percent. A normal $Petco_2$, indicating adequate alveolar ventilation (with a normal pH) ranges from 35 to 43 mm Hg. Expressed as a percentage, this normal value equates to approximately 4.6% to 5.6% CO_2.

Since the $Petco_2$ in normal subjects is equivalent to the $Paco_2$, and since $Paco_2$ levels closely approximate the $Paco_2$ in the normally ventilated and perfused lung, the end-tidal CO_2 represents a useful and noninvasive index of the adequacy of ventilation. Fig. 31-11 demonstrates the relationship between end-expired CO_2 concentrations and $Paco_2$ levels as related to changes in alveolar ventilation in normal subjects.

In terms of partial pressures, a normal gradient of 2 to 3

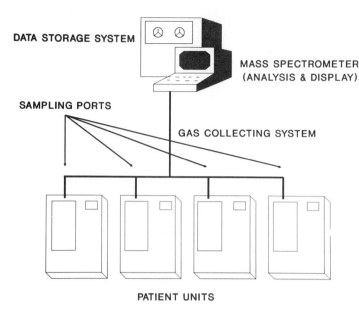

Fig. 31-9   Capnagraph system using mass spectrometer and multiple sampling ports for monitoring expired CO_2 levels in critically ill patients.

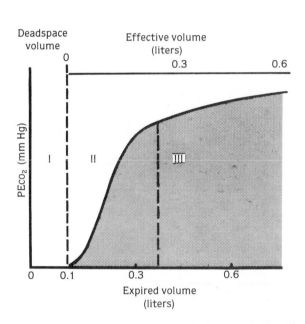

Fig. 31-10   Single-breath tracing for exhaled carbon dioxide. (From Wilkins RL, Sheldon RL, and Krider SJ: Clinical assessment in respiratory care, St Louis, 1985, The CV Mosby Co.)

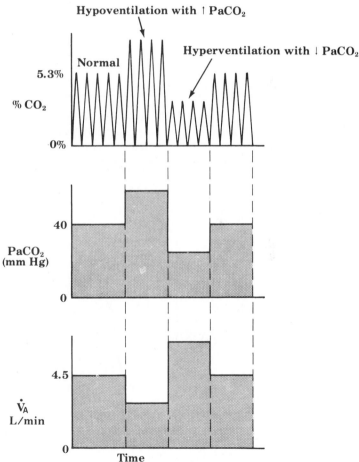

Fig. 31-11   Shows the changes in end-tidal CO_2 with changes in ventilation. During normal alveolar ventilation ($\dot{V}A$), Pa_{CO_2} and end-tidal CO_2 are normal. During hypoventilation, Pa_{CO_2} and end-tidal CO_2 increase. During hyperventilation, Pa_{CO_2} and end-tidal CO_2 decrease. (From Pilbeam SP: Mechanical ventilation: physiological and clinical applications, St Louis, 1986, The CV Mosby Co.)

mm Hg exists between the end-tidal and arterial P_{CO_2} levels. This small gradient between the PET_{CO_2} and Pa_{CO_2} is due to normal dilution of pure alveolar gas with residual deadspace gas (low in CO_2). Therefore, accurate estimates of the use of Pa_{CO_2} using capnography should account for this normal gradient.

In patients with abnormal distribution of ventilation and perfusion, visible changes in the expired CO_2 tracing are observed, particularly in Phases II and III (see Fig. 31-12). Typically, these changes include a slower and more irregular rise in CO_2 levels during phase II, and/or a lower than normal end-tidal CO_2 levels during Phase III. The slow and irregular rise in CO_2 levels during phase II is indicative of a ventilation-perfusion imbalance, specifically a high $\dot{V}_A/\dot{Q}_C$ ratio. The lower than normal Phase III CO_2 levels suggest the presence of a abnormally high $P(a-ET)co_2$ gradient, also indicative of a high $\dot{V}_A/\dot{Q}_C$ ratio.

Conditions such as COPD, pulmonary embolism, and low perfusion states caused by shock or left ventricular failure may all decrease perfusion to ventilated areas of the lung, thereby raising the $\dot{V}_A/\dot{Q}_C$ ratio and altering the expired CO_2 waveform. As illustrated in Fig. 31-13, these conditions tend to manifest themselves differently on analysis of a single breath capnographic tracing, especially when the patient exhales maximally below the resting FRC. Such patterns, while not diagnostic in themselves,

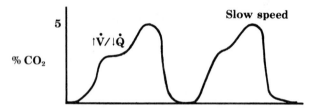

Fig. 31-12   With a slow tracing it is possible to pick up abnormalities in the CO_2 curve. A sloping expiratory curve may indicate a $\dot{V}_A/\dot{Q}_C$ abnormality. (From Pilbeam SP: Mechanical ventilation: physiological and clinical applications, St Louis, 1986, The CV Mosby Co.)

provide a useful indication of the degree of $\dot{V}_A/\dot{Q}_C$ disturbance, and can warn of developing problems, such as acute pulmonary embolization.

Efficiency of ventilation. The efficiency of ventilation is best assessed by measurement of the patient's physiologic dead space and dead space to tidal volume ratio, or V_D/V_T. Other useful, but less sophisticated indices of the efficiency of ventilation include clinical rules of thumb, assessment nomograms, and the ventilation quotient.

Physiologic dead space measurement. As described in Chapter 8, the physiologic dead space is calculated using the Enghoff modification of the Bohr equation:

$$V_{Dphy} = [V_T \times (Paco_2 - P\bar{E}co_2/Paco_2)] - V_{Dmec}$$

where V_{Dphy} is the physiologic dead space, V_T is the average tidal volume, $Paco_2$ is the partial pressure of CO_2 in the arterial blood, $P\bar{E}co_2$ is the average partial pressure of CO_2 in the mixed expired air. V_{Dmec}, or the mechanical dead space, represents a correction factor for that portion of the patient's expired air that is rebreathed through the connecting apparatus.

Rearranging the equation to calculate the physiologic dead space to tidal volume ratio, or V_D/V_T, we derive the following formula:

$$V_D/V_T = \frac{Paco_2 - P\bar{E}co_2}{Paco_2} - \frac{V_{Dmec}}{V_T}$$

If the patient is being supported by positive-pressure ventilation, an additional correction is required. This is because the compressed volume of the ventilator contributes

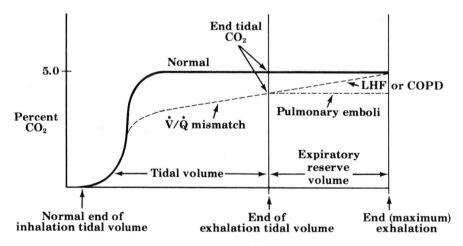

Fig. 31-13   This graph represents the percentage of CO_2 at varying exhaled lung volumes. For a normal individual (solid line) the end-tidal CO_2 at the end of normal tidal exhalation is equal to that at maximum exhalation. With left ventricular failure (LVF) and chronic obstructive pulmonary disease (COPD), the end-tidal CO_2 is less than normal at the end of a normal exhalation and may rise slightly at the end of a maximum exhalation. With pulmonary emboli present, a low end-tidal CO_2 will not rise in value at the end of a maximum exhalation. (From Pilbeam SP: Mechanical ventilation: physiological and clinical applications, St Louis, 1986, The CV Mosby Co.)

to the expired gas, without raising its CO_2 content. Therefore, the mixed expired partial pressure of carbon dioxide collected from a patient being supported by positive-pressure ventilation will be lowered by an amount equivalent to the magnitude of the compressed volume. Correction of the $P\bar{E}CO_2$ is accomplished using the following formula:

$$\text{Corrected } P\bar{E}CO_2 = \text{Measured } P\bar{E}CO_2 \times V_T/(V_T - V_C)$$

where V_C is the calculated compressed volume of the ventilator system.

Alternatively, a special ventilator circuit may be used to eliminate contamination of the patient's expired gases with the ventilator's compressed volume (Fig. 31-14). By incorporating a second exhalation port and one-way valve at the patient airway connection, the expired gas is diverted to the collection system, with the compressed volume being evacuated through the normal exhalation port.

In either case, exhaled gas is collected in a Douglas bag or similar large volume (greater than 10 L) collection device (see Fig. 31-14), with the volume measured by an in-line mechanical or electronic respirometer. Exhaled gas should be collected for a period of at least three minutes, with an arterial blood sample drawn during collection. The gas and blood samples are analyzed, and the respective PCO_2 values applied in the above formula.

In lieu of measuring the V_D/V_T ratio by intermittent collection of expired gases and arterial blood gas sampling, capnography can be used to provide an ongoing estimate of physiologic dead space. In this approach, the peak expired CO_2 (P_{ETCO_2}) is substituted for the P_{aCO_2}, and the mean expired CO_2 level used instead of that obtained from the collection bag. As with the intermittent method, correction must be made for both mechanical deadspace and compressed gas volume.

Ventilation is considered efficient if the V_D/V_T falls within the 0.2 to 0.4 range. However, since intermittent positive-pressure ventilation tends to increase physiologic dead space, this normal range will seldom be observed in patients receiving this mode of ventilatory support. For this reason, V_D/V_T ratios in the 0.4 to 0.6 range are clinically acceptable. A V_D/V_T ratio above 0.7 generally indicates that ventilation is so inefficient as to preclude the patient from maintaining adequate CO_2 removal at tolerable levels of minute ventilation.

Estimates of ventilation efficiency. Although the efficiency of ventilation is best assessed by actual measurement of the V_D/V_T, this approach is not always feasible or necessary. Instead, the practitioner may estimate the efficiency of ventilation using clinical rules of thumb, nomograms, or computed indices.

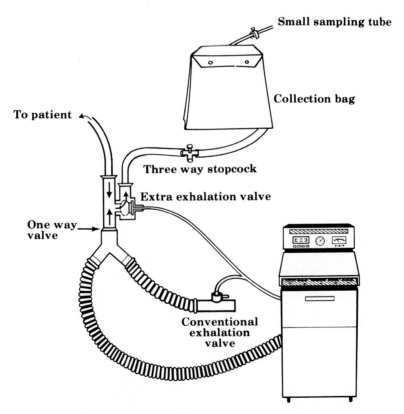

Fig. 31-14 Equipment used for collecting mixed gases from a patient on mechanical ventilation. (From Pilbeam SP: Mechanical ventilation: physiological and clinical applications, St Louis, 1986, The CV Mosby Co.)

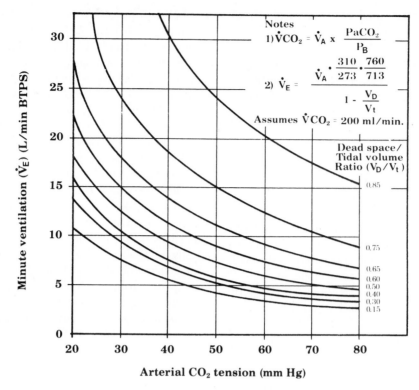

Fig. 31-15 This graph shows the relationship between minute ventilation and Pa_{CO_2} for various isopleths of the ratio of dead space to tidal volume (V_D/V_T). The upper right hand corner contains the basic assumptions for this relationship. $\dot{V}_{CO_2} = CO_2$ output, $\dot{V}_A$ = alveolar ventilation, P_B = barometric pressure. To obtain the V_D/V_T, measure the $\dot{V}_E$ and the Pa_{CO_2} and plot these points on the graph. The V_D/V_T is obtained by noting the isopleth that coincides with this point. To obtain the $\dot{V}_E$ required to achieve a desired Pa_{CO_2}, draw a vertical line from the desired Pa_{CO_2} on the abscissa to the V_D/V_T isopleth obtained in the first step above. Draw a horizontal line from this point to the ordinate to obtain the required $\dot{V}_E$. (Reproduced with permission from Selecky PA et al: Am Rev Respir Dis 117:181, 1978; in Pilbeam SP: Mechanical ventilation: physiological and clinical applications, St Louis, 1986, The CV Mosby Co.)

As a rule of thumb for adult patients, ventilation is inefficient if the minute ventilation exceeds 10 L/min and the P_{CO_2} is normal or high. Exceptions to this rule are patients with increased ventilatory demands due to high metabolic rates, as described earlier.

This clinical rule of thumb is based on assessment nomograms like that shown in Fig. 31-15. On this nomogram, the V_D/V_T is estimated as the point of intersection between the minute ventilation (y-axis) and the Pa_{CO_2} (x-axis) lines. Alternatively, this nomogram can also be used to determine the $\dot{V}_E$ required to maintain a desired Pa_{CO_2} if the physiologic dead space is known. However, this nomogram assumes a normal CO_2 production and is inappropriate for use on patients with higher than normal metabolic rates.

Alternatively, a derived index called the ventilation quotient, or Vq, has been suggested as a measure of the efficiency of ventilation. To compute the ventilation quotient, one must measure the patient's minute ventilation, body weight, and arterial P_{CO_2}:

$$Vq = \frac{\dot{V}_E \text{ (L/min)}}{\text{Weight (kg)}} \times \frac{Pa_{CO_2}}{3.6}$$

According to this formula, a normal Vq ranges between 0.9 and 1.0. Ventilation quotients between 1.5 and 3.0 indicate an abnormal increase in physiologic deadspace or wasted ventilation, with values in excess of 3.0 indicating grossly inefficient ventilation.

As an estimate of the relative efficiency of ventilation, the ventilation quotient is more precise than the "rule of thumb" previously described; it accounts for differences in ventilatory demand based on the patient's weight. Like the assessment nomogram, however, it assumes normal CO_2 production and does not account for the increases in metabolic rate so common among critically ill patients.

Assessment of ventilatory mechanics. Early emphasis on the physiologic parameters of gas exchange as related to respiratory failure has recently been supplemented with increasingly sophisticated assessment of the mechanical properties of the ventilatory apparatus. The importance of

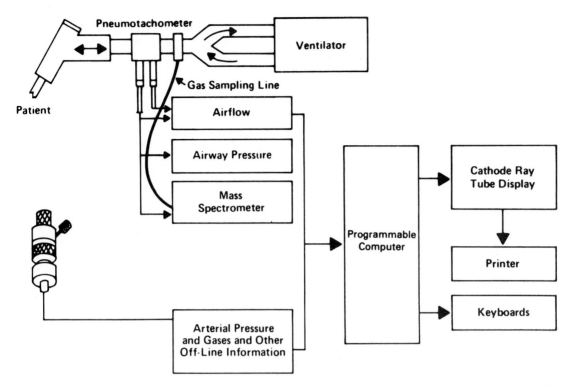

Fig. 31-16   Respiratory monitoring system. Airflow, pressure, and gas concentrations are measured simultaneously. Calculations are made by a computer utilizing these signals and off-line information. (From Bone RC: Respir Care 28(5):602, 1983.)

monitoring ventilatory mechanics is based on the knowledge that excessive work of breathing can lead to respiratory muscle fatigue. In turn, respiratory muscle fatigue may serve as a primary cause of respiratory failure, or, alternatively, exacerbate an existing insufficiency due to other causes.

Our analysis of techniques used to assess ventilatory mechanics will focus first on direct and indirect measures of the work of breathing, followed by approaches used to evaluate the strength, load capability, and fatigue level of the respiratory muscles. Although emphasis will be placed on the relatively simple and proven methods of bedside assessment, recent research on new and more sophisticated approaches to evaluating ventilatory mechanics also will be described.

Assessing the work of breathing. A patient's work of breathing may be assessed by either direct measurement (see Chapter 8) or by indirect evaluation of its major components, compliance and resistance.

Direct measurement. In terms of direct measurement, the work required for a patient to breathe is measured as the area of the pressure-volume curve. If pressure is measured in kilogram-meters (kg-m) and volume in liters (L), then the work of breathing is expressed in kg-m/L. Alternatively, the work of breathing can be expressed in joules per liter (j/L), with 1 kg-m equal to approximately 10 joules.

The total work of breathing consists of the work of the lung and the work of the thorax, plus any additional work imposed by the breathing apparatus, such as a ventilator tubing system or artificial airway. Total work of breathing (lung + thorax + imposed) can only be measured when the subject is not breathing spontaneously; all the work is being done by a mechanical ventilator. Of course, these conditions often apply in the critical care setting, allowing for bedside measurement of the total work of breathing.

In practice, measurement of the total work of breathing can be accomplished using a differential pressure pneumotachometer attached between the ventilator and patient at the proximal airway (Fig. 31-16). Changes in "mouth" or airway pressure are measured directly by the pneumotachometer pressure line closest to the airway. In Fig. 31-16, changes in volume (delivered by the ventilator) are also measured by the pneumotachometer, as the integral of the flow signal over time (flow × time = volume). A computer or microprocessor then calculates the product of P × V, yielding a measure in either kg-m/L or j/L.

For normal individuals, the average total work of breathing is about 0.073 kg-m/L, or 0.73 j/L. Patients with obstructive or restrictive lung disease may exhibit two to three times this normal value at rest, with marked increases in work at higher minute ventilations.

How much work is too much, that is how much work a patient is able to tolerate before the respiratory muscles fatigue, is not entirely clear. Maintenance of adequate spontaneous ventilation over a long term is probably not possible when work loads exceed 0.20 kg-m/L, or 2.0 j/L, although this threshold level surely varies according to patient condition. For this reason, and because bedside measurement of the work of breathing is currently a relatively complex and expensive procedure, other indirect measures of work, such as compliance and resistance estimates, are more commonly used.

Indirect measurement. Since the work of breathing varies directly with the total impedance to ventilation, and since the pressure change required to ventilate a patient is a measure of the total force required to overcome this impedance, the peak airway pressure (P_{peak}) may be used as a rough estimate of the mechanical properties of the lungs and thorax. Of course, if the baseline airway pressure is above zero, as occurs during CMV with PEEP, the pressure change required to ventilate the lungs is the difference between the peak pressure and the PEEP pressure.

If the patient is being ventilated by a volume ventilator, the corrected tidal volume can be divided by the change in airway pressure to yield a measure called the dynamic characteristic of the respiratory system:

$$\text{Dynamic characteristic} = \frac{(\text{Tidal volume} - \text{Compressed volume})}{(P_{peak} - \text{PEEP})}$$

Like the measurement of compliance, this dynamic characteristic is measured in ml/cm H_2O. Normal values for an intubated adult are between 35 and 50 ml/cm H_2O. Indeed, some authors refer to this measure as "dynamic" compliance. However, this label is misleading, since, unlike compliance, the dynamic characteristic of the respiratory system is a measure of the total impedance to ventilation, including both its elastic (compliance) and frictional (resistance) components.

To partition, or separate out, the elastic and frictional components of total impedance, the practitioner can institute an end-inspiratory pause maneuver (EIP). As shown in Fig. 31-17, the EIP momentarily holds the delivered volume in the lungs under static conditions. If held long enough to ensure equilibration of pressures throughout the lung units, an EIP will result in a pressure plateau (P_{stat}), equivalent to the force necessary to maintain the lungs and thorax at the delivered volume under static conditions.

By dividing the corrected tidal volume by the plateau pressure, we derive a close approximation of total compliance of the lungs and chest wall, called effective compliance (C_{eff}):

$$\text{effective compliance } (C_{eff}) = \frac{(\text{Tidal volume} - \text{Compressed volume})}{(P_{stat} - \text{PEEP})}$$

Normal effective compliance ranges between 60 and 100 ml/cm H_2O. Diseases of the lung parenchyma such as pneumonia, pulmonary edema, and pulmonary fibrosis, or any chronic diseases with a fibrotic component, are all as-

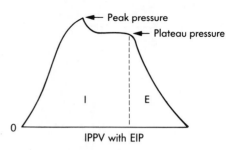

Fig. 31-17   Effect of EIP. The difference between peak pressure and plateau pressure is caused by airways resistance. The difference between plateau pressure and end-expiratory pressure is that amount of pressure needed to distend the system (tubing, lungs, chest wall), and the difference can be used to calculate system compliance. See text for further discussion. (From Martin L: Pulmonary physiology in clinical practice, St Louis, 1987, The CV Mosby Co.)

sociated with an effective compliance below this normal range. Acute changes, such as atelectasis, pulmonary edema, or lung compression because of a tension pneumothorax will cause a rapid drop in C_{eff}. When C_{eff} is less than 25 to 30 ml/cm H_2O, as may occur in severe ARDS, the amount of work necessary to maintain adequate ventilation is inordinately high and can quickly lead to muscle fatigue. C_{eff} values less than 25 to 30 ml/cm H_2O make weaning from ventilatory support difficult.

Measured on a regular basis, C_{eff} data may be used to establish trends in pulmonary status and can help guide the application of PEEP or CPAP therapy. This will be discussed in a subsequent section.

An estimate of the frictional component opposing ventilation, or airway resistance, can also be obtained using the end-inspiratory pause maneuver. Since the peak pressure reflects total impedance, and the plateau pressure corresponds to the elastic component of opposition to ventilation (compliance), then the difference between the peak and plateau pressures must be caused by airway resistance (Raw).

If the inspiratory flow is constant and known with accuracy, then the airway resistance may be estimated according to the following formula:

$$\text{Estimated Raw (cm } H_2O/L/sec) = \frac{(P_{peak} - P_{stat})}{\dot{V} \text{ (L/min)}/60}$$

Normal adult airway resistance ranges from about 0.5 to 2.5 cm H_2O/L/sec. In a normal adult intubated with an 8.0 mm endotracheal tube, we would expect the airway resistance to be about 4 to 6 cm H_2O higher than this normal range because of the additional resistance imposed by the artificial airway. An increase in Raw above 10 to 15 cm H_2O/L/sec in an intubated patient with otherwise normal lungs signals abnormal airway narrowing caused by factors such as increased secretions, bronchospasm, pulmonary

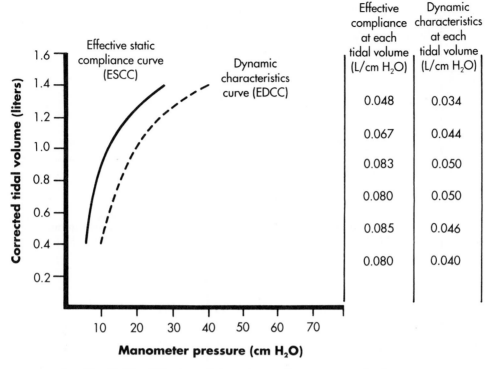

Effective compliance at each tidal volume (L/cm H₂O)	Dynamic characteristics at each tidal volume (L/cm H₂O)
0.048	0.034
0.067	0.044
0.083	0.050
0.080	0.050
0.085	0.046
0.080	0.040

Fig. 31-18   Effective and dynamic compliance curves and values.

vascular congestion, or partial occlusion of the artificial airway.

Some new generation ventilators, such as the Bear 5, Puritan-Bennett 7200a, and the Hamilton Veolar, automate the calculation of C_{eff} and estimated Raw upon operator selection of an end-inspiratory pause. These automated calculations are valid only if the EIP is long enough to allow complete pressure equilibration throughout the lung, and the device is set in the constant flow mode. Most clinicians suggest that an EIP of at least 1 to 2 seconds may be necessary to ensure pressure equilibration throughout the lung. Even longer time intervals may be necessary in severe obstructive lung disease.

Whether using manual or automated methods, the practitioner should simultaneously observe the patient's breathing pattern to be certain that a normal exhalation precedes the pressure measurements. Failure to do so will cause inaccurate measurements of pressure and affect the calculated values. Plateau pressure readings are particularly susceptible to fluctuations caused by spontaneous breathing.

As an alternative to single-point computation of C_{eff} and Raw, some clinicians suggest multipoint curve analysis of the mechanical properties of the respiratory apparatus. This approach involves calculating and plotting the dynamic characteristics and effective compliance points over a series of standardized tidal volumes, such as 7,

10, 13, and 16 ml/kg. As shown in Fig. 31-18, this results in two curves: the effective static compliance curve (ESCC) and the effective dynamic characteristics curve (EDCC).

Comparison of these curves over time provides an easily interpreted graphic portrayal of changing pulmonary mechanics. As can be seen in Fig. 31-19, conditions that are associated with increased airway resistance cause a shift in the EDCC downward and to the right. On the other hand, conditions that are associated with decreased lung or chest wall compliance shift both the EDCC and ESCC downward and to the right. If the condition of the patient acutely worsens without a change in either the EDCC or ESCC, the clinician should suspect a problem not directly affecting the lung parenchyma or airways, such as a pulmonary embolism.

Assessing respiratory muscle function. Whereas work of breathing and compliance and resistance measurements provide an indication of the load being encountered by the respiratory muscles, they do not necessarily indicate how well these muscles can respond to the imposed load. The ability of the respiratory muscles to respond to imposed work loads may be assessed in two ways. First, we can use bedside measurement techniques to indirectly quantify muscle strength or endurance. Alternatively, we may determine the fatigue level of muscle, either by observation or direct measurement.

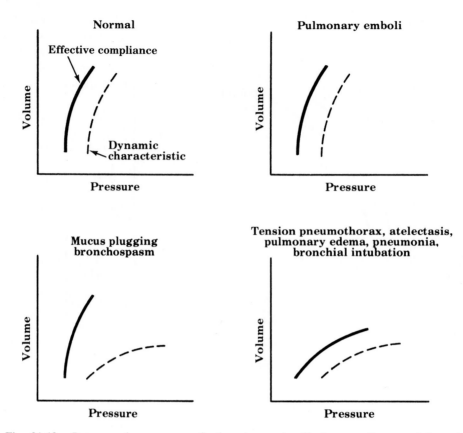

Fig. 31-19   Pressure-volume curves reflecting changes in effective compliance and dynamic characteristics (dynamic compliance) during mechanical ventilation. Under normal conditions the effective and dynamic characteristic curves will be similar. Since pulmonary emboli does not affect resistance or compliance, neither curve will change in this condition. With mucus plugging, airway resistance increases and the dynamic curve shifts to the right and flattens (more pressure is required) while the static compliance curve does not change. In conditions which reduce lung compliance, both curves will shift to the right and flatten. (From Pilbeam SP: Mechanical ventilation: physiological and clinical applications, St Louis, 1986, The CV Mosby Co.)

Quantifying muscle strength or endurance. The three most common methods currently used for bedside assessment of respiratory muscle strength, or endurance, are the forced vital capacity (VC), the maximum voluntary ventilation (MVV), and the maximum inspiratory force (MIF). A fourth measure, called the effort index (EI), quantifies the MIF against the effective compliance of the patient at a standardized lung volume.

The VC maneuver can be performed at the bedside using a mechanical or electronic spirometer attached directly to the patient's airway. Since the VC maneuver is effort dependent, accurate measurements can be obtained only with conscious and cooperative patients. Given the inherent variability in bedside results, it is probably best to repeat the maneuver two to three times, taking the best measure as the final result.

The VC maneuver represents an integrated measure of coordinated inspiratory and expiratory muscle function as related to the compliance of the lungs and chest wall. Normal individuals are able to generate a VC of approximately

65 to 75 ml/kg. Values below 65 to 75 ml/kg in conscious and cooperative patients indicate a generalized restrictive process, which may be due to neuromuscular weakness, acutely decreased lung volumes, or chronic parenchymal disease. When the VC drops below 10 to 15 ml/kg, it is unlikely that the patient has sufficient reserve capacity to support spontaneous ventilation for prolonged time periods.

Whereas the VC assesses the patient's coordinated muscle function on a single breath, the maximum voluntary ventilation determines the ability of the alert and cooperative patient to sustain an increased respiratory load over a period of time. As with the VC maneuver, the MVV procedure can be performed at the bedside using a hand-held spirometer attached to the patient's airway. The patient is encouraged to breathe as deep and as fast as possible over a predefined time interval, such as 15 or 20 seconds. The value is then extrapolated to a full minute.

Normal MVV values for adults range from about 120 to 180 L/min. When the MVV values fall below 20 L/min, or

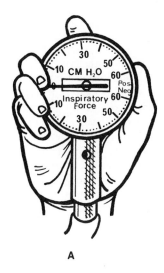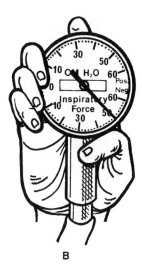

Fig. 31-20   An inspiratory force measurement. The gauge is attached to the patient's endotracheal tube, **A.** The patient is instructed to take in a deep breath while the clinician obstructs the airway by closing the open port on the gauge, **B.** The negative pressure detection, measured here as -50 cm H_2O, is the patient's inspiratory force or peak inspiratory pressure. (From Pilbeam SP: Mechanical ventilation: physiological and clinical applications, St Louis, 1986, The CV Mosby Co.)

if the MVV is less than twice the resting minute ventilation, it is unlikely that the patient will be able to spontaneously maintain an adequate level of ventilation without mechanical assistance. Some critically ill patients may not be able to perform this procedure.

The maximum inspiratory force (MIF), also known as the negative inspiratory force (NIF), or maximum inspiratory pressure (PImax), is a more specific measure than the VC, providing information solely on the output of the inspiratory muscles against a maximum stimulus. The maximum stimulus is provided either by total occlusion of the airway or by preventing inspiratory gas flow. Unlike the VC maneuver, the MIF can be performed on unconscious or uncooperative patients.

Measurement of MIF at the bedside is normally accomplished using a aneroid manometer equipped with a maximum value indicator (Fig. 31-20). To assure maximum stimulation, one of two procedures is used. In the first, the practitioner completely occludes the airway for a full 20 seconds, observing and recording the maximum deflection of the manometer. Alternatively, the practitioner uses a one-way valve that allows exhalation but not inspiration. With this device, the patient will "buck down" toward residual volume on each successive breath, at which point a maximum inspiratory effort is assured.

Both techniques can cause extreme anxiety in alert patients and should be preceded by a careful and reassuring explanation. Moreover, if using the one-way valve method, the practitioner should ensure restoration of lung volume after the test by providing several large tidal volumes, either via the ventilator sigh mechanism or with a manual resuscitator.

As indicated in Table 31-6, normal MIF values vary by patient age and sex. Values less than these norms indicate either inspiratory neuromuscular weakness or an abnormal ventilatory drive. When the MIF drops below -20 to -30 cm H_2O, it is unlikely that the patient has sufficient muscle strength to support adequate spontaneous ventilation.

The effort index (EI) represents a standardized estimate of the fraction of the MIF that would be necessary to breathe a tidal volume of 400 ml at the patient's measured effective compliance, or C_{eff}:

$$Effort\ index\ (EI) = 400/C_{eff}/MIF$$

A normal effort index is below 0.30. Values between 0.30 and 0.55 indicate that the patient must exert an abnormally high effort to generate an average tidal volume, thereby increasing the work of breathing. An EI of greater than 0.55 suggests that the effort to generate an average tidal volume is so excessive as to require ventilatory support.

Table 31-6   Normal Maximum Inspiratory Force (cm H_2O) By Age and Sex

Age group	Mean (+/− SD) PImax from residual volume	
	Male	Female
9-18	−96 +/−35	−90 +/−25
19-50	−127 +/−28	−91 +/−25
51-70	−112 +/−20	−77 +/−18
>70	−76 +/−27	−66 +/−18

From Rochester DF and Hyatt RE: Respiratory muscle failure, Med Clin North Am 67:573-579, 1983.

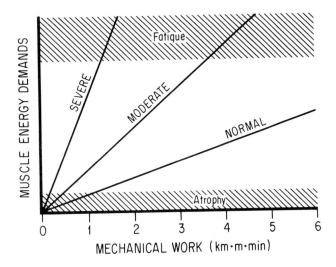

Fig. 31-21 Schematic relationship between ventilatory muscle loads (horizontal axis) and energy demands (vertical axis). As loads increase (either from impedance changes or ventilation requirements), energy demands increase, and when energy demands exceed muscle capabilities, fatigue develops. Disease states steepen the relationship between loads and energy (ie, the muscles become less efficient), and fatigue occurs at a lower load. If a muscle is totally unloaded with mechanical ventilatory support for an excessive period of time, atrophy develops. (From MacIntyre NR: Respir Care 33(2):121, 1988.)

Assessing muscle fatigue. Fatigue represents a reversible decrease in the force a muscle can develop during sustained or repeated contraction. Respiratory muscles fatigue when the work load imposed on them exceeds their energy utilization capabilities. As illustrated in Fig. 31-21, diseased states steepen the relationship between imposed loads and energy demands, causing fatigue to develop faster and at a lower load. Clinically, respiratory muscle load may increase because of either (1) an increase in total impedance resulting from decreased compliance and/or increased airway resistance or (2) an increase in ventilatory demand, such as would occur with an increase in physiologic deadspace, or with hypoxic stimulation of the peripheral chemoreceptors.

Respiratory muscle fatigue may be either a cause or effect of respiratory failure. As cause, muscle fatigue can lead to a decreased minute ventilation, respiratory acidosis, and, ultimately, respiratory and cardiac arrest. As an effect, respiratory muscle fatigue is simply a manifestation of other primary problems causing either increased impedance or increased ventilatory demand. Whether cause or effect, fatigued respiratory muscles may take anywhere from 24 to 48 hours to fully recover. The need for this recovery period should be considered by the practitioner when selecting the type and length of ventilatory support needed by a given patient.

The early stages of respiratory muscle fatigue may be associated with a variety of clinical signs and symptoms, including dyspnea, tachypnea, and asychronous or paradoxical breathing. These latter observable changes in the pattern of breathing may serve as an "early warning" of impending respiratory failure and are currently the only readily available means for bedside assessment of this problem. Supplementing observational assessment of respiratory muscle fatigue are a variety of new quantitative research methods, some of which may soon be available at the bedside.

Observational assessment of respiratory muscle function. Until more objective measurements of respiratory muscle function are available at the bedside, the subjective observation of respiratory muscle activity can provide valuable information on the relative state of fatigue of these muscles. This information, combined with other more objective indicators, can help guide patient management decisions.

In order to assess respiratory muscle function, the practitioner should observe the patient's use of both the primary and accessory muscles groups. Since observation of the accessory muscle groups was discussed under general patient assessment, we will focus here on observing the action of the primary muscles.

Observation of the action of the primary muscles should focus on a comparative assessment of diaphragmatic and chest wall excursion. Fig. 31-22 differentiates the three major patterns of diaphragmatic and chest wall excursion.

In normal patients in the supine position, the descent of the diaphragm will cause outward movement of the abdomen, and the intercostals will cause outward movement of the rib cage. As evident in Fig. 31-22, these normal events are coordinated and occur simultaneously with the increment in inspired tidal volume.

If the rib cage and abdomen do not move outward at the same time, the breathing pattern is described as asynchronous (see Fig. 31-22). For example, if the abdomen moves outward noticeably faster than the rib cage, this indicates that the respiratory muscles are not working in synchrony. This pattern often serves as an early indicator of an excessive respiratory muscle load.

Asynchronous breathing may progress to a more severe pattern called paradoxical breathing (see Fig. 31-22). In this pattern, the abdomen is observed to move outward while the lower rib cage moves inward during inspiration. As with asynchrony, paradoxical breathing indicates an excessive respiratory muscle load and probably serves notice of impending respiratory failure.

Not shown in Fig. 31-22, but also indicative of end-

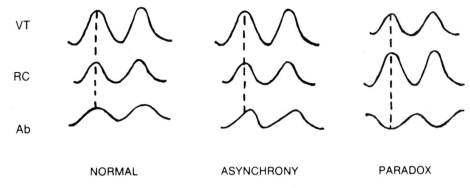

VT

RC

Ab

NORMAL   ASYNCHRONY   PARADOX

Fig. 31-22   Schema of motion of the rib cage *(RC)* and abdomen *(Ab),* and the calibrated sum of these signals, which is tidal volume (VT). In normal subjects the RC and Ab signals increase and decrease in synchrony. The rate of motion of the two compartments differs during asynchronous breathing, while during paradoxical breathing one compartment moves in an opposite direction to the VT signal. (From Dantzker DR and Tobin MJ: Respir Care 30(6):423, 1985.)

stage respiratory muscle fatigue, is a breathing pattern called respiratory alternans. Respiratory alternans is a phenomenon in which the patient is observed to switch back and forth between mainly diaphragmatic and mainly intercostal muscle activity, perhaps attempting to conserve the strength of each group.

Quantitative assessment of respiratory muscle function. Newer quantitative approaches to assessing respiratory muscle function include the use of inductance plethysmography, electromyography, and transdiaphragmatic tension measurements. These methods are providing new understandings of the importance of respiratory muscle function in respiratory failure, but are presently limited to investigational, as opposed to routine use.

Inductance plethysmography uses a principle of electrical circuitry (a series LC circuit) to measure relative displacement of the abdomen and rib cage. Two separate bands, each containing an electrical coil through which a small current is passed, are wrapped around the abdomen and rib cage. Expansion of the bands stretches the electrical coils, thereby causing a change in circuit inductance. Changes in circuit inductance cause a reciprocal change in current flow, proportional to the magnitude of stretch or expansion.

The inductance plethysmograph can display relative motion of the abdomen and rib cage simultaneously against a time axis, as previously shown in Fig. 31-22. Alternatively, abdominal and rib cage motion may be plotted against each other on an X-Y recorder or oscilloscope. Data from this x-y plot, when combined with tidal volume information, is used to derive measures such as the percentage of abdominal paradox and the average asynchrony index. Fig. 31-23 demonstrates the close relationship between these newer measures of respiratory muscle function and the deterioration in minute ventilation and pH observed after removal of a patient from a ventilator.

Electromyography (EMG) measures the electrical activity of muscles in much the same way that an ECG measures the electrical activity of the heart. However, unlike the ECG, the EMG of large muscle groups like the diaphragm or intercostals is extremely complex and difficult to interpret. However, recent work using the analysis of EMG frequency domains has shown that the onset of muscle fatigue is accompanied by a distinct shift in the mean power frequency of the EMG from high to low. Specifically, EMG analysis indicates muscle fatigue when the high to low frequency ratio (H-to-L ratio) falls to below 80% of control values. Fig. 31-24 demonstrates the close relationship between the drop in H-to-L ratio below 80% of control and the subsequent deterioration in ventilatory parameters.

Transdiaphragmatic tension measurements require concurrent measurement of pressure changes across the diaphragm, using both esophageal and gastric balloons, as compared to volume and time parameters. Using this method, one can calculate a diaphragmatic tension-time index, or TTdi, equivalent to the mean transdiaphragmatic pressure difference (Pdi) times the ratio of inspiratory time to total breath cycle duration (TI/Ttot):

$$\text{Tension-time Index (TTdi)} = \text{Pdi} \times \text{TI/Ttot}$$

Studies using this measure have shown a good correlation between the time-tension index and the H-to-L ratio obtained by more complex EMG methods. Moreover, research has shown that a critical time-tension index exists (0.15), above which a particular breathing pattern cannot be sustained for more than 45 minutes.

Assessment of hemodynamics. Hemodynamic monitoring methods allow the clinician to obtain information on various pressure and flow parameters in both the systemic and pulmonary circulations. This data can serve both diagnostic and therapeutic purposes. Diagnostically, hemodynamic information can help the clinician differentiate between various cardiovascular and pulmonary problems.

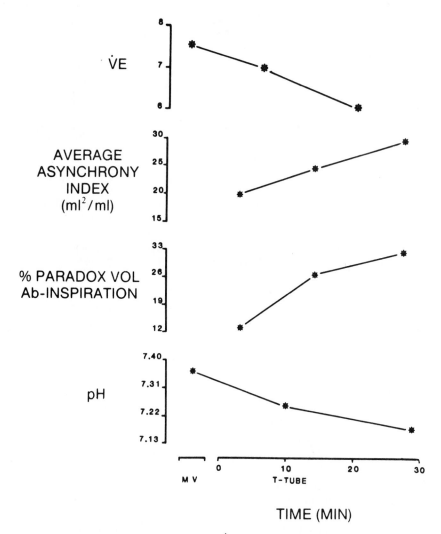

Fig. 31-23 Alterations in minute ventilation (V̇E), average asynchrony index, percent paradox volume of the abdomen *(Ab)* during inspiration, and arterial blood pH in a patient who failed a T-tube trial of weaning from mechanical ventilation (MV). (From Dantzker DR and Tobin MJ: Respir Care 30(6):428, 1985.)

Therapeutically, pressure and flow data can serve as a guide to selecting and changing therapeutic interventions.

As with previous methods of assessment, hemodynamic monitoring can be invasive or noninvasive. Noninvasive methods, such as the physical examination, vital signs, and the ECG have already been discussed in detail in prior chapters. Our focus here will be on invasive hemodynamic monitoring techniques, in particular the use of systemic and pulmonary arterial catheterization to obtain measurements of blood pressures and flow.

Arterial pressure monitoring. Systemic arterial blood pressure is the most commonly measured hemodynamic parameter. Just as with blood gas tensions, blood pressure can be measured invasively by arterial cannulation or noninvasively by use of a blood pressure cuff and mercury or aneroid sphygmomanometer. Each method has its advantages, but the invasive technique tends to be more accurate as the pressures are sampled directly. In addition, invasive

monitoring allows for display of the pressure pattern on a bedside station, usually in conjunction with the electrocardiogram. In combination, display of these two parameters simultaneously provides the clinician with considerable information regarding the electrical and mechanical functions of the left heart, as related to the status of the peripheral vasculature.

Sites for systemic arterial cannulation are the radial, brachial, and femoral arteries. As with arterial puncture, the radial site is preferred because of the extra safety provided by collateral circulation through the ulnar artery. Patency of this artery is always determined by performing the Allen test before catheter placement. Placement of a catheter is by percutaneous puncture or surgical cutdown. In addition to providing hemodynamic monitoring data, an arterial catheter, or arterial "line", provides a direct source for obtaining arterial blood samples without the discomfort associated with percutaneous arterial puncture.

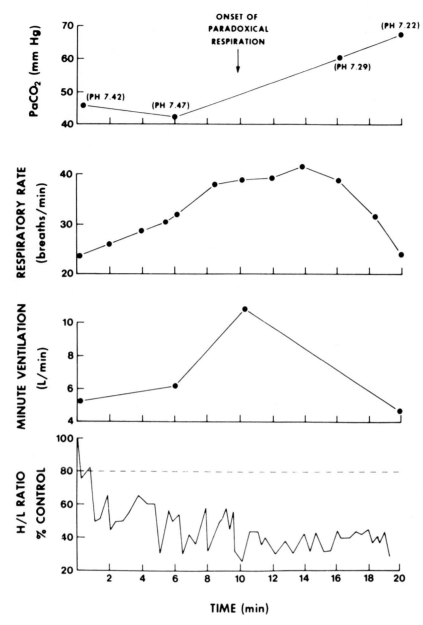

Fig. 31-24   Sequence of changes in Pa$_{CO_2}$, respiratory rate, minute ventilation ($\dot{V}_E$), and high/ low (H/L) ratio of the diaphragm in patient 1 during a 20-minute attempt at discontinuation. The initial change was the fall in H/L ratio, followed by a progressive increase in respiratory rate. The Pa$_{CO_2}$ initially fell, and the patient became alkalemic. Paradoxic abdominal displacements were not noted until after there had been a substantial increase in respiratory rate and minute ventilation. Hypercapnia and respiratory acidosis did not develop until after abdominal paradox and alternation between rib cage and abdominal breaths were noted. Just before artificial ventilation was reinstituted, there was a sharp fall in respiratory frequency and minute ventilation. (From Hudson LD: Respir Care 28(5):548, 1983.)

Equipment. Fig. 31-25 shows the typical equipment setup for invasive monitoring of arterial blood pressure. The arterial catheter is connected to a disposable continuous flush (Intraflow) device that maintains patency of the system by providing a small but continuous flow of IV fluid (2 to 4 ml/hr) through the system. Because arterial pressures are significantly higher than venous pressures, gravity infusion is insufficient to drive the IV fluid into the artery. Therefore, the IV bag containing the infusion fluid must be pressurized, usually with a hand bulb pressure pump.

Normally, stopcocks placed in line with the continuous

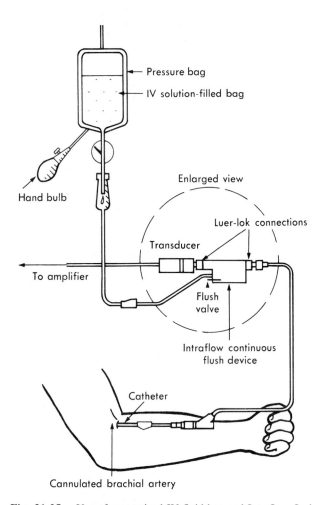

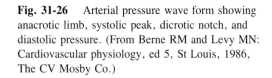

Fig. 31-25   Use of pressurized IV fluid bag and Intraflow flush device for optimal maintenance of arterial catheter patency. Stopcocks may be placed on each side of the flush device for room air reference and blood sampling. (From Schroeder JS and Daily EK: Techniques in bedside hemodynamic monitoring, St Louis, 1976, The CV Mosby Co.)

flush device allow calibration of the system against atmospheric pressure and arterial sampling. A strain gauge pressure transducer, connected to the flush device, provides an analog electrical signal to the amplifier/monitor, which displays the corresponding pressure waveform.

Waveform analysis. Fig. 31-26 illustrates a normal arterial pressure waveform for a single cardiac cycle, with time on the x-axis and pressure on the y-axis. For clarity, this waveform is wider than that normally observed on a pressure monitor, which generally operates at a slower "sweep" speed.

As with the cardiac cycle, the arterial pressure waveform is divided into two phases: systole and diastole. In terms of pressure events, systole begins with opening of the aortic valve. Arterial pressure rises to its peak systolic level, then begins to taper off as the stroke volume is fully ejected into the aorta. Once ventricular pressure drops sufficiently below that in the aorta, ventricular systole ends and the aortic valve closes, an event marked on the waveform by the dicrotic notch. Thereafter, arterial pressure gradually declines until the next systole. The potential energy stored as a result of the elastic expansion of the aorta and large arteries provides for continuous blood flow during diastole.

The pressure components of this normal arterial waveform include the systolic pressure, diastolic pressure, pulse pressure, and mean arterial pressure (see Fig. 31-26). The systolic pressure (SP) is equivalent to the peak of the arterial pressure waveform and normally ranges between 90 and 140 mm Hg (brachial). The diastolic pressure (DP), is measured as the low point of the arterial pressure waveform, and normally ranges between 60 and 90 mm Hg. The pulse pressure (PP) represents the difference between the systolic and diastolic pressures and averages about 40 mm Hg in healthy adults. The mean arterial pressure (MAP) is the average pressure throughout the cardiac cy-

Fig. 31-26   Arterial pressure wave form showing anacrotic limb, systolic peak, dicrotic notch, and diastolic pressure. (From Berne RM and Levy MN: Cardiovascular physiology, ed 5, St Louis, 1986, The CV Mosby Co.)

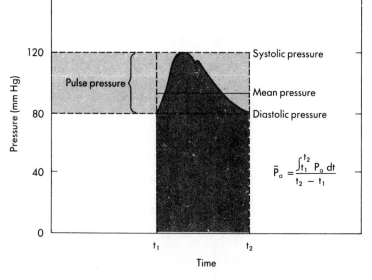

$$\bar{P}_a = \frac{\int_{t_1}^{t_2} P_a \, dt}{t_2 - t_1}$$

cle and averages between 80 to 100 mm Hg in adults. MAP is calculated by integration of the arterial pressure waveform signal over time, as performed by an electronic integrator or microprocessor. Lacking this capability, the MAP can be estimated using the following formula:

$$MAP = \frac{SP + (DP \times 2)}{3}$$

The box on p. 814 summarizes the normal values for arterial pressures obtained by arterial cannulation.

Most modern arterial pressure monitors provide continuous digital display of these pressures, also allowing output

to be diverted to a strip-chart recorder for permanent record keeping. Fig. 31-27 compares and contrasts strip-chart recordings of a normal arterial waveform, *A*, with those observed in patients with aortic insufficiency, *B*, cardiogenic shock, *C*, pulsus alternans caused by CHF, *D*, a bigeminal arrhythmia, *E*, and pulsus paradoxus caused by pericardial tamponade, *F*.

Maintenance and troubleshooting. In many settings, the respiratory care practitioner assumes full or partial responsibility for the operation of arterial pressure lines. This responsibility includes ensuring the optimum ongoing function of the system and troubleshooting problems in pres-

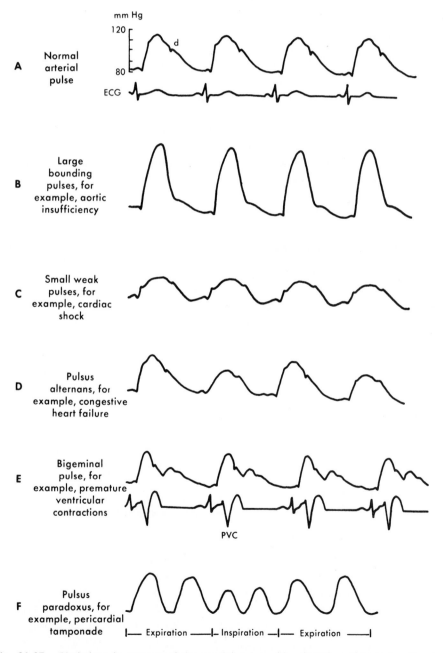

Fig. 31-27 Variations in contour of the arterial pulse with selected cardiovascular disorders. (From Andreoli KG et al: Comprehensive cardiac care, ed 6, St Louis, 1987, The CV Mosby Co.)

NORMAL ADULT SYSTEMIC ARTERIAL PRESSURES

PRESSURE	NORMAL RANGE
Systolic	100 to 140 mm Hg
Diastolic	60 to 90 mm Hg
Mean	70 to 105 mm Hg

sure measurement. Table 31-7 provides common-sense guidelines to optimize arterial pressure monitoring, while Table 31-8 outlines the cause, prevention, and treatment of several of the most common reasons for obtaining inaccurate arterial pressure measurements.

Complications. Invasive monitoring of arterial pressures carries a significant risk of complications. Hemorrhage is always a possibility with arterial cannulation and can be avoided only by careful equipment setup and scrupulous monitoring. Infection is another major risk, as this may lead to systemic sepsis. Thrombi may form on the catheter and lead to embolization of peripheral arteries. In the worst case, tissue necrosis may develop distal to the inser-

Table 31-7   Guide for Optimal Arterial Monitoring

Procedure	Reason
Label IV tubing of arterial line as "artery" or "arterial line."	Visual aid may help to avoid confusion with venous lines
Keep pressure bag inflated to pressure greater than patient's arterial pressure.	Slow deflation of bag will result in blood flow back into tubing
Maintain constant fluid flow with continuous flush device (2 to 4 ml/hr).	Constant fluid flow maintains patency and prevents clotting
Check all connections.	Loose connections can introduce air or allow blood loss
Immobilize extremity.	Extremity movement can result in needle or catheter displacement
Keep all connectors and puncture sites visible.	Possible bleeding may be observed
Frequently check pulse distal to puncture site.	Weakening or loss of pulse may indicate thrombosis
Check circulation, movement, and sensation of extremity distal to puncture site.	Any changes in circulation, movement, or sensation may indicate hematoma formation
Label date of catheter insertion on dressing.	Removal of catheter after 72 to 96 hr may reduce risk of infection

From Daily EK and Schroeder JS: Techniques in bedside hemodynamic monitoring, ed 4, St Louis, 1989, The CV Mosby Co.

tion site, requiring amputation of the involved area. This latter complication is of particular concern when large artery sites are used with small infants. Care must also be taken on insertion to prevent nerve damage, which may lead to paralysis or chronic pain syndromes.

Pulmonary artery monitoring. To obtain a complete bedside picture of a patient's hemodynamic status, arterial pressure measurements need to be supplemented with data obtained by invasive catheterization of the pulmonary arterial system.

Equipment. Equipment necessary to obtain data via pulmonary artery catheterization include a specialized flow-directed balloon-tipped pulmonary artery catheter (commonly called a Swan-Ganz catheter), a continuous flush pressure transducer system like that used for arterial monitoring, a pressure amplifier/monitor with continuous display capabilities, and a bedside cardiac output computer.

First used in the 1970s, the Swan-Ganz catheter provides information useful in differentiating between right and left ventricular failure and other cardiopulmonary disorders. Moreover, pressure measurements obtained with this catheter are an important adjunct in fluid management and drug therapy. Finally, the Swan-Ganz catheter provides a mechanism to directly measure cardiac output.

The Swan-Ganz catheter (Fig. 31-28) is made of pliable, radiopaque polyvinyl chloride. The catheter most commonly used has four lumens or channels: (1) a distal channel or distal injection port which terminates at the tip of the catheter, thereby permitting both the measurement of pulmonary artery pressures and the withdrawal of mixed venous blood; (2) a balloon inflation channel, used to inflate or deflate a small balloon located about 1 cm from the tip of the catheter, thereby allowing determination of pulmonary capillary "wedge" pressures; (3) a proximal channel or injection port located 30 cm from the catheter tip, which permits measurement of right atrial or central venous pressures and allows injection of solutions for cardiac output determination; and (4) an extra injection port to provide continuous infusion capabilities. Also running the length of the catheter is a wire connected to a thermistor bead, located approximately 4 cm from the catheter tip. Connection of this thermistor sensor system to a cardiac output computer allows bedside measurement of cardiac output using the thermal dilution technique.

Indications. Given the numerous risks and complications associated with its use, a pulmonary artery catheter is indicated only when the information available via this technique is required for effective patient management. Among the conditions for which effective patient management depends on data obtainable only via a pulmonary artery catheter are the following:

- Shock states (cardiogenic, hypovolemic, septic, etc);
- Myocardial infarction causing cardiovascular instability;
- Pulmonary vascular disease;

- Pulmonary edema (cardiogenic and noncardiogenic); and
- Adult respiratory distress syndrome.

Insertion. Assuming ECG and pressure monitoring is available, Swan-Ganz catheterization can be performed by a physician at the bedside. The distal port of the catheter is hooked up to a pressure transducer that is connected to the bedside display monitor. The basilic, brachial, femoral, subclavian, or internal jugular veins may be used as insertion sites, with the latter two being the most common.

After entry into the selected vein, the catheter is advanced until the tip is in the right atrium. At this time the balloon is inflated to the recommended volume of air (1.5 cc) and the catheter is advanced further. As shown in Fig. 31-29, the catheter pressure reading and waveform is continuously observed as the catheter proceeds from the right atrium, *RA*, through the tricuspid valve, into the right ven-

tricle, *RV*, through the pulmonary semilunar valve, into the pulmonary artery, *PA*, and finally into a "wedge" position, *PAWP*. After insertion and stabilization, the catheter position in the pulmonary circulation is confirmed with a chest x-ray.

Immediately after pulmonary capillary wedge pressure is obtained, the balloon is deflated, allowing blood to flow past the catheter and exposing the tip to pulmonary artery pressures for continuous monitoring. It is important to note that the wedge position should not be maintained for longer than 15 consecutive seconds to prevent pulmonary infarction.

Pressure measurements. Table 31-9 summarizes the pressures that can be measured with the four-channel pulmonary artery catheter, including their normal ranges.

RA pressures normally are the lowest of all heart chambers, ranging from 0 to 10 mm Hg. The normal RA pres-

Table 31-8   Inaccurate Arterial Pressure Measurements

Problem	Cause	Prevention	Treatment
Damped pressure tracing	Catheter tip against vessel wall	Usually cannot be avoided	Pull back, rotate, or reposition catheter while observing pressure waveform
	Partial occlusion of catheter tip by clot	Use continuous drip under pressure	Aspirate clot with syringe and flush with heparinized saline (<2 to 4 ml)
		Briefly "fast flush" after blood withdrawal (<2 to 4 ml)	
		Adding 1 unit heparin/1 ml IV fluid may help	
	Clot in stopcock or transducer	Carefully flush catheter after blood withdrawal and re-establish IV drip	Flush stopcock and transducer; if no improvement, change stopcock and transducer
		Use continuous flush device	
Abnormally high or low readings	Change in transducer reference level	Maintain air-reference port of transducer at midchest and/or catheter tip level for serial pressure measurements	Recheck patient and transducer positions
Damped pressure without improvement after flushing	Air bubbles in transducer or connector tubing	Carefully flush transducer and tubing when setting up system and attaching to catheter	Check system; flush rapidly; disconnect transducer and flush out air bubbles
	Compliant tubing	Use stiff, short tubing	Shorten tubing or replace softer tubing with stiffer tubing
No pressure available	Transducer not open to catheter	Follow routine, systematic steps for setting up system and turning stopcocks	Check system—stopcocks, monitor, and amplifier setup
	Settings on monitor amplifiers incorrect—still on *zero, cal,* or *off*		
	Incorrect scale selection	Select scale appropriate to expected range of physiologic signal	Select appropriate scale

From Daily EK and Schroeder JS: Techniques in bedside hemodynamic monitoring, ed 4, St Louis, 1989, The CV Mosby Co.

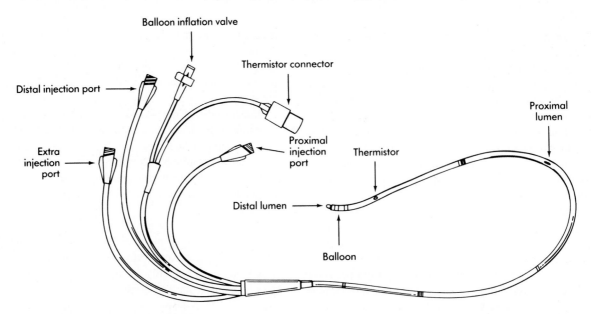

Fig. 31-28   The quadruple-channel Swan-Ganz catheter. The most distal channel (distal injection port) is for pulmonary artery pressure measurement; blood can also be aspirated from this channel for mixed venous oxygen measurements. A second channel (balloon inflation valve) is used to inflate-deflate the distal balloon. A third channel (proximal injection port), which exits 30 cm from the catheter tip, is used for central venous (right atrial) pressure monitoring and fluid infusion. The fourth channel (extra injection port), which is not present on all catheters, can be used for continuous infusion of hyperalimentation fluids. The thermistor connector plugs into a bedside cardiac output computer. (From Martin L: Pulmonary physiology in clinical practice, St Louis, 1987, The CV Mosby Co.)

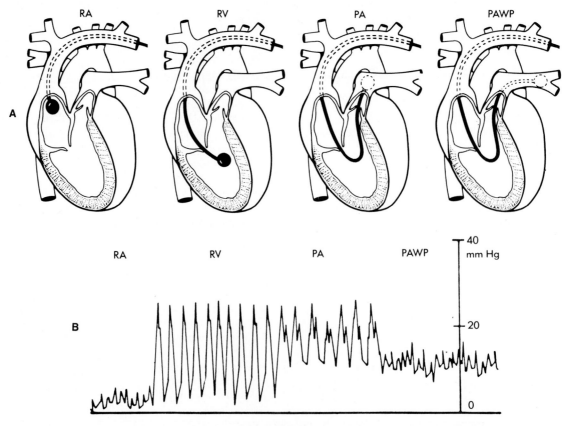

Fig. 31-29   **A,** Swan-Ganz catheter position in heart. **B,** As monitored by pressure tracings. *RA,* Pressure tracing from right atrium; *RV,* pressure tracing from right ventricle; *PA,* pressure tracing from pulmonary artery; *PAWP,* pulmonary artery wedge pressure tracing.) (From Martin L: Pulmonary physiology in clinical practice, St Louis, 1987, The CV Mosby Co.)

sure waveform, although sometimes difficult to visualize on a monitor, includes the a, c, and v waves representing, respectively, atrial contraction, ventricular contraction, and atrial filling against a closed tricuspid valve. Mean RA pressure is equivalent to central venous pressure (CVP), which reflects atrial preload, as determined by the balance between the capacity of the cardiovascular system, its circulating volume, and the efficacy of venous return to the heart (see Chapter 7). The causes of abnormal RA pressures, both high and low, are summarized in the box opposite.

The PA pressure waveform resembles that in the systemic arterial circulation, but with pressures averaging one-sixth those observed in the large systemic arteries. PA systolic pressure normally is equivalent to right ventricular systolic pressure (15 to 30 mm Hg) and reflects the volume of blood ejected from the right ventricule as compared with the resistance to flow in the pulmonary circuit. With diastole, closure of the pulmonic valve (also marked by a dicrotic notch) keeps PA diastolic pressures above those of right ventricular diastole. PA diastolic pressures normally range between 5 to 16 mm Hg. The mean PA pressure, abbreviated as MPAP or PAP, is calculated in the same manner as the mean systemic arterial pressure, and ranges between 10 to 22 mm Hg. PAP is an indicator of right ventricular afterload.

PA pressures will tend to increase with increased right ventricular stroke volumes, increased pulmonary vascular resistance, or with elevated left atrial pressures, as would occur in mitral stenosis, or left ventricular failure. PA pressures will tend to decrease when blood volume decreases or pulmonary vascular resistance decreases, as with vasodilation.

The pulmonary artery wedge pressure, abbreviated by various authors as PAWP, PCWP (pulmonary capillary wedge pressure), or PAo (pulmonary artery occluded pressure), normally ranges between 6 to 12 mm Hg. When properly measured, the PAWP reflects the downstream

---

ALTERATIONS IN RIGHT ATRIAL (RA) PRESSURES

ELEVATIONS OF RA PRESSURE MEASUREMENTS OCCUR WITH THE FOLLOWING:

1. Right ventricular failure (myocardial infarction, cardiomyopathy)
2. Pulmonary valvular stenosis
3. Tricuspid stenosis and regurgitation
4. Pulmonary hypertension
5. Pulmonary embolism
6. Volume overload
7. Compressions around the heart; constrictive pericarditis, cardiac tamponade
8. Increased large vessel tone throughout the body, resulting in venoconstriction
9. Arteriolar vasodilation that increases the blood supply to the venous system
10. Increased intrathoracic pressure (positive pressure breath or pneumothorax)
11. Placement of the transducer below the patient's right atrial level; raising the patient above the transducer
12. Infusion of solution (especially by pressure infusion pumps) into the central venous pressure line
13. Left heart failure

CAUSES OF DECREASED RA PRESSURE MEASUREMENTS INCLUDE THE FOLLOWING:

1. Vasodilation (by drug or increase in body temperature)
2. Inadequate circulating blood volume (hypovolemia) caused by dehydration; actual blood loss; and large amounts of gastrointestinal loss, wound drainage, perspiration, urine output (diuresis), insensible losses (high temperature, low humidity), and losses to the interstitial space (edema, "third spacing")
3. Spontaneous inspiration
4. Placement of the transducer above the patient's right atrial level
5. Air bubbles or leaks in the pressure line

Table 31-9 Basic Pressure Measurements from Swan-Ganz Catheterization

Measurement	Normal range
Central venous pressure	<10 mm Hg
Right atrial pressure	<10 mm Hg
Right ventricular pressure, systolic	15 to 30 mm Hg
Right ventricular pressure, diastolic	0 to 8 mm Hg
Pulmonary artery pressure, systolic	15 to 30 mm Hg
Pulmonary artery pressure, diastolic	5 to 16 mm Hg
Pulmonary artery pressure, mean	10 to 22 mm Hg
Pulmonary artery wedge pressure, mean	6 to 12 mm Hg

From Martin L: Pulmonary physiology in clinical practice: the essentials for patient care and evaluation, St Louis, 1987, The CV Mosby Co.

pressure in the pulmonary circulation, that is the pulmonary venous pressure. Pulmonary venous pressure, in turn, reflects left atrial pressure, which under optimum conditions, gives an indication of the left ventricular end-diastolic pressure (LVEDP), or left ventricular preload. Thus the pulmonary artery wedge pressure can provide a "window" on the events occurring in the left side of the heart.

There are, however, several situations in which the PAWP does not accurately reflect left ventricular preload. As summarized in the box on p. 818, these may be categorized into situations where (1) PAWP is less than LVEDP, (2) PAWP is greater than LVEDP, and (3) PAWP equals LVEDP, but the LVEDP does not correlate with the left ventricular end-diastolic volume.

Of particular importance to the respiratory care practi-

SITUATIONS WHERE PAWP MAY NOT ACCURATELY REFLECT LEFT VENTRICULAR PRELOAD*

1. PAWP IS LESS THAN LVEDP.

Aortic regurgitations

Reduced left ventricular compliance (see number 3)

2. PAWP IS GREATER THAN LVEDP.

When catheter tip is in zone 1 or 2; may occur from artificial ventilation, with or without peep, or from volume depletion

Atrial myxoma

Thoracic tumors pressing on pulmonary veins

Mitral stenosis or regurgitation

Increased left ventricular compliance (see number 3)

3. PAWP EQUALS LVEDP, BUT LVEDP DOES NOT CORRELATE WITH LVEDV.

Decreased left ventricular compliance	*Increased left ventricular compliance*
Increased right ventricular volume	Decreased right ventricular volume
Pericardial tamponade	Removal of pericardium
Some drugs, eg, isoproterenol	Some drugs, eg, nitroglycerin
High LVEDV	Low LVEDV
Tachycardia	Bradycardia
PEEP	
Myocardial ischemia and infarction	
Myocardial hypertrophy	

*Ideal Situation—PAWP equals LAP equals LVEDP, and LVEDP is proportional to LVEDV. When this is true, PAWP can be used as a measure of left ventricular preload.

From Martin L: Pulmonary physiology in clinical practice: the essentials for patient care and evaluation, St Louis, 1987, The CV Mosby Co.

tioner involved in PAWP measurements is the effect of positive-pressure ventilation on the accuracy of the data obtained. Whether positive-pressure ventilation will affect PAWP accuracy depends on several factors, including the fluid status of the patient, the level of airway pressure, and the position of the catheter in the lungs. As long as the patient has a normal circulating blood volume and the catheter tip is located in an area of the lung where pulmonary blood flow is uninterrupted by changes in alveolar pressure ("zone 3"), then the PAWP, if measured at the end of exhalation, probably reflects true downstream pressures. Moreover, PEEP levels of 10 cm H_2O or less in normal volemic patients do not significantly influence PAWP, as measured in zone 3 of the lung. For this reason, and because we normally need to know the PAWP under conditions of treatment, removal of a patient from positive-pressure ventilation to measure the PAWP is generally unnecessary.

Cardiac output determinations. The pulmonary artery pressure catheter also can be used to measure cardiac output (CO) by the thermodilution method. As shown in Fig. 31-30, cardiac output is obtained by injecting either a dextrose or saline solution at 0°C (or room temperature) into the proximal port (RA lumen) of the pulmonary artery catheter. The resulting heat loss between this port and the thermistor bead near the tip of the catheter is a function of the rate of blood flow and is measured by a cardiac output computer.

Hemodynamic profiles. In combination with the pressure measurements previously described, knowledge of the patient's cardiac output allows the clinician to calculate a variety of important hemodynamic parameters, such as the cardiac index, stroke volume, left and right ventricular stroke work indices, and systemic and pulmonary vascular resistance. Formulas and normal values for these important hemodynamic parameters are summarized in Table 31-10. Based on this derived information, it is possible to differ-

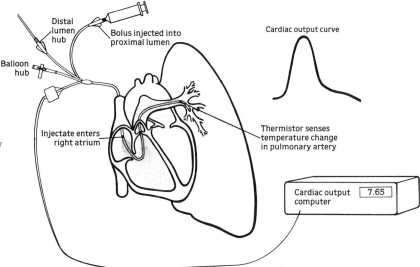

Fig. 31-30   Thermodilution cardiac output measurement. (From Wilkins RL, Sheldon RL, and Kirder SJ: Clinical assessment in respiratory care, St Louis, 1985, The CV Mosby Co.)

entiate between a variety of common conditions encountered in critical care, as delineated in Table 31-11. As always, such quantitative analysis can serve to complement and refine, but never replace, traditional methods of patient assessment.

Pitfalls and complications. Pulmonary artery catheterization is among the most hazardous forms of monitoring currently used in the critical care setting. These hazards are attributable to both errors in judgment or management associated with data collection or interpretation and the numerous technical complications that accompany use of the pulmonary artery catheter. The box on p. 820 summarizes the most common pitfalls and complications associated with pulmonary artery catheterization. Although many of

Table 31-10   Common Values Calculated from Hemodynamic Measurements

Value	Formula*	Normal range
Cardiac index	$\dfrac{\dot{Q}_T \text{ (L/min)}}{\text{Body surface area (m}^2)}$	2.8 to 4.2 L/min/m^2
Stroke volume	$\dfrac{\dot{Q}_T \text{ (ml/min)}}{\text{Heart rate (beats/min)}}$	50 to 80 ml/beat
Stroke index (SI)	$\dfrac{\text{Stroke volume (ml/beat)}}{\text{m}^2}$	30 to 65 ml/beat/m^2
Left ventricular stroke work index	$SI \times (MSAP - PAWP) \times 0.0136$	43 to 61 gm-meters/m^2
Right ventricular stroke work index	$SI \times (MPAP - CVP) \times 0.0136$	7 to 12 gm-meters/m^2
Systemic vascular resistance†	$\dfrac{MSAP - CVP \text{ (mm Hg)}}{\dot{Q}_T \text{ (L/min)}}$	11 to 18 mm Hg/L/min
Pulmonary vascular resistance†	$\dfrac{MPAP - PAWP \text{ (mm Hg)}}{\dot{Q}_T \text{ (L/min)}}$	1.5 to 3.0 mm Hg/L/min
% Shunt	$\dfrac{Cc'_{O_2} - Ca_{O_2}}{Cc'_{O_2} - C\overline{v}_{O_2}}$	<5%
Oxygen uptake	$Q_T \times (Ca_{O_2} - C\overline{v}_{O_2})$	150 to 300 ml O$_2$/min

*MSAP, mean systemic arterial pressure; CVP, central venous pressure; MPAP, mean pulmonary artery pressure; PAWP, pulmonary artery wedge pressure (mean); m^2, square meters of body surface area; Q$_T$, cardiac output; Cc'$_{O_2}$, Ca$_{O_2}$, and Cv$_{O_2}$, oxygen content in end-capillary blood, arterial blood, and mixed venous blood, respectively.

†In many textbooks, the resistance formula is multiplied by a conversion factor of 80 to obtain resistance units of dynes $\times$ sec $\times$ cm^{-5}. Either formula is correct. When dynes $\times$ sec $\times$ cm^{-5} is used, the normal range for systemic vascular resistance (SVR) is approximately 880 to 1440 and for pulmonary vascular resistance (PVR) is approximately 150 to 240.

From Martin L: Pulmonary physiology in clinical practice: the essentials for patient care and evaluation, St Louis, 1987, The CV Mosby Co.

Table 31-11   Some Hemodynamic Changes in Common Clinical Conditions*

Condition	Chest x-ray infiltrates	SAP	SVR	$\dot{Q}_T$	PAP	PAWP
Adult respiratory distress syndrome	Both sides	Variable	Variable	Variable	Variable	Normal to decreased
Left-sided heart failure	One or both sides	Normal to decreased	Increased	Decreased	Increased	Increased
Septic shock	None, one, or both sides	Decreased	Decreased	Increased	Normal to decreased	Normal to decreased
Dehydration	None	Decreased	Increased	Normal to decreased	Normal to decreased	Decreased
Pulmonary hypertension	None	Normal	Normal	Normal	Increased	Normal

*Many conditions overlap so that the typical hemodynamic changes may not manifest in an individual patient. For example, a patient with sepsis and heart failure may have decreased cardiac output; a patient with adult respiratory distress syndrome and heart failure may have an increased PAWP, SAP, systemic arterial pressure; SVR, systemic vascular resistance; QT, cardiac output; PAP, pulmonary arterial pressure; PAWP, pulmonary artery wedge pressure.

From Martin L: Pulmonary physiology in clinical practice: the essentials for patient care and evaluation, St Louis, 1987, The CV Mosby Co.

these pitfalls and complications fall within the purview of the physician responsible for catheter insertion or overall patient management, respiratory care practitioners involved in pulmonary artery monitoring procedures can take an active role in minimizing patient risk by recognizing common management problems and taking appropriate corrective action, as specified by institutional protocols.

Composite indices. Given the complexity of problems underlying respiratory failure and the numerous measures currently available to assess a patient's status, recent efforts have focused on the development and validation of composite indices designed to predict patient outcomes. Typically, these indices combine two or more discrete physiologic parameters associated with the severity of illness and use a scoring system to yield a combined measure with greater predictive power.

Table 31-12 provides an example of a composite index currently under investigation by Hicks and associates. This respiratory assessment index (RAI) weighs selected ventilatory, mechanical, oxygenation, and hemodynamic parameters (previously discussed) to obtain a composite score, ranging from 0.0 to 1.0.

The RAI score correlates well with the length of ventilatory support required. In a study of 87 patients requiring ventilatory support, those with RAIs greater than 0.7 required, on average, 37 hours of support, whereas those with RAIs below 0.51 required an average 126 hours on a ventilator. Moreover, of the six patients in the study who died, all had RAI scores markedly lower than 0.4 prior to death.

Because these results are preliminary in nature, it is premature to adopt such a tool for widespread use. Nonetheless, the potential utility of composite indices such as the RAI is clear, reiterating the importance of a multisystem

---

PITFALLS AND COMPLICATIONS IN HEMODYNAMIC MONITORING

PITFALLS (ERRORS IN JUDGMENT OR MANAGEMENT)

1. Inappropriate indications (when less invasive methods are just as good and when data will not change therapy)
2. Obtaining data incorrectly (inaccurate machine calibration and incorrect transducer placement)
3. Misusing data (improper interpretation of data obtained)
4. Not checking all relevant or related data before making therapeutic decisions (data such as chest x-ray, serum albumin, and urine output)
5. Not removing catheter when hemodynamic data are no longer used or are no longer useful in patient management

COMPLICATIONS FROM THE TECHNIQUE

1. Ruptured or torn pulmonary or tricuspid valve
2. Pneumothorax (usually from subclavian insertion)
3. Pulmonary thrombosis and hemorrhage, including rupture of pulmonary artery
4. Right-sided endocardial damage (including hemorrhage, thrombus, and infection)
5. Knotting or kinking of catheter
6. Thrombosis in venous site of insertion
7. Cardiac arrhythmias, including heart block
8. Infection at site of insertion or at catheter tip
9. Balloon rupture
10. Loss of guide wire or portion of catheter within the venous system

From Martin L: Pulmonary physiology in clinical practice: the essentials for patient care and evaluation, St Louis, 1987, The CV Mosby Co.

Table 31-12 Respiratory Assessment Index (RAI), Score Ranges, and Calculation Based on Values Reported in the Literature.

Variable	Weight			
	3	2	1	0
C_{eff} (ml/cm H_2O)	>50	40-49	30-39	<30
Pao_2/Fio_2	>300	250-299	150-249	<150
$\dot{V}q$*	<1.5	1.5-1.9	2.0-3.0	>3.0
pH	7.35-7.45	7.34-7.30 or 7.46-7.50	7.29-7.20 or 7.51-7.60	<7.20 or >7.60
MAP (mm Hg)	80-100	101-120 or 65-79	121-150 or 50-64	>150 or <50

$$RAI = \frac{Sum\ of\ individual\ scores}{15}, \text{ where 15 is highest possible sum of individual scores.}$$

RAI range = 0.00 − 1.0.

$$*\dot{V}q = \text{ventilation quotient. } Vq = \frac{\dot{V}E}{Wt\ in\ kg} \times \frac{PaCO_2}{3.6}$$

From Capps JS and Hicks GH: Monitoring non-gas variables during mechanical ventilation, Respir Care 32(7):566, 1987.

perspective in assessing and managing the patient in respiratory failure.

Troubleshooting

Troubleshooting is a learned skill that involves the identification and correction of mechanical and patient-related problems occurring during ventilatory support. The ultimate goal of troubleshooting is to detect potential problems before they occur or before they can cause any stress or harm to the patient. Troubleshooting is an ongoing process that requires foreknowledge of what problems can occur and how best to solve them.

Potential problems which may occur during ventilatory support include leaks or malfunctions in the ventilator system and changes in the clinical condition of the patient. Table 31-13 lists common clues to ventilator troubleshooting, possible reasons for the observed problems, and advice on correcting the problems. The reader is encouraged to become familiar with these situations by replicating them in a simulated laboratory setting.

When a potential problem is discovered, the first priority is to assure that the patient is being adequately ventilated and oxygenated. If there is any doubt about the proper function of the ventilatory support system, the patient should be disconnected from the device and ventilated with 100% oxygen via a manual resuscitator until the problem is resolved.

Routine checks and documentation

Given the number of patient-ventilator system parameters which must be verified and the importance of sequential data in patient management, a flow sheet should be used to document both routine monitoring checks and parameter changes (Fig. 31-31). Although the format of the flow sheet may vary, and each institution will have its own documentation requirements, all flow sheets should have a number of common characteristics.

Table 31-13   Troubleshooting the Ventilator

Clue	Possible reason	Advice
Decreased minute or tidal volume	Leak around endotracheal tube, from the system, or through the chest tube	Check all connections for leaks
	Decreased patient-triggered respiratory rate	Check respiratory rate
	Decreased lung compliance	Evaluate patient
	Airway secretions	Clear airway of secretions
	Altered settings	Check patient-ventilator system
	Malfunctioning spirometer	Calibrate spirometer
Increased minute or tidal volume	Increased patient-triggered respiratory rate	Check respiratory rate
	Altered settings	Check patient-ventilator system
	Hypoxia	Evaluate patient; consider ABG findings
	Increased lung compliance	*Good news*
	Malfunctioning spirometer	Calibrate spirometer
Change in respiratory rate	Altered setting	Check patient-ventilator system
	Increased metabolic demand	Evaluate patient
	Hypoxia	Evaluate patient; consider ABG findings
Sudden increase in maximum inspiratory pressure	Coughing	Alleviate uncontrolled coughing
	Airway secretions or plugs	Clear airway secretions
	Ventilator tubing kinked or filled with water	Check for kinks and water
	Kinked endotracheal tube	Check for kinks
	Changes in patient position	Consider repositioning
	Endotracheal tube in right mainstem bronchus	Verify position
	Patient-ventilator asynchrony	Correct asynchrony
	Bronchospasm	Identify cause and treat
	Pneumothorax	Decompress chest

From Martz KV, Joiner JW, and Shepherd RM: Management of the patient-ventilator system: a team approach, ed 2, 1984, St Louis, The CV Mosby Co.

Continued on p. 822, bottom.

Space should be provided for charting ventilator settings including the mode of ventilation, frequency of mechanical and spontaneous breaths, tidal volume, airway pressures, peak flow, I:E ratio, F_{IO_2}, system temperature, and alarm settings. In addition, there should be ample space for documentation of clinical data, including patient assessment, measured values such as arterial blood gases, dynamic characteristics and effective compliance, respiratory mechanics, and other parameters which are being monitored to assess respiratory function.

Several of the newer microprocessor-controlled ventilators now have the capability of outputing much of this data to a printer. Although such computerized output can save recording time, the practitioner always should verify the accuracy of this data by checking each parameter manually.

Other than in the control mode, any significant change (>10%) in the rate of breathing from prior values must be assessed. Moreover, since in the IMV, PSV, and MMV modes a larger responsibility for ventilation is placed on the patient, greater care must be taken to look for signs of excessive work of breathing such as tachypnea, asynchronous breathing, paradoxical breathing, or respiratory alterans.

In assessing the frequency of breathing, the clinician should determine both the rate at which the ventilator is set to deliver breaths, as well as the rate of patient initiated, or spontaneous, breaths. Preferably the flow sheet should provide separate columns for each so that the patient's contribution can be evaluated. The machine rate must be verified by actually counting the number of breaths delivered per minute. Analog and digital read-outs, while generally accurate, should not be depended on to verify these values. If in the assist/control mode, the ventilator will generally have an indicator of patient initiated breaths. In the IMV mode, the spontaneous breaths may be indicated,

Table 31-13   Troubleshooting the Ventilator—cont'd

Clue	Possible reason	Advice
Gradual increase in maximum inspiratory pressure	Increased lung stiffness	Measure static pressure
	Diffuse obstructive process	Evaluate for reversible problems: Atelectasis Increased lung water Bronchospasm
Sudden decrease in maximum inspiratory pressure	Volume loss from leaks in system	Check patient-ventilator system for leaks
	Clearing of secretions; relief of bronchospasm; increasing compliance	*Good news*
F_{IO_2} drift	O_2 analyzer error	Calibrate analyzer
	Blender piping failure	Correct failure
	O_2 source failure	Correct failure
	O_2 reservoir leak	Check ventilator reservoir
I:E ratio < 1:3 or > 1:1½	Altered inspiratory flow rate	Check flow setting and correct
	Alteration in other settings that control I:E ratio	Check settings and correct
	Alteration in sensitivity setting	Check and correct
	Airway secretions (pressure ventilator)	Clear airway of secretions
	Subtle leaks	Measure minute ventilation
Inspired gas temperature inappropriate	Addition of cool water to humidifier	Wait
	Altered settings	Correct temperature control setting
	Thermostat failure	Replace heater
Changes in delivered PEEP	If ventilator control used: Changes in compliance Changes in tidal volume	Correct problem if possible; if not, increase PEEP setting to deliver desired level of PEEP
	If external PEEP source used: Evaporation of water Disconnection of expiratory tubing from PEEP device	Add water; check and reconnect
Changes in static pressure	Changes in lung compliance	Evaluate patient and correct cause if possible
Changes in inspiratory flow rate, sigh volume, assist or control mode, alarm status, dead-space volume	Changes in these settings resulting from deliberate or accidental adjustment of dials or knobs	Check to determine whether current settings are the ones intended

B.S.A. _____

DATE	ARTERIAL LINE						SG DISTAL						FLUSH	ICP	INT.	PROCEDURES		
SHIFT 7 3 11 / TIME	INSERTION SITE	EXTREMITY TEMPERATURE	EXTREMITY COLOR	DISTAL PULSE	WAVE FORM	CALIBRATION	INSERTION SITE	WAVE FORM	CALIBRATION	TIME C.O. DONE	C.O. L/MIN	C.I. L/MIN/M²	500 ML NS 1000U HEPARIN	WAVE FORM	CALIBRATION	TIME	PROCEDURE #	INT.

TIME	MODE	RATE (PER MIN)	TIDAL VOLUME (CC)			PRESSURE (cmH₂O)				MISCELLANEOUS				BLOOD GAS VALUES						INT.	PROCEDURE CODE
	INVERSE I:E ASSIST CONT IMV SIMV & PS SIMV CPAP	MECHANICAL / SPONTANEOUS	MACHINE DELIVERED	EXHALED MEASURED	SPONTANEOUS	PEAK / EQUAL SYSTEM	PEEP CPAP / SET LIMIT	PS / I:E RATIO	FIO2 (ANALYZED)	FLOW RATE (L MIN) / INSP TIME (SEC)	H₂O LEVEL / ALARM FUNCT.	GAS TEMP.	PH	PCO₂	PO₂	O₂ SAT.	OXIMETER SAT.	B.E.		1. INTUBATION

The procedure code column (right side) reads:

1. INTUBATION
2. EXTUBATION
3. TRACH △
4. HEMO-PROFILE
5. CARDIO-PROFILE
6. A-LINE INITIAL SET UP
7. ARTERIAL CANNULATION
8. A-LINE, TRANS, LINE, FLUSH △
9. SG TRANS, LINE, FLUSH
10. SG TRANS, LINE FLUSH △
11. FEMORAL SHEATH INITIAL SET UP
12. FLUSH △
13. DRESSING △
14. PORT — O2
15. IABP △
16. VENT △
17. VENT TUBING △

PROC. IN MIN. NEEDED

18. VENT TRANSPORT
19. IABP TO SURGERY
20. IABP TRANSPORT
21. CARDIO VERSION
22. CODE 90
23. AIRWAY MAINT.
24. SG INSERTION STANDBY
25. IABP INSERTION

ENDO-TRACH TUBES

LOCATION -

SIZE -   mm

TAPE MARK -   cm

CUFF PRESS-   cmH₂O

OXIMETER ALARM SETTINGS

HIGH-

LOW-

TIME	PROGRESS NOTES

INT.	SIGNATURE	PATIENT STAMP
PAGE #		

GP-40952

RESPIRATORY CARE FLOWSHEET

FLORIDA HOSPITAL
763-1 (288 REV.)

Fig. 31-31   Respiratory care flowsheet. (Reprinted with permission from the Department of Respiratory Care Services, Florida Hospital Medical Center, Orlando.)   *Continued.*

DATE	PROGRESS NOTES
/ /	
SHIFT 7 3 11	
TIME	

	INTRA AORTIC BALLOON PUMP DATA							PATIENT PRESSURES				PATIENT DATA			INT.
TIME	ARTERIAL TIMING SITE	TRIGGER MODE	RATIO	HELIUM PRESSURE (PSI)	ALARM ON	PURGE	AEDP	PSP	PDP	BAEDP	APSP	HEART RATE	HEART RHYTHM	PAD WEDGE (mmHg)	

TIME	INTRA AORTIC BALLOON PUMP PROGRESS NOTES

BALLOON INFORMATION

SIZE -

TYPE -

VOLUME -   ML

INT.	SIGNATURE	PATIENT STAMP

PAGE #

GP-40952

FLORIDA HOSPITAL   **RESPIRATORY CARE FLOWSHEET**

763-1 (288 REV.)

Fig. 31-31, cont'd

but should be observed and verified by observing the patient's chest expansion, in conjunction with either the negative deflections occurring on the pressure manometer or actual recording of spontaneous exhalations.

Volumes documented as part of the ventilator check should include the set tidal volume, the delivered tidal volume, the compressed volume loss, the set and delivered sigh volume (if used), and the patient's spontaneous tidal volume (if in the IMV mode). Spontaneous tidal volume is measured in order to determine the patient's ability to breathe independently in both modes of ventilation, especially during the weaning process.

There are several methods of measuring volume. The most basic is the bellows-type exhaled gas spirometer, which collects and fills in proportion to the volume exhaled. This system is prone to leaks and inaccuracies in the presence of continuous flows. Many of the newer ventilators incorporate a pneumotachometer to measure exhaled flow. This flow signal is integrated in time to provide a digital read-out of volume. The practitioner can also use a hand held respirometer to measure and verify volumes.

Since volume settings may be out of calibration, the set volume should be verified at the machine outlet. The delivered volume is checked after the exhalation valve. The compression factor of the tubing should be taken into consideration; this factor multiplied by the peak pressure is the volume which is "lost" in the circuit. Spontaneous tidal volumes are best measured with the patient off the ventilator, especially in the assist/control and continuous-flow IMV modes.

Peak inspiratory pressure should be checked and monitored regularly. Monitoring alerts the practitioner to changes in pulmonary mechanics. Peak pressure will increase as V_T and flow are increased, if compliance decreases, or if resistance increases. The peak pressure will usually increase if the airway is occluded by secretions or obstructed by compression because of patient biting or tubing misplacement.

Oxygen concentrations are normally provided by a blending mechanism, either built-in or attached to the ventilator. Accuracy of such devices cannot be assumed and should be confirmed by analysis with each ventilator check and setting change. This is accomplished by placing a calibrated analyzer probe in the inspiratory side of the circuit, proximal to the humidifier and bacteria filter, to prevent contamination of the circuit and moisture damage to the probe.

Airway temperature should be kept near normal body temperature and the humidifier regularly checked for adequate water levels. Caution must be taken against overfilling the humidifier as this may significantly increase circuit resistance and interfere with spontaneous breathing. The most aseptic and convenient means of assuring adequate water levels are with a continuous feed system connected to the humidifier, although this may prove to be expensive and/or unreliable.

When performing a ventilator check, any discrepancies in settings must be investigated. This can be accomplished by consulting with the patient's nurse or physician and checking the chart for appropriate orders. Some authors suggest that parameters should always be returned to those indicated on the flow chart. However, careful investigation may reveal extenuating circumstances which justify the changes made. Nonetheless, if in the judgment of the practitioner undocumented changes endanger the patient, parameters should be restored to their previously documented values while the matter is resolved.

As discussed in Chapter 14, the entire circuit should be changed every 24 to 48 hours to prevent bacterial growth. External air filters should be cleaned, changed regularly, and also changed between patients. The ventilator should be wiped down periodically to prevent the accumulation of dust and spills. Special caution should be taken when this is done to prevent the inadvertent change of parameters. If a ventilator is being used on the same patient for a prolonged period of time, the entire ventilator should be replaced periodically to allow for thorough cleaning and safety checks.

ADJUSTING VENTILATORY SUPPORT PARAMETERS

Once appropriate data has been gathered and analyzed, key support parameters should be adjusted according to the goals of ventilatory support. Primary adjustments made by the respiratory care practitioner are those designed to stabilize or normalize both ventilation and oxygenation.

Adjusting ventilatory parameters

The goal of adjusting ventilatory parameters is to restore adequate and efficient ventilation. Since the adequacy of ventilation is assessed by measurement of the arterial or alveolar P_{CO_2} as related to the patient's pH, ventilatory parameters should be adjusted to achieve a Pa_{CO_2} which normalizes the pH.

Adjustments in the patient's Pa_{CO_2} are made mainly by altering the total minute ventilation. The following formula provides a rough estimate of the change in minute ventilation necessary to achieve a desired Pa_{CO_2}:

$$\text{New } \dot{V}_E = \text{Current } \dot{V}_E \times \frac{\text{Current } Pa_{CO_2}}{\text{Desired } Pa_{CO_2}}$$

Obviously, the $\dot{V}_E$ can be altered by changing the rate, changing the tidal volume, or both. When the need exists to increase the $\dot{V}_E$, it is generally more desirable to increase the tidal volume rather than the rate, as this will also increase the efficiency of ventilation (the proportion of alveolar ventilation to total ventilation per minute). However, since low tidal volumes are associated with progressive atelectasis, decreasing the $\dot{V}_E$ is generally accomplished by lowering the rate (if tolerable) rather than the tidal volume.

In the assist/control mode of ventilation, simple lowering of the $\dot{V}_E$ may not result in the desired rise in Pa_{CO_2}. In these cases it may be necessary to add mechanical dead space to the ventilator circuit. As rebreathed volume, mechanical dead space increases the inspired partial pressure of CO_2, thereby raising the alveolar and arterial CO_2 tensions. Although nomograms exist to estimate the amount of deadspace necessary to achieve a given Pa_{CO_2}, most clinicians suggest incremental trials with 50 cc segments until the desired Pa_{CO_2} is achieved. The use of added mechanical dead space in the IMV mode is generally contraindicated because of the smaller patient tidal volumes characterizing this mode of ventilatory support.

In most patients the Pa_{CO_2} should be kept in the normal range of 35 to 45 mm Hg and the pH within the normal range of 7.35 to 7.45. However, it should be remembered that the patient with chronic CO_2 retention may have normal Pa_{CO_2} values in the 50 to 60 mm Hg range, and that lowering the P_{CO_2} by mechanical ventilation may result in an iatrogenic alkalosis. There may also be cases in which hyperventilation is one of the goals of ventilatory support, as when it is used to decrease cerebral edema.

If the efficiency of ventilation is poor, as indicated by a high physiologic dead space, the clinician must attempt to identify the underlying cause. If the cause is patient-related, such as pulmonary embolization or airway obstruction, appropriate treatment should be instituted. On the other hand, inefficient ventilation may be caused by the pattern of ventilation that has been established, in which case adjustments in the ventilatory rate or inspiratory flow or the use of an end-inspiratory pause may be considered.

Adjusting oxygenation

In adjusting patient oxygenation, the ultimate goal is to maintain adequate oxygen delivery to the tissues, while keeping the F_{IO_2} under potentially toxic levels. To this end, each patient must be evaluated individually, taking into consideration age and normal Pa_{O_2}.

Adjusting the F_{IO_2}. For patients with normal oxygen carrying capacities and cardiovascular performance, an acceptable target Pa_{O_2} range is 60 to 100 mm Hg. This level achieves near maximal oxygen saturation, although some COPD patients may be accustomed to Pa_{O_2} values in the 50 to 60 mm Hg range. The response to a change in F_{IO_2} depends on the underlying disease process. The patient with normal lungs will have adequate Pa_{O_2} values with low concentrations of oxygen. Patients who are hypoventilating or have a minor ventilation-perfusion mismatch will also respond well to small increments in the F_{IO_2}. In contrast, a patient with a large physiologic shunt will exhibit little improvement in Pa_{O_2} as F_{IO_2} values are increased.

In the absence of significant intrapulmonary shunting, the following formula is helpful in estimating F_{IO_2} needs:

$$\text{New } F_{IO_2} = Pa_{O_2} \text{ desired} \times \frac{\text{Current } F_{IO_2}}{\text{Current } Pa_{O_2}}$$

On the other hand, if the presence of significant intrapulmonary shunting has been established, the following formula is more appropriate:

$$F_{IO_2} \text{ needed} = \frac{P(A-a)_{O_2} + 100}{760}$$

where the $P(A-a)_{O_2}$ is the alveolar-arterial oxygen tension gradient, as measured on 100% oxygen. Thereafter, the lowest F_{IO_2} possible is chosen, which will provide a Pa_{O_2} in a range determined to be adequate by the care team.

Adjusting PEEP or CPAP. Positive end expiratory pressure (PEEP) and continuous positive airway pressure (CPAP) are generally indicated in situations where arterial hypoxemia is refractory to traditional oxygen therapy. Clinically, this is evident when the Pa_{O_2} cannot be maintained above 60 mm Hg on greater than 60% oxygen.

Because both modes of ventilatory support can compromise cardiovascular function and are associated with an increased incidence of pulmonary barotrauma, it is important to carefully monitor the levels being used and the effect on the patient.

When PEEP or CPAP are instituted, the goal should be to achieve adequate oxygenation, with an acceptable F_{IO_2}, without compromising the patient's cardiovascular function. In principle, this "optimum" level of PEEP or CPAP is indicated when oxygen delivery to the tissues is maximized. Precise determination of the optimum PEEP or CPAP level can be accomplished only when hemodynamic data, specifically cardiac output and mixed venous P_{O_2} measures, are available.

This approach to optimizing PEEP or CPAP involves applying incremental levels of distending pressure, while monitoring the patient's cardiopulmonary response. Fig. 31-32 provides an example of a PEEP "study" using this empirical method. As distending pressures are elevated, careful attention is given to changes in arterial and mixed venous oxygenation as related to cardiac output and blood pressure. Total oxygen delivery is calculated at each incremental level of pressure, with the "optimum" pressure level corresponding to the point at which these parameters indicate the best effect. In the example provided, PEEP levels of 20 and 25 appear equally satisfactory. However, in this case, the lower level (20 cm H_2O) is chosen to minimize the potential for barotrauma.

Obviously, this approach can only be used when the patient has a pulmonary artery catheter in place. An alternative approach to selecting the optimum level of distending pressure, when pulmonary artery monitoring is not available, is to assess Pa_{O_2} levels as related to effective compli-

	0	5	10	15	20	25	30
Minutes/time	15	30	45	60	75	90	105
Blood Pressure (mm Hg)	117/80	120/85	120/80	110/70	115/75	115/75	90/65
P_{Peak} (cm H_2O)	33	39	43	51	51	53	60
P_{PL} (cm H_2O) (plateau)	28	33	37	48	45	47	58
V_t spontantous/V_t ventilator	200/1000	200/1000	250/1000	250/1000	250/1000	250/1000	250/1000
$f_{spontaneous}$/$f_{ventilator}$	4/10	4/10	3/10	4/10	3/10	5/10	4/10
$\dot{V}_E$ Total (l/min)	10.8	10.8	10.8	11.0	10.8	11.3	11.5
C_s (ml/cm H_2O)	36	36	37	35	40	45	36
PaO_2 (F_IO_2 = 1.0)	43	59	65	73	103	152	167
CaO_2 (vol %)	15.3	17.8	18.3	18.9	19.2	19.4	19.6
$PaCO_2$ (mm Hg)	37	37	38	37	39	37	38
pH	7.41	7.42	7.42	7.42	7.40	7.41	7.41
$P(A-a)O_2$ (mm Hg)	607	591	585	577	547	498	483
$PaCO_2$ - $P_{ET}CO_2$ (mm Hg)	16	15	13	10	9	8	15
$P\bar{v}O_2$ (or $S\bar{v}O_2$) (mm Hg or %)	27	37	38	38	39	40	34
C.O. L/min	4.1	4.2	4.0	4.5	4.4	4.4	3.3
$C(A-\bar{V})O_2$ (vol %)	5.3	5.2	5.4	5.0	4.9	4.9	6.7
PCWP (mm Hg)	3	5	8	11	12	13	18
PAP (mm Hg)	37/21	39/25	41/24	43/25	40/21	38/24	45/30
C.O. x CaO_2 Oxygen transport	790	811	772	869	854	854	776

Comments: Bilateral scattered crackles present in both lungs.

Fig. 31-32 Example of a PEEP study flow sheet including ventilation, oxygenation, and hemodynamic data. Key points to observe when first reviewing a PEEP study are (1) blood pressure, (2) mixed venous oxygen, and (3) oxygen transport. Notice that these three values decline at a PEEP of 30 cm H_2O. Blood pressure drops to 90/65, Pvo_2 drops to 34 mm Hg, and oxygen transport drops to 776 ml/min. A more optimum PEEP level is +20 cm H_2O where these parameters and others indicate that oxygen transport is improving without significant cardiovascular side effects. (From Pilbeam SP: Mechanical ventilation: physiological and clinical applications, St Louis, 1986, The CV Mosby Co.)

ance and arterial blood pressure at various PEEP or CPAP increments. As shown in Fig. 31-33, increasing levels of distending pressure are normally associated with an increase in both the FRC and the compliance of the lung, as well as an increase in Pao_2. This phenomenon is a result of recruitment of additional alveoli and the characteristic steepening of the pressure-volume curve that occurs at higher lung volumes.

In principle, a point is reached at which lung compliance is maximized, beyond which alveoli become overdistended and compliance begins to taper off. As long as arterial blood pressure remains stable, this point may be taken as a rough estimate of the optimum PEEP level, to be confirmed by observational assessment of the adequacy of perfusion and oxygenation.

DISCONTINUING VENTILATORY SUPPORT (WEANING)

As with all aspects of respiratory care, the process of discontinuation of ventilatory support, or weaning, must be tailored to the needs of each patient. The ease with which ventilatory support can be discontinued varies substantially among patients, according to their underlying pathophysiologic disorder and their psychologic readiness. Some patients develop a psychologic dependence on ventilators, even after they are physiologically capable of doing without support. For this reason, two basic principles should guide clinicians in the weaning process. First, patients should be removed from ventilatory support as soon as possible. Second, patients should be carefully prepared prior to their removal from ventilatory support.

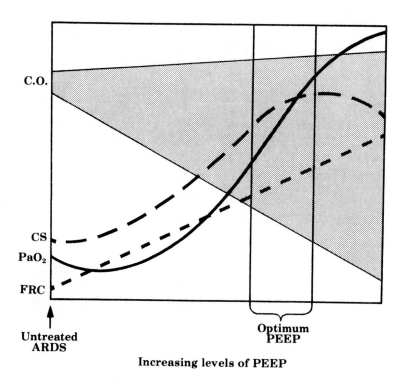

Fig. 31-33 The curves above represent the physiologic factors that change during the application of PEEP or CPAP. As the PEEP level is increased Pao_2 FRC, and static compliance (Cs) normally increase. Cardiac output (CO), represented by the shaded area, can increase slightly, stay the same, or decrease. The optimum PEEP level can be expected to occur where Pao_2, FRC, and Cs are high. Cardiac output should be maintained near normal so that oxygen transport to the tissues remains high. (From Pilbeam SP: Mechanical ventilation: physiological and clinical applications, St Louis, 1986, The CV Mosby Co.)

General approaches

There are two general weaning techniques, each with many possible variations (Fig. 31-34). In the first, or traditional approach, all ventilation is supplied by the ventilator in the assist/control mode until physiologic measures indicate patient readiness for spontaneous support of ventilation and oxygenation. Two variations of this method are common. In many instances, weaning begins and ends simultaneously, as illustrated in Fig. 31-34, *A*. Those who object to this method often refer to it as the "sink or swim" approach. Alternatively, traditional weaning may occur gradually, with the patient breathing spontaneously for intervals between periods of total ventilatory support (Fig. 31-34, *B*). In either case, the clinician relies on some set of physiologic measures to predict patient readiness for weaning.

The second general approach to weaning a patient from ventilatory support employs intermittent mandatory ventilation (IMV). As with the traditional approach, two variations are common. IMV may be introduced after a period of total ventilatory support, as shown in Fig. 31-34, *C*. Alternatively, ventilatory support may be initiated with IMV, as demonstrated in Fig. 31-34, *D*. In either case, the number of machine-supplied breaths is progressively reduced

until the patient can meet all ventilatory needs via spontaneous breathing. Unlike the traditional approach, this method of gradual withdrawal deemphasizes predictions of patient capabilities, placing emphasis on the empirical results of progressive reductions in ventilatory support.

More recently, a third general approach to discontinuing ventilatory support, pressure support ventilation (PSV), has been proposed as a viable alternative to traditional and IMV methods.

Prerequisites for weaning

Regardless of which weaning approach is chosen, success is unlikely unless certain conditions are previously established. The box on p. 829 summarizes factors that can hamper the weaning process. Generally, the patient should be awake, alert, and able to follow instructions. Also, the patient should be rested, not fatigued and sleep deprived as is commonly seen in the intensive care unit. As long as major problems, such as shock, cardiac arrhythmias, severe gastrointestinal bleeding, and acute renal failure exist, the likelihood of success is small. Ideally, the patient should be receiving adequate nutritional support, preferably a high protein diet (high carbohydrate loads increase the respiratory quotient and CO_2 production). If the patient

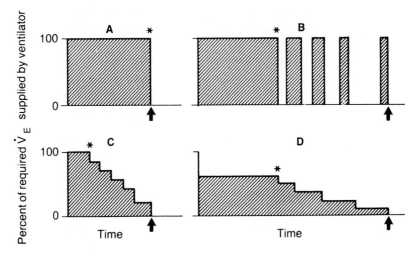

Fig. 31-34 Conceptual representation of weaning by traditional (upper) and intermittent mandatory ventilation (IMV, lower) techniques. Asterisks indicate the points at which weaning is begun, and arrows indicate when it is completed. With traditional weaning from the assist-control mode, all ventilation is supplied by the ventilator until weaning is attempted as guided by measurements of physiological readiness. In most instances weaning begins and ends at the same moment (upper left). With gradual or slow traditional weaning (upper right), the patient breathes spontaneously for intervals between periods of total ventilatory support. When IMV is used to wean patients from total ventilatory support (lower left), the number of ventilator breaths is progressively reduced, beginning before the patient can meet all ventilatory needs spontaneously and ending as soon as this point is reached. Slow IMV weaning, often from IMV as the primary ventilator mode (lower right), consists of gradually reducing the ventilator's contribution as long as the patient's spontaneous efforts keep the arterial pH above a predetermined minimum value. Theoretically, as shown here, both techniques permit discontinuation of mechanical ventilation at the same moment in a patient's recovery from acute respiratory failure, although weaning is begun earlier with IMV. (From Pierson DJ: Respir Care 28:646-660, 1983.

PROBLEMS IN WEANING

Cardiovascular collapse (shock, heart failure)
Poor muscle strength or atrophy
Increased work of breathing
Excessive secretions
Patient not psychologically or physiologically ready
Primary illness not resolved
Improper weaning procedure or patient cannot be weaned (terminal illness)
Pulmonary complications (eg, atelectasis, pulmonary infection, bronchospasm)
Poor nutrition
Continued use of sedatives or analgesics
Acid-base imbalance
Electrolyte imbalance
Abdominal distention
Anemia
Fluid overload
Renal failure
Malfunction of equipment

From Pilbeam SP: Mechanical ventilation: physiological and clinical applications, Denver, 1986, Multimedia Publishing, Inc.

experiences pain with breathing, weaning may be difficult. Other important clinical problems to resolve before weaning include anemia, fever (infection), and electrolyte imbalances, especially phosphate deficiencies (seen primarily in alcoholic patients, severely diabetic patients, and those receiving total parenteral nutritional support).

The timing of the weaning should also be considered. It is generally unwise to start weaning during a night shift. Physicians, allied health personnel, and patients are more rested in the morning. If a patient in the midst of weaning were to "crash," it would be better to have it happen during the day than at night.

Predicting a patient's ability to spontaneously support breathing

As summarized in Table 31-14, the results of clinical research over many years have provided the clinician with well-validated indicators of a patient's ability to adequately support their own breathing. These indicators include multiple measures of ventilation, oxygenation, and mechanics (as previously discussed), and other relevant factors related to the patient's general condition. As is evident, these indicators are essentially the same as those used in determining the need for mechanical ventilation.

The emphasis on objective physiologic criteria as a basis for determining patient readiness for weaning is not shared by all clinicians. Indeed, as previously discussed, proponents of the IMV method of weaning tend to deemphasize the quantitative approach, relying more on actual empirical results. In support of this opinion, evidence has been garnered showing that many ambulatory COPD patients do not meet the strict physiologic criteria for weaning. Some even argue that reliance on these measures only delays the weaning process. Clearly, a middle ground exists. This combined approach, emphasizing both objective data analysis and astute clinical observational skills, is probably the most useful for the clinician and is readily adaptable to both the traditional and IMV approaches to weaning.

The traditional approach

The traditional approach is the older of the two techniques and consists of one or more trials of removal from ventilator support. Generally, the longer a patient is ventilated, the more difficult and longer the weaning period. Moreover, because ventilatory support is an unnatural process, the longer it persists, the greater its risks. Therefore, under the assumptions of the traditional approach, the objective of mechanical ventilation is to support the patient through acute respiratory failure and to restore the patient to spontaneous unassisted breathing as soon as possible.

Rapid weaning. Rapid weaning is common place when ventilatory support is applied for prophylactic reason, such as after thoracic or cardiac surgery. This procedure is also common when ventilatory support is applied for short periods of time solely to maintain alveolar ventilation, which may occur after heavy anesthesia or in uncomplicated cases of narcotic drug overdose. The following box outlines a traditional rapid weaning protocol that may apply under such circumstances.

Gradual weaning. The gradual weaning approach is more common when ventilatory support is prolonged, as in the management of acute exacerbations of COPD or with neuromuscular disorders resulting in respiratory failure. Conditioning of these patients for weaning should start well in advance, by giving them encouraging reports of their progress and emphasizing that the mechanical ventilator represents a temporary measure only, designed to give them "rest" from the stress of breathing until they are better.

It is helpful to carefully watch the patient's behavior when he or she is removed from the ventilator for short periods, such as those required for suctioning, airway man-

Table 31-14   Criteria for Weaning from Mechanical Ventilation.

Parameter	Acceptable results
Level of consciousness	Awake, oriented, alert
Drive to breathe	Present and normal
Cardiopulmonary stability	Blood pressure, heart rate, temperature, respiratory rate and urine output normal
Airway secretions	Normal in amount and quality
Respiratory strength:	
Vital capacity	More than 15 ml/kg or 1-1/2 to 2 times normal tidal volume
Inspiratory force	−20 to −100 cm H_2O
Respiratory rate	Less than 25 breaths/min (adult)
Minute ventilation	Less than 10 L/min and can be doubled on command
Tidal volume	Three times body weight in kg
Dead space	V_D/V_T less than 0.6
Shunt	Less than 15%
Arterial blood gases	Within the patient's normal limits at an F_{IO_2} less than 0.4
$P(A-a)O_2$ on F_{IO_2} of 1.0	<300 to 350 mm Hg

From Pilbeam SP: Mechanical ventilation: physiological and clinical applications, Denver, 1986, Multimedia Publishing, Inc.

TRADITIONAL WEANING PROTOCOL

1. Fulfill predetermined objective criteria for initiating weaning
   a. Primary respiratory process improved
   b. Oxygenation adequate on F_{IO_2} 0.5 or less
   c. Ventilatory needs manageable: $\dot{V}_E$ < 10 L/min (for Pa_{CO_2} 40 mm Hg)
   d. Ventilatory mechanics adequate for needs:
      VC > 10 ml/kg
      MIF > 20 cm H_2O
      (MVV > 2 × resting $\dot{V}_E$ requirement)
2. Choose appropriate time for attempt
   a. Adequate personnel available
   b. No other ongoing procedures or other major activities
3. Eliminate or minimize respiratory depressants
   a. Narcotics; other analgesics
   b. Sedatives
4. Suction airway as needed
5. Place patient in head-elevated or semi-upright position
6. Switch from mechanical to spontaneous ventilation at same or slightly higher F_{IO_2}
   a. T-piece (blow-by) circuit
   b. Via ventilator if applicable
7. Observe patient continuously
8. Measure arterial blood gases in 20 to 30 min; continue spontaneous ventilation if:
   a. Pa_{O_2} acceptable (>80% of preweaning value)
   b. pH >7.30 and stable

F_{IO_2} = Fraction of inspired oxygen; VC = vital capacity; MIF = maximum inspiratory force; MVV = maximum voluntary ventilation.
From Pierson DJ: Weaning from mechanical ventilation in acute respiratory failure: concepts, indications, and techniques, Respir Care 28(5):650, 1983.

agement, or servicing the ventilator. If spontaneous breathing is evident at these times, some estimate of its adequacy can be noted. Certainly, such spontaneous breathing must return before weaning can even be considered; it is often helpful to have the patient take occasional breaths while not connected to the machine. In the control and assist/control modes, some patients may have to be urged to make this effort, since it is so easy for them to allow the ventilator to perform all the work of breathing. However, most patients accept as reasonable this need to try breathing on their own; such periods can be extended for long as is it acceptable.

Once a patient's spontaneous breathing has been demonstrated, he or she is ready for the next step. While disconnected from the ventilator, the patient can be encouraged to breathe on his or her own for a few minutes with the practitioner in attendance. The patient should be provided with an appropriate level of humidified oxygen (about 10% higher than had been delivered by the ventilator) via a T tube or other comparable delivery device. Supported ventilation should be resumed before the patient tires, with the intervals of spontaneous breathing gradually increased, allowing occasional periods of restful support. In patients who exhibit extreme anxiety when the ventilator is physically disconnected from their airway, the practitioner may initially use the "zero" rate control setting (spontaneous breathing) on the ventilator, if available. However, this approach has its own problems, since the imposed work of breathing through some ventilator circuits is very high.

The practitioner should look for certain signs to determine the need for reconnecting the patient to the ventilator. These signs include agitation, tachypnea, tachycardia, bradycardia, hypotension, cyanosis, asynchronous or paradoxical breathing, angina, and cardiac arrhythmias. Generally, the occurrence of these signs indicates that the patient is not tolerating the procedure and should be reconnected to the ventilator. However, strict adherence to this protocol would lead to failure in most weaning attempts. Indeed, clinical studies have shown that successfully weaned patients may exhibit heart rate increases of 15 to 20 per minute, increases in respiratory rates of up to 14 per minute, and 5 to 10 mm Hg "swings" in their $Paco_2$ and Pao_2 values, without deleterious results. Therefore the practitioner must exercise sound clinical judgment in deciding when or whether to continue or terminate the weaning effort. This decision can be aided by blood gas results obtained during the attempt to withdrawal ventilatory support.

The reader will find that some authors speak deprecatingly of this "trial-and-error" method of removing patients from ventilator support for periods of time and at intervals that are quite arbitrary. Still, this is a time-tested method that has been successful when supervised by conscientious and knowledgeable respiratory care personnel. It does not take an experienced practitioner long to evaluate a patient's ventilatory stamina and to set up a gradual program of ventilator withdrawal that is safe and effective. Some experts advocate removing the patient from the ventilator for a fixed short period of time and gradually shortening the intervals between. As an example, this might mean letting the patient breathe unassisted for 2 minutes of an hour, then 2 minutes each half hour, quarter hour, and so on, until mechanical aid is discontinued. When weaning has started in earnest, oxygenation and humidification in the free-breathing intervals are important.

The IMV approach

In prior chapters we looked at the physiologic and technical aspects of IMV and only touched on its role in weaning. IMV was originally intended as a weaning device, to be activated in the ventilator circuit as the patient improved. We have already learned, however, that IMV has become accepted by many clinicians as a primary mode of ventilation.

Because current approaches to weaning by IMV are intended to progress as quickly as possible, the distinction between rapid and gradual methods used with the traditional approach does not apply. Indeed, those who use IMV as the primary mode of ventilation generally do not consider weaning a phase of ventilatory support.

Proponents of IMV argue that this approach helps prevent asynchronous breathing, prevents respiratory alkalosis, shortens weaning time, allows for weaning with patients who have failed other weaning techniques, maintains respiratory muscle function, reduces the cardiovascular effects of mechanical ventilation with PEEP, and has psychologic benefits for the patient.

On the other hand, those opposed to this method argue that, by definition, the IMV mode cannot respond to changes in patient status and requires more monitoring. They also suggest that IMV increases the work of breathing, prolongs weaning (and cost) if not used properly, and may increase the risk of barotrauma (if SIMV is not available). Nonetheless, even those generally opposed to the widespread application of IMV as a primary mode of ventilation will agree that the method can be helpful in patients who have consistently failed the traditional approach.

No technique is foolproof, and IMV is no exception. IMV is less desirable than traditional approaches to weaning in patients who are unstable and cannot be monitored closely, those with CNS depression or impaired respiratory drive, or those in shock. Moreover, even under the best of circumstances, weaning with IMV often "stalls" at rates of 2 to 4 per minute, with further reductions resulting in unacceptable respiratory acidosis. This common clinical problem is probably associated with the high work of breathing imposed by the artificial airway, the ventilator circuit, or both. Indeed, if the resistance of the ventilator circuit is at fault, patients may still require trials off the ventilator on a T piece, even though they have been on an IMV system. These considerations do not negate the value of IMV, since perhaps without it, weaning would be impossible in some patients. There is little doubt that IMV has given a tremendous option in the choices of managing the critically ill patient.

Pressure support ventilation as a weaning tool

As previously discussed, pressure support ventilation (PSV) augments spontaneous breathing with a set amount of positive airway pressure. At low pressure levels, pressure support helps unload the respiratory muscles from the imposed work of breathing caused by artificial airways and/or ventilator circuitry, a problem characteristic of some ventilators in the IMV mode. At higher levels of pressure support, essentially all the work of breathing can be assumed by the ventilator.

Those who advocate pressure support as a means of weaning cite research showing that spontaneous breaths during IMV occur at the expense of high diaphragmatic tensions because of the impedances caused by both the underlying disease process and the artificial airway. Indeed, recent studies indicate that pressure support ventilation counteracts the work of breathing imposed by artificial airways, ventilator circuits, and demand systems. Moreover, pressure support ventilation may actually change the nature, or "quality", of respiratory work, enhance respiratory muscle endurance, and improve patient synchrony and comfort. Table 31-15 provides a tentative comparison of IMV and pressure support ventilation as weaning tools.

To the extent that the claims surrounding pressure support ventilation prove to be true, this mode of ventilation may indeed represent an improvement over both IMV and traditional approaches to discontinuing ventilatory support. However, more clinical research is needed before any definitive conclusions as to which, if any, of the currently available modes for discontinuing ventilatory support are "best." Indeed, with historical experience on research into other modes of medical intervention serving as a guide, we

should probably not be asking which mode is best, but under what conditions a given mode produces the best results.

Choice of approaches

Until such answers are available, selection of the most appropriate weaning approach in a given circumstance should be guided by sound knowledge of the relative advantages and disadvantages of each of these methods, as related to the patient's underlying pathology and individual needs. Slavish adherence to uniform protocols on patients as different as those regularly encountered by the respiratory care practitioner should be avoided. Indeed, consideration of alternative methods of achieving similar ends according to different patient needs represents the highest form of clinical judgment, that is, the "art" of respiratory care.

SUMMARY

The management of critically ill patients is among the most complex and demanding aspects of respiratory care. Effective patient management requires that the respiratory care practitioner integrate technical knowledge with assessment skills to draw conclusions, make recommendations, and take appropriate action. By definition, successful management of the critically ill also requires a multisystems approach.

Management of patients requiring ventilatory support is a cyclical and ongoing process involving three major components: data collection, data analysis and interpretation, and decision-making. The effective application of the management process should be founded on tangible clinical goals. Goals provide clear and consistent direction to those involved in the patient's management, yet allow for tailoring the respiratory care plan according to the patient's condition and individual needs.

Applied as an interim measure only, the primary goal of ventilatory support is to discontinue its use as soon as the

Table 31-15   Comparison of IMV and PSV Weaning

	IMV	PSV
Quantity of patient work	Adjust by mandatory rate Guide by spontaneous respiratory rate, P_{CO_2}	Adjust by pressure support Guide by spontaneous rate, P_{CO_2}
Quality of patient work	Lung mechanics and endotracheal tube = high tension-volume ratio	Pressure assisting lowers tension-volume ratio
Patient ventilator synchrony	Irregular support Clinician-set $\dot{V}$ and V_T may be difficult to synchronize	Regular support Patient interaction with clinician-set pressure allows for $\dot{V}$ and V_T that may synchronize more easily

From MacIntyre NR: Weaning from mechanical ventilatory support: volume-assisting intermittent breaths versus pressure-assisting every breath, Respir Care 33(2):124, 1988.

underlying problem is resolved. Once the initial ventilatory parameters are established, the clinician should conduct a preliminary assessment of the patient and patient-ventilator system to assure that all parameters are well tolerated and the patient is stable and as comfortable as possible.

Thereafter, meticulous ongoing monitoring of the patient and patient-ventilator system is essential. In general, ongoing monitoring involves skill in general patient assessment, physiologic data gathering and interpretation, and patient-ventilator system troubleshooting.

Once appropriate data has been gathered and analyzed, key ventilatory support parameters should be adjusted according to the previously established goals. This process continues until the underlying need for ventilatory support has diminished to the point where its removal can be considered and implemented.

BIBLIOGRAPHY

Abramson RS et al: Adverse occurrences in intensive care units, JAMA 244:1582-1588, 1980.

Armstrong PW and Baigrie RS: Hemodynamic monitoring in the critically ill, Philadelphia, 1978, Harper & Row.

Ashutosh K et al: Asynchronous breathing movements in patients with chronic obstructive pulmonary disease, Chest 67:553-567, 1975.

Barrocas A, Tretola R, and Alonso A: Nutrition and the critically ill patient, Respir Care 28:50-59, 1983.

Bassili HR and Deitel M: Effect of nutritional support on weaning patients off mechanical ventilators, JPEN 5:161, 1981.

Bassili HR and Deitel M: Nutritional support in long term intensive care with special reference to ventilator patients: a review, Can Anaesth Soc J 28:17, 1981.

Benotti P and Blackburn GL: Protein and caloric or macronutrient metabolic management of the critically ill patient, Crit Care Med 7:520, 1979.

Bone RC: Monitoring ventilatory mechanics in acute respiratory failure, Respir Care 28:597-607, 1983.

Bone RC: Monitoring patients in acute respiratory failure, Respir Care 27:700-701, 1982.

Borman KR, Weigelt JA, and Aurbakken CM: Guidelines for weaning from positive end-expiratory pressure in ventilated patient, Am J Surg 152(6):687-690, 1986.

Bowser MA et al: A systematic approach to ventilator weaning, Respir Care 20:959, 1975.

Branson RD and Hurst JM: Laboratory evaluation of moisture output of seven airway heat and moisture exchangers, Respir Care 32:741-747, 1987.

Brochard L et al: Pressure support (PS) decreases work of breathing and oxygen consumption during weaning from mechanical ventilation, Am Rev Respir Dis 135:A51, 1987 (abstract).

Buchbinder N and Ganz W: Hemodynamic monitoring: invasive techniques, Anesthesiology 45(2):146-155, 1976.

Burton GG and Hodgkin JE, editors: Respiratory care: a guide to clinical practice, ed 2, Philadelphia, 1984, JB Lippincott Co.

Bustin D: Hemodynamic monitoring for critical care, Norwalk, Conn, 1986, Appleton-Century-Crofts.

Calhoon S et al: Efficacy of chest radiographs in a respiratory intensive care unit, Chest 80:379, 1981.

Capps JS and Hicks GH: Monitoring non-gas respiratory variables during mechanical ventilation, Respir Care 32:558-568, 1987.

Carlon GC et al: Evaluation of an "in vivo" Pao$_2$ and Paco$_2$ monitor in the management of respiratory failure, Crit Care Med 8(7):410-413, 1980.

Chatburn RL: Dynamic respiratory mechanics, Respir Care 31:703-711, 1986.

Cherniak RM and Cherniak L: Respiration in health and disease, ed 3, Philadelphia, 1983, WB Saunders Co.

Cohen CA et al: Clinical manifestations of inspiratory muscle fatigue, Am J Med 73:308-316, 1982.

Collee GG et al: Bedside measurement of pulmonary capillary pressure in patients with acute respiratory failure, Anesthesiology 66:614-620, 1987.

Craig KC, Pierson DJ, and Carrico CJ: The clinical application of PEEP in ARDS, Respir Care 30:184-201, 1985.

Danek SJ, Lynch JP, and Dantzker DR: The dependence of oxygen uptake on oxygen delivery in the adult respiratory distress syndrome, Am Rev Respir Dis 122:387, 1980.

Dantzker DR, editor: Cardiopulmonary critical care, New York, 1986, Grune & Stratton.

Dantzker DR and Gutierrez G: The assessment of tissue oxygenation, Respir Care 30:456-461, 1985.

Dantzker DR and Tobin MJ: Monitoring respiratory muscle function, Respir Care 30:422-429, 1985.

DeHaven CB, Hurst JM, and Branson RD: Evaluation of two different extubation criteria: attributes contributing to success, Crit Care Med 14:92-94, 1986.

Demers RR, Sullivan MJ, and Paliotta J: Airflow resistances of endotracheal tubes, JAMA 237:1362, 1977.

Downs JB et al: Intermittent mandatory ventilation: a new approach to weaning patients from mechanical ventilators, Chest 64:331, 1973.

Downs JB and Douglas ME: In Kirby RR and Graybar GB: Intermittent mandatory ventilation, Int Anesthesiol Clin 18:81, 1980.

Fahey PJ, editor: Theory and practice in monitoring mixed venous oxygen saturation, vol 2, San Diego, 1985, Abbott Laboratories.

Fahey PJ, Harris K, and Vanderwarf C: Clinical experience with continuous monitoring of mixed venous oxygen saturation in respiratory failure, Chest 86(5):748-752, 1984.

Fairley HB: Monitoring respiratory mechanics, Respir Care 30:406-410, 1985.

Fallat RJ: Respiratory monitoring. In Bone RC, editor: Critical care: a comprehensive approach, Park Ridge, Ill, 1984, American College of Chest Physicians.

Feeley TW and Hedley-White J: Weaning from controlled ventilation and supplemental oxygen, N Engl J Med 292:903, 1975.

Field S, Sanci S, and Grassino A: Respiratory muscle oxygen consumption estimated by the diaphragm pressure-time index, J Appl Physiol 57:44-51, 1984.

Gallagher CG, Hof VIM, and Younes M: Effect of inspiratory muscle fatigue on breathing pattern, J Appl Physiol 59:1152-1158, 1985.

Gallagher TJ and Civetta JM: Goal-directed therapy of acute respiratory failure, Anesth Analg 59:831, 1980.

Gilbert R et al: The first few hours off a respirator, Chest 65:152, 1974.

Gilbert R and Keighley JF: The arterial-alveolar oxygen tension ratio: an index of gas exchange applicable to varying inspired oxygen concentrations, Am Rev Respir Dis 109:142-5, 1974.

Goeckenjan G: Continuous measurement of arterial Po$_2$: significance and indications in intensive care, Biotel Patient Montitg 6:51, 1979.

Goldfarb MA et al: Tracking respiratory therapy in the trauma patient, Am J Surg 129:255-258, 1975.

Gore JM et al: Handbook of hemodynamic monitoring, Boston, 1985, Little, Brown & Co.

Grassino A, Bellemare F, and Laporte D: Diaphragm fatigue and the strategy of breathing in COPD, Chest 83(suppl):85-89, 1984.

Grossbach I: Troubleshooting ventilator and patient-related problems, Crit Care Nurse 6(5):64-79, 1986.

Grossman GD: Nutritional assessment of critically ill patients, Respir Care 30:463-468, 1985.

Harris K: Noninvasive monitoring of gas exchange, Respir Care 32:544-552, 1987.

Hess D et al: The validity of assessing arterial blood gases 10 minutes after an F_{IO_2} change in mechanically ventilated patients without chronic pulmonary disease, Respir Care 10:1037-1041, 1985.

Hess D, Maxwell C, and Dganit S: Determination of intrapulmonary shunt: comparison of an estimated shunt equation and a modified equation with the classic equation, Respir Care 32:268-273, 1987.

Hicks GH et al: A prognostic index for assessment of mechanical ventilation, Respir Care 31:931, 1986 (abstract).

Hodgkin JE, Bowser MA, and Burton GG: Respirator weaning. In Shoemaker WC: The lung in the critically ill patient: pathophysiology and therapy of acute respiratory failure, Baltimore, 1976, Williams & Wilkins Co.

Hubmayr RD, Gay PC, and Tayyab M: Respiratory system mechanics in ventilated patients: techniques and indications, Mayo Clin Proc 62(5):358-368, 1987.

Hudson LD: Evaluation of the patient with acute respiratory failure, Respir Care 28:542-550, 1983.

Hylkema BS et al: Lung mechanical profiles in acute respiratory failure: diagnostic and prognostic value of compliance at different tidal volumes, Crit Care Med 13:637-640, 1985.

Kacmarek RM: Systematic modification of ventilatory support. In Barnes TA, editor: Respiratory care practice, Chicago, 1988, Year Book Medical Publishers.

Kacmarek RM and Venegar JV: Mechanical ventilatory rates and tidal volumes, Respir Care 32:466-474, 1987.

Kram HB et al: Determination of optimal positive end-expiratory pressure by means of conjunctival monitoring, Surgery 101(3):329-334, 1987.

Kram HB et al: Conjunctival oxygen monitoring in postoperative respiratory failure shock, Int J Clin Monit Comput 1(3):165-170, 1984.

Ledingham IM, MacDonald AM, and Douglas HS: Monitoring of ventilation. In Shoemaker WC, THompson WL, and Holbrook PR, editors: Textbook of critical care, Philadelphia, 1984, WB Saunders Co.

Low GGJ: Ongoing patient assessment. In Barnes TA, editor: Respiratory care practice, Chicago, 1988, Year Book Medical Publishers.

MacIntyre NR: Weaning from mechanical ventilatory support: volume-assisting intermittent breaths versus pressure-assisting every breath, Respir Care 33:121-125, 1988.

Macklem PT: The clinical relevance of respiratory muscle research, Am Rev Respir Dis 134:812-815, 1986.

Mancebo J, Calaf NN, and Benito S: Pulmonary compliance measurement in acute respiratory failure, Crit Care Med 13:589-594, 1985.

Marini JJ: Obtaining meaningful data from the Swan-Ganz catheter, Respir Care 30:572-581, 1987.

Martin L: Abbreviating the alveolar gas equation: an argument for simplicity, Respir Care 31:40-44, 1986.

Martin L: Pulmonary physiology in clinical practice: the essentials for patient care and evaluation, St Louis, 1987, The CV Mosby Co.

Martz KV, Joiner JW, and Shepherd RM: Management of the patient-ventilator system: a team approach, ed 2, St Louis, 1984, The CV Mosby Co.

Matthay RA, Weidman HP, and Matthay MA: Cardiovascular function in the intensive care unit: invasive and noninvasive monitoring, Respir Care 30:432-449, 1985.

Maunder RJ et al: Managing PEEP: the Harborview approach, Respir Care 31:1059-1068, 1986.

McPherson SP et al: A circuit that combines ventilator weaning methods using continuous flow ventilation (CFV), Respir Care 20:261, 1975.

Melic EJ and Ploysongsang Y: Respiratory mechanics in the adult respiratory distress syndrome, Crit Care Clin 2:573, 1986.

Milic EJ, Gottfried SB, and Rossi A: Noninvasive measurement of respiratory mechanics in ICU patients, Int J Clin Monit Comput 4(1):11-20, 1987.

Mitchell RR, Wilson RM, and Sierra D: ICU monitoring of ventilation distribution, Int J Clin Monit Comput 2(4):199-206, 1986.

Mithoefer JC: Assessment of tissue oxygenation. In Simmons DH, editor: Current pulmonology, vol 4, New York, 1982, John Wiley & Sons.

Modell JH: Weaning patients from mechanical ventilation, Respir Care 20:373, 1975.

Mohsenifar Z et al: Relationship between O_2 delivery and O_2 consumption in the adult respiratory distress syndrome, Chest 83:267, 1983.

Neff TA: Monitoring alveolar ventilation and respiratory gas exchange, Respir Care 30:413-419, 1985.

Osborn JJ: Monitoring respiratory function. In Shoemaker WC: The lung in the critically ill patient: pathophysiology and therapy of acute respiratory failure, Baltimore, 1976, Williams & Wilkins Co.

Osgood CF et al: Hemodynamic monitoring in respiratory care, Respir Care 29:25-34, 1984.

Pardee NE, Winterbauer RH, and Allen JD: Bedside evaluation of respiratory distress, Chest 85:203-6, 1984.

Paulus DA: Invasive monitoring of gas exchange: continuous measurement of mixed venous oxygen saturation, Respir Care 32:535-541, 1987.

Peters JA and Burke KI: Nutritional assessment of the patient with respiratory disease. In Wilkins RL, Sheldon RL, and Krider SJ, editors: Clinical assessment in respiratory care, St Louis, 1985, The CV Mosby Co.

Peters RM: Work of breathing and abnormal mechanics, Surg Clin North Am 54:955-966, 1974.

Petty TL and Nett LM: In Shoemaker WC and Thompson WL, editors: Critical care: state of the art, vol 2, Fullerton, Calif, 1981, The Society of Critical Care Medicine.

Pierson DJ: Weaning from mechanical ventilation in acute respiratory failure: concepts, indications, and techniques, Respir Care 28:646-660, 1983.

Pierson DJ and Lakshminarayan S: Postoperative ventilatory management, Respir Care 29:603-609, 1984.

Pilbeam SP: Mechanical ventilation: physiological and clinical applications, St Louis, 1986, Multimedia Publishing.

Proctor HJ and Woolson R: Prediction of respiratory muscle fatigue by measurement of the work of breathing, Surg Gynecol Obstet 136:367-370, 1973.

Puri VK et al: Complications of vascular catheterization in the critically ill: a prospective study, Crit Care Med 8:495, 1980.

Radford EP: Ventilation standards for use in artificial respiration, J Appl Physiol 7:451, 1955.

Robin ED: Dysoxia: abnormal tissue oxygen utilization, Arch Int Med 137:905, 1977.

Robinson J, editor: Using monitors, Horsham, PA, 1981, Intermed Communications.

Rochester DF and Hyatt RE: Respiratory muscle failure, Med Clin North Am 67:573-579, 1983.

Rossi A et al: Measurement of static compliance of the total respiratory system in patients with acute respiratory failure during mechanical ventilation, Am Rev Respir Dis 131:672-677, 1985.

Roussos C and Macklem PT: Inspiratory muscle fatigue. In Handbook of physiology, Sec 3, Respiration, 1986, American Physiologic Society.

Sackner MA et al: Assessment of asynchronous and paradoxic motion between rib cage and abdomen in normal subjects and in patients with chronic obstructive pulmonary disease, Am Rev Respir Dis 130:588-593, 1984.

Sahn SA and Lalshminarayan MB: Bedside criteria for discontinuation of mechanical ventilation, Chest 63:1002-1005, 1975.

Schweiss JF, editor: Continuous measurement of blood oxygen saturation in the high risk patient, vol 1, San Diego, 1986, Abbott Laboratories.

Selecky PA et al: A graphic approach to assessing interrelationships among minute ventilation, arterial carbon dioxide tension, and ratio of physiologic deadspace to tidal volume in patients on respirators, Am Rev Respir Dis 117:181, 1978.

Shapiro BA et al: Changes in intrapulmonary shunting with administration of 100% oxygen, Chest 77:138, 1980.

Shapiro BA, Harrison RA, and Walton JR: Clinical application of blood gases, ed 3, Chicago, 1982, Year Book Medical Publishers.

Sharp JT: Respiratory muscles: a review of old and newer concepts, Lung 157:185, 1980.

Sharp JT et al: The total work of breathing in normal and obese men, J Clin Invest 43:728-739, 1964.

Thys DM, Cohen E, and Girard D: The pulse oximeter, a noninvasive monitor of oxygenation during thoracic surgery, Thorac Cardiovasc Surg 34(6):380-383, 1986.

Tilkian SM, Conover MB, and Tilkian AG: Clinical implications of laboratory tests, St Louis, 1983, The CV Mosby Co.

Tobin MJ et al: Validation of respiratory inductive plethysmography in patients with pulmonary disease, Chest 83:615-620, 1983.

Tobin MJ et al: Breathing patterns, Chest 84:202-205, 1983.

Tobin MJ et al: The pattern of breathing during successful and unsuccessful trials of weaning from mechanical ventilation, Am Rev Respir Dis 134:1111-1118, 1986.

Tremper KK and Shoemaker W: Transcutaneous oxygen monitoring of critically ill adults, with and without low flow shock, Crit Care Med 9:709, 1981.

Weil MH and Afifi AA: Experimental and clinical studies on lactate and pyruvate as indicators of the severity of acute circulatory failure (shock), Circulation 41:989, 1970.

Weil MH et al: Relationship between colloid osmotic pressure and pulmonary artery wedge pressure in patients with acute cardiorespiratory failure, Am J Med 64(4):643-650, 1978.

Weinger MB and Brimm JE: End-tidal carbon dioxide as a measure of arterial carbon dioxide during intermittent mandatory ventilation, J Clin Monit 3(2):73-79, 1987.

Wilkins RL, Sheldon RL, and Krider SJ: Clinical assessment in respiratory care, St Louis, 1985, The CV Mosby Co.

Wilson RS and Pontoppidan H: Acute respiratory failure: diagnostic and therapeutic criteria. In Shoemaker WC: The lung in the critically ill patient: pathophysiology and therapy of acute respiratory failure, Baltimore, 1976, Williams & Wilkins Co.

Zwillich CW et al: Complications of assisted ventilation: a prospective study of 354 consecutive episodes, Am J Med 57:161-169, 1974.

32

Neonatal and Pediatric Intensive Care

Norman C. Schussler
Craig. L. Scanlan

One of the most challenging but rewarding areas of clinical activity for the practitioner is providing respiratory care to infants and children. Neonatal and pediatric respiratory care has evolved to be among the most sophisticated and complex speciality areas in the field, demanding from the practitioner the utmost in skill and knowledge.

Competent practice in this area requires a firm understanding of the many anatomic and physiologic differences between the infant, child, and adult as well as the unique pathophysiology involved in common neonatal and pediatric respiratory disorders. Only by being equipped with such knowledge can the practitioner anticipate and provide the treatment regimens necessary to decrease the overall morbidity and mortality of this special category of patients.

OBJECTIVES

This chapter focuses on the unique needs and special considerations characterizing the care of infants and children. Specifically, on completion of the chapter, the reader will be able to:

1. Describe the key elements of the normal fetal circulation;

2. Describe the anatomic and physiologic events associated with the normal transition of the fetus from uterine to extrauterine life;

3. List and describe the key anatomic and physiologic differences between the neonate, child, and adult;

4. Differentiate the various methods of assessing the newborn, including maternal and fetal factors;

5. Describe the indications, hazards, and special tools and techniques involved in applying selected respiratory care modalities to infants and children, with a special emphasis on ventilatory support modes;

6. Describe the etiology, pathophysiology, clinical manifestations, and treatment regimens for the following neonatal disease processes:
   Meconium aspiration syndrome;
   Hyaline membrane disease;
   Transient tachypnea of the newborn;
   Apnea of prematurity;
   Wilson-Mikity syndrome;
   Bronchopulmonary dysplasia.

7. Describe the etiology, pathophysiology, clinical manifestations, and treatment regimens for the following common pediatric disorders:
   Sudden infant death syndrome (SIDS);
   Bronchiolitis;
   Croup;
   Epiglottitis;
   Cystic fibrosis;
   Foreign body aspiration;
   Near drowning.

KEY TERMS

Most terms used in this chapter are defined in context. The following terms are introduced without explicit definition but may be found in the text glossary:

abruptio placenta	opacification
allantois	parturition
amnion	placenta previa
autosomal recessive	preeclampsia
bilirubin	prolapsed cord
bracheocephalic trunk	radiolucent
choanal atresia	retinopathy
congenital	ultrasonography
dysplasia	uteroplacental
gestation	insufficiency
hypotonia	

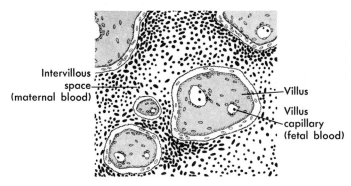

Fig. 32-1 Microscopic appearance of the villi in an intervillous space. Fetal capillaries permeate the villi, which are immersed in maternal blood within the intervillous spaces. (From Korones SB: High-risk newborn infants: the basis for intensive nursing care, ed 4, St Louis, 1986, The CV Mosby Co.)

TRANSITION FROM UTERINE TO EXTRAUTERINE LIFE

Many of the cardiopulmonary problems that occur in the perinatal period are associated with difficulties in the fetus's transition from uterine to extrauterine life. Understanding the origin of these problems and their resolution requires a firm grasp of how the fetus survives in utero and how the amazing transition from a watery environment to air breathing is made.

Fetal circulation

Survival of the fetus in utero is based on the successful development of a circulatory link between the mother and evolving embryo. Within a week of implantation, finger-like projections called *chorionic villi* arise from the primitive aorta and invade the uterine endometrium.[1-3] These projections consist of an outer epithelial layer and a connective tissue center containing the fetal capilllaries. As the villi increase in size and number, they further erode the endometrial tissues, creating irregular pockets called *intervillous spaces*. Ultimately, maternal blood fills these intervillous spaces, continually "bathing" the fetal capillaries in an oxygen- and nutrient-rich environment (Fig. 32-1).

As gestation progresses, the villi decrease in size but increase in number. In this manner, the surface area available for maternal-fetal exchange increases exponentially throughout pregnancy, to about 14 m^3 at term. Maternal-fetal exchange also improves over time as the villous connective tissue layer thins, thereby decreasing the distance between the maternal blood and fetal capillaries.

The placental circulation. Combined, the uterine endometrial tissues and blood vessels of the mother and chorionic villi (anchored to a chorionic plate) of the fetus constitute the *placenta*. Fig. 32-2 provides a cross-sectional view of a well-developed placenta. Maternal blood flows into the intervillus space through the spiral arteries. At the intervillus space, the maternal and fetal blood come into close proximity, facilitating diffusion of oxygen, carbon dioxide, and metabolic products. After this exchange takes place, maternal blood leaves the intervillus space through venous channels, returning to the maternal circula-

tion. Freshly oxygenated fetal blood leaves the chorionic villi capillaries to join placental venules, which eventually merge to form a single umbilical vein.

On the fetal side of the fully developed placenta, the chorionic and amnionic layers give rise to the allantois, or umbilical cord. As evident in cross-section (Fig. 32-3), the umbilical cord contains the single umbilical vein (returning to the fetus) and two umbilical arteries (coursing toward the placenta). Generally, the umbilical vein is larger than the arteries but thinner-walled. Surrounding all three blood vessels is a white gelatinous material called Wharton's jelly. For a short period after birth (up to 24 hours in some infants), the umbilical arteries remain patent and may be used as both an infusion site and a source for arterial blood sampling (to be discussed subsequently).

Abnormal implantation of the placenta (abruptio placenta, placenta previa) or decreased blood flow to the placenta (uteroplacental insufficiency) is a significant cause of intrauterine growth retardation and fetal asphyxia. The detrimental affects of such conditions can cause respiratory distress in the immediate postnatal period.

Factors affecting placental exchange. Although in close proximity, maternal blood and fetal blood never physically mix. Nonetheless, certain maternal drugs, bacteria, and viruses may move across intervillus space and cause immediate or delayed problems only evident later.

In the intervillus space, various factors favor gaseous diffusion of oxygen to the fetus.[3] Maternal oxygen, with its Pao$_2$ of 80 to 100 mm Hg, readily diffuses to fetal blood, with its Pao$_2$ of approximately 16 mm Hg. Oxygen uptake by the fetus also is assisted by the Bohr effect, as described in Chapter 9. Moreover, the hemoglobin content of the fetus is generally greater than that of adults, thereby increasing oxygen-carrying capacity. However, the major factor responsible for survival of the fetus in what would otherwise be an intolerably hypoxic environment is the existence of fetal hemoglobin (HbF).[3-6]

Compared with adult hemoglobin, HbF combine less readily with 2,3 DPG and thereby exhibits an increased affinity for oxygen. As depicted in Fig. 32-4, this increased affinity for oxygen is manifested by a left shift of the HbF

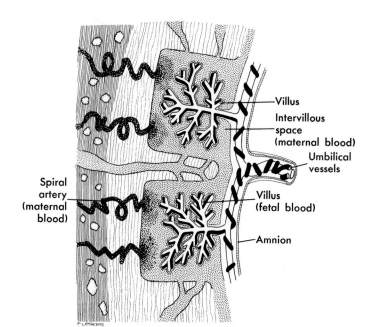

Fig. 32-2 Section through the placenta showing the spiral arteries that supply maternal blood to the intervillous space, the branching villi immersed in the intervillous space, and the umbilical vessels that branch repeatedly to terminate as villous capillaries. (Modified from Netter. In Oppenheim E, editor: Ciba collection of medical illustrations, vol 2, Reproductive system, 1965. From Korones SB: High-risk newborn infants: the basis for intensive nursing care, ed 4, St Louis, 1986, The CV Mosby Co.)

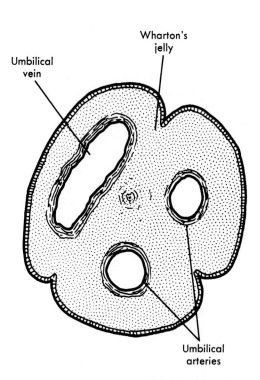

Fig. 32-3 Cross-section of umbilical cord. The arteries have thick walls; the lumen of the vein is larger than those of the arteries, and its wall is thin. (From Korones SB: High-risk newborn infants: the basis for intensive nursing care, ed 4, St Louis, 1986, The CV Mosby Co.)

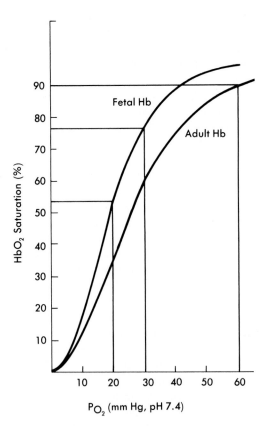

Fig. 32-4 Fetal hemoglobin produces left shift of oxyhemoglobin curve. (From Koff PB, Eitzman DV, and Neu J: Neonatal and pediatric respiratory care, St Louis, 1988, The CV Mosby Co.)

dissociation curve, with a P_{50} some 6 to 8 mm Hg less than that of adult hemoglobin (HbA). For example, at a Po_2 of 30 mm Hg, HbF is over 85% saturated with oxygen compared with about 60% for HbA.

Fetal hemoglobin is normally completely replaced by adult hemoglobin within the first 4 to 6 months of life. During this time, the clinician should be aware that cyanosis will appear later and at lower Po_2 values than in the adult. As indicated in Chapter 15, cyanosis generally becomes apparent only when the Sao_2 drops to between 75% and 85%. In the infant with a high proportion of HbF, this level of saturation will not occur until the Pao_2 is about 30 to 40 mm Hg.

Despite these factors, the Po_2 of the blood returning to the fetus through the umbilical vein is only about 30 mm Hg.[3,4] This high maternal-fetal diffusion gradient results from variations in diffusing capacity throughout the placenta, the uneven distribution of maternal blood flow, the

presence of shunts on both sides of the placenta, and the high oxygen consumption of the placenta itself. The box on p. 840 summarizes the normal blood gas values of a term fetus in both the umbilical arteries and veins.

Fetal circulation. Oxygenated blood from the placenta is carried in the umbilical vein to the fetal circulatory system through the hepatic system (Fig. 32-5). Approximately one third of this blood flows to the lower trunk and extremities. The other two thirds is shunted past the liver through the *ductus venosus* toward the inferior vena cava. This stream of oxygenated blood mixes with the venous blood returning from the lower trunk and extremities and enters the right atrium.

About 50% of this blood, still relatively well oxygenated, is shunted from the right atrium to the left atrium through the *foramen ovale*. This blood then goes to the left ventricle and ascending aorta, where it continues on to perfuse the brain, brachiocephalic trunk, and descending aorta.

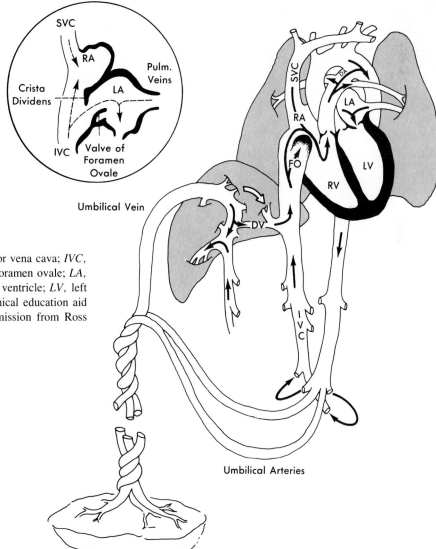

Fig. 32-5 Fetal circulation. *SVC,* Superior vena cava; *IVC,* inferior vena cava; *RA,* right atrium; *FO,* foramen ovale; *LA,* left atrium; *DV,* ductus venosus; *RV,* right ventricle; *LV,* left ventricle; *DA,* ductus arteriosus. (From Clinical education aid 7, Ross Laboratories. Reprinted with permission from Ross Laboratories, Columbus, Ohio.)

BLOOD GAS VALUES OF TERM FETUS

UMBILICAL ARTERIES	UMBILICAL VEIN
Po_2 16 mm Hg	Po_2 29 mm Hg
Pco_2 46 mm Hg	Pco_2 42 mm Hg
pH 7.33	pH 7.35

Adapted from Seeds AE: Pediatr Clin North Am 17:811, 1970. From Koff PB, Eitzman DV, and Neu J: Neonatal and pediatric respiratory care, St Louis, 1988, The CV Mosby Co.

Venous blood from the superior vena cava is directed downward into the right ventricle, then into the main pulmonary artery. Because of the low Po_2 values characterizing the fetal environment, pulmonary vascular resistance in the fetus is high. For this reason, the mean pulmonary artery pressure in the fetus is higher than the mean aortic pressure. Since blood will follow the path of least resistance, less than 10% of the blood entering the pulmonary artery actually goes on into the pulmonary vasculature.[3,4] The remainder is shunted from the main pulmonary artery to the descending aorta through the *ductus arteriosus*. This shunted flow then mixes with the blood ejected from the left ventricle. A portion of this less well oxygenated blood circulates to the gut and lower extremities, with the remainder returning to the placenta for reoxygenation through the two umbilical arteries.

In contrast to the adult heart, in which the right and left ventricles pump in series, the fetal ventricles pump in parallel, with both contributing flow to the systemic circulation. In the normal fetus, three factors account for the proper distribution of this combined ventricular output: (1) a low systemic resistance, (2) a high pulmonary resistance, and (3) the three circulatory shunts previously described.

Cardiopulmonary events at birth

Before birth, the placenta acts as the nutritive, respiratory, digestive, and renal organ of the fetus. The fetal circulation is adapted to serve these functions of the placenta, and when the fetus and placenta are separated at birth, rapid and dramatic changes must occur before adequate gas exchange can take place in the lungs. Continued survival demands that the infant quickly establish effective pulmonary gas exchange.

First, the lung liquid must be cleared and the lungs inflated with air. The fetal lung does not exist in a collapsed state but is normally distended with a liquid ultrafiltrate of the plasma to a volume equivalent to the functional residual capacity (FRC), or about 30 ml/kg. In a normal vagi-

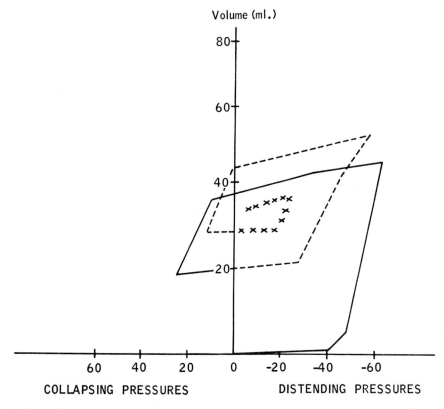

Fig. 32-6   Transpulmonary pressures developed in the human neonate during the first three breaths after birth. (From Avery ME: The lung and its disorders in the newborn infant, ed 2, Philadelphia, 1964, WB Saunders Co.)

nal delivery, about one third of this fluid is cleared by compression of the thorax in passage through the birth canal. The remainder of the lung fluid is cleared by the pulmonary capillaries and lymphatics during the first few breaths.

To replace the remaining lung fluid with air and establish a stable FRC, the newborn must develop very high transpulmonary pressure (PL) gradients during the first few breaths. These high pressure gradients are necessary to overcome the opposing forces of fluid viscosity in the airways and surface tension in the alveoli.

The stimulus for these initial efforts is both peripheral and central. First, the newborn is bombarded by new tactile and thermal stimuli, all of which stimulate breathing. Moreover, as gas transfer across the placenta is suddenly interrupted, the newborn quickly becomes hypoxemic, hypercapnic, and acidotic.

As depicted in Fig. 32-6, essentially no air enters the newborn lung until the PL exceeds -40 cm H_2O. As the lung volume increases in a stepwise fashion with each breath, less and less pressure is necessary to overcome these opposing forces, and within three to four breaths, the resting FRC is achieved. This stepwise establishment of the FRC is aided by the vagally mediated paradoxical reflex of Head and is probably enhanced by expiration against a partially closed glottis.[5]

As depicted in Fig. 32-7, with initiation of breathing and proper lung expansion, the Pa_{O_2} increases, the Pa_{CO_2} decreases, and the pH begins to rise back toward normal. These factors result in a dramatic decrease in pulmonary vascular resistance and constriction of the ductus arteriosus. Together, the decrease in pulmonary vascular resis-

tance and constriction of the ductus arteriosus increase blood flow through the pulmonary circulation. The decrease in pulmonary vascular resistance also lowers pulmonary artery pressures, facilitating complete fluid reabsorption in the pulmonary capillaries.

At about the same time, the cessation of umbilical flow results in a rapid increase in systemic vascular resistance, which in turn causes a rise in left ventricular pressures. With right ventricular pressures now lower than those on the left, the foramen ovale closes, eliminating the final right to left shunt and thus marking functional completion of the transition between the fetal and normal extrauterine circulations. Full transition occurs later, as the ductus arteriosus and foramen ovale anatomically close. Anatomic closure (through fibrosis) of the ductus arteriosus normally occurs within 3 weeks, although permanent adherence of the tissue flap covering the foramen ovale may take several months.

All these changes normally occur during the first few minutes after birth and allow the newborn to achieve essentially normal gas exchange within the first 12 to 24 hours of life. However, a number of abnormal conditions can interfere with the events of this critical transitional stage, thereby leading to insufficiency or failure of the respiratory or cardiovascular systems.

ANATOMIC AND PHYSIOLOGIC DIFFERENCES

Effective neonatal and pediatric respiratory care must be based on a firm understanding of several key anatomic and physiologic differences between the infant, child, and adult. Of course, these differences are most pronounced

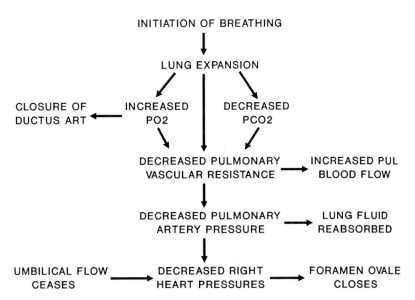

Fig. 32-7 Newborn respiratory and circulatory changes. (From Kirby RR, Smith RA, and Desautels DD, editors: Mechanical ventilation, New York, 1985, Churchill Livingstone.)

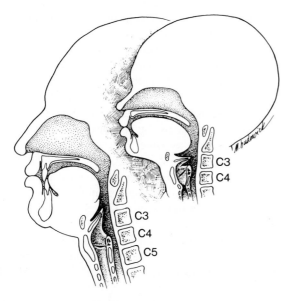

between the newborn and adult, with a gradual development toward adult characteristics occurring over time.

Anatomic differences

The anatomic differences between the newborn, child, and adult are not only in obvious physical size but also in the position and function of key respiratory structures.[7-10]

Head and upper airway. As depicted in Fig. 32-8, the head of the infant is proportionately larger than the adult's. Therefore, in infants with poor muscle tone, the weight of the head can cause an acute flexion of the cervical spine, a position that may cause airway obstruction.

Although the head is proportionately larger, the nasal passages of an infant are proportionately smaller than the adult's. This fact, combined with the relatively large and highly vascular adenoid tissue found in infants and children, makes nasal intubation more difficult and risky in these patients. Moreover, the infant jaw is much rounder and the tongue is much larger in relation to the overall oral cavity, increasing the likelihood of airway obstruction with loss of muscle tone.

Interestingly, infants tend to be obligate nose breathers. Even in the face of partial or complete obstruction, such as choanal atresia, most infants will not attempt oral breathing. The primary exception to this observation occurs during crying, when infants tend to inhale through the mouth. Infants retain nose breathing until 4 to 5 months of age, when they begin oral respiration.[8]

Larynx and epiglottis. The infant larynx lies higher in the neck than in later years, with the glottis being located between the third and fourth cervical vertebrae. In addi-

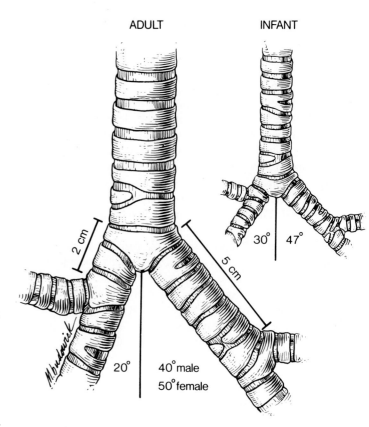

tion, the larynx of the infant is more funnel shaped than the adult's, with the narrowest point being the interior diameter of the cricoid cartilage, rather than the glottis, as in adults.[7,8]

The infant epiglottis is longer and less flexible than the adult's and, due to the position of the larynx and hyoid bone, lies higher and in a more horizontal position. During swallowing, the positioning of the infant larynx provides a direct connection to the nasopharynx. This creates two essentially separate pathways, one for breathing and one for swallowing, and helps explains why the infant can breath and suckle simultaneously. Anatomic descent of the epiglottis begins between 2-½ and 3 months of age.

The mucosa of the infant's upper airway, especially the larynx, is thin and easily traumatized. For this reason, continuous attempts at intubation or suctioning can easily cause swelling and obstruction in these areas.

Conducting airways. The large conducting airways of the infant are both shorter and narrower than those of the adult. The normal newborn trachea, for example, averages some 5 to 6 cm long and about 4 mm in diameter, but it may be only 2 cm long and 2 to 3 mm wide in some small preterm infants. As a result, the anatomic dead space of the newborn is proportionately smaller than the adult's, being about 0.75 ml/lb of body weight.

As shown in Fig. 32-9, the division of the infant trachea into mainstem bronchi occurs at more acute angles than in the adult, particularly on the right side.[10] Nonetheless, the right mainstem bronchi of the infant are still more in line with the trachea than the left, as in the adult.

The tracheobronchial tree of the newborn is more compliant than its adult counterpart. In children under 5 months of age, the bronchiolar structure has few elastic fibers. Lacking the normal supportive structures found in the adult, the infant airway is more prone to collapse, both during inspiration and expiration. Airway collapse can result in air trapping, overdistention, and atelectasis.[6,7]

Respiratory zone. Although the infant's airway is smaller than the adult's, the primary respiratory units (ie, those parts of the lung consisting of the respiratory bronchioles and alveolar ducts and sacs) have the same volume. Respiratory units increase in number, whereas airways increase in size as the infants ages. However, by 5 to 8 years of age, the number of gas exchange units in the child's lung is comparable to that in the adult. Thereafter, increased gas exchange ability occurs by growth in the size, rather than number, of alveoli.[8,9]

Chest wall and musculature. Consisting mainly of cartilage, the chest cage of the newborn is highly compliant. For this reason, when an infant increases negative intrapleural pressure (P_{pl}) during periods of respiratory distress, the chest wall is more readily drawn inward.[11] This phenomenon is observed clinically as suprasternal, substernal, and intercostal retractions.

Also unlike that of the adult, the musculature of the infant's thoracic cage is immature, providing little structural support and minimally contributing to ventilation.[11] Furthermore, the shape of the infant thoracic cage is relatively round, with the ribs being horizontally orientated.[6,7] For these reasons, the anteroposterior diameter of the infant thorax remains almost unchanged during inspiration. This places a greater burden on the infant's diaphragm as the primary inspiratory muscle.

The diaphragm itself lies higher in the newborn (T8-9) than in the adult (T9-10), and its movement is generally limited to vertical displacement. Even this motion is restricted by a proportionately larger liver, spleen, and abdominal visera. Gastric insufflation, common in infants, can further compromise diaphragmatic excursions.

Physiologic differences

Table 32-1 summarizes some of the key physiologic differences between the newborn and adult.[6] We will highlight the clinical significance of these differences, particularly as they relate to the control of breathing, metabolic, and ventilatory requirements and mechanics of ventilation.

Control of breathing. Newborns, particularly those less than 35 to 37 weeks' gestation, have frequent periods of short duration apnea and periodic breathing. Apneic spells and episodes of periodic breathing are most commonly observed during sleep or oral feeding and may be accompa-

nied by bradycardia, especially in preterm infants. This phenomenon is attributable to a decreased ventilatory responsiveness to CO_2 common among premature infants.[13]

Although peripheral chemoreceptors are active in the neonate, both premature infants and full-term babies exhibit a paradoxical response to hypoxemia. Unlike adults, a newborn exposed to significant arterial hypoxemia (a Pao_2 below 30 to 40 mm Hg) responds with either a decrease in ventilation or apnea. Central nervous system (CNS) depression is the most likely explanation for this phenomenon.[14,15]

As already described, the full-term infant has an active inflation reflex, which facilitates initial lung expansion. Although it diminishes progressively after birth, this reflex contributes to the increased inspiratory efforts that characterize a full-term infant's response to airway obstruction or atelectasis. On the other hand, infants less than 32 weeks' gestation often become apneic when faced with increased respiratory workloads, suggesting that this reflex is not fully developed.

Metabolism and ventilatory requirements. The basal metabolic rate of a full-term, 3 kg infant is about 2 cal/kg/hour, nearly twice that of a full-grown adult. This means that the infant's oxygen consumption and carbon dioxide production per kilogram of body weight are also double that of the adult, necessitating twice the equivalent adult minute ventilation ($\dot{V}_E$).

Since tidal volume (V_T) values adjusted for body weight are comparable with those observed in the adult (6 to 7 ml/kg), the neonate must achieve this proportionately greater ventilatory demand by increasing the frequency of breathing to an average of 30 to 40 breaths/minute. This high rate of breathing, in turn, results in a greater proportion of the ventilation per minute being wasted, that is, an increased $\dot{V}_D$. This occurs despite the fact that the anatomic dead space of an infant is proportionately smaller than that of an adult.

Table 32-1 Physiologic Differences Between Neonate and Adult

Variable	Newborn	Adult
Body weight (kg)	3	70
Tidal volume (V_T) (ml/kg)	6	6
Respiratory rate (breaths/min)	35	15
Volume expired (ml/kg/min)	210	90
Physiologic dead space/V_T ratio	0.30	0.33
O_2 consumption (ml/kg/min)	6.4	3.5
CO_2 consumption (ml/kg/min)	6.0	3.0
Calories (kg/hr)	2	1
Total lung capacity (TLC) (ml/kg)	63	86
Functional residual capacity (FRC) (ml/kg)	30	35
Vital capacity (VC) (ml/kg)	35	70

Modified from Godinez RI: Special problems in pediatric anesthesia, International Anesthesiology Clinics, Boston, 1985, Little, Brown & Co, p 88.

Mechanics of breathing. The absolute compliance of the neonatal lung is substantially less than that of an adult. However, if we correct the compliance value for lung volume at FRC (a measure called specific compliance), we find the newborn infant's lung compliance to be comparable with an adult's, or about 60 ml/cm H_2O/L.

However, since the neonatal chest wall is highly compliant, little opposition is offered to the recoil tendency of the lungs, which assume a smaller resting volume.[16] Thus the infant FRC averages only 30 ml/kg, compared with about 35 ml/kg for the adult. Because the FRC is smaller than in the adult, airway closure and atelectasis can occur more easily, resulting in lowered $\dot{V}_A/\dot{Q}_C$ ratios and increased physiologic shunting. Moreover, a small FRC means that alterations in ventilation will cause more rapid changes in blood gas values.[17-19] Finally, with a small FRC providing less oxygen reserve, and with double the adult metabolic rate, an infant deprived of adequate inspired oxygen can become severely hypoxemic within seconds.

ASSESSMENT OF THE NEWBORN INFANT

A comprehensive analysis of methods of clinical assessment of the newborn and child is beyond the scope of this chapter. We will simply highlight some of the key elements of assessment as related to the recognition and management of common respiratory problems occurring in the perinatal period. More comprehensive reviews of clinical assessment of both the neonate and child can be found in other sources.[20-22]

General assessment

Ideally, general assessment of the newborn begins before birth and involves consideration of both the maternal history and condition and the fetal and newborn status.

Maternal factors. Among the most important maternal factors related to the health of the fetus and the outcomes of pregnancy are the mother's age, parity, history of previous births, prior or existing maternal disease, and the use of drugs, alcohol, or tobacco during pregnancy.[23] In terms of maternal history, the risk of problems is highest with either very young mothers (less than 16 years old) or older women (greater than 40), first pregnancies (primagravida) or grand multiparity (more than five prior pregnancies), or a recurrent history of difficult pregnancies.

Prior or existing maternal disease, especially hypertensive disorders, diabetes mellitus, and viral or bacterial infections during pregnancy, all increase risk to the fetus. For example, diabetes increases the risk of both congenital heart defects and hyaline membrane disease. On the other hand, renal disease, toxemia of pregnancy, and primary hypertension all increase the likelihood of placental insufficiency and the associated risk of fetal distress during labor and delivery.[22] Infectious disorders may be passed to the fetus across the placenta or, more commonly, during

labor and delivery. At a minimum, these disorders can result in a congenitally acquired infection. Unfortunately, some maternal infections, such as rubella, may cause severe developmental abnormalities.

Recently, the effect of various drug agents has gained substantial attention as a factor affecting the outcomes of pregnancy. We have known for many years that the administration of analgesic or anesthetic agents to the mother during labor and delivery increases the risk of newborn respiratory distress. More recently, it has become evident that maternal addiction to narcotics may result in intrauterine growth retardation and severe neonatal withdrawal symptoms after birth. Excessive use of alcohol during pregnancy is now associated with the development of the fetal alcohol syndrome (FAS), and we now know that mothers with a history of smoking typically give birth to low birthweight babies.

Fetal assessment. In years gone by, evaluation of the fetus was limited to simple physical assessment methods, including transabdominal palpation and auscultation. Modern technology has made available several sophisticated approaches for assessing fetal status before birth. These methods include ultrasonography, amniocentesis, fetal heart rate monitoring, and fetal blood gas analysis.[23,24]

Ultrasonography. Ultrasonography uses high-frequency sound waves to obtain a "picture" of the infant in utero. This allows the physician to determine with accuracy the position of the fetus and placenta, to make quantitative measures of fetal growth (thereby helping to determine gestational age), to determine the presence or absence of major anatomic anomalies, and to assess the amniotic fluid qualitatively.

Amniocentesis. Amniocentesis is the process of direct sampling and quantitative assessment of the amniotic fluid. Amniotic fluid may be inspected for meconium (fetal bowel contents) or blood, and sloughed fetal cells may be analyzed for genetic normality. Of critical importance to the respiratory care practitioner, however, is the ability to assess fetal pulmonary maturation with amniocentesis. This test, called the L/S ratio, involves quantitative analysis of the relative amount of two phospholipids, lethicin and sphingomyelin, synthesized by the fetus in utero. As shown in Fig. 32-10, with increasing gestational age, the ratio of lethicin to sphingomyelin increases. At about 34 to 35 weeks' gestation, the ratio abruptly rises above 2:1, indicating the existence of a stable pathway for surfactant production.

Fetal heart rate monitoring. Fetal heart rate monitoring is an assessment tool used during labor and delivery that can help the physician determine the existence, severity, and nature of fetal distress. Fetal heart rate monitoring involves simultaneous measurement of the fetal heart rate and the strength of uterine contractions.

As portrayed in Fig. 32-11, there are three major patterns of change in fetal heart rate during labor: early deceleration, late deceleration, and variable deceleration. Early

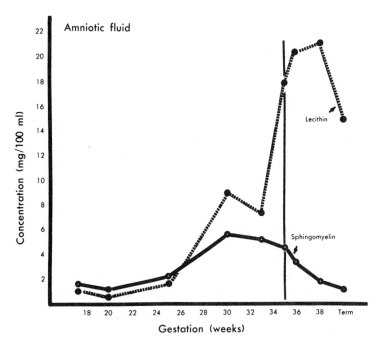

Fig. 32-10   Lecithin (broken line) and sphingomyelin (solid line) concentrations plotted against gestational age. L/S ratio rises to 1.2 at 28 weeks and to 2 or more at 35 weeks, indicating little chance of hyaline membrane disease postnatally. (From Gluck L et al: Am J Obstet Gynecol 109:440, 1971.)

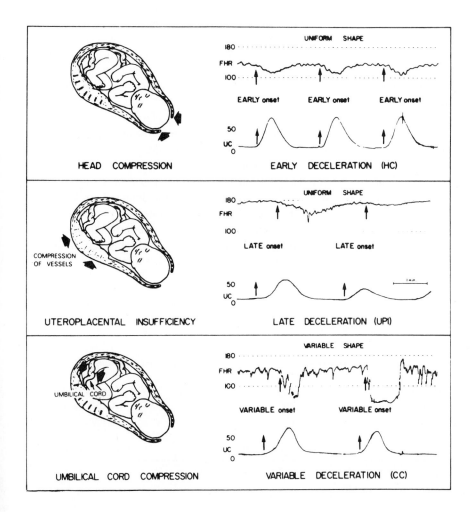

Fig. 32-11   Fetal heart rate patterns. (From Avery GB, editor: Neonatology: pathophysiology and management of the newborn, ed 2, Philadelphia, 1981, JB Lippincott Co.)

deceleration occurs in the early phase of contractions and is believed to be caused by vagal stimulation associated with compression of the head. Early deceleration does not appear to be associated with fetal compromise. Late deceleration occurs well after the onset of contractions and is associated with impaired maternal blood flow to the placenta and the potential for fetal asphyxia. With variable deceleration, there is no clear relationship between uterine activity and fetal heart rate. This pattern is the most common of the three and is believed to be caused by compression of the umbilical cord. Short periods of umbilical cord compression have little effect on the outcome of labor and delivery and are therefore not of major concern. However, longer period of compromised umbilical blood flow are worrisome and can lead to hypoxic fetal distress. Often, umbilical cord compression can be relieved by repositioning the mother.

Fetal blood gas analysis. The assessment of fetal blood gases during labor and delivery can help ascertain the extent of fetal compromise when other factors indicate potential problems. Normally, fetal blood gases are obtained from a capillary sample taken from the presenting part, usually the scalp, and analyzed mainly for the pH. The normal fetal capillary pH ranges from 7.35 to 7.25, with the lower values occurring during the later stages of labor. A pH below 7.20 indicates a combined respiratory and metabolic acidosis, with the metabolic component suggesting tissue hypoxia, anaerobic metabolism, and lactic acidosis.

Assessment of the newborn. Assessment of the neonate begins immediately following delivery. Two components of neonatal assessment are of particular significant to the respiratory care practitioner: the Apgar score and the determination of gestational age versus growth.[23]

Apgar score. The Apgar system represents a standardized assessment routine that allows rapid evaluation of both the presence and degree of neonatal distress. Results of this assessment also provide guidance on the appropriate level and type of intervention.

As indicated in Table 32-2, the newborn's heart rate, respiratory effort, muscle tone, reflex irritability, and skin color are individually assessed according to preestablished definitions, resulting in a composite "score." Typically, to establish trends, this assessment is conducted at 1 and 5 minutes after delivery. At 1 minute, an Apgar score of 2 or less indicates the need for immediate resuscitation, including ventilatory assistance. Infants scoring between 3 and 6 at 1 minute typically require stimulation and supplemental oxygen. A score of 7 or higher is considered normal, indicating the need for only routine care and observation. An infant exhibiting an Apgar score of 6 or less after 5 minutes is still severely depressed and at risk of developing major complications. Such infants are normally placed in intensive care, where appropriate therapeutic interventions are initiated.

Large-scale studies of infants during their first year of life clearly demonstrate the use of the 5-minute Apgar score (in combination with birthweight) in predicting subsequent neurologic status. On average, less than 2% of normal birthweight infants with 5-minute Apgar scores between 7 and 10 exhibit neurologic abnormalities at 1 year of age. Similar-sized infants with 5-minute Apgar scores of 3 or less have three times the incidence of neurologic abnormalities. This incidence of apparent neurologic damage increases to nearly 20% among smaller infants with low (0 to 3) Apgar scores.

Determination of gestational age versus growth. Determination of gestational age is a complex process involving the assessment of multiple physical characteristics and neurologic signs. Of more primary concern to the respiratory care practitioner is the relationship between estimated gestational age and the infant's prenatal growth, as determined by body weight.

As shown in Fig. 32-12, by plotting the infant's estimated gestational age against body weight on a chart with normal growth curves, it is possible to classify more precisely the newborn's relative developmental status. In terms of gestational age, *term* infants are those born between 38 and 42 weeks' gestation. Infants born before 38 weeks are classified as *preterm,* while those born after 42 weeks are categorized as *postterm.* In terms of weight, infants falling between the 10th and 90th percentiles of nor-

Table 32-2   Apgar Table

Sign	Score		
	0	1	2
Heart rate	Absent	Slow (<100/min)	>100/min
Respirations	Absent	Slow, irregular	Good, crying
Muscle tone	Limp	Some flexion	Active motion
Reflex irritability (catheter in nares, tactile stimulation)	No response	Grimace	Cough, sneeze, cry
Color	Blue or pale	Pink body with blue extremities	Completely pink

From Koff PB, Eitzman DV, and Neu J: Neonatal and pediatric respiratory care, St Louis, 1988, The CV Mosby Co.

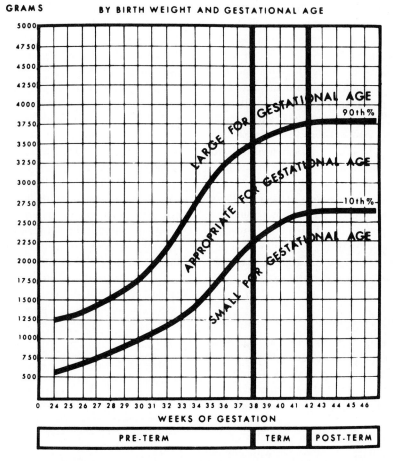

UNIVERSITY OF COLORADO MEDICAL CENTER

CLASSIFICATION OF NEWBORNS

BY BIRTH WEIGHT AND GESTATIONAL AGE

Fig. 32-12   Colorado intrauterine growth chart. (From Avery GB, editor: Neonatology: pathophysiology and management of the newborn, ed 2, Philadelphia, 1981, JB Lippincott Co.)

mality are considered appropriate for gestational age, or AGA. Those above the 90th percentile are termed large for gestational age (LGA), while those falling below the 10th percentile are termed small for gestational age (SGA). By classifying infants into one of the resulting nine categories—such as "preterm, AGA"—the clinician can help identify those at highest risk and predict both the nature of the risks involved and the likely mortality.

Table 32-3 provides summary data on the relationship between neonatal birthweight, gestational age, and mortality. Because of their limited ability to withstand the stresses of extrauterine life, preterm infants have the highest mortality. As Table 32-3 shows, death rates among preterm babies increase with decreasing birthweight, such that only about 30% of infants weighing 1500 g or less at birth (all of whom are preterm) survive. Compared with term babies, the lungs of these small infants are not yet fully prepared for gas exchange, the digestive tract cannot absorb fat as well, and the immune system is not yet capable of defending effectively against infection. Moreover,

Table 32-3   The Relationship of Birthweight and Gestational Age to Neonatal Mortality

Weight (gs)	Age (wk)	Mortality (%)	Increase mortality (%)
More than 2500	37 or more	0.5	
More than 2500	less than 37	1.4	×2.8
1501 to 2500	37 or more	3.2	×6.4
1501 to 2500	less than 37	10.5	×21.0
Less than 1500	All	70.7	×141.0

Adapted from Yerushalmy JJ: The classification of newborn infants by birth weight and gestational age, J Pediatr 71:164, 1967.

the large ratio of surface area to body weight characterizing these infants predisposes to increased heat loss and problems in thermoregulation. Finally, the vasculature of these small, premature infants tends to be less well developed, increasing the likelihood of hemorrhage (especially in the ventricles of the brain).

Interestingly, LGA infants (those weighing over 4000 g at birth) also have higher mortality than normal-sized term babies. This higher death rate has been attributed to a number of factors, including the obvious mechanical problems associated with labor and delivery. These problems may explain, in part, why these LGA infants tend to have lower Apgar scores than their normal-sized term counterparts.

LGA infants are more common among diabetic mothers (except those with advanced disease), but this population represents only a small proportion of all LGA births. In many cases, high birthweight may simply be based on genetic factors. Alternatively, the categorization of many infants as LGA may be a result of underestimation of actual gestational age.

Respiratory assessment of the infant

Of course, not all respiratory problems occur acutely at birth. As indicated in Table 32-4, only a small number of the numerous conditions leading to respiratory distress are immediately apparent at this time.[24] More commonly, respiratory-related disorders become apparent sometime after birth, by either sudden onset or progressive development. Indeed, knowledge of the time and nature of onset of the respiratory distress can provide the physician with important diagnostic clues on the cause of the underlying problem.

Although many respiratory care practitioners are involved in the events preceding and surrounding birth, they are more commonly called on to help assess and treat an infant who develops respiratory difficulties after delivery. In this regard, many of the adult physical assessment techniques discussed in Chapter 16 either must be modified or simply do not apply. Moreover, both the technical aspects of arterial blood gas sampling and the interpretation of blood gas results differ substantially from what the practitioner is accustomed to with adults patients.[25] Proper assessment of the infant demands an understanding of the these critical differences.

Physical assessment. As applied to the infant, traditional auscultation, palpation, and percussion methods are more difficult to perform and their results are more difficult to interpret than in the adult. This difficulty is due to both the size of the neonatal chest and the tendency for breath sounds to be widely transmitted throughout it.

More useful in clinical practice is the observational component of physical assessment. Respiratory distress in the infant is typically accompanied by one or more of six key signs: nasal flaring, cyanosis, expiratory grunting, tachypnea, retractions, and paradoxical breathing.

Nasal flaring is apparent as dilation of the alar nasi on inspiration and represents an early sign of an increase in ventilatory demands and the work of breathing. In concept, flaring of the alar nasi decreases the resistance to nasal airflow. The ease with which nasal flaring can be observed varies substantially according to facial structure of the infant.

Chapter 15 described both the usefulness and limitations of cyanosis as an indicator of hypoxemia in adults. As with adults, cyanosis may be absent in the infant who is anemic, even though his or her arterial oxygen tension may be relatively low. Moreover, in the infant with a high proportion of HbF, cyanosis may not occur until the Pa_{O_2} is about 30 to 40 mm Hg. Also creating difficulties in identification and interpretation is hyperbilirubinemia, a common condition in preterm infants. In this condition, levels of bilirubin in the blood and tissues are increased, causing a yellow discoloration of the skin that may mask the presence of cyanosis.

Grunting occurs when the infant attempts to exhale against a partially closed glottis. In concept, grunting increases airway pressure during expiration, thereby prevent-

Table 32-4   Causes of Respiratory Distress Grouped by Characteristics of Onset

Onset	Sudden	Gradual or progressive
At birth	Pneumothorax	HMD
	Apnea	TTNB
	Asphyxia	Pneumonia (eg, group B
	Maternal drugs	streptococci)
	Choanal atresia	Meconium aspiration
	Diaphragmatic hernia	Congenital heart disease
		Hypoplastic left heart
		syndrome
		Transposition
		Pulmonary atresia
0 to 7 days	Pneumothorax	Pneumonia
	Pneumomediastinum	T-E fistula
	Apnea	Congenital intrathoracic
	Prematurity	lesions
	CNS hemorrhage	Congenital heart disease
	Sepsis	Hypoplastic left heart
	Hypoglycemia	syndrome
	Pulmonary hemorrhage	Coarctation
	Aspiration	Ventricular defect
		Tetralogy of Fallot
		Patent ductus arteriosus
		Endocardial cushion
		defect
		Malposition
		Distended abdomen

From Guthrie R and Hodson WP: Clinical diagnosis of pulmonary insufficiency. In Thibeault DW and Gregory GA: Neonatal pulmonary care, Norwalk Conn, 1986, Appleton Century-Crofts.
HMD, Hyaline membrane disease; *TTNB,* transient tachypnea of the newborn; *T-E,* tracheoesophageal; *CNS,* central nervous system.

ing airway closure and alveolar collapse. Grunting may vary from mild (audible only by stethoscope) to severe (audible with the naked ear). Although typical of the infant with hyaline membrane disease, grunting can be present in other respiratory disorders of the newborn, especially those associated with alveolar collapse.

Tachypnea is present in newborns breathing at frequencies greater than 60/min. Since it is the most common of all signs of respiratory distress in the infant, tachypnea is a very nonspecific indicator. Although the practitioner should always be on the lookout for tachypnea in infants, periods of apnea lasting 20 seconds or more are a more ominous sign of newborn distress.

Retractions represent the indrawing of chest wall muscle and tissue between bony chest wall structures. Retractions can occur alone or in combination in the suprasternal, substernal, and intercostal regions. Their presence indicates an increase in total impedance and work of breathing, especially due to decreased pulmonary compliance.

As a symptom of respiratory distress, paradoxical breathing in infants is substantially different in presentation from that occurring in adults. Instead of the abdomen's being drawn in during inspiration, paradoxical breathing in the infant is characterized by inward movement of the chest wall. This paradoxical inward movement of the chest wall may range in severity from a simple time lag in chest excursions during inspiration to a full-blown "see-saw" motion in which the chest caves inward while the abdomen moves out. As with retractions, the presence of this paradoxical breathing indicates an increase in total impedance and work of breathing.

All these signs of respiratory distress, except for tachypnea, have been combined into an assessment system comparable to the Apgar score but designed for postpartum use (Fig. 32-13). This Silverman Index (named after its developer) can be used by the practitioner to help grade and track the severity of the underlying cause of respiratory distress.[26] Compared with the Apgar system, however, Silverman scoring is reversed. Low scores, in the range of 0 to 3, indicates minimal distress, whereas higher scores indicate significantly compromised respiratory function.

Arterial blood gas analysis. As with adults, arterial blood gas analysis is the single most important and reliable tool for assessing the severity of respiratory impairment in the infant. Also as with adults, many noninvasive techniques—such as transcutaneous P_{O_2} and P_{CO_2} electrodes and pulse oximeters—are being employed to obtain comparable data.[25] Nonetheless, arterial blood gas analysis remains the principle approach when precise results are critical.

Methods. As with adults, arterial blood samples may be obtained from infants by intermittent arterial puncture or an indwelling peripheral arterial line. However, the application of these procedures to the neonate is fraught with technical difficulties. Alternate means for obtaining arterial blood samples in the infant are (1) umbilical artery catheterization and (2) the use of arterialized capillary blood, usually from the heel. The advantages, disadvantages, and possible complications of these various methods of blood gas sampling are summarized in Table 32-5.[25]

Particular caution should be taken in assessing the results of capillary sampling.[27] First, variations in method make this the least reliable of all sampling approaches. Second, even when samples are properly obtained, useful analysis of a capillary sample is usually limited to the carbon dioxide tension and pH. As with transcutaneous monitoring, the presence of peripheral vasoconstriction or hypoperfusion makes capillary oxygen tensions unreliable.

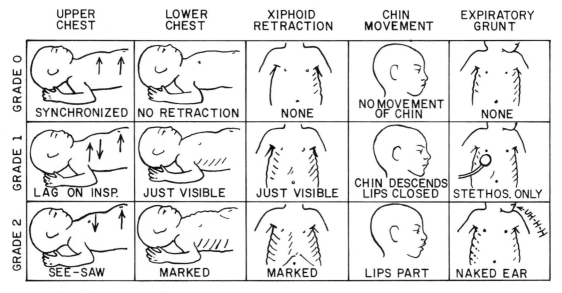

Fig. 32-13 Silverman score—a system for grading severity of underlying lung disease. (Reproduced with permission from Silverman WA and Andersen DH: Pediatrics 17:1, 1956.)

Table 32-5   Advantages, Disadvantages, and Complications of Invasive Blood Gas-Sampling Techniques

	Peripheral artery catheterization	Umbilical artery catheterization	Peripheral artery puncture	Capillary sampling
ADVANTAGES	Provides frequent blood gas sampling with minimum discomfort; provides accurate ABG values; is rapid to perform (if arterial puncture is easy); provides continuous blood pressure monitoring; artery may be identified with cutaneous transillumination or by Doppler ultrasound techniques	Provides frequent blood gas sampling with minimum discomfort; is usually simple and rapid to perform; provides large vessel for access in small infants; may be used for certain infusions; provides continuous blood pressure monitoring	Provides accurate ABG values; is rapid to perform on older child; has less risk of infection or embolism; provides sampling from different sites to diagnose heart anomalies; artery may be identified with cutaneous transillumination or by Doppler ultrasound techniques	Provides least invasive sampling technique; provides least risk of infection or embolism; is able to be repeated frequently; is suitable for long-term follow-up care of chronic respiratory infant
DISADVANTAGES	Often is technically difficult to place catheter without surgical "cutdown"; fluid overload can occur from infusion fluid; volume depletion can occur from frequent blood sampling; requires collateral circulation	Fluid overload can occur from infusion fluid; volume depletion can occur from frequent blood sampling; postductal admixture results in lower Po_2 values than are delivered to retina	Often is technically difficult to obtain (especially with frequent sampling or from patient in shock); crying or pain alters reported values; requires collateral circulation	Is not reliable for older infant or child; is usually imprecise and not used for critically ill infant: Po_2 may not reflect arterial trends; crying or pain alters reported values
COMPLICATIONS	Infection; embolism (thromboembolism or air embolism); infiltration of infusion fluid; nerve damage; severe bleeding around catheter or around tubing connections; vasospasm	Infection; embolism (thromboembolism or air embolism); abdominal organ necrosis can occur from hypertonic infusion; severe bleeding around catheter or around tubing connection; vasospasm	Risk of infection can occur without aseptic technique; severe bleeding; risk of embolism; nerve damage; hematoma	Increased work of breathing and possibly fatigue; cutaneous fibrosis of heel; bone spurs from deep punctures; puncture of posterior tibial artery

Adapted from Burton GG and Hodgkin JE: Respiratory care: a guide to clinical practice, ed 2, Philadelphia, 1984, JB Lippincott Co, p. 264; Fletcher MA, MacDonald MG, and Avery GB: Atlas of procedures in neonatology, Philadelphia, 1983, JB Lippincott Co, p. 146; Merenstein GB and Gardner SL: Handbook of neonatal intensive care, St Louis, 1985, The CV Mosby Co. p 99. From Koff PB, Eitzman DV, and Neu J: Neonatal and pediatric respiratory care, St Louis, 1988, The CV Mosby Co.
ABG, arterial blood gas.

Regardless of method used, the practitioner must remember that the infant's total blood volume is vastly smaller than the adult's. Too frequent drawing of blood samples, or taking unnecessarily large samples, can critically deplete an infant's blood volume in a relatively short time. It is therefore necessary to maintain carefully an ongoing record of all "blood-outs."

Assessment. To properly assess arterial blood gas results in the immediate postnatal period, the practitioner must be aware of the differences in normal values at this early stage of life. As indicated in Table 32-6, soon after delivery normal-term infants typically exhibit a mild metabolic acidosis, whereas normal preterm infants tend to have a slightly greater acidemia (resulting mainly from an additional respiratory component) with a moderate hypoxemia.[28] This moderate hypoxemia is probably a result of both inefficiencies in pulmonary oxygen transfer across the preterm infant's less well developed lung and some persistence of the fetal circulatory pathways, particularly some right-to-left shunting through the ductus arteriosus.

These variations from normal values reflect both the stressful events of birth and a small underlying differences in the buffering capacity of fetal blood, neither of which requires treatment. Within 5 days of parturition, the normal infant's blood gas values begin to approximate those of the adult, except for a slightly lower P_{O_2}.

Finally, a right-to-left shunt through a patent ductus arteriosus—regardless of the cause—can result in a lower Pa_{O_2} in the umbilical artery (a common site for arterial blood gas sampling) than in the right radial and temporal arteries.[27] This phenomenon is due to the fact that blood flowing through a patent ductus arteriosus normally enters the aorta distal to both the brachiocephalic and left common carotid arteries but usually proximal to the left subclavian. Thus blood gathered from the umbilical artery

(and often from the left arm) is "postductal," being somewhat lower in oxygen content and Pa_{O_2} than the preductal flow going to the brain and right arm. In these cases, when oxygenation status is marginal, clinical judgment should be based on samples obtained from the right radial artery, since this Pa_{O_2} best reflects oxygen delivery to the brain.

GENERAL MANAGEMENT OF THE CRITICALLY ILL NEONATE

Many of the general principles of management of the critically ill newborn are similar to those previously discussed for adults. However, several special considerations apply to the treatment of neonates. Key management considerations that apply to neonate care are temperature regulation, fluid and electrolyte balance, nutrition, and infection control.[12,20,21,29]

Temperature regulation

Because of their proportionately greater body surface area, newborns lose body heat to the environment much more easily and quickly than do adults. Moreover, unlike adults, their thermal regulatory mechanisms may not be fully developed. Under such circumstances, the infant cannot readily adapt to changing environmental temperatures, especially conditions predisposing to hypothermia. Neonatal hypothermia can result in increased oxygen consumption, hypoglycemia, metabolic acidosis, pulmonary vascular hypertension, increased right-to-left shunting, and apnea (Fig. 32-14).

For this reason, the infant's body temperature must be maintained between 36.5° and 36.8°C.[30] This is accomplished by keeping the neonate in a *neutral thermal environment* (NTE). Depending on infant size, the ambient temperature corresponding to an NTE for newborns varies

---

Table 32-6   Age-Related Values Commonly Reported for Normal Arterial Blood Gases

	Normal preterm infants (at 1 to 5 hours)	Normal term infants (at 5 hours)	Normal preterm infants and term infants (at 5 days)	Children, adolescents, and adults
pH	7.33	7.34	7.38	7.40
range	7.29 to 7.37	7.31 to 7.37	7.34 to 7.42	7.35 to 7.45
P_{CO_2}	47	35	36	40
range	39 to 56	32 to 39	32 to 41	35 to 45
P_{O_2}	60	74	76	95
range	52 to 67	62 to 86	62 to 92	85 to 100
HCO_3^-	25	19	21	24
range	22 to 23	18 to 21	19 to 23	22 to 26
BE	−4	−5	−3	0
range	−5 to −2.2	−6 to −2	−5.8 to −1.2	−2 to +2

Adapted from Orzalesi MM, et al: Arch Dis Child 42:174, 1967; Koch G and Wendel H: Biol Neonate 12:136, 1968. From Koff PB, Eitzman DV, and Neu J: Neonatal and pediatric respiratory care, St Louis, 1988, The CV Mosby Co.
HCO_3^- bicarbonate; *BE,* base excess.

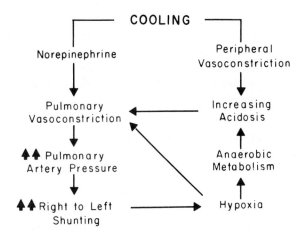

Fig. 32-14   The vicious circle resulting from cooling in the neonate. (From WB Saunders Co.)

between 32° and 35°C. In general, the smaller the infant, the higher the NTE within this range. The NTE also increases over time. For example, the NTE for a newborn weighing between 1500 and 2500 g is between 32.8° and 33.8°C. Six weeks later, the same infant can be maintained at temperatures between 29.0° and 31.8°C. Either incubators or radiant warmers are used to achieve these conditions. In addition to these methods, application of a layered thermal hat to small neonates can significantly reduce oxygen consumption and extend the NTE range by as much as 1°C.

Fluid and electrolyte balance

Maintenance of appropriate fluid balance in the newborn is more difficult than in the adult. Factors contributing to this problem are the newborn's small total body fluid volume, proportionately larger body surface area, increased skin permeability, and immature renal function. For these reasons, fluid balance must take into account gestational age, postpartum age, environmental temperature and humidity, and underlying pathologic problem(s).

In terms of acid-base balance, the functional development of the kidneys is not complete until about 1 month of age. Thus the newborn has a limited ability to compensate for ventilatory acid-base derangements. Moreover, the extracellular fluid "compartment" of newborns is about twice as large (as a proportion of body weight) as that in adults. Given the comparatively large volume of extracellular water, fluid and electrolyte shifts from one body compartment to another can occur readily, and the acid-base status of the blood can quickly fluctuate. It is not unusual for a neonate to exhibit a base excess at one time and, half an hour later—without any intervention, to show a deficit of buffer base.

Nutrition

Because of their high metabolic rates, infants' basal caloric requirements per kilogram are twice those of an adult. As with adults, certain illnesses, especially those resulting in tissue damage and repair, infection, and fever, increase metabolic rates substantially.

Since sick infants generally cannot be fed orally, the parenteral route must be used to satisfy their nutritional requirements. In most centers, 10% dextrose, administered at the rate of 150 ml/kg/day, is used initially to meet basic caloric requirements. However, if oral feedings cannot be initiated within 3 to 5 days, this pure carbohydrate support must be supplanted with either oral or parenteral administration of amino acids and fats.[12]

Infection control

Because of their immature immune response, critically ill newborns tend to be more susceptible to developing nosocomial infections than adults.[31] Many of these begin as localized infections of areas such as the skin and conjunctiva but can rapidly progress to a more serious and life-threatening systemic infections.

Staphyloccocus aureus and group B beta-hemolytic *Streptococcus* are the major gram-positive offenders, with colonization occurring mainly through contaminated hands. Gram-negative infections, such as those caused by *Pseudomonas aeruginosa,* are more likely caused by contaminated equipment, particularly that used in respiratory care. Only strict adherence to infection control procedures, as delineated in Chapter 14, can minimize the likelihood of acquired newborn infections.

RESPIRATORY CARE MANAGEMENT

Respiratory care management of the infant and child involves most of the approaches used with adults. However, given the significant anatomic and physiologic differences between adult and infant, and the uniqueness of some of the respiratory disorders characterizing the neonatal and pediatric patient, substantial variations are required in the tools and techniques of respiratory care. We will focus primarily on the special tools and techniques used in the provision of oxygen therapy, chest physical therapy, airway management, continuous positive airway pressure (CPAP), and ventilatory support in infants, with mention made, where applicable, of unique concerns in the older child.

Oxygen therapy

The goal of oxygen therapy in infants is to provide adequate tissue oxygenation at a safe concentration of inspired oxygen, that is, an FIO_2 low enough to prevent either retinal or lung tissue damage.[32-34] Nonetheless, oxygen must never be deprived from an infant in need. Indeed, with some critically ill neonates it is impossible to maintain an acceptable level arterial oxygenation without dangerously high oxygen concentrations.

Unfortunately, there is as yet no agreement on the exact upper limit of either FIO_2 or PaO_2. Acceptable levels of arterial oxygenation differ from institution to institution.

Some hospitals strictly apply a range of 50 to 70 mm Hg as the criterion, but levels slightly above 70 mm Hg are acceptable.[35,36] Certain conditions, such as persistent fetal circulation, may necessitate even higher Po_2s.

Methods of administration. Supplemental oxygen may be administered to infants through a mask, cannula or catheter, isolette, or oxyhood. Table 32-7 compares the advantages and disadvantages of these various oxygen delivery methods.[23]

As with adults, the mask is the device of choice in emergency situations. It is also useful when infants are transported or when they must be removed from an oxygen enclosure for special procedures. However, masks are generally not well tolerated by infants and can easily result in pressure necrosis of the delicate neonatal skin.

Because of its relative simplicity and ability to provide controlled and stable FIO_2 values, the oxyhood is generally the device of choice for long-term oxygen administration. Table 32-8 compares the equipment needs and procedures used to delivery oxygen through an oxyhood with and without an oxygen blending system.[32]

The FIO_2 administered through an oxyhood is delivered either through a heated humidifier or heated nebulizer. In either case, to ensure removal of exhaled carbon dioxide, the minimum flow through the system should be no less than 7 L/min.[37] The delivery of dry gas is strictly contraindicated. Dry gas can damage the respiratory tract mucosa and will increase the infant's insensible water loss. Unheated gas delivery is also contraindicated, since it can cause hypothermia, with its associated problems. If a heated jet nebulizer is used without a blending system, care must be taken to reduce the amount of rainout in the tubing. An excessive amount of water in the tubing will increase flow resistance and slowly increase the FIO_2. Excessive noise levels in the hood must be avoided, since subsequent hearing loss can ensue.[38,39]

Nasal cannula or catheters may also be used for long-term administration of low concentrations of oxygen to the larger neonatal or pediatric patient.[40] The major drawback of cannula and catheters is that the FIO_2 can only be measured at the source and estimated at the patient. Moreover, too high a flow may irritate the nasal mucosa, cause gastric distension, or unknowingly create CPAP. For neonates, the cannula may need to be shortened.

Hazards and complications. In addition to the problem of oxygen toxicity, oxygen therapy in infants carries the risk of retrolental fibroplasia. Thus it is imperative that the FIO_2 and the Pao_2 be carefully monitored.[36]

In terms of oxygen toxicity, some evidence suggests that the growing lung is more sensitive to oxygen than the adult lung. High partial pressures of oxygen may also be a contributing factor in the development of bronchopulmonary dysplasia, to be discussed subsequently.

Retrolental fibroplasia (RLF) affects neonates up to about 1 month of age, by which the time the retinal arteries will have matured sufficiently so that it is no longer a problem. There is evidence that retinal damage is most likely in infants weighing less than 1500 g and can occur even on brief exposure to high Pao_2 values, as may occur when bagging before suctioning. It is recommended that when bagging is necessary, it be carried out at the same FIO_2 that the patient is breathing. It is even suspected that in extremely premature infants, the oxygen concentration of room air is sufficient to cause retinopathies.[41]

Another consideration in newborn oxygen therapy is a phenomenon known as "flip-flop." Flip-flop refers to a larger than expected drop in the Pao_2 when the FIO_2 is lowered and the failure of the Pao_2 to return to its original level when the FIO_2 is raised back to its original level.

The cause for this phenomenon is not known. In some infants, the pulmonary vessels are particularly sensitive to changes in the oxygen tension, and lowering the FIO_2 re-

Table 32-7 Oxygen Delivery Devices

Device	Advantages	Disadvantages
Mask	Ease of application	CO_2 buildup with inadequate flow; pressure necrosis; inaccurate FIO_2, difficult to fit and maintain on infant
Cannula/catheter	Good for long-term care in chronic disease; usually tolerated well	Inaccurate FIO_2; insufficient humidity; insertion difficulties with catheter
Isolette	Warmed and humidified gas; good for low oxygen levels in stable infants	Varying FIO_2; long stabilization time; risk of bacterial contamination
Oxyhood	Warmed and humidified gas at any FIO_2 when used with oxygen blender. Stable FIO_2 not interrupted by routine care of infant	Overheating can cause apnea and dehydration; underheating will cause increased oxygen consumption; inadequate flow will cause CO_2 buildup; noise may lead to hearing loss

From Aloan CA: Respiratory care of the newborn: a clinical manual, Philadelphia, 1987, JB Lippincott Co.

sults in pulmonary vasoconstriction and decreased regional $\dot{V}/\dot{Q}$ ratios or intrapulmonary right-to-left shunt. Under these conditions, the Pao_2 would drop out of proportion to the reduction in Fio_2. Flip-flop can usually be prevented by making Fio_2 changes in small, as opposed to large, increments.

Monitoring. Ideally, delivered Fio_2 values should be analyzed continuously. Lacking this capability, the Fio_2 should be sampled and confirmed at least every 2 hours with a properly calibrated oxygen analyzer.[36] Arterial blood gas analysis should be conducted as often as necessary to ensure adequacy of both oxygenation and ventilation and whenever a change is made in the Fio_2.

Chest physical therapy

The basic concepts underlying chest physical therapy (CPT) in infants and children are essentially the same as those applicable to adults.[23,42] Variations in the tools and techniques of infant and pediatric CPT relate mainly to differences in the anatomic size and location of the airways and lung segments and lobes.

Indications. Properly performed CPT can be effective in infants and children whose airways are obstructed secondary to the accumulation of normal or abnormal respiratory tract secretions.[43-46] This need is apparent in newborns with meconium aspiration, pneumonia, and atelectasis. In children, CPT is indicated in cystic fibrosis, bronchiectasis, pneumonia, and a variety of neuromuscular disorders resulting in impaired clearance mechanisms.

Methods. As with adults, postural drainage, percussion, and vibration techniques are the basic tools of CPT in infants and children. Secretion removal by suctioning may complement these methods and is discussed separately in this chapter in the section on airway management.

In terms of postural drainage and percussion, the practitioner will find that infants and small children are best managed by holding them on one's lap or shoulder. This provides more comfort and security for the child and facilitates achievement of the treatment objectives.

As delineated in Fig. 32-15, anatomic differences in the location of the lobes and segments of the lung and the configuration of the tracheobronchial tree in infants and children require minor modifications in both the positioning for postural drainage and the identification of areas for percussion.[47]

In regard to percussion and vibration techniques, extreme care should be taken to avoid percussion below the rib margins, since this could damage the kidneys, stomach, liver, or spleen. This potential problem is greatest in small infants because of the relative size of the abdominal and thoracic cavities and their contents.

Table 32-8 Setup Procedure for Oxyhood Administration

Equipment needed	Procedure
With blender	
1. Air/oxygen blender with flowmeter and nebulizer (heater if indicated)	1. Connect nebulizer to blender and set nebulizer collar at 100%. Dial blender to desired Fio_2
2. Large-bore tubing and water trap	2. Attach large-bore tubing to water trap and nebulizer and attach more tubing from the water trap to oxyhood
3. Oxyhood of appropriate size	3. Place oxyhood in Isolette or radiant warmer
4. Nebulizer	4. Turn on flow to minimum of 7 L/min (check for aerosol production—should see a mist)
	5. Analyze Fio_2
	6. Monitor temperature if nebulizer is heated.
	7. Chart on appropriate respiratory progress notes
Without blender	
5. Air and oxygen flowmeters and nebulizer	1. Connect nebulizer to air flowmeter. Set nebulize collar at 100%.
6. Bleed-in adapter and oxygen connective tubing	2. Connect oxygen connective tubing to bleed-in adapter and to nipple on oxygen/air flowmeter
7. Oxygen flowmeter nipple adapter	3. Connect bleed-in adapter to nebulizer port
8. Large bore tubing and water traps	4. Adjust air and oxygen flowmeters to desired Fio_2 ensuring that combined flow is greater than 7 L/min
	5. Attach large bore tubing to bleed-in adapter and water trap. Attach second piece from water trap to oxygen hood.
	6. Analyze Fio_2 as above; note: it will take a few minutes for desired Fio_2 concentration to stabilize
	7. Chart as above

From Koff PB, Eitzman DV, and Neu J: Neonatal and pediatric respiratory care, St Louis, 1988, The CV Mosby Co.

Also for this reason, cupped hands or adult-sized mechanical percussors cannot be used in infants. "Tenting" of the middle three fingers of the hand may suffice in larger infants and small children, but small, commercially available percussion cups may be necessary in neonates. Likewise, special "downsized" mechanical vibrators are necessary to provide this mode of CPT to small infants.

Unlike adults, infants and small children cannot generate a spontaneous cough on command. Therefore, adjunctive methods to clear secretions mobilized with CPT must be employed, including pharyngeal and tracheal suctioning. In some situations, these techniques will not be effective, and therapeutic bronchoscopy may need to be considered. In older children, demonstration of effective coughing technique by the practitioner may help encourage proper clearance, as will incorporation of incentive spirometry as a component of the coughing routine.

Complications. Complications of CPT in infants and children are generally similar to those encountered in adults. Infants in particular are more prone to regurgitate gastric contents if CPT is conducted too close to a feeding. This problem, and its associated potential for aspiration, can be avoided if a nasogastric tube is already in place. Of particular concern in neonates is the effect of CPT positioning on intracranial pressures.[48] For this reason, the use of the Trendelenburg position in newborns or, for that

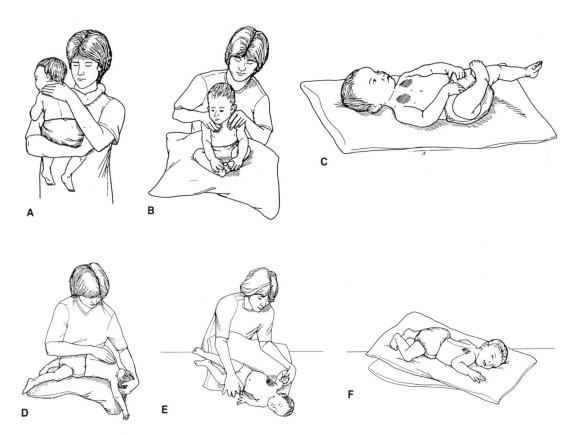

Fig. 32-15 Postural drainage and percussion positions for infant and child. Angles of drainage for infant are not as obtuse as those for child. **A,** Posterior segments of right and left upper lobes are drained with patient in upright position at 30-degree angle forward. Percuss over upper posterior thorax. **B,** Apical segments of right and left upper lobes are drained with patient in upright position, leaning forward 30 degrees. Percuss over area between clavicle and top of scapula on each side. **C,** Anterior segments of right and left upper lobes are drained with patient in flat, supine position. Percuss anterior side of chest directly under clavicles to around nipple area (shaded). Avoid direct pressure on sternum. **D,** Right and left lateral basal segments of lower lobes are drained at 30 degrees Trendelenburg. Patient lies on appropriate side, rotated 30 degrees forward. Percuss over uppermost portions of lower ribs. **E,** Right and left anterior basal segments of lower lobes are drained at 30 degrees Trendelenburg. Patient lies on appropriate side with 20-degree turn backward. Percuss above anterior lower margin of ribs. **F,** Right and left superior segments of lower lobes are drained at 15 degrees Trendelenburg, with patient in prone position. Percuss below scapula in midback area. (From Levin DL, Morriss FC, and Moore GC, editors: A practical guide to pediatric intensive care, ed 2, St Louis, 1984, The CV Mosby Co.)

matter, any child in whom intracranial pressures are of concern is generally contraindicated. The Trendelenburg position may also be problematic in children suffering from status asthmaticus or congestive heart failure.

Monitoring. Given the inherent instability of the critically ill infant or child and the potential hazards associated with CPT, both a thorough preliminary assessment and ongoing patient evaluation during and after treatment are mandatory. Traditional assessment of the respiratory rate, color, pulse, and blood pressure before, during, and after treatment should be supplemented with either continuous transcutaneous P_{O_2} or pulse oximetry monitoring, especially if the patient's oxygenation status is marginal or unstable.[49,50] In such patients, an increased FI_{O_2} during therapy may be necessary to offset the decrease in PaO_2 that can occur with this type of treatment. Restoration of the P_{O_2} to at least pretreatment levels must be ensured before ending a treatment session.

Airway management

Because of the significant anatomic differences between the neonate and adult, the tools and techniques of infant airway management are somewhat unique. Specifically, the selection and use of airway equipment and the methods of airway management must be individually tailored to the infant according to size, weight, and postpartum age.[51]

Equipment. A wide selection of infant- and pediatric-sized masks, oral airways, suction catheters, laryngoscope blades, and endotracheal tubes is necessary to accommodate variations in patient age and weight. Table 32-9 provides recommendations regarding endotracheal tube and suction catheter sizes for infants and children.[51,52]

Using oral airways and masks. When using an oral airway in infants, a Guedal type (with a central passageway) is probably the best choice, since the infant tongue may easily occlude the lateral slots of other designs, thereby worsening the obstruction. When using a mask on an infant, the practitioner should be careful not to overextend the head, since this may flatten the trachea and worsen airway obstruction. Furthermore, one should never raise the mandible forcefully to close the mouth (as sometimes done with adults), since the tongue will then press on the soft palate and occlude the nasopharynx. At times, especially in the neonate, the jaw should be gently advanced and the mouth kept open beneath the mask to establish a good airway.

Endotracheal intubation. As previously indicated in Table 32-9, proper endotracheal tube size and depth of insertion can be estimated by the infant's age or height. If the tube is too small, a considerable volume leak may result, making positive pressure ventilation ineffective. On the other hand, too large a tube can cause mucosal trauma and damage to the larynx. Moreover, too large a tube may result in inward sloughing of the laryngeal membranes after extubation, resulting in severe upper airway obstruction.

Table 32-9   Endotracheal Tube and Suction Catheter Sizes For Infants and Children

Age or weight	ET tube ID (mm)	Tube length (cm) oral	Tube length (cm) nasal	Suction cath (F)
NEWBORN				
Less than 1000 g	2.5	9-11	11-12	5
1000 to 2000 g	3.0	9-11	11-12	6
2000 to 3000 g	3.5	10-12	12-14	6
More than 3000 g	4.0	11-12	13-14	8
CHILDREN				
6 months	3.0-4.0	11-12	12-14	6-8
18 months	3.5-4.5	11-13	13-15	8
2 years	4.0-5.0	12-14	14-16	8-10
3 years	4.5-5.0	12-14	14-16	8-10
4 years	4.5-5.5	13-15	15-17	8-10
5 years	4.5-5.5	13-15	15-17	8-10
6 years	5.5-6.0	14-16	16-18	10
8 years	6.0-6.5	15-17	17-19	10
12 years	6.0-7.0	17-19	19-21	10
16 years	6.5-7.5	19-21	21-23	10-12

Estimating formula for tube internal diameter (ID) in mm:
   (1) Tube ID = (Age + 16)/4
   (2) Tube ID = Height(cm)/20
Estimating formula for tube length (cm):
   (1) Oral: 12 + (Age/2)
   (2) Nasal: 15 + (Age/2)

Infant endotracheal tubes are generally uncuffed. As applied to infants, cuffs may quickly erode the relatively softer and unsupported tracheal walls. Even without cuffs, the tube diameter is very small and the tube can be very easily kinked or obstructed; thus positioning of the head, avoidance of cumbersome connecting apparatus, and extreme care in suctioning to avoid mucus plugs become very important.[51,53]

Because of the size of the tongue and position of the epiglottis, most practitioners find the Miller (straight) laryngoscope blade best for intubating infants. Since even small amounts of edema can cause serious airway obstruction in infants, great care must be taken to avoid trauma to the mucosa during the intubation procedure. The distance between the cords and carina is much smaller in infants, making endobronchial intubation more likely. Because tube movement of only a few millimeters can result in a mainstem intubation or extubation, the practitioner must confirm tube placement after intubation and prevent tube movement during the course of treatment using an appropriate stabilization technique. Fig. 32-16 demonstrates a traditional approach to stabilization of an oral endotracheal tube using tape and tincture of Benzoin. Fig. 32-17 depicts

an orotracheal tube holder designed specifically for this purpose.

Suctioning. Oral and pharyngeal suctioning in infants is best accomplished with a bulb syringe. Either a DeLee trap or a mechanical vacuum source with attached catheter may be used for nasopharyngeal and nasotracheal suctioning of the neonate. Equipment for suctioning larger infants and children is the same as that used with adults (see Chapter 21), with appropriate modifications in the amount of vacuum pressure used and catheter size.[53] Recommended vacuum pressures for neonates range from -60 to -80 mm Hg, although copious and thick secretions may require lower pressures. With large infants and children, vacuum pressures in the -80 to -100 mm Hg range are generally safe and effective. Catheter sizes are selected according to the patient's age and, where applicable, the size of the tracheal airway (Table 32-9).

Procedure. The procedure for nasopharyngeal and nasotracheal suctioning in infants and children is comparable to that described for adults in Chapter 21, with a few key exceptions. In infants less than 6 months old, preoxygenation with 100% oxygen is not recommended because of the risk of retinopathies.[53] Instead, most clinicians recommend elevating the F_{IO_2} by no more than 10% above that being delivered before suctioning.

Hyperinflation of infants should always be accomplished with an appropriate-sized manual resuscitator with an airway pressure manometer.[54] The pressure used to hyperinflate an infant's lungs should be carefully monitored and should never be more than 25% greater than that being used for mechanical ventilation, if applicable.

Given an infant's small lung volume and airway size, suctioning can quickly and easily cause atelectasis unless

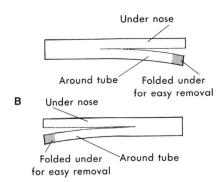
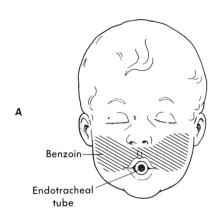

Fig. 32-16   Method for taping endotracheal tube. **A,** Benzoin is applied to cheeks and upper lip. Skin bond cement may also be used. **B,** Split tape is applied. (From Koff PB, Eitzman DV, and Neu J: Neonatal and pediatric respiratory care, St Louis, 1988, The CV Mosby Co.)

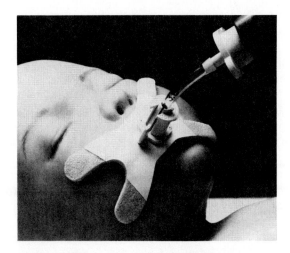

Fig. 32-17   Method for securing endotracheal tube using tube holder from Respiratory Support Products. (Courtesy of Respiratory Support Products, Costa Mesa, Calif; from Koff PB, Eitzman DV, and Neu J: Neonatal and pediatric respiratory care, St Louis, 1988, The CV Mosby Co.)

close attention is paid to detail. Catheter insertion to the point of resistance without partial withdrawal will obstruct a distal airway and quickly result in lobar or segmental collapse once vacuum is applied. For this reason, some clinicians recommend limiting insertion depth to just beyond the tip of the endotracheal tube, as based on knowledge of tube length and external marking of the catheter.[23] Time limits for suctioning infants should also be reduced; most recommend that actual suction application be strictly limited to no more than 5 seconds.

Finally, saline irrigation, if used, should be limited to no more than 0.5 ml in neonates. In larger infants and children, 0.5 to 3.0 ml of saline may be used.

Monitoring. As with CPT, assessment of the patient's respiratory rate, color, pulse, and blood pressure should be supplemented with either continuous transcutaneous P_{O_2} or pulse oximetry monitoring, especially if the patient's oxygenation status is marginal or unstable. Where available, the practitioner should also observe the electrocardiogram (ECG) on the bedside monitor, since cardiac arrhythmias—particularly bradycardia—represent common complications of suctioning neonates.[55] Suctioning can also raise intracranial pressures, presumably by cough stimulation.[56]

On completion of the suctioning procedure, the practitioner must ensure that the patient is stable and that adequate ventilation is occurring. Careful auscultation should be conducted to verify proper endotracheal tube placement, since accidental extubation or endobronchial intubation are common complications of suctioning small infants.

Continuous positive airway pressure

The primary therapeutic indication for CPAP in critically ill infants is similar to that applied to adults. Specifically, CPAP is indicated when the Pa_{O_2} is unsatisfactory while spontaneously breathing a high FI_{O_2}.[57-59] For infants, this generally means a Pa_{O_2} less than 50 mm Hg while breathing an oxygen concentration of 50% or more, or an a/A ratio of less than 0.2 to 0.4.

As with adults, CPAP increases the FRC and recruits additional alveoli for gas exchange. In infants prone to alveolar collapse, this maneuver will usually decrease the amount of right-to-left shunting. However, unlike the adult response, CPAP may decrease lung compliance (CL) in some infants, especially in those with hyaline membrane disease. This paradoxical response probably results from overdistention of otherwise normal alveoli.[12]

Since a decrease in CL is associated with an increased work of breathing, CPAP should be used cautiously in infants with CO_2 retention, unless this is related to obstruction of the small airways. In these cases, such as might occur with meconium aspiration, a small amount of CPAP may decrease airway resistance (Raw) and actually improve $\dot{V}_E$, thereby lowering the Pa_{CO_2}.[12] On the other

hand, if too much CPAP is applied to infants with meconium aspiration, hyperinflation and air trapping may only worsen.

Since this mode of therapy is most successful when implemented early in the progression of a hypoxemic respiratory disorder, many physicians will begin CPAP administration as soon as an infant exhibits clear signs of respiratory distress. Among the signs of respiratory distress indicating a potential need for CPAP are marked tachypnea, severe retractions, grunting, cyanosis breathing 50% or more oxygen, periodic breathing or recurrent apnea, and x-ray manifestations of severe parenchymal lung disease.[58,59]

In addition to its therapeutic use, infant CPAP may also be applied for supportive purposes. Supportive indications for CPAP include apnea, tracheobronchial malacia, and small airways obstruction. The box below differentiates among the therapeutic, supportive and combined uses of infant CPAP.[57]

Methods of administration. Most modern infant CPAP systems consist of a continuous-flow Y circuit with a flow or threshold resistor connected to the expiratory limb.[60] Fig. 32-18 shows the classic CPAP device described by Gregory in 1971, which used a simple screw clamp on an anesthesia bag as an expiratory flow resistor. In 1974, the Carden valve, a simple reverse venturi that approximated the characteristics of a threshold resistor, was introduced

---

NEONATAL AND PEDIATRIC SITUATIONS WHEN CONTINUOUS POSITIVE AIRWAY PRESSURE MAY BE INDICATED

THERAPEUTIC CPAP

RDS (respiratory distress syndrome)
High permeability pulmonary edema
Cardiogenic pulmonary edema
Pneumonia with respiratory failure
Multilobe atelectasis
Smoke inhalation injury
Aspiration pneumonitis
Chemical pneumonitis

SUPPORTIVE CPAP

Apnea of prematurity
Obstructive sleep apnea
Tracheobronchial malacia

COMBINED—THERAPEUTIC CPAP AND SUPPORTIVE CPAP

Bronchiolitis with pneumonia
Artificial airways (maintaining physiologic CPAP)
Weaning from mechanical ventilation

From Koff PB, Eitzman DV, and Neu J: Neonatal and pediatric respiratory care, St Louis, 1988, The CV Mosby Co.

as a means to deliver CPAP. At about the same time, the use of underwater seals as CPAP threshold resistor became popular.

Today, specially calibrated spring-loaded disks, gravity-weighted valves, or electronic solenoids generally have replaced these early methods of creating CPAP.[60] Moreover, CPAP is incorporated as a mode option on essentially all newer-generation infant ventilators. Such systems take advantage of the built-in F_{IO_2} control, humidification, and safety and alarm features of these ventilators. Regardless of design or features, a CPAP system should impose as little additional work of breathing on the infant as possible.[61,62]

The major difficulty with infant CPAP is not how to generate the pressure, but how to apply it to the airway. The five major methods by which CPAP can be applied include (1) head chambers, (2) face masks, (3) endotracheal tubes, (4) nasopharyngeal tubes, and (5) nasal prongs. Table 32-10 compares and contrasts these modes of CPAP application in regard to their various design features.[23] Because of the many hazards associated with the head chamber and the difficulties inherent in mask application, these two approaches are seldom used anymore, having been supplanted by the nasal or tracheal routes.

Administration of CPAP by either a nasopharyngeal tube or nasal prongs can cause gastric distension, thereby

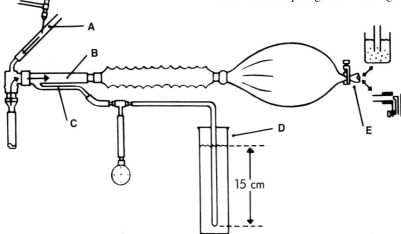

Fig. 32-18   Continuous-flow CPAP system using orificial resistor as originally described by Gregory. **A,** Premixed and humidified source gas to patient connector inlet. **B,** Expiratory line. **C,** Attachment to pressure manometer and to **D,** underwater-seal pressure pop-off system. **E,** Screw clamp on tail of anesthesia bag used to vary size of orifice and adjust PEEP level. (From Blodgett D: Manual of pediatric respiratory care procedures, Philadelphia, 1982, JB Lippincott Co.)

Table 32-10   Comparison of CPAP Methods

Method	Advantages	Disadvantages
Endotracheal tube	Patent airway; easy attachment to resuscitator or mechanical ventilator; easily stabilized and controlled	Hazards associated with intubation
Nasal prongs	Eliminates need for intubation; easily applied	Pressure necrosis and trauma; loss of CPAP with crying or leaks; false pressure reading with high flows; positioning difficult to maintain
Nasopharyngeal tube	Eliminates need for intubation; easily inserted	Pressure necrosis and trauma; loss of CPAP with crying or leaks
Mask	Eliminates need for intubation; easily applied	Mouth care difficult; leaks; danger of increasing CO_2 with inadequate flow; pressure necrosis; danger of aspiration
Head chamber	Eliminates need for intubation; easily applied	Leaks; compression of neck vessels; tissue necrosis; excessive noise levels; access for resuscitation difficult; mouth and head care difficult

From Aloan CA: Respiratory care of the newborn: a clinical manual, Philadelphia, 1987, JB Lippincott Co.

necessitating insertion of a gastric tube. Moreover, both these approaches are based on the fact that neonates normally breathe through the nose. However, a crying infant is likely to inspire substantial volumes of air through the mouth. For this reason, infants receiving CPAP by either nasopharyngeal tube or nasal prongs should also be enclosed in an oxyhood delivering an F_{IO_2} comparable with that being received through the nasal route. This will ensure a stable F_{IO_2} regardless of the infant's breathing pattern.[12]

Initiating CPAP. When initiating infant CPAP, the practitioner should carefully check both the circuit pressure and flow before attaching the device to the patient. Once the infant is attached to the patient connector, the proximal airway pressure should be checked to ensure that the prescribed pressure is being delivered. Pressure requirements generally are in the 2 to 8 cm H_2O range. Flow should be sufficient to meet patient needs but not be so excessive as to cause inadvertent CPAP in the system.[63] An initial flow of three times the infant's estimated $\dot{V}_E$ is a good starting point, with subsequent adjustments made to keep airway pressure deflections to 1 cm H_2O or less during inspiration.

Monitoring and adjustment. Many of the sophisticated monitoring approaches used with critically ill adults, such as pulmonary artery catheterization, are not readily applicable to infants. For this reason, the monitoring and adjustment of infant CPAP levels is more "trial and error" oriented. The usual routine is to determine empirically the effect of small increments (2 cm H_2O) of CPAP pressure on arterial blood oxygenation while carefully observe the infant's clinical response.[12,57]

With successful application of CPAP, the infant's respiratory rate usually drops toward normal and the grunting and retractions that usually accompany respiratory distress tend to lessen or cease. Arterial blood gas analysis will reveal an improved Pao_2, usually allowing a subsequent reduction in the F_{IO_2} to safer levels.

Persistence of grunting, sternal retractions, and cyanosis (if present) usually indicates the need for additional CPAP pressure. On the other hand, worsening hypoxemia or hypercapnea, and the active use of the abdominal muscles during expiration, suggests excessive levels of CPAP. Too high a level of CPAP may also cause a reduction in cardiac output, as manifested by a decreased arterial blood pressure, peripheral vasoconstriction, and metabolic acidosis.[64]

If oxygenation cannot be maintained at a satisfactory level with CPAP, if prolonged apneic spells continue, or if hypercapnea persists or worsens, mechanical ventilation is indicated.

Discontinuation. Discontinuation of infant CPAP should be considered when the results of arterial blood gas analysis, chest x-ray films, and clinical assessment indicate resolution of the underlying pathologic problem. First

consideration is given to decreasing the F_{IO_2} to nontoxic levels, followed by lowering the CPAP level. Since simultaneous changes in pressure level and F_{IO_2} tend to confound interpretation of the infant's response to therapy, only one parameter should be changed at a time.

When an infant can maintain adequate arterial blood gases without signs of respiratory distress on 2 to 3 cm H_2O CPAP while breathing 40% oxygen or less, the endotracheal or nasal tube should be removed and the infant placed in an oxyhood at an equivalent or slightly higher F_{IO_2}. Leaving an endotracheal tube in place without CPAP is contraindicated in these infants, since it increases the work of breathing and prevents glottic closure, potentially causing a decrease in FRC and worsening of arterial oxygenation.

Hazards and complications. Many of the hazards and complications of infant CPAP are similar to those encountered in adults.[64] As previously mentioned, CPAP can cause overdistension of normal lung units, thereby decreasing C_L as a whole. Overdistension also increases the risk of pulmonary barotrauma and may increase the physiologic dead space. CPAP also increases P_{pl}, thereby impeding venous return to the right heart. Increased impedance to venous return can potentially lower cardiac output and increase intracranial pressures. Increased intracranial pressures in the infant can contribute to intraventricular hemorrhage.

As with adults, CPAP can increase pulmonary vascular resistance, mainly by compressing the pulmonary capillaries in areas of the lung that are overdistended. However, an increase in pulmonary vascular resistance in infants can worsen arterial hypoxemia by increasing right-to-left shunting through the foramen ovale and ductus arteriosus. This problem becomes evident when increments of CPAP pressure worsen, instead of improve, arterial oxygenation.

Other hazards and complications unique to infant CPAP relate to its common modes of application, especially the use of nasal or nasopharyngeal tubes, as previously discussed.

Mechanical ventilation

The approach taken to mechanical ventilation of the infant and small child differs in significant ways from that applied to adults. This difference is most evident in the neonatal period, when the anatomic and physiologic disparities are greatest. As the infant grows toward adulthood, these differences begin to dwindle, such that mechanical ventilation of the older child becomes comparable in most respects to that used with adults.

Indications. The box on p. 861 summarizes the major indications for mechanical ventilation of newborns. As with adults, acute respiratory failure is the primary indication for mechanical ventilation. Also as with adults, acute respiratory failure in infants has many potential causes but can be broadly classified as either hypoxemic or hypercapneic.

INDICATIONS FOR MECHANICAL VENTILATION OF NEONATES

RESPIRATORY FAILURE

$Paco_2 > 55$ mm Hg

$Pao_2 < 50$ mm Hg

DEPRESSION OF RESPIRATORY DRIVE

Apnea of prematurity

Intracranial hemorrhage

Drug depression

IMPAIRED PULMONARY FUNCTION

RDS

Meconium aspiration

Pneumonia

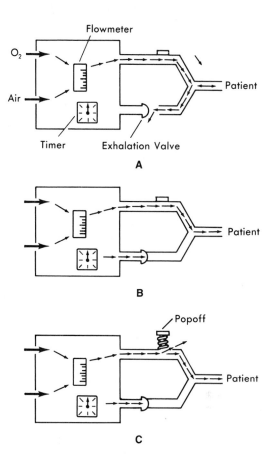

Fig. 32-19 Schema of neonatal ventilator. **A,** Spontaneous phase. **B,** Inspiratory phase. **C,** Pressure-limiting phase. (From Koff PB, Eitzman DV, and Neu J: Neonatal and pediatric respiratory care, St Louis, 1988, The CV Mosby Co.)

Hypoxemic respiratory failure is present when the signs of respiratory distress and hypoxemia persist despite treatment with CPAP and supplemental oxygen. Indeed, in some clinical centers, mechanical ventilation is instituted whenever an infant's Pao_2 drops below 50 mm Hg while breathing 50% or more oxygen.[12,65]

Hypercapneic respiratory failure in newborns in usually due to depression of the central respiratory drive. Common conditions associated with depression of the central respiratory drive in neonates include neonatal asphyxia, apnea of prematurity, intracranial hemorrhage, and the influence of certain narcotic or analgesic drugs transmitted from the mother during labor and delivery.

Ventilatory support may also be required when alterations in lung function create $\dot{V}/\dot{Q}$ imbalances or increase the work of breathing. These conditions occur together when the FRC is decreased, as in hyaline membrane disease and interstitial pneumonia. On the other hand, small airway obstruction, such as occurs with meconium aspiration, increases Raw and causes hyperinflation yet also results in a mismatching of ventilation and perfusion and increased work of breathing.[12]

Basic principles. The predominant approach to infant ventilatory support is time-cycled, pressure-limited, continuous-flow IMV. Infants and small children up to 10 kg in weight are best ventilated using this approach, with larger children being supported with true volume-cycled ventilation (with or without IMV).[17,65-67]

Functional characteristics. Fig. 32-19 portrays the operational and functional characteristics of a modern time-cycled, pressure-limited continuous-flow IMV infant ventilator. In Fig. 32-19, *A* the ventilator is in its expiratory phase. Air and oxygen under pressure are blended and delivered continuously and at a constant rate of flow through a calibrated flowmeter directly into the patient circuit (sin-

gle-circuit system). A pneumatic, fluidic, or electronic timer mechanism controls the function of an expiratory valve, which may consist of a gas-powered diaphragm or electronic solenoid valve. During the expiratory phase of the ventilator cycle, this valve remains open, allowing the infant to spontaneously draw fresh inspired gas from that being circulated through the system. During spontaneous expiration, the continuous flow flushes exhaled gas out the expiratory valve to the atmosphere. Adjustment of flow or threshold resistance through the expiratory valve allows regulation of CPAP (spontaneous breathing only) or positive end-expiratory pressure (PEEP) (with IMV) levels.

On completion of the selected expiratory time interval, the expiratory valve closes, cycling the ventilator to inspiration (see Fig. 32-19, *B*). With the expiratory valve closed, gas now must flow into the infant's lungs.

As gas continues to flow into the infant's lungs, pressure in the system rises until the preset pressure limit is reached (see Fig. 32-19, *C*). At this point a mechanical or electronically controlled pressure "pop-off" or relief valve opens. With the exhalation valve still closed but the pressure pop-off open, gas now follows the path of least resis-

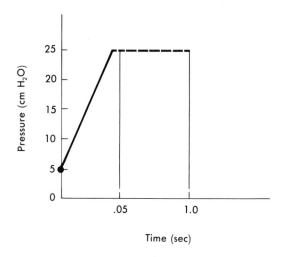

Fig. 32-20 Prolonging inspiration increases plateau period. (From Koff PB, Eitzman DV, and Neu J: Neonatal and pediatric respiratory care, St Louis, 1988, The CV Mosby Co.)

tance, escaping out the pressure relief valve instead of further inflating the infant's lungs. As long as the exhalation valve remains closed and the pressure relief valve open, pressure in the system will remain constant at the preset pressure limit.

As shown in Fig. 32-20, the duration of this pressure hold or pressure plateau is determined by the preset inspiratory time. Once the preset inspiratory lapses, the exhalation valve opens and a new expiratory phase begins, allowing the infant to again breathe spontaneously.

Advantages and disadvantages. The primary advantages of the time-cycled, pressure-limited mode of ventilatory support for infants are (1) user control over mechanical rate, inspiratory and expiratory times, and mean airway pressure and (2) elimination of breath stacking. On the other hand, with time-cycled, pressure-limited ventilatory support both the V_T and $\dot{V}_E$ vary with changes in the mechanical properties of the infant's lungs.

As long as the mechanical properties of the infant's lungs remain stable, the delivered V_T depends solely on the preset gas flow, inspiratory time, and pressure limit and will remain relatively constant. However, with a preset pressure limit, should the infant's C_L or R_{aw} change, V_T and $\dot{V}_E$ will increase or decrease accordingly.

In this respect, time-cycled, pressure-limited ventilation is comparable to pressure-cycled ventilation, requiring closer and more scrupulous patient assessment and ventilator monitoring. As an example, if the endotracheal tube of an infant receiving this mode of ventilatory support becomes kinked or plugged, the preset pressure limit will still be reached and the ventilator will continue to cycle on its preset time intervals, but no volume will be transmitted to the lungs.

Although recent improvements in technology have made it possible to monitor infant V_T and $\dot{V}_E$ accurately, these new devices should serve only to alert the practitioner to potential problems. As always, there is no substitute for the astute observational skills of an experience clinician.

Volume-limiting inspiration. By setting the pressure limit *above* that required to deliver the gas flow over the duration of inspiration, the constant flow time-cycled infant ventilator may be "volume limited." As an example, if the gas flow is preset at 6.0 L/min (100 ml/sec) and the inspiratory time is preset to 0.5 seconds, then the V_T delivered by the ventilator is calculated as the product of flow ($\dot{V}$) times inspiratory time (t_I):

$$V_T = \dot{V} \times t_I$$
$$VT = 100 \text{ ml/sec} \times 0.5 \text{ sec}$$
$$= 50 \text{ ml}$$

Of course, not all this volume will actually enter the patient's lungs. As with adult ventilators, a component of the delivered volume will be compressed in the ventilator circuitry, thus effectively lowering that actually available to the patient.

Volume limiting clearly allows more precise control over the infant's $\dot{V}_E$ than does the time-cycled, pressure-limited mode. However, volume limiting allows breath stacking to occur. Moreover, depending on the pressure limit setting, airway pressures in the volume-limited mode can rise to dangerous levels without warning, thereby increasing the possibility of pulmonary barotrauma. Last, since volume limiting with small infants generally requires lower flows than those used in the time-cycled, pressure-limited mode, the imposed work of breathing through the circuit may be increased. For these reasons, the time-cycled, pressure-limited mode is generally preferred.

Key design considerations. The box on p. 863 outlines the key design considerations characterizing an "ideal" infant ventilator.[12] Other than reliability and ease of use, the most important general characteristics of an infant ventilator relate to its circuitry. Because of the extremely small V_T values typical in neonatal mechanical ventilation, both circuit dead space and compressed volume must be minimal.[68] Moreover, changes in the internal volume of the circuit, as might occur with fluctuations in humidifier water level, are unacceptable.[69] Patient circuits are thus made of relatively noncompliant materials, and humidification systems are designed with small internal volumes and (ideally) the means to maintain a constant water level. Condensation in infant ventilator circuits is a particularly vexing problem that can result in grave hazards to the infant if the water finds its way to the airway.[69]

Table 32-11 compares and contrast a number of currently available infant ventilators according to selected operational characteristics. The reader interested in more detail regarding actual use and operation of these ventilators should consult either the manufacturer's operation manuals or standard equipment reference texts.[12,60,70]

DESIRED CHARACTERISTICS FOR NEONATAL VENTILATORS

General characteristics
  Designed specifically for neonatal use
  Reliable and easy to operate
  Simple, inexpensive, and readily accessible calibration
    and repair
  100% Relative humidity of inspired gas
  Minimal dead space
  Minimal internal compressible and distensible volume;
    nondistensible ventilator circuit tubing
  Minimal noise
  Low cost
Functional characteristics
  Precisely controlled F_{IO_2}
  Cycling rate 0 to 200/min
  Continuous flow system for IMV
  V_Ts 5 to 100 ml
  CPAP or PEEP, 0 to 15 cm H_2O (independent of flow,
    peak inspiratory pressures, or rate)
  Independently adjusted inspiratory and expiratory times
    (inspiratory time 0.2 to 1.5 sec)
  Adjustable inspiratory flow rate 0 to 20 L/min
  Manual cycling device
  Adjustable inspiratory time-limiting device
  Adjustable pressure-limiting valve
  Failsafe valve in case of ventilator malfunction

Alarms
  Visual, audible, adjustable, and battery-powered
  High and low pressure for PEEP and peak inspiratory
    pressure (based on proximal airway pressure)
  High and low rate
  High and low F_{IO_2}
  Prolonged inspiratory time
  Inspired gas temperature
  Electrical or pneumatic power failure
Monitoring capability
  F_{IO_2}
  Inspiratory and expiratory time
  I:E ratio
  Proximal airway pressure
  Duration of positive pressure
  Respiratory rate
  Mean airway pressure

From Kirby RR, Smith RA, and Desautels DD, editors: Mechanical ventilation, New York, 1985, Churchill Livingstone.

Table 32-11 Functional Comparison of Infant Ventilators

Ventilator*	Control mechanism	Ventilator rate	Inspiration time	Expiration time	I:E ratio
Babybird	Pneumatic	Resultant	Preset	Preset	Resultant
Babybird 2A	Electronic	Preset	Preset	Resultant	Resultant
Bourns BP-200	Electronic	Preset	Resultant	Resultant	Preset
Bourns Bear Cub	Electronic	Preset	Preset	Resultant	Resultant
Bio-Med MVP-10	Fluidic	Resultant	Preset	Preset	Resultant
Sechrist IV-100B	Fluidic	Resultant	Preset	Preset	Resultant
Healthdyne 102/105	Electronic	Preset	Preset	Resultant	Resultant
Infrasonics Infant Star	Electronic	Preset	Preset	Resultant	Resultant

*Except for the Infrasonics Infant Star, all the above ventilators are based on the continuous-flow IMV principle of operation and are normally used in the pressure-limited time-cycled mode. The Infrasonic Infant Star provides an alternative demand flow mode. Note: a preset parameter is user selectable through a ventilator control; a resultant parameter cannot be set by the user but derives from the interaction of two or more preset values.

That over a dozen infant ventilators are currently in use attests to the fact that there is as yet no one ideal ventilator on the market. Nonetheless, current limitations in the field of neonatal mechanical ventilation are less attributable to shortcomings in equipment performance than to our lack of understanding on how best to use our existing technology.[12] Recognizing the limits of our current knowledge and experience, the following section provides general guidance on the use and application of infant mechanical ventilation.

Setting and adjusting ventilator parameters. Modern time-cycled, pressure-limited ventilators make the adjustment of ventilatory parameters relatively easy. However, the "best" combination of parameters for the neonate remains controversial.

Nonetheless, all clinicians agree that ventilatory parameters must be set and adjusted according to each patient's individual needs and response. Key parameters include the frequency of breathing (f), the t_I, the I:E ratio, the pressure limit or peak inspiratory pressure (PIP), the flow ($\dot{V}$), the F_{IO_2}, and the level of continuous distending pressure (PEEP). Related to the time and pressure parameters is the concept of mean airway pressure, or MAP. Although not a valve that can be preset, MAP has been identified as a composite measure by which both the effectiveness and complications of infant mechanical ventilation can be judged.

These parameters are initially set to "average" values using clinical rules of thumb. Later, the clinician makes adjustments in the parameters to ensure adequate ventilation and oxygenation while attempting to minimize the likelihood of associated complications.

Frequency. On some infant ventilators, such as the Bear Cub and Healthdyne 102/105, the rate or frequency of breathing is a preset parameter in which care the clinician simply selects the desired value. On other ventilators, such as the Sechrist IV-100B and BioMed MVP-10, the frequency of breathing is a resultant, established by independent adjustment of the inspiratory and expiratory time controls.

In either case, the frequency of breathing is the major determinate of alveolar ventilation and thus the infant's $Paco_2$. IMV rates of 30 to 40 breaths/minute generally provide adequate alveolar ventilation and elimination of carbon dioxide in most infants.[65] If the $Paco_2$ cannot be maintained at the desired level within this frequency range, consideration should be given to altering the pressure limit or inspiratory time. Higher rates are sometimes used to induce hypocapnea and respiratory alkalemia in infants with persistent fetal circulation.[12] This can reduce pulmonary vascular resistance and right-to-left shunting.

Inspiratory time and I:E ratio. By definition, all time-cycled infant ventilators provide user control over t_I. If the frequency of breathing is a preset parameter, then the time available for expiration (t_E) will simply be the remainder

of the total cycle time. In this case, changes in t_I will not affect the rate of breathing but will alter the I:E ratio.

On the other hand, when the frequency of breathing is established by adjustment of separate inspiratory and expiratory time controls, alterations in t_I will alter both the rate and the I:E ratio. For a constant t_E, an increase in t_I will lower the rate and raise the I:E ratio, whereas a decrease in t_I will increase the rate and lower the I:E ratio.

Initially, an inspiratory time between 0.3 and 0.5 seconds is satisfactory for most situations, with adjustment made according to both the nature of the underlying pathologic problem and the results of clinical assessment and arterial blood gas analysis.

For example, it is generally accepted that prolongation of the t_I above 0.5 will improve arterial oxygenation in infants with conditions that lower the FRC. In these cases, prolongation of inspiration increases the time that the alveoli are distended, thereby increasing the opportunity for oxygen transfer into the blood.[19,71] Moreover, a lower PIP can be used when the t_I is increased, especially when the I:E ratio is prolonged to the point where inspiration is equal to or actually longer than expiration (a "reverse" I:E ratio).[72]

However, recent research indicates that the risks of long inspiratory times, especially the increased potential for pulmonary barotrauma, generally outweigh the benefits. For this reason, t_I in infants is usually maintained below 0.7 seconds, with the I:E ratio adjusted to approximately 1:2.[73,74]

Of course, there are also times when a faster than normal t_I may be desired. For example, if the underlying pathologic problem is small airway obstruction with hyperinflation, as may occur with meconium aspiration, a t_I less than 0.3 seconds (with a proportionately longer expiratory phase) may help allow complete exhalation and prevent further hyperinflation. Short t_I values may also be desirable when attempting to minimize the cardiovascular effects of intermittent positive pressure ventilation, as in infants with persistent fetal circulation.

Peak inspiratory pressure. The peak inspiratory pressure, (PIP) represents the preset pressure limit that is sustained during the inspiratory phase of mechanical ventilation. For a given set of lung characteristics, the PIP, in conjunction with the t_I and $\dot{V}$, will determine the V_T delivered to the patient.

Although the initial pressure limit setting varies among institutions and according to patient needs, a starting value of between 20 and 25 cm H_2O is generally satisfactory.[12,65] Thereafter, the PIP should be adjusted accordingly, with the goal being the lowest value necessary to obtain satisfactory ventilation and oxygenation.

Gas flow. Since the typical infant ventilator operates in the continuous flow IMV mode, gas flow must be sufficient to (1) meet the infant's ventilatory demands during spontaneous breathing and (2) provide an adequate V_T at the PIP and t_I selected during the mechanical inspiratory phase.

An initial flow setting of between 6 to 10 L/min generally meets these needs and, in most cases, provides the typical pressure plateau characterizing time-cycled, pressure-limited ventilation (Fig. 32-21, *A*).[65] Lower flows result in a slowing of the pressure rise during inspiration, such that the pressure limit may not be reached until toward the end of the inspiratory phase (Fig. 32-21, *B*). Thus, changes in flow may be used to alter the pressure wave pattern and adjust the time necessary to reach the preset pressure limit. However, if the flow is set too low, the spontaneous demands of the infant will not be met. Clinically, this situation is evident when spontaneous inspiration causes a negative deflection on the airway pressure manometer. If this occurs, the flow should be increased.

As previously described, if the pressure limit is set above that required to deliver the gas flow over the duration of inspiration, the ventilator will function in a volume-limited mode. In this case, increases in either flow or inspiratory time will increase the V_T delivered to the infant, and changes in C_L and Raw will result in changes in the PIP.[75]

Finally, if the device used to generate PEEP or CPAP in the system has flow-resistive properties, increases in flow will raise, and decreases in flow will lower, system pressure.[60]

Inspired oxygen concentration. During mechanical ventilation the FIO_2 should be kept as low as tolerated to avoid the risk of retinopathies and pulmonary oxygen toxicity. Oxygen may also be a contributing factor in the development of bronchopulmonary dysplasia (BPD) in the neonate (as discussed subsequently).

Positive end-expiratory pressure. As in adults, PEEP is indicated in infants whose arterial oxygenation is unsatis-

factory due to alveolar instability and a decreased FRC.[59] The resulting increase in FRC and alveolar oxygen tensions also can reduce pulmonary vascular resistance, thereby decreasing intrapulmonary as well as cardiac shunting in the neonate. PEEP may also be of use in de-

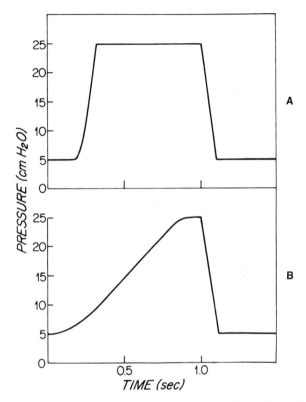

Fig. 32-21 Pressure wave pattern of neonatal ventilator. **A,** High flow rate. **B,** Low flow rate. (From Koff PB, Eitzman DV, and Neu J: Neonatal and pediatric respiratory care, St Louis, 1988, The CV Mosby Co.)

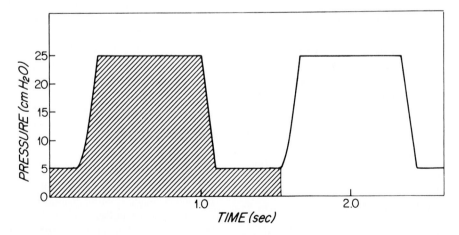

Fig. 32-22 Pressure wave pattern of neonatal ventilator, with shaded area representing calculated mean airway pressure (MAP). (From Koff PB, Eitzman DV, and Neu J: Neonatal and pediatric respiratory care, St Louis, 1988, The CV Mosby Co.)

creasing flow resistance and improving ventilation in infants with small airway obstruction.[12]

Levels of PEEP between 4 to 10 cm H_2O are most commonly used.[65] Higher levels of PEEP are poorly tolerated in patients with obstructed airways because further overdistention can suppress venous return and increase dead space ventilation and CO_2 retention.[12] Too high a level of PEEP can also increase pulmonary vascular resistance and right-to-left shunting, resulting in a deterioration, rather than an improvement, in oxygenation status.

Mean airway pressure. MAP is defined as the average pressure applied to the lungs over a defined period. As depicted in Fig. 32-22, this represents the total area under the curve of pressure over time. Parameters that affect MAP include the f, the PIP, the PIP waveform, the t_I, the I:E ratio, and the PEEP level.

Clinical research shows that higher levels of MAP are associated with better arterial oxygenation.[17,72] However, the likelihood of pulmonary barotrauma also correlates directly with the magnitude of MAP, with the incidence of air leaks increasing dramatically when the MAP rises above 12 cm H_2O.[12]

The most appropriate MAP is the one that enhances oxygenation and ventilation and minimizes the risks of barotrauma and cardiovascular depression in the individual patient under care. Thus the "optimum" MAP must be individualized according to the unique clinical presentation and underlying pathologic problem of the infant receiving ventilatory support.[18] Moreover, the practitioner must realize that the same MAP may be achieved by different combinations of the various time and pressure parameters.

Of course, it is control over these individual time and pressure parameters that gives the clinician flexibility in patient management. Lumping these parameters together into a single measure can help us to understand their combined impact on cardiopulmonary function. However, establishing "normal" or desired MAP levels should be discouraged.[12]

Weaning and discontinuation. As with adult mechanical ventilation, the primary goal of infant ventilatory support is to discontinue it as soon as possible. However, unlike the formal weaning criteria and protocols that have been developed for adults, the process of discontinuing mechanical ventilation in infants is less well established and significantly different from center to center.

Fig. 32-23 provides an example of one such general framework for weaning infants from mechanical ventilation. Underlying this approach is early emphasis on eliminating or lessening those support components that pose the greatest patient risk, that is, F_{IO_2} values greater than 0.7, PIPs greater than 30 cm H_2O, PEEP levels greater than 8 cm H_2O, and t_Is greater than 0.7 seconds.[12] After these parameters are brought into more acceptable ranges, the rate of breathing is decreased as tolerated, with a switch made to CPAP once the F_{IO_2} is below 0.5 and the PIP is

below 25 cm H_2O. CPAP pressures and oxygen concentrations are then reduced until the infant is able to maintain satisfactory arterial blood gases on less than 40% oxygen and 2 cm H_2O CPAP, at which point extubation is indicated. Some infants may require a small amount of nasal CPAP after extubation to keep alveoli from collapsing until grunting returns.

Complications. The box on p. 867 summarizes the most common complications associated with mechanical ventilation of the newborn.[12,18,65] Barotrauma, bronchopulmonary dysplasia, and Wilson-Mikity syndrome have all been linked to mechanical ventilation of the newborn and will be discussed subsequently. RLF and retinopathy of prematurity (ROP) are complications not so much of mechanical ventilation itself but of the accompanying oxygen administration. Likewise, airway complications occur independently of positive pressure ventilation.

As with adults, positive pressure can cause a rise in pulmonary vascular resistance. However, in neonates and infants with certain congenital cardiovascular defects, this rise in pulmonary vascular resistance can worsen preexist-

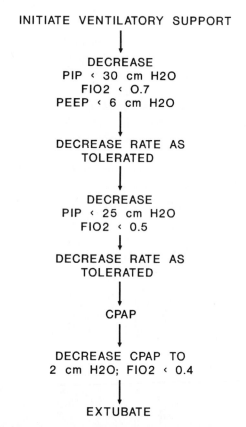

INITIATE VENTILATORY SUPPORT

↓

DECREASE
PIP ‹ 30 cm H2O
FIO2 ‹ 0.7
PEEP ‹ 6 cm H2O

↓

DECREASE RATE AS TOLERATED

↓

DECREASE
PIP ‹ 25 cm H2O
FIO2 ‹ 0.5

↓

DECREASE RATE AS TOLERATED

↓

CPAP

↓

DECREASE CPAP TO
2 cm H2O; FIO2 ‹ 0.4

↓

EXTUBATE

Fig. 32-23 General guidelines for weaning infants with acute respiratory failure from mechanical ventilatory support. At each step, try to maintain Pa_{O_2} between 50 and 70 mm Hg and Pa_{CO_2} between 35 and 45 mm Hg. If possible, make only one change at a time. (From Kirby RR, Smith RA, and Desautels DD, editors: Mechanical ventilation, New York, 1985, Churchill Livingstone.)

From Koff PB, Eitzman DV, and Neu J: Neonatal and pediatric respiratory care, St Louis, 1988, The CV Mosby Co.

ing extrapulmonary right-to-left shunts. In any congenital defect in which there is a right-to-left shunting, the benefits from positive pressure on the lungs will be moderated by this increase in shunting.

As with the adult, positive pressure also can overinflate more compliant alveoli, compress the pulmonary capillaries, and direct pulmonary blood flow to more poorly ventilated alveoli.[17] This phenomenon increases the number of lung units with low $\dot{V}/\dot{Q}$ ratios, further contributing to hypoxemia.

Should an increase in CPAP or PEEP cause a fall in Pa_{O_2}, it is likely that the pressure level is causing an increase in either intrapulmonary or extrapulmonary right-to-left shunting. This situation can be rectified by simply decreasing the CPAP or PEEP.[59,71]

Of course, the use of appropriate levels of positive pressure almost always improves arterial oxygenation, and the beneficial effects of applying mechanical ventilation, PEEP, or CPAP to critically ill infants usually far outweigh their possible consequences.[66]

COMMON DISORDERS OF THE NEWBORN

There are literally dozens of cardiopulmonary disorders associated with the perinatal period. Some of these repre-

sent congenital anatomic malformations of the heart, lungs, or airways due to developmental abnormalities and are beyond the scope of this chapter. Others conditions are related to simple prematurity, while some disorders occur as a result of problems during labor and delivery. Yet other problems appear to occur as a result of treatment and are termed iatrogenic.

We will focus mainly on the more common disorders of prematurity and labor and delivery, to include meconium aspiration syndrome, hyaline membrane disease, transient tachypnea of the newborn, apnea of prematurity, and the Wilson-Mikity syndrome. Concluding this section will be a discussion of an apparently preventable iatrogenic problem called bronchopulmonary dysplasia.

Meconium aspiration syndrome

Toward the end of gestation, the normal fetus exhibits respiratory movements at rates ranging from 30 to 70/min. Short incidents of fetal asphyxia cause these respiratory movements to cease. However, if the asphyxia is prolonged, the fetus may exhibit large gasping movements, thereby inhaling surrounding liquid material into the lungs.

Pathophysiology. Normally, the liquid surrounding the fetus is pure amniotic fluid, consisting mainly of fetal lung fluid and some fetal urine. Aspiration of amniotic fluid, although not without consequences, is a relatively benign phenomenon, since it can be readily cleared during initial extrauterine breathing. More problematic is aspiration of the contents of the fetal bowel, called *meconium*. Meconium is a sterile mixture of swallowed amniotic fluid, mucopolysaccharides, cholesterol, bile acids and salts, intestinal enzymes, and other substances.

Traditionally, the passage of meconium was thought to indicate a significant incident of fetal asphyxia. Indeed, the passage of meconium is more common when fetal umbilical venous blood oxygen saturation falls below 30%. However, some infants who were never subject to intrauterine hypoxia also pass meconium, suggesting that other mechanisms may be responsible.[76]

As many as 8% to 10% of all births are accompanied by meconium-stained amniotic fluid.[77] The incidence of meconium in the amniotic fluid is highest when gestation exceeds 37 weeks' duration, in breech deliveries, and with SGA infants. Although about 30% of infants born with meconium-stained amniotic fluid exhibit abnormal x-ray findings, only about one in five goes on to develop the true clinical signs of meconium aspiration syndrome. The syndrome is most likely when the meconium is of a thick consistency and can be recovered from the neonate's trachea.

Meconium aspiration syndrome generally involves two primary pathophysiologic problems: pulmonary obstruction and parenchymal lung damage.[76] As shown in Fig. 32-24, the obstructive component—resulting from plug-

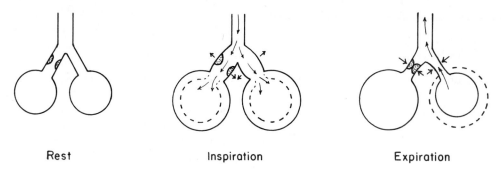

Rest   Inspiration   Expiration

Fig. 32-24   Demonstration of ball-valve effect. At rest, airway lumen is partially obstructed; with inspiration, negative intrathoracic pressure opens airway and relieves obstruction. Gas enters and expands alveoli. On expiration, intrathoracic pressure changes to positive force that narrows airway, causing total occlusion. Gas cannot be expelled and is trapped within alveoli. (From Koff PB, Eitzman DV, and Neu J: Neonatal and pediatric respiratory care, St Louis, 1988, The CV Mosby Co.)

ging of the airways with aspirated meconium—is often of the "ball-valve" type. This problem can lead to air trapping and an increased incidence of pneumothorax and pneumomediastinum. The parenchymal component is comparable to the chemical pneumonitis found in adult aspiration syndromes. Frequently complicating the syndrome, especially when it is associated with severe hypoxemia, is pulmonary hypertension and intracardiac right-to-left shunting.

Clinical manifestations. Infants with meconium aspiration syndrome typically exhibit low Apgar scores, gasping respirations, tachypnea, grunting, and retractions. Radiologic examination (Fig. 32-25) usually shows irregular pulmonary densities (representing areas of atelectasis) combined with hyperlucent areas (representing hyperinflation due to air trapping). Arterial blood gas analysis typically reveals hypoxemia with a mixed respiratory and metabolic acidosis.[76]

Treatment. When meconium-stained amniotic fluid is present, the likelihood of meconium aspiration syndrome can be minimized by vigorous oropharyngeal suctioning during vaginal delivery and before the first breath is taken (as the head is presented). Alternatively, infants born through thick meconium should immediately be intubated and suctioned.[78]

Should the clinical signs of meconium aspiration syndrome develop, oxygen therapy should be instituted and vigorous chest physical therapy with frequent suctioning performed. Should the infant deteriorate, CPAP or mechanical ventilation may be indicated. CPAP is indicated if the primary problem is hypoxemic and respiratory acidosis is either not present or of only moderate severity. By distending the small airways, CPAP can help overcome the ball-valve obstruction characterizing this disorder and actually improve both oxygenation and ventilation.[79] On the other hand, if the respiratory acidosis is severe and the clinical assessment demonstrates an inordinate work of breathing, mechanical ventilation should be instituted.

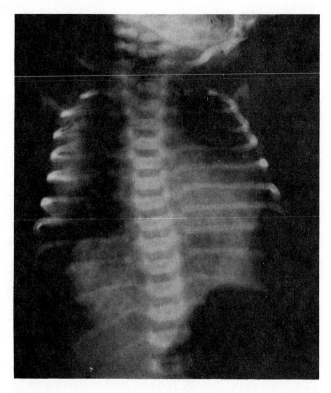

Fig. 32-25   Meconium aspiration is severe in this chest film. Broad areas of density represent atelectasis and interstitial fluid. Regional emphysema is seen in the remaining radiolucent areas. The overall effect of diffuse airway obstruction is overexpansion of the lungs, as indicated by the low position of the diaphragm. (From Korones SB: High-risk newborn infants: the basis for intensive nursing care, ed 4, St. Louis, 1986, The CV Mosby Co.)

Infants with severe meconium aspiration syndrome are among the most difficult to ventilate. They frequently retain CO_2, thereby requiring high rates and peak pressures.[12] Unfortunately, given the underlying problems of airway closure and air trapping characterizing this syndrome, this combination of parameters simply increases the possibility of pulmonary barotrauma. High mean airway pressures may also help worsen a preexisting pulmonary hypertension, thereby aggravating any right-to-left cardiac shunting. For these reasons, most clinicians recommend that infants with meconium aspiration syndrome be ventilated with the shortest t_I values and lowest peak pressures possible, with an I:E ratio sufficiently long to ensure adequate exhalation from obstructed lung units.[12]

Hyaline membrane disease

Hyaline membrane disease, or respiratory distress syndrome of the newborn, is a disease of prematurity. The major contributing factor in the development of hyaline membrane disease is a lack of adequate surfactant production.[80-84] Not until the 34th to 36th week of gestation is surfactant available in adequate quantities for extrauterine life.

Besides the relative state of pulmonary maturity, proper surfactant production also depends on the adequacy of fetal perfusion. Thus maternal factors that compromise fetal blood flow, such as abruptio placenta, preeclampsia, and maternal diabetes, may contribute to the incidence of this disease.

Another contributing factor to the development or aggravation of hyaline membrane disease may be the persistence of high pulmonary vascular resistance after birth. If the fetus is stressed and develops acidosis and severe hypoxemia, pulmonary vascular resistance will increase. This can lead to areas of pulmonary ischemia and further interference with surfactant production.

Pathophysiology. Fig. 32-26 outlines the pathophysiologic events associated with the progression of hyaline membrane disease. A decrease in surfactant production causes an increase in surface tension forces in the alveoli. This causes alveoli to become unstable and collapse, leading to atelectasis and an increased work of breathing. At the same time, the increase in surface tension forces increases the tendency for fluid to move from the pulmonary capillaries into the alveoli. Together, these factors impair oxygen exchange with the pulmonary capillary blood, leading to a severe hypoxemia.

The severe hypoxemia and developing acidemia increase pulmonary vascular resistance, which can reopen or aggravate existing extrapulmonary right-to-left shunting, and only worsen the hypoxemia. The effects of hypoxia and acidosis also directly impair further surfactant production.

At autopsy of the infant who dies of hyaline membrane disease, the lungs are found to be dark red, hypoinflated, and liverlike in texture. If the infant was treated with mechanical ventilation, the terminal air sacs may be hyperinflated and damaged from barotrauma. Alveolar ducts and air sacs remain collapsed. Hyaline membranes are often found lining the alveolar ducts and air sacs. These membranes have a waxy appearance and are thought to be composed of debris of destroyed cells, fibrin, and other blood

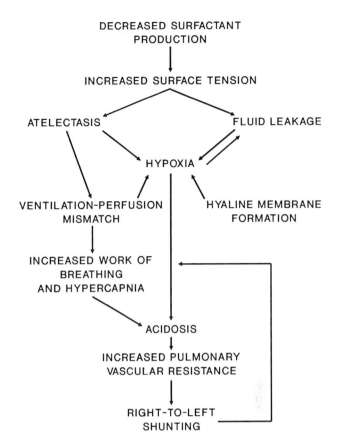

Fig. 32-26 Clinical progression of hyaline membrane disease. (From Aloan CA: Respiratory care of the newborn: a clinical manual, Philadelphia, 1987, JB Lippincott Co.)

components. In infants recovering from this disease, the hyaline membranes are destroyed by macrophagic action.

Clinical manifestations. The first signs of respiratory distress observed in the infant with hyaline membrane disease are usually present immediately or soon after birth. Although most of the physical signs follow closely on one another, tachypnea is usually the first to appear. The increased respiratory rate is accompanied by progressively worsening retractions, the development of a paradoxical breathing pattern, and audible grunting. Nasal flaring may also be observed. Chest auscultation often reveals a dry, uneven, crackling sound.

Cyanosis may or may not be present. Without the aid of blood gas analysis, it is difficult to determine the effects of temperature, perfusion, skin pigment, and lighting on arterial oxygenation. However, if the child has pale or cyanotic mucus membranes or is cyanotic around the eyes, lips, or nail beds, this indicates severe hypoxemia.

As with ARDS, the hypoxemia caused by hyaline membrane disease typically is refractory to treatment, meaning that increased oxygen concentrations do little to improve the arterial oxygenation.[19,72,84] However, certain other pulmonary conditions, as well as hypotension, hypothermia, and poor perfusion, will mimic this aspect of hyaline membrane disease.

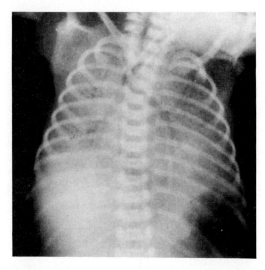

Fig. 32-27 Radiolucent appearance of severe hyaline membrane disease. The lungs are dense. The cardiac shadow is barely discernible in left chest. Prominent black streaks emanating from both hilar areas are air bronchograms. (From Korones SB: High-risk newborn infants: the basis for intensive nursing care, ed 4, St. Louis, 1986, The CV Mosby Co.)

Given the relative nonspecificity of these signs, definitive diagnosis of hyaline membrane disease is usually made by chest x-ray film (Fig. 32-27). Reticulogranular densities and the presence of air bronchograms are typical of this disorder and important in "staging" its degree of severity. The reticulogranular pattern is caused by the aeration of the respiratory bronchioles and the collapse of the alveoli. Air bronchograms appear as aerated, dark, major bronchi delineated by the collapsed or consolidated lung tissue surrounding them.

Hyaline membrane disease is staged by chest x-ray findings in the following manner:

- *Stage I* is marked by a generalized reticulogranular density over all lung fields. The cardiac shadow is sharp. The diaphragms are noted to be down to approximately the eighth rib.
- *Stage II* shows an increase in reticulogranular densities and air bronchograms over the medial two thirds of the lung fields. The lungs are not as well expanded, and the diaphragms are higher than the eighth rib.
- *Stage III* shows increasing reticulogranular densities and more prominent air bronchograms. Inflation of the lungs is only down to the seventh rib. The chest wall may be distorted and have a "bell-shape" appearance. The cardiac shadow is indistinct.
- *Stage IV* shows the characteristic "whiteout" appearance, with extreme opacification. There is an exaggerated "bell shaping" of the chest wall. The cardiac shadow is obliterated, and the diaphragms are indistinct above the seventh rib.

Treatment. Continuous distending pressure (CPAP or PEEP) is the primary supportive tool in the management of hyaline membrane disease. Criteria for treatment vary from hospitals to hospital and even physician to physician, but the application of various regimens are geared toward the same pathophysiologic processes.

CPAP. Unless the infant's condition is considered severe, a trial with nasal CPAP is indicated. Nasal prongs offer the advantage of applying CPAP without the hazards inherent in an endotracheal tube. Once CPAP is initiated, the persistence of the clinical signs of respiratory distress, especially grunting and retractions, suggests that the airway pressure is insufficient and should be raised by a small increment (1 to 2 cm H_2O). If the infant's clinical condition deteriorates rapidly, a more aggressive form of therapy is required.

Intubation should be performed under controlled conditions and, ideally, as an elective procedure. A trial of endotracheal CPAP with the settings comparable to that used with the nasal route should be tried before considering mechanical ventilation. Often endotracheal CPAP results in an improvement in Pao_2 over that obtained through the nasal route, presumable due to less pressure leakage. If oxygenation is not improved on maximum levels of CPAP and Fio_2, or if the patient is apneic, mechanical ventilation with PEEP must be instituted.

Mechanical ventilation. The aim of mechanical ventilation in hyaline membrane disease is to overcome the tendency of the lungs to collapse and maintain alveolar inflation. In severe HMD, the alveoli collapse on each expiration, requiring an increased intra-alveolar pressure (P_{alv}) to reinflate them. To maintain this pressure for an adequate time, a constant pressure pattern is desirable. With sufficiently high inspiratory flows, a time-cycled pressure-limited constant flow generator provides such a pattern.

Some centers prefer low PIP levels combined with "reversed" I:E ratios, that is, inspiratory-expiratory time ratios greater than 1:1. Studies show that reversing the I:E ratio is a more effective way of improving oxygenation than increasing PIP.[19,71,72] This approach improves oxygenation by increasing the overall amount of time the alveoli are inflated, but it may be associated with higher incidences of pulmonary barotrauma than more traditional methods.[12,73,74]

Arterial Pco_2 is not normally affected when PEEP and reversed I:E ratios are used. Because of the short time constant of the lung in hyaline membrane disease, the lung empties very quickly. Unless the $Paco_2$ is high at the onset of parameter changes, CO_2 retention is not a common complication of high mean airway pressure. However, if hypercapnea is present and alveolar ventilation is inadequate, the practitioner should consider increasing the rate of breathing, the inspiratory pressure, or both. Intermittent mechanical ventilation rates of up to 30 to 40 breaths/min can be used to lower $Paco_2$ without derangements of the

Pao$_2$. If possible, increases in the PIP beyond 30 cm H$_2$O should be avoided because of the increased potential for barotrauma.[12]

High mean airway pressures do not usually affect blood pressure and cardiac output in infants with hyaline membrane disease.[18,72] Combined, the low compliance of the lungs and high compliance of the chest wall minimize pressure transmission to the pleural and thoracic cavities. Alveolar expansion is limited, as is compression of pulmonary blood vessels. Nonetheless, as an infant with hyaline membrane disease begins to recover, compliance increases, making high mean airway pressure more hazardous. Common complications associated with management of the disease with mechanical ventilation include bronchopulmonary dysplasia, patent ductus arteriosus, pulmonary barotrauma, and intracranial hemorrhage.

Artificial surfactant. Recently, FDA-approved clinical trials of an artificial surfactant instilled directly into the lungs of infants with HMD have shown promising results in decreasing both morbidity and mortality rates. As of this writing, however, this method is still considered experimental. Moreover, current protocols for use of this substance demand rigorous respiratory care, including either CPAP or mechanical ventilation with PEEP (as indicated).

Transient tachypnea of the newborn

Transient tachypnea of the newborn is often referred to as type II respiratory distress syndrome. Its etiology is still unclear but is most likely caused by a delay in the resorption of fetal lung liquid.[85,86] During most births, about two thirds of this lung fluid is expelled by a "thoracic squeeze" in the birth canal, with the remainder being reabsorbed through the lymphatics during initial breathing. However, these mechanisms are impaired in infants born by cesarean section or those with incomplete development of the pulmonary lymphatics (preterm or SGA infants).[86]

The residual lung fluid is quite viscous and causes an increase in airway pressure and an overall decrease in C$_L$, which explains the characteristic tachypnea. The decrease in C$_L$ requires the infant to generate more negative P$_{pl}$ values, which may result in hyperinflation of some areas and air trapping in others.

Infants who develop transient tachypnea are usually born at term without any specific predisposing antenatal events in common. Often there is a history of delivery by cesarean section without labor, prolapsed umbilical cord, maternal diabetes, maternal bleeding, or maternal medication with meperidine (Demerol). In many cases, however, the maternal history and labor and delivery are completely normal.

Clinical manifestations. During the first few hours of life respiratory rates are elevated; however, alveolar ventilation, as measured by arterial pH and Pco$_2$, is usually normal. The chest x-ray film, which may initially be confused with hyaline membrane disease, shows hyperinfla-

tion secondary to air trapping with perihilar streaking. The perihilar streaking probably representing engorgement of the periarterial lymphatics. Pleural effusions may be evident in the costophrenic angles and interlobar fissues.

Treatment. Infants with transient tachypnea usually exhibit a benign course, responding readily to low concentrations of oxygen given by hood. Infants in need of higher F$_{IO_2}$ may benefit from CPAP. Because the retention of lung fluid may be gravity dependent, frequent changes in the infant's position may help speed clearance and minimize $\dot{V}/\dot{Q}$ imbalances. Since the tachypnea cannot always be distinguished from neonatal pneumonia, the administration of intravenous antibiotics for at least 3 days after obtaining appropriate cultures should be considered. The need for mechanical ventilation is rare and probably signifies a complicating factor. Clearing of the lungs, as indicated by both the chest x-ray film and clinical improvement, is usually evident within 24 and 48 hours, although some infants may take as long as a week to show dramatic improvements.

A small percentage of infants with transient tachypnea will go on to develop persistent pulmonary hypertension. This possibility should be considered if the arterial Po$_2$ does not increase as expected with supplemental oxygen administration.

Apnea of prematurity

Definition. Apnea represents the complete cessation ventilatory air flow. Cessation of any effort to breathe is termed central apnea, while unsuccessful efforts to breathe against upper airway obstruction are called obstructive apnea. So-called mixed apnea represents a combination of obstructive central apneic events.[87]

Apnea of prematurity is usually of the central variety. Short central apneic pauses of 15 seconds or less are normal at all ages. Apneic pauses are considered abnormal if they (1) last more than 20 seconds or (2) are associated with cyanosis, pallor, hypotonia, or bradycardia.

Etiology. The incidence of apnea of prematurity is inversely proportional to gestational age. Over half of all preterm and SGA infants exhibit one or more clinically significant apneic episodes, many of which are associated with bradycardia. This finding suggests that apnea of prematurity is associated with an immature respiratory control system.

In addition to prematurity, apnea in infants may also be caused by underlying pathologic conditions such as bacterial sepsis, hypothermia, seizures, intraventricular hemorrhage, anemia, and hypoxia.

Treatment. Care of infants with confirmed or suspected apnea must include continuous respiratory and heart rate monitoring. Some infants may also warrant continuous noninvasive monitoring of oxygenation, as provided by either transcutaneous Po$_2$ electrode or pulse oximetry. Most apneic incidents can be quickly terminated by gentle mechanical stimulation, such as picking the infant up, flicking the soles of the feet, or rubbing the skin.[87]

If the cause of the apnea is other than prematurity, treatment must be directed at resolving the underlying condition. Apnea due to prematurity responds well to the methylxanthines, especially theophylline and caffeine.[88] These agents stimulate the CNS and increase the infant's responsiveness to carbon dioxide. CPAP is also used to treat apnea of prematurity. Although the mechanism of its action is not clearly established, CPAP probably stimulates vagal receptors in the lung, thereby reflexly increasing the output of the brain stem respiratory centers. Severe or recurrent apnea that is not responsive to these interventions may require mechanical ventilatory support.

As the respiratory response mechanisms mature, apnea of prematurity normally resolves itself. Apneic spells begin to disappear by the 37th to 44th week of postconceptual age, with no apparent long-term effects. Infants who exhibited apnea of prematurity are not at any higher risk for SIDS.[87]

Wilson-Mikity syndrome

The Wilson-Mikity syndrome, also known as chronic pulmonary insufficiency of prematurity, is a relatively rare condition seen almost exclusively in low birthweight infants.[89] Since the lung does not develop homogeneously, the infant with Wilson-Mikity syndrome exhibits areas of underdevelopment, which are less compliant, and areas of more advanced lung development, which are more compliant.

Pathophysiology. To maintain airway patency in areas of decreased compliance, the infant attempts to increase intrathoracic pressure. This easily collapses the nonsupported bronchial tree and causes atelectasis and air trapping. This results in unequal distribution of ventilation, hypoxia, hypercapnia, and $\dot{V}/\dot{Q}$ mismatch.

Clinical manifestations. The infant with Wilson-Mikity syndrome can have a relatively unremarkable first few days of life. In distinction to bronchopulmonary dysplasia, some infants who develop Wilson-Mikity syndrome have not received supplementary oxygen or positive pressure ventilatory support. Eventually, the infant shows signs of tachypnea, periods of apnea, and slight cyanosis. The syndrome follows a pattern of increased severity and lasts anywhere from 2 to 6 weeks after onset.

As in other chronic pulmonary conditions, the Pa_{CO_2} rises and the infant may be cyanotic at times. The chest x-ray film may show a very diffuse opacification, much like a lace pattern with areas of hyperinflation secondary to air trapping. From 6 months to 2 years of age, the chest x-ray film may appear normal or may contain cystic foci, which may be mistaken for bronchopulmonary dysplasia. Signs and symptoms slowly improve in survivors, with most clearing between 6 months and 2 years of age.

Treatment. The treatment of the infant with Wilson-Mikity syndrome is supportive as necessary with positive pressure ventilation and supplementary oxygen.

Bronchopulmonary dysplasia

Infants with respiratory failure in the first few weeks of life may develop a chronic pulmonary condition called bronchopulmonary dysplasia.[90-99] Immaturity, oxygen toxicity, and positive pressure ventilation have all been implicated in its pathogenesis, although the exact origin is unknown.

Pathophysiology. The formation of a hyaline membrane occurs acutely, often complicated by a left-to-right shunt through a patent ductus arteriosus or patent foramen ovale. Pulmonary edema occurs next, followed by interstitial fibrosis and finally by emphysematous changes. A delay in normal lung growth and development is often present, along with episodes of pulmonary insufficiency and chronic pulmonary infections. As with hyaline membrane disease, bronchopulmonary dysplasia manifests itself in a series of progressive stages, both pathologic and radiologic. However, it develops over a much longer course than does hyaline membrane disease.[90-99]

Stage I, lasting over the first 2 to 3 days, represents the period of acute respiratory distress. This stage of bronchopulmonary dysplasia may be indistinguishable from severe hyaline membrane disease.

Stage II, beginning around day 4 and lasting up to day 10, represents a period of regeneration. Hyaline membrane disease may be present but is beginning to resolve. Necrosis and repair of the alveolar epithelium is evident. Regeneration and proliferation of the bronchial epithelium occurs. Ulceration and membrane formation in bronchioles is also present, but fibrosis is not. X-ray films during stage II are similar to those seen in hyaline membrane disease, with opacification of the lungs obscuring the heart border and air bronchograms.

Stage III, beginning around day 10 and lasting up to day 20, is the transitional period to chronic disease. As depicted in Fig. 32-28, the x-ray film at this stage shows interstitial edema and focal areas of atelectasis combined with cystic areas of radiolucency. These areas of radiolucency (usually appearing at about 9 days) represent localized emphysema and tend to be most prominent in the perihilar region. These areas often increase in size and number for 3 to 4 months until they fill the entire lung fields. Over this time, the lungs become increasingly hyperexpanded. Since this clinical picture resembles that observed with the Wilson-Mikity syndrome, differentiation between the two is on the basis of pathologic findings or the early clinical course.

Stage IV (usually beginning after 1 month) represents the period of chronic disease. The pathologic changes show obliterative bronchiolitis, bronchiolar fibrosis, and

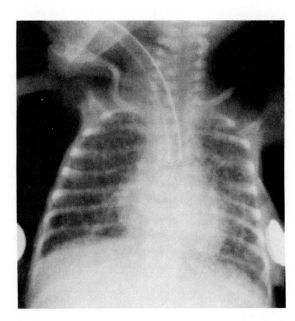

Fig. 32-28   Moderate BPD: interstitial edema and focal atelectasis produce a diffuse density in both lungs. A few small, round radiolucencies represent early regional emphysema. (From Korones SB: High-risk newborn infants: the basis for intensive nursing care, ed 4, St. Louis, 1986, The CV Mosby Co.)

ulceration. Metaplasia of bronchiolar epithelium with narrowing of the bronchioles may also occur. The x-ray appearance shows that resolution has started in this stage (Fig. 32-29). The cystic areas are replaced by hyperlucency at the bases and streaky infiltrates toward the apices. The hyperlucency and the streaky areas finally resolve over a period of months.

Clinical manifestations. Initially the infant may have only required a small amount of supplemental oxygen. As the Pao$_2$ drops, additional oxygen is necessary. This cycle progresses until the infant arterial oxygenation can no longer be maintained without a dangerously high Fio$_2$.

The lungs have areas of atelectasis and areas of air trapping from variable obstruction of the airways. Pulmonary function tests reveal varying degrees of hypoxemia and hypercapnia secondary to airway obstruction, air trapping, pulmonary fibrosis, and areas of atelectasis. There is a marked increase in Raw with an overall decrease in dynamic compliance.

Treatment. The best treatment of BPD is prevention. Modern methods of neonatal intensive care apparently are contributing to a decreased incidence of this chronic disabling disorder, but its manifestations are still a common outcome in low birthweight infants treated for respiratory distress.

Management of infants with bronchopulmonary dysplasia involves steps to minimize further lung damage and the

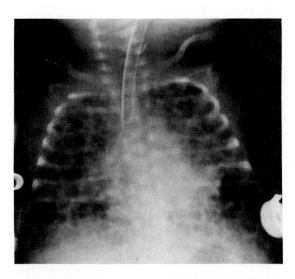

Fig. 32-29   Radiologic appearance of bronchopulmonary dysplasia in advanced stage. White strands are seen throughout both lung fields, representing fibrosis. Lungs are overexpanded in the extreme; diaphragms are at a very low level, and intercostal spaces bulge. (From Korones SB: High-risk newborn infants: the basis for intensive nursing care, ed 4, St. Louis, 1986, The CV Mosby Co.)

development of pulmonary hypertension and cor pulmonale. These infants may depend on supplemental oxygen or mechanical ventilation for months and have symptoms of airway obstruction for years.[90]

Therapy is usually supportive throughout the course of the disease, since the dysplasia tends to be self-limiting in surviving infants.[96] The infant with bronchopulmonary dysplasia is given respiratory support as necessary. Supplemental oxygen has been shown to decrease the pulmonary hypertension that is common with this disorder.[97] Diuretics are administered as necessary to decrease pulmonary edema (which effectively increases lung compliance), with antibiotics given to treat existing pulmonary infections.[98] Chest physical therapy may help mobilize secretions and prevent further atelectasis. Bronchodilator therapy may be useful in decreasing Raw.[99] Recent research indicates that steroid and antioxidant therapy may help prevent or slow the progress of this disorder.

PEDIATRIC RESPIRATORY CARE

Compared with the common cardiopulmonary diseases in the neonatal period, the more common conditions in the older infant and child result from airway obstruction caused by bacterial or viral infections, genetic disorders, and, sadly, preventable accidents. In addition, a disorder of unknown etiology, SIDS, continues to exacts a large toll in unexpected infant deaths.

Sudden infant death syndrome

SIDS, or crib death, is the leading cause of death in infants less than 1 year old in the US. It is estimated that nearly 2 out of every 1000 infants will die of SIDS, accounting for between 5000 and 10,000 infant deaths each year in the US alone.[100] A presumptive diagnosis is based on the conditions of death, in which a previously healthy infant dies suddenly and unexpected, usually during sleep. Although about two thirds of the infants dying of SIDS show some evidence of repeated incidents of hypoxia or ischemia on autopsy, no precise cause of death can be identified.[87,101]

Etiology. The cause of SIDS remains unknown. Apnea of prematurity is not a predisposing factor, and no evidence exists to date to suggest immaturity of the respiratory centers as a cause. Despite the fact that infants in families where two or more preceding SIDS deaths have occurred are at slightly higher risk, there is no convincing evidence of a genetic link. Where three or more SIDS deaths have occurred in the same family, the possibility of child abuse (purposeful asphyxia) must be considered.[102]

Epidemiologic analysis. Currently, our best knowledge of SIDS comes from epidemiologic studies.[103] These studies reveal a statistical patterns of risk factors associated with the incidence of this perplexing problem (see box below).

Typically, the infant who dies of SIDS is a preterm black male born to a poor mother less than 20 years old who received inadequate prenatal care. Moreover, the incident is most likely to happen to an infant between 1 to 3 months of age who is sleeping at night during the winter months. The risk of SIDS is also higher among infants who have previously experienced an apparent life-threatening event (ALTE).[87] An ALTE is an incident characterized by some combination of apnea, pallor, cyanosis, and limpness that is considered frightening to the observer.

Prevention. Given its unknown etiology and sudden and unexpected occurrence, there is no treatment for SIDS. Prevention aims at identifying infants at high risk and providing, where appropriate, home monitoring and training of family members in cardiopulmonary resuscitation (CPR).

With the potential for parental fear of SIDS extremely high, the possibility for abuse of home monitoring is great. To better define the need and appropriate approach for home monitoring of infants, the National Institutes of

---

FACTORS ASSOCIATED WITH INCREASED FREQUENCY OF SIDS IN VICTIMS AND THEIR FAMILIES

MATERNAL CHARACTERISTICS

Less than 20 years old
Poor
Black, Native American, or Alaskan native
Previous fetal loss
Cigarette smoking
Narcotic abuse
Ill during pregnancy
Inadequate prenatal care

INFANT CHARACTERISTICS AT BIRTH

Male
Premature birth
Small for gestational age
Low APGAR scores
Resuscitation with oxygen and ventilation
Second or third in birth order or of a multiple birth pregnancy
Previous siblings SIDS victims

INFANT CHARACTERISTICS NEAR TIME OF DEATH

Age less than 6 months (peak between 1 and 3 months)
Winter season
Asleep at night
Mild illness in week before death
History of apparent life-threatening event (ALTE)

From Koff PB, Eitzman DV, and Neu J: Neonatal and pediatric respiratory care, St Louis, 1988, The CV Mosby Co.

Health (NIH) recently developed a consensus statement on infantile apnea and home monitoring. The eight specific NIH recommendations regarding the need for and use of home monitoring are summarized in the box below.[104]

Bronchiolitis

Bronchiolitis is an acute infection of the lower respiratory tract, usually caused by the respiratory syncytial virus, or RSV.[105,106] Nearly one in ten infants under the age of 2 will acquire a bronchiolitis infection, with the greatest incidence in those around 6 months of age. Outcomes are generally good, although about 1% of infants hospitalized for bronchiolitis die of respiratory failure. Those most prone to develop respiratory failure as a consequence of bronchiolitis are the very young, those who are immunodeficient, and those with congenital heart disease, bronchopulmonary dysplasia, cystic fibrosis, or childhood asthma.

Clinical manifestations. The clinical manifestations of bronchiolitis are those associated with inflammation of the small bronchi and bronchioles. Bronchiolitis commonly occurs soon after an ordinary upper respiratory infection. The infant may have a slight fever with an intermittent cough. After a few days, signs of respiratory distress develop, particularly dyspnea and tachypnea. Progressive inflammation and narrowing of the airways causes both inspiratory and expiratory wheezing and increased Raw. The chest x-ray film may show signs of hyperinflation with areas of consolidation.

The diagnosis of RSV can be established by immunoflourescent assay, or IFA. IFA can confirm the infection the same day and therefore assists in the implementation of a valid treatment plan.

Treatment. As depicted in Fig. 32-30, treatment of the patient with bronchiolitis varies with the severity of the infection and the observed clinical picture.[106] Many patients can be treated at home with humidification and oral decongestants. Patients with more severe symptoms are generally hospitalized, with treatment directed at relieving the airway obstruction and associated hypoxemia.[107,108]

The hospitalized child is frequently treated with systemic hydration and oxygen by oxyhood or croup tent and assistance with airway clearance as needed. Because bronchiolitis and childhood asthma have similar symptomatology, a trial course of bronchodilator therapy with a beta$_2$-adrenergic agent may be useful. If the underlying problem is bronchiolitis, such therapy is generally ineffective. Antibiotics may be administered to treat secondary bacterial infections.

If the respiratory distress persists, ribavirin treatment can decrease the overall severity and duration of the disease.[109-112] Ribavirin is a broad-spectrum virustatic agent active against a wide range of DNA and RNA viruses, including the retrovirus known to cause acquired immune deficiency syndrome (AIDS). In addition to its use against the respiratory syncytial virus, ribavirin has proved useful in the treatment of influenza infections (both type A and B) in young adults.

NIH CONSENSUS STATEMENT ON INFANTILE APNEA AND HOME MONITORING

1. Home cardiorespiratory monitoring is medically indicated in certain groups of infants at high risk for sudden death, including the following:
   a. Infants with one or more severe ALTEs requiring vigorous stimulation, mouth-to-mouth resuscitation, or CPR.
   b. Siblings of two or more victims of SIDS.
   c. Preterm infants with apnea of prematurity who are otherwise ready for discharge.
   d. Infants with conditions such as central hypoventilation or tracheostomy.
2. It is not clear from existing evidence whether the potential benefits of monitoring outweigh the risk for other groups of infants in whom the risk of sudden death is elevated. These groups include the following:
   a. Siblings of one SIDS victim.
   b. Infants with less severe ALTEs.
   c. Infants of opiate-abusing or cocaine-abusing mothers.
3. Cardiorespiratory monitoring is not medically indicated for normal infants or asymptomatic preterm infants.

4. Caregivers must be trained and demonstrate proficiency in infant CPR and must understand that cardiorespiratory monitoring does not guarantee survival.
5. Pneumocardiograms are not useful in screening infants in an attempt to predict SIDS victims or victims of infantile apnea.
6. Decisions for stopping home monitoring should be based on clinical criteria: It is reasonable to discontinue the monitor when the infant has had 2 or 3 months free of events requiring vigorous stimulation, mouth-to-mouth resuscitation, or CPR.
7. Effective home monitoring requires a coordinated, interdisciplinary effort from physicians, nursing and social work services, health care agencies, and medical equipment vendors.
8. In the rare infant with recurrent severe apnea of infancy requiring resuscitation, prolonged hospitalization may be necessary. The vast majority of infants with an ALTE and apnea of infancy have an excellent prognosis without sequelae.

BRONCHIOLITIS

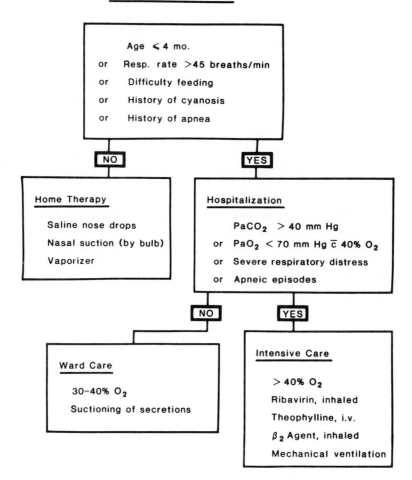

Fig. 32-30   Schema of bronchiolitis therapy shows criteria for and elements of therapy in home versus hospital and hospital ward versus intensive care unit. (From Koff PB, Eitzman DV, and Neu J: Neonatal and pediatric respiratory care, St Louis, 1988, The CV Mosby Co.)

Ribavirin is nebulized with a specially designed small-particle aerosol generator, or SPAG (see Chapter 23). Normally, the aerosol is directed into an oxyhood or croup tent and administered for 12 to 18 hours per day for 3 to 7 days.[112] Administration to ventilator-dependent children must be done with caution. Precipitation of the aerosol clogs the expiratory valve and causes inadvertent high PEEP. However, use of a one-way valve on the inspiratory side and a bacterial filter on the expiratory side of the ventilator circuit is useful in preventing these problems.[113] Should the child progress to true respiratory failure, mechanical ventilation must be instituted.[108] Because of the obstructive nature of this disorder, low rates and long expiratory times may be necessary to prevent air trapping. Vigorous bronchial hygiene, including tracheobronchial aspiration, is usually needed to maintain a patent airway.

Croup

Common croup is an infectious disorder of the upper airway that normally results in subglottic swelling and ob-

struction. Rather than a single clinical entity, croup may manifest itself as one of three different syndromes: (1) laryngotrachitis, also called "classic" croup, (2) "spasmodic" croup, or (3) laryngotracheobronchitis.[106,114] We will emphasize the clinical manifestations and treatment of classic croup.

Clinical manifestations. *Classic croup* occurs most frequently in children under the age of 3, with most cases caused by the parainfluenza virus. Less common as causative agents are the respiratory syncytial and influenza viruses.[115-117]

Signs and symptoms of the disease become evident after 2 or 3 days of nasal congestion, fever, and coughing.[106] Typically, the child presents with a slow, progressive inspiratory and expiratory stridor and a croupy "barking" cough. As the disease progresses, dyspnea, cyanosis, exhaustion, and agitation become evident.

X-ray examination can be helpful in confirming the diagnosis and in ruling out epiglottitis. Classic croup manifests itself on the anteroposterior film with a characteristic subglottic narrowing of the trachea, called the *steeple sign.* Lateral films typically show ballooning of the hypopharynx.

Treatment. The evaluation and treatment of the child with croup must focus on the degree of respiratory distress and associated findings. Table 32-12 presents a scoring system by which the degree of respiratory distress can be reliably quantified.

If stridor is mild or occurs only on exertion and cyanosis is not present (croup "score" of 3 or less), hospitalization is generally not required, and the child is treated at home. If the combined signs total to a score above 4—indicating stridor at rest accompanied by harsh breath sounds, suprasternal retractions, and cyanosis when breathing room air—hospitalization is indicated. Management of the child with mild to moderate croup includes cool mist therapy with or without supplemental oxygen. Aerosolized racemic epinephrine and corticosteroid administration are helpful in decreasing laryngeal swelling.

Progressive worsening of these signs, combined with arterial blood gas results indicating severe hypercapnea and hypoxemia, indicate the need for intubation and mechanical ventilation. As with bronchiolitis, tracheobronchial aspiration is usually needed to maintain a patent airway.

Spasmodic croup differs from classic croup mainly in rapidity of onset.[106,114,115] Spasmodic croup develops very quickly, often resolving just as abruptly. The etiology of spasmodic croup is unknown, but an allergic response is suspected. Along with the associated signs of airway swelling, gagging and vomiting are common. Because many patients show a significant improvement after vomiting, some clinicians treat spasmodic croup with ipecac. With the persistence of respiratory distress, the treatment regimen is similar to that for classic croup. Considering its sudden onset, the differential diagnosis of spasmodic croup must include epiglottitis and foreign body aspiration.[115,117]

Laryngotracheobronchitis, or bacterial tracheitis, is clinically similar to classic croup in its early stages. However, laryngotracheobronchitis tends to progress to a more incapacitating and, at times, life-threatening condition.

Laryngotracheobronchitis probably occurs as a bacteria supra-infection of classic croup, with *Staphylococcus aureus,* group A *Streptococcus pyogenes,* or *Haemophilus influenzae* as the most common infectious agents.[106] Diagnosis is confirmed by culture of the respiratory tract secretions, which tend to be more copious than with classic croup. Treatment is similar to classic croup but with an emphasis on appropriate antibiotic therapy.

Epiglottitis

Epiglottitis represents an acute and often life-threatening infection of the upper airway that causes severe obstruction secondary to supraglottic swelling.[106,118,119] Although not as common as croup, epiglottitis tends to affect a similar age group, that is, children under the age of 5. The etiologic agent is *H influenzae,* type B.

Clinical manifestations. The child usually presents with a high fever, cyanosis, and labored breathing.[118,119] The patient does not have a croupy "bark" but instead exhibits a muffled voice. Older children may complain of sore throat and difficulty in swallowing with a resulting drooling, which is almost always diagnostic of epiglottitis. Visual examination of the upper airway should always be performed in a controlled setting. Inadvertent traction of the tongue can cause further and immediate swelling of the epiglottis with an abrupt and total upper airway obstruction. On lateral neck x-ray film, the epiglottis is markedly thickened and flattened (the "thumb" sign), the aryepiglottic folds are swollen, and the valecula may not be visualized. As with croup, the hypopharynx may be ballooned out.[106]

Treatment. Once the diagnosis is confirmed, the child should be accompanied by a clinician skilled in airway management who is prepared to intervene in the case of acute airway obstruction. Optimally, children with epiglottitis should be electively intubated under general anesthesia in the operating room. Nasal or orotracheal intubation is commonly performed, but a tracheostomy may be necessary if the patient's condition warrants it. There should be no attempt to lie the child down, nor attempts to intubate until the patient is sedated, since this may precipitate acute airway obstruction and respiratory arrest. Once an airway is secured, bacterial culture should be taken and antibiotic therapy started.[106,118,119]

Table 32-12   Clinical Croup Score

	Score		
	0	1	2
Inspiratory breath sounds	Normal	Harsh with rhonchi	Delayed
Stridor	None	Inspiratory	Inspiratory and expiratory
Cough	None	Hoarse cry	Bark
Retractions and flaring	None	Flaring and supersternal retractions	As under 1, plus subcostal, retractions
Cyanosis	None	In air	In 40% O_2

From Downs JJ: Pediatric intensive care: annual refresher course lectures, ASA, 1974.

Cystic fibrosis

Cystic fibrosis is an autosomal recessive disease characterized by pancreatic insufficiency, abnormally thick secretions from the endocrine glands, and an increased concentration of sodium and chloride in the sweat glands.[120-122] In Europe, cystic fibrosis is known as mucoviscidosis.

Clinical manifestations. The clinical features observed in cystic fibrosis are related to pancreatic dysfunction and to a chronic, diffuse, obstructive, and infectious pulmonary process. The earliest defects include secretion of thick mucus that partially obstructs the bronchioles and infection.[120-122] Infections are persistent, initially from *S aureus* but later from *Pseudomonas aeruginosa*. The patient has a frequent cough, tachypnea, and wheezing. There is a progressive thickening of the bronchi, bronchioles, and alveoli. The chest x-ray film typically reveals a patchy atelectasis, irregular aeration, and air trapping.

Later pulmonary complications include bronchitis and bronchiolitis. Recurrent infections eventually destroy the small airways, with a resulting bronchiectasis. In older children, cor pulmonale is evident as an associated cardiac involvement.[120-122]

In addition to pulmonary problems, the highly viscous endocrine glands secretions cause pancreatic duct obstruction. The liver and intestines are also involved. Digestive juices are hindered, and the person cannot digest fats or break down nutrients. There is an inability to break down fat, and thus there is increased fat loss in the stool (steatorrhea). Because of their inability to absorb fat, patients have difficulty in absorbing fat-soluble vitamins (A, D, E, and K). These patients have difficulty in gaining weight because they cannot digest their food properly, and therefore they are treated with pancreatic enzymes and vitamin supplements.[120-122]

Treatment. Treatment for cystic fibrosis is a daily and ongoing regimen. A low-fat diet, vitamin supplements, and pancreatic enzymes are taken to minimize digestive problems. Antibiotic therapy is based on culture and sensitivity results. Ribavirin treatment may be of some use, since respiratory syncytial virus has been shown to be a contributing factor in the destruction of the pulmonary parenchyma.

Respiratory therapy measures should be geared toward decreasing the amount of airway obstruction. Humidification, bronchodilators, mucolytic agents, expectorants, and vigorous chest physiotherapy all assist in airway clearance. Breathing and muscle training techniques should include resistive breathing and manipulations of breathing pattern.[120] Measures are usually supportive until the patient progresses to respiratory failure. Patients eventually die of chronic and devastating pulmonary infections or cor pulmonale.

Accidents

Accidents are the leading cause of death in children and adolescents.[123] Motor vehicle accidents are the most common cause of childhood mortality, with multiple organ system trauma or neurologic injury being the major cause of death. However, the treatment of trauma in children and adolescents is a complex topic beyond the scope of this chapter.

Instead, we will focus on two other types of accidents common to this age group, that is, foreign body aspiration and near drowning. Respiratory care practitioners typically see a large number of victims of these accidents, both within and outside the hospital. Of course, prevention is the best treatment for these accidents. Nonetheless, the practitioner must be prepared to deal with such emergencies, regardless of where or when they occur.

Foreign body aspiration. The major incidence of foreign body aspiration occurs in children between 6 months to 6 years of age.[124] This is invariably due to the fact that young children are always placing things in their mouth. The signs and symptoms observed depend on the size and shape of the material as well as its deposition within the respiratory system.

Manifestations. Foreign body aspiration usually results in immediate and severe respiratory distress.[125] Coughing, gagging, choking, and wheezing are common signs. Since similar signs are observed in croup and epiglottitis, these conditions must be ruled out as a possible diagnosis. Radiologic studies are particularly useful in this regard.

Treatment. The treatment of airway obstruction due to foreign body aspiration depends on the degree of obstruction, the child's state of consciousness, and whether the incident was witnessed.[51]

Complete airway obstruction is treated initially with back blows and chest thrusts in infants, or the Heimlich maneuver in older children (see Chapter 22). Should these maneuvers fail in the clinical setting, laryngoscopy or bronchoscopy may be necessary (Fig. 32-31). Subsequently, endotracheal intubation, tracheostomy, or cricothyrotomy may be indicated.[126]

A common complication of foreign body aspiration below the larynx is infection distal to the point of obstruction, leading to atelectasis, pneumonia, abscess, or even bronchiectasis. For this reason, following removal, bronchodilators and vigorous chest physiotherapy should be given for approximately one week.

Drowning and near drowning. One of the more preventable of childhood accidents is drowning and near drowning.[127] It is not only those who cannot swim who drown. Indeed, under certain conditions, even a good swimmer may drown. Initial aspiration of even a small amount of water can cause bradycardia and hypotension due to vagal stimulation and result in some type of submersion injury.[128,129]

Pathophysiology. The misconception in drowning is that the individual falls victim to extreme aspiration of fluid. The traditional thought is that if a large amount of fresh water is swallowed, the person undergoes dilutional changes in plasma protein as well as red blood cell lysis

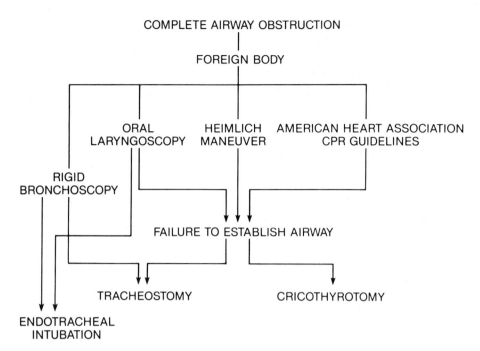

Fig. 32-31   Management of complete airway obstruction. (Modified from Badgwell et al: Can J Anaesth 34:90, 1987; from Finucane BT and Santora AH: Principles of airway management, Philadelphia, 1988, FA Davis Co.)

due to osmotic disruption. Salt water aspiration was thought to cause intravascular hypertonicity, drawing water from the capillaries, with a resulting pulmonary edema.

Usually drowning victims do not aspirate amounts of water large enough to cause these changes. Instead, a reflex laryngeal spasm causes airway closure and prevents such aspiration. Indeed, a person may "dry drown" or "wet drown."[127] In dry drowning, the initial reflex laryngospasm persists until respiratory paralysis sets in. Therefore, the victim aspirates little water. On the other hand, while the wet drowned person experiences the same initial laryngospasm, the continual buildup of carbon dioxide causes an attempt to breathe, after which the victim aspirates.

Although submersion injuries affects multiple systems, the effect on the lung is most notably, involving severe $\dot{V}/\dot{Q}$ mismatching and intrapulmonary shunting, with a resultant hypoxemia, acidosis, and generalized anoxic injury.[127-129]

Treatment. One of the controversies surrounding the treatment of drowning is the appropriateness of the Heimlich maneuver. This may be of little use and wastes valuable time. Resuscitative measures should be immediate and directed toward reversing the hypoxemia and acidosis.[128,129] If the patient has aspirated fresh water, then it is difficult to remove because it has been absorbed into the lymphatics. Salt water aspiration causes copious secretions, the flow of which does not cease after the Heimlich maneuver. What is needed is the early administration of positive pressure to stabilize the alveoli and slow the development of pulmonary edema.[128,129]

Aggressive measures should be taken for all near-drowning victims, regardless of the time submerged. This is especially true for young patients and those who were submerged in cold water. Nonetheless, even with prompt and vigorous resuscitative measures, irreversible neurologic problems may result. Hypothermia, should it occur, should be treated according to severity and duration. Active rewarming is adequate for mild hypothermia, while active core rewarming may be necessary for the long-term and severely hypothermic victim. In the long run, the recuperation from submersion injuries depends on the extent of anoxic and neurologic damage incurred from such incidents.

SUMMARY

Neonatal and pediatric respiratory care is among the most sophisticated speciality areas in the field. Competent practice in this area requires a firm understanding of the many anatomic and physiologic differences between the infant, child, and adult as well as the unique pathophysiology involved in common neonatal and pediatric respiratory disorders.

Many of the cardiopulmonary problems that occur in the perinatal period are associated with difficulties in the fetus' transition from uterine to extrauterine life. Others conditions are related to simple prematurity, while some problems appear to iatrogenic. On the other hand, pulmonary problems in the older infant and child result mainly from airway obstruction due to bacterial or viral infections, genetic disorders, and preventable accidents.

A critical component in the respiratory care management of infants and children is thorough clinical assessment. Because of the significant anatomic and physiologic differences between adult and infant, many of the assessment techniques useful with older patients simply cannot apply in the young infant. Ideally, general assessment of the infant begins before birth and involves consideration of both the maternal history and condition and the fetal and newborn status. As the child grows and develops, more of the assessment methods used with adults begin to apply.

Many of the general principles of management of the critically ill newborn are similar to those for adults. However, special considerations that apply to neonate care are include temperature regulation, fluid and electrolyte balance, nutrition, and infection control. In terms of respiratory care management, substantial variations are required in the tools and techniques applied to the critically ill infant. These special tools and techniques provide the practitioner with the basis for anticipating the unique needs of critically ill infants and children and for planning and implementing their treatment regimens.

REFERENCES

1. Moore KL: The developing human—clinically oriented embryology, ed 3, Philadelphia, 1982, WB Saunders Co.
2. Sadler TW: Langman's medical embryology, ed 5, Philadelphia, 1985, Williams & Wilkins.
3. Koff PB: Development of cardiopulmonary system. In Koff PB, Eitzman DV, and Neu J: Neonatal and pediatric respiratory care, St Louis, 1988, The CV Mosby Co.
4. Escobedo MB: Fetal and neonatal cardiopulmonary physiology. In Schreiner RL and Kisling JA, editors: Practical neonatal respiratory care, New York, 1982, Raven Press.
5. Eitzman DV: Physiologic development. In Koff PB, Eitzman DV, and Neu J: Neonatal and pediatric respiratory care, St Louis, 1988, The CV Mosby Co.
6. Stave U, editor: Perinatal physiology, New York, 1978, Plenum Medical Books Co.
7. Crelin ES: Functional anatomy of the newborn, New Haven, 1973, Yale University Press.
8. Laitman JT and Crelin ES: Developmental changes in the upper respiratory system of human infants, Perinatol Neonatol 4:15-21, 1980.
9. Thyurlbeck WM: Postnatal growth and development of the lung, Am Rev Respir Dis 111:803, 1975.
10. Kubota Y et al.: Tracheobronchial angles in infants and children, Anesthesiology 64:374, 1986.
11. Muller N and Bryan AC: Chest wall mechanics and respiratory muscles in infants, Pediatr Clin North Am 26:503-516, 1979.
12. Bancalari E and Eisler E: Neonatal respiratory support. In Kirby RR, Smith RA, and Desautels DD, editors: Mechanical ventilation, New York, 1985, Churchill Livingstone.
13. Rigatto H, Brady JP, and de la Torre Verduzco R: Chemoreceptor reflexes in preterm infants. II. The effect of gestational age on the ventilatory response to inhaled CO_2, Pediatrics 55:614, 1975.
14. Rigatto H, Brady JP, and de la Torre Verduzco R: Chemoreceptor reflexes in preterm infants. I. The effect of gestational age and postnatal age on the ventilatory response to inhalation of 100% and 15% oxygen, Pediatrics 55:604, 1975.
15. Brady JP and Ceruti E: Chemoreceptor reflexes in the newborn infant: effect of varying degrees of hypoxia on heart rate and ventilation in a warm environment, J Physiol (Br) 184:631, 1966.
16. Gerhardt T and Bancalari E: Chest wall compliance in full-term and premature infants, Acta Paediatr Scand 69:359, 1980.
17. Carlo WA and Martin RJ: Principles of neonatal assisted ventilation, Pediatr Clin North Am 33:221-237, 1985.
18. Greenbough A and Roberton NR: Neonatal ventilation, Early Hum Develop 13:127-136, 1986.
19. Herman S and Reynolds EOR: Methods for improving oxygenation in infants mechanically ventilated for hyaline membrane disease, Arch Dis Child 48:612-617, 1973.
20. Klaus MH and Fanaroff AA, editors: Care of the high-risk neonate, ed 3, Philadelphia, 1986, WB Saunders Co.
21. Thibeault DW and Gregory GA, editors: Neonatal pulmonary care, ed 2, Norwalk, Conn, 1986, Appleton-Century-Crofts.
22. Kendig EL and Chernick V, editors: Disorders of the respiratory tract in children, ed 4, Philadelphia, 1983, WB Saunders Co.
23. Aloan CA: Respiratory care of the newborn: a clinical manual, Philadelphia, 1987, JB Lippincott Co.
24. Behnke M: Patient assessment. In Koff PB, Eitzman DV, and Neu J: Neonatal and pediatric respiratory care, St Louis, 1988, The CV Mosby Co.
25. Czervinske MP: Arterial blood gas analysis and other monitoring. In Koff PB, Eitzman DV, and Neu J: Neonatal and pediatric respiratory care, St Louis, 1988, The CV Mosby Co.
26. Silverman WA and Anderson DH: A controlled clinical trial of effects of water mist on obstructive respiratory signs, death rate and necropsy findings among premature infants, Pediatrics 17:1, 1956.
27. Fan LL, Dellinger KT, Mills AL et al: Potential errors in neonatal blood gas measurements, J Pediatr 97:650, 1980.
28. Koch G and Wendel H: Adjustment of arterial blood gases and acid base balance in the normal newborn infant during the first week of life, Biol Neonate 12:136, 1968.
29. Korones SB: High-risk newborn infants, ed 3, St Louis, 1981, The CV Mosby Co.
30. Scopes J and Ahmed I: Ranges of critical temperatures in sick and premature newborn babies, Arch Dis Child 41:417, 1966.
31. Quie PG: Lung defense against infection, J Pediatr 108:813-816, 1986.
32. Bakken E and Desautels DA: Oxygen therapy. In Koff PB, Eitzman DV, and Neu J: Neonatal and pediatric respiratory care, St Louis, 1988, The CV Mosby Co.
33. Lough MD, Doershuck CF, and Stern RC: Pediatric respiratory therapy, ed 3, Chicago, 1985, Year Book Medical Publishers, Inc.
34. Burgess WR and Chernick V: Respiratory therapy in newborn infants and children, ed 2, New York, 1986, Thieme-Stratton, Inc.
35. Kinsey VE, Arnold HJ, Kalina RE et al: Pao_2 levels and retrolental fibroplasia: a report of the cooperative study, Pediatrics 60:655, 1977.
36. American Academy of Pediatrics: Standards and Recommendations for Hospital Care of Newborn Infants, ed 6, Evanston, Ill, 1977, The Academy.
37. Gale R, Redner-Carmi R, and Gale J: Accumulation of carbon dioxide in oxygen hoods, infant cots, and incubators, Pediatrics 60:453, 1977.
38. Dawes GW and Williams TJ: The oxygen hood as a noise factor in infant care, Respir Care 24:12, 1979 (abstract).
39. Blennow G, Svenningsen NW, and Almquist B: Noise levels in infant incubators, Pediatrics 53:29, 1974.
40. Guilfoile T and Dabe K: Nasal catheter oxygen therapy for infants, Respir Care 26:35, 1981.
41. Payne JW: Diseases of the eye. In Avery ME and Taeusch H Jr, editors: Schaeffer's diseases of the newborn, ed 5, Philadelphia, 1984, WB Saunders Co.
42. Scott AA and Koff PB: Airway care and chest physiotherapy. In Koff PB, Eitzman DV, and Neu J: Neonatal and pediatric respiratory care, St Louis, 1988, The CV Mosby Co.
43. Curran C and Kachoyeanos M: The effects on neonates of two methods of chest physical therapy, MCN 4:309, 1979.

44. Etches PC and Scott B: Chest physiotherapy in the newborn: effects on secretion removal, Pediatrics 62:713, 1978.

45. Finer NN: Chest physiotherapy in the neonate: a controlled study, Pediatrics 61:2, 1978.

46. Sutton PP, Lopez-Vidriero MT, Pavia D et al: Assessment of percussion, vibratory-shaking and breathing exercises in chest physiotherapy, Eur J Respir Dis 66:147-152, 1985.

47. Levin D: Postural drainage and percussion for the infant and child. In Pediatric intensive care, ed 2, St Louis, 1984, The CV Mosby Co.

48. Emery JR and Peabody JL: Head position affects intracranial pressure in newborn infants, J Pediatr 103:950, 1983.

49. Raval D et al: Changes in Tc_{PO_2} during tracheobronchial hygiene in neonates, J Pediatr 96:1118, 1980.

50. Barnes CA, Asonye UO, and Vidyasagar D: Effects of bronchopulmonary hygiene on $P_{tc_{O_2}}$ values in critically ill neonates, Crit Care Med 9:819, 1981.

51. Finucane BT and Santora AH: Principles of airway management, Philadelphia, 1988, FA Davis Co.

52. Keep PJ and Manford ML: Endotracheal tube sizes for children, Anesthesiology 29:181, 1974.

53. Scott AA and Koff PB: Airway care and chest physiotherapy. In Koff PB, Eitzman DV, and Neu J: Neonatal and pediatric respiratory care, St Louis, 1988, The CV Mosby Co.

54. Evaluation: manually operated infant resuscitators, Health Devices 3:164, 1974.

55. Cordero L and Hon EH: Neonatal bradycardia following nasopharyngeal stimulation, J Pediatr 78:441, 1971.

56. Perlman JM and Volpe JJ: Suctioning in the preterm infant: effects on cerebral blood flow velocity, intracranial pressure, and arterial blood pressure, Pediatrics 72:3, 1983.

57. Czervinske MP: Continuous positive airway pressure. In Koff PB, Eitzman DV, and Neu J: Neonatal and pediatric respiratory care, St Louis, 1988, The CV Mosby Co.

58. Finer NN and Kelly MA: Optimal ventilation for the neonate. I. Continuous positive airway pressure, Perinatol Neonatol 7:95-100, 1983.

59. Duncan AW, Oh TE, and Hillman DR: PEEP and CPAP, Anaesth Intens Care 14:236-250, 1986.

60. McPherson SP: Respiratory therapy equipment, ed 3, St Louis, 1985, The CV Mosby Co.

61. Weinstein MM and Weinstein MR: Increased airway resistance complicating respiratory distress syndrome, Crit Care Med 15:76-77, 1987.

62. Czervinske MP, Durbin CG, and Gale TJ: Resistance to gas flow across 14 CPAP devices for newborns, Respir Care 31:18, 1986.

63. Simbruner G: Inadvertent positive pressure in mechanical ventilation of the newborn with detection and effects on lung mechanics and gas exchange, J Pediatr 168:589-595, 1986.

64. Turney T et al: Complications of constant positive airway pressure, Arch Dis Child 50:128, 1975.

65. Betit P and Thompson JE: Mechanical ventilation. In Koff PB, Eitzman DV, and Neu J: Neonatal and pediatric respiratory care, St Louis, 1988, The CV Mosby Co.

66. Gottschalk SK, King B, and Schuth C: Basic concepts in positive pressure ventilation of the newborn, Perinatol Neonatol 4:15-19, 1980.

67. Goldsmith JP and Karotkin EH, editors: Assisted ventilation of the neonate, Philadelphia, 1981, WB Saunders Co.

68. Pirie GE and Cain DL: Options for ventilating the pediatric patient. III. Circuits and humidification systems, Perinatol Neonatol 75-83, 1984.

69. Nelson D and McDonald JS: Heated humidification, temperature control, and "rain-out" in neonatal ventilation, Respir Ther 7:41, 1977.

70. Desautels DA: Mechanical ventilators. In Koff PB, Eitzman DV, and Neu J: Neonatal and pediatric respiratory care, St Louis, 1988, The CV Mosby Co.

71. Donahue LA and Thibeault DW: Alveolar gas trapping and ventilator therapy in infants, Perinatol Neonatol 3:35-37, 1979.

72. Boros SJ et al: The effect of independent variations in inspiratory-expiratory ratio and end-expiratory pressure during mechanical ventilation in hyaline membrane disease: the significance of mean airway pressure, J Pediatr 94:114-117, 1979.

73. Heicher DA, Kasting DS, and Harrod JR: Prospective clinical comparison of two methods for mechanical ventilation of neonates: rapid rate and short inspiratory time versus slow rate and long inspiratory time, J Pediatr 98:957, 1981.

74. Bancalari E, Feller R, and Gerhardt T: Prospective evaluation of IPPV settings in infants with RDS, Clin Res 28:879A, 1980.

75. Simbruner G and Gregory GA: Performance of neonatal ventilators: the effect of changes in resistance and compliance, Crit Care Med 9:509, 1981.

76. Burchfield DJ and Neu J: Neonatal parenchymal diseases. In Koff PB, Eitzman DV, and Neu J: Neonatal and pediatric respiratory care, St Louis, 1988, The CV Mosby Co.

77. Gregory GA: Meconium aspiration in infants: a prospective study, J Pediatr 85:848, 1974.

78. Ting P and Brady J: Tracheal suction in meconium aspiration, Am J Obstet Gynecol 122:767, 1975.

79. Fox WW et al: The therapeutic application of end-expiratory pressure in the meconium aspiration syndrome, Pediatrics 56:214, 1975.

80. Farrell PM and Avery ME: State of the art—hyaline membrane disease, Am Rev Respir Dis 111:657-688, 1975.

81. Hyaline membrane disease. In Avery ME and Taeusch H Jr, editors: Schaeffer's disease of the newborn, ed 5, Philadelphia, 1984, WB Saunders Co.

82. Martin RJ, Fanaroff AA, and Skalina ML: The respiratory distress syndrome and its management. In Fanaroff AA and Martin RJ, editors: Behrman's neonatal and perinatal medicine—diseases of the fetus and infant, ed 3, St Louis, 1982, The CV Mosby Co.

83. Stahlman M: Acute respiratory disorders in the newborn. In Avery, G, editor: Neonatology—pathophysiology and management of the newborn, ed 3, Philadelphia, 1987, JB Lippincott Co.

84. Reynolds EOR: Management of hyaline membrane disease, Br Med Bull 31:18-24, 1975.

85. Avery ME et al: Transient tachypnea of the newborn, Am J Dis Child 111:380, 1966.

86. Rawlings JS and Smith FR: Transient tachypnea of the newborn: an analysis of neonatal and obstetrical risk factors, Am J Dis Child 138:869-871, 1984.

87. Chesrown SE: Sudden infant death syndrome and apnea disorders. In Koff PB, Eitzman DV, and Neu J: Neonatal and pediatric respiratory care, St Louis, 1988, The CV Mosby Co.

88. Gerhardt T, McCarthy J, and Bancalari E: Effect of aminophylline on the respiratory center activity and metabolic rate in premature infants with idiopathic apnea, Pediatrics 63:537, 1979.

89. Mikity VG: Respiratory distress in the premature infant (Wilson-Mikity syndrome). In Kendig EL and Chernick V, editors: Disorders of the respiratory tract in children, ed 4, Philadelphia, 1983, WB Saunders Co.

90. Nickerman BG: Bronchopulmonary dysplasia: chronic pulmonary disease following neonatal respiratory failure, Chest 87:528-535, 1985.

91. Hodgman JE: Chronic lung disease. in Avery G, editor: Neonatology—pathophysiology and management of the newborn, ed 3, Philadelphia, 1987, JB Lippincott Co.

92. Fox WW, Morray JP, and Martin RJ: Chronic pulmonary disease of the neonate. In Fanaroff AA and Martin RJ, editors: Behrman's neonatal and perinatal medicine—diseases of the fetus and infant, ed 3, St Louis, 1982, The CV Mosby Co.

93. Bancalari E and Gerhardt T: Bronchopulmonary dysplasia, Pediatr Clin North Am 33:1-23, 1986.

94. Taghizadeh A and Reynolds EOR: Pathogenesis of bronchopulmonary dysplasia following hyaline membrane disease, Am J Pathol 22:243-256, 1976.

95. Kirkpatrick BV and Mueller DG: Bronchopulmonary dysplasia. In Kendig EL and Chernick V, editors: Disorders of the respiratory tract in children, ed 4, Philadelphia, 1983, WB Saunders Co.

96. Morray JP, Fox WW, Kettrick RG, and Downes JJ: Improvement in lung mechanics as a function of age in the infant with bronchopulmonary dysplasia, Pediatr Res 16:290-294, 1982.

97. Abman SW, Wolfe RR, Accurso FJ et al: Pulmonary vascular response to oxygen in infants with severe bronchopulmonary dysplasia, Pediatrics 75:80-84, 1985.

98. Logvinoff MM, Leman RJ, Taussig LM, and Lamont BA: Bronchodilators and diuretics in children with bronchopulmonary dysplasia, Pediatr Pulmonol 1:198-203, 1985.

99. Wilkie RA and Bryan MH: Effects of bronchodilators on airway resistance in ventilator dependent neonates with chronic lung disease, J Pediatr 111:278-282, 1987.

100. National Institutes of Health, National Institute of Child Health and Human Development: Sudden infant death syndrome (SIDS), April 1986, Special Report to Congress.

101. Hunt CE and Brouillette RT: Sudden infant death syndrome, 1987 perspective, J Pediatr 110:669, 1987.

102. Rosen CL, Frost JD Jr, and Glaze DG: Child abuse and recurrent infant apnea, J Pediatr 109:1065, 1986.

103. Kraus JF: Methodologic considerations in the search for risk factors unique to sudden infant death syndrome. In Tilden RJ, Roeden LM, and Steinschneider A, editors: Sudden infant death syndrome, Proceedings of the 1982 international conference, Baltimore, 1983, Academic Press.

104. Consensus statement: NIH consensus development conference on infantile apnea and home monitoring, Pediatrics 79:292, 1987.

105. Tercier JA: Bronchiolitis: a clinical review, J Emerg Med 1:119-123, 1983.

106. Kurth CD and Goodwin SR: Obstructive airway diseases in infants and children. In Koff PB, Eitzman DV, and Neu J: Neonatal and pediatric respiratory care, St Louis, 1988, The CV Mosby Co.

107. Nahata MC, Johnson JA, and Powell DA: Management of bronchiolitis, Clin Pharmacol 4:297-303, 1985.

108. Outwater KM and Crone RK: Management of respiratory failure in infants with acute viral bronchiolitis, Am J Dis Child 138:1071-1075, 1984.

109. Eggleston M: Clinical review of ribavirin, Infect Control 8:215-216, 1987.

110. Barry W, Cockburn F, Cornall R et al: Ribavirin aerosol for acute bronchiolitis, Arch Dis Child 61:593-597, 1986.

111. Fernandez H, Banks G, and Smith R: Ribavirin: a clinical review, Eur J Epidemiol 2:1-14, 1986.

112. Hall CB, McBride JT, Sala CL et al: Ribavirin treatment of respiratory syncytial viral infection in infants with underlying cardiopulmonary disease, JAMA 254:3047-3051, 1985.

113. Demers RR, Parker J, Frankel LR, and Smith DW: Administration of ribavirin to neonatal and pediatric patients during mechanical ventilation, Respir Care 31:1188-1196, 1986.

114. Cherry JD: The treatment of croup: continued controversy due to failure of recognition of historic, ecological, etiologic, and clinical perspectives, J Pediatr 94:352, 1979.

115. Ryckman F and Rodgers SM: Obstructive airway disease in infants and children, Surg Clin North Am 65:1663-1687, 1985.

116. Goldhagen JL: Croup: pathogenesis and management, J Emerg Med 1:3-11, 1983.

117. Broniatowski M: Respiratory distress in children, Ear Nose Throat J 64:13-19, 1985.

118. Grodin MA: Epiglottitis, J Emerg Med 1:13-19, 1983.

119. Barker GA: Current management of croup and epiglottitis, Pediatr Clin North Am 26:565, 1979.

120. Beckerman RC and Berdan ML: Overview of a lethal genetic disease: cystic fibrosis, Respir Ther 20-26, 1980.

121. Lloyd-Still JD: Clinical manifestations. In Lloyd-Still JD, editor: Textbook of cystic fibrosis, Boston, 1983, John Wright PSG Inc.

122. Taussig LM, Landau LI, and Marks MI: Cystic fibrosis—respiratory system. In Taussig LM, editor: Cystic fibrosis, New York, 1984, Thieme-Stratton Inc.

123. National Safety Council: Accident facts, Chicago, 1984, The Council.

124. Harris CS et al: Children asphyxiation by food: a national analysis and overview, JAMA 251:2231, 1984.

125. Wiseman NE: The diagnosis of foreign body aspiration in childhood, J Pediatr Surg 19:531-535, 1984.

126. Black RE, Choi KJ, Syme WC et al: Bronchoscopic removal of aspirated foreign bodies in children, Am J Surg 148:778-781, 1984.

127. Sarnail AP and Vohra MP: Near drowning: fresh, salt, and cold water immersion, Clin Sports Med 5:33-45, 1986.

128. Kizer KW: Resuscitation of submersion casualties, Emerg Med Clin North Am 1:543-552, 1983.

129. Kram JA and Kizer KW: Submersion injury, Emerg Med Clin North Am 2:545-552, 1984.

New Horizons in Respiratory Care

33

Health Education and Health Promotion

Ann W. Tucker

As the conclusion of the twentieth century approaches, Americans have many reasons to be proud of our health care system. Although problems of access to care continue (see Chapter 1), the health status of the American people has never been better.[1] For example, most of the infectious diseases that ravaged American communities at the beginning of this century have been eradicated. Moreover, mortality rates in all age groups have declined, and the longevity of the population has improved dramatically.

With these important advances has come the recognition that the health status of the population as a whole has become largely dependent on life-style behaviors.[2-4] Not surprisingly, diseases related to life-style are now the leading cause of death in the United States. Heart disease, cancer, cerebrovascular disease, and accidents/trauma—all highly related to personal life-style patterns—now account for more than 50% of all deaths in the United States annually.

The increasing recognition that life-style behaviors are the leading cause of death and disability in the United States is having a major impact on the scope and nature of the delivery of health care. Reduction of premature morbidity and mortality requires efforts from health care providers, the government, individuals, communities, and the private sector. In addition, it requires a new approach to health care delivery—an approach that emphasizes the promotion of health and the prevention of disease.

In this context, all health professionals, including respiratory care practitioners, will be expected to expand their roles beyond that required to simply treat disease and disability. They will be expected to provide education to individuals for the purpose of preventing the onset of diseases or disability and enhancing the quality of life.

Moreover, assumption of these key leadership roles in the health promotion movement will demand that health professionals function within a variety of new and alternative health care delivery settings, including community institutions and the home.

OBJECTIVES

For respiratory care practitioners, providing bedside education to patients receiving treatment is not an unfamiliar role. For many practitioners and students, however, educating individuals in the prevention of disease and promotion of health may be a new concept. In order to help develop these skills, this chapter will provide the respiratory care practitioner with an overview of health promotion and health education. Specifically, after completion of the chapter, the reader will be able to:

1. Relate life-style behaviors to selected indicators of the health status of individuals and groups;

2. Compare and contrast the medical model of health care delivery with alternative approaches to health services;

3. Identify the major priorities and objectives underlying national efforts to improve the health status of the American people;

4. Differentiate the concepts of health promotion and health education;

5. Compare and contrast the role of the consumer and the health care professional in health education efforts;

6. Describe the components of a systematic model for the development of health education programming;

7. Identify and describe the various settings in which respiratory care practitioners can assume a role in providing health education activities;

8. Relate the role of the family to the successful provision of health promotion services;

9. Describe specific ways in which respiratory care practitioners can contribute to the improvement of the health status of the nation.

Most terms used in this chapter are defined in context. The following terms are introduced without explicit definition but may be found in the text glossary:

acronym	ethnicity
authoritarian	holistic
behavioral	life span
cerebrovascular	life-style
cholesterol	morbidity
DHHS	nonjudgmental
didactic	surveillance
epidemiology	synergistic
eradicate	taxonomy

CONTEXT FOR HEALTH EDUCATION AND HEALTH PROMOTION

To demonstrate why this new approach to health care delivery has become so important, we will first examine the evidence linking a population's life-style behaviors with its health status. Then we will analyze the limitations of the current medical model of health care delivery. Finally, we will look at alternative approaches to improving the health status of the US population, as developed by the US government.

Relationship between life-style behaviors and health status

In the early 1970s, the Canadian government examined the major causes of disease and disability affecting its population. This landmark study clearly demonstrated that the many causes of disease and disability could be grouped into four major categories: (1) inadequacies in the existing health care system, (2) behavioral factors or unhealthy life-styles, (3) environmental hazards, and (4) human biologic factors. Fig. 33-1 shows these factors and their relative impact on health status.

These broad categories were then applied to a study of the risk factors associated with the 10 leading causes of death in the United States. The researchers found that approximately 50% of all deaths could be attributed directly to those causes grouped in the behavioral factors or unhealthy life-styles category.[1]

More recently, a study conducted in California found that individual life expectancy could be increased significantly by the practice of seven simple behaviors: eating breakfast, eating moderately and regularly, not smoking cigarettes, engaging in exercise, drinking only moderate amounts of alcohol, and obtaining 7 to 8 hours of sleep nightly. For males, the practice of these behaviors increased life expectancy an average of 11 years. Females following these practices could expect an average increase in life span of 7 years.[5]

Such studies have increasingly drawn public attention to the impact that such factors as cigarette smoking, nutri-

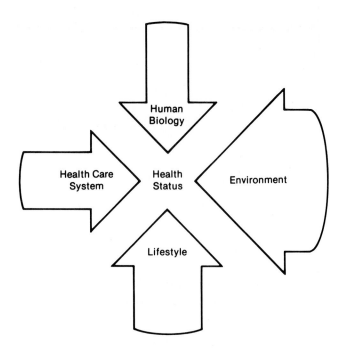

Fig. 33-1   Determinants of health status. (This figure is similar to one developed by Blum HL: Planning for health, development and application of social change theory, New York, 1973, Human Sciences Press, p 3. Reprinted with permission.)

tional practices, and exercise have on health status. That the public is becoming more aware of the implications of poor health habits on individual health and quality of life is clear. A Harris poll taken in 1978 revealed that more than 90% of Americans understand the impact of various life-style behaviors on their health status. Despite this awareness, at least one third of American adults smoke cigarettes, are overweight, and/or do not exercise regularly.[4] The disparity between the public's knowledge of good and bad health habits and its tendency toward less-than-healthy life-styles stems, in part, from the general approach taken toward health care throughout the twentieth century.

Medical model of health care delivery

Throughout this century, the organization and delivery of health care have been based mainly on the medical model. Under this model, primary responsibility for preserving, maintaining, and restoring health rests with the health care delivery system. Consequently, both consumers and health care providers have developed a dependency on this system.

Three assumptions underlying the medical model encourage this dependency relationship. First, the medical model asserts that disease and disability arise outside the individual. Second, it is assumed that, because external factors are responsible for the development of illness, victims of disease and disability are not responsible for their conditions. Third, the medical model asserts that, under these circumstances, patients should turn to the medical care system for diagnosis and treatment.[6]

On the basis of this model, the health care delivery system has become increasingly characterized by specialization of health care providers, a high reliance on medical technology, and the use of treatment approaches that focus on curing disease and disability. In addition, the model has fostered social expectations regarding the importance of the health care delivery system. As a result, many consumers tend to view the health care delivery system as the solution for all matters pertaining to the prevention and maintenance of health and the treatment and rehabilitation of persons with disease and other disorders.[6]

Many critics of the medical model contend that the model has contributed to a number of serious flaws in the existing health care delivery system. The system has become fragmented, health care resources have been unevenly distributed, and health care costs have increased at a pace greater than the general rate of inflation.[7] As the American population's reliance on the health care system has grown, it has become increasingly difficult for individuals to maintain personal independence regarding decisions pertaining to health. Furthermore, critics note that the health status of the American population has not improved in proportion to the number of resources devoted to health care.[6]

An alternative approach

Increasing concern with the limits of a system based mainly on curative health care, in combination with a growing awareness of the importance of healthy behavior, led the US government to search for alternative ways to affect the health status of the nation. The focus of this effort was founded on three basic questions:

1. How could the emerging body of research on lifestyle behaviors be used to establish national health care policies?
2. What types of achievable and measurable health goals should be established?
3. What types of strategies could be developed to prevent premature death and disability?

After several years of research and recommendations from various health care providers and the public, the US Department of Health, Education, and Welfare (DHEW)—now the Department of Health and Human Services (DHHS)—released the 1979 landmark report entitled *Healthy People.*[1] That report and a companion volume entitled *Promoting Health/Preventing Disease: Objectives for the Nation* set out the key steps necessary for the nation to change its health care orientation and to reduce premature death and disability in its population.[8]

Both reports emphasize that the most effective means of reducing premature mortality and morbidity is prevention of disease and promotion of health. In the introduction to the report *Healthy People,* the secretary of the DHEW stressed that the nation's health strategy must be dramati-

cally reoriented to emphasize the prevention of diseases, rather than relying entirely on their treatment after they have struck.[1] This changing philosophy toward health care has recently been reemphasized by the United States Public Health Service. According to that agency, health promotion and disease prevention hold the key to further improvements in the health status of the American people.[9]

The 1979 reports established both national health goals and objectives and time lines for their achievement. Five public health goals and fifteen priority areas were delineated. As listed in the following box, the public health goals established, in measurable terms, the rate of reduction in mortality to be achieved among each of five major age groups. The reports further recommended that the nation be held accountable for achieving these goals by the year 1990.

To achieve these goals, the 1979 report recommended that health care efforts be directed toward 15 priority areas, which were grouped into three categories: (1) preventive services, (2) health protection, and (3) health promotion. As defined by the US government, preventive services include health care services that are provided to individuals by health care professionals. Health protection includes measures that can be used by the government and other agencies, as well as by industry, to protect people from harm. Health promotion involves activities for individuals and communities to promote healthy life-styles. A listing of these priority areas is provided in the box on p. 888.[1]

In addition, the DHHS established objectives for each of these 15 priority areas under five specific headings: improving health status, reducing risk factors, increasing public or professional awareness, improving services or protection, and improving surveillance or evaluation systems.[9]

Currently, the Department of Health and Human Ser-

PUBLIC HEALTH GOALS BY AGE GROUP

- A 35% reduction in infant mortality
- A 20% reduction in deaths of children aged 1 to 14 to fewer than 34 per 100,000
- A 20% reduction of deaths among adolescents and young adults 24 years of age and younger, to fewer than 93 per 100,000
- A 25% reduction in deaths among the 25- to 64-year age group
- A major improvement in health, mobility, and independence in older persons, to be achieved largely by reducing by 20% the average number of days of illness among this age group

From US Department of Health, Education, and Welfare: Healthy people: the surgeon general's report on health promotion and disease prevention, DHEW [PHS] Publication No. 79-55071, Washington DC, 1979, US Government Printing Office.

FIFTEEN PRIORITY AREA "OBJECTIVES FOR THE NATION"

A. PREVENTIVE SERVICES

1. High blood pressure control
2. Family planning
3. Pregnancy and infant health
4. Immunization
5. Sexually transmitted diseases

B. HEALTH PROTECTION

6. Toxic agent control
7. Occupational safety and health
8. Accident prevention and injury control
9. Fluoridation and dental health
10. Surveillance and control of infectious disease

C. HEALTH PROMOTION

11. Smoking and health
12. Misuse of alcohol and drugs
13. Nutrition
14. Physical fitness and exercise
15. Control of stress and violent behavior

From McTernan EJ and Rice NC: An overview of the role of allied health professionals in the health promotion and disease prevention movement, J Allied Health 15: 289-294, 1986.

vices is reviewing the progress made toward achievement of these 1990 goals and objectives. Pending completion of this analysis, the DHHS will update these national expectations and, on the basis of a series of regional conferences, issue a revised set of goals and objectives for the year 2000.

An examination of the current five goals and 15 priority areas reveals that achievement of a "healthy people" requires a collaborative effort among multiple health-related disciplines.[2] By virtue of their training, credibility in the health care delivery system, and large numbers, allied health professionals such as respiratory care practitioners are among the best prepared to assume leadership positions in the health promotion movement.[3] The recognition that allied health professionals have an important role to play in the prevention of diseases has catalyzed a change in the way these providers view their roles and responsibilities in the delivery of health services. As a result, in the early 1980s many health-related professional organizations began to reformulate their standards for education and practice, and they have developed formal policy statements regarding health promotion and disease prevention. Professional organizations or related accrediting agencies that have adopted formal policy statements include respiratory care professionals, occupational therapists, physical therapists, clinical laboratory personnel, registered dietitians, physician assistants, and radiologic technologists.[11] The

HEALTH PROMOTION AND DISEASE PREVENTION POSITION STATEMENT AMERICAN ASSOCIATION FOR RESPIRATORY CARE

The American Association for Respiratory Care (AARC) submits this paper to identify and illustrate the involvement of the respiratory care practitioner in the promotion of health and the prevention of disease and supports these activities.

The AARC realizes that respiratory care practitioners are integral members of the health care team, hospitals, home health care settings, pulmonary laboratories, rehabilitation programs, and all other environments where respiratory care is practiced as outlined in the AARC Statement of Principles.

The AARC recognizes that education and training of the respiratory care practitioner is the best method by which to instill awareness for the opportunity to improve the patient's quality and longevity of life and that such information should be included in their formal education and training.

The AARC recognizes the respiratory care practitioner's responsibility to participate in pulmonary disease training, smoking cessation programs, pulmonary function studies for the public, air pollution alerts, allergy warnings, and sulfite warnings in restaurants, as well as research in those and other areas where efforts could promote improved health and disease prevention.

Furthermore, the respiratory care practitioner is in a unique position to provide leadership in determining health promotion and disease prevention activities for students, faculty, practitioners, patients, and the general public.

The AARC recognizes the need to provide and promote consumer education related to the prevention and control of pulmonary disease to establish a strong working relationship with other health agencies, educational institutions, federal and state government, businesses and other community organizations and to monitor such.

Furthermore, the AARC supports efforts to develop personal and professional wellness models and action plans that will inspire and encourage all members and nonmembers alike to cooperate on health promotion and disease prevention.

From American Association for Respiratory Care: Position statements, Dallas, American Association for Respiratory Care, undated.

formal policy statement of the American Association for Respiratory Care on health promotion and disease prevention appears in the box above.

More recently, educators in various disciplines have begun to reformulate their curricula to include activities directly related to the role of allied health professionals in health promotion and disease prevention. For example, the

State University of New York at Stony Brook has developed a core course and discipline-specific professional modules designed to introduce students to methods and practices useful in the promotion of health and the prevention of disease.[12] Similar curricular changes are now under way in many respiratory care educational programs.

HEALTH PROMOTION AND HEALTH EDUCATION CONCEPTS

How can allied health professionals, such as respiratory care practitioners, support the goals of a *Healthy People*? Health professionals can contribute to the prevention of disease and disability both by helping patients and the public develop more healthy life-styles and by working to effect changes in the environment.[2]

However, if health professionals are to help people develop more healthy life-styles, they must begin taking a different attitude toward health care delivery. Health professionals will be expected to provide individuals with services that are directed toward both preventing the onset of disease or disability and promoting the quality of life through healthier behaviors. Although assuming greater responsibility for their own health, consumers will continue to depend on health professionals to assist them in assessing their health needs, developing health-enhancement strategies, and monitoring and modifying their progress.

Clearly, with societal expectations regarding the health care delivery system changing, health promotion and health education are becoming increasingly important components of one's role as a health professional.

Health promotion

Assumptions. As discussed earlier, the relationship between a person's life-style and health status is well documented. Health promotion focuses on this relationship. Unlike the traditional medical model, health promotion assumes that a person's health status is highly dependent on personal factors arising within that person. In other words, the way people live and the decisions they make regarding individual life-style behaviors often predispose individuals to specific diseases or disabilities.[6] For example, persons who choose to smoke cigarettes are at higher risk of contracting diseases such as lung cancer, chronic obstructive pulmonary diseases, respiratory infections, and high blood pressure. Although consumers will be held increasingly accountable for promoting and maintaining their own health, health care professionals will continue to help individuals develop and maintain life-styles that are conducive to good health.

Definition. Health promotion is a broad concept that has been applied in many contexts and for many purposes. For consumer and health care provider alike, much confusion exists as to the meaning and nature of this term. Such confusion is intensified when the term becomes overused or misapplied. According to Duncan and Gold[13]:

> The term health promotion has gained wide popularity in recent years. This widespread usage has been accompanied by a wide diversity of definitions. . . . In many cases health promotion seems to have become an all-inclusive umbrella term under which any health service may find coverage. Health services have become health promotion services; outpatient clinics have become health promotion centers. In these cases, "health promotion" has become a fad or a gimmick—as meaningless as labelling certain cereals and other foods as natural.

Although still broad in concept, Lawrence Green has defined health promotion as that combination of educational, organizational, economic, and environmental supports necessary for behavior conducive to health. Mullen proposed that health promotion consists of two components: (1) disease prevention and (2) wellness.[13]

Components. Regardless of the definition employed, health promotion begins with healthy persons and applies methods designed to contribute to the growth, enlargement, or excellence of the health status of these persons.[13] Included are activities that focus on holistic health care, high-level wellness, and disease prevention.

Holistic health care. The term holistic is derived from the Greek word *holos,* meaning whole. In the context of health, the phrase holistic health means more than the physical state of being or the absence of disease. Holistic health asserts that health is a dynamic process that comprises many dimensions, each contributing synergistically to a person's health or quality of life.[14,15]

Supporters of holistic health care have proposed a multidimensional model of health.[14,15] According to this framework, health is composed of six dimensions: physical, social, emotional, mental, spiritual, and vocational. The model assumes that each dimension interacts with the other dimensions while contributing to the "whole." The box on p. 890 provides a brief definition of each of these six dimensions.

Within this framework, holistic health care involves promotion of health and prevention of disease in all six dimensions. Emphasis on one or more dimensions to the detriment to others may result in an imbalance in a person's health.

High-level wellness. As first defined in 1961, high-level wellness is oriented toward maximizing the potential of which the individual is capable.[16] High-level wellness includes the integration of all six dimensions of health. When persons experience high-level wellness, they have achieved and are maintaining a balance in integrating all six dimensions.

Disease prevention. Disease prevention as a component of health promotion was originally emphasized by Levall and Clark in 1965.[16] Levall and Clark developed a taxonomy whereby disease prevention was classified into three levels: primary, secondary, and tertiary. Each level is dis-

SIX DIMENSIONS OF HEALTH

Physical. Physical health is the dimension with which most individuals are familiar. Physical health includes the level of physical fitness, the existence of disease or predisposing risk factors, and the level of biologic functioning.

Social. Social health is the ability of individuals to function in and interact with society. This dimension of health is concerned with the quality of the interaction and the level of satisfaction with interpersonal relationships.

Mental. Mental health is concerned with the level of intelligence and ability to learn.

Emotional. The level of ability to express feelings when appropriate is indicative of an individual's emotional health.

Spiritual. Spiritual health is a difficult dimension to define. Generally, attributes such as honesty, integrity, purpose, or ambition in life are all considered elements of this dimension. In addition, spiritual health includes the belief in some unifying source.

Vocational. Vocational health expands the conception of health to include the integration between social (community) and personal health components. Vocational health includes financial success and advancement, recognition for contributions, sharing of work experience with others, contribution (sacrifice) to humankind, improving the quality of lives of others, meeting nonrecreational challenges, expanding "professional" horizons, gaining new perspectives to problem solutions, and giving oneself to goals or objectives related to the greater good.

From Eberst RM: Defining health: a multidimensional model, J School Health 54: 99-104, 1984; Greenberg JS: Health and wellness: a conceptual differentiation, J School Health 55: 403-406, 1985.

tinguished by the type of activities employed to improve, prevent, or restore health.[17]

Primary prevention focuses on enhancement of the well-being of healthy persons or groups of persons. Primary responsibility for enhancement of health rests with the individual. Choosing not to smoke, wearing seat belts, and eating a balanced diet are examples of primary prevention behaviors.

Secondary prevention includes early diagnosis and periodic screening for disease. The purpose of secondary prevention is to find and treat disease before it becomes a permanent disability or results in premature death. Both the consumer and the health care provider share responsibility for secondary prevention. Examples of secondary prevention include pulmonary function screening, hypertension screening, breast self-examination, Papanicolaou smears, oral cancer examinations, and periodic eye testing.

Tertiary prevention includes rehabilitation and restoration of function for an individual, as well as efforts to minimize any further consequences of disease or disability. The primary responsibility for tertiary prevention rests

with the health care delivery system. Examples of prevention at this level that are familiar to most respiratory care practitioners are pulmonary and cardiac rehabilitation programs (see Chapter 34).

Health education

At the core of health promotion (holistic health care, high-level wellness, and prevention) are the principles of health education. Health education is a process of planned learning opportunities designed to enable individuals to make and act upon informed decisions about things affecting their health.[18]

Basic requirements. This definition sets forth several criteria for health education. First, health education is a planned activity. Planning of health education programs requires a comprehensive assessment of factors and values that predispose, enable, or reinforce persons to adopt behaviors conducive to health. Second, health education programs use multiple educational and behavioral methods, which are reinforced over time. Third, the primary goal of health education is behavioral change. This change must be voluntary and occur with the full knowledge and personal decision making of the participants.[3] Fourth, health education activities are directed toward individuals and/or individuals acting collectively.[18]

Health education strives to promote, maintain, and improve individual and community health through the educational process.[19] This goal establishes an important link between health and education. It implies that health education covers the continuum between health and disease and the continuum between prevention and treatment. The educational activities suggested in this goal are those that relate to the promotion, maintenance, and enhancement of health.[18]

Health education programs are aimed at individuals and at groups. Moreover, health education can occur in several settings, including health care institutions, the community, homes, schools, and the workplace. Regardless of the setting, effective improvement of health requires that health education be combined with related strategies for health promotion.[2] Development and implementation of these strategies require collaborative efforts between health care professionals and consumers.

Role of consumer. Education for health, rather than treating and curing disease and disability, requires a shift in philosophy regarding responsibility for health. The burden of responsibility is shifted from the health care delivery system to the consumer.[16]

However, health is just one of many factors competing for attention in a person's life. As discussed earlier, the holistic concept of health consists of at least six major dimensions (physical, social, emotional, mental, spiritual, and vocational). Moreover, family, cultural, community, and societal norms, as well as economic and political factors, have a major influence on the level of wellness achieved in each of these major dimensions. In addition, the value that persons place on health will determine the extent to which they follow a recommended health regimen.

Consumers as well as health professionals must know and understand the variety of forces that have an impact on a person's health behaviors. Once these influences are recognized, there is great potential to facilitate the adoption and maintenance of behaviors conducive to health.

Role of the health professional. Despite the fact that the ultimate responsibility for health rests with the individual, facilitation of the development of health promoting behaviors through education is an important function of health personnel. In this capacity, health professionals must, first and foremost, serve as role models for the public. Successful outcomes in health education cannot be expected unless the professionals involved model healthful behaviors and life-styles. To this end, the American Association for Respiratory Care has established a role model statement to help practitioners set good examples for the public (see box opposite).

Although provision of a good example is necessary for successful health education programming, it does not, of and by itself, provide a sufficient basis for achieving desired outcomes. For this process to be effective, health professionals must assure that certain conditions are established. Among the key conditions prerequisite to effective health education efforts are the following[3]:

1. Program participants must be actively engaged in the learning process. The educational process is impeded if participants are just passive recipients of information.
2. Health education activities must incorporate the values and health beliefs of the learners. Therefore family, cultural, societal, and economic barriers must be considered when opportunities are provided for individuals to make decisions regarding their health.
3. The role of the health educator is to facilitate behavioral change. Therefore the learning process should be approached collaboratively.
4. Predisposing, enabling, and reinforcing health attitudes and behaviors require effort, which will take place only over time.
5. The health care professional must be willing to listen nonjudgmentally to the concerns of the learners. The health care provider must have empathy and understanding to effectively overcome social, economic, political, and cultural barriers.
6. The level of a learner's self-concept and self-esteem may act to facilitate or inhibit that person's ability to make decisions and to act on those decisions. Therefore the health professional should be willing to provide emotional support and assurance when warranted.
7. The characteristics of the health educator make a significant difference in the outcome of the education program. Generally, a successful outcome will be facilitated if the educator exudes confidence but is not overly didactic and authoritarian.

ROLE MODEL STATEMENT AMERICAN ASSOCIATION FOR RESPIRATORY CARE

As health professionals engaged in the performance of cardiopulmonary care, the practitioners of this profession must strive to maintain the highest personal and professional standards. A most important standard in the profession is for the practitioner to serve as a role model in matters concerning health.

In addition to upholding the code of ethics of this profession by continually striving to render the highest quality of patient care possible, the respiratory care practitioner shall set himself apart as a leader and advocate of public respiratory health.

The respiratory care practitioner shall participate in activities leading to awareness of the causes and prevention of pulmonary disease and the problems associated with the cardiopulmonary system.

The respiratory care practitioner shall support the development and promotion of pulmonary disease awareness programs, to include smoking cessation programs, pulmonary function screenings, air pollution monitoring, allergy warnings, and other public education programs.

The respiratory care practitioner shall support research in all areas where efforts could promote improved health and could prevent disease.

The respiratory care practitioner shall provide leadership in determining health promotion and disease prevention activities for students, faculty, practitioners, patients, and the general public.

The respiratory care practitioner shall serve as a physical example of cardiopulmonary health by abstaining from tobacco use and shall make a special personal effort to eliminate smoking and the use of other tobacco products from his home and work environment.

The respiratory care practitioner shall uphold himself as a model for all members of the health care team by demonstrating his responsibilities and shall cooperate with other health care professionals to meet the health needs of the public.

From American Association for Respiratory Care: Position statements, Dallas, American Association for Respiratory Care, undated.

How health education efforts can be organized effectively to meet these conditions is the subject of the next section of the chapter.

A MODEL FOR HEALTH PROMOTION AND HEALTH EDUCATION PROGRAMMING

There are many approaches to health promotion and health education. Some of these methods are based solely on experience, whereas others are founded on a strong behavioral and social science base. For purposes of illustration, we have chosen to focus on the latter type of model.

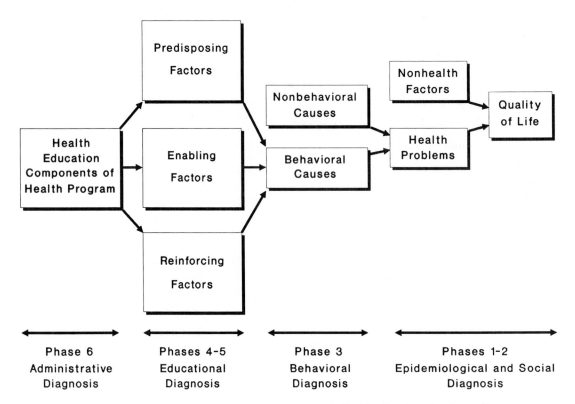

Fig. 33-2   The PRECEDE model. (From Green LW et al: Health education planning: a diagnostic approach, Mountain View, Calif, 1980, Mayfield Publishing Co.)

In 1980 Green and associates[20] developed a systematic approach to planning, implementing, and evaluating health education programs called the PRECEDE model. The PRECEDE model (an acronym for *p*redisposing, *r*einforcing, and *e*nabling *c*auses in *e*ducational *d*iagnosis and *e*valuation) is based on the premise that health education is used to intervene in development and change for the purpose of promoting health or preventing disease.

The model recognizes that behavioral change is complex. In order to affect change, the model uses theoretical foundations from four disciplines: epidemiology, social and behavioral sciences, administration, and education.

Consistent with the philosophy of health education, developers of the model assert that behavioral change must be voluntary. Indeed, voluntary change is the cornerstone of the PRECEDE model. In other words, change must occur with the full knowledge and consent of the individual. Only when the health of others is threatened should health behaviors be compelled. In addition, the model's developers insist that recommended behavioral change must correspond with the value system of the individual and of society; otherwise, there must be an opportunity to adjust the value system.[20]

As shown in Fig. 33-2, the PRECEDE model uses a deductive approach for development of health education programs. Using this model, the health practitioner first diagnoses the intended behavioral outcomes of the program

and then works backward to identify the causes of desirable and undesirable health behavior.

Green and associates have divided this process into seven phases, with each phase using specific diagnostic strategies from epidemiology, the social and behavioral sciences, education, and administration. A brief description of each phase follows.

Phase 1. Quality-of-life assessment

The first phase assesses the quality of life in the population. In this assessment, consideration is given to general problems in the society. Such problems are defined both subjectively and objectively—subjectively by the community and by individuals themselves and objectively by specific social indicators. Social indicators include such factors as population statistics; rates of illegitimacy, unemployment, and absenteeism; welfare data; and information on such conditions as alienation, hostility, discrimination, voting, riots, crime, and crowding.

Phase 2. Differentiating health and nonhealth problems

The second phase diagnoses specific problems that contribute to the quality of life as identified in phase 1. These specific problems are grouped into nonhealth factors and health problems that have an impact on the quality of life. Among the nonhealth factors are underemployment, education, lack of industry, race, age, sex, social disintegration, geography, and transportation. Health problems may involve malnutrition, overpopulation, ill health, alcoholism, cardiovascular diseases, respiratory diseases, cancers, and accidents. Vital indicators such as morbidity, mortality, fertility, and disability statistics facilitate epidemiologic and social diagnosis.

Phase 3. Behavioral diagnosis

This phase analyzes behavioral and nonbehavioral causes of the health problems observed in the population. To differentiate between behavioral and nonbehavioral causes of a health problem, the health care provider should first list all of the causes of the problem.

For example, if chronic obstructive pulmonary disease (COPD) is identified as a major health problem in a given population, the health care provider would identify all known risk factors:

- Occupational exposure (cotton fiber, coal dust, asbestos)
- Socioeconomic status
- Cigarette smoking (duration, depth of inhalation, number of cigarettes smoked)
- Family history of disease
- Air pollution
- α_1-antitrypsin defect
- Age

Clearly, the behavioral causes of COPD are cigarette smoking and associated cigarette behaviors. Age, family history, the genetic defect, and air pollution are nonbehavioral. Socioeconomic status and occupational exposure are more difficult to categorize, since both of them have a behavioral as well as a nonbehavioral component. The importance of identifying nonbehavioral factors must be emphasized, because it provides program planners with more realistic expectations regarding the ultimate effectiveness of the program.

Phases 4 and 5. Educational diagnosis

Phases 4 and 5 are concerned with the educational diagnosis. Green and associates have identified three major categories of factors that have an impact on health behavior: (1) predisposing, (2) enabling, and (3) reinforcing factors.

Predisposing factors include such variables as individuals' knowledge, attitudes, values, and perceptions regarding health behaviors. Enabling factors involve availability of resources, accessibility of resources, and requisite skills and knowledge. Reinforcing factors, crucial during any change process, include the attitudes and behavior of health personnel or "significant others," such as peers, parents, and employers.

During phase 4 all the factors that may predispose, enable, or reinforce voluntary change in behavior are identified. In phase 5 these factors are analyzed and decisions are made as to which factors will receive intervention.

Phase 6. Administration

Phase 6 is considered the administrative component of the model. During this phase, the health education program is planned and implemented.

Phase 7. Evaluation

The final phase of the PRECEDE model is evaluation. Specific levels include evaluation of the process of the health education program; evaluation of the impact of predisposing, enabling, reinforcing, and behavioral factors; and evaluation of program outcomes, such as health and social benefits. Program planners should be aware that evaluation should be a continuous process throughout all phases of the development and implementation of the health education program.

Health education programs are effective only to the extent that they influence health practices that research shows to be causally related to desired health outcomes.[18] By providing a systematic approach to diagnosis of cause-and-effect relationships between behavior and health, the PRECEDE model provides key direction and guidance to health education program planners.

IMPLICATIONS FOR RESPIRATORY CARE PRACTITIONERS

Factors that contributed to the expanded roles and responsibilities of health professionals were examined in the first half of this chapter. As a result of these broadened roles, health-related professionals are providing services beyond the traditional curing function. These additional services include health-promotion, disease-prevention, and health education activities.

In the field of respiratory care, these new services and responsibilities are allowing respiratory care professionals to expand the scope and nature of their practice. In addition, respiratory care practitioners are delivering health care in a variety of new settings, such as the work site, the home, and the community. Provision of health care in these new and alternative settings also has had an impact on the nature of health care practice; respiratory care practitioners, as well as other health professionals, now have the opportunity to offer preventive services as well as rehabilitative services.

Setting for services

In analyzing the manner in which health care professionals are providing such care to various segments of the population, it is often useful to organize health promotion and health education services according to the settings in which these services are provided. The settings range from health care institutions to the work site and the home, the community, and educational institutions.[11,21]

Respiratory care practitioners provide important health-promotion and health education services in all of those settings.[22] The following is a brief summary of the types of service provided by respiratory care practitioners in each setting.

Health care institutions. The health care institutions in which respiratory care professionals practice health promotion and health education services include inpatient facilities (hospitals and nursing homes) and ambulatory care facilities (physicians' offices, clinics, health maintenance organizations, prison health services, surgical care centers). Within these health care institutions, respiratory care practitioners perform a variety of vital primary, secondary, and tertiary health promotion services.

In the area of primary prevention, respiratory care professionals organize smoking-awareness and smoking-cessation programs for staff, employees, and patients. In this role, respiratory care practitioners provide multiple opportunities for program participants to receive appropriate information and develop requisite skills to resist or cease smoking.[21]

Secondary prevention involves early diagnosis and further prevention of the debilitating consequences of a disease. Respiratory care professionals are involved in a variety of diagnostic procedures. These include early detection of small-airway dysfunction, pulmonary function screening, and hypertension screening. If pulmonary diseases are detected, it is the responsibility of the respiratory care practitioner to provide appropriate health care information and to develop a health promotion/education program based on the patient's needs and values.[21-23]

Tertiary prevention programs, also known as rehabilitation programs, are concerned with instruction of patients in rehabilitation techniques, exercise tolerance, bronchial hygiene, breathing retraining, and disease education.[21] Chapter 34 provides details on the goals, objectives, and methods of cardiopulmonary rehabilitation programs.

Work site. Health promotion at the work site is being advocated as a cost-effective approach to controlling health care costs (direct costs and insurance costs), preventing employee absenteeism, increasing job satisfaction, and increasing productivity.[11] As a member of an interdisciplinary health care team at the work site, the respiratory care practitioner's responsibilities may include (1) pulmonary function and hypertension screening, (2) development of smoking-cessation and stress-management programs, and (3) acting as a consultant in development of policies at the work site related to smoking on the job and exposure to occupational hazards (asbestos, cotton, and other fibers).[21-23]

Home. Home health care is one of the fastest-growing segments of health care delivery. Home care is defined as the provision of health and related social support services to physically and mentally impaired persons in their places of residence.[24] Advocates of this approach emphasize its cost effectiveness and its humane approach to delivery of health care services. According to Barhydt-Wezenaar[24]:

By bringing health care services to people in their own homes, hospitalization can often be prevented and residential health care facility placement can be delayed. Cost savings resulting from the provision of home care services, which can be offered at a cost well below the costs of institutional health care, provide added incentive for the use of home care services. . . . Making available care in one's own home or in an alternative home setting is a realistic and often more humane approach to cultivating the health and well-being of people.

A variety of health care services can be provided in the home. Such services range from chronic care for totally dependent patients to care for patients whose needs are temporary. In the home, respiratory care practitioners perform traditional functions, such as pulmonary screening and provision of comprehensive pulmonary rehabilitation services. In addition to therapeutic care, respiratory care practitioners provide essential education services for smokers, nonsmokers who reside with smokers, persons with asthma, and persons with cystic fibrosis.[21-23] Chapter 35 gives details on the role of respiratory care practitioners in the provision of home care.

Community. Health promotion and health education services performed in health care facilities, at the work site, and in the home generally focus on health care for individuals. At the community level, health promotion activities are usually directed toward groups of persons. Some health promotion services that may be performed by respiratory care practitioners at the community level include the development of community smoking-cessation programs, development and implementation of family asthma programs, sponsorship of community better-breathing clubs, and development of community group sessions for persons with COPD. In addition, respiratory care practitioners may provide important services as volunteers for the American Lung Association, the American Heart Association, and the American Red Cross. They also may serve as educators and exhibitors at community health fairs.[21,22]

Educational institutions. Given the fact that the development of many unhealthy behaviors can begin in childhood, educational institutions (particularly the elementary and secondary schools) provide an ideal setting in which to begin health education activities. Tobacco education programs are a good example of this type of activity.

As noted in the first half of this chapter, cigarette smoking is considered the primary risk factor of many of today's leading causes of death. An ever-increasing body of research is documenting that the development of this behavior generally occurs in late childhood or during adolescence. Consequently, it is necessary to educate our youth about the hazards of cigarettes. Educational institutions provide the best setting in which to offer tobacco education programs, and respiratory care practitioners are among the best-equipped health professionals to provide such learning experiences.

Successful tobacco education programs have several key characteristics. The programs should be initiated while children are in elementary school, preferably in kindergarten or first grade. Even in these early grades, children are aware of cigarettes and have begun to formulate beliefs and values regarding their use or nonuse. These factors should be considered in the development of any health education program.[25]

At very early ages, family factors appear to be a strong and consistent influence on children's smoking behaviors, knowledge, and attitudes. Because of this, parents also should be educated in the ways they can best promote the development of antismoking values in their children.[25]

Program planners must recognize that children's and adolescents' beliefs and behaviors are shaped by influences outside the school and family environment. Consequently, children and adolescents should be educated regarding the impact that their peers and the media have on the development of behaviors that are detrimental to their health.[25]

The role of the family

Regardless of the setting chosen for the delivery of health promotion services, it must be recognized that the family plays a crucial role in developing and maintaining the well-being of its members. The family has unique characteristics that have a bearing on the health knowledge and behaviors of its members and on the family's use of the health care delivery system. These characteristics include ethnicity, socioeconomic status, level of education, culture and traditions, and family structure. Thus, respiratory care practitioners should be sensitive to the needs and values of the family in order to develop and implement effective health promotion programs.[26]

Many health care institutions are becoming involved in family health care. Health care facilities are developing internal support systems by offering disease-specific family support services, family wellness programs, and exercise and health promotion programs. Hospitals are forming family support systems with community and religious organizations. In addition, they are providing referral services to social service agencies.[27]

Persons who provide health care in the home have recognized that the presence of family members or other care givers provides an opportunity for the patient to remain in his or her home while receiving health care. Family members can be trained in many of the maintenance functions performed by health care providers. As a result of family involvement, persons who need such services as ventilator therapy are able to receive requisite health care in the comfort of their own homes.[27]

The role of the family will receive increasing attention as the government, health care providers, and the public work together to reduce the costs and consequences of the leading causes of premature morbidity and mortality.

SUPPORTING THE GOALS OF *HEALTHY PEOPLE*

As noted earlier, the US government believes that the key to reducing premature morbidity and mortality is the adoption of prevention services, health protection services, and health promotion services. Within these broad categories, fifteen priority areas and 226 measurable objectives have been identified to facilitate achievement of the national health goals.

Achievement of these national health goals requires a concerted effort from a multitude of health care providers; one group of health care professionals alone cannot be expected to assume responsibility for accomplishment of these goals. Consequently, allied health professional organizations should determine where they can most effectively channel their energies and resources toward the achievement of these goals.

Three of the fifteen priority areas and several of the objectives within these priority areas are particularly important for respiratory care practitioners. These include high blood pressure control (preventive services), accident prevention and injury control (health protection services), and smoking control (health promotion services).

High blood pressure control

If left untreated, hypertension becomes the leading cause of cerebrovascular disease and a major risk factor of cardiovascular disease and renal failure. It is estimated that approximately 60 million Americans have blood pressure high enough to increase their risk of premature morbidity and mortality. Of these persons, more than 50% require medical treatment, with the remainder requiring regular medical surveillance.[9]

Objectives in this priority area with which the respiratory care professional should be familiar include the following[9]:

- *Improved health status.* By 1990 at least 60% of the estimated population with definite high blood pressure (160/95 or higher) should have attained successful long-term blood pressure control (ie, a blood pressure at or below 140/90 for 2 or more years).
- *Increased public-professional awareness.* By 1990 at least 50% of adults should be able to state the principal risk factors for coronary heart disease and stroke (ie, high blood pressure, cigarette smoking, elevated blood cholesterol levels, diabetes).

   By 1990 at least 90% of adults should be able to state whether their current blood pressure is normal (below 140/90) or elevated on the basis of a reading taken at the most recent visit to a medical or dental professional or other trained reader.
- *Improved services protection.* By 1990 no geopolitical area of the US should be without an effective public program to identify persons with high blood pressure and to follow up on their treatment.

A variety of activities have been identified to facilitate achievement of these objectives. These activities include the development, implementation, and evaluation of public information and education campaigns, risk-reduction programs, relaxation therapy, screening and surveillance programs, and dietary changes (ie, reduction of sodium intake).[9]

Accident prevention and injury control

The number one cause of death among the 1- to 44-year age group is accidents, generally motor vehicle accidents. However, of particular importance to the respiratory care practitioner is the risk of accidental injury and death due to acute airway obstruction, which is especially high among young children.

Objectives in this priority area with which respiratory care professionals should be familiar include the following[9]:

- *Improved health status.* By 1990 the home accident fatality rate for children under 15 should be no greater than 5.0 per 100,000 children.

  By 1990 the mortality rate for drowning should be reduced to no more than 3.0 per 100,000.
- *Reduced risk factors.* By 1990 at least 110 million functional smoke alarm systems should be installed in residential units.
- *Improved services protection.* By 1990 virtually all injured persons in need should have access to regionalized systems of trauma centers.

Prevention of accidental injury and death involves the development and implementation of a variety of activities. These range from development of public safety education campaigns to modification of environmental hazards (including those in the home and the community). In addition, legislation should be introduced to reduce the risk of manufacturing items that may contribute to acute airway obstruction among small children.

Smoking control

Cigarette smoking is the number one determinant of mortality and morbidity in the US. Persons who smoke have a 70% higher rate of premature death than those who do not smoke. The consequences and costs of smoking cigarettes are delineated below.

Consequences. Cigarette smokers are at great risk of premature mortality and morbidity from emphysema, chronic bronchitis, cancers of the respiratory tract, and coronary heart disease. It is estimated that 350,000 deaths each year can be directly attributed to cigarette smoking; 20,000 of these deaths are caused by COPD.[9,28] According to Romer[29]:

The relationship between cigarette smoking and COPD was among the first recognized and is the best understood of the dis-

eases caused by smoking. Investigation into the role of cigarette smoking is that the development of COPD leaves no room for reasonable doubt based on the experimental epidemiological evidence—cigarette smoking is the major cause of COPD in the US.

Even in the absence of clinical manifestations of COPD, the following respiratory complications have been observed more frequently among smokers than among nonsmokers: respiratory tract infections, more protracted respiratory symptoms following mild viral illnesses, and postoperative respiratory complications.[28] It has long been known that cigarette smoking contributes to low infant birth weight, and research is now documenting an increased incidence of respiratory disorders in children of cigarette smokers.[29]

Costs. In 1984 a study was conducted for the purpose of estimating the costs of major illnesses created by cigarette smoking for the years 1964 through 1983. The costs resulting from cancer, heart disease, and COPD were estimated. These costs were evaluated in terms of direct health care costs and lost productivity due to cigarette-related illness and premature death. It was ascertained that over this 20-year period, cigarette-induced illnesses had cost our economy nearly $932 billion in lost productivity and direct health care costs. Of the $932 billion, about one third ($315 billion) was attributed to illnesses related to COPD.[30]

Since 1964 more than 30 million Americans have quit smoking and the proportion of smokers has declined from 42% to less than 30% of the adult population. Although these figures are encouraging, millions of Americans continue to smoke, contributing to the high toll of premature death and disability and exorbitant health-related costs.

To combat the effects of smoking, the US Public Health Service identified the following priority objectives[9]:

- *Reduced risk factors.* By 1990 the proportion of adults who smoke should be reduced to below 25%.

  By 1990 the proportion of children and youth 12 to 18 years of age who smoke should be reduced to below 6%.
- *Increased public-professional awareness.* By 1990 at least 85% of the adult population should be aware of the special risk of developing and worsening chronic obstructive lung disease, including bronchitis and emphysema, among smokers.

As with high blood pressure control and accident and injury control, the activities that have been identified for the control of smoking include education campaigns in the schools and community at large, the development and implementation of risk-reduction programs, the implementation of smoking-cessation programs,[31] and the introduction of legislation to curtail smoking in public places.

SUMMARY

There is a revolution in health care. This revolution is based on the increasing recognition that the health status of the American population is determined mostly by factors over which individuals have control: their health behaviors and life-style patterns. However, the philosophy underlying our current health care delivery system is that responsibility for the health status of Americans rests with health care providers. In the context of this new recognition of individual responsibility, improvement of the health status of Americans requires redirection of the health care delivery system.

Since at least 1979, the US government has maintained the position that one of the most effective methods of reducing premature morbidity and mortality is to implement health promotion activities at the national, state, and local levels. To this end, the US government, through the Department of Health and Human Services, identified national health goals and delineated several steps necessary to achieve these goals.

On the basis of these governmental initiatives, many health professions have reformulated their roles and responsibilities for delivering health care. Reformulation of these roles and responsibilities has occurred through the establishment of official standards regarding health promotion and disease-prevention practices. To that end, this chapter has explored the changing nature of health care delivery for health-related professionals.

Health promotion was viewed as consisting of three interrelated concepts: holistic health care, high-level wellness, and disease prevention. Health education was considered the core of health promotion efforts.

Ideally, health education efforts should be directed at the introduction and strengthening of desirable health behaviors while eliminating or weakening behaviors that may be detrimental to a person's health. To illustrate how health professionals may develop health education programs aimed at voluntarily changing undesirable health behaviors, the seven-phase PRECEDE model was presented.

For the respiratory care practitioner, health promotion services can be delivered in a variety of settings, including health care institutions, the work site, the home, the community, and educational institutions. In each of these settings, respiratory care professionals may provide a variety of educational and therapeutic health care services.

However, respiratory care practitioners represent only one of several groups of health professionals who can effectively help to reduce premature morbidity and mortality. This requires collaboration from many sectors: health care providers, governmental agencies, and the American people. Efforts directed toward preventing the onset of disease appear to offer the best means of eliminating the costs and consequences of our major killers. Clearly, prevention is an idea whose time has come.

REFERENCES

1. US Department of Health, Education, and Welfare: Healthy people: the surgeon general's report on health promotion and disease prevention (DHEW-PHS pub no 79-55071), Washington, DC, 1979, US Government Printing Office.
2. Bunker JF et al: Curricular implications of health promotion and disease prevention in allied health education, J Allied Health 15: 329-338, 1986.
3. Hamburg MV: Health education: a tool for preventive care in allied health, J Allied Health 15: 305-308, 1986.
4. Martin-Peterson J and Cottrell RR: Self-concept, values, and health behavior, Health Educ 18:6-9, 1987.
5. Breslow L: A positive strategy for the nation's health, JAMA 242: 2093-2095, 1979.
6. Du Val MK: Mary Switzer memorial lecture: health education, health promotion, and the allied health professions, J Allied Health 11:13-20, 1982.
7. Torrens PR: Historical evolution and overview of health services in the United States. In Williams SJ and Torrens PR, editors: Introduction to health services, ed 2, New York, 1984, John Wiley & Sons.
8. US Dept of Health and Human Services: Promoting health/preventing disease: objectives for the nation, Washington, DC, 1980, US Government Printing Office.
9. US Dept of Health and Human Services, Public Health Service: Implementation plans for attaining the objectives for the nation, Washington, DC, 1983, US Government Printing Office.
10. McTernan EJ and Rice NC: An overview of the role of allied health professionals in the health promotion and disease prevention movement, J Allied Health 15:289-294, 1986.
11. Douglas PD: Practice implications of health promotion and disease prevention in allied health, J Allied Health 15:323-328, 1986.
12. Axton KL and Rice NC: Planning for health promotion in the RC curriculum, AARC Times 12(6):20, 22, 24, 1988.
13. Duncan DF and Gold RS: Reflections: health promotion—what is it? Health Values 10:47-48, 1986.
14. Eberst RM: Defining health: a multidimensional model, J School Health 54:99-104, 1984.
15. Greenberg JS: Health and wellness: a conceptual differentiation, J School Health 55:403-406, 1985.
16. Green K: Health promotion: its terminology, concepts, and modes of practice, Health Values 9: 8-14, 1985.
17. Alles WF, Rubinson L, and Monismith S: Health promotion. In Rubinson L and Alles W, editors: Health education: foundations for the future, St Louis, 1984, Times Mirror/Mosby College Publishing.
18. Shirreffs JA: The nature and meaning of health education. In Rubinson L and Alles W, editors: Health education: foundations for the future, St Louis, 1984, Times Mirror/Mosby College Publishing.
19. National Task Force on the Preparation and Practice of Health Educators, Inc: A framework for the development of competency-based curricula for entry level health educators, New York, 1986, National Task Force on the Preparation and Practice of Health Educators, Inc.
20. Green LW et al: Health education planning: a diagnostic approach, Palo Alto, Calif, 1980, Mayfield Publishing Co.
21. Beckett RG: The respiratory care practitioner role in health promotion. In Kra E, editor: Proceedings of allied health leadership in health promotion and disease prevention, University of Connecticut at Storrs and State University of New York at Stony Brook, 1986.
22. Bunch D: RTs take the lead in health promotion, AARC Times 12(6):26-33, 66, 1988.
23. Axton KL: Implications of health promotion and disease prevention for the practice of respiratory care. In Kra E, editor: Proceedings of allied health leadership in health promotion and disease prevention, University of Connecticut at Storrs and State University of New York at Stony Brook, 1986.

24. Barhydt-Wezenaar N: Home care and hospice. In Jonas S, editor: Health care delivery in the United States, ed 3, New York, 1986, Springer Publishing Co, p 237.

25. Tucker AW: Elementary school children and cigarette smoking: a review of the literature, Health Educ 18(3):18-27, 1987.

26. Crooks CE, Iammarino NK, and Weinberg AD: The family's role in health promotion, Health Values 11(2):7-12, 1987.

27. Robinson PD, Roe H, and Boys LJ: The focus of hospitals on family care, Health Values 11(2): 19-24, 1987.

28. US Dept of Health, Education, and Welfare: Smoking and health: a report of the Surgeon General (DHEW-PHS pub no 79-50066), Washington, DC, 1979, US Government Printing Office.

29. Romer K: Smoking and health: health promotion/disease prevention curriculum modules for allied health professionals (no. 11), Dallas, 1986, The University of Texas Health Science Center at Dallas, p 18.

30. National Interagency Council on Smoking and Health: Cigarette-induced medical costs exceed $930 billion, Smoking and Health Reporter, Bloomington, Ind, 1984, Indiana University.

31. Nett L: Respiratory care and lung health promotion: a perfect union for the 1990s, AARC Times 12(6):41-42, 1988.

34

Cardiopulmonary Rehabilitation

Kenneth A. Wyka

Steady improvements in acute care are presenting new medical and social problems. As more survive the acute phases of various illnesses, there are increasing numbers of persons with chronic disorders that manifest themselves in a wide spectrum of physiologic, psychological, and social disabilities.

Foremost among these persons are those with chronic cardiopulmonary disease. Although differences in the original diagnosis can affect treatment outcomes and long-term survival, patients with chronic cardiopulmonary disorders have much in common. All tend to share an inability to cope effectively with the physiologic limitations that characterize their disease process. As a consequence of this physiologic disability, they commonly exhibit an array of psychosocial problems. The end result is all too often a less-than-desirable quality of life.

The high incidence of repeated hospitalizations and the progressive disability of these patients necessitate concerted efforts to establish purposeful and supervised programs of chronic care. Ideally, such programs should address both the physiologic impairment and its psychosocial consequences. This approach requires both a holistic and a long-term perspective for which trained personnel and physical facilities are currently in short supply. Part of the solution to this problem lies in the provision of comprehensive home care (see Chapter 35). Many chronically handicapped patients require daily care, some of which can be provided in ambulatory centers but the bulk of which must be provided and carried out within the home environment.

However, comprehensive home care cannot succeed without complementary efforts to facilitate patients' physical, mental, and social readaptation to their disability. We are in desperate need of both better facilities and more highly skilled manpower capable of offering a full spectrum of cardiopulmonary rehabilitation services.

Clearly, respiratory care can and should play an important role in the provision of cardiopulmonary rehabilitation services. Until recently, however, respiratory care educa-

tion has focused almost exclusively on development of the skills necessary to provide acute-care services. If respiratory care practitioners are to take a more active role in the long-term care and rehabilitation of patients with chronic disorders of the cardiopulmonary system, greater emphasis must be placed on development of the special knowledge and skills needed to assist patients in adapting to and living with their disability.

OBJECTIVES

This chapter provides foundation knowledge on the goals, methods, and current issues involved in organizing, implementing, and evaluating planned programs of rehabilitation for persons with chronic cardiopulmonary disorders. Because the scope of this text relates primarily to respiratory care, greater emphasis will be given to pulmonary rehabilitation programming. Specifically, on completion of this chapter, the reader will be able to:

1. Define the concept of pulmonary rehabilitation on the basis of position statements of the American College of Chest Physicians (ACCP) and the American Thoracic Society (ATS);

2. Differentiate between the physical and psychosocial bases of pulmonary rehabilitation;

3. Compare and contrast the potential benefits of pulmonary rehabilitation according to their current acceptability and probability;

4. Describe the patient-selection process, including criteria for entry, for a pulmonary rehabilitation program;

5. Discuss the importance of cardiopulmonary exercise evaluation in terms of patient selection and pulmonary rehabilitation program evaluation;

6. Describe the process of pulmonary rehabilitation on the basis of format, content, and program implementation;

7. Explain the importance of aerobic exercises and inspiratory muscle resistance training in the physical reconditioning process;

8. Differentiate pulmonary and cardiac rehabilitation on the basis of focus, procedure, and outcomes.

KEY TERMS

Most terms used in this chapter are defined in context. The following terms are introduced without explicit definition but may be found in the text glossary:

ACCP	ergometer
ADL	holistic
ATS	hypoglycemia
ambulation	METS
anaerobic threshold	multicompetent
contracture	multidisciplinary
CORF	psychosocial
disability	readaptation
	vocational

GOALS OF CARDIOPULMONARY REHABILITATION

Rehabilitation was defined by the Council on Rehabilitation in 1942 as "the restoration of the individual to the fullest medical, mental, emotional, social and vocational potential of which he/she is capable."[1] The overall goal is to maximize functional ability and to minimize the impact of the disability on the individual, the family, and the community.

In 1974 the American College of Chest Physicians' Committee on Pulmonary Rehabilitation defined pulmonary rehabilitation as follows[2]:

an art of medical practice wherein an individually tailored, multidisciplinary program is formulated which through accurate diagnosis, therapy, emotional support and education, stabilizes or reverses both the physio- and psychopathology of pulmonary diseases and attempts to return the patient to the highest possible functional capacity allowed by his/her pulmonary handicap and overall life situation.

In an official statement adopted in 1981, the American Thoracic Society Executive Committee delineated two principal objectives of pulmonary rehabilitation[3]:

1. To control and alleviate as much as possible the symptoms and pathophysiologic complications of respiratory impairment; and

2. To teach the patient how to achieve optimal capability for carrying out his/her activities of daily living.

Depending on the needs of the specific patient, comprehensive care may include the delivery of a structured, defined program of rehabilitation as an element of the patient's care. In the broadest sense, however, pulmonary re-

habilitation represents any method designed to improve the quality of life experienced by patients with disabling pulmonary disease.[4]

In the same sense, cardiac rehabilitation involves good, comprehensive cardiac care for patients with cardiovascular disease. In many ways, the philosophy, objectives, and methods of both pulmonary and cardiac rehabilitation share much in common. Key differences in the two approaches will be considered later in this chapter.

HISTORICAL PERSPECTIVE

Pulmonary rehabilitation is not a new concept. In 1951 Alvan Barach and associates[5] commented on the need for training programs for chronic lung patients with regard to "reconditioning" efforts to improve the ability to walk without dyspnea. Our apparent ignorance of the problem persisted into the 1960s, as the recommended treatment for patients with chronic lung disease included the administration of oxygen as well as rest and avoidance of stress. This produced a vicious cycle in the patient, resulting in skeletal muscle deterioration, progressive weakness and fatigue, and increasing levels of dyspnea, even at rest. Patients became homebound, then roombound, and eventually bedbound. Improved avenues of therapy and rehabilitation as suggested by Barach and associates were direly needed.

In 1962 Pierce and associates[6] published results that demonstrated Barach's insight into the value of pulmonary reconditioning. They observed that rehabilitative efforts in patients with chronic obstructive pulmonary disease (COPD) permitted them to perform exercises with lower pulse rates, respiratory rates, minute volumes, and CO_2 production. However, these benefits were achieved without significant changes in pulmonary function.

In 1964 Paez and associates[7] indicated that efficiency of motion and oxygen use were both improved in patients with chronic lung disorders as the result of reconditioning techniques. Some 4 years later, Christie[8] demonstrated that these rehabilitative benefits could be acquired on an outpatient basis with minimal supervision.

More recently, Hudson and associates[9] demonstrated a significant reduction in the days of hospitalization of 44 patients after they had begun participation in an outpatient pulmonary rehabilitation program. A shorter-term inpatient program conducted by Moser and associates[10] at the University of California (San Diego) School of Medicine showed significant postprogram reductions in participants' O_2 consumption, minute ventilation, heart rate, and respiratory rate during exercise. Moreover, of the 29 patients who completed the program, 16 improved in terms of their dyspnea class and 11 demonstrated a significant gain with regard to their activities of daily living.

Although long-term results of pulmonary rehabilitation are contradictory and often difficult to interpret, recent evidence suggests that program deficiencies may be a contributing factor in cases in which no improvements in pertinent physical or psychosocial measures are obtained. Specifically, insufficient theoretical and practical training of health professionals in rehabilitation methods, a lack of uniformity in rehabilitation teams, and treatment courses that are too few in number or too short in duration have been implicated as reasons for less-than-satisfactory outcomes.[11]

These investigations have changed the ways in which patients with chronic lung disease are being managed. With increasing evidence of its efficacy in improving patients' exercise tolerance, decreasing the frequency and duration of their acute care and enhancing their quality of life and sense of well-being, well-planned and comprehensive programs of pulmonary rehabilitation are being organized in a variety of settings. Regardless of setting or design, such programs must be founded on the sound application of current knowledge in the clinical and social sciences.

SCIENTIFIC BASES

Rehabilitation must focus on the patient as a whole and not solely on the underlying pathophysiologic disturbance. For this reason, effective rehabilitation programming must combine knowledge from both the clinical and the social sciences. Knowledge from the clinical sciences is useful in quantifying the extent of physiologic impairment and in setting reasonable expectations regarding the improvements that can and cannot be expected from physical reconditioning. Knowledge from the social sciences is helpful in determining the psychological, social, and vocational impact of the disability on the patient and his or her family and in establishing ways to improve the patient's quality of life.

This combined approach is substantiated by recent evidence demonstrating a high degree of correlation between objective measures of patients' physiologic impairment and their quality of life.[12] Indeed, in these patients, social and psychological indicators better predict both the frequency and the length of subsequent acute care rehospitalizations than do traditional measures of pulmonary dysfunction.[13]

Physical reconditioning

At rest, a person maintains homeostasis by balancing external, internal, and cellular respiration. External respiration is gas exchange effected by the lungs, internal respiration is gas exchange effected at the tissue level, and cellular respiration represents the oxidative process that occurs in the mitochondria for the production of energy in the form of adenosine triphosphate (ATP).

Physical activity, such as exercise, increases these processes, and to maintain homeostasis the cardiorespiratory system must keep pace. As illustrated in Fig. 34-1, this is

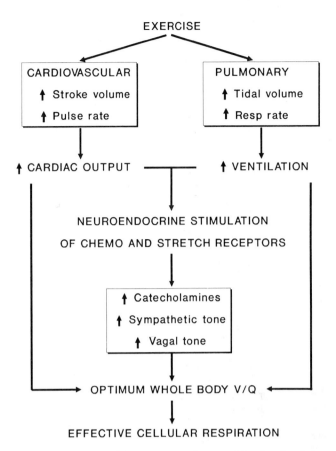

Fig. 34-1   The body's response to increased levels of activity such as exercise.

accomplished in a number of ways.[14] Ventilation and circulation increase to supply tissues and cells with necessary oxygen and to eliminate the increased levels of carbon dioxide that result from oxidative metabolism. This production by the cells of carbon dioxide ($\dot{V}CO_2$) and consumption of oxygen ($\dot{V}O_2$) are frequently expressed as a ratio and referred to as the respiratory quotient (RQ). Normally, at rest, a person consumes about 250 ml of O_2 per minute and, in the process, produces approximately 200 ml of CO_2 per minute. The normal RQ is therefore about 0.8. Although the final pathway for carbohydrate, protein, and fat metabolism is shared, there are differences in the respiratory quotient for each. The RQ of carbohydrate is 1.0, that of protein is 0.8, and that of fat is 0.7.

As shown in Fig. 34-2, oxygen consumption and carbon dioxide production also increase in linear fashion as exercise levels increase. If the body is unable to deliver adequate oxygen for the demands of energy metabolism, blood lactate levels increase. The buffering of lactic acid results in increased carbon dioxide production. This provides an added stimulus to ventilation. The point at which increased levels of lactic acid result in an increased $\dot{V}CO_2$ and $\dot{V}E$ is referred to as the anaerobic threshold.[14] The RQ at this point is equal to or greater than 1.0, indicating that

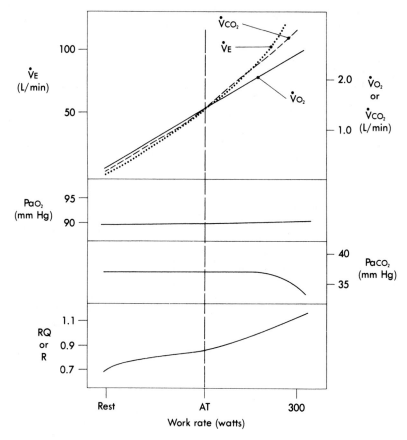

Fig. 34-2   Schematized data representing the relationship between ventilation and O_2 uptake and CO_2 output and the changes in gas tension during incremental exercise. *AT,* Anaerobic threshold. (From Lane EE and Walker JF: Clinical arterial blood gas analysis, St Louis, 1987, The CV Mosby Co.)

carbon dioxide production has equaled or surpassed oxygen consumption. When the anaerobic threshold is exceeded, metabolism becomes anaerobic, thus decreasing energy production and increasing fatigue.

Increases in physical activity result in increases in ventilation. This, coupled with an increased cardiac output, provides a ventilation/perfusion ratio that is optimal for adequate gas exchange (see Fig. 34-1).

The maximum voluntary ventilation appears to be a good indicator of the respiratory system's ability to handle increased levels of physical activity. It can be measured directly or estimated by multiplying the forced expiratory volume in 1 second (FEV_1) by a factor of 35. Normally, a person can achieve 60% to 70% of the maximum voluntary ventilation value on maximum exercise. This indicates that sufficient reserve still exists in the respiratory system and that ventilation is not the primary limiting factor for the termination of exercise.[14]

The exercise capabilities of patients with chronic pulmonary disorders who lack this reserve will be severely limited. In these patients the high rate of CO_2 production during exercise results in respiratory acidosis and a sensation

of breathlessness or dyspnea out of proportion to the level of activity. In addition, muscles (both skeletal and respiratory) use higher percentages of the total oxygen consumption as work levels in these patients increase (Fig. 34-3). In combination, these factors contribute to a high degree of patient intolerance for any significant increase in the level of physical activity.

Pulmonary rehabilitation must therefore include efforts to recondition patients physically and reduce exercise intolerance by strengthening essential muscle groups, improving overall oxygen use, and enhancing the body's cardiovascular response to physical activity.

Psychosocial support

If the overall goal of pulmonary rehabilitation is to improve the quality of patients' lives, then physical reconditioning alone provides an insufficient basis for successful programming. Indeed, attrition in pulmonary rehabilitation programs is associated more with the degree to which patients' psychological and social needs are met than with the success or failure of physical reconditioning efforts.[15,16]

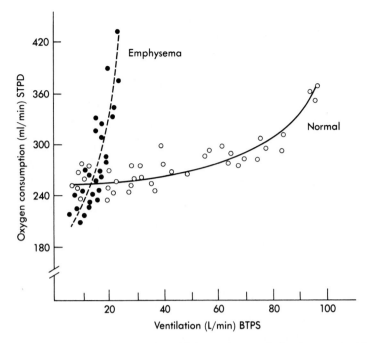

Fig. 34-3 The changes in O_2 consumption with increasing ventilation in normal subject (○) and in patient with emphysema (●). *BTPS,* Body temperature, saturated with water vapor, body pressure; *STPD,* volume of dry gas at 0°C and 760 mm Hg atmospheric pressure. (From Cherniack RM, Cherniack L, and Naimark A: Respiration in health and disease, ed 3, Philadelphia, 1984, WB Saunders Co.)

That a relationship exists between patients' physical, mental, and social well-being has been clearly established.[17] The term psychosomatic refers to the relationship between the emotional state or outlook of a person (psyche) and the physical responses of the person's body (soma). Everyday life is full of relationships such as, for example, the physical fatigue that follows a period of emotional tension. Many of these associations are considered part of normal human behavior. However, emotional states such as stress can cause or aggravate an existing physical problem. Likewise, physical manifestations of disease, such as recurrent dyspnea, can exacerbate stress.

Moreover, the characteristic progressiveness of chronic pulmonary disease can negatively affect patients' overall outlook on their disease and thus their motivation to adapt to its consequences. Respiratory care practitioners must realize that all their skilled technical services, as well as the best pharmacologic therapy, can be negated and a patient driven to a steadily downhill course because of an unfavorable mental orientation. Of course, emotional problems are not unique to patients with respiratory disease. Depression and hostility are common correlates of many acute and chronic diseases. In chronic respiratory disease, however, this may be a double-edged sword. Not only can emotional disturbances affect the general well-being of the patient, but they may also directly aggravate the very defects that are responsible for the underlying disability.[18]

The role of emotional and personality problems in the genesis of childhood bronchial asthma is well known and has been extensively recorded in the medical literature. It is probable that certain cases of adult (intrinsic) asthma, for which no specific allergic basis can be found, are attributable, in part, to psychological or emotional disorders. In chronic pulmonary disease, however, psychological factors are more effect than cause.[17] Often the patient with progressive emphysema has severe anxiety, hostility, and stress as a direct consequence of the disability. Because patients are fearful of economic loss and death, they can also develop hostility toward the disease and often toward those with whom they come into close contact.

Unfortunately, proper attention to the psychological component of chronic lung disease has been largely neglected.[17-19] Although the reasons for this neglect are many, a disproportionate emphasis on the physical basis of diseases and associated methods of therapy in the education of health professionals is a major factor. The fact that psychological therapy has been used successfully in the management of bronchial asthma justifies its wider application to nonasthmatic diseases as well.

In regard to the social needs of patients with chronic lung disease, one commonly observes patients spontaneously deriving support and encouragement from simple association with each other. This informal observation suggests that the presence or absence of social support mechanisms may be a factor in determining how well patients who lack a strong social support structure are at higher risk of rehospitalization than those who have such networks in place.[13] Clearly, well-designed pulmonary rehabilitation programming should take advantage of this knowledge and address the social support needs of participating patients.

In terms of social function, the physiologic impairment of chronic lung disease can severely restrict a patient's ability to perform even the most routine tasks that require physical exertion. Obviously, intolerance for physical exertion delimits the scope of a patient's social activity. More important, however, is the potential loss of confidence in the ability to care for oneself that can accompany such impairments and the resultant loss of feelings of dignity and self-worth. These self-perceptions are only worsened when family, friends, or health care professionals "label" the patient as a pulmonary cripple. Such factors can establish a cycle of further social withdrawal and intensified psychological depression with an increased frequency of acute exacerbations of the underlying disease.

It is here that the link between the physical reconditioning and psychosocial support components of pulmonary rehabilitation becomes most evident. By reducing exercise intolerance and enhancing the body's cardiovascular response to physical activity, patients can achieve a more independent and active life-style. For some, simply being able to walk to the market or play with their grandchildren will contribute to a greater feeling of social importance and self-worth. For others, physical conditioning may allow a return to near normal levels of activity, despite recurrent periods of dyspnea. Among those for whom physical reconditioning gives a level of normalcy to daily activities, opportunities exist to address vocational needs and expectations.

Many disabled patients with pulmonary disorders are in their economically productive years and are anxious to return to economic self-sufficiency. For them, occupational retraining and job placement are necessary ingredients of a purposeful rehabilitation program. Such a program should be based on the individual needs and expectations of each patient.[20] Much study is yet needed to categorize occupations in terms of energy requirements of the respiratory system and to derive simple but informative tests of the work of breathing to enable the rehabilitation team to match patients to those jobs in which they would have the greatest chance of success. Not only must the patient's physical status be considered, but education, past experience, aptitude, and personality must be considered as well.[20-22] Obviously, this requires both the skills of health-related professionals, such as vocational counselors and occupational therapists,[23] and the cooperation of business and industry in the community. Successful vocational rehabilitation efforts have already been made in cases of disability resulting from such conditions as incapacitating

trauma and stroke; only recently have similar approaches been applied in behalf of patients with pulmonary disability.[22,23]

PULMONARY REHABILITATION PROGRAMMING

Program goals and objectives

Pulmonary rehabilitation programs vary in their design and implementation but generally share common goals. Typically, these shared goals include the following[24-30]:
- Control of respiratory infections;
- Basic airway management;
- Improvement in ventilation and cardiac status;
- Improvement in ambulation and other types of physical activity;
- Reduction in overall medical costs;
- Reduction in hospitalizations;
- Psychosocial support;
- Occupational retraining and placement (when and where possible); and
- Family education, counseling, and support.

These general goals assist planners in formulating more specific program objectives. Depending on the specific needs of the participants, such objectives can include the following:
- Development of diaphragmatic breathing skills;
- Development of stress management and relaxation techniques;
- Involvement in a daily physical exercise regimen to condition both skeletal and respiration-related muscles;
- Adherence to proper hygiene, diet, and nutrition;
- Proper use of medications, oxygen, and breathing equipment (if applicable);
- Application of postural drainage with chest percussion/vibration (when indicated);
- Focus on group support; and
- Provisions for individual and family counseling.

When program objectives are specifically defined and structured in a measurable way, strategies can be tailored to ensure the maximum results and benefit. Demonstration of program efficacy also becomes easier and more acceptable to the medical community. However, benefits realized by participating patients are not always easy to identify and may be controversial.

Benefits and potential hazards

Benefits. An underlying assumption of all pulmonary rehabilitation programs designed for those with chronic lung disorders is that the disease process is progressive and irreversible. On the basis of this assumption, it is inappropriate to expect long-term improvements in objective indicators of pulmonary function, such as those obtained by means of spirometry or blood gas analysis. Indeed, the research literature clearly demonstrates that rehabilitation cannot affect the progressive deterioration in lung function that characterizes chronic pulmonary disorders.[11,31]

However, the evidence is just as convincing that properly implemented programs of pulmonary rehabilitation can improve a patient's overall use of oxygen by increasing the efficiency of muscle use and by promoting more effective breathing techniques. We know that exercise ventilation in patients with COPD is inefficient in that the oxygen cost for a given amount of ventilation is excessive.[32] We also know that training of specific skeletal muscle groups alone may not produce an improvement in exercise tolerance but that training of respiration-related muscles can improve exercise tolerance.[33,34]

Therefore, to maximize the desired results of pulmonary rehabilitation, any program must include an effort to recondition and retrain both the respiration-related and skeletal muscle groups. The box below classifies the benefits of exercise reconditioning for patients with chronic lung disorders on the basis of current knowledge of their acceptability and probability.[35]

As previously indicated, reconditioning provides more than just physiologic benefits. However, achievement of the related social, psychological, and vocational outcomes

---

POTENTIAL BENEFITS FROM EXERCISE RECONDITIONING

I. ACCEPTED BENEFITS

Increased physical endurance
Increased maximum oxygen consumption
Increased skill in performance with
    Decreased ventilation
    Decreased oxygen consumption
    Decreased heart rate
    Increased anaerobic threshold

II. POTENTIAL BENEFITS

Increased sense of well-being
Increased clearance of secretions
Increased hypoxic drive
Increased left ventricular function

III. UNLIKELY OR UNKNOWN BENEFITS

Prolonged survival
Improved pulmonary function tests
Lowered pulmonary artery pressure
Improved arterial blood gas results
Improved blood lipids
Change in muscle oxygen extraction
Change in step desaturation or apnea

From Hughes RL and Davison R: Limitations of exercise reconditioning in COLD, Chest 83:241-249, 1983.

---

requires a complementary and multidisciplinary focus on psychosocial readaptation. For this reason, programs that attend solely to physical reconditioning efforts are not truly rehabilitative in nature. Only those that address both physical and psychosocial needs should be considered true rehabilitation programs.

Naturally, physiologic benefits currently are more acceptable to the medical community and are easier to determine, measure, and document. Psychosocial benefits, on the other hand, tend to be both more controversial and more difficult to substantiate. Nonetheless, participants in comprehensive rehabilitation programs tend to feel better, experience less dyspnea, and have fewer infections and hospitalizations, and they usually are able to lead more active and productive lives than those who are not involved in or availed of such services. Ultimately, these benefits may be the best indicators of a program's success. However, continued work and investigation are still required to better define and quantify these potential benefits and thereby improve the content and delivery of pulmonary rehabilitation programming.

Potential hazards. While benefits to physical reconditioning and pulmonary rehabilitation can be expected and realized by a significant number of patients with chronic respiratory disorders, certain potential hazards do exist. These may be outlined as follows:

A. Cardiovascular abnormalities
    1. Arrhythmias (especially life-threatening ones) can be reduced through the administration of supplemental oxygen during exercise;
    2. Systemic hypotension.
B. Blood gas abnormalities
    1. Arterial desaturation;
    2. Hypercapnia.
C. Muscular abnormalities
    1. Functional or structural injuries;
    2. Diaphragmatic fatigue and failure;
    3. Exercise-induced muscle contracture.
D. Miscellaneous
    1. Exercise-induced asthma may be present in young patients with asthma but is rarely encountered in COPD;
    2. Hypoglycemia;
    3. Dehydration.

Although short-term and long-term hazards to pulmonary rehabilitation do exist, they can be minimized or eliminated. Proper patient selection, education, supervision, and monitoring are key factors in the reduction of possible hazards. It is to these methods that we now turn.

Patient evaluation and selection

Before a program of comprehensive pulmonary rehabilitation is begun, criteria for proper patient selection and inclusion into the program need to be defined and established. This should be done through extensive testing, evaluation, and assessment of patients.

Patient evaluation. Patient evaluation should begin with a complete patient history—medical, psychological, vocational, and social. A well-designed questionnaire and interview form will assist with this step.

The patient's history should be followed by a complete physical examination. A recent chest film, a resting electrocardiogram, a complete blood count, determination of serum electrolytes, and urinalysis will provide additional information on the patient's current medical status.

To ascertain the patient's cardiopulmonary status, a complete series of pulmonary function and cardiopulmonary stress tests should be performed. The pulmonary function testing should include assessment of pulmonary ventilation, lung volume determinations, diffusing capacity (D_{LCO}), and spirometry before and after bronchodilation. The cardiopulmonary stress test should include an electrocardiogram and should measure blood pressure, heart rate, respiratory rate, O_2 saturation, maximum ventilation ($\dot{V}_{E_{max}}$), O_2 consumption (either absolute $\dot{V}_{O_2}$ or METS, the multiple equivalents of resting O_2 consumption), CO_2 production ($\dot{V}_{CO_2}$), respiratory quotient (R), and the O_2 pulse during various graded levels of exercise on either an ergometer or a treadmill. These stages are usually spaced at 1- to 2-minute intervals, depending on the protocol selected and followed. In addition, an arterial line may be inserted to allow serial determinations of blood gases during the course of the evaluation. While this will provide the most accurate reflection of oxygenation and ventilation during graded activity, oximetry and transcutaneous membrane measurements are better tolerated and provide acceptable equivalent data.

It should be noted that evaluations of cardiopulmonary exercise are also useful in differentiating between primary respiratory or cardiac causes of exercise limitations.[36] Table 34-1 summarizes these key similarities and differences. Obviously, besides helping to differentiate between the underlying causes of exercise intolerance, application of cardiopulmonary exercise evaluation data assists practitioners in the proper placement of qualifying candidates into either pulmonary or cardiac rehabilitation programs.

For a cardiopulmonary exercise evaluation to be performed properly and safely, certain measures must be adhered to. A physician must be present during the entire test, and a cardiac "crash cart" with monitor, defibrillator, oxygen, cardiac drugs, and suction and airway equipment must be readily available. Staff members who conduct and assist with the procedure must be certified in basic and advanced life-support techniques, following either the American Heart Association or the American Red Cross standards. Just before the test the patient should have a physical examination including a resting electrocardiogram. The exercise test should be terminated promptly if the patient exhibits any major arrhythmias or experiences any angina or severe dyspnea.

The patient should fast for 8 hours before the procedure and should not take any medications that could alter test results. The patient should wear comfortable, loose-fitting clothing and footwear with adequate traction for treadmill or ergometer activity. The mouthpiece or face mask used during the test should be sized properly and fit comfortably, with no leaks. Test conditions should be as standardized as possible to allow for comparison of results before and after rehabilitation and those obtained periodically from year to year as the patient is treated and followed.

Emphasis is being placed on the value of exercise testing because it provides objective criteria for demonstrating the benefits of physical reconditioning and pulmonary rehabilitation in patients with chronic pulmonary disorders. Although improvement in pulmonary functions and arterial blood gases may not be evident, improvement in parameters measured during a cardiopulmonary exercise evaluation is demonstrable. Generally, exercise tolerance is enhanced and the anaerobic threshold is increased. In many persons oxygen consumption is increased with an improved METS at all levels of activity, especially at or near the anaerobic threshold. An improved cardiovascular response (heart rate, blood pressure, and cardiac output) has also been identified. Therefore, this type of testing is of definite value and should be included in the patient evaluation process before and after any pulmonary rehabilitation endeavor.

All of the procedures and tests identified here are necessary because they evaluate the patient's current cardiopulmonary condition. This will assist in proper patient selection, help to reduce the incidence of any patient injury or cardiopulmonary accident during the course of the rehabilitation program, assure that the patient can exercise and recondition safely, and serve as a basis for postprogram evaluation in determining acquired cardiopulmonary benefits and overall improvement in the patient's condition.

Table 34-1 Exercise Parameters Distinguishing Cardiac and Ventilatory (COPD) Limitations*

Parameter*	Cardiac†	COPD†
Max $\dot{V}_{O_2}$	↓	↓
Max HR	N or ↓	↓
O_2 pulse	↓	N
Max $\dot{Q}$	↓	↓
$\dot{Q}/\dot{V}_{O_2}$	↓	N
Pa_{O_2}	N	↓
Pa_{CO_2}	↓	↑
$\dot{V}_E/\dot{V}_{CO_2}$	↑	↑
AT	↓	N

*$\dot{V}_{O_2}$, Oxygen consumption; HR, heart rate; $\dot{Q}$, cardiac output; $\dot{V}_E/\dot{V}_{CO_2}$, ratio of ventilation to CO_2 production; AT, anaerobic threshold.
†N, Normal; ↑, increased; ↓, decreased.
From Lane EE and Walker JF: Clinical arterial blood gas analysis, St Louis, 1987, The CV Mosby Co.

Patient selection and rejection. Patients should be selected for pulmonary rehabilitation programs on the basis of the likelihood of their benefiting from such participation and activity. General indications and contraindications for inclusion in a comprehensive pulmonary rehabilitation program appear in the box below. Naturally, not all patients with chronic lung disorders are candidates for pulmonary rehabilitation. Those patients with end-stage disease who have little or no cardiopulmonary reserve probably would not be able to participate in the program activities and would therefore not benefit to any meaningful degree.

In addition, groups or classes should be kept homogeneous. Placing in a program persons who are at different stages of cardiopulmonary disability can prove to be very defeating. Those with mild to moderate impairment may become discouraged about how severe lung disease can become, and those with severe impairment will feel they cannot keep up with or maintain the level of activity exhibited by those with less severe impairment. It is best to group patients on the basis of severity and overall ability. In this way, they can participate, compete, and progress together in the program without frustration, fear, or loss of motivation.

Objectively, candidates considered for inclusion in a pulmonary rehabilitation program generally fall into one of the following groups:

- Patients in whom there is a respiratory limitation to exercise resulting in termination at a level less than 75% of the predicted maximum oxygen consumption ($\dot{V}_{O_{2max}}$);
- Patients in whom there is significant irreversible airway obstruction with a forced expiratory volume in 1 second (FEV_1) of less than 2 L or an FEV_1/FVC of less than 60%;
- Patients in whom there is a significant restrictive lung disease with a total lung capacity (TLC) of less than

80% of predicted and single-breath carbon monoxide diffusing capacity (D_{LCO}) of less than 80% of predicted;
- Patients with pulmonary vascular disease in whom the single-breath carbon monoxide diffusing capacity (D_{LCO}) is less than 80% of predicted or in whom exercise is limited to less than 75% of maximum predicted oxygen consumption (predicted $\dot{V}_{O_{2max}}$).

Patients may be excluded from pulmonary reconditioning or rehabilitation programs if they do not meet the criteria for inclusion. In addition, patients may also be rejected if there is a significant cardiovascular component to exercise limitation (with exclusion of pulmonary vascular disease) or there is an adverse cardiovascular response to exercise. Cardiac monitoring may be required during their reconditioning. As a result, these patients should be placed in an appropriate cardiac rehabilitation program and followed accordingly.

Program design and implementation

Having identified program objectives in an earlier section of this chapter and having just reviewed the patient-selection process, we can now take a serious look at program format, content, and implementation.

Format. Essentially, programs can have either an open-ended or a closed design, with or without planned follow-up sessions.[31,37-39] With an open-ended format, patients enter the program and progress through it until certain predetermined objectives are achieved. There is no set time frame. An individual patient can complete the program in weeks or in months, depending on his or her condition, needs, motivation, and performance. If the clinical objectives are not reached, the patient continues on with the program. This type of format is good for the patient who is self-directed, has scheduling difficulties, and requires certain specific individual attention. The major drawback is the lack of group support and involvement. This may be minimal at best or totally lacking. Program content can be presented on an individual basis by the course facilitator or through the use of audiovisual aids.

On the other hand, the closed design is more traditional and uses a set time period in which program content is covered. These pulmonary rehabilitation programs usually run for 8, 10, 12, or 16 weeks and classes may meet anywhere from one to three times a week. Class sessions are usually 1 to 3 hours long. Presentations are more formal, and group support and involvement are encouraged. Patients finish the program when the scheduled sessions are completed, not when predetermined clinical objectives are necessarily met. This can be a drawback. However, patients can enroll again if the anticipated improvements have not been realized. In addition, class size may prevent or reduce the amount of individualized attention a patient may receive.

Regardless of the format used, the overall aim of any pulmonary rehabilitation program is to present the essen-

---

INDICATIONS AND CONTRAINDICATIONS FOR PULMONARY REHABILITATION

INDICATIONS

Moderate to severe obstructive lung disease
Bronchial asthma and associated bronchitis (asthmatic bronchitis)
Combined obstructive and restrictive ventilatory defects
Chronic mucociliary clearance problems
Exercise limitations because of severe dyspnea

CONTRAINDICATIONS

Cardiovascular instability requiring cardiac monitoring (consider cardiac rehabilitation)
Malignant neoplasms involving the respiratory system
Severe arthritis or neuromuscular abnormalities (consider aquatic exercises for rehabilitation)

tial material to its patients, to have them complete a reconditioning regimen safely, and to demonstrate as much physical and psychosocial improvement as possible. In order for any results to be lasting, these programs must include periodic follow-up sessions and activities for reinforcement. Follow-up must be ongoing and available to all patients who complete pulmonary rehabilitation. Frequently this essential element of the process is difficult, but program coordinators must ensure that it is routinely scheduled. Follow-up or reinforcement could be open-ended (available during regular rehabilitation sessions and offering open attendance) or could be scheduled monthly, bimonthly, or quarterly. The important thing is to have some type of follow-up available.

Content. The actual content of any pulmonary rehabilitation effort is based on the identified or stated program objectives. Before patients are admitted to the formal program, however, they must be nonsmokers. Reconditioning and rehabilitation will have little or no value if the patient still smokes.[31] Consequently, some form of smoking-cessation program must be provided as a prerequisite for smokers. This could be achieved through group sessions, individualized counseling, hypnosis, use of pharmacologic aids, or programs conducted through the American Lung Association, the American Cancer Society, the American Heart Association, or any private concern. Smoking cessation can be conducted at the facility where reconditioning and rehabilitation sessions are held, or patients can be referred to outside programs. Results are not guaranteed, however, and many patients who smoke will find it difficult, if not impossible, to quit. Desire and motivation, along with reinforcement, are key elements in the elimination of tobacco from one's life-style.

The content provided during a rehabilitation program can be divided into educational and physical reconditioning components. To illustrate, Table 34-2 outlines a sample session that incorporates these two key components. One without the other will result in a less-than-effective program. Both components are needed to rehabilitate the patient with chronic pulmonary disease to a state of improved physical condition and psychosocial outlook.

As shown in Table 34-2, rehabilitation sessions ideally should run for 2 hours. However, shorter (60 to 90 minutes) or longer (150 minutes or more) sessions may be necessary, depending on group size, available equipment, and group interaction. It is advisable to have patients arrive 10 to 15 minutes before a scheduled session to allow for informal group interaction and support. Classes should begin on time and conclude promptly as scheduled. Educational presentations should be brief and to the point, with liberal use of audiovisuals or demonstrations to enhance understanding. To facilitate patient comprehension, the language should be simple and unnecessary technical terms or concepts should be avoided. Handouts that enhance certain points made during a presentation are both

useful and desirable. A folder or a notebook should be used by each patient to maintain all program materials and to keep a record of all related activities.

The physical reconditioning component of the pulmonary rehabilitation program consists primarily of an exercise prescription based on the results of the patient's pre-program cardiopulmonary evaluation. This prescription should include the following activities:

- Aerobic exercises for the lower extremity involving either walking on a flat, smooth surface for a specified period of time, walking on a treadmill for a specified distance or time, or pedaling a stationary bicycle for a specified distance or period of time. Patients with significant orthopedic deformities or disabilities should participate in aerobic aquatic exercises.
- Exercises for the upper extremity, with the use of either an ergometer or a rowing machine. This type of activity increases accessory muscle endurance by progressive exercise. Weights and/or calisthenics (including isometrics) may also be used if upper extremity ergometers and rowing machines are unavailable.
- Inspiratory resistance exercises to increase exercise capacity by reconditioning the inspiratory muscles. Patients should be trained in the proper use of this or any other inspiratory muscle trainer selected. Resistance will be increased gradually until completion of the pulmonary rehabilitation program.

To ensure success with the physical reconditioning part of the program, patients must actively participate at the facility during each session and also at home. This means that each patient must obtain for home use a treadmill or a stationary bicycle (exercycle) and identify a location where daily walking activities can be accomplished. In addition, to help ensure compliance with the program, a daily log or diary sheet must be completed. Fig. 34-4 shows a sample

Table 34-2   Sample Pulmonary Rehabilitation Session

Component	Focus	Time (minutes) frame
Educational	Welcome (group interaction)	5
	Review of program diaries (past week activities)	20
	Presentation of educational topic	20
	Questions, answers, and group discussion	15
Physical reconditioning	Physical activity and reconditioning	45
	Individual goal-setting and session summary	15
TOTAL		120 (2 hours)

Patient Log   Week Number_____

Day	PFLEX	Twelve Minute Walk	Exercycle	Remarks
	No._____ Duration____	Distance _____ No. of stops____	Distance_____ Duration_____	
	No._____ Duration____	Distance_____ No. of stops____	Distance_____ Duration_____	
	No._____ Duration____	Distance_____ No. of stops____	Distance_____ Duration_____	
	No._____ Duration_____	Distance_____ No. of stops _____	Distance_____ Duration_____	
	No._____ Duration_____	Distance_____ No. of stops____	Distance_____ Duration_____	
	No._____ Duration_____	Distance_____ No. of stops____	Distance_____ Duration_____	
	No._____ Duration_____	Distance_____ No. of stops____	Distance/_____ Duration_____	

Other comments/questions from this week:

Fig. 34-4   Sample log or diary form on which a patient in a pulmonary rehabilitation program records daily physical reconditioning activities and exercises.

log sheet, which is a section of the patient's manual. These log or diary forms are reviewed each time the patient attends a session and, on the basis of this information, further individualized reconditioning goals are set.

With the treadmill or stationary bicycle, patients are required to cover a certain distance or exercise for a certain time period every day they are in the program. If distance is the focus, then patients are required to cover greater and greater distances with increasing tension or resistance as they progress through the program. If the focus is on duration, then patients must go for longer periods of time on either the stationary bicycle or the treadmill. Commonly, the duration is set (30 minutes per session twice a day) and the patients are asked to gradually cover more distance within each 30-minute segment as tension or resistance on the equipment is also gradually increased. Daily results are recorded in each patient's log or manual. The overall result should be a strengthening of the lower extremities, with increasing endurance to perform physical activities.

Walking on a flat, smooth surface is another integral part of the reconditioning process. It usually takes the form of a "12-minute walk" performed once a day for the duration of pulmonary rehabilitation. The 12-minute walk is a convenient way for a patient to carry out a well-defined amount of activity with increasing vigor and results over a number of weeks. During the 12 minutes, patients are asked to walk on flat ground (zero grade) for as long as they can. When dyspnea becomes uncomfortable, they are instructed to stop and rest (however, the 12-minute interval still continues). After resting briefly, walking should be continued at a pace comfortable to each individual patient.

The objective is for each patient to walk as far as possible during the 12 minutes, stopping as necessary and quantifying the total distance covered, including number of stops and rest periods. Landmarks such as telephone poles, city blocks, or actual measurements may be used in quantifying distance. Patients are encouraged to increase distances covered each time (if possible) and to record their progress in their manuals or diaries. Some patients will double or triple their walking distance from the beginning of the program to its end and will realize a decrease in the number of stops or rest periods needed.

Upper-body strength can be achieved through the use of exercise bicycles, rowing machines, weight lifting, and/or calisthenics with isometrics. These are usually performed during class sessions but may be carried out at home if the necessary equipment is available and if proper supervision exists. Upper-body conditioning will help patients perform a number of useful activities at home and will also help to increase their overall physical endurance.

Inspiratory muscle resistance training completes the program of physical reconditioning.[34,40-44] Using inexpensive, commercially available devices, patients are instructed to breathe at increasing levels of resistance during the course of the program, thus increasing the strength of their inspiratory muscles. Inspiratory resistance breathing exercises may take place once or twice a day for at least 30 minutes per session. Resistance is increased gradually (as tolerated by the patient), usually once a week or once every 2 weeks. Patients are also encouraged to practice their diaphragmatic breathing techniques, another essential component of rehabilitation, during inspiratory muscle training. Once again, the activity and related results and/or problems should be documented in the patient's diary or manual.

To complement the physical reconditioning aspect of the pulmonary rehabilitation effort, the educational portion of the program should cover topics that are both useful and necessary to the patient.[45] The box below reviews a sequential listing of topics covered during a 10-week rehabilitation program of my design. Naturally other topics can be included and covered but, in terms of relative importance, the ones mentioned are generally given the highest priority. The actual content of these sessions includes the following:

- **Respiratory structure, function, and disease,** including a discussion of dyspnea. This presentation lays the groundwork for the program and gives each patient some basic information about the cardiorespiratory system and related disorders. This particular session can be presented by a physician or a respiratory therapist.
- **Diaphragmatic and pursed-lip breathing techniques,** including a section on avoidance or reduction of panic

---

A LISTING OF TOPICS COVERED DURING THE EDUCATIONAL PORTION OF A 10-WEEK PULMONARY REHABILITATION PROGRAM

Session 1: Introduction and welcome
Program orientation
Respiratory structure, function, and disease

Session 2: Diaphragmatic and pursed-lip breathing techniques

Session 3: Methods of relaxation and stress management

Session 4: Proper exercise techniques and personal routines

Session 5: Aspects of postural drainage, chest percussion, and vibration

Session 6: Administration of oxygen and aerosol therapy (respiratory therapy procedures and home care)

Session 7: Medications: their use and abuse

Session 8: Dietary guidelines and good nutrition

Session 9: Recreation and vocational counseling

Session 10: Program conclusion and evaluation graduation

breathing. This topic can be presented by a physical or a respiratory therapist and serves as a cornerstone for the physical reconditioning effort. Patients must learn how to control their breathing efforts to ensure maximum result (ventilation) at a minimum of effort (energy expenditure). Diaphragmatic breathing with pursed lips will help to accomplish this, but the technique will require daily practice on the part of the patient and continued reinforcement throughout the entire program by the group facilitator.

- **Methods of relaxation and stress management.** This session is best conducted by a psychologist with experience in lung diseases and breathing disorders. Patients must learn to avoid aggravation and upsetting circumstances and to adopt, instead, a more relaxed attitude about their particular life circumstances. This will help to reduce unnecessary oxygen use, will help to conserve energy, and will help to avoid undesirable cardiovascular and nervous responses to stress.

- **Exercise techniques and personal routines.** The rationale for and the value of exercise should be covered and discussed along with suggestions for the adoption of personal exercise routines after the rehabilitation program is over. This topic can be presented by a physical therapist or a respiratory therapist with experience in exercise physiology.

- **Postural drainage, chest percussion, and vibration.** This topic is especially helpful to those patients who have secretion-clearing problems associated with chronic bronchitis and bronchiectasis. Family members and friends may be invited to attend this session in order to acquire some basic skills with these procedures. This area should be taught by either a respiratory therapist or a physical therapist.

- **Respiratory home care (oxygen and aerosol therapy).** A careful review of home care equipment, procedures, and self-administered therapy should be undertaken by a respiratory therapist who has had home care exposure. Safety and equipment-cleaning procedures should also be covered for each type of therapy. This is a very important topic, especially when patients are using home oxygen, aerosol, or IPPB therapy. Those patients who are not yet on this type of therapeutic regimen may have questions or fears and be unreceptive to the concept. Presentation of the modalities available and other patients' discussions of their positive experiences with respiratory home care will help to alleviate the fears and anxieties of nonusers.

- **Medications.** This is another key topic about which patients have numerous questions and concerns. It is best presented by a physician or a pharmacist but may also be covered by a respiratory therapist or a respiratory nurse clinician. Proper use of medications should be addressed along with possible abuses and adverse effects. Attention should be focused on adrenergic and anticholinergic agents, steroids, metered-dose inhalers (MDI), diuretics, theophylline compounds, and pharmaceuticals that affect the cardiovascular system. Sufficient time should also be allotted for questions and answers.

- **Dietary guidelines.** This subject focuses on weight management and good nutrition as it relates to cardiopulmonary health. The topic belongs to the realm of the dietitian or nutritionist. Key elements of a good diet, including high protein to build up atrophied muscles, must be considered. The facilitator should cover proper eating habits, methods of gaining and losing weight, foods to avoid, ways to increase appetite, and daily menu planning. This session will stimulate patients to eat better and thus supply their bodies with the necessary fuel for increased energy production.

- **Recreation and vocational counseling.** This topic can be presented by an occupational therapist or a social worker with experience in work counseling. This session should motivate participants to seek out various types of recreational activities and even part-time work if they are able. The topic is often presented at the end of the pulmonary rehabilitation program, when patients should have acquired some physical endurance and should be preparing for a more active and productive life-style. The class may "brainstorm" ideas for recreational or physical activities, and from this plans for action can be formulated. Changes in attitudes toward physical activity should be perceived by the group facilitator. Patients should no longer think that they cannot walk, exercise, or even be left alone at home. Their overall psychological outlook can definitely change for the better if they have been successful in the program.

These topics need to be presented in an orderly, coherent fashion with the use of supplementary audiovisual materials and demonstrations, where appropriate. The program facilitator or leader must ensure that rehabilitation sessions are conducted on time and in a way that permits maximum involvement and participation on the part of each patient. This facilitator can be a physician, a respiratory care practitioner, a physical therapist, or a respiratory nurse clinician. However, regardless of who takes the lead, it is indeed important for that person to have group-facilitating skills, to be able to motivate, to instill confidence, and to have complete knowledge and familiarity with cardiopulmonary diseases and the rehabilitation process.

Motivation of the patient to attend class sessions, to participate both in class and at home, to adhere to program guidelines, and to persist with the program's regimen falls on the shoulders of the group facilitator. This person must constantly encourage, correct, and direct patients toward the achievement of program and personal goals. The task is not an easy one but, with patience and persistence, it can be accomplished. The result will be effective pulmonary rehabilitation, with patients doing more with less dyspnea and leading more productive lives with decreased hospitalization and lower overall medical costs.

Implementation. This section will explore various aspects of program implementation. One concern already alluded to is that of staffing or personnel. Pulmonary rehabilitation should be a multidisciplinary endeavor. Team care is enhanced by involvement of a variety of health care professionals in the planning, implementation, and evaluation components of the program. The ideal pulmonary rehabilitation program would include the services of a pulmonologist, a respiratory care practitioner, a physical therapist, an occupational therapist, a dietitian, a social worker, a respiratory nurse clinician, a pharmacist, and a psychologist. When any of these specialists are not available, then duties or responsibilities for conducting the sessions must be shared. A person who is competent in a number of disciplines would be an asset and might even function as a program facilitator or director. Institutional policy usually dictates the level of compensation, if any, that professionals receive for participation in the program. Job descriptions and scheduling are other issues that require consideration, but these are usually handled through effective program administration.

In addition to staffing, facilities are another concern that must be addressed. Patient attendance and participation will be discouraged if the program is conducted in uncomfortable or unreachable facilities. Basically, two separate rooms would be ideal—one room for the educational portion of the program, including room for group interaction and support, and one room for physical reconditioning. Rooms should be spacious and comfortable, with adequate lighting, ventilation, and temperature control. Chairs should be comfortable, with good back support. Restroom facilities should be in or adjacent to the rehabilitation area. An area for individual counseling is also desirable, but any private office would help to meet this need. If space is used by other departments for other functions, then proper scheduling of rehabilitation sessions needs to be considered. Adequate time should be allotted for each class session and for necessary setup and breakdown of equipment. Finally, the area designated for pulmonary rehabilitation should be accessible to the patient, with parking spaces set aside for those who drive to the sessions.

Another aspect of program implementation involves timely scheduling of the rehabilitation sessions. This has already been mentioned in terms of scheduling of meeting space and staff participation. The third factor involves patient attendance. With the open-ended format, patients can more or less attend rehabilitation at any time that is convenient for them, as long as the facility is open and staffed accordingly. With the closed format, sessions are scheduled one to three times per week, for 1 to 3 hours, with programs running 8 to 16 weeks. Class times need to be scheduled when the largest number of patients can attend. Traffic patterns, bus schedules, and availability of rides are concerns that need to be discussed. The ideal situation involves a separate area set totally aside for pulmonary re-

habilitation, with a dedicated staff of professionals conducting the program. Then scheduling of either open-ended or closed-design programs becomes easier and more manageable. Sessions can be conducted in the morning, afternoon, or evening hours and even on weekends if necessary. Proper scheduling helps to encourage participation and removes potential stumbling blocks that could undermine the rehabilitation process.

Class size is another issue that must be addressed. Theoretically, a rehabilitation program could be conducted with as few as one participant up to 15 or more, depending on available space, equipment, and staff. However, to foster group identity, interaction, and support, small-group discussions are encouraged. The ideal class size should range from three to 10 participants. Keeping the class size manageable facilitates vital group interaction processes and allows for more individualized attention. These factors help sustain motivation, thereby reducing the likelihood of participant attrition.

Naturally, economic concerns surface when class size is considered. Although it is clear that program quality must be the first priority, program viability realistically depends on the number of participants. As a general guideline, programs should be conducted with a class size that is comfortable with regard to space and staffing and one that is also economically feasible. Such an approach will help ensure that programs are both economically feasible and capable of producing meaningful outcomes for patients.

In addition, equipment is needed for the didactic and reconditioning aspects of the rehabilitation program. To meet the educational needs of the program, a blackboard or a flipchart, a 35 mm slide projector, a screen, an overhead projector, and a cassette tape player are necessary. A videotape player with monitor may be helpful, especially if the program involves the use of individualized instruction or commercially available material. Also, slides, tapes and formal learning packages dealing with the educational topics covered during the rehabilitation program should be available for group and individualized presentation. These can be purchased from outside sources or designed and developed in-house.

For physical reconditioning, stationary bicycles, treadmills, rowing machines, upper-extremity ergometers, weights, pulse oximeters, and inspiratory resistance breathing devices represent the minimum equipment requirements. The actual quantity of equipment needed depends on class size, scheduling, and available space. There should be enough equipment on hand to keep all patients exercising and to monitor their activity. Emergency oxygen and bronchodilator medications should also be maintained in the rehabilitation area. Equipment guidelines for a class of six to ten participants include the following:

- 5 stationary bicycles
- 2 treadmills
- 1 rowing machine

- 2 upper-extremity ergometers
- 5 pulse oximeters for monitoring pulse rate and oxygen saturation
- 1 emergency oxygen cylinder (E) and bronchodilator medications

In addition, each patient should be supplied with an inspiratory resistance breathing device.

Because equipment can be expensive, care must be taken in its selection and purchase. Devices and appliances should be durable, easy and safe to use, simple to maintain, and not overly expensive. Initially, basic items are purchased. As a program develops and expands, equipment resources can be enhanced.

Finally, other program needs should be reviewed and considered. These include the following:

- Patient manual, including daily log forms or activity diary.
- Provision of light refreshments for program participants.
- Development of a communication network between facility and program participants in the event of schedule changes because of emergencies or cancellation of class sessions due to illness, weather, etc.
- Identification of a home care provider for home oxygen, respiratory therapy equipment, and stationary bicycles. Although this is not absolutely necessary, it is helpful in standardizing the type of equipment used within the program.
- Development of a system of charges and mechanisms for patient payment. This will be considered further in the next section of this chapter.

When all of the factors needed for effective implementation of pulmonary rehabilitation are considered, programs will have lower patient attrition and a greater chance for overall success. As programs are conducted, regular evaluations by both patient and staff must be made. Needed changes should be implemented on an ongoing basis. Only in this manner can one expect continued refinement of the process and improvement in outcomes.

Cost and reimbursement. The costs of pulmonary rehabilitation programs are generally based on the average cost per participating patient. This will vary throughout the country and will be dependent on a number of factors, as indicated in the box opposite. Obviously, the larger the class size and the more participants involved in the overall program, the lower will be the cost per patient. The Loma Linda University Medical Center Pulmonary Rehabilitation Program reported for the fiscal year July 1981 to June 1982 that the average cost per patient was $452. This was based on total expenses of $519,942 for the year, with 1150 patients participating.[46]

When patient charges are being determined, consideration must also be given to the type and amount of funding received to offset program expenses and available insurance reimbursement. Testing and evaluations before and after the program will naturally generate revenues but should not be included in the formulation of program charges. However, payments for pulmonary function testing, exercise testing, arterial blood gas analysis and other evaluations may help to keep a pulmonary rehabilitation program financially viable.

Charges for an entire program or for each session must be structured in a way that does not deter patient attendance. Many pulmonary patients are on a fixed income and have other living and medical expenses to account for. A happy medium between a patient's ability to pay and program expenses (charge) must be identified. Any scholarships or funding from local charitable organizations, foundations, or agencies (such as the American Lung Association) will help make any financial responsibility easier to bear. The most comprehensive and effective program available will have no impact if patients are unwilling or unable to attend and participate because of financial limitations.

My own experience with pulmonary rehabilitation program charges is similar to that at Loma Linda University. Expenses for two different 10-week programs in New Jersey (Lung Diagnostics and Better Breathing) averaged $400 per patient. This would result in a program fee ranging from $400 to $500 per participant and, in the case of a 10-week session, $40 to $50 per class.

Reimbursement policies for inpatient rehabilitation vary throughout the country, as do charges for participation in these programs. In 1982, the Health Care Financing Administration (HCFA) published the final rules for Medicare reimbursement guidelines for comprehensive outpatient rehabilitative facilities (CORFs). Under part B of Medicare, the scope of services of a CORF now include reimbursement for outpatient activities and one home visit. Reimbursement is dependent on the CORF's meeting the conditions of participation established in section 933 of PL 96-499. This also includes provisions for certification of the

---

FACTORS AFFECTING PULMONARY REHABILITATION PROGRAM CHARGES TO PATIENTS

1. Marketing and program promotion
2. Number of personnel involved in program facilitation and administration
3. Space and utility expenses
4. Audiovisual, exercise, and monitoring equipment (purchase and maintenance)
5. Production and duplication of course materials
6. Patient supplies
7. Office supplies
8. Refreshments
9. Miscellaneous expenses

program. Each CORF must present its program description and anticipated results to local third-party payers to establish both payment and cost-reimbursement policies.[46]

By following these guidelines, Medicare will establish an allowable charge for the program and reimburse 80% of this rate after the patient meets the annual prescribed deductible. Other programs, both inpatient and outpatient in nature, have obtained reimbursement from third-party payers by charging for rehabilitation sessions as physical therapy exercises for COPD, reconditioning exercise sessions, office visit with therapeutic exercises, or physician office visit—intermediate. The goal is to obtain as much insurance reimbursement as possible, thereby decreasing the financial burden on the patient.

Legal issues. In the past, reimbursement for respiratory rehabilitation services provided on an outpatient basis by a respiratory care practitioner was not available. The role of the respiratory practitioner was poorly defined. Efforts at recognition for reimbursement were frustrated by both legislative and regulatory omissions. The creation of the Medicare and Medicaid programs in 1965 under the Social Security Act failed to recognize respiratory therapy, then a growing and emerging health care profession.[47]

In 1980 Medicare proposed creation of CORFs, which mentioned respiratory care services as reimbursable. This was the first statute to recognize respiratory therapy as such. These regulations were published in 1982. Although the CORF ruling allows for reimbursement for outpatient services provided by a respiratory care practitioner, including one home care visit, more is needed. Respiratory home care has been demonstrated as a cost saver with regard to health care expenditures.[48] In conjunction with a pulmonary rehabilitation program, even more meaningful patient and budgetary outcomes are possible. The profession as a whole must continue to seek legal recognition and acceptable reimbursement policies and practices for both rehabilitation and home care activities.

Program results

As previously indicated, pulmonary rehabilitation has not been able to produce any meaningful improvements in the traditional objective measures of lung function. In addition, improved survival, changes in muscle O_2 extraction, enhanced mucociliary clearance, and a more positive psychological outlook are other controversial outcomes for the patient that result from participation in pulmonary rehabilitation.[31]

Actual or accepted outcomes include improved exercise tolerance, increased maximum oxygen consumption ($\dot{V}_{O_{2max}}$), and higher levels of physical activity with positive changes in pulse, ventilation, and anaerobic threshold.[10,34,49-51] Table 34-3 shows representative patient results, based on cardiopulmonary exercise evaluations, after a 10-week pulmonary rehabilitation program. Note the improved METS levels, increased anaerobic thresholds, and maximum oxygen consumptions recorded at the conclusion of each patient's test. In this group, patients were able to sustain higher levels of activity for longer periods of time. However, because of the small size of this sample, care should be taken in generalizing these results. Nonetheless, similar physiologic results have been reported in the literature along with correlated improvements in patients' functional abilities, as measured by ADL scores.

It must be stated that pulmonary rehabilitation cannot eliminate the occurrence of dyspnea in these patients. However, pulmonary rehabilitation can make shortness of breath less debilitating and more manageable. Thus, although patients still become dyspneic, they do so after greater amounts of exercise or other physical activity and are able to have more confidence in themselves. They recognize that lack of activity is destructive and that perhaps their only hope for an improved life-style is to adhere to program guidelines and to follow through with the prescribed educational and reconditioning regimen.

CARDIAC REHABILITATION

Before this section of the chapter is concluded, some consideration will be given to cardiac rehabilitation. Cardiac rehabilitation is defined as a comprehensive exercise and educational program designed for patients with cardio-

Table 34-3 Physiologic Results in Six Patients, Based on Cardiopulmonary Exercise Testing, After a 10-Week Intensive Pulmonary Rehabilitation Program

Patient	Sex	Age	Before rehabilitation			Following rehabilitation		
			METS	RQ	$\dot{V}_{O_{2max}}$ % pred.	METS	RQ	$\dot{V}_{O_{2max}}$ % pred.
A	M	75	4.9	0.98	65%	5.8	0.80	87%
B	F	59	4.1	1.03	45%	4.7	0.83	56%
C	M	69	5.0	1.18	52%	5.9	1.49	62%
D	F	65	4.8	0.93	53%	6.2	0.92	71%
E	M	62	5.4	1.11	72%	9.3	1.03	113%
F	F	67	3.0	0.98	50%	4.8	0.81	77%

Courtesy of The Breathing Center.

vascular diseases. Like pulmonary rehabilitation, good cardiac rehabilitation programs are multidisciplinary in approach and focus. Goals include patient education (which fosters prudent heart living), physical reconditioning (which can result in improved work capacity), weight loss, and a return to work.

Enrollment is based on a cardiovascular evaluation and related parameters. Because cardiovascular rehabilitation programming has been in existence longer than pulmonary rehabilitation, and because its outcomes tend to have greater validity and acceptance, reimbursement is more readily available at the current time.

The goal of any structured cardiac rehabilitation program is to help patients develop a regular pattern of safe exercise in order to achieve greater cardiovascular performance during activity. Programs are usually divided into monitored and maintenance segments, with home care options available. Exercise prescriptions are individualized for participating patients in an effort to maximize outcomes and reduce the chances of adverse effects.

Pulmonary and cardiac rehabilitation share a number of similarities and differences. Some of them have already been briefly discussed. Table 34-4 summarizes these programs by comparing a number of key characteristics.

In essence, the two programs are similar in many ways, differing only in their rehabilitative focus and type of patient monitoring. It should be added that the average age of patients involved in pulmonary and cardiac rehabilitation programs may differ to some extent. Patients with chronic pulmonary disease, especially COPD, will be in their 60s and 70s. Patients with restrictive diseases will range in age from the teens to the 70s. Patients who are dependent on ventilators present other specialized concerns, including a very broad range in age.[52] On the other hand, patients with cardiac problems will probably range from their late 30s on up to their 60s or 70s. Again, one of the keys to motivation and program success is to keep the programs homogeneous with respect to age, degree of impairment, and level of preprogram functional activity and ability. This pertains to either pulmonary or cardiac rehabilitation efforts.

Finally, respiratory care involvement in cardiac rehabilitation will probably be significantly less. For the most part, respiratory care practitioners, unless multicompetent, will be involved with instruction on oxygen use and assistance with patients' exercise sessions. Most often, the cardiologist and the cardiac nurse specialist or clinician are involved with program facilitation and administration. Other health professionals who may be involved include the dietitian, the physical therapist, the occupational therapist, the pharmacist, the social worker, and the psychologist.

SUMMARY

It is safe to say that properly planned pulmonary rehabilitation programs can produce certain positive, measurable outcomes for patients. The success of such efforts depends on careful application of current clinical and social science knowledge and the use of a multidisciplinary approach throughout all phases of program organization, implementation, and evaluation. Within this context, respiratory care practitioners are playing an increasingly important role.

Although these efforts can bring hope to patients for a more active and productive existence, we must remember that the need for pulmonary rehabilitation stems, in part, from the lack of attention currently given to the promotion of healthy life-styles and the prevention of pulmonary disease (see Chapter 33). Ultimately, success in health promotion and disease prevention activities should lessen the need for long-term and rehabilitative care. Until this ideal is achieved, pulmonary rehabilitation will continue to represent a necessary and growing component of respiratory care.

REFERENCES

1. Council on Rehabilitation: Definition of rehabilitation, Chicago, 1942, Council on Rehabilitation.
2. Petty TL: Pulmonary rehabilitation, Basics RD 4:1, 1975.
3. American Thoracic Society Executive Committee: Pulmonary rehabilitation: an official statement of the American Thoracic Society, Am Rev Respir Dis 124:663-666, 1981.

Table 34-4 A Comparison of Pulmonary and Cardiac Rehabilitation Programs

Characteristic	Pulmonary	Cardiac
Use of an exercise stress test for patient evaluation	Yes (cardiopulmonary)	Yes (cardiac)
Primary focus of program	On breathing techniques and exercise tolerance	On cardiovascular fitness
Use of education and exercise as key program components	Yes	Yes
Patient monitoring during exercise	Sao_2 and pulse	ECG, blood pressure, and pulse
Multidisciplinary approach	Yes	Yes
Reimbursable	Yes	Yes

4. Harris PL: A guide to prescribing pulmonary rehabilitation, Prim Care 12:253-266, 1985.

5. Barach AL, Bickerman HA, and Beck G: Advances in the treatment of nontuberculous pulmonary disease, Bull NY Acad Med 28:353-384, 1952.

6. Pierce AK et al: Responses to exercise training in patients with emphysema, Arch Intern Med 113:28-36, 1964.

7. Paez PN et al: The physiologic basis of training patients with emphysema, Am Rev Respir Dis 95:944-953, 1967.

8. Christie D: Physical training in chronic obstructive lung disease, Br Med J 2:150-151, 1968.

9. Hudson LD, Tyler ML, and Petty TL: Hospitalization needs during an outpatient rehabilitation program for severe chronic airway obstruction, Chest 70:606-610, 1976.

10. Moser KM et al: Results of a comprehensive rehabilitation program, Arch Intern Med 140:1596-1601, 1980.

11. Gimenez M: Technics and results in respiratory kinesitherapy of chronic obstructive bronchopneumopathies, Rev Fr Mal Respir 11:525-543, 1983.

12. Daughton D et al: Relationship between a pulmonary function test (FEV_1) and the ADAPT quality-of-life scale, Percept Mot Skills 1983, 57:359-62.

13. Jensen PS: Risk, protective factors, and supportive interventions in chronic airway obstruction, Arch Gen Psychiatry 40:1203-1207, 1983.

14. Zaltzman M and Steinberg H: Normal and abnormal cardiopulmonary responses to exercise, Appl Cardiol 14:19-21, 1986.

15. Fix AJ et al: Emotional, intellectual and physiological predictors of vocational outcome of pulmonary rehabilitation patients, Psychol Rep 46:379-382, 1980.

16. Shenkman B: Factors contributing to attrition rates in a pulmonary rehabilitation program, Heart Lung 14:53-58, 1985.

17. Dudley DL et al: Psychosocial concomitants to rehabilitation in chronic obstructive pulmonary disease. I. Psychosocial and psychological considerations, Chest 77:413-420, 1980.

18. Dudley DL et al: Psychosocial concomitants to rehabilitation in chronic obstructive pulmonary disease. III. Dealing with psychiatric disease (as distinguished from psychosocial or psychophysiologic problems), Chest 77:677-684, 1980.

19. Dudley DL et al: Psychosocial concomitants to rehabilitation in chronic obstructive pulmonary disease. II. Psychosocial treatment, Chest 77:544-551, 1980.

20. Fix AJ et al: Personality traits affecting vocational rehabilitation success in patients with chronic obstructive pulmonary disease, Psychol Rep 43:939-944, 1978.

21. Kass I et al: Correlation of psychophysiologic variables with vocational rehabilitation outcome in patients with chronic obstructive pulmonary disease, Chest 67:433-440, 1975.

22. Dyksterhuis JE: Vocational rehabilitation of chronic obstructive pulmonary disease patients, Rehab Lit 33:136-138, 1972.

23. Pomerantz P, Flannery EL, and Findling PK: Occupational therapy for chronic obstructive lung disease, Am J Occup Ther 29:407-411, 1975.

24. Putnam JS and Beechler CR: Comprehensive care in chronic obstructive pulmonary disease, Prim Care 3:593-608, 1976.

25. Faling LJ: Pulmonary rehabilitation—physical modalities, Clin Chest Med 7:599-618, 1986.

26. Paine R and Make BJ: Pulmonary rehabilitation for the elderly, Clin Geriatr Med 2:313-335, 1986.

27. Hodgkin JE et al: American Thoracic Society, Medical Section of the American Lung Association, Pulmonary rehabilitation, Am Rev Respir Dis 124:663-666, 1981.

28. Young A: Rehabilitation of patients with pulmonary disease, Ann Acad Med Singapore 12:410-416, 1983.

29. Levi-Valensi P et al: Rehabilitation of chronic pulmonary patients: critical study of objectives and methods: current state of the problem, Poumon Coeur 33:7-14, 1977.

30. Fergus LC and Cordasco EM: Pulmonary rehabilitation of the patient with COPD, Postgrad Med 62:141-144, 1977.

31. Alkalay I et al: Chronic obstructive pulmonary disease: rehabilitation program with continuation on an outpatient basis, J Am Geriatr Soc 28:88-92, 1980.

32. Spiro SG et al: Cardiorespiratory adaptations at the start of exercise in normal subjects and in patients with chronic obstructive bronchitis, Clin Sci Mol Med 47:165-172, 1974.

33. Casciari RJ et al: Effects of breathing retraining in patients with chronic obstructive pulmonary disease, Chest 79:393-398, 1981.

34. Sonne LJ and Davis JA: Increased exercise performances in patients with severe COPD following inspiratory resistive training, Chest 81:436-439, 1982.

35. Hughes RL and Davison R: Limitations of exercise reconditioning in COLD, Chest, 83:241-249, 1983.

36. Sue D: Exercise testing and the patient with cardiopulmonary disease, Probl Pulmon Dis 2:1-8, 1986.

37. Hodgkin JE: Organization of a pulmonary rehabilitation program, Clin Chest Med 7:541-549, 1986.

38. Gilmartin ME: Pulmonary rehabilitation—patient and family education, Clin Chest Med 7:619-627, 1986.

39. White B and Andrews JL: Pulmonary rehabilitation in an ambulatory group practice setting, Med Clin North Am 63:379, 1979.

40. Ries AL and Moser KM: Comparison of isocapnic hyperventilation and walking exercise training at home in pulmonary rehabilitation, Chest 90:285-289, 1986.

41. Levine S, Weiser P, and Gillen J: Evaluation of a ventilatory muscle endurance training program in the rehabilitation of patients with chronic obstructive pulmonary disease, Am Rev Respir Dis 133:400-406, 1986.

42. Chen H, Dukes R, and Martin BJ: Inspiratory muscle training in patients with chronic obstructive pulmonary disease, Am Rev Respir Dis 131:251-255, 1985.

43. Belman M and Mittman C: Ventilatory muscle training improves exercise capacity in chronic obstructive pulmonary disease patients, Am Rev Respir Dis 121:273-280, 1980.

44. Pardy R: The effects of inspiratory muscle training on exercise performance in chronic airflow limitation, Am Rev Respir Dis 123:421-425, 1981.

45. Hanak M: Patient and family education: teaching programs for managing chronic disease and disability, New York, 1986, Springer Publishing Co.

46. Nicol J et al: Strategies for developing a cost effective pulmonary rehabilitation program, Respir Care 28:1451-1455, 1983.

47. Porte P: Legislation and respiratory rehabilitation, Respir Care 28:1498-1502, 1983.

48. Roselle S and D'Amico FS: The effect of home respiratory therapy on hospital readmission rates of patients with chronic obstructive pulmonary disease, Respir Care 27:1194-1199, 1982.

49. Haas A and Cardon H: Rehabilitation in chronic obstructive pulmonary disease: a five-year study of 252 male patients, Med Clin North Am 53:593-606, 1969.

50. Mohsenifar KM et al: Sensitive indices of improvement in a pulmonary rehabilitation program, Chest 83:189-192, 1983.

51. Make BJ: Pulmonary rehabilitation: myth or reality? Clin Chest Med 7:519-540, 1986.

52. Make BJ et al: Rehabilitation of ventilator-dependent subjects with lung disease, Chest 86:358-365, 1984.

35

Respiratory Home Care

Kenneth A. Wyka

Respiratory or pulmonary home care represents one of the fastest growing and most dynamic segments of respiratory care. With changes in hospitalization brought about by the advent of diagnosis-related groups (DRGs) and peer review organizations (PROs), and with an ever-increasing elderly population, the need for comprehensive home health services has become more keenly felt and recognized.

Since most home care currently is initiated after an acute-care hospitalization, a well-designed program must be carefully integrated with the discharge-planning process. Moreover, because home care is normally a multidisciplinary effort, coordinated teamwork is an essential component of effective home health programming.

Among the key areas of practitioner involvement in modern respiratory home care are continuous oxygen therapy, long-term mechanical ventilation, and in-home continuation of planned pulmonary rehabilitation. These and other aspects of respiratory home care are the major focus of this chapter.

OBJECTIVES

After completion of this chapter, the reader should be able to:

1. Define the concept of respiratory home care;

2. State the standards for respiratory therapy home care as adopted by the American Association for Respiratory Care (AARC);

3. Describe the guidelines for home care of the ventilator-dependent patient as proposed by the American College of Chest Physicians (ACCP);

4. Identify current Medicare criteria for reimbursement of home oxygen therapy;

5. Differentiate the appropriate use, advantages, and disadvantages of the various systems for home oxygen delivery;

6. Discuss the delivery of respiratory care in the home on the basis of patient selection and discharge, prescribed therapeutic modalities, factors ensuring success, and potential problems or difficulties;

7. Discuss the current reimbursement mechanism(s) available for respiratory equipment and related services provided in the home setting.

KEY TERMS

Most terms used in this chapter are defined in context. The following terms are introduced without explicit definition but may be found in the text glossary:

angina pectoris	NBRC
AARC	obstructive sleep apnea
ACCP	oximetry
CORF	pneumocardiography
conjunctivitis	polysomnography
cryogenic	PRO
DRG	psychosocial
erythrocythemia	rhinitis
erythrocytosis	SIDS
HCFA	sinusitis
hypersomnolence	SNF
inspissated	zeolite

HISTORICAL PERSPECTIVE

The use of respiratory therapy in the home for the management of patients with chronic cardiorespiratory conditions is an accepted and necessary practice today. However, its widespread application, including "high-tech" levels of care, are relatively new and the health care industry is only beginning to appreciate the positive impact respiratory home care can have on patient management and related health care costs.

Respiratory care became a formal health care discipline in the late 1940s and developed rapidly in the 1950s with the advent of intermittent positive pressure breathing (IPPB) therapy and devices. Other types of therapy administered during this period of time were oxygen, aerosol and mist treatments, and mechanical ventilation (positive and negative pressure). As other therapeutic modalities were added over the following years, the discipline eventually became a profession.

Before 1970, however, respiratory therapy procedures were almost exclusively administered within the hospital. There were isolated cases of patients receiving oxygen, IPPB, aerosol therapy, and even negative-pressure ventilation in the home, but, for the most part, respiratory care for the homebound patient was unavailable. Some of the reasons for this were as follows:

- Technology: Equipment was pneumatic, complicated, and cumbersome. Portability needed to be resolved. Also, disposable materials were not readily available.
- Personnel: Few trained and credentialed respiratory care practitioners were in existence before 1970. Almost all qualified practitioners were employed by hospitals in supervisory and managerial roles.
- Attitudes: Many health care professionals did not believe that patients could adhere to prescribed therapeutic routines in the home. They believed that the best place for ongoing therapy was the hospital. As a result, many respiratory therapy departments had outpatient clinics treating patients anywhere from one to five times per week or more.
- Home care equipment providers: These were small in number and offered limited services at best.
- Reimbursement: Reimbursement was not available for respiratory care delivered by a respiratory technician or therapist. When Medicare and Medicaid came into existence in 1965, respiratory therapy was not mentioned in the reimbursement policies and was therefore excluded. However, oxygen and related equipment became reimbursable under part B of Medicare in 1967, and this reimbursement would have a significant impact on the growth of home care in the years to come.
- Regulatory standards: Until 1988, all standards related to provision of home care were based on federal reimbursement criteria or state licensing regulations. In 1986 the Joint Commission on Accreditation of Healthcare Organizations (JCAHO) began working on a set of standards for the home health care industry, to include all companies and organizations that provide equipment and/or care for patients outside the hospital setting. These standards were implemented in 1988.

After 1970, respiratory home care began to emerge as a speciality with its own identity. Electrically driven IPPB units became available, as did small-volume liquid oxygen systems, oxygen concentrators, portable ventilators, and disposable supplies. At the same time, the number of accredited respiratory therapy programs grew steadily, producing greater numbers of practitioners who became credentialed through the National Board for Respiratory Care (NBRC). Although Medicare and other insurance carriers did not directly reimburse respiratory care practitioners for the services they provided, reimbursement for oxygen and other equipment rented or purchased by patients was supported. As a result, the number of companies and organizations providing respiratory home care increased dramatically, as did the competition for patients.[1]

More recently, DRG and PRO legislation have made home care in general and respiratory home care in particular a practical alternative to certain forms of hospital care. Essentially all of the necessary elements (technology, provider standards, qualified personnel, equipment suppliers, home care providers, and attitudes) are now in place to shape the current and future practice of respiratory home care. The final key element—direct reimbursement for respiratory care services—is on the horizon and will help to attract even more qualified professionals into this important new area of patient care.

GOALS, OBJECTIVES, AND STANDARDS FOR HOME CARE

The American Association for Respiratory Care (AARC) defines respiratory home care as those specific forms of respiratory care provided in the patient's place of residence by personnel trained in respiratory therapy working under medical supervision.[2]

Goals and objectives

The primary goal of home care is to provide quality health care services to patients or clients in their home setting, thereby minimizing dependence on hospitalization in acute-care facilities as the basis for ongoing treatment.

In regard to respiratory home care, several specific objectives are evident. Respiratory home care can contribute to:

- Supporting and maintaining life;
- Improving patients' physical, emotional, and social well being;
- Promoting patient and family self-sufficiency;
- Ensuring cost-effective delivery of care.

Most patients for whom respiratory home care is considered have chronic diseases that affect the respiratory system. Categories of disorders for which respiratory home care may be appropriate include the following:

- Chronic obstructive pulmonary disease (COPD);
- Cystic fibrosis;
- Chronic neuromuscular disorders;
- Chronic restrictive conditions;
- Carcinomas of the lung.

In addition, some acute conditions may best be treated in a home care setting. These disorders include respiratory tract infections that do not require hospitalization, such as certain forms of pneumonia, croup, and bronchiolitis, and mild forms of asthma.

Although some aspects of respiratory home care have

yet to demonstrate their efficacy, various studies over the years have shown that certain carefully selected treatment regimens can play an important role in maintaining patients' lives, in improving their quality of life, in increasing their functional performance, and in reducing the individual and societal costs associated with hospitalization.[3-7]

Standards for home care

Unlike those in the acute care sector, standards for the provision of home care have evolved somewhat sporadically. Federal regulations have tended to focus on reimbursement criteria for selected home medical equipment and services. State efforts, where applicable, have addressed general licensing regulations for certain categories of home care provider. Until recently, private sector initiatives have been limited to promulgation of position statements by relevant professional organizations, such as the AARC. Not until 1988 was a comprehensive effort made to provide general accreditation standards for providers of home care.

Federal regulations. Federal regulation of respiratory home care began in 1967 with recognition of oxygen and related equipment as reimbursable under part B of the Medicare program. Since that time, several changes in these provisions have occurred, with the general tendency toward more objective criteria for documenting patient eligibility and significantly stricter limitations on total costs. Details on these regulations—current as of this writing—will be provided later in this chapter. However, given the rapidity of changes occurring in this area, the reader should consult sources such as the *Federal Register* for the most up-to-date information on federal home care reimbursement policies.

State efforts. Many states have statutory or administrative regulations that govern licensing of home health care providers, such as home health agencies (HHAs) or visiting nurse associations (VNAs). Since these regulations may differ substantially among the applicable states, readers should contact their state health departments for details.

Private sector initiatives. Typical of many health profession organizations with an interest in quality home care, the American Association for Respiratory Care (AARC) recognized early on the need for standards in the provision of these services. Toward this end, the AARC was among the first to develop and promulgate a set of home care standards. Originally published in 1979, these AARC standards include the following provisions[2]:

- **Standard I:** The need for therapy must be clearly established. There must be criteria and therapeutic objectives for program entry requirements. A unified approach should exist between the physician and the therapist for the objectives and modalities of therapy.
- **Standard II:** A medical record that includes the prescription must be established and maintained on all patients receiving any form of respiratory therapy home care.
- **Standard III:** Respiratory therapy equipment used must be safe and appropriate. The patient must demonstrate its effective use, and he or she or the family must demonstrate its proper maintenance, including sterilization or appropriate cleanliness.
- **Standard IV:** There must be evidence that patients are receiving follow-up evaluations at least once per month, and more often if necessary, by some member of the home care team.

In 1986, the Joint Commission on Accreditation of Healthcare Organizations (JCAHO) initiated a 2-year project to develop a comprehensive set of accreditation standards for the home health care providers. This project included field reviews, pilot surveys, and input from such groups as the American Association of Retired Persons, the American Federation of Home Health Agencies, the American Hospital Association, the American Medical Association, the American Nurses Association, the American Occupational Therapy Association, the American Physical Therapy Association, the National Association for Home Care, the National Association for Social Workers, the Blue Cross and Blue Shield Association, and the American Association for Respiratory Care. The proposed standards were drafted and revised on the basis of comments from the home care industry in general and from other reviewers. Evaluation of the proposed standards considered the effect of implementation on quality of care, costs, and the possibility of improving care.

Disseminated in 1988, the final *Standards for the Accreditation of Home Care* consist of nearly 80 primary standards and some 180 "required characteristics" divided into two major sections.[8] Section I contains generic standards applicable to all home care organizations. As depicted in the box on pp. 920-921, these generic standards focus on seven major areas: (1) patient/client rights and responsibilities, (2) patient/client care, (3) safety management and infection control, (4) the home care record, (5) quality assurance, (6) management and administration, and (7) the governing body.

Whereas Section I standards apply to all home health care providers, Section II standards are specific to the type of service(s) delivered. In this section separate standards are delineated for home health services, pharmaceutical services, personal care and support services, and equipment management. For example, the major standards applicable to home care organizations providing equipment management services are as follows:

EM.1: Organizations providing equipment directly or by contract effectively manage the selection, setup, and maintenance of equipment and educate patients/clients in its use.

EM.2: Equipment and related medical supplies provided are appropriate to the care delivered and to the home environment.

JOINT COMMISSION ON ACCREDITATION OF HEALTHCARE ORGANIZATIONS GENERIC STANDARDS FOR THE ACCREDITATION OF HOME CARE

PATIENT/CLIENT RIGHTS AND RESPONSIBILITIES (PR)

PR.1* The patient/client has the right to make informed decisions regarding his/her care.

PR.2* There is continuity in the care provided by the home care organization.

PR.3* All information concerning patient/client care is treated confidentially.

PR.4* The patient/client is informed upon admission of the home care organization's mechanism for receiving, reviewing, and resolving patient/client complaints.

PR.5* The home care organization honors patient/client rights and informs the patients/clients of their responsibilities, if any, in the care process.

PATIENT/CLIENT CARE (PC)

PC.1* A home care organization admits only patients/clients whose needs can be met by the services it provides.

PC.2* An individual plan of care or service is developed and implemented for each patient/client.

PC.3* Care coordination+ is provided in order to assure continuity of care for the patient/client.

PC.4 The patient/client is appropriately transferred, referred, or discharged.

SAFETY MANAGEMENT AND INFECTION CONTROL (SI)

SI.1* The home care organization has a program designed to educate appropriate staff and patients/clients in safety measures in the home to minimize hazards related to the care or service provided.

SI.2* Measures are taken to prevent, identify, and control infections.

SI.3 The organization has an emergency preparedness plan designed to provide continuing care and support appropriate to the care or service provided in the event of an emergency that would result in interruption of patient/client services.

SI.4 The safety management, infection control, and emergency preparedness plan are monitored and evaluated.

HOME CARE RECORD (CR)

CR. 1* An accurate home care record is maintained to document the home care or service provided to each patient/client.

CR. 2 A standardized format is used in the home care record for documenting all care or service provided to patients/clients.

CR. 3 When care or service is not provided directly by the home care organization, documentation of the contracted service is included in the home care record.

CR. 4 The organization has a written policy that delineates who has the authority to make entries in and review the home care record.

CR. 5 An explanatory legend defines any abbreviations or symbols used in records.

CR. 6 The home care record of a patient/client discharged from a home health service is completed within a reasonable time period, as specified in home care organization policy.

CR. 7 The length of time home care records are to be retained is recorded in policies and procedures of the home care organization and is in accordance with applicable law and regulation.

CR. 8 Reasonable security measures are taken to safeguard both the home care record and its content, whether in hard copy, on film, or in computer form, against loss, defacement, tampering, and unauthorized disclosure or use.

CR. 9 There are home care organization policies regarding the confidentiality of records and release of health information.

CR.10 There is a policy regarding the documentation of incidents.

CR.11 Organizations providing home health services review at least quarterly a representative sample of records in order to assure the records reflect the care or service provided, the condition and progress of the patient/client, and the condition of the patient/client at discharge.

*Key factors denoted with asterisk.

Accreditation surveys are conducted by practicing professionals with extensive experience in home care. Accreditation of a home care organization is based on the demonstration of compliance with the JCAHO home care standards. The rating scale used is as follows:

- Substantial compliance: Organization meets all major provisions of the standard
- Significant compliance: Organization meets most provisions of the standard
- Partial compliance: Organization meets some provisions of the standard
- Minimal compliance: Organization meets few provisions of the standard
- Noncompliance: Organization fails to meet the provisions of the standard

JOINT COMMISSION ON ACCREDITATION OF HEALTHCARE ORGANIZATIONS GENERIC STANDARDS FOR THE ACCREDITATION OF HOME CARE—cont'd

QUALITY ASSURANCE (QA)

QA.1* There is an ongoing quality assurance program designed to objectively and systematically monitor and evaluate the quality and appropriateness of patient/client care, resolve identified problems, and pursue opportunities to improve patient/client care.

MANAGEMENT AND ADMINISTRATION (MA)

MA. 1* There is an executive officer.

MA. 2* There is a director(s) of patient/client services.

MA. 3* The policies and procedures established by the governing body are implemented.

MA. 4* Policies and procedures addressing the delivery of care or service are developed, implemented, reviewed, and, as appropriate, revised.

MA. 5* Lines of responsibilities and accountability are clearly established for all staff.

MA. 6* There are written personnel policies and procedures.

MA. 7 When volunteer services are used, volunteers are selected, regularly trained, and supervised according to guidelines established by the organization.

MA. 8* Home care staff providing home health or support services participate in orientation, in-service training, and continuing education programs.

MA. 9 There are financial management policies and procedures.

MA.10* When any home care service offered by the organization is not provided directly by employees or volunteers, there is a written agreement defining the nature and scope of services provided.

GOVERNING BODY (GB)

GB. 1* The governing body, whether an individual, a group, or a government agency, has ultimate responsibility and legal authority for the home care organization.

GB. 2 The members of the governing body and the management and administration of the home care organization communicate systematically.

GB. 3 There is an annual operating budget as required by applicable law and regulation.

GB. 4 An executive officer, responsible for the day-to-day operations of the agency, is appointed through a procedure established by the governing body.

GB. 5 There is a process approved by the governing body to assure that all individuals who provide patient/client care or service are competent to provide such care or service.

GB. 6 The governing body receives reports at least annually on the quality and appropriateness of patient/client care and the allocation of resources.

GB. 7 The governing body annually evaluates the home care organization's performance in relation to its written statement of purposes and objectives.

GB. 8* The governing body of a corporate entity that has the responsibility for more than one home care organization delineates the level(s) of authority and responsibility for each home care organization.

GB. 9* The governing body implements a written conflict-of-interest policy that includes guidelines for the disclosure of any existing or potential conflict of interest.

GB.10 All members of the governing body fulfill their responsibilities as provided in the organization's policies.

Accreditation is not up to the surveyor. Instead, findings are sent to the JCAHO for further analysis and comparison with the national standards. Notification of the decision comes 2 to 3 months later, with accreditation status assigned to one of three categories: accreditation, accreditation with contingencies, or nonaccreditation. Contingencies must be corrected or resolved within a given time frame and all home care accreditation, as with hospital accreditation, must be periodically renewed.

With both the AARC and JCAHO standards now providing a sound basis for the organization and delivery of quality home care, health professionals and consumers alike can now expect home care providers to comply with these professional expectations. Of course, the ultimate goal should always be to place the patient's needs first in an effort to provide an optimum level of professional service.

HOME CARE PLANNING

Most patients with chronic pulmonary disorders are referred for respiratory home care after an acute-care hospitalization. Others are placed in a home care service from a physician's office or an outpatient facility. In almost all of these instances, the patient's physician identifies the need for ongoing care and writes an order for some form of respiratory home care to be implemented.

The home care team

Although the attending physician normally is responsible for initiating the home care order, a number of health care professionals can and should be involved in the discharge process. The following box identifies the key members that comprise this team, along with their key responsibilities. As with pulmonary rehabilitation (Chapter 34), a team approach in home care produces the best patient results. Communication and mutual respect for each member's talents and abilities are two key elements in making the discharge and home care process work. Any breakdown in the system may delay or affect the patient's discharge, home care, and/or follow-up.

The decision concerning discharge can be made by one member of this team (usually the physician) or by any number of team members. With difficult cases, family members and the hospital chaplain (pastoral body) may also be involved in the decision-making process. The decision to discharge the patient to the home environment frequently means that established criteria for discharge (education and training, patient status, and home conditions) have been satisfactorily met and that sufficient family or neighbor support exists at home. Most often, these criteria pertain to home mechanical ventilation. Other forms of respiratory home care require far less planning, patient education, and patient support and are much easier to provide and follow-up.

The discharge plan

The discharge plan should consider the following key points:
- Date of discharge;
- Therapeutic goals for home care;
- Therapeutic modalities to be administered, including frequency;
- Necessary equipment for implementation;
- Patient instruction and setup;
- Selection of home care agency;
- Plans for patient follow-up and evaluation.

Therapeutic objectives, as related to patient care, may include any of the following:
- To support ventilation (life support);
- To improve oxygenation (at rest, with activity, or during sleep);
- To reverse bronchospasm;
- To promote mucociliary clearance;
- To assist with bronchopulmonary toilet and promote bronchial hygiene;

MEMBERS OF THE RESPIRATORY HOME HEALTH CARE TEAM

DISCIPLINE	RESPONSIBILITIES
Utilization review	Advises and/or recommends consideration of patient discharge. Documents patient's in-hospital care.
Discharge planning (social service or community/public health)	Brings all the needed home care elements together and ensures that a patient can be discharged home. Makes contacts with outside agencies that may assist with patient care.
Physician	Writes order for patient discharge. Evaluates patient's condition and prescribes respiratory home care. Establishes therapeutic objectives.
Respiratory care	Recommends types of home care modalities. May set up therapeutic regimen at home and follow up accordingly. May suggest home care provider for necessary equipment and supplies.
Nursing	Writes home care plan for patient. Assesses patient's status and provides necessary home care follow-up.
Dietary	Assesses patient's nutritional needs and writes dietary plan for patient. Makes arrangements for meals as may be necessary.
Physical therapy	Provides necessary physical therapy and recommends any additional modalities or procedures.
Psychiatry/psychology	Assesses patient's emotional status and provides any needed counseling or support.
Durable medical equipment (DME) supplier/ home care company	Provides necessary home care equipment and supplies and handles any emergency situations involving delivery or equipment operation.

- To help maintain upper airway patency;
- To promote effective breathing techniques and avoid panic breathing.

By keeping objectivity in the plan, the effectiveness of the total discharge plan will be enhanced and patient outcomes will be easier to assess and achieve.

Patients may be referred directly to a visiting nurse service (VNA), a home health agency (HHA), or an equipment-management company. Regardless of the manner of referral, when respiratory equipment is needed and prescribed for home use, a supplier must be chosen. Hospitals, home health agencies, nursing services, physician offices, or outpatient facilities can use one of the following methods:

- Use one specific supplier;
- Use a number of reliable suppliers on a rotating basis;
- Use their own company;
- Joint venture with a supplier and use the resources of that partnership;
- Use a supplier with whom some contractual relationship exists for equipment rentals.

Regardless of method used, the selection of a home care supplier should be based on consideration of several factors. These include cost, scope of services, dependability, location, personnel, past track record, and availability. Patient referrals almost always go to suppliers who offer 24-hour service 7 days a week. This service must be problem free and provided by a reliable, professional, and courteous staff. Charges should be reasonable and competitive, and other patient services such as initial and follow-up visits by respiratory care practitioners with appropriate credentials are helpful in the selection process.

Since rental of home care equipment, including oxygen, can be a lucrative business, many institutions, agencies, and facilities have become involved with it. For this reason, a closer look at home care equipment suppliers is warranted.

Home care equipment (DME) suppliers

Home care equipment is commonly referred to as durable medical equipment (DME). Most DME suppliers provide a spectrum of equipment services, from oxygen and aerosol equipment to wheelchairs and hospital beds. For purposes of our discussion, we will focus on DME suppliers that provide respiration-related equipment and services.

DME suppliers range in size from multimillion dollar corporations offering a broad range of services on a nationwide basis to small local companies that specialize in one facet of home care, such as respiratory home care. With the advent of oxygen reimbursement under Medicare part B in 1967, the number and diversity of DME companies proliferated. These companies, both large and small, usually provide the following respiratory home care services:

- 24-hour service 7 days a week;

- Acceptance of insurance coverage (private, Medicare, and Medicaid);
- Home instruction and follow-up by a respiratory care practitioner;
- Most forms of respiratory care modalities.

Home care equipment can also be provided through HHAs, VNAs, hospitals, outpatient facilities, charitable organizations (American Cancer Society, American Lung Association, etc.), hospice groups, and private concerns (physician offices, respiratory practitioners in private practice, and other related entities). Often, because of the financial rewards involved in establishing a DME service, agencies, hospitals, and physician groups have established joint ventures with companies in an attempt to enter the home care business. Such partnerships are legal if the following conditions exist:

- All parties are at "risk" when entering into the agreement;
- A legal contractual arrangement that identifies responsibilities for all involved parties is written;
- The joint venture is not based on patient referrals alone.

Usually institutions, agencies, or physicians become involved in the DME business for the following reasons:

- For potential economic rewards;
- To maintain tighter control over patient monitoring and care provided within the home environment;
- To improve level of service and communication with the home care team;
- To provide continuity of care between hospital and home;
- To facilitate pulmonary rehabilitation efforts;
- To help control patients' consumption of home care resources and related costs;
- To provide an expert level of care and follow-up as may be deemed necessary.

The potential economic rewards associated with the DME business are listed first because many individuals have entered such ventures explicitly to reap a profit. However, with the passage of the Omnibus Budget Reconciliation Act of 1987, there occurred a substantial change in the method used in determining reimbursement rates for home medical equipment. Commonly referred to as the "six-point plan," this law took effect on Jan. 1, 1989.

Although this law does not change the Medicare requirements for reimbursement for medical equipment, it does significantly alter payment schedules, thereby forcing DME suppliers to seek the most cost-efficient means of providing their equipment and services. The six-point plan also eliminates many highly profitable but dubious practices, such as long-term rentals of inexpensive equipment that could easily be purchased. Included in the plan are the following provisions:

- Inexpensive equipment (items costing $150 or less) may be rented or purchased on a "lump-sum" basis. However, the rental payments may not exceed the purchase price of the item.

- Items that require frequent and extensive servicing, such as mechanical ventilators, suction apparatus, and IPPB or compressor/nebulizer units, will be rented for as long as medically necessary in order to avoid any risk to the patients.
- Reimbursement for customized equipment will be on a "lump-sum" basis, with this amount being based on the insurance carrier's individual consideration. Maintenance not covered by a warranty may also be reimbursed, provided it is reasonable and necessary.
- Reimbursement for expensive home medical equipment (items costing more than $150) will be on a rental basis, but payments will be capped at 15 months. After the 15-month time limit is reached, the patient will be entitled to use the equipment as long as it is medically necessary. Suppliers will not be entitled to further rental payments during months 16 to 21. If the patient still has need for the item after the 22nd month of use, a service and maintenance fee may be charged. (The fee will be the lower of the reasonable and necessary fee established by the carrier or the monthly rental fee schedule amount.) Title to any equipment remains with the supplier.
- Payment for items other than durable medical equipment (defined as prostheses, orthoses, and medical supplies not described in the law, excluding parenteral and enteral nutrition) will be made on a "lump-sum" basis for the recognized purchase price, which will be determined by the same process as described for inexpensive equipment.
- Reimbursement for oxygen and oxygen equipment will be on a monthly basis. The basic payment rate for oxygen equipment, excluding portable equipment, will be calculated by dividing the total reasonable charges for oxygen and oxygen equipment during the 12-month period ending December 1986 by the total number of months patients were on oxygen therapy. A similar but separate calculation will be made for portable equipment. Beginning with 1989, the monthly payment will be 95% of the basic payment rate increased by the percentage increase in the consumer price index for the 12-month period ending December 1987. After 1989, the payment rate will be increased by the percentage increase in the consumer price index for the 12-month period ending in June of the previous year. Special payment rates will be allowed for high and low liter flow. For patients using more than 4 L/min, the basic payment rate will be increased by 50%. For patients using less than 1 L/min, the basic payment rate will be decreased by 50%. For patients using oxygen at between 1 L/min and 4 L/min, the basic payment rate will be applied. For patients who require portable oxygen equipment, reim-

bursement will be 95% of the basic payment rate plus the payment calculated for portable equipment (at the time of publication of this text, oxygen reimbursement rates remain controversial, and in some states are being appealed and revised).

RESPIRATORY HOME CARE SERVICES

Oxygen therapy

The use of supplemental oxygen in the home remains the most common and popular respiratory home care modality. In 1987 it was estimated that more than 600,000 patients in the United States were receiving some form of home oxygen therapy.[9] This high rate of usage is based, in part, on the fact that the application of home oxygen (in continuous or intermittent fashion) improves survival in selected patient groups, especially those with advanced chronic obstructive pulmonary disease (COPD).[4,10]

Documentation of need. Home oxygen therapy also has been the most improperly prescribed and abused form of respiratory home care. However, these abuses drastically decreased in 1985 when the Health Care Financing Administration (HCFA) published national uniform medical criteria for coverage of home oxygen therapy under the federal Medicare program.[11]

These new regulations mandated that prescriptions for home oxygen therapy be based on documented hypoxemia, as determined by either blood gas analysis or oximetry. Oxygen prescriptions could no longer be based indirectly on the patient's diagnosis and related signs and symptoms, such as dyspnea, orthopnea, or mental confusion. In addition, "prn" oxygen was no longer acceptable. Included in these regulations are the following key provisions[11]:

1. Coverage is provided for patients with significant hypoxemia in the chronic stable states, if the following conditions are met:
   a. The patient has appropriately tried other treatment measures without success.
   b. The patient has one of the following covered health conditions:
      (1) Chronic obstructive pulmonary disease (COPD)
      (2) Diffuse interstitial lung disease
      (3) Cystic fibrosis
      (4) Bronchiectasis
      (5) Pulmonary neoplasm (primary or metastatic)
   c. The patient has conditions or symptoms related to hypoxia that may improve with oxygen, such as:
      (1) Pulmonary hypertension
      (2) Recurring congestive heart failure (CHF)
      (3) Chronic cor pulmonale
      (4) Erythrocytosis
      (5) Impairment of cognitive processes
      (6) Nocturnal restlessness
      (7) Morning headache

d. Noncovered conditions are as follows:
   (1) Angina pectoris in the absence of hypoxemia
   (2) Dyspnea without cor pulmonale or evidence of hypoxemia
   (3) Severe peripheral vascular disease resulting in desaturation in one or more extremities
   (4) Terminal illnesses that do not affect the lungs

2. Clinical evidence of hypoxemia must be documented in the following ways:
   a. Arterial Po_2 value at or below 55 mm Hg or an arterial oxygen saturation at or below 88%, taken at rest with patient breathing room air. Coverage is provided for home oxygen by Medicare.
   b. Arterial Po_2 value at or below 55 mm Hg or an arterial saturation at or below 88% taken during sleep for a patient who demonstrates higher values (56 mm Hg or more or 89% or more) while awake. A fall in arterial Po_2 level of more than 10 mm Hg or a decrease in arterial saturation of more than 5% associated with symptoms or signs attributable to hypoxemia (impairment of cognitive processes, insomnia, or nocturnal restlessness) are also acceptable. In any of these cases, coverage is provided for nocturnal use of oxygen.
   c. Coverage for the use of supplemental oxygen during exercise is provided for patients who demonstrate an improvement in hypoxemia during physical activity. There must be clinical evidence of an arterial Po_2 level at or below 55 mm Hg or an arterial saturation at or below 88% as determined during exercise for a patient who demonstrates higher values (56 mm Hg or more or 89% or more saturation) during the day at rest. There must also be evidence of clinical improvement with improved blood oxygenation during exercise with oxygen in use and an increase in ability to perform exercise and physical activities.

3. Coverage for home oxygen is also provided for patients whose arterial Po_2 value is 56 to 59 mm Hg or whose arterial oxygen saturation is 89% if there is evidence of:
   a. Dependent edema suggesting congestive failure
   b. "P" pulmonale on electrocardiogram (p wave greater than 3 mm in standard leads II, III, or AVF)
   c. Erythrocytosis or erythrocythemia with a hematocrit greater than 56%

4. For patients with an arterial Po_2 value at or above 60 mm Hg or arterial oxygen saturation at or above 90%, carriers must apply a rebuttal presumption that home oxygen is not medically necessary. In order for claims for home oxygen to be reimbursed, the carrier's reviewing physician must:
   a. Review documentation submitted in rebuttal of this presumption
   b. Grant specific approval of the claims

5. For portable oxygen systems, coverage is provided if the following conditions are met:
   a. The claim must meet the requirements specified for medical documentation, laboratory evidence, and health conditions for coverage of home oxygen therapy
   b. The medical documentation must include a description of the activities or exercise routine (distance and/or duration and frequency) that a patient undertakes for which a portable system is required
   c. The claim must include documentation that use of the portable system during the prescribed physical routine or exercise results in clinical improvement as evidenced by an increase in ability to perform exercise or physical activities

In addition, the prescription for home oxygen therapy *must* include the following information:
- Flow rate in liters per minute and/or concentration;
- Frequency of home use in hours per day and minutes per hour (if applicable);
- Duration of need—a specific number of months up to lifetime/indefinite (this will vary according to the Medicare carrier for each different geographical area);
- Diagnosis of severe primary lung disease, secondary conditions related to lung disease, and hypoxia-related conditions or symptoms that may improve with oxygen;
- Laboratory evidence in the form of arterial blood gas analysis or oximetry under the appropriate testing conditions;
- Additional medical documentation that there are no acceptable alternatives to home oxygen therapy.

The physician must authorize home oxygen in this fashion and recertify the need on an ongoing basis, usually once a year.

Supply methods. Today home oxygen is commonly supplied by one or more of the following systems:
- Compressed-oxygen cylinders;
- Liquid oxygen (LOX) systems;
- Oxygen concentrators or enrichers.

A closer look at the use of these systems follows. Table 35-1 provides a summary of their major advantages and disadvantages.

Compressed-oxygen cylinders. When oxygen was first prescribed for home use, large gaseous oxygen cylinders (H or K) were the primary supply containers. For the high-volume user, or for the patient on mechanical ventilation, these large cylinders were commonly yolked together to provide greater storage capacity.

Advantages of the use of compressed-oxygen cylinders in the home include the absence of any waste (even when the cylinder is not used), the availability of portable oxygen in the form of size D and E cylinders, and its ability to meet the home oxygen needs of small-volume users.

The primary disadvantage of this supply approach is the relatively small amount of available oxygen in the space occupied by the tank, even though the cylinder is pressurized. Other disadvantages include the high pressures used for gaseous oxygen storage, the weight of large cylinders, and their bulkiness and cost. To minimize the problem of bulkiness and weight, most cylinders manufactured today are aluminized. This adds to their portability, both in and out of a patient's residence.

Safety measures for cylinder oxygen are the same as those covered in Chapter 24. The cylinder should be secured with a stand or "donut" base; the unit should not be placed near sources of extreme heat or cold. Smoking is not permitted in any area where oxygen is being administered, and oil should not be used to lubricate regulator or flowmeter valves or connections. These safety measures should be thoroughly reviewed by the respiratory care practitioner with both the patient and the family, and their ability to use the system safely should be documented.

In addition, a pressure-reducing valve with a flowmeter is needed to reduce the high cylinder pressure to a lower, safer working pressure and to deliver the oxygen at the prescribed rate of flow. Flowmeters can deliver flows of 0 to 15 L/min; however, some newer devices have 5 to 8 L/min flow limits. Bubble humidifiers are used to humidify the dry oxygen. Because the mineral content of tap water may be high ("hard water"), water used in these humidifiers should be distilled. Otherwise, the porous diffusing element through which the oxygen passes may become occluded. Although complete blockage is not likely, occlusion of the diffusing element results in the production of larger bubbles in smaller numbers, thereby reducing the effectiveness of humidification.

Liquid oxygen systems. Because 1 cubic foot of liquid oxygen is equivalent to 860 cubic feet of gaseous oxygen, liquid oxygen systems make possible the storage of large quantities of oxygen in a substantially smaller space. This is ideal for the high-volume user, who would require a large number of gaseous oxygen cylinders (10 or more per month) to meet therapeutic needs.

As depicted in Fig. 35-1, a typical home liquid-oxygen system is a miniaturized version of that used to supply a hospital. Like its larger counterpart, the home system consists of a reservoir unit similar in design to a Thermos bottle. The inner container of liquid oxygen (LOX) is suspended in an outer container, with the space between a vacuum. The liquid oxygen in the inner reservoir is maintained at a temperature of approximately $-300°F$. Because of constant vaporization, oxygen exists in the gaseous form above the liquid. When not in use, this vaporization maintains the pressure in the container between 20 and 25 psi. Pressure above this level is vented by the primary pressure-relief valve.

When the flow is turned on, gaseous oxygen leaves the container through a vaporizing coil, where it is heated by exposure to ambient temperatures. It then leaves the system through a standardized oxygen outlet connection and is metered by a flow-control valve. If the cylinder pressure drops below a preset level (usually about 20 psig) during use, an economizer valve closes, causing the liquid oxygen to move up the center siphon tube and directly into the vaporizing coil, where ambient temperatures convert the liquid oxygen to a gas. Because of the extensive use of low-flow and oxygen-conserving delivery systems, many newer liquid-oxygen cylinders have flow-metering devices calibrated in 0.5 L/min units and are limited to a maximum flow of between 5 and 8 L/min.

Depending on manufacturer and model, small liquid-oxygen cylinders hold anywhere from 45 to 100 pounds of LOX (18 to 40 L of *liquid* oxygen). To calculate the dura-

Table 35-1 Advantages and Disadvantages of the Three Major Home Oxygen Supply Systems

System	Advantages	Disadvantages
Compressed-oxygen cylinder	Good for small-volume user No waste or loss Stores oxygen indefinitely Widespread availability	Large cylinders are heavy and bulky High pressures may represent a safety hazard (2200 psi) Provides limited volume of oxygen Frequent deliveries may be necessary
Liquid oxygen system	Provides large quantities of oxygen Low pressure system (20 to 25 psi) Portable units can be refilled from reservoir (up to 8-hour supply at 2 LPM) Valuable for rehabilitation	Loss of oxygen due to venting when system is not in use LOX must be delivered as needed Low temperature of LOX may represent a safety hazard
Oxygen concentrator	No waste or loss Low-pressure system (15 psi) Cost effective when continual supply of oxygen is needed Eliminates need for oxygen delivery	Disruption in electrical service renders system inoperable Back-up oxygen is necessary Cannot operate ventilators or other high-pressure devices Concentration of oxygen decreases with flow rate Electrical costs for operating system may be substantial

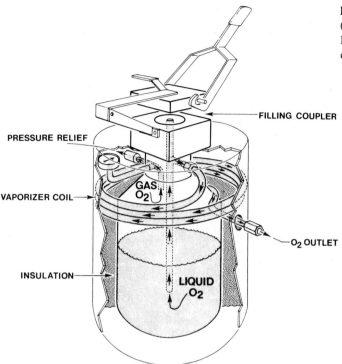

Fig. 35-1   Diagram of a home liquid oxygen supply system. (From Lampton LM: Home and outpatient oxygen therapy; in Brashear RE and Rhodes ML, editors: Chronic obstructive lung disease, St Louis, 1978, The CV Mosby Co.)

FILLING COUPLER

PRESSURE RELIEF

VAPORIZER COIL

GAS O₂

O₂ OUTLET

INSULATION

LIQUID O₂

tion of flow available from a liquid-oxygen system, one must first convert the weight of liquid oxygen in pounds to the equivalent volume of gaseous oxygen in liters. At normal liquid cylinder operating pressures, 1 pound of stored liquid oxygen equals approximately 344 L of gaseous oxygen (average ambient temperature and pressure).

For example, given a 100-pound liquid-oxygen system with a gauge reading indicating a half-full cylinder, one would compute the available gaseous oxygen (in liters) as follows:

Step 1

$$\text{Available LOX (lb)} = 100 \times 0.5$$
$$= 50 \text{ lb}$$

Step 2

$$\text{Available gaseous oxygen} = \text{Weight (lb) remaining} \times$$
$$\text{Conversion factor}$$
$$= 50 \text{ lb} \times 344 \text{ L/lb}$$
$$= 17,200 \text{ L}$$

Finally, to compute the actual duration of flow, one simply divides the available volume of gaseous oxygen by the prescribed liter flow. Assuming a prescribed flow of 2 L/min, the duration of flow for a half-full 100-pound cylinder would be calculated as follows:

Step 3

$$\text{Duration of flow} = \frac{\text{Available gaseous oxygen (L)}}{\text{Prescribed liter flow (L/min)}}$$

$$\text{Duration of flow} = \frac{17,200 \text{ L}}{2 \text{ L/min}}$$
$$= 8600 \text{ minutes}$$
$$= 143.3 \text{ hours}$$
$$\cong 6 \text{ days}$$

In order to minimize the work involved in computing the duration of flow of home liquid-oxygen systems, many manufacturers provide simple conversion charts for this purpose. Table 35-2 gives an example of a conversion chart for a typical 100-pound home liquid-oxygen system.

Many home liquid-oxygen systems also come equipped with smaller portable units (Fig. 35-2). Depending on the manufacturer and the model, these portable units may weigh between 5 and 11 pounds and can be refilled directly from the stationary reservoir as needed. This system meets the needs of many ambulatory patients who are capable of exercise or other physical activities conducted outside the home environment. Although design characteristics vary, most portable LOX units come with a carrying case or a small cart and can provide 5 to 8 hours of oxygen at a flow of 2 L/min.

One problem with liquid oxygen relates to the loss of gas as a result of venting. Since liquid oxygen is stored at cryogenic temperatures, ambient temperatures accelerate evaporation of the liquid to a gas. If the system, including portable equipment, is not in use, pressure will build up and actuate the pressure-relief valve. This causes gaseous oxygen to be wasted. Although most systems are designed to minimize this loss, intermittent use of a liquid-oxygen

Fig. 35-2 Diagram of a portable liquid oxygen unit. (From Lampton LM: Home and outpatient oxygen therapy; in Brashear RE and Rhodes ML, editors: Chronic obstructive lung disease, St Louis, 1978, The CV Mosby Co.)

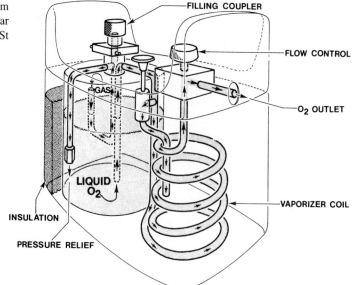

system will always result in some wastage. Continual use of oxygen will eliminate this problem, since system pressures will never build up to activate the pressure-relief valve.

Since most home liquid-oxygen systems operate at pressures below 50 psi, they cannot be used to drive equipment needing this standard pressure, such as pneumatically powered ventilators. However, since the typical home ventilator is electrically powered and uses a flow-metering device to provide supplementary oxygen, this limitation is generally not a problem. Nonetheless, when oxygen at 50 psi is needed, large gaseous cylinders usually constitute the storage system of choice.

Oxygen concentrators (enrichers). An oxygen concentrator is an electrically powered device that is capable of physically separating the oxygen in room air from nitrogen, thereby providing an enriched flow of oxygen for therapeutic use. Currently, there are two types of oxygen concentrator: (1) the "molecular sieve" oxygen concentrator and (2) the membrane oxygen concentrator.

The molecular sieve oxygen concentrator (Fig. 35-3) uses an electrically powered pump to compress and deliver filtered room air to one of two sets of sieves. These sieves contain zeolite pellets (inorganic sodium-aluminum silicate), which are capable of absorbing both gaseous nitrogen and water vapor. Because these pellets need to be

Table 35-2 Conversion Chart for Computing Duration of Flow 100 lb (40 L) Home Liquid-Oxygen Reservoir

Gauge reading	1	2	3	4	5
Weight (lb)	12.5	25	50	75	100
Liquid liters	5	10	20	30	40
Gaseous liters	4303	8606	17,212	25,818	34,424

DURATION OF FLOW (HOURS)

Flow (L/min)					
0.5	143	287	574	861	1147
1	72	143	287	430	574
1.5	48	96	191	287	382
2	36	72	143	215	287
2.5	29	57	115	172	229
3	24	48	96	143	191
3.5	20	41	82	123	164
4	18	36	72	108	143
4.5	16	32	64	96	127
5	14	29	57	86	115
6	12	24	48	72	96
7	10	20	41	61	82
8	9	18	36	54	72

Note: All figures are estimates based on continuous use.

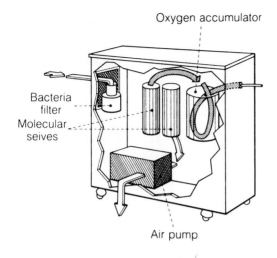

Oxygen accumulator

Bacteria filter

Molecular seives

Air pump

Fig. 35-3 A molecular sieve-type oxygen concentration. (Courtesy DeVilbis Co, Toledo, Ohio.)

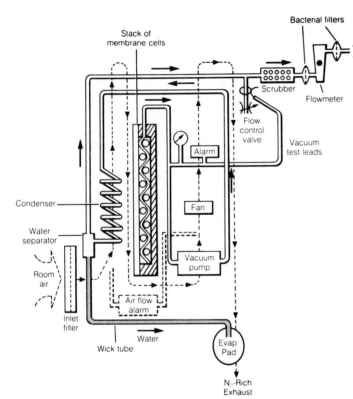

Stack of membrane cells

Bacterial filters

Scrubber

Flowmeter

Humid O₂-rich air to patient

Flow control valve

Alarm

Vacuum test leads

Fan

Condenser

Water separator

Vacuum pump

Room air

Air flow alarm

Inlet filter

Wick tube

Water

Evap Pad

N₂-Rich Exhaust

Fig. 35-4 A membrane-type oxygen concentrator. (Courtesy Oxygen Enricher Co, Schenectady, NY.)

purged of nitrogen and water vapor periodically, an automatic system intermittently switches between sieves, reversing flow through the one previously used.

Gas leaving the molecular sieves is stored in a small oxygen accumulator. At flows of between 1 and 2 L/min, the molecular sieve oxygen concentrator can provide more than 90% oxygen. At higher flows, however, the process becomes less efficient. At a 2 to 5 L/min flow oxygen concentrations fall to between 80% and 90%, and at 10 L/min most oxygen concentrators can provide only 50% oxygen.[12] Since the sieve pellets eventually become exhausted, they must be changed periodically. If the pellets

do become exhausted, the oxygen concentrations delivered will drop significantly, regardless of liter flow.

Membrane oxygen concentrators employ a thin gas-permeable plastic polymer membrane to separate oxygen from room air (Fig. 35-4). A vacuum pump (diaphragm compressor) provides a negative pressure gradient across the membrane. The design of the membrane is such that the rate of gaseous diffusion for oxygen and water vapor is greater than that for nitrogen, yielding an enriched mixture of approximately 40% oxygen at flows of up to 10 L/min.[13] Although providing a lower oxygen concentration than that available with oxygen concentrators of the molecular sieve type, the F_{IO_2} provided by membrane concentrators remains relatively stable throughout the normal range of flows.

Since water molecules readily diffuse through the membrane, the enriched oxygen mixture delivered by membrane concentrators to the patient is saturated with water vapor at ambient temperatures, thereby eliminating the need for a humidification device. However, excess water vapor generated in this process must be removed. This is accomplished by a simple condenser system, with the water condensate evaporated into the nitrogen-rich exhaust (see Fig. 35-4).

Oxygen concentrators are among the most cost-efficient means of supplying oxygen to patients who require continuous home oxygen at low liter flows. Depending on local utility rates, a concentrator running 24 hours a day will increase the average monthly electric bill by only 5% to 10%. Of course, back-up cylinder gas should be available in the event of an electric power failure. Alternatively, an emergency home generator may provide a back-up power supply to the concentrator.

Like most liquid-oxygen systems, oxygen concentrators cannot be used to operate devices that require a high-pressure (50 psi) gas source. Routine monthly maintenance should include cleaning and replacement of internal and external filters and confirmation of the concentration of delivered oxygen with a calibrated oxygen analyzer. Molecular sieve concentrators also may need periodic replacement of the zeolite pellet canisters.

In terms of therapeutic effectiveness, oxygen concentrators can provide blood gas levels of oxygen comparable with those achieved with more traditional supply systems (eg, 100% cylinder gas with a cannula), especially when used to supply patients with low inspired oxygen concentrations.[14,15] Moreover, current reimbursement regulations (see the "six-point plan" previously discussed) favor use of the most effective and cost-efficient home oxygen systems available. As a result, the use of oxygen concentrators and conserving systems (discussed next) will become increasingly important and popular.

Delivery methods. Oxygen delivery systems most commonly used at home include the nasal cannula, the simple oxygen (medium-concentration) mask, and the entrainment mask. In general, nasal catheters and partial rebreathing and nonrebreathing masks are not recommended for home oxygen administration.

Normally, oxygen is not an expensive commodity, but overuse, inappropriate prescription practices, and other abuses related to billing have made its use expensive. In addition, the popularity of oxygen as a home care modality, the cost of providing this service, and recent changes in reimbursement policies have all helped to alter attitudes regarding the economics of home oxygen. Medicare and other insurance carriers have taken a closer look at oxygen consumption and related payments.

In an effort to keep oxygen use and costs down, and in anticipation of further changes in reimbursement practices, a number of oxygen-conserving devices have been developed and marketed. Since the more traditional methods of oxygen administration are covered in detail in Chapter 25, we will focus here on the application of these newer oxygen-conserving devices, including the transtracheal oxygen catheter, the reservoir cannula, and the demand-flow oxygen delivery system.[16,17]

Transtracheal catheter. The transtracheal catheter is a new modality developed for long-term administration of oxygen. First described by Heimlich[18] in 1982, the tech-

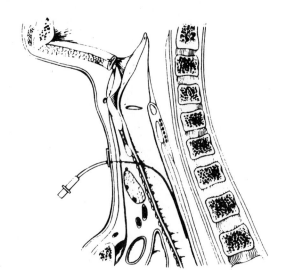

Fig. 35-5   Transtracheal oxygen catheter in position. (Courtesy Erie Medical, Milwaukee, Wisc.)

nique involves administration of oxygen directly into the trachea through a small Teflon catheter inserted surgically between the second and third tracheal rings (Fig. 35-5). The catheter is secured on the outside by a custom-sized chain necklace and receives oxygen through standard tubing connected to a flowmeter.[18] Because it is delivered to the middle portion of the trachea, oxygen accumulates in both the upper airways and the trachea during expiration. The effect is to expand the anatomic reservoir, thereby increasing the F_{IO_2} at any given flow. Specifically, anywhere from 50% to 72% less oxygen flow is required to achieve a given Pa_{O_2} with a transtracheal catheter than with a nasal cannula.[18,19] In some patients, adequate oxygenation may be achieved with flow rates as low as 0.25 L/min.

This can be of great economic benefit to a person who requires oxygen at home 24 hours a day, at costs ranging from $400 to $500 per month. Other frequently reported benefits of the transtracheal catheter include increased patient mobility, avoidance of nasal and ear irritation from drying of mucous membranes, improved compliance with continuous use of oxygen, improved oxygenation in cases of hypoxemia that is nonresponsive (refractory) to nasal cannula therapy, and improved satisfaction with physical appearance when a cannula is not worn on the face. Improvements in sleep, senses of smell and taste, appetite, and dyspnea are observed in some patients.[19]

Transtracheal catheters and their tubing should be replaced every 3 months to avoid product failure. Inflammation and other abnormalities should be promptly reported to the prescribing physician. Health checkups by a physician are recommended once every 3 months. Routine removing and cleaning of the catheter should be performed by the patient. With transtracheal oxygen therapy, the respiratory care practitioner should assume primary responsi-

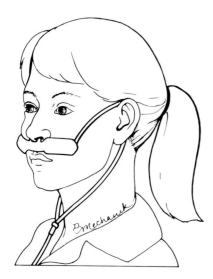

Fig. 35-6   Reservoir cannula.

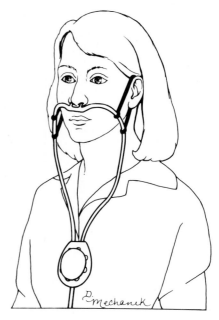

Fig. 35-7   Pendant reservoir oxygen-delivery system.

bility for (1) providing patient education, (2) coordinating communication among members of the home health team, (3) arranging for equipment and supplies, and (4) recognition and referral of any potential abnormalities and problems.[19]

Because of these benefits in cases in which oxygen therapy is needed continuously for very long periods of time, the technique of transtracheal administration should gain wide acceptance as experience with its use grows.

Reservoir cannula. The reservoir cannula (Fig. 35-6) represents a hybrid device, combining the concepts of a low-flow and reservoir delivery system.[16,17] The reservoir cannula operates by storing about 20 ml of oxygen in a small reservoir during exhalation.[20] This stored oxygen is then added to the normal flow during early inspiration, thereby enhancing the amount available at the alveolar level and decreasing the flow requirements for a given FIO_2. As an example, a reservoir cannula set at 0.5 L/min can provide arterial oxygen saturations equivalent to that available with a regular cannula set at 2 L/min.[20]

Because some patients objected to the cosmetic appearance of the reservoir cannula, a "pendant" reservoir system was developed (Fig. 35-7). In this configuration, the reservoir is situated on the anterior chest wall, where it can easily be hidden from view. Performance characteristics of the pendant reservoir system are comparable to those of the reservoir cannula.[21]

For oxygen-conserving devices that use an external reservoir to save oxygen during exhalation, the delivered FIO_2 will vary with the reservoir volume, oxygen flow, and ventilatory pattern. Fig. 35-8 portrays these relationships under a steady-state condition, demonstrating the relative efficiency of the oxygen-conserving device over a simple low-flow system without a reservoir.[16] Obviously, any

change in ventilatory pattern would change the estimated oxygen concentrations delivered by both types of device.

Demand-flow oxygen-delivery systems. Rather than using a reservoir to conserve oxygen during expiration, a demand-flow oxygen-delivery device employs a sensor and valve system to eliminate expiratory oxygen flow altogether (Fig. 35-9).[22-24] The sensing device (usually a fluidic or electromechanical valve) determines the beginning of inspiration, immediately actuating a valve to deliver a quick "pulse" of oxygen. Closure of the actuator valve prevents delivery of oxygen during exhalation. Variations in the amount of oxygen delivered are achieved in two different ways. Either the length of the oxygen pulse is varied or the oxygen is delivered on a variable breath schedule, such as every second or third inhalation. In concept, the demand-flow oxygen delivery should provide the greatest savings in oxygen usage for a given level of arterial saturation, but it is also the most prone to mechanical failure.

Table 35-3 compares and contrasts these oxygen-conserving devices according to their principles of operation, performance characteristics, and advantages and disadvantages.[16]

In summary, oxygen therapy is an essential component of the respiratory home care regimen. All patients with chronic cardiopulmonary diseases who require home oxygen therapy should be able to obtain it in the most effective and efficient way possible. The problem is to match each patient's specific condition and related needs to the most appropriate delivery system. It is here that the respiratory care practitioner can play an essential role. By considering the therapeutic objectives, patient condition, labo-

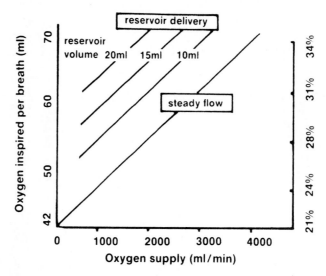

Fig. 35-8   Oxygen-delivery model for reservoir-storage cannulas as compared with steady-flow cannulas. The model is based on the assumptions that the patient is breathing 20 breaths/per minute, I:E is 1:2, critical delivery volume is the first 200 ml of inhalation, and the time required to deliver that volume is 0.5 second. The effective inspired oxygen volumes received by the patient are shown for steady-flow conditions and storage reflux conditions using 10, 15, and 20 ml oxygen boluses. (From Tiep BL: Respir Care 32(2):109, 1987.)

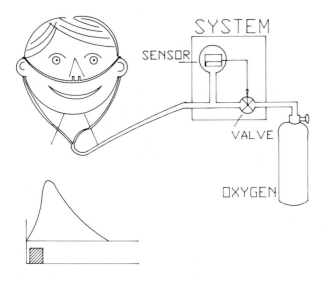

Fig. 35-9   Demand-flow oxygen delivery. As the patient begins to inhale, subatmospheric pressure causes the solenoid to open immediately for a brief time and to deliver oxygen during early inspiration. (From Tiep BL: Respir Care 32(2):110, 1987.)

ratory values (at rest, during sleep, and/or with exercise), projected use (delivery system, flow, and/or concentration), and other variables, the respiratory care practitioner can and should assume primary responsibility for determining the most appropriate approach for home oxygen therapy.

Mechanical ventilation

Mechanical ventilation represents true high technology within the home care environment. Mechanical ventilation is now a recognized and useful form of respiratory home care—for both humane and financial reasons. The advent

of diagnosis related groups (DRGs) and other regulatory efforts pertaining to hospitalization have made mechanical ventilation in the home a necessary measure in the management and treatment of selected patients. In 1986 at least 3000 ventilator-dependent patients were being successfully cared for at home.[25] On the basis of current estimates, this number will continue to grow at a steady pace.

Patient groups. Patients requiring mechanical ventilation in the home fall into three broad groups or categories:

1. Patients who are unable to maintain adequate ventilation over prolonged periods of time (daytime or nocturnal use in particular)
2. Patients who require continuous ventilatory support for long-term survival
3. Patients who are terminally ill with short life expectancies

The box on p. 933 provides additional information regarding these patient groups.[25] As is evident, the primary patient groups best served by mechanical ventilation in the home are those with neuromuscular diseases or injuries, chest wall deformities, severe chronic obstructive lung diseases, and malignant conditions involving the respiratory system.

General criteria. Regardless of the underlying problem, certain criteria must be met before home mechanical ventilation should be considered:

- Willingness of family to accept responsibility for mechanical ventilation in the home;
- Presence of adequate family and professional support;
- Overall viability of the home care plan;
- Patient stability;
- Layout and available resources in the home or alternate site.

Planning. Mechanical ventilation within the home or alternate site can be a successful endeavor, but extensive planning, education, and follow-up are essential. Members of the discharge and home care team include the physician, the discharge planner, the respiratory care practitioner, the psychologist, the DME provider, and the home health care (visiting) nurse. Other disciplines that may be involved include physical therapy, occupational therapy, dietary therapy, and pharmacy—depending on the patient's condition and related needs. Basic steps in the patient-discharge process include the following:

1. Family is consulted regarding feasibility of patient's discharge;
2. Physician writes appropriate orders;

Table 35-3   Comparison of Oxygen-Conserving Methods

	Method		
Characteristic	Transtracheal catheter	Reservoir cannula	Demand delivery
Conservation mechanism	Reduction of dead space	Storage of oxygen during exhalation	Delivery only during early inhalation
Unique advantages	Unobtrusive; possible improved patient compliance	Disposable. Probably least subject to mechanical failure	Maintains O_2 savings over usual delivery ranges
Oxygen required (expressed as a fraction of continuous-flow requirement)	$\frac{1}{3}$ to $\frac{1}{2}$	$\frac{1}{4}$ to $\frac{1}{2}$	$\frac{1}{7}$ to $\frac{1}{3}$
Need for humidification*	None	None	None
Obtrusiveness	Least obtrusive	Most obtrusive	Comparable to steady flow
Unique disadvantages	Catheter clogging, surgical complications (e.g., infection, subcutaneous emphysema)	Most obtrusive	Theoretically most vulnerable to mechanical failure*

*No incidents reported.

PROFILES OF PATIENT GROUPS REQUIRING MECHANICAL VENTILATION WITHIN THE HOME ENVIRONMENT

	GROUP DESCRIPTION	DISEASES INVOLVED
Profile 1	Mainly composed of neuromuscular and thoracic wall disorders; particular stage of disease process allows patient certain periods of spontaneous breathing time during day; generally requires only nocturnal mechanical support	Amyotrophic lateral sclerosis Multiple sclerosis Kyphoscoliosis and related chest wall deformities Diaphragmatic paralysis Myasthenia gravis
Profile 2	Requires continuous mechanical ventilatory support associated with long-term survival rates	High spinal cord injuries Apneic encephalopathies Severe chronic obstructive lung disease Late-stage muscular dystrophy
Profile 3	Usually returns home at request of patient and family; patient's condition is terminal, life expectancy is short, and patient and family wish to spend remaining time at home; patients usually pose management problems in the home because of their rapidly deteriorating conditions	Lung cancer End-stage chronic obstructive pulmonary disease

3. Discharge planner coordinates efforts of team members and discharge plan is formulated;
4. Physician and other team members discuss plan with family and/or care givers;
5. Education and training are initiated and completed;
6. Patient and family are prepared for discharge;
7. Equipment and supplies are readied;
8. Discharge planner meets with team and makes final preparations;
9. Patient is discharged (with trial period, if necessary);
10. Ongoing and follow-up care is provided by visiting nurse, respiratory care practitioner, and other health care professionals (as necessary).

To properly prepare the patient and the family for discharge, a comprehensive educational program needs to be undertaken and completed. Areas that should be covered in such an educational program include the following:

- Anatomy and pathophysiology of the cardiopulmonary system;
- Medical terminology;
- Aspects of ventilatory support;
- Equipment operation;
- Airway management;
- Equipment maintenance and disinfection;
- Patient monitoring;
- Emergency procedures.

All primary and secondary patient care givers should attend and successfully complete this educational process. This may take anywhere from 1 to 2 weeks of instruction, demonstration, and return demonstration. Before discharge, the patient should be placed on the actual ventilator that will be employed in the home setting. In the early stages after discharge, patient follow-up by a respiratory care practitioner may need to occur every day, but as patient and family become familiar with the equipment and related procedures, follow-up can decrease in frequency to weekly or biweekly visitations as needed.

Goals and standards of care. To help ensure the highest level of respiratory home care for the ventilator-dependent patient, a number of standards and guidelines have been established. In particular, there are the American College of Chest Physicians (ACCP) Guidelines for Mechanical Ventilation in the Home Setting and Standards for the Provision of Care to Ventilator-Assisted Patients in an Alternative Site as approved by the American Association for Respiratory Care.[26,27] The ACCP guidelines suggest the following goals be considered in caring for the ventilator-dependent patient on a long-term basis:

Goal I   To extend life
Goal II   To enhance the quality of life
Goal III   To reduce morbidity
Goal IV   To improve the physical, physiologic, social, and psychosocial functions of ventilator-assisted patients
Goal V   To provide cost benefits

These guidelines also identify the best candidates for home ventilation, namely, patients with neuromuscular or skeletal disorders such as muscular dystrophy or kyphoscoliosis. Patients with restrictive lung diseases involving the pulmonary parenchyma are almost never candidates for home mechanical ventilation. Most of these patients are acutely ill, often are not clinically stable, and usually remain severely dyspneic even with ventilatory support.

The ACCP guidelines further suggest criteria by which to assess the clinical stability of patients under consideration for home mechanical ventilation[26]:

- Absence of severe dyspnea while on a ventilator;
- Acceptable arterial blood gas results;
- Inspired oxygen concentrations that are relatively low;
- Psychological stability;
- Evidence of developmental progress (for pediatric/adolescent candidates);
- Absence of life-limiting cardiac dysfunction and arrhythmias;
- If possible, no use of positive end expiratory pressure (PEEP); if needed, PEEP should not exceed +10 cm H_2O;
- Ability to clear airway secretions—either by cough or by use of tracheobronchial suction;
- A tracheostomy tube as opposed to an endotracheal tube;
- No readmissions expected for more than 1 month.

Finally, the guidelines address such issues and concerns as the availability of an adequate financial reimbursement mechanism, an assessment of resources within the home or alternative site, necessary equipment and supplies to provide the prescribed home care, and the formulation of a workable discharge plan.

The Standards of Care approved by the American Association for Respiratory Care (AARC) are as follows[27]:

Standard I: The provision of care to a ventilator-assisted patient located in an alternative site* shall be defined and guided by established written policies and procedures accepted by both the discharging institution and the alternative care site.

Standard II: The services provided to ventilator-assisted patients shall be dispensed in accordance with a prescription written by the physician responsible for the care of that particular patient.

Standard III: Participants shall be prepared for their responsibilities in the provision of services through appropriate training and education.

Standard IV: The ventilator-assisted patient shall be provided with safe and effective equipment appropriate for that patient's physiologic needs.

Standard V: There shall be established recording and reporting mechanisms for the program.

---

*An alternative site may be defined as any identifiable location outside the acute care hospital setting, such as the home, convalescent center, nursing facility, or retirement center where ventilator-assisted patients receive care.

Standard VI: The quality and appropriateness of care provided under the auspices of the program must be monitored and evaluated by the program's medical director, and identified problems must be resolved.

The guidelines and standards discussed here provide a basis for any effective discharge and home care plan that involves ventilator-dependent patients. They help to identify members of the discharge and home care team, identify criteria for patient assessment before discharge, review education and training protocols, establish equipment standards, and formulate protocols for ongoing and follow-up care. In essence, they identify who and what are needed, when and how discharge and home care should be done, and who is responsible for overseeing the entire process.

Role of DME supplier. In this process, the role of the DME supplier should not be overlooked or underestimated. The DME supplier often provides the follow-up services of the respiratory care practitioner assigned to the case. All of the equipment and home care supplies needed fall under the responsibility of the DME supplier. Besides the mechanical ventilator and back-up unit (if necessary), the DME supplier normally provides other essential equipment and supplies. A typical listing of these essentials includes the following:

- Oxygen;
- Hospital bed;
- Patient lift;
- Portable suction;
- Bag-valve-mask unit or portable resuscitator;
- Disposable supplies (circuits, catheters, pads);
- Monitoring devices such as pulse oximeter;
- Tracheal tubes and related care kits.

Equipment considerations. The single most important item of equipment provided is the mechanical ventilator. Depending on the patient's disease, condition, and related therapeutic need, the device will be either a negative-pressure or a positive-pressure unit. In most instances, positive-pressure ventilators are used within the home environment. However, negative-pressure devices have experienced a rebirth. They are being used to provide long-term ventilatory support for patients with neuromuscular or neurologic problems and in maintaining patients with chronic lung diseases who require support periodically or on a nocturnal basis.[28] Negative-pressure ventilation is very useful in patients who need limited ventilatory support and who have essentially clear, patent airways with little or no respiratory secretions. In general, this type of ventilation is contraindicated in the treatment and management of obstructive sleep apnea (OSA). Negative-pressure ventilators that are currently available for home use include the following:

- Porta-Lung chamber (Massachusetts Rehabilitation Services);
- Iron lung (J.H. Emerson Company);
- Chest cuirass (Lifecare)—used in conjunction with a negative-pressure generator;

- Raincoat (J.H. Emerson) and pneumosuit with leggings (New Tech Associates)—also used in conjunction with negative-pressure generators;
- Negative-pressure generators:
  - Emerson 33-CRE;
  - Emerson 33-CRX;
  - Emerson 33-CRA;
  - Thompson Maxivent (Puritan-Bennett);
  - Lifecare 170C;
- Pneumobelt (Lifecare);
- Rocking bed (J.H. Emerson Company).

However, the ventilators most commonly encountered in the home are still those of the positive-pressure type. These units can range from very simplistic devices, such as the Puritan-Bennett Thompson portable units, to the more sophisticated Bear 33, Life Products LP-6, and Puritan Bennett C-2800 units. Most positive-pressure units are volume-cycled, although some can also be pressure-cycled. Most are piston-driven devices that produce a sine-wave flow pattern. Depending on manufacturer and model, available volumes typically vary from 0 to 3000 ml and respiratory rates can range from 1 to 69 breaths/min. IMV/SIMV is a feature on most, along with various audio and visual alarms. A number of devices have an internal battery that can provide up to 1 hour of operation (depending on established ventilatory parameters) in the event of an electrical power failure. Many of these ventilators can also be connected to an external power source, such as a marine battery.

Positive-pressure ventilators can be used for most types of patients who require mechanical ventilation in the home, from pediatric to adult levels. Some of the units currently available for home use include the following:

- Life Products models LP-3, LP-4, LP-5, and LP-6;
- Thompson Maxivent (Puritan-Bennett)—can provide both positive- and negative-pressure ventilation;
- Thompson Bantam-GS (Puritan-Bennett);
- Thompson M25B (Puritan-Bennett);
- Thompson M3000XA (Puritan-Bennett);
- Puritan-Bennett Companion 2800;
- Lifecare 170C — provides both positive- and negative-pressure ventilation;
- Lifecare models PLV-100 and PLV-102;
- Bear 33 (Bear Medical).

When one is deciding which ventilator to use, a number of factors need to be considered. These include portability, alarms, reliability, patient's condition and inspired oxygen requirement, space available for unit, and competence of family and other care givers. Ventilators used within the home or an alternative site should have the following characteristics[28]:

- Trouble-free operation for extended periods of time;
- Easy patient cycling (assist/control, IMV, SIMV);
- An adequate alarm system (pressure limits, patient disconnect, etc);

HOME CONSULTATION REPORT - VENTILATOR-DEPENDENT PATIENT

Date_____

Patient_____   Diagnosis_____

Address_____   _____

Doctor_____   Referral_____

Address_____   Therapist_____

VENTILATOR SETTINGS   ### TREATMENTS

type_____ V_{sigh}_____   Bronchodilator Therapy:_____

mode_____ R_{sigh}_____   _____

V_T_____ P_{sigh}_____   CPT/Other_____

FIO_2_____   Daily hours on   _____

P_{sys}_____   ventilator_____

P_{limit}_____

EQUIPMENT REVIEW AND CHECK

_____ventilator settings #1   _____resuscitator bag

_____ventilator settings #2   _____suction machine

_____alarms   _____oxygen supply

PATIENT EVALUATION

Suctioning:_____

Auscultation:_____

Blood Pressure_____Pulse_____Respirations_____

Patient Assessment:_____

_____

_____

Comments/Plan_____

_____

_____

_____

_____

Director Respiratory Services

Fig. 35-10   Home care visitation report form for a ventilator-dependent patient. (Courtesy Abbey-Foster Medical Corp.)

- Portability with internal battery and means of being connected to an external power source;
- User-friendly controls that are easy to understand and a circuit that is easy to change.

Evaluation and follow-up. Routine follow-up visits by a respiratory care practitioner help to ensure the success of patient management within the home. Equipment must be checked and cleaned as necessary. The patient's status should be carefully assessed, and appropriate recommendations for change should be made to the primary or prescribing physician. Any prescribed respiratory therapy should be administered during the visit, and all necessary

supply items should be left with the patient's care givers. After each visit, a report form must be completed (Fig. 35-10) and kept on record as part of the documentation process. Subsequent follow-up visits should take place regularly (weekly or biweekly) and whenever necessary.

Benefits. Although mechanical ventilation in the home represents an enormous undertaking, it can bring about substantial benefits to the patient and cut medical costs. Patients have more positive psychological outlooks when they are at home, even while on mechanical ventilation. There appears to be more freedom and more motivation to live and to become involved in productive activities. In addition, the cost savings are significant. Care in a hospital may cost as much as $250,000 per year. Similar care at home may range from $15,000 to $30,000 per year, depending on equipment and professional support provided. When discharge is executed properly, the hospital readmission rates can be extremely low, with the duration of home care continuing for years.[28]

Other modes of respiratory home care

In addition to home oxygen therapy and mechanical ventilation, other modes of respiratory care are now common in the home setting. These interventions may constitute the primary in-home therapy, or they may be used to supplement or enhance other modes of care. Included for discussion here are aerosol therapy, intermittent positive pressure breathing, airway care, nasal CPAP, and monitoring of apnea.

Aerosol therapy. The administration of bland and medicated aerosols is a common respiratory home care practice. Aerosol therapy may be continuous or intermittent, depending on the patient's condition and the therapeutic objectives:

- **Continuous Aerosol:** This form of therapy may be indicated for patients with tracheostomies, patients with thick inspissated secretions, or pediatric patients placed within cool-mist tents (for treatment of croup, cystic fibrosis, etc.). Most often, normal saline solution or distilled water is aerosolized. Ultrasonic devices or 50 psi compressors are used in aerosol production. The major problem is that of infection from contaminated equipment. To reduce the incidence of infections, equipment and the delivery system must be cleaned and changed routinely. Additional discussion of disinfection procedures can be found later in this chapter.

- **Intermittent Aerosol:** this type of home therapy involves the administration of bland aerosols (distilled water or normal saline solution) in cool-mist or heated forms and medicated aerosol treatments for patients with asthma, bronchitis, and other chronic lung disorders. Medications frequently nebulized are isoetharine (Bronkosol), metaproterenol (Alupent), albuterol (Proventil or Ventolin), atropine, and n-acetylcysteine (Mucomyst).

Medicated aerosols require a small compressor with a hand-held nebulizer that has either a mouthpiece or an aerosol mask. Cool-mist and heated aerosols require an ultrasonic nebulizer or a 50 psi compressor with a nebulizer, such as a Puritan heated nebulizer or a comparable Ohio unit. Disposable systems have also become popular for home use.

Proper instruction and follow-up are necessary for patients receiving any form of home aerosol therapy. Equipment must be properly checked, cleaned, and maintained to ensure proper compliance with the physician's prescription and stated therapeutic objectives.

Intermittent positive pressure breathing (IPPB). This therapy, although not as widely used as in the past, still has useful home care applications. It is most useful in the administration of bronchodilators to patients with certain obstructive lung diseases and in the treatment of restrictive lung diseases, such as multiple sclerosis, pulmonary fibrosis, and kyphoscoliosis, and certain neuromuscular defects (see Chapter 26). The most common type of equipment used to deliver home IPPB therapy is a small electrically driven unit such as the Bennett AP-5 unit. However, pneumatic devices, such as the Bennett TV-2P, Bennett PR-1 and PR-2, and Bird Mark 7 and 8 units, are also in use. Again, as with aerosol therapy, the major concerns revolve around education of the patient and compliance with the prescribed regimen of therapy and equipment disinfection.

Postural drainage, percussion, and vibration. These forms of chest physical therapy can be applied manually or mechanically with the aid of a percussor/vibrator (see Chapter 27). Medicare will reimburse for this type of equipment if no one is available or able to provide manual percussion and vibration at home. Postural drainage, percussion, and vibration should be administered as directed by the physician's prescription and are best applied after any aerosol or IPPB therapy. Patients with cystic fibrosis, bronchiectasis, chronic bronchitis, and any pulmonary conditions in which secretions are a problem find this therapeutic regimen most beneficial. Family members can usually be instructed in the proper delivery of postural drainage, percussion, and vibration. The presence of any mechanical device will make the therapy session easier for the family member. Patients may also be able to apply the percussion and vibration to themselves with this equipment. Most devices are light in weight and easy to handle, with variable speed controls.

Airway care. Small portable suction units have been available for home use since the 1960s. Pressure is measured in inches of mercury (Hg) and care must be taken to adjust this suction pressure properly for each patient. For infants, 5 to 7 inches Hg is recommended; 7 to 12 inches Hg is recommended for children, and 12 to 15 inches Hg for adults. The equipment consists of a suction pump, a collection bottle, and suction tubing with catheter. Instruction of patient and family is usually carried out in the hospital before the patient is discharged. Home reinforcement and follow-up are also necessary. Maintenance and cleaning need to be followed on a daily basis. In many cases, suction catheters are used for a day and then discarded. This measure is followed in an effort to control supply costs. Catheters are placed in a disinfecting solution, such as hydrogen peroxide or 2.5% acetic acid, between suctioning attempts. Patients with tracheostomies receive care from a trained family member, a visiting nurse, or an assigned respiratory care practitioner. Tracheal tube changes are usually performed by the physician, the respiratory care practitioner, or the home health care nurse.

Nasal CPAP (continuous positive airway pressure). Nasal CPAP is a relatively new form of respiratory home care used in the treatment of obstructive sleep apnea (see Chapter 28). In 1987, Medicare approved reimbursement for the rental of nasal CPAP equipment, provided there was sufficient documentation establishing the diagnosis of the sleep apnea syndrome. This documentation must be obtained by means of a sleep study (polysomnography) that demonstrated the occurrence of at least 30 episodes of apnea 10 seconds or more in duration during sleep.

Nasal CPAP equipment consists of a flow-generating device, a one-way valve or reservoir bag, a nasal mask, and a pressure valve. CPAP pressures range from 5 cm H_2O to 15 cm H_2O (or higher, depending on the system used). After the patient is properly fitted with a nasal mask and the prescribed pressure set and verified, the unit is turned on and checked for leaks.

If the system operates correctly and if the patient complies with the therapy, the problems associated with sleep apnea (morning headaches, daytime hypersomnolence, etc.) should be resolved. Problems associated with nasal CPAP include conjunctivitis, rhinitis, sinusitis, and skin irritation. The mask should be cleaned daily to remove facial oils and replaced, along with the head gear, at least twice a year. Respiratory follow-up should focus on an evaluation of the patient and of his or her compliance with therapy, on equipment operation, and on recognition and referral of any patient-related problems.

Apnea monitoring. Sudden infant death syndrome (SIDS) is another disorder frequently associated with sleep with which a respiratory care practitioner may become involved. High-risk infants are frequently kept on apnea monitors in the hospital setting and are discharged with this equipment after extensive instruction of the family in equipment use and in infant cardiopulmonary resuscitation (CPR). Most monitors detect respirations and heart rate and activate audio and visual alarms when established high or low alarm limits are reached. Follow-up visits by a respiratory care practitioner or a nurse are frequent at first but occur less often as the family develops a familiarity with the equipment and monitoring routine. The use of apnea monitors is usually discontinued after an infant's pneumocardiograms have become negative. Guidelines for home apnea monitoring, recently developed by the National Institutes of Health (NIH), are discussed in Chapter 32.

Equipment disinfection and maintenance

Because of the increasing numbers of respiratory patients being cared for in the home environment, the danger of infection from contaminated equipment has also increased. To give direction to home care providers and respiratory care practitioners regarding the cleaning and processing of home care equipment, the American Respiratory Care Foundation recently disseminated a set of guidelines for disinfection of respiratory care equipment in the home care setting.[29]

These standards, endorsed by the American Association for Respiratory Care, are intended to enhance and complement the home care standards now promulgated by the JCAHO for home care company and organization accreditation (as previously discussed). The standards address the sources of infection, the basic principles of infection control, patients at particular risk, disinfection methods, equipment processing, and care of solutions and medications.

With regard to basic principles of infection control, the ARCF recommends standard emphasis on proper handwashing technique by care givers, in conjunction with avoidance of visits to the patient by friends or relatives who have respiratory infections.

With regard to DME suppliers, the ARCF guidelines require that all permanent equipment, such as ventilator circuits, oxygen-delivery equipment, and medication-delivery components, be sterilized or receive high-level disinfection before being supplied to another patient. Equipment that is designated as disposable or "single-patient use" must be used by one patient only and must not be supplied to another patient, regardless of the sterilization or disinfection methods available by the home care provider.

In terms of the cleaning process, the ARCF recommends that all equipment be completely disassembled and washed initially in cool water to soften and loosen dried material. This initial wash should be followed by a soak in warm soapy water for several minutes, with equipment scrubbed as necessary to remove any remaining organic material. After this step, the equipment must be thoroughly rinsed to remove any residual soap and then drained of excess water.

According to the ARCF guidelines, quaternary ammonium compounds and various dilutions of acetic acid are not recommended for the disinfection of respiratory home care equipment. Instead, "high" disinfection with activated glutaraldehyde is considered the method of choice. Nonetheless, it is my opinion that issues such as availability, cost, and other potential problems (such as skin irritation) must be considered by both the home care provider and the patient before a final determination is made as to which disinfectant solution best meets the patient's individual needs.

With regard to the use of water as a diluent or for humidification or nebulization, the ARCF guidelines recommend that it be boiled, stored in a refrigerator, and discarded after 24 hours. The ARCF also recommends that manufacturers' guidelines for the proper handling of specific medications be strictly followed.

In addition to these general guidelines, the ARCF has provided specific sets of instructions for patients and care givers regarding the cleaning and disinfection of selected types of home care equipment, including continuous me-

PATIENT AND CARE GIVER INSTRUCTIONS FOR CLEANING AND DISINFECTION OF VENTILATOR CIRCUITS

Before you start to clean and disinfect your equipment, be sure that:

- Your work area is clear and clean.
- You have all of your supplies out and ready for use.
- Your hands are clean.
- Clean gloves are available in case you need them.
- You have a clean apron or a clean old shirt to put over your clothes to protect them from splashes and spills of dirty water that may contain germs.

CONSIDERATIONS

1. The outer surface of the ventilator may be wiped off as necessary with a clean, damp (not wet) cloth. You do not need to worry about cleaning the inside of the machine, but it should be checked and necessary maintenance should be done according to the manufacturer's recommendations by someone from the company that supplied the machine.

2. The patient circuit must be taken completely apart and cleaned and disinfected every 24 hours.

PROCEDURE

1. Take the circuit completely apart. Wipe the outer surface of the small tubes with a clean, damp cloth. Hang from line with clips or clothespins.

Take large-bore tubings, connectors, nebulizer or humidifier, and exhalation valve apart. Wash first in cool water to soften and loosen dried material. Then soak in warm soapy water for several minutes. Scrub with brush to remove any phlegm or secretions or other material that should not be there. Rinse until all soap is gone. Drain off as much water as you can.

2. Place the parts in the disinfectant solution. Be certain that all of the inside and outside surfaces of the parts are covered with the disinfectant. Leave the parts in the disinfectant for at least 15 minutes or the manufacturer's recommended length of time. Check the clock or use a timer.

3. Be sure that your hands or gloves are clean. Rinse all of the parts thoroughly under running water.

4. Drain off as much water as you can and hang tubings to dry. Put small parts on a clean, dry surface.

5. When all parts are completely dry, put the exhalation valve and nebulizer back together; then put the circuit back together, ready for use. Be sure that your hands are clean before you start to put the circuit back together. Store the circuit in a clean plastic bag.

6. It is best to have at least three complete ventilatory circuits—one in use, one being cleaned or drying, and one in reserve.

---

chanical ventilator circuits, intermittent positive pressure breathing circuits, suction equipment, and aerosol- and oxygen-delivery systems. The box above provides an example of patient instructions for cleaning and disinfecting a mechanical ventilator circuit.[29]

PATIENT ASSESSMENT AND FOLLOW-UP

As indicated in the American Association for Respiratory Care's standards for respiratory home care, there must be evidence that patients are receiving follow-up evaluations at least once a month, and more often if necessary, by some member of the home health care team.[2] This person could be the attending physician, the visiting public health nurse, a physical therapist, or a respiratory care practitioner. Although some DME suppliers may argue the economics involved with monthly visitations by respiratory technicians or therapists, many do provide and cover the cost of such visits.

Initially, on being discharged from the hospital and settling in at home, patients may require more frequent follow-up, as in the case of ventilator-dependent patients. With time and experience, however, visits can be less frequent. Nonetheless, some type of periodic follow-up in the

home by a respiratory specialist is needed. The frequency of visits should be determined by the following factors:

- The patient's condition, clinical status, and therapeutic needs (objectives);
- Family or care giver support available;
- Type and complexity of home care equipment set up in the home;
- The overall environment in which the patient lives;
- The degree to which the patient is able to provide self-care.

When a visit is made by a respiratory care practitioner, a number of functions must be performed. These include the following:

- Patient assessment (objective and subjective data), including pretreatment and posttreatment measurements of pulse, respiratory rate, blood pressure, and peak expiratory flow rate (or FVC, FEV_1 and $FEV_1\%$ if appropriate);
- Evaluation of patient's compliance with prescribed respiratory home care;
- Equipment assessment (operation, cleanliness, and need for related supplies);
- Identification of any problem areas or patient concerns;

PATIENT HOME VISITATION REPORT

NAME_____ AGE_____

ADDRESS_____ TELEPHONE_____

PHYSICIAN_____REFERRAL_____

PATIENT DIAGNOSIS/HISTORY_____

THERAPEUTIC OBJECTIVE(S)_____

PRESCRIBED HOME CARE_____

HOME CARE EQUIPMENT_____

PATIENT EVALUATION:

AUSCULTATION NOTES:

CLINICAL MEASUREMENTS:

	PULSE	RESPIRATIONS	B/P	PEFR	% OF PRED.
PRE-TREATMENT -	_____	_____	_____	_____LPM	_____%
POST-TREATMENT-	_____	_____	_____	_____LPM	_____%

PRED. PEFR =   _____LPM   % OF IMPROVEMENT = _____%

THERAPEUTIC PLAN AND RELATED COMMENTS:

NEXT SCHEDULED VISIT:

_____   _____
         Visiting Therapist   Date

Fig. 35-11 Home care visitation report form for a patient receiving respiratory home care other than mechanical ventilation. (Courtesy Jarvis and Jarvis Home Healthcare.)

▪ Statement related to patient's goals and therapeutic plan.

A standardized written report, such as that depicted in Fig. 35-11, should be completed by the visiting therapist, with copies sent to the patient's physician, the home care referral source, and any other interested member of the home health care team. This report should become part of the patient's medical record and should be referred to when one is following the course of the patient's disease and overall progress. Policies and procedures regarding patient setup and follow-up in the home should be established and kept on file by each DME supplier who provides any type of oxygen and/or respiratory therapy within the home setting.

ISSUES IN RESPIRATORY HOME CARE

Reimbursement

Although respiratory care services are fully reimbursed in the hospital, they are not in the home environment. Some reimbursement is available in certain skilled nursing facilities (SNF), through home health agencies, in the home for ventilator-dependent patients, and through chronic outpatient rehabilitation facilities (CORFs) with regard to pulmonary rehabilitation. This reimbursement, however, is minimal and inconsistent and varies geographically throughout the United States.

While reimbursement for home oxygen and respiratory home care equipment is available through Medicare and other insurance carriers, services and visits performed by respiratory care practitioners generally are not. The reasons for this are political, economic, and clinical.

When reimbursements for home care services were first developed, respiratory care was a relatively new profession and not fully understood or appreciated by the medical community. While the profession has grown and achieved due recognition, the reimbursement picture has not. Today Medicare expenditures are closely scrutinized and tightly controlled. Other health care professions are not willing or ready to relinquish what they have acquired over the years regarding home care involvement and related payments. Therefore any changes with respect to reimbursement for respiratory home care services will have to come about through legislative measures. Other developments that will have an impact on the reimbursement issue include the following[30]:

- A reduction in the number of allied health professions and professionals;
- A tendency toward the evolution of multicompetency in health care;
- Legal credentialing of all respiratory care practitioners;
- Raising of the minimum education and entry requirements for practitioners in the field;
- Increased stature and importance of the respiratory care profession as a result of performance and public awareness.

Ethical and legal issues

As respiratory home care has increased, so too has the potential for fraud and abuse. Among the most common areas of potential ethical or legal impropriety are the following[31]:

1. *"Finders' fees."* Payment to a practitioner for patients referred to a particular DME supplier.
2. *Hiring of hospital staff.* Respiratory care practitioners in a particular department are hired or contracted to perform home visits in return for patient referrals from that hospital.
3. *Consultation services.* This practice (including payment for services) is legal so long as it is not tied to patient referrals.
4. *Inducements to the patient.* The offer of "free, noncovered" items induces a patient to use a particular DME provider.
5. *Free equipment.* Instead of cash payments, free equipment is offered in return for patient referrals.
6. *Payment of electric bills.* This is considered another inducement for patient referrals.

Under the Medicare/Medicaid Anti-Fraud and Abuse Amendments of 1977 (PL 95-142) such actions can result in criminal prosecution and very stiff penalties. For example, if a respiratory care practitioner is found guilty of fraud or abuse under this law, he or she can be fined $25,000 and/or imprisoned for up to 5 years for each offense.

To discourage such improprieties, the AARC has adopted a statement on the ethical performance of respiratory home care (see Chapter 12). In addition, the AARC has taken the position that[32]:

1. Profit or revenue generation must not influence the selection, evaluation, or continuation of any respiratory home care services. Fees, kickbacks, or other remunerations paid or offered by DME providers or received or solicited by respiratory care practitioners for referral of patients are considered unethical and illegal.
2. Persons who are either employed by or receive remuneration from both health care institutions that may refer patients and DME suppliers who offer respiratory home care must openly disclose this relationship to both parties.
3. Institutionally based respiratory care practitioners who have significant ownership interest in a DME company that provides respiratory home care must openly disclose this relationship to the employing institution, Medicare part B carriers, and all others who may be involved in the referral process. The practitioner must remove himself from the process of patient referrals to that provider.

It is hoped that these legal and ethical standards will minimize fraud and abuse in the delivery of respiratory home care. However, only the active involvement of practitioners in supporting and upholding these governmental and professional expectations can assure that the occasional unscrupulous provider is exposed and prosecuted to the fullest extent possible. As discussed in Chapter 12, this is the least we can expect from a field that seeks recognition as a true profession.

SUMMARY

In less than 20 years, respiratory home care has evolved from an isolated and often neglected responsibility to a key component in the provision of comprehensive health care. Frankly, much of this rapid growth was associated with an early lack of regulatory control and profiteering. However, as both the government and private agencies began seeking ways to lower health care costs, home care became a practical alternative to prolonged hospitalization in the acute care setting.

Today, legitimate uses for respiratory home care include long-term oxygen therapy and home care of the ventilator-dependent patient. Other respiratory care modalities may be employed, either by themselves or to supplement these forms of care.

The success of these undertakings depends on careful team planning, effective patient and family education, and coordinated and ongoing assessment and follow-up.[33] The respiratory care practitioner is a vital member of the home health care team and should play a primary role in several elements of the planning, implementation, and evaluation process. With other health care providers and governmental agencies beginning to appreciate the important role filled by respiratory care practitioners in the home, an increase in their utilization is assured. Practitioners can facilitate this acceptance by becoming more skilled and knowledgeable in the special methods needed to implement effective respiratory services in the home and in delivering these services ethically and in cost-effective ways.

REFERENCES

1. Wyka KA: A review of respiratory home care, RX Home Care 6:41-49, 1984.
2. American Association for Respiratory Care: Standards for respiratory therapy home care: an official statement by the American Association for Respiratory Care, Respir Care 24:1080-1082, 1979.
3. Fischer DA and Prentice WS: Feasibility of home care for certain respiratory-dependent restrictive or obstructive lung disease patients, Chest 82:739, 1982.
4. The Medical Research Council Working Party: Long-term domiciliary oxygen therapy in chronic hypoxic cor pulmonale complicating chronic bronchitis and emphysema, Lancet 1:681-686, 1981.
5. Sivak ED et al: Home care ventilation: the Cleveland Clinic experience from 1977 to 1985, Respir Care 31:294-302, 1986.
6. Goldberg AJ and Faure EAM: Home care for life-supported persons in England: the Responaut Program, Chest 86:910, 1984.
7. Make BJ et al: Long-term management of ventilator-assisted individuals: the Boston University experience, Respir Care 31:303, 1986.
8. Joint Commission on Accreditation of Health Care Organizations: Standards for the accreditation of home care, Chicago, 1988, Joint Commission on Accreditation of Health Care Organizations.
9. Petty TL: New developments in home oxygen therapy, Respir Mgmt 17:24-29, 1987.
10. Nocturnal Oxygen Therapy Trial Group: Continuous or nocturnal oxygen therapy in hypoxemic chronic obstructive lung disease, Ann Intern Med 93:391-398, 1980.
11. Transmittal 702: Final regulations released on home use of oxygen, AARTimes 9:27-30, 1985.
12. Chusid EL: Oxygen concentrators, Int Anesthesiol Clin 20:235-247, 1982.
13. McPherson SP: Respiratory therapy equipment, ed 3, St Louis, 1985, The CV Mosby Co.
14. Brown HV and Ziment I: Evaluation of an oxygen concentrator in patients with COPD, Respir Ther 5(6):55, 1978.
15. Chusid EL et al: Treatment of hypoxemia with an oxygen enricher, Chest 76:268, 1979.
16. Tiep BL: New portable oxygen devices, Respir Care 32:106-112, 1987.
17. Myers RJ: Oxygen-conservation devices, RX Home Care 8:35-38, 1986.
18. Heimlich HJ: Respiratory rehabilitation with transtracheal oxygen system, Ann Otol Rhinol Laryngol 91:643, 1982.
19. Spofford B et al: Transtracheal oxygen therapy: a guide for the respiratory therapist, Respir Care 32:5, 1987.
20. Tiep BL et al: Evaluation of an oxygen conserving nasal cannula, Respir Care 30:19-25, 1985.
21. Tiep BL et al: A new pendant storage oxygen-conserving nasal cannula, Chest 87:381-383, 1985.
22. Pflug AE, Cheney FW, and Butler J: Evaluation of an intermittent oxygen flow system, Am Rev Respir Dis 105:449-452, 1972.
23. Anderson WM, Ryerson G, and Block AJ: Evaluation of an intermittent demand nasal oxygen flow system with a fluidic valve, Chest 86:313-318, 1984.
24. Franco MA et al: Pulse dose oxygen delivery system, Respir Care 29:1034, 1985.
25. O'Ryan JA: An overview of mechanical ventilation in the home, Respir Mgmt 17:27-36, 1987.
26. Make B: ACCP guidelines for mechanical ventilation in the home setting, AARC Times 11:56-68, 1987.
27. American Association for Respiratory Care: Standards for the provision of care to ventilator-assisted patients in an alternative site, AARC Times 11:45-47, 1987.
28. Kacmarek RM and Spearman CB: Equipment used for ventilatory support in the home, Respir Care 31:311-328, 1986.
29. American Respiratory Care Foundation: Guidelines for disinfection of respiratory care equipment used in the home, Respir Care 33:801-808, 1988.
30. Giordano SP: Why aren't the respiratory care professional's services reimbursed? AARC Times 11:53-57, 1987.
31. Larson K: DME referrals: what's legal and what's not, AARTimes 10:28-31, 1986.
32. American Association for Respiratory Care: Statement of principles on fraud and abuse in home care, Dallas, undated, American Association for Respiratory Care.
33. American Association for Respiratory Care: Final report of the consensus meeting on home respiratory care equipment, September 1988 (co-sponsored by the US Food and Drug Administration and Health Resources and Services Administration), Dallas, 1989, The Association.

36

Computer Applications in Respiratory Care

Craig L. Scanlan

Computer and information technologies are bringing about a fundamental transformation in our society. Although first evident in the business sector, this trend is now beginning to dramatically affect the delivery of health services. Nowhere is this effect likely to be greater than in the area of respiratory care.

Although first used for managing information, computers have also been applied to support clinical aspects of respiratory care for many years. Computer-aided blood gas analysis and pulmonary function testing were developed in the late 1960s and early 1970s. More recently, computer-aided bedside monitoring has become commonplace in many clinical facilities. The use of computer technology to assist clinicians in interpreting data, reaching diagnoses, and planning patient care is just beginning. Also on the horizon is the use of closed-loop computer systems to control certain aspects of patient management, including mechanical ventilation.

Clearly, the involvement of respiratory care practitioners with computer technology will increase dramatically in the coming decade. To take full advantage of the computer, all practitioners must develop a basic understanding of both the strengths and limitations of this important clinical tool, and how it currently is and will be applied to enhance the quality of patient care.

OBJECTIVES

This chapter will provide an overview of the history, current status, and future trends in computer and information technology. Special emphasis will be given to the use of these technologies in the delivery of respiratory care services. Specifically, after completion of this chapter, the reader will be able to:

1. Differentiate what computers can and cannot do;
2. Describe the historical evolution of computer technology;
3. Identify the components of a modern digital computer and the various types of software applications in current use;
4. Describe the importance of and means by which computers can communicate with each other;
5. Identify the common uses of computer and information technology in the delivery of health care services, including those provided by respiratory care practitioners.

TERMS

Most terms used in this chapter are defined in context. However, because of its unique content, a separate glossary of computer terms appears at the chapter end.

CAPABILITIES AND LIMITATIONS OF COMPUTERS

Regardless of size or expense, a modern digital computer is simply a tool that is useful in improving and extending our human capabilities. However, the computer has substantially more power and versatility than most other tools currently available to us. Because, in part, of its power and versatility, the computer has caused a fundamental change in the way we go about living and working. Effective use of this tool requires an understanding of both its strengths and limitations.

What computers can do

Whether a large mainframe or desktop version, the modern digital computer is an extremely versatile tool. Although most people think of computers only in terms of their ability to quickly perform mathematical computations, these devices are actually capable of a host of other important functions.

As delineated in the box below, these functions include mathematical computations, logical operations, the storage and rapid retrieval of numeric and text data, the translation of numeric and text data from one form into another, the reordering of data according to prespecified instructions, the editing of existing data, conditional decision-making, the monitoring of external events, and the control of external devices.

Although all such functions can be performed manually by humans, many represent mundane or repetitive tasks requiring a minimal amount of thought or creativity. A good example of such a task would be the sorting of 10,000 admitting forms according to the patient's date and time of admission. Even those processes which demand human talents can often be performed much more quickly and accurately with the aid of a computer. An example of this type of process would be the computation of a patient's hemodynamic parameters at the bedside.

What computers cannot do

Nonetheless, there are many things that people can do much better than computers. Currently, computers cannot discover new methods, use intuition, innovate or be creative, understand human language, program themselves, reason about input or output values, or decide if a problem is solvable. Computers are very fast and accurate, but thinking is still uniquely human.

Computers can be programmed to correct small errors that may occur during their operation. For example, a computer can decide if a number is too large or too small for it to process. However, a computer cannot decide if it has been given the "correct" information or if the answers it provides make sense. Only a human operator can determine the meaning of such data.

A computer can simulate some intellectual processes that resemble human thought, but no computer currently understands humans. For example, computers may communicate in English, but a computer does not know what the English words mean. Computers also have difficulty handling "fuzzy" problems. Fuzzy problems are those which cannot be reduced to objective numeric or logical equations. They often require value judgments and intuitive or creative reasoning. As an example, the decision of how to get a patient to comply with a treatment regimen represents a fuzzy problem, for which current computer technology is ill suited.

HISTORY OF COMPUTERS

Early developments

Digital computing probably began some 7000 years ago with the invention of the abacus. Still used extensively in Asia, the abacus consists of a set of rods on which beads may be moved up or down. Since each abacus rod or column represents a multiplier of ten, the abacus is considered a digital computing machine based on the decimal, or base 10 system.

The next major advance in digital computation occurred in 1617. John Napier, of Scotland, introduced a computation device consisting of variable length sticks of bone, called "Napier's bones." This ingenious tool automated several arithmetic processes, including multiplication and division. Napier subsequently developed logarithmic functions to assist in mathematical computations.

In 1642, a French scientist and philosopher, Blaise Pascal, developed a digital "calculating engine." This device looked somewhat like a mechanical automobile odometer. Geared wheels with numbers appeared in windows. To enter a number one turned the wheel. Addition of a new number would increment the wheels in sequence, yielding a simple sum.

In 1671, a German diplomat, Gottfried Wilhelm Leibniz, introduced a device called the "Stepped Reckoner." This device extended Pascal's calculating engine by automating both multiplication and division. Leibniz later developed a system of logic and computation called *binary arithmetic,* which would become the cornerstone of digital computing (see box on p. 945).

In the early 1800s, a Frenchman, Joseph Marie Jacquard, developed an automated weaving machine called the "Jacquard Loom." Designed to avoid errors and reduce the cost of woven goods, the loom was activated by perforated cards pressed against an array of rods. Several of these cards were chained together to "program" the ma-

---

HOW COMPUTERS PROCESS DATA

THE PROCESS	THE MANIPULATION
Calculate	Perform mathematical operations such as add, subtract, multiply, divide, square root, etc. Solve formulas.
Logic	Perform logical operations such as AND, OR, invert, etc.
Store	Remember facts and figures in files.
Retrieve	Access data stored in files as required.
Translate	Convert data from one form to another.
Sort	Examine data and put it into some desired order or format.
Edit	Make changes, additions, and deletions to data and change its sequence.
Make Decisions	Reach simple conclusions based on internal or external conditions.
Monitor	Observe external or internal events and take action if certain conditions are met.
Control	Take charge of or operate external devices.

chine to weave consistent and complicated patterns. The Jacquard Loom was so successful that it put many skilled weavers out of work. These displaced weavers tried to thwart this technological change by destroying the looms.

At about the same time, Charles Babbage, in conjunction with Ada Byron (Lord Byron's daughter), developed and refined a device called the "Analytical Engine." The Analytical Engine was probably the first device to mimic the major functions of modern digital computers. In addition to performing simple arithmetic functions, the Analyt-

ical Engine could actually analyze data and make conditional decisions based on the results of its computations. Punched cards, like those used in the Jacquard Loom, were used both to "input" data into the machine and to perform operations on this data. The device was first used to compute and print ocean tide tables. This latter function was probably the first example of automated "word processing."

Wide-scale use of automated computing occurred in conjunction with the 1890 US Census. A Census Bureau employee, Herman Hollerith, instituted automated census data collection and analysis using a modified form of the Jacquard Loom punched card. Demographic information punched on these data cards was "read" electronically by passing the cards over a bath of mercury. As each card passed over this liquid metal, needles would snap down through the holes, thereby closing an electrical circuit and registering the appropriate data for further analysis. These "Hollerith cards" ultimately became the standard means to input and store computer data and instructions. Only in the 1970s did direct terminal input and tape and disk storage take over these functions. Hollerith later merged with two companies to form the Computing Tabulating Records Company, which, in 1924, became the International Business Machine Company (IBM).

The modern era

Toward the end of the 1930s, two major developments heralded the modern era of digital computing. In Germany, Konrad Zuse developed a seven-foot square maze of electronic relays and circuits called the "Z1" computing machine. A keyboard was used to input problems to the Z1. At the end of a calculation, results were flashed on a board composed of several small lights. Later, Zuse used instructions punched as holes on a strip of 35 mm film to replace keyboard data entry.

The Z1 was the first device to use binary electromechanical logic circuits, or "on/off" switches. This approach avoided use of the cumbersome decimal system, instead applying Leibniz's binary arithmetic. These logic circuits also made possible the electronic application of Boolean algebra (see box on p. 946). Boolean algebra is a system of logical comparison applicable to anything from numbers and letters, to objects and statements. This system has become the cornerstone of all symbolic logical operations in modern digital computers.

World War II provided a major stimulus for rapid progression of digital computing technology. In Germany, Zuse refined his binary digital computer to help solve engineering problems associated with aircraft and missile design. He also proposed to develop a computer based on vacuum tubes rather than electromechanical relays. This use of purely electronic components would have increased computational speed by over a thousand fold. As fate would have it, his proposal was turned down by the Third Reich.

BINARY NUMBER SYSTEM

In decimal notation, each position to the left of the decimal indicates an increased power of 10. In the binary, or base 2 system, each place to the left signifies an increased power of 2. Therefore 2 to the zeroeth power is one, 2 to the first power is two, 2 to the second power is four, and so on. As illustrated below, finding the decimal equivalent of a binary number is simply a matter of noting which place columns the binary 1s occupy and adding up their values:

DECIMAL		BINARY			
Place 10	Place 1	Place 8	Place 4	Place 2	Place 1
	0	0	0	0	0
	1	0	0	0	1
	2	0	0	1	0
	3	0	0	1	1
	4	0	1	0	0
	5	0	1	0	1
	6	0	1	1	0
	7	0	1	1	1
	8	1	0	0	0
	9	1	0	0	1
1	0	1	0	1	0

Numbers larger than 16 require more than four binary columns, such that the decimal number 238 is expressed in binary as:

11101110   or:

0 in the 1s	0
1 in the 2s	2
1 in the 4s	4
1 in the 8s	8
0 in the 16s	0
1 in the 32s	32
1 in the 64s	64
1 in the 128s	128
	238

Addition of binary numbers is the same as with decimal numbers except $1 + 1$ in binary equals 0, with the one carried to the next column:

0	0	1
+0	+1	+1
0	1	10

BOOLEAN ALGEBRA

In 1854, the British mathematician George Boole published a work entitled "An Investigation of the Laws of Thought" which revolutionized the science of logic. In these essays, Boole proposed a form of algebra applicable to anything from numbers and letters to objects and statements. In Boole's system, propositions or statements that were either true or false could be encoded in symbolic language and then manipulated in much the same manner as ordinary numbers.

With all propositions and manipulations reduced to true/false or either/or results, Boolean algebra was ideally suited to binary computation. For this reason, Boole's system of logical comparison quickly became the cornerstone of all symbolic logical operations in the digital computer.

Today, Boolean algebra is used extensively in most software applications. The following is a list of the most common logical operators in use:

SYMBOL	MEANING
= or EQ	Equals
<> or NE	Not equal to
> or GT	Greater than
>= or GE	Greater than or equal to
< or LT	Less than
<= or LE	Less than or equal to

For numeric manipulations, the above operations and the Boolean result of the manipulation are very straightforward, as in the following examples:

OPERATION	BOOLEAN RESULT
7 = 7	True
7 = 6	False
5 < 8	True
8 <> 5	True

For comparison of letters, alphabetic order is the basis for most comparisons, such that B is greater than A (B > A), and Y is less than Z (Y < Z). Comparison of groups of letters, called "strings," is accomplished in a similar manner, as follows:

OPERATION	BOOLEAN RESULT
"Terry" = "Terry"	True
"Terry" = "Terri"	False
"ABC" > "ADC"	False

Not to be outdone by their counterparts overseas, American engineers and scientists, supported by both IBM and the US Navy, developed the Mark 1 computer. Introduced at Harvard University in 1944, the Mark 1 computer was over fifty feet long and eight feet high, and contained some 750,000 electromechanical relays strung together with over 500 miles of wiring. The Mark 1 used binary arithmetic to solve complex ballistic problems, whipping through calculations in one day that formerly took over six months to compute manually.

Also during the war, the British secretly developed the first vacuum tube binary digital computer. This device, called "Colossus," was capable of scanning and interpreting some 25,000 characters per second. Colossus was used primarily to decipher and break the German war codes and has been credited with helping bring an early end to the war.

Toward the end of the war, the US Army awarded a contract to the University of Pennsylvania's Moore School of Engineering to develop a new vacuum tube computer like Colossus. This device, called the Electronic Numerical Integrator and Computer, or "ENIAC" for short, weighed over 30 tons. Using some 17,000 vacuum tubes and 100,000 electrical components, ENIAC was able to process numeric calculations a thousand times faster than the Navy's Mark 1. However, ENIAC was not completed until after the end of the war. Once completed, ENIAC was used to perform critical calculations necessary to develop the hydrogen bomb.

Computer generations

As the first true, fully electronic digital computers, ENIAC and Colossus together are now considered examples of "First Generation" computers (Table 36-1). First generation computers were based on vacuum tube technology and used huge manual plug boards (like an old-fashion

Table 36-1   The Computer Generations

Generation	Hardware	Software
FIRST 1945-1957	Vacuum tubes Delay line, CRT and drum memories	Machine code Plug boards
SECOND 1957-1963	Transistors Magnetic core memories	Higher level languages (COBOL, FORTRAN)
THIRD 1963-1971	Integrated circuits Semiconductor memory Minicomputers Magnetic disk storage	Operating systems Multitasking Virtual memory
FOURTH 1971-1989	Microprocessors & personal computers VLSI Faster, denser RAM Networking	Database Management Systems (DBMS) 4th generation languages
FIFTH 1989-2000	VHSIC Parallel processing architectures RISC architectures	Computer-Aided Software Engineering Expert systems Natural language processing
SIXTH 2000-?	Optical processors and storage	Automated programming

telephone operator) to input instructions or "programs." Crude "memory" capabilities were achieved using electro-mechanical drums holding data as punched holes. Later improvements included true electronic memory based on mercury filled tubes called "delay lines." Toward the end of this first generation, programming via manual plug boards was replaced by the use of binary instructions stamped on paper tape (not unlike Zuse's 35 mm film). This process of providing binary instruction to a computer became known as "machine coding."

Common to all first generation computers was a design structure called the stored program concept. Developed in 1945 by John von Neumann at Princeton University, this "von Neumann architecture" still provides the foundation for most modern digital computers.

According to von Neumann, an efficient all-purpose computer must have five key components: (1) a *central control unit* designed to "orchestrate" overall operations; (2) an *arithmetic logic* unit (ALU) capable of arithmetic and logical functions; (3) an *input mechanism* by which the user can provide both data and instructions to the computer; (4) a *memory* to store data and instructions; and (5) an *output mechanism* by which the results of data analysis can be provided back to the user.

The next major advance in computer technology was an outgrowth of the invention of the transistor in 1948. Transistors, like vacuum tubes, can serve as electronic on/off switches. However, unlike vacuum tubes, transistors are highly dependable, produce little heat, are very small, and extremely inexpensive to produce.

The introduction of the first transistorized computer, the IBM 1620, heralded the beginning of the Second Generation of computer technology (1957 to 1963). Also introduced during this period was the wire loop magnetic core memory. This magnetic core memory greatly enhanced the ability of the computer to store and quickly retrieve both instructions (programs) and data.

Perhaps just as important was the development of new and easier methods for providing programming instructions to the computer. Prior to this time, programming a computer required use of the same on/off codes used by the machine itself, that is "machine code." With the advent of the second generation of computer hardware came "higher-level" programming languages, such as COBOL and FORTRAN. These programming languages allowed the user to write computer instructions in more human-oriented terms, such as "SUM" and "AVER" (instructions to add and find the mean, respectively). Such languages would then translate each of these simple statements into a series of complex binary machine codes.

Several major hardware developments foreshadowed the beginning of the Third Generation of computer technology (1963 to 1971). By far, the most important of these was the development of the *integrated circuit*, or IC. An IC is a small silicon-base semiconductor "chip," upon which thousands of miniaturized transistors can be placed. Early ICs lowered the cost and increased the dependability of computer circuitry by a factor of 10 over conventional transistor technology. Modern ICs, no larger than a matchbook, may have over a million transistor components, providing a thousand-fold improvement in both cost and relative computational power over their early counterparts. The development of the integrated circuit also led to the introduction of the minicomputer, a scaled-down workhorse that brought modern computer technology within the reach of both small businesses and clinical research facilities.

During this phase, semiconductors also became the primary mode for storing data and instructions for immediate use by the computer (primary memory). Enhancements in mass storage technology (secondary memory) also occurred with IBM's development of the magnetic disk.

Software developments during this Third Generation of computer technology were equally important. Up until this time, a computer could only attend to a single task or serve a single user at a given time. The development of specialized software, called *operating systems*, changed this limited approach by allowing the computer's time to be divided into extremely small "slices," each as short as 1/30,000 of a second.

Although still capable of performing only a single task during each individual time slice, computers with this new capability could switch rapidly between separate intervals, giving the appearance of doing two or more things simultaneously. This capability to rapidly "juggle" two or more activities using separate time allocations is called *multitasking*. Multitasking capabilities allow a single user to have the computer appear to perform two or more tasks at the same time, such as sorting data and performing numeric computations. Alternatively, multitasking allows a single computer to concurrently serve more than one user, a concept called *timesharing*.

Operating systems developed during this third generation also allowed the computer's memory to be "partitioned" into separate virtual memories, each capable of storing and acting on different programs and data. The development of this virtual memory thus allowed a single computer to act as though it were many computers.

Currently we are marking the end of the Fourth Generation of computer technology. Begun in 1971, this generation has been characterized by continued miniaturization of components. Such components, based on a concept called Very Large Scale Integration (VLSI), combine many diverse functions, previously requiring multiple ICs, into a single computer chip. These developments made possible the modern personal computer, which now relies heavily on VLSI technology. Software developments during this era include sophisticated database management systems and fourth generation programming languages, such as PASCAL, FORTH, and C.

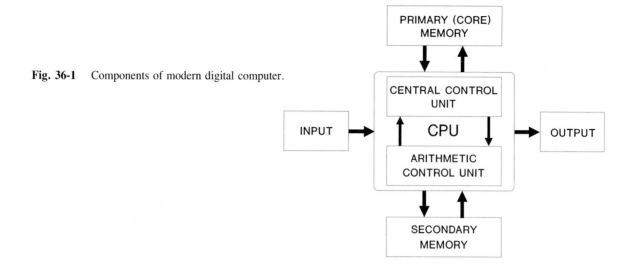

Fig. 36-1   Components of modern digital computer.

The Fifth Generation of computer technology, which is just beginning, will see further refinements in IC technology, while also exploring alternatives to the classical von Neumann architecture. Such alternatives include parallel processing and Reduced Instruction Set Computers (RISCs). Both of these developments are designed to challenge the computational "speed limits" currently characterizing conventional computer designs.

Parallel processing is designed to speed computations by dividing a single large task into many smaller tasks, each performed by a separate microprocessor. For example, using a single microprocessor, a traditional computer must go through 15 steps to find the product of 16 times 2 (sequentially adding 2 + 2 fifteen times). On the other hand, a computer using just eight microprocessors working in parallel could perform the same task in just four steps, or nearly 400% faster!

Reduced Instruction Set Computers apply a different principle to increase computational speed. They use a very limited and simple set of machine instructions. Because the instruction set is limited, the microprocessor has to "know" fewer commands, thereby increasing the speed of command processing. Moreover, simple instructions can be processed faster than complex ones, allowing the microprocessor to perform more activities in a given time interval.

Also characterizing the Fifth Generation of computer technology are new advances in software, including computer-aided software engineering (CASE) applications, natural language processors, and expert systems (to be discussed later).

Although difficult to predict, future developments in computer technology (the "Sixth Generation") will probably include greater use of optical storage and processing methods. Also likely is true automated programming, where the computer itself, given a description of the task at hand, will "write" its own instructions.

HOW COMPUTERS WORK

Respiratory care practitioners who want to take full advantage of computer technology should have a basic understanding of how these tools function. Toward this end, the following discussion provides a brief overview of modern computer hardware and software. Based on this overview of current technology, we then look at how computers are being used to enhance communication.

Hardware

As described earlier, a modern digital computer consists of five key hardware components: (1) a central control unit, (2) an arithmetic logic unit, (3) an input mechanism, (4) a memory to store data and instructions, and (5) an output mechanism. Fig. 36-1 is a schematic illustration of these key elements constituting a modern digital computer.

Central processing unit. Together, the arithmetic logic unit and central control unit constitute what is commonly referred to as the central processing unit (CPU). The "core" of most microprocessors, such as those found in personal computers, is nothing more than a single integrated circuit CPU chip.

The central control unit contains a logic decoder which "translates" sequenced instructions and directs the operation of the rest of the CPU. The arithmetic logic unit, or ALU, performs basic arithmetic and logical operations, such as addition and Boolean comparisons (greater than, less than, etc). In addition to these two components, a typical CPU also has a number of registers used to temporarily store and transfer data elements, or "point to" their location in memory. A special purpose register, called the accumulator, holds the output of the arithmetic logic unit.

Memory. A computer's memory, representing electronic "space" where the computer can store data or instructions, consists entirely of data encoded into 0s and 1s. Data and instructions are stored in the form of binary digits, or *bits*. Each bit represents an on or off signal, symbolized as either a 0 or 1. Eight bits combine to form a *byte*. A byte represents a collection of data bits which function as one. Typically, one byte may be used to represent a character, such as the letter "A." In order to represent a word, several bytes are needed.

A modern computer typically has two general types of memory: primary and secondary. Primary memory is in physical proximity to and is immediately available to the CPU. Secondary memory is located external to the CPU itself and accessible only through the use of special mass storage devices.

Primary memory. Primary, or core memory, typically consists of two components: Read Only Memory and Random Access Memory. *Read Only Memory* (ROM) normally consists of preprogrammed instructions that help the central control unit fulfill its "housekeeping" functions. For example, the ROM in a personal computer contains the basic instructions necessary to get the computer up and operating once it is powered on. Also in ROM is a "kernel" of the operating system used to deal with simple input and output functions (called the Basic Input/Output System, or BIOS).

Instructions in ROM are permanently stored within the physical structure of one or more semiconductor chips. Since they are stored physically (as opposed to electronically), these instructions remain in ROM regardless of the power status of the computer. Also, as the name implies, ROM instructions can only be "read" by the CPU and cannot normally be altered by the user.

Random access Memory (RAM) physically consists of one or more "banks" of semiconductor chips that store binary data or instructions for use by the CPU. Unlike the computer's ROM, random access memory is normally empty unless data or instructions are fed to it. Typically, initiation of a program signals the CPU to feed a program's instructions and its associated data into RAM for subsequent use.

Unlike the instructions stored in ROM, the data stored in random access memory is maintained electronically. Thus a loss of electrical power will cause all data stored in the computer's RAM to be lost. For this reason, RAM is also referred to as "volatile" memory.

Secondary memory. To avoid having to keep all data and instructions in RAM, most computers possess secondary memory, or "mass storage", capabilities. Secondary memory is not directly accessible to the computer's CPU. Instead, data is stored externally to the computer itself, usually on magnetic tapes or disks. These tapes or disks are impregnated with magnetized material such as iron oxide. Application of electrical current to this material causes it to polarize either in one direction (off) or another (on), thereby creating an electronic bit of information. Sensitive electronic reading "heads" can discern the polarity of these bits of data, thereby translating them into binary code for use by the CPU. More recently, optical storage methods are being used to provide computers with enhanced secondary memory capabilities (see below).

The *storage capacity* of tape and disk media varies according to the density of the magnetized material on its surface. Plastic disks (also called "floppy" disks) and tapes have relatively low storage capacities per unit area, while hard metal disks (often called "fixed disks") have greater storage ability. For example, a typical 3-1/2 inch floppy disk is capable of storing about 1440 kilobytes of data (1,440,000 bytes), equivalent to over 700 double-spaced pages of typewritten information. However, a hard disk of similar size can hold over 40 *mega*bytes (40 million bytes) of data, equivalent to some 20,000 pages of information!

Newer optical storage methods, similar in concept to the compact laser disks used in the audio recording industry, are extending this storage capacity more than ten-fold. Recently, single 5-1/4 inch compact disks have been developed that can hold some 400 megabytes of data, more than enough to store the full Encyclopedia Britannica and a dozen other reference texts!

Input and output devices. For a computer to interact with its user or the environment, two conditions are necessary. First, there must be a means to provide data or instruction to the CPU (input). Second, there must be a means to transmit the results of processor activity back to the user or environment (output).

Input devices. Input data may consist of either a program of computer instructions, or the words, numbers, or graphic information needed by the program to complete its task. This data may be provided directly from the computer's memory, from the user, or from the environment. Common input devices include the keyboard, optical scanners, digitizing pads or graphics tablets, and analog/digital converters.

Keyboard. The most common means for a user to enter data into a computer is through a keyboard. As shown in Fig. 36-2, a typical computer keyboard consists of three major components: (1) a typewriter-like section of alphanumeric keys, (2) a numeric/cursor control keypad, and (3) special-purpose function keys.

The typewriter-like section of the key board is used to input individual letters or strings of characters that form words. The numeric/cursor keypad can serve one of two functions: numeric data entry (like a desktop calculator) or cursor control (moving the cursor around the computer screen). Which function the numeric/cursor control keypad performs is determined by a toggle switch. In the "Off" position, the toggle switch causes the numeric/cursor control keypad to function in the cursor control mode; in the

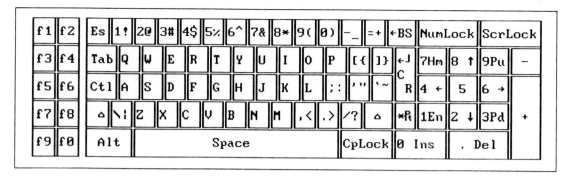

Fig. 36-2   Representative computer keyboard.

"On" position, the toggle switch causes this keypad to function as a numeric input device. Alternatively, especially in graphic-intensive applications, cursor control may be separately provided by an additional input device, such as a mouse or lightpen.

Function keys are used by application programs to perform special operations. For example, pressing a function key in a word processing program may save the document to a disk file. Alternatively, the same function key in a statistical application may be used to calculate the mean of a group of numbers. What a particular function key does is determined by the programmer responsible for writing the application program.

In order for keyboard input to be meaningful to a computer, it must be converted into binary machine code. In most systems, this is accomplished using a standard coding system, called the American Standard Code for Information Interchange, or ASCII (pronounced as "ask-key"). Developed by the American National Standards Institute (ANSI), the ASCII system represents all number, letter, and symbol input from the keyboard as a seven bit code, with an eighth "parity" bit used for error checking. For example, the capital letter "A" is represented in binary ASCII as 0100 0001. This code was designed to make various types of data processing and communication machines compatible.

Optical scanners. Optical scanners are devices which scan visual information, translate it into digital form, and input it into the computer. An optical mark reader (OMR) is the simplest optical scanning input device. The optical mark reader simply identifies shaded areas on a form, such as those placed by a student on a specially designed test answer sheet. An optical character reader (OCR) is a scanning device which uses special software to recognize printed characters. These characters are then converted to ASCII code for direct input into the computer. A graphics scanner is an input device that converts a graphic image, such as an anatomic drawing or x-ray, into a digitized format. Typically, a scanned graphic image is converted into thousands or hundreds of thousands of binary picture elements, called pixels. Each pixel represents a tiny dot of

light that can be turned either on or off on the visual screen display.

Digitizing pads (graphics tablets). A digitizing pad, or graphics tablet, is a specialized input device designed to convert the freehand movements of a pen or mouse on a flat surface into a digital image. Digitizing pads have been used extensively for some time in commercial art production and engineering design. In health care, the digitizing pad is beginning to find extensive use in graphics-intensive applications, such as anatomy and kinesiology. Moreover, when used in conjunction with an overlaying template, a digitizing pad can be an effective means of providing simplified data input. For example, a digitizing pad with a template of a child's body could be used by the child to "point to" the location of pain or discomfort. Likewise, a patient with an artificial airway who is unable to speak could use a digitizing pad with graphic icons and letters of the alphabet to help communicate.

Analog to digital converters. In scientific applications, including medicine and respiratory care, much of the input data we would like to analyze by computer is in *analog,* as opposed to digital format. Analog information is data which corresponds or is analogous to a physical measurement. A mercury thermometer is a good example of a simple analog measurement device. In this case, the height of the column of mercury is physically analogous to the heat intensity or temperature.

More commonly, analog information is provided electronically as either a change in voltage or current. A good example of electronically acquired analog data is that obtained from a spirographic tracing of a flow-volume loop. Assuming that we use an electronic pneumotachygraph to obtain the flow-volume loop, the resulting data is provided as either a voltage or current change over time. Although such analog data can be used to "drive" an X-Y recorder, and thereby display the signal on paper, it cannot be directly analyzed by a digital computer.

For this reason, the analog signal must be converted to digital format. This is accomplished using a special input device called an *analog-to-digital converter* (ADC). An ADC transforms the varying analog input (such as voltage)

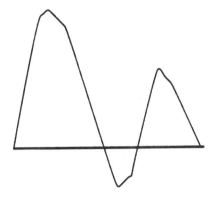 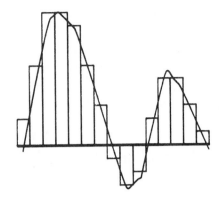

Fig. 36-3 Analog-to-digital conversion. The analog signal (left) is converted to digital format (right) by sampling at high frequency.

into a series of rapid on-off pulses (binary code) by sampling the signal received at an extremely rapid rate. As illustrated in Fig. 36-3, as soon as the converter takes its sample reading, it assigns a number to each segment. At best, the raw digital value at any given time can only approximate the analog original. However, using lightning fast techniques such as successive approximation, the final digital value will be equivalent to that of the original analog signal. Only after the continuous analog signal has been transformed to discrete digital data may it be used by a computer.

Output devices. Output data, like input data, may be in the form of words, numbers, or graphic information. Common output devices include the computer monitor or screen, a variety of printers, and plotters. Output data may also consist of digital or analog signals designed to activate or control specialized equipment. Finally, output data may be used as subsequent input to the computer for further processing.

Computer monitor. The computer monitor is the most common output device. Results of input and processing typically are displayed on a monitor screen. This display may take the form of words, numbers, or graphic information. Traditionally, most computer monitors were simple cathode ray tubes (CRTs), designed much like the home television. More recently, new display technologies, such as liquid crystal (LCDs) and gas plasma displays, are providing alternatives to the CRT. The resolution available with output display devices has increased substantially over the past decade. This increased resolution is making possible graphic image output that approaches photographic quality.

Printers. The printer is the primary means for converting computer output into *hard copy*. Hard copy represents words, numbers, and/or graphic information which is transferred to paper. Printers fall into three major categories: simple impact printers, dot-matrix printers, and laser (or page) printers.

Simple impact printers operate much like a typewriter,

using a ball or wheel of characters ("daisy wheel"), a hammer, and an ink ribbon to transfer letters, numbers, and symbols to paper. Output quality is high, but simple impact printers are slow and cannot readily reproduce graphic images. Moreover, impact printers can be very noisy.

Dot-matrix printers use a print head consisting of heated wires or "pins" arranged in one or more vertical columns. As the print head moves across the paper, the pins are "fired" hundreds of times in different combinations to form the dot pattern of the individual characters or graphic image. As compared to simple impact printers, dot-matrix printers can produce printed output much more rapidly and are capable of graphics reproduction. However, since the characters produced consist of small discrete dots, the output quality of most dot-matrix printers is not as good as that produced by simple impact printers. Newer dot-matrix printers partially overcome this problem by using a print head with a larger number of pins (24 instead of the traditional 9).

The laser printer uses electrophotographic technology to print a full page of characters or graphics at a time. A small laser beam, turned on or off millions of times each second, bounces a light stream off a mirror. The reflected light neutralizes portions of the surface of a positively charged drum, creating a reverse image. The drum is then dusted with a positively charged ink powder, or "toner," which sticks to the neutral areas of the drum. When the negatively charged paper contacts the drum, the toner is attracted to it, forming the desired image. The image is fused to the paper by a combination of heat and pressure. As the finished page is produced, the drum is cleared of its charge, cleaned, and recharged for the next cycle.

Typical laser printers can produce images with resolutions of about 300 dots per inch (dpi). Moreover, the laser printer is a relatively fast output device, capable of "printing" between 8 and 50 pages per minute. New laser printers are now being developed to provide color, as opposed to simple black-and-white images.

Plotters. A plotter is a specialized X-Y recorder used as

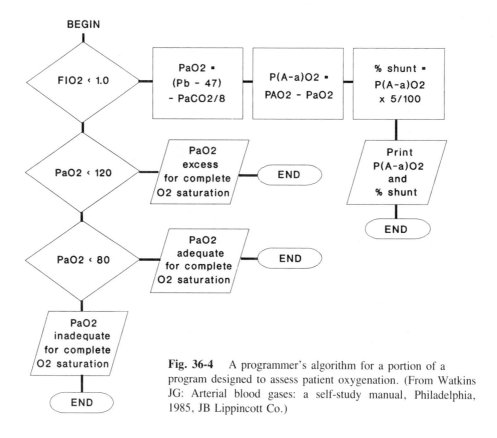

Fig. 36-4 A programmer's algorithm for a portion of a program designed to assess patient oxygenation. (From Watkins JG: Arterial blood gases: a self-study manual, Philadelphia, 1985, JB Lippincott Co.)

an output device for a computer. They are used mainly to produce complex line images, such as those used in computer-aided design (CAD). A plotter translates digital computer output into the motion of a drawing pen and/or the underlying paper. Special codes sent to the plotter can cause it to switch pens, thereby allowing for varying line thicknesses and different colors.

Output control signals. Output data may also consist of digital or analog signals designed to activate or control specialized equipment. For example, a home microprocessor may receive an input signal corresponding to temperature (via analog-to-digital conversion), compare this signal to a predetermined setting (say 68°F), and use this information to turn on or off the home's heating system. Likewise, a microprocessor-based IV system may use an optical input device to "count" the drops per minute through the tubing and either signal an alarm or vary the infusion rate by an appropriate output signal. In respiratory care, a microprocessor-based ventilator can take an input signal, such as flow, convert it to volume, and send an output signal telling the exhalation to open when the desired volume is achieved.

Software

Software represents the means by which a human operator instructs a computer what to do and how to do it. Without software, a computer is useless. A complete set of such instructions, designed to accomplish a specific task,

is called a *program.* Individuals who develop and test computer software programs are called programmers. Although one need not be a programmer to use a computer, it is useful to understand both the basic concepts underlying computer programming and the various types of software used in modern digital computers.

Computer programs. Conventional computer programs are based on an *algorithm.* An algorithm is a clearly defined, step-by-step procedure for solving a specific problem. Fig. 36-4 uses a flow chart to illustrate one such algorithm, designed to assess the oxygenation status of a patient breathing supplemental oxygen.

Once the programmer has developed the algorithm, it is converted into a sequential list of instructions or commands, called a program. This program tells the computer exactly what operations to carry out. The box shows a portion of the actual computer program (written in BASIC) used to carry out the operations necessary to assess the oxygenation status of a patient breathing supplemental oxygen. In this case, the program uses input data such as the patient's age and F_{IO_2} to solve the problem. Of course, new data can be used from a different patient to repeat the process and again solve the problem.

There are three basic concepts underlying all conventional computer algorithms:
1. *Simple sequence:* Each step in the algorithm is performed in sequence, one after another.
2. *Conditional Branching:* Based on the value of a

A PORTION OF A BASIC LANGUAGE PROGRAM DESIGNED TO ASSESS PATIENT OXYGENATION

```
2010   IF F>.21 THEN 3000
2020   IF PO>85 THEN 4000
2030   IF AGE>40 THEN 2070
2040   IF PO>79 THEN OP$ = RP$(15): GOTO 1000
2050   IF PO<80 THEN OP$ = RP$(21): GOTO 1000
2070   Y = 94−(AGE−10)* 4
2080   IF PO>=Y THEN OP$ = RPS$(15): GOTO 1000
2090   IF PO<Y THEN OP$ = RP$(21): GOTO 10000
2999   REM * FLOW CHART 9−8 *
3000   IF F>= 1 THEN 3010
3005   IF F<1 THEN 3070
3010   PA = (PB−47)−(C/.8)
3020   A = PA−PO
3030   SH = (A*5)/100
3035   SH$ = STR$(SH)
3036   A$ = STR$(A)
3037   GOTO 10000
3038   PRINT#DV, "A-aD02 = ":A
3070   IF PO>120 THEN OP$ = RP$(18): GOTO 10000
3080   IF PO>79 THEN OP$ = RP$(19): GOTO 10000
3090   IF PO<80 THEN OP$ = RP$(20): GOTO 10000
4000   IF PO<110 THEN OP$ = RP$(15): GOTO 10000
4010 Z = PB 47
4020   PA = (Z*F)−(C/.8)
4030   IF PA>PO THEN OP$ = RP$(15): GOTO 10000
4040   IF PA<PO THEN OP$ = RP$(16): GOTO 10000
10001  PRINT#DV CHR$(12): FOR ZZ = 1T079: PRINT
       #DV, """..NEXT ZZ: PRINT#

10002  OV$     =     "OXYGEN     STATUS"     PRINT#
       TAB(35−LEN(OV$)/2); OV$DV.
10005  IF SH$$ <>"" THEN PRINT#DV,
       "% SHUNT =". SH$
10006  IF A$ <>"" THEN PRINT#DV, "A-aD02 = ". A$
10020  PRINT #DV, TAB(35− LEN(OP$)/2); OP$
10025  FOR ZZ = 1T079: PRINT#DV, "*";;NEXTZZ:
       PRINT#DV
10026  PRINT#DV: PRINT#DV
10027  FOR ZZ = 1T079: PRINT#DV, "";; NEXTZZ:
       PRINT#DV
10028  BG$'= "ACID BASE STATUS":
       PRINT#DV.TAB(35−LEN(BG$)/2): BG
10030  PRINT#DV.TAB(35−LEN(RP$)/2; RP$
10040  FOR ZZ = 1T079: PRINT#DV, "*";;NEXTZZ:
       PRINT#DV
10045  PRINT#DV: PRINT#DV
10046  RP$ = ""
10050  END
20000  X = 43:Y = 55
20005  PRINT CHR$(12)
20010  PT$ = CHR$(27) + CHR$(89) + CHR$(X) +
       CHR$(Y)
20020  PRINT PT$; "ERRONEOUS DATA RERUN
       AGB'S"
20030  END.
```

From Watkins JG: Arterial blood gases: a self-study manual, Philadelphia, 1985, JB Lippincott Co.

given conditional statement, the program will either branch to other portions of the algorithm or continue in the programmed sequence, but not both.

3. *Looping:* An operation or sequence of operations is done over and over again until some condition is satisfied.

In our example program (see box), lines 3010 through 3030 illustrate simple sequencing, in which the patient's alveolar Po_2, $P(A-a)o_2$, and percent shunt are computed. Branching in this program is accomplished by conditional IF/THEN statements, such as that appearing in line 2030 (IF AGE>40 THEN 2070). This statement tells the computer that if the patient is over 40-years-old, go to line 2070. Of course, line 2070 contains the estimation formula for calculating a patient's normal Po_2 based on their age, that is $Y=94-(AGE-10)*.4$. On the other hand, if the patient is 40-years-old or less, the program statement "IF AGE>40 THEN 2070" tells the computer to simply ignore this branch and go on to the next line (line 2040).

An example of looping within this BASIC program appears in line 10025:

```
FOR ZZ = 1T079: PRINT#DV,"*";;NEXTZZ:PRINT#DV
```

This program statement uses the FOR/NEXT convention to repeat the printing of an asterisk 79 times (the full width of standard computer paper). This simple task is used to enhance the look of the report printout.

Types of software. Software, or computer programs, may be best thought of as existing at various levels (Fig. 36-5). The "lowest" level of computer instructions occurs within the machine itself. This level consists of the pure binary code (1s and 0s) we call *machine language.* Early computers required humans to write programs directly in this machine language. Fortunately, higher level computer languages are now available to make communication with computers less frustrating.

Assembly language. One step above machine language is assembly language. Assembly language uses short mne-

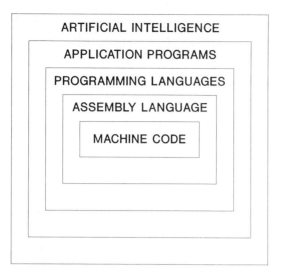

Fig. 36-5 The "layers" or levels of computer instructions, with machine code being the innermost.

AN EXAMPLE OF A SMALL ASSEMBLY PROGRAM WRITTEN FOR THE INTEL 80286 MICROPROCESSOR	
A100	
MOV	CL,[0080]
XOR	CH,CH
MOV	AX,0040
MOV	ES,AX
MOV	DI,001E
CMP	CL,00
JZ	012A
SUB	CL,01
CMP	CL,0F
JBE	001D
MOV	CL,0F
MOV	SI,0082
LODSB	
CMP	AL,7E
JNZ	0127
MOV	AL,0D
STOSW	
LOOP	0120
ES:	
MOV	WORD PTR [001A],001E
ES:	
MOV	[001C],DI
MOV	AH,4C
INT	21

monic symbols instead of 1s and 0s. The mnemonic symbols used in an assembly language program are unique to both the design and the specific instruction set used by a given microprocessor. The box shows a short assembly language program written for the Intel 20286 microprocessor. This program is designed to collect input from the user and pass it on to an application program at start-up. As evident in the program listing, assembly language bears little resemblance to human language, and, except for the programmer responsible for the code, is difficult to understand.

Once written, an assembly language program (in symbolic form) is translated into a machine language program (in binary form) by a special type of software called an *assembler.* The original symbolic assembly language program is called the *source program,* while the final binary machine language program is called the *object program.*

Thus, assembly language source programs are essentially one-to-one translations of machine language object programs. Being so close in form to machine language, assembly language programs can be processed or "run" very quickly.

True programming languages. The next level of computer software are "true" programming languages. A true programming language consists of a set of English-like instructions which generally describe the task they perform. Moreover, each single instruction translates into many machine language statements. For example, a single statement in the BASIC programming language may translate into five or more binary code object instructions. Examples of true programming languages other than BASIC are FORTRAN, COBOL, PASCAL, LISP, Forth and C. Unlike assembly language, these true programming languages

are not directly dependent on the design of the microprocessor and can be used on many different computers.

Application generators. An application generator lies halfway between a programming language and an application program. Like a programming language, an application generator is used to develop a set of instructions by which the computer can perform some specific task. However, these instructions are created by the application generator, rather than by a programmer. The technique of using an application generator to assist in software design is often referred to as *computer-aided software engineering* or "CASE" for short.

Typically, an application generator queries the user regarding specific data or data processing requirements necessary to accomplish a given task. Based on this input, the application generator creates an appropriate program. Ideally, then, an application generator can create a specific application program without the need for a programmer. However, current application generators still fall far short of this ideal, with most application programs created by this method still requiring substantial "fine-tuning" by an experienced programmer.

Application programs. An application program is simply a set of preprogrammed instructions which enable a computer to perform a specific function. Common functions provided by application programs include word processing, database management, and statistical computation.

There are literally tens of thousands of commercial application programs available for modern digital computers. These programs range in scope and function from large scale multisite, multiuser information systems, such as those used by the airlines to book and confirm reservations, to simple "utility packages," designed to print an address sideways on an envelope. Wherever there is a problem amenable to solution by computer, one is likely to find an application program in use or development.

Given this range of scope and function, it is generally easier to categorize application programs according to the type of information they deal with, rather than their specific function. In this context, we may identify six broad categories of application programs:

1. Those that deal with the integration of hardware and software, thereby providing control over how the computer operates (operating systems);
2. Those that deal primarily with text and documents;
3. Those that deal primarily with the manipulation of numeric data;
4. Those that deal primarily with categorical data (either text or numeric);
5. Those that deal primarily with graphic data and images; and
6. Those that deal with knowledge representation (artificial intelligence applications).

Operating systems. Operating systems are the most basic yet essential type of application program. An operating system simply oversees the many needed "housekeeping" functions of a computer. A typical operating system provides five key functions, all of which are necessary to use other application programs. These functions include the following:

- Command and program execution,
- Input and output (I/O) control,
- Memory management,
- Multitasking, and
- Applications interface.

The command and program execution function determines both the sequencing and time that certain functions will be executed by the CPU. I/O control directs the operations of both the input and output devices, such as the keyboard and screen. The memory management component controls the use of and access to the computer's primary and secondary memory, including the use of virtual memory. Multitasking, if provided, allows the computer to divide CPU time among many different tasks, as previously described. Lastly, the applications interface provides the basis for other application programs to effectively use these functions, serving as a "platform" for controlling other programs.

There are two basic forms of operating systems: command-driven and graphics-based. A command-driven

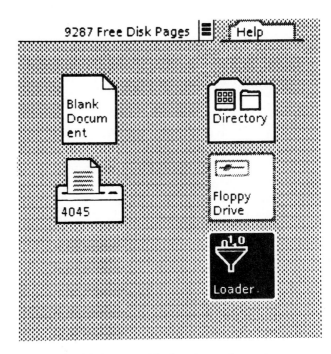

Fig. 36-6 A graphics-based operating system.

operating system uses English-like commands such as "COPY" (to copy a file) or "EXEC" (to execute a program). Several such commands may be grouped together to perform a series of operating system tasks in sequence. A series of operating system commands designed to function in sequence is called a *batch file*. For example, a batch file could direct the computer to (1) list a directory of files, (2) sort the files by date of creation, and (3) send the sorted list of files to an output device, such as a printer.

The most common command-driven operating systems used in micro and minicomputers are DOS, OS/2, and Unix. DOS (for *Disk Operating System*) is a single user, single tasking operating system that gained popularity with the introduction of the IBM Personal Computer in 1982. OS/2 is a second generation microcomputer operating system for IBM PCs and compatibles that provides the single user with multitasking capabilities and an optional graphics oriented user interface (the "Presentation Manager"). Unix (originally developed by AT&T) is a multitasking, multiuser operating system used extensively in engineering and scientific workstation applications. Common mainframe command-driven operating systems include VMS (for Digital Equipment Corporation's VAX line of computers) and VM-370 (for the IBM 370 mainframes).

As shown in Fig. 36-6, a graphics-based operating system uses symbols or "icons" to represent various functions. In this example, icons representing a document, directory of files, printer ("4045"), floppy drive, program loader, and help folder appear on the screen. With this type of operating system, the user could have the computer print the document simply by pointing to it with a mouse or lightpen, and then copying it to the printer.

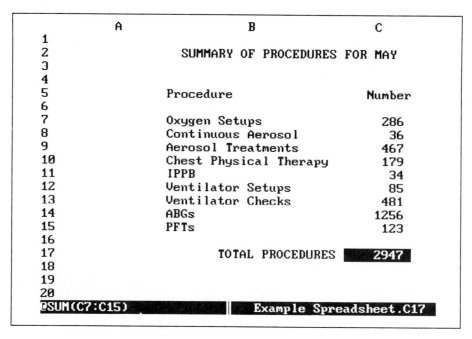

Fig. 36-7   A simple spreadsheet for manipulation of numeric data.

Originally developed at Xerox Corporation's Palo Alto Research Center (PARC), this graphics-based approach gained popularity with the introduction of the Apple MacIntosh Series of personal computers. Generally, graphics-based operating systems are easier for new users to master, but provide a more delimited range of functions than their command-based counterparts. Nonetheless, there is a growing tendency toward the use of this type of graphics-based user interface.

Text and documents. Application programs that deal primarily with text and documents are commonly referred to as word processors. Word processors may operate on a mainframe, microcomputers, or minicomputers. These application programs have the ability to create, edit, store, and retrieve text files, called *documents*. Multipurpose word processing software generally includes a variety of editing functions, including margin control, justification, search and replacement of text strings, block copy and move operations, and spell checking. This book was written using a multipurpose word processing application program. Single purpose word processing applications are more delimited in scope, being used for specific applications, such as the preparation of scientific documents (with various mathematical and scientific symbols).

Manipulation of numeric data. Application software used to manipulate numeric data provides computers with their "number-crunching" capability. All such programs use mathematical algorithms called formulas to handle numeric computations.

Perhaps the most common multipurpose application program designed specifically for numeric manipulation is the *spreadsheet*. Fig. 36-7 illustrates a simple spreadsheet being used to total the procedures performed by a Respiratory Care Department in a given month. As can be seen, a spreadsheet is divided into horizontal rows (typically labeled as numbers) and vertical columns (typically labeled as letters). The intersection of one row and column represents a cell, into which either numeric data or a formula can be placed. By referencing other cells of numeric data, a formula can automatically perform any one of many standard mathematical operations on that data. For example, the formula in the cell represented by the intersection of Column C, Row 17 (C17) is as follows:

$$@SUM(C7:C15)$$

This formula tells the program to calculate the sum of all the numbers in Column C, specifically those in the cells C7 through C15. The result is the total number of monthly procedures.

Of course, spreadsheet programs typically are much more complicated than this example, and can be used to perform a broad range of mathematical functions. Complex spreadsheets can look up data from another source, perform logarithmic and statistical operations, and provide "what-if" modeling of numeric data to predict the effect of changing assumptions.

Other common multipurpose numeric-based application programs include those designed to perform statistical analysis of data and those used to compute complex scientific equations using differential or integral calculus.

Single purpose numeric-based software applications are preprogrammed to conduct a more delimited set of compu-

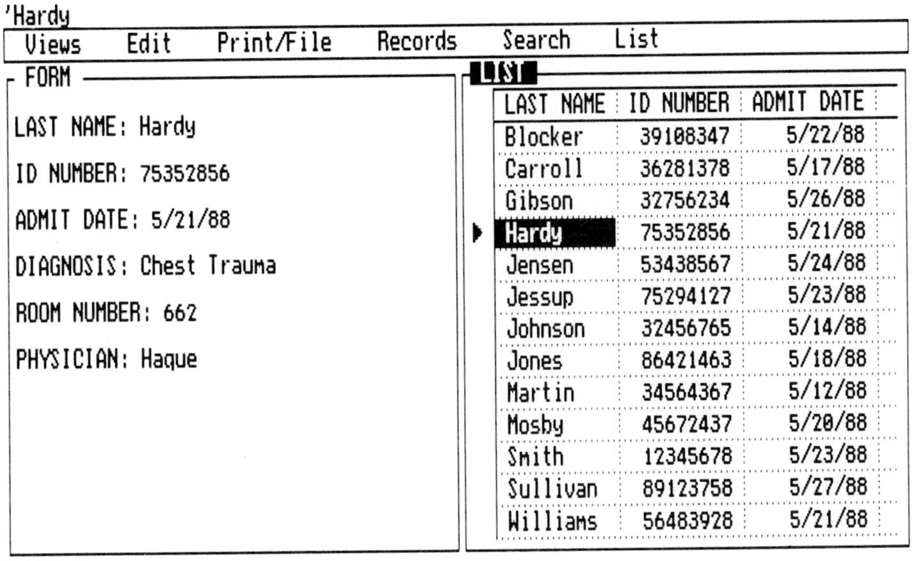

'Hardy

| Views | Edit | Print/File | Records | Search | List |

FORM

LAST NAME: Hardy

ID NUMBER: 75352856

ADMIT DATE: 5/21/88

DIAGNOSIS: Chest Trauma

ROOM NUMBER: 662

PHYSICIAN: Haque

LIST

LAST NAME	ID NUMBER	ADMIT DATE
Blocker	39108347	5/22/88
Carroll	36281378	5/17/88
Gibson	32756234	5/26/88
Hardy	75352856	5/21/88
Jensen	53438567	5/24/88
Jessup	75294127	5/23/88
Johnson	32456765	5/14/88
Jones	86421463	5/18/88
Martin	34564367	5/12/88
Mosby	45672437	5/20/88
Smith	12345678	5/23/88
Sullivan	89123758	5/27/88
Williams	56483928	5/21/88

Fig. 36-8   A simple patient database. The list view appears on the right, with the form view on the left.

tations on input provided either by the user or by analog to digital conversion (ADC) of electrical signals from diagnostic, monitoring, or therapeutic equipment. Good examples of this type of application are commercial software packages that compute the numeric results of pulmonary function tests or arterial blood gas analyses.

Categorical data. In order to handle large volumes of data, it is necessary to establish specific categories of information. For example, a patient's last name, admitting date, diagnosis, and attending physician are all categories of information. By applying these categories to many observations, large volumes of text and numeric data can be logically organized, stored, retrieved, and manipulated according to one's specific information needs.

A system for organizing text and numeric data in such a way that it can be easily stored, retrieved, and manipulated is called a *database management system.* A database management system consists of two related components: an underlying program of computer instructions that provide the storage, retrieval, and manipulation functions, and one or more databases.

A database is simply a collection of *records.* A record represents a collection of categorical data describing either a single person, object, or event. Each "piece" of categorical information within a record is called a *field.*

Fig. 36-8 shows a simple patient database. On the right, a portion of the full database is portrayed in what is often referred to as the list view. This format shows a number of patient records, organized by columns and rows. Each row represents a single patient record, whereas each column represents a field of specific information. The database "pointer" is currently directed at one of these patient records.

The left side of Fig. 36-8 illustrates that single record, including all its information fields. This type of display is often referred to as the form view. As is evident, the form view shows all the fields for this specific patient, including last name, identification number, date of admission, admitting diagnosis, room number, and attending physician.

The power of a database management system lies in its ability to quickly and accurately search for, sort, and report on specific categories of information. For example, suppose we want to prepare a report on the respiratory care given to all patients admitted in a given year according to their diagnosis. A database management system could quickly search for and sort these records, and, with the appropriate instruction, prepare our report in less time than it would take to make a cup of coffee.

Recent advances in database management systems simplify this process by allowing the user to retrieve data by using commands very similar to spoken English (called Structured Query Language, or SQL) or by giving examples (called Query By Example, or QBE). Both methods are designed to facilitate data retrieval and reporting. The following is an example of SQL used to prepare a report of respiratory treatments given to all patients during calendar year 1988, grouped by their admitting diagnoses:

```
SELECT      patient.name,
            patient.id,
            patient.dx,
            resp.rx
FROM        patient, resp
WHERE       patient.id = resp.id
            AND
            patient.admitdate between "880101"
                and "881231"
ORDER BY    patient.dx;
```

Natural language processors take this process a step further, allowing plain English commands to be interpreted by the computer. For example, the above SQL report instructions might look like this in a database management system that incorporates a natural language processor:

- Prepare a report of patient names, IDs, diagnoses, and respiratory treatments for all patients admitted during 1988 from the patient and respiratory databases.
- Group the patients by their diagnoses.

Some database management systems also provide for extensive manipulation of numeric data within their fields. Numeric fields that use data from other fields for computation are called derived fields. For example, a "procedure charge" field on a patient record could be totaled by a derived field called "total charges" to compute the daily charges for that patient. Likewise, two fields on a practitioner reporting form, called "procedure numbers" and "time units" could be multiplied to create a derived field called "total work units" (procedure numbers × time units for the indicated procedure). Further, this "total work units" field could be divided by an "hours worked" field to derive a new "productivity index" field.

The most sophisticated database systems are called *relational* databases. In simple terms, relational databases allow the user to work concurrently with more than one database at a time. This capacity allows one to "relate" or link data in a file with relevant data in another file.

Fig. 36-9 schematically portrays the ability of a database management system to work simultaneously with more than one database. Here, a practitioner is working with a patient treatment record, part of which is called the transaction database. The transaction database is "linked" with a hospital-wide master database of patient information via a common link field, such as the patient's identification number. Once the link is established, relevant information from the master database (such as the patient's name) is automatically "looked-up" and transferred to the patient record in the transaction database. On the other hand, the "procedure charge" field in the treatment record can automatically be added to the "total charges" field in the master database, a process called *updating*. Finally, different fields from both databases could be combined in the formulation of a report. Once established, these linkages not only minimize the need to re-enter data, but also decrease the likelihood of input error.

Graphics and imaging. Application programs that deal primarily with images, as opposed to words or numbers, are referred to as graphics or imaging applications. In business, graphics applications are used primarily to create charts of numeric data for presentation (presentation graphics). In commercial art production, graphics software can provide freehand drawing capabilities and sophisticated computer animation. In the biomedical setting, graphics applications are used mainly to produce, enhance, or help interpret digitalized images of human structure or function.

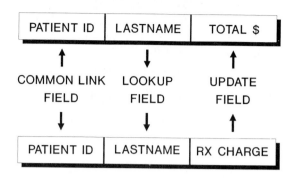

MASTER DATABASE

Fig. 36-9   A relational database management system can work with more than one database at the same time. See text for details.

The most familiar computer-based imaging application in biomedicine is probably computerized axial tomography, or CAT scanning. A CAT scanner uses a minicomputer and sophisticated imaging software to digitize, analyze, and enhance information derived from a series of axial x-ray tomograms. The result is a high resolution, two dimensional image of a transverse "section" through the human body.

In cardiopulmonary diagnostics, computer-based imaging is becoming commonplace in both echocardiography and angiography. In these applications, real-time three dimensional views of the heart and/or its coronary circulation can be generated. Enhancement to these images can be provided by "filtering out" unnecessary surrounding structures, thereby providing a detailed portrayal of only the pertinent anatomy.

Artificial intelligence. Artificial intelligence (AI) is a subdivision of computer science devoted to creating computer software that imitates, or mimics, certain functions of the human mind. The goal of AI is to give computers added capabilities and allow them to exhibit more intelligent behavior. The intent is not to replace human beings, but to provide us with more powerful tools that can better assist us in our work.

Intelligence represents the *human* ability to acquire and apply knowledge and is founded on both rational thinking and reasoning processes. To a limited degree, artificial intelligence permits computers to accept knowledge from human input, then use that knowledge through simulated thought and reasoning processes to solve problems.

Knowledge consists of facts, concepts, theories, procedures, and relationships. Knowledge also represents information that has been organized and analyzed to make it understandable and applicable to solving a problem or making a decision. Human knowledge, or an understanding of some subject area, is obtained through education and experience. Although a computer cannot learn like a human being, it can "acquire" knowledge from human experts. This acquired knowledge, provided to the computer by humans, is termed a *knowledge base*.

Once a knowledge base is built, artificial intelligence techniques give the computer the ability to simulate human thought and reasoning processes. Specifically, artificial intelligence techniques allow the computer to make inferences and draw judgments based on the facts and relationships contained in the knowledge base. Artificial intelligence gives a computer the ability to solve a wider range of problems than that possible with simple calculation, data storage and retrieval, or control. As a result, the computer becomes a far more useful tool, supplementing and enhancing our human capabilities.

AI software can be written in virtually any computer language, such as BASIC, FORTRAN, PASCAL, and C. However, AI programming languages have been developed especially for AI applications. The two most popular AI programming languages are LISP and Prolog.

Regardless of which language is used, the techniques for creating AI programs vary considerably from the conventional software used with digital computers. Conventional software tells the computer how to solve the problem, whereas AI software tells the computer what the problem is but not how to solve it. Instead of giving the computer step-by-step procedural instructions, we give it knowledge about the problem area and some inferencing capability. We then allow the computer to determine the best method of arriving at a solution.

For this reason, most AI software does not employ the traditional algorithmic process used in conventional programming. Instead, AI software uses symbolic representation and manipulation. As in conventional software, these symbols consist of letters, words, or numbers. However, AI software can use these symbols to represent both objects and the relationships among them. Objects can be people, things, ideas, concepts, events, or statements of fact. Various processes are then used to manipulate these objects and analyze their relationships, thereby solving a particular problem.

The most common problem-solving processes used by AI software are search and pattern matching. Given some initial start-up information, the AI program searches the knowledge base and looks for specific conditions or patterns. It attempts to identify "match-ups" that satisfy the criteria set up to solve the problem. The computer literally hunts around until it finds the best answer it can give based on the knowledge it has.

Currently, there are three categories of problem-solving applications for artificial intelligence software. These applications are:

1. Natural language processing,
2. Robotics and computer vision, and
3. Expert systems.

Natural language processing employs artificial intelligence methods to allow humans to communicate with a

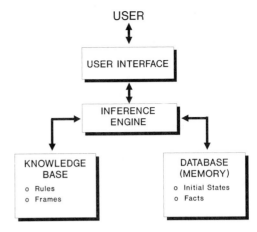

Fig. 36-10   Block diagram of an expert system.

computer in native languages, such as English (refer to the example given previously for querying a database). Speech recognition is an extension of natural language processing that uses AI concepts to accept and recognize spoken, as opposed to written language. Robotics is that branch of AI dedicated to the design and use of intelligent robots. An intelligent robot is a reprogrammable, multifunctional manipulator that can perform a variety of manual tasks normally done by humans. The most sophisticated of these robots can use a variety of electronic sensors to mimic human-like "senses." In industry, the two most important senses are computerized "touch" and "vision."

By far the most important category of AI software in health care is the expert system. Like other forms of AI, an expert system incorporates a knowledge base and an inferencing system. However, unlike natural language processing or robotic applications, an expert system captures and makes available the knowledge of one or more experts in a particular domain of interest. In this manner, an expert system can serve as an intelligent consultant to nonexperts, helping them to answer questions, solve problems, and make decisions in the applicable knowledge domain.

Like all AI software, expert system software is knowledge-based, containing a set of facts, data, and relationships pertaining to a problem area. However, unlike other forms of AI, expert systems take advantage of *heuristic* knowledge. As opposed to simple factual or textbook knowledge, heuristic knowledge is derived primarily from real world experiences. As such, it is the most practical kind of knowledge available to humans, being specifically related to the solution of everyday problems.

A general block diagram of an expert system is illustrated in Fig. 36-10. The key components are (1) a knowledge base, (2) an inference system, (3) a data base, and (4) a user interface.

The heart of any expert system is its knowledge base. There are many different methods for representing knowledge in an expert system. The most common method is by using production rules. Production rules usually take the form of an IF-THEN statement. The (IF) component states some premise, condition, or antecedent. The (THEN) component states a conclusion, action, or consequence that will take place if the premise or condition stated in the (IF) side of the rule is met. Thus, if the premise or condition is met, the conclusion, action, or consequence is also true. In this case, the rule is said to be "triggered." The following examples of production rules show how certain types of respiratory care knowledge can be expressed:

IF	the peak pressure rises
AND	the delivered volume remains constant
AND	the peak-plateau pressure remains constant
THEN	the effective compliance is decreased, CF 1.0
IF	the rate is >100 and <160
AND	the rhythm is regular
AND	P waves are present
AND	the P-R interval is normal
AND	the QRS complex is normal
THEN	the arrhythmia is sinus tachycardia, CF 0.9

Each rule is made up of what we call clauses. Like a sentence, a clause states some fact and contains a subject, a verb, and an object. Typically, a single production rule contains only one (IF) clause and only one (THEN) clause. However, as seen above, the (IF) component of the rule may contain more than one premise.

Also associated with each conclusion may be a certainty factor, or "CF." The CF simply indicates the degree of confidence we have in the validity of the conclusion. Certainty factors can vary between 0 (no likelihood) and 1 (a "sure thing"). They provide expert systems with the capacity to handle the "fuzzy" types of problems previously discussed.

Of course, each rule represents only a small bit of knowledge. Large numbers of rules are usually linked together to establish a line of reasoning. For example, the conclusion of one rule may become the premise of another. This collection, or network, of rules forms the expert system knowledge base, commonly referred to as a rule base.

Although the knowledge or rule base is essential, an expert system cannot function without an inference system. This system, called the "inference engine," applies sophisticated search and pattern matching techniques to the knowledge base. As this process proceeds, and as various rules are triggered, the system accumulates additional facts in its working database, using this newly acquired data to refine its search for a solution. The system continues to apply the rules until it either finds a satisfactory solution or exhausts all possibilities, thereby "failing" to reach a conclusion.

Using this general approach, expert systems can be broadly categorized according to the primary function they perform (see box below). Currently, there are six major applications of expert systems: diagnosis, interpretation, monitoring and control, prediction, planning, and instruction.

Diagnosis is the most common application of expert systems. Diagnostic expert systems are used extensively in industry to identify and troubleshoot equipment malfunctions. In health care, the most frequent application of diagnostic expert systems is to diagnose medical illnesses.

For a diagnostic expert system to be effective, the relationship between symptoms and causes must be identifiable and consistent. Primary difficulties in the development of diagnostic expert systems are the masking of symptoms by other symptoms, intermittent symptoms, inaccessible data, and lack of knowledge about relationships of symptoms to causes.

Interpretive expert systems analyze data to determine their meaning. For example, in the industrial sector, interpretive expert systems are used extensively to analyze mass spectrometry data and determine the presence or absence of various chemical structures. In health care, examples of interpretive expert systems include those used to assess the result of blood gas analysis and those designed to interpret the meaning of pulmonary function test data.

For an interpretive expert system to be effective, there must be a known and consistent interpretation of a given set of data. Moreover, the system must provide a solution only when a definitive interpretation is apparent. Primary problems in the development and use of interpretive expert systems are incomplete data, unreliable data, and conflicting data.

In complex systems such as nuclear power plants, aircraft traffic control, and medical monitoring, the need often exists to make quick decisions based on complex data. Often, a human cannot analyze the data fast enough to make an appropriate response. In other cases, round-the-

---

GENERIC EXPERT SYSTEM CATEGORIES

CATEGORY	DESCRIPTION
Diagnosis	Identifying the cause of problems
Interpretation	Analyzing data to determine its meaning
Monitoring and control	Intelligent automation of complex tasks
Planning	Developing goal-oriented schemes
Prediction	Intelligent guessing of outcomes
Instruction	Optimizing computer-based instruction

clock monitoring is necessary, and experts are not always available to provide needed consultation.

In these situations, a monitoring and control expert system can continuously assess complex input data and either suggest an appropriate action or take such action automatically. In the former case, the expert system is operating as an *open loop,* with human input necessary to complete the control action. In the latter case, when the system automatically takes action based on sensor-provided input data, it is said to be operating as a *closed loop,* that is without the need for operator input.

Prediction, or modeling, represents the capacity to use currently available data to determine some future outcome or state of affairs. The most common example of the use of expert systems for prediction is the complex modeling employed by the US Weather Bureau to predict the weather. Economic modeling is also commonplace in the business sector.

In health care, the current use of expert systems for prediction is less widespread. However, systems have been developed to predict the prognosis of patients undergoing certain surgical procedures or those afflicted with some specific combination of clinical disorders. In these systems, large volumes of prior patient data are used to develop statistical indices of severity of illness or condition. These indices are then incorporated into a prediction equation which computes the likelihood of survival or the degree of morbidity to be expected.

A plan is a procedure, or course of action, designed to achieve a specific goal. A planning, or decision-making, expert system produces an optimum plan of action based on the input of pertinent variables. For example, in the industrial setting, expert systems are commonly used to plan the configuration of complex computer systems, based on the individual needs and expectations of the purchaser. In health care, expert planning systems may assist dietitians in the development of nutritional plans for their patients or support psychiatrists in providing appropriate counseling. Although the need exists, there are currently no clinical expert planning systems for the respiratory care practitioner.

Instructional expert systems represent the last major category of this type of software. In general, the best way to learn about something is to get instruction from an expert. In the same manner, an expert system that stores expert knowledge can be used to teach others this knowledge. However, beyond being the repository for knowledge in a subject area, an ideal instructional expert system should be able to assess the learner's prior level of knowledge, individually adjust the instruction according to that level, and verify the learner's mastery of the new knowledge.

More detail on the application of these various types of expert systems in respiratory care will be provided later in this chapter.

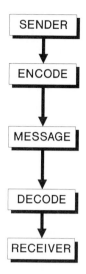

Fig. 36-11   Basic elements of a data communication process.

DATA COMMUNICATION

Recent advances in technology have made digital computing available to individual users at extremely low cost. However, the rapid growth of information technologies demands that computers, and the people that use them, be able to share data and communicate with each other.

The process of sharing data among computers is called *data communication.* Fig. 36-11 portrays the basic elements of the data communication process. A message (consisting of words, numbers, and/or graphic images) is generated by a sender. Before transmission, the message must be structured in such a way that it can be sent quickly and accurately. This process is called encoding. The encoded message is sent over a transmission route to a given destination (called the receiver). Once received, the message must be decoded into a form that the receiver can comprehend.

Host-remote telecommunication systems (Fig. 36-12)

The simplest example of data communication using digital computers is the linkage commonly established between a mainframe computer, called the host, and a microcomputer, called the remote, over standard voice telephone lines. The purpose of this type of linkage is usually to access and transmit data stored on the host to the remote microcomputer, a process called downloading. For example, a pharmacist might need to frequently access a host computer that maintains a large database that stores drug interaction information.

In this example, two ingredients are necessary for these computers to "talk" to each other. First, there must be a mechanism to rapidly transmit binary data back and forth over the telephone lines. Second, there must be a common "language" by which each computer can understand the other's actions and commands.

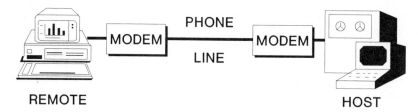

Fig. 36-12 Host-remote telecommunication system over telephone lines.

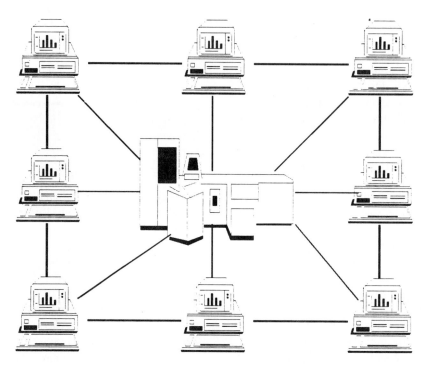

Fig. 36-13 A computer network.

Since telephone line transmission is based on analog acoustic signals, there must be a means to convert the computers' digital data to and from this analog format. This is accomplished by a device called a *modem*. A modem, or *mod*ulator-*dem*odulator, is simply a special type of analog-to-digital converter specifically designed to work with analog acoustic signals. The speed of transmission of computer data via modem is measured via the baud rate (roughly equivalent to the number of bits transmitted per second). For example, a three hundred baud modem (slow by current standards) would take approximately 66 seconds to transmit a full page of double-spaced characters. This same task can be accomplished in about 10 seconds with a modern 2400 baud modem.

However, simple transmission of the data alone cannot ensure effective communication between the computers. There must exist a common communication protocol, or set of rules which dictates exactly how communication will occur between the two systems. Examples of commonly used communication protocols include XMODEM and KERMIT.

These protocols provide a means for the computers to exchange "status signals." Status signals allow the computers to notify each other when data has been sent, when it is ready to be accepted, or when it has been accepted. This exchange is called handshaking. Most communication protocols also provide what is referred to as an automatic error correction mechanism. Automatic error correction helps identify errors occurring during data transmission. If an error is detected, the correction mechanism will usually attempt to retransmit the data until accuracy is verified. Although not critical for the communication of text-based data, error correction is essential in the transmission of binary data files, where an error in just one data bit could make a whole software program inoperable.

Computer networks

A computer network (Fig. 36-13) represents a system of one or more computers connected through transmission lines for purposes of data communication. There are two general types of computer networks: the local area network or LAN, and the wide area network (WAN). A LAN is simply a small group of computers and/or terminals linked together by specialized hardware and software, usually localized within a particular work area, such as an office or building. A WAN is an extension of the LAN concept, whereby computers may communicate with each other across long distances, such as between cities or between continents.

Regardless of size, computer networks differ from simple host-remote systems in two major respects. First, a computer network allows all linked computers to communicate with each other. In this manner, a message from any one computer could readily be sent to all other computers on the network. Second, most networks use high speed communication lines designed solely for data transmission. As compared to standard telephone lines, special coaxial cables can provide a hundred-fold increase in the rate of data transmission. Newer fiberoptic cables can transmit data at least a million times faster than standard telephone lines!

When a large number of terminals or computers are linked to a central mainframe system, it is inefficient to have separate transmission lines for each remote station. Instead, a single transmission line may be used to link several remote stations to the mainframe. A technique called multiplexing allows multiple streams of data to be transmitted over the same line.

COMPUTER APPLICATIONS IN RESPIRATORY CARE

Digital computers have been used in respiratory care for well over 20 years. The early use of computers in this field coincided with the introduction of hospital-wide financial and patient information management systems. At about the same time, research clinicians were beginning to apply the computer to help increase the speed and accuracy of testing procedures, particularly those amenable to solution by mathematical algorithms, such as pulmonary function computations. More recently, computers are being applied to assist clinicians in interpreting data, reaching diagnoses, and automating selected aspects of patient care.

Information management

Hospital-wide information systems. The first widescale use of computers in the hospital setting was limited to the business end of health care. Hospitals developed and incorporated computerized patient billing systems to replace their antiquated manual bookkeeping methods. Initially, most of this activity occurred via batch processing of keypunched data from charge slips provided by the various service departments. The direct involvement of clinicians with the computer system was only minimal.

The next logical step was to incorporate clinical data as a component of the hospital information system. This was accomplished after patient discharge, at which time selected elements of patient data, such as the admitting diagnosis and discharge status, were incorporated into the database and used primarily for reimbursement reporting.

Toward the end of the 1970s, advances in technology made possible true interactive patient information management systems. Typically, these systems incorporate a large mainframe database with a remote terminal network. These remote terminals provide concurrent access by hospital staff and clinicians to relevant patient data.

In its most basic form, a patient information management system allows access to commonly needed data elements, such as the admitting diagnosis, the attending physician, or the physician orders. More sophisticated patient information management systems have the capacity to supplant some or all of the manual medical recordkeeping functions. For example, a sophisticated patient information management system not only can provide physician order entry, but also allow users to enter progress and treatment notes, chart selected data (such as vital signs), and maintain and review a cumulative record of diagnostic test results. To minimize user training and facilitate data inputting, such systems typically are menu driven, providing a selection of the most common treatment options or data needs. When combined with specialized input devices, such as a lightpen, the clinician need only point to a selection in order to enter it into the record.

Whether such systems will totally supplant the traditional medical record remains to be seen. Clearly, the technology already exists. However, such technology will only succeed if it is accepted by end-users as meeting their information needs.

Departmental management. Recently, many respiratory care departments have incorporated their own computer-based management systems. In the absence of a hospital-wide patient information system, departmental computing is commonly used to log and track physician orders, record patient treatments, and create billing and procedural summaries. However, where a hospital-wide patient information system exists, departmental computing tends to focus more on the management of personnel and material resources. In this case, departmental computing may be used to facilitate scheduling of staff, monitor their productivity, maintain the supply inventory, and track equipment preventive maintenance schedules.

When departmental computing is used to log and track physician orders and record patient treatments, two approaches are common. In the first approach, practitioners simply enter relevant data into the departmental computer after completion of their rounds. Unfortunately, this mechanism is relatively time consuming, requiring both transcription of notes on the floors and their manual transferal into the computer. With a single computer and a large number of staff, access also becomes problematic.

Recent advances in technology provide a means to overcome this problem. Instead of manually recording notes on the floors, practitioners use small hand-held computers for "remote" data entry. In this manner, selected patient information, new orders, order changes, treatment times, and verification of treatments can be logged directly into the hand-held unit. At the completion of rounds, this information is quickly downloaded into the base computer, or "manager." Software operating on the base computer combines this information with that downloaded by other staff practitioners, allowing for compilation of all data for a given shift.

Clinical applications

Although first used for managing information, computers have also been applied to support clinical aspects of respiratory care for many years. Computer-aided blood gas analysis and pulmonary function testing were developed in the late 1960s and early 1970s. More recently, computer-aided bedside monitoring has become commonplace in many clinical facilities. The use of computer technology to assist clinicians in interpreting data, reaching diagnoses, and planning patient care is just beginning. Also on the horizon is the use of closed-loop computer systems to control certain aspects of patient management, including mechanical ventilation.

Computer-aided testing. The first major application of computers in respiratory care was in the area of computer-aided testing. By using a computer and associated software to gather and compute diagnostic data, clinicians were able to increase the speed and accuracy of their testing procedures, particularly in the areas of blood gas analysis and pulmonary function testing. Subsequently, computer-aided testing also became widespread in hemodynamic assessment, where small bedside devices took over the role of computing complex cardiac output equations, using either the dye or the thermal dilution method.

In concept, all computer-aided testing is similar. An input signal, usually in analog format, is converted into binary digital data. Using a program of mathematical algorithms, the computer performs the necessary calculations and outputs the information to either a display device or a printer.

The set of instructions for these computations may reside in primary memory in the form of a ROM program or be available through secondary mass storage via magnetic disk. For example, the programs used by microprocessor-based arterial blood gas analyzers to compute blood gas parameters and those incorporated into a cardiac output computer, are usually stored in ROM. A program of instructions residing in ROM is often called "firmware," as opposed to software. However, most computerized pulmonary function systems use software programs that are stored in secondary memory on disk. In either case, if the system is to electronically store records of test results, some means of secondary storage is necessary.

Recently, support software has been developed to assist the clinician in maintaining a quality assurance program for diagnostic testing equipment. At the present time, such software is used mainly in computer-aided arterial blood gas analysis, where it can automate machine testing, calibration procedures and maintain verification logs for quality assurance documentation.

Computer-aided monitoring. The next logical step was to take the computer to the bedside and use it to assist in the acquisition and computation of cardiopulmonary monitoring data. Early on, simple electronic integrators and timing accumulators were used to compute variables such as tidal volume, mean airway and vascular pressures, and breathing and heart rates. The next step was to incorporate true microprocessors with appropriate ROM-based algorithms to compute derived variables. For example, the analog-to-digital conversion of a tidal volume signal from a ventilator can be combined with an electronically measured breathing rate to compute a minute ventilation. Likewise, ADC input of cardiac output, mean arterial and pulmonary artery pressures, and right atrial and pulmonary capillary wedge pressures to a computer can be used to quickly derive a complete hemodynamic profile.

Such techniques, now commonplace in many clinical centers, expedite the processing of complex information, thereby giving the physician, nurse, or respiratory practitioner more time to spend in the care of the patient. However, the use of the computer simply to derive monitoring data represents only a small step toward exploiting its full potential in patient management. Extension of these capacities, including the ability of the computer to assist clinicians in interpreting data, reaching diagnoses, and planning patient care is now beginning.

Computer-based interpretation and diagnosis. Use of the digital computer to interpret clinical data and help diagnose patient conditions represents a natural extension of its unique capabilities. However, whereas simple algorithmic processes are satisfactory for data acquisition, retrieval, and computation, computer-based interpretation and diagnosis must employ AI software concepts. Current computer-based AI applications used in respiratory care focus on the interpretation of pulmonary function, blood gas analysis, and hemodynamic data; and on the diagnosis of patient conditions.

Pulmonary function test interpretation. The first true computer-based AI application developed in respiratory care, called "PUFF," was developed in the late 1970s at Stanford University. PUFF is a rule-based expert system designed to provide highly accurate and repeatable interpretations of pulmonary function test results. PUFF queries the user regarding both selected pulmonary function test results and patient signs and symptoms. PUFF then derives a series of standard test values and concludes with a detailed interpretation and pulmonary function diagnosis. An example of a pulmonary function report generated by the PDP-11 minicomputer version of PUFF is shown in Fig. 36-14. That PUFF results are highly consistent with the interpretations provided by expert pulmonary physiologists is evident. In clinical practice, approximately 95% of its reports are accepted without modification.

PRESBYTERIAN HOSPITAL OF PMC
CLAY AND BUCHANAN, BOX 7999
SAN FRANCISCO, CA 94120
PULMONARY FUNCTION LAB

WT 40.8 KG, HT 161 CM, AGE 69, SEX F
REFERRAL DX-

TEST DATE 05/13/80

| | | | PREDICTED | | | POST DILATION | |
			(+/−SD)	OBSER	(%PRED)	OBSER	(%PRED)
INSPIR VITAL CAP	(IVC)	L	2.7	2.3	(86)	2.4	(90)
RESIDUAL VOL	(RV)	L	2.0	3.8	(188)	3.0	(148)
TOTAL LUNG CAP	(TLC)	L	4.7	6.1	(130)	5.4	(115)
RV/TLC		%	43.	62.		56.	(115)
FORCED EXPIR VOL	(FEV1)	L	2.2	1.5	(68)	1.6	(73)
FORCED VITAL CAP	(FVC)	L	2.7	2.3	(86)	2.4	(90)
FEV1/FVC		%	73.	65.		67.	
PEAK EXPIR FLOW	(PEF)	L/S	7.1	1.8	(25)	1.9	(26)
FORCED EXPIR FLOW 25-75%		L/S	1.8	0.7	(39)	0.7	(39)
AIRWAY RESIST (RAW)							
(TLC = 6.1)			0.0 (0.0)	1.5		2.2	
DF CAP-HGB = 14.5							
(TLC = 4.8)			24.	17.4	(72)	(14% IF TLC = 4.7)	

INTERPRETATION

Elevated lung volumes indicate overinflation. In addition, the RV/TLC ratio is increased, suggesting a moderately severe degree of air trapping. The forced vital capacity is normal. The FEV1/FVC ratio and mid-expiratory flow are reduced and the airway resistance is increased, suggesting moderately severe airway obstruction. Following bronchodilation, the expired flows show moderate improvement. However, the resistance did not improve. The low diffusing capacity indicates a loss of alveolar capillary surface, which is mild.

Conclusions: The low diffusing capacity, in combination with obstruction and a high total lung capacity is consistent with a diagnosis of emphysema. Although bronchodilators were only slightly useful in this one case, prolonged use may prove to be beneficial to the patient.

PULMONARY FUNCTION DIAGNOSIS: 1. MODERATELY SEVERE OBSTRUCTIVE AIRWAYS DISEASE. EMPHYSEMATOUS TYPE.

Fig. 36-14 Pulmonary function report generated by PDP-11 version of PUFF.

Arterial blood gas interpretation. Despite its importance in the management of a wide variety of patient conditions, the interpretation of arterial blood gas test results by both physicians and other health related professionals remains highly unreliable. Based on this fact, and the knowledge that arterial blood gas interpretation employs a delimited set of concrete rules, it should come as no surprise that expert system software has been successfully developed and applied in this area.

Fig. 36-15 is an example of the report provided by one such expert system. As is evident, measured values, including the patient's temperature and F_{IO_2}, are provided as input by the user. The system then uses standard algorithmic processes to derive the P_{AO_2}, $P(A-a)O_2$, hemoglobin saturation, HCO_3^-, and the $[H^+]$ (in nanometers per liter). Then, using a knowledge base consisting of known rules, it provides both a acid-base and respiratory interpretation. Further analysis, provided on request, would allow the

user to compare these results to expected acid-base responses to chronic conditions, such as chronic hypercapnea. Like the PUFF expert system, the results of such analyses are highly consistent with the interpretations provided by experts, with most reports accepted without modification.

Hemodynamic assessments. Given the number and complexity of hemodynamic measures and the difficulty in their interpretation by all but the most experienced clinicians, hemodynamic assessment represents an ideal area in which to apply clinical expert systems. An example of the dialog between a clinician and one such expert system, developed by the author, appears in the box on p. 967.

Based on input data, this expert system quickly performs all pertinent calculations, thereby deriving a standard hemodynamic profile for the patient. Using this derived data, the system then consults its knowledge base, consisting of some eighty production rules. If all premises

---

EXAMPLE OF INTERACTION WITH A HEMODYNAMIC MONITORING EXPERT SYSTEM

What is the patient's first name?
→Mary
What is the patient's last name?
→Smith
What is Mary Smith's patient number?
→123456789
There is no record of Mary Smith, #123456789, on file. Do you wish to establish a file for this patient (Y/N)?
→Y
What is Mary Smith's height (in inches)?
→65
What is Mary Smith's weight (in pounds)?
→160
What is Mary Smith's heart rate (in beats/min)?
→90
What is Mary Smith's cardiac output (in L/min)?
→3.0
What is Mary Smith's CVP or right atrial pressure (in mm Hg)?
→−1
What is Mary Smith's mean pulmonary artery pressure (in mm Hg)?
→10
What is Mary Smith's mean pulmonary wedge pressure (in mm Hg)?
→5
What is Mary Smith's mean arterial pressure (in mm Hg)?
→50
Which of the following clinical signs does Mary Smith exhibit?
(check all that apply):

postural hypotension	altered sensorium
skin pallor*	cool skin*
oliguria	concentrated urine*
weak pulse*	flat neck veins*

---

fitting a specific conclusion are proven true, the system provides a definitive hemodynamic interpretation. As an example, Fig. 36-16 illustrates the outcome of the consultation shown in the box, including both the hemodynamic profile and its interpretation. In this case, the system concludes that Mary Smith is suffering from hypovolemic shock.

Should a definitive assessment be impossible, the system notifies the clinician of the inconclusiveness of the data presented and provides suggestions to help refine the diagnosis, as in the following example:

> Based on the data provided, a conclusive diagnosis of the patient's cardiovascular status is not possible;

however, the high wedge pressure and low LVSWI suggest cardiogenic shock. A 50 cc fluid challenge over 10 minutes may help to confirm the diagnosis.

General diagnostic systems. Up to this point, all the expert system examples have focused on a relatively narrow domain of clinical knowledge. However, expert systems designed to support general clinical diagnosis have to be much broader in scope, encompassing a larger number of possible clinical disorders and supporting a substantially greater number of clinical signs and symptoms. The first and best developed general medical diagnostic expert system is CADUCEUS.

Originally developed at Carnegie-Mellon University and now undergoing clinical trials at the National Institute of Health, CADUCEUS's expertise derives from one of the largest knowledge bases ever developed. This knowledge base consists of a broad spectrum of hand-crafted facts and rules, including some 500 diseases, 350 disease manifestations, and over 100,000 symptom associations that together cover about 85% of the possible diagnoses in internal medicine.

Using a disease tree or taxonomy approach, CADUCEUS builds up disease models as it proceeds. Patient data is first used to predict plausible hypotheses, equivalent to differential diagnoses. These preliminary hypotheses are then used to predict other clinical manifestations that must be either confirmed or used to alter the original hypotheses.

A simplified microprocessor-based form of the CADUCEUS system, called INTERNIST-PLUS, provides insight into the power of this type of expert system. The knowledge base underlying INTERNIST-PLUS consists of a large number of disease entities, each associated with a list of clinical signs and symptoms, called attributes.

Using a traditional physiologic systems approach, the user selects observed patient attributes from a menu of possible choices. For example, Fig. 36-17 provides the listing of available attributes for the respiratory system. We will assume, for purposes of demonstration, that the clinician selects the following attributes from the Respiratory System menu:

    1 (Cough)
    6 (Dullness to percussion-chest)
    7 (Dyspnea)
    10 (Friction rub-pleural)
    17 (Sputum-purulent)
    18 (Tachypnea)

Further, assume that the clinician enters chills, fever, chest pain, tachycardia, cyanosis, and leukocytosis from other selected system menus. As illustrated in Fig. 36-18, once all attributes for all pertinent systems are entered, INTERNIST-PLUS provides an analysis of the data by delineating a list of possible diagnoses, ordered according to

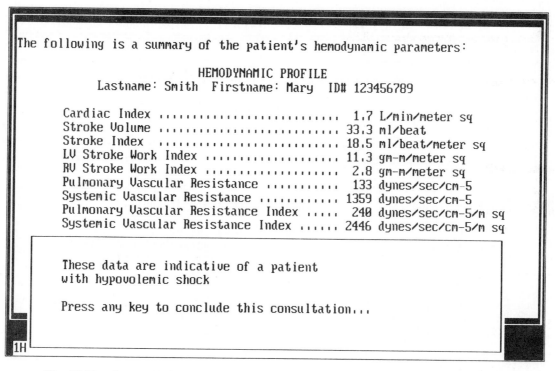

```
~~~~~~~~~~~~~~~~~~~~ 10-31-1988   UMDNJ-SHRP   09:28:43 ~~~~~~~~~~~~~~~~~~~~
                  ARTERIAL BLOOD GAS:  TABLE OF VALUES
Measured:    PaO2         %O2          PaCO2        pH           T(F)
             53           21           67           7.31         98.6

Derived:     PAO2    AaD      %SAT     [HCO3~]      [H+]         H!
             66      13       73       33           49           1.2


~~~~~~~~~~~~~~~~~~~~~~ ACID BASE INTERPRETATION: ~~~~~~~~~~~~~~~~~~~~~~~~
                         MILD ACIDEMIA due to
       Coexistant Primary Processes: RESPIRATORY ACIDOSIS and METABOLIC ALKALOSIS


~~~~~~~~~~~~~~~~~~~~~~ RESPIRATORY INTERPRETATION: ~~~~~~~~~~~~~~~~~~~~~~~
        The Patient  is HYPOXEMIC which is due PRIMARILY to HYPOVENTILATION




PRESS 'ESC' for MAIN MENU, 'R' to RUN ANOTHER, or 'C' for CHRONIC COMPARISON
```

Fig. 36-15 Summary interpretation of expert system analysis of arterial blood gas data. (From Wears RL and Kamen DR: Blood gas consultant, Copyright 1984.)

```
The following is a summary of the patient's hemodynamic parameters:

                       HEMODYNAMIC PROFILE
            Lastname: Smith  Firstname: Mary  ID# 123456789

      Cardiac Index .......................... 1.7 L/min/meter sq
      Stroke Volume .......................... 33.3 ml/beat
      Stroke Index  .......................... 18.5 ml/beat/meter sq
      LV Stroke Work Index ................... 11.3 gm-m/meter sq
      RV Stroke Work Index ...................  2.8 gm-m/meter sq
      Pulmonary Vascular Resistance ..........  133 dynes/sec/cm-5
      Systemic Vascular Resistance .......... 1359 dynes/sec/cm-5
      Pulmonary Vascular Resistance Index .....  240 dynes/sec/cm-5/m sq
      Systemic Vascular Resistance Index ...... 2446 dynes/sec/cm-5/m sq


      These data are indicative of a patient
      with hypovolemic shock

      Press any key to conclude this consultation...

1H
```

Fig. 36-16 Outcomes of a consultation with an expert system designed to assess hemodynamic parameters.

their "level of support" (equivalent to a confidence factor). In this case, the best supported diagnosis is pneumonia (93% support), followed in order of confidence by such conditions as pericarditis, chronic bronchitis, plague, lung abscess, and so on.

Closed-loop control of mechanical ventilation. As previously discussed, expert systems designed for monitor-

ing and control can continuously assess complex input data and either suggest appropriate actions (open-loop systems) or take such actions automatically (closed-loop systems). Thus far, all discussion has focused on open-loop computer systems (ie, those which provide clinical data or advice, but defer to the user for appropriate actions). Unlike open-loop systems, closed-loop computerized control sys-

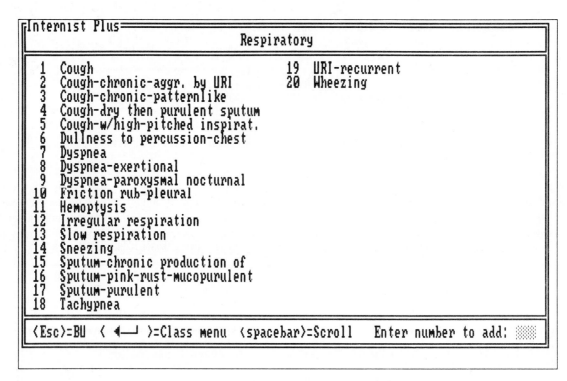

Fig. 36-17 Menu of patient attributes for the respiratory system in a general diagnostic expert system. (Internist-Plus, N^2 Computing, Silverton, Ore.)

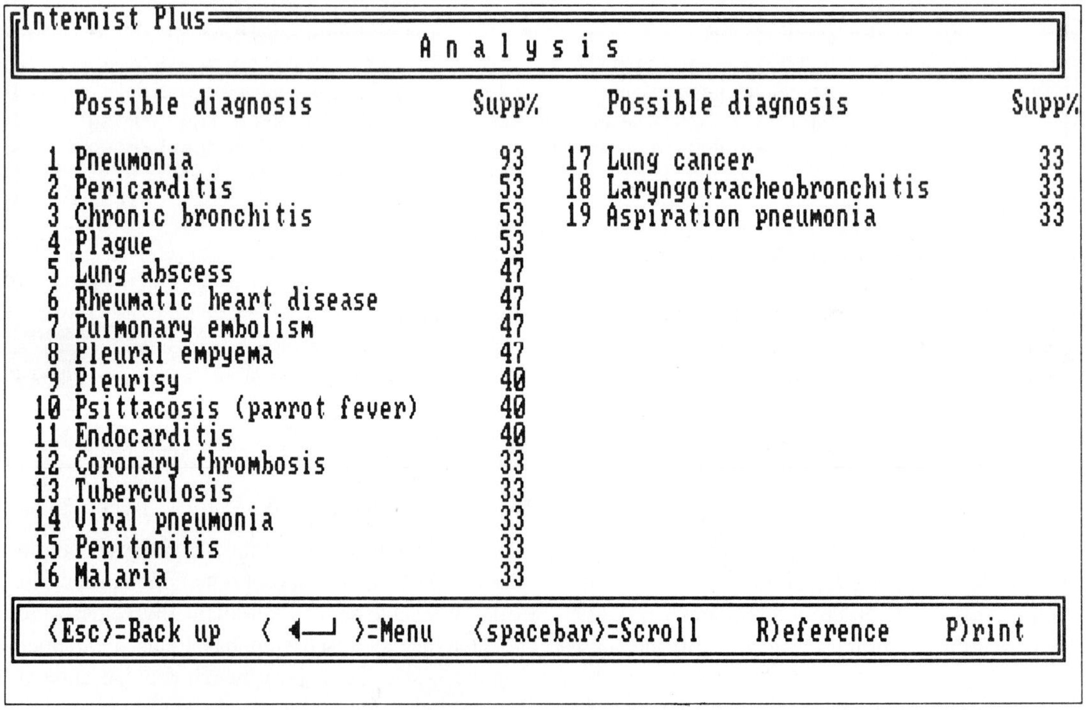

Fig. 36-18 Results of analysis of selected patient attributes in a general diagnostic expert system. (Internist-Plus, N^2 Computing, Silverton, Ore.)

tems employ sensor-provided input data as the basis for automatically taking predefined actions, without the need for user decision-making. In this manner, a predefined result is achieved by continuously monitoring one or more responses and constantly adjusting the process to achieve the desired end.

The most common example of a closed-loop control system used in respiratory care is the servo-controlled heated gas humidifier. To control this device, the clinician sets the desired gas temperature. Based on continuous input provided by an electronic temperature sensor, the automatic control mechanism then increases or decreases the power output to the heating element to maintain the desired airway temperature.

In its simplest form, this type of closed-loop control can be accomplished without a microprocessor, using only a simple electromechanical mechanism. However, by incorporating a microprocessor circuit with appropriate ROM-based software, the humidifier system can be made more "intelligent," thereby providing such additional functions as default temperature control in the event of sensor failure and recognition of common problems in operation (automated troubleshooting).

Obviously, the concept of closed-loop computerized control need not be limited to simple devices such as a ventilator's heated humidifier. The next logical step in the management of patients requiring mechanical ventilation is closed-loop control of the ventilator itself.

The clinical application of closed-loop ventilator control actually preceded the advent of digital computers in medicine. In 1957, a closed-loop ventilator designed to obtain an appropriate minute ventilation and O_2/N_2O concentrations in patients undergoing general anesthesia was first reported in the literature. In this system, the inspiratory time and rate of breathing were fixed, with the patient's minute ventilation automatically varied by an electromechanically controlled pressure regulator linked to an infrared CO_2 analyzer.

Not until 1973 was a ventilator linked to a digital computer for purposes of ventilator control. This closed-loop system was applied successfully in animal anesthesia experiments to regulate minute ventilation, and oxygen, nitrous oxide, and halothane concentrations. As in the earlier example, minute ventilation was varied according to end-expired CO_2 measurements.

Because of the inaccuracies associated with equating end-expired CO_2 measurements to actual arterial CO_2 levels, clinicians later adapted an existing servo-controlled ventilator (the Siemens Servo 900) to respond automatically to changes in the arterial blood pH, as measured by microelectrodes placed in the femoral artery of paralyzed dogs. Notwithstanding problems associated with the calibration drift of the pH electrode, this closed-loop system was deemed successful in maintaining the desired pH in the animal models used (as reported in 1978 by Coon and others—see bibliography).

Subsequent clinical research has focused on refining these mechanisms to provide computerized closed-loop control of minute ventilation and PEEP levels. The major technical obstacles impeding wide-spread clinical application of these closed-loop control mechanisms include the unreliability of end-expired CO_2 measurements as an indicator of arterial P_{CO_2} (especially in patients with unstable $\dot{V}/\dot{Q}$ ratios and metabolic rates) and ongoing difficulties in the continuous assessment of intra-arterial blood gas parameters.

The only true application of closed-loop ventilatory control to have reached the bedside, mandatory minute ventilation (MMV), does not employ either expired or arterial gas analysis as a basis for adjusting ventilatory parameters. Instead, the expired minute ventilation itself is used as input to the microprocessor. As discussed in Chapter 30, this approach has significant limitations and will require substantial refinements before clinicians can confidently apply it.

Most clinicians agree that if the closed-loop control of mechanical ventilation is to ever succeed, emphasis must be placed on the use of multiple data inputs, as opposed to the current trend to focus on a single control variable, such as pH, P_{CO_2}, or minute ventilation. Given that the gathering and interpretation of multiple data inputs are technically feasible, the biggest obstacle to the wide-spread application of closed-loop control of mechanical ventilation may well be the clinicians themselves.

Currently, physicians and respiratory care practitioners look upon this approach to ventilatory support with considerable caution and, in some cases, downright fear. Nonetheless, just as airline pilots have come to accept and even praise the sophisticated computerized control mechanisms now available on today's commercial aircraft, so too will clinicians learn to effectively use computer controlled mechanical ventilation.

Integrated approaches

In some respects, one may argue that the clinical use of the computer has actually made patient care more difficult. This argument is based on the observation that the large amounts of patient data made available by the computer can be overwhelming and are seldom integrated into a unified whole. Thus, a hospital-wide patient system may maintain one sort of information, a departmental database may focus on another aspect of relevant data, and a computer-based ICU system may emphasize still a different set of clinical information.

Since certain elements of all this diverse information may be pertinent to providing quality care to the patient, current efforts are directing attention to the development of more integrated approaches to the acquisition, storage, and retrieval of relevant clinical data. Fig. 36-19 portrays a schematic model of this integrated approach, focusing on the department level of data usage.

Here, the department's computer resources are linked to

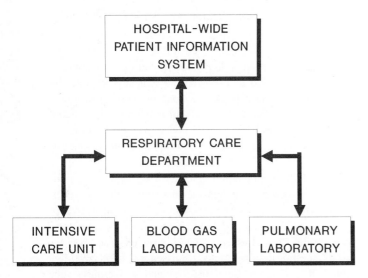

Fig. 36-19   Schema of an integrated clinical information system at the department level.

both the hospital-wide patient information system and selected clinical patient management systems, including the blood gas laboratory, pulmonary function laboratory, and the ICU monitoring system. Based on this framework, both general patient information and pertinent clinical data can be integrated and continuously updated across all systems, allowing clinicians full and immediate access to the information needed to plan, provide, and evaluate patient care.

As of this writing, no fully integrated system like that described is operational in respiratory care or in any hospital service department. Nonetheless, a variety of such systems are under development and will begin to see extensive usage throughout the coming decade.

SUMMARY

Whether a large mainframe or desktop version, the modern digital computer is an extremely versatile tool. Computers can quickly and accurately perform complex mathematical and logical operations, store and retrieve numeric and text data, translate numeric and text data from one form into another, reorder data according to prespecified instructions, edit existing data, make conditional decisions, monitor external events, and control external devices. However, computers are not currently able to discover new methods, use intuition, innovate or be creative, understand natural language, program themselves, catch input errors, reason about output values, or decide if a problem is solvable. Computers are very fast, accurate, and patient, but thinking is still uniquely human.

Modern computer technology involves both hardware and software. There are five key hardware components in a contemporary digital computer: (1) a central control unit, (2) an arithmetic logic unit, (3) an input mechanism, (4) a memory to store data and instructions, and (5) an output mechanism. Computer software represents the means by which a human operator instructs a computer what to do and how to do it. A complete set of such instructions, designed to accomplish a specific task, is called a program. Conventional computer programs are based on a clearly defined, step-by-step procedure for solving a specific problem, called an algorithm.

Preprogrammed instructions which enable a computer to perform a specific function are called application programs. Application programs may be categorized into six broad groups: (1) those that deal with the integration of hardware and software (operating systems); (2) those that deal primarily with text and documents; (3) those that deal primarily with the manipulation of numeric data; (4) those that deal primarily with categorical data (either text or numeric); (5) those that deal primarily with graphic data and images; and (6) those that deal with knowledge representation, that is, artificial intelligence (AI) applications.

By far the most important category of AI software is the expert system. An expert system incorporates a knowledge base and an inferencing system to capture and make available the knowledge of one or more experts in a particular domain of interest. In this manner, an expert system can help nonexperts answer questions, solve problems, and make decisions in the applicable knowledge domain. Currently, there are six major applications of expert systems: diagnosis, interpretation, monitoring and control, prediction, planning, and instruction.

Digital computers have been used in respiratory care for over 20 years. The early use of computers in this field coincided with the introduction of hospital-wide financial and patient information management systems. At about the same time, research clinicians were beginning to apply the computer to help increase the speed and accuracy of testing procedures, particularly those amenable to solution by mathematical algorithms, such as pulmonary function computations. More recently, computers are being applied to assist clinicians in interpreting data, reaching diagnoses, and automating selected aspects of patient care.

Notwithstanding the continuing growth in the use of computers in medicine and health care, it is important to remember that patient care in general and respiratory care in particular, are at the same time both human and humane endeavors. Although the computer can assist in our role as health care providers, it cannot take the place of a caring and empathetic practitioner. Indeed, like any good clinical tool, the computer should be used only to help free us from the mundane and repetitive tasks that tend to take so much time away from the direct care of our patients. To the extent that the computer furthers the distance between patient and clinician, its use must be vigorously avoided.

GLOSSARY OF COMPUTER TERMINOLOGY

abort to abandon program execution and to reestablish control at the operating system.

access to place data for storage, or to ascertain data for use, in a system.

access time the amount of time required to store or retrieve data between main memory and an external storage instrument. Access time is usually measured in milliseconds.

accumulator the register in a computer which houses the results of arithmetic computations or loads and stores data between the CPU and main memory.

algorithm a predetermined group of directions to solve a problem in a finite number of steps.

alphanumeric data composed of alphabetic and/or numeric characters.

ALU Arithmetic Logic Unit, the segment of the CPU which carries out arithmetic and logic functions.

analog a representation of numerical quantities by an output signal which measures continuous physical variables (such as voltage, length, pressure, flow) proportionate to the input.

analog computer a computer which functions by way of measuring continuous physical variables, manipulating the variables to arrive at a solution, and generating the numerical equivalent of that solution for output. Analog computers are generally engineered for specific applications in the scientific or technical fields.

analog data representation of continuous data by physical variables.

analog-to-digital converter (ADC) an instrument measuring an analog signal and converting it to digital form, thus enabling the data to be fed to a computer.

append to add on to the end, such as adding further data to the end of a file.

application software software to enable the computer to perform specific functions, such as word processing, data processing, etc.

archive to store data in such a way that supports retrieval, or the collection of data itself which is stored in this manner.

arithmetic operator a symbol used to dictate the particular operation to be executed in a mathematical expression $(+, *, /, \text{etc})$.

arithmetic register the register housed in the ALU which handles arithmetic and logic computations.

arithmetic relation a set of two mathematical expressions separated by a relational operator, such as $7 > 4$.

array a set of elements related in a logical manner that are indicated by one label. Such sets are usually stored sequentially in main memory locations.

artificial intelligence (AI) a synthetically created intellect which is capable of engaging in humanoid thought processes. The key factors in such an intellect are the ability to absorb new data, understand new input, solve problems via logical reasoning, and especially, to "remember," to learn from past errors and experiences so that it can adapt itself accordingly.

ASCII American Standard Code for Information Interchange, an ANSI developed code with seven bits which are sufficient to represent all the characters of a typewriter keyboard. An eighth parity bit for error checking is included in the transmission. This code was developed to make various types of data processing and communication machines compatible.

assemble translating symbolic code into its equivalent counterpart in machine code; the direct results can be executed by the computer.

assembler a program capable of assembling and commonly generating an assembly listing.

assembly language a low level programming language which utilizes memory aiding directives (STO for store, etc.) as opposed to binary numbers equal to the machine language directive counterpart. These

languages are written for use with the machine language of a particular computer.

automatic error correction a technique for the perception of errors during data transmission so that the data can be transmitted again or another correction can be implemented to assure accuracy.

backup a system for saving data should a computer failure (such as caused by power outages) occur.

BASIC Beginners All-purpose Symbolic Instruction Code, an easily learned and simple to use programming language. It is the main language in most microcomputers. It uses mnemonic devices for commands (RUN, PRINT, etc.) and possesses a wide variety of features.

batch a set of data and directives processed by the computer as a single unit in one run.

baud a measurement of speed in telecommunications. The measure is of each discrete signal element transmitted in one second. Assuming each signal element is one bit, then the number of bits transmitted per second is the baud rate.

binary 1. a condition where one of only two alternatives must exist (on or off, is or isn't, etc.) 2. a numerical system utilizing only the digits 1 and 0.

bit *bi*nary dig*it*, a quantum of data in computer storage.

Boolean algebra a method for representing principles of logic mathematically for the manipulation of logical variables.

branch the part of a program where the flow of directives is split and the computer is presented with multiple paths from which to choose.

bug a defect, or error, in a program which inhibits its operation. When programs are in the developing stages, several bugs are usually present which must be worked out.

byte a collection of data bits which function as one. Normally, a byte is comprised of eight bits. One byte could represent a character, and several bytes together could represent a word.

CAI Computer assisted instruction.

capacity the amount of data which can be stored in a memory device.

carrier a continuous, stable signal wave transmitted by a public utility for use as a communication channel for users.

Cathode Ray Tube (CRT) a television like screen generally having 24 rows and 80 columns for viewing data.

Central Processing Unit (CPU) the primary component of the computer. The CPU houses the core memory, the control component to manage computer system operations, and the arithmetic and logic unit (ALU).

channel a communications pathway along which signals can be sent.

character a single alphanumeric data bit. The word "horse" contains five characters.

character string any grouped sequence of characters.

chip a very small integrated circuit, generally a few centimeters in length, which can handle a large amount of data relative to its size.

C-Language a programming language for microcomputers developed in the United States by Bell Laboratories.

COBOL COmmon Business Oriented Language, a high-level programming language developed for handling business data.

command a directive from a program or directly entered into a terminal for the performance of a function.

command language a programming language with a limited range of commands to facilitate interaction between a user and the computer.

communication the act of transferring data from one storage device to another.

compile to translate a high-level programming language into a set of machine language directives for use by the computer.

compiler a program which compiles.

conditional an if-then type arrangement where current status of a situation determines future action.

constant an element such as in a mathematical expression with a value that does not change when the expression is solved.

cursor a light indicator displayed on a CRT for the purpose of indicating where the next character will be generated.

cycles per second the number of repeated signal waves transmitted in one second, the same as the measurement of the wavelength (hertz).

Selected definitions excerpted with permission from the IBM Software Directory, New York, 1984, RR Bowker Co. Copyright Reed Publishing (USA) Inc.

data any information or arrangement of character sets meant to represent information.

database a group of related records and files on a direct access storage device, stored in such a structure that appending, manipulating, and retrieving data from the base is a simple, naturally expected operation.

data processing the storing and manipulating of data for constant retrieval and updating.

debug the process of testing computer programs for inherent errors and removing those errors.

default the act a computer takes to automatically assign a predetermined value to a variable in the event that certain directives concerning a different value for the variable are not presented beforehand.

encode to use the rules of a code for transforming data into a coded message.

error 1. a malfunction in a program or piece of equipment. 2. a status word which indicates that an error has been detected, and the system is standing by for correction.

execute to perform the required functions on the selected data as dictated by programming directives.

field a unit of data comprised of adjacent alphanumeric characters or bits.

file a group of related records forming a data structure. For example, a group of records in which each contain an address in a particular state would be a file of addresses for that state.

flowchart a symbolic chart which describes the flow of events of an entire program, such as the branching alternatives to be selected or the path taken after the occurrence of the last event.

font the full selection of characters which can be printed at a certain style and size.

FORTRAN FORmula TRANslator, a high-level programming language mainly for the execution of mathematical programs. It is a compact language with many capabilities for a variety of mathematical problems, which facilitates the creation of such programs.

function 1. a coded directive or set of directives designed to produce a specific method of response when performed. 2. In multiplication, a set of ordered pairs in which the value of X is multiplied to give the value of Y. For example, $Y=5 (X)$.

giga (G) prefix denoting one billion (one thousand million) such as gigacycles, gigahertz, etc.

GIGO Garbage In, Garbage Out, a catch phrase among all programmers. This slogan signifies the fact that when incorrect, meaningless data or garbage is put into a system, the same will be ejected through the output.

handshaking the exchange of status signals between a transmitting and a receiving device to signify that data has been sent, is ready to be accepted, or has been accepted.

hardcopy computer output which is physically represented on paper such as graphs or printouts.

hard disk a magnetic disk for storing data which is more delicate and not as portable as a soft or floppy disk (diskette) but with far greater storage capacity and far greater access speed.

head an electronic instrument which reads data from, writes data onto, or erases data from a magnetic storage medium.

hertz (Hz) a measure of the frequency of carrier wave cycles referring to the number of completed cycles each second.

heuristic referring to a method of solving problems through repeated trial and error, applying the experimental results gained along the way to arrive at the correct solution.

high level language a programming language such as COBOL, FORTRAN, BASIC, or PASCAL which can accommodate a variety of functions and is not dependent on the machine language of a computer. One of the prime advantages of a high level language is that the commands used are forms of English words which are descriptive of the task they perform.

host 1. the primary or controlling computer which directs the operations of a group of other computers. 2. a central information system or database which can be accessed by multiple users.

image processing the use of a computer's capabilities to perform operations on visual images, such as storing them in data form, making special enhancements on them, etc.

input the data fed into a computer or program which is used to generate the output. For example, if a program is designed to add a value of four to the data entered into the routine, the user might enter a value of five as the input. The program would utilize that input to compute the value of nine, which would be the output.

instruction a command which orders the computer to perform a specific task.

instruction set the scope of all the instructions which can be used with a specific computer system.

integrated circuit (IC) a circuit residing on a small silicon chip within which all the electronic components of the entire circuit are contained. The size, reliability of internal connections, and reduced power consumption make such circuits quite advantageous.

interactive where the operator utilizes the computer in such a manner that the operations of the computer are directly controlled by the operator.

interpreter a program which can translate a source program into machine language for execution by the computer.

I/O input/output.

iteration the repetition of a specific function or set of instructions.

job a group of functions for the computer to perform, such as a program or set of programs, for a specific application.

Job Control Language (JCL) the language of a computer used for directing the operating system, such as preparing the system to interpret the language in which a program is written or to take instructions directly from the user.

kilo (K) prefix denoting one thousand. 48K memory in a computer would refer to forty-eight thousand bytes (kilobytes) of available storage.

keyboard a device arranged similarly to a typewriter for entering alphanumeric data into the computer or program.

kilohertz (KHz) referring to the frequency of a radio wave, kilohertz denoting one thousand completed cycles of wave movement each second.

Light Emitting Diode (LED) a semiconductor diode which emits light when a current is passed through it. Several such bars or diodes are used to make alphanumeric displays for digital watches, calculators, and other computer devices, much like the liquid crystal display.

lightpen a hand held, electronic stylus which senses light from and transmits signals to positions on a computer video screen.

line number a number in BASIC programming which is placed at the beginning of a programming line, enabling the computer to execute the lines in ascending values of the numbers, or to go to the line specified in another line.

Liquid Crystal Display (LCD) a display device to represent alphanumeric data. A liquid crystal is contained in glass, and an external light source affects the optical density of the crystal so as to make it visible or invisible to the naked eye. Such displays are used in calculators and digital watches and other computer devices.

LISP LISt Processing, a high level programming language primarily for list processing and for the manipulation of text.

load to transfer a data or programs from an auxiliary storage medium (such as a disk or tape) into the computer's working memory for immediate use.

logoff to enter specific data which will terminate access to a computer system.

logon to enter specific data which will initiate access to a computer system.

loop a series of instructions arranged so that it will be repeated until a certain condition has been reached.

low level language any programming language of limited commands which is expressed symbolically and which is limited in its complexity of possible procedures.

machine code the basic pattern of bits which forms the code used in machine language, sometimes used to refer to machine language.

machine language the programming language to which the computer directly responds. Each computer has its own machine language, dependent upon the systems configuration. As machine language is comprised of a binary code, programs are not generally written in this language, but rather, in higher level languages which can be translated into machine language for the computer.

magnetic tape a plastic tape with a magnetized surface which can store data.

mainframe the largest of computer types, sometimes filling several rooms. The storage capacity and operating speed of a mainframe computer is far greater than mini or microcomputers.

mass storage an external (secondary) storage device which can be connected to and accessed by the computer; used for storing mass data.

megabyte (MB) one million bytes.

megahertz (MHz) a measure of the frequency of wave cycles, indicating one million cycles per second.

memory a device which can record data and store it for retrieval.

memory bank a continuous arrangement of storage locations.

menu a visual display of possible options and functions of a program from which a user can choose.

microcomputer also referred to as a personal computer, a small, inexpensive computer which can fit on a table top and run complex programs for a variety of applications.

minicomputer an intermediate sized more expensive computer with capabilities between that of a microcomputer and a mainframe computer.

modem MODulator DEModulator, a device which uses modulation to convert a digital signal to an analog signal for transmission across a standard telephone line. The receiving device is equipped with a modem to reconvert the signal back into digital form for use by the computer.

monitor the video display screen with which the user observes the actions of the computer.

mouse a hand held device which a user can move. The movements are recorded and the cursor on screen moves to mark the corresponding point on the screen.

move to transfer data from one storage location to another.

network a system of one of more computers connected through communication lines to various terminals or computers.

nonvolatile memory memory in a computer which saves data in the event of a power loss or a system shutdown. ROM is usually considered nonvolatile.

numeric data data which is represented by the digits zero through nine.

numeric pad a group of numeric data keys on a terminal or other such device to make numeric data entry more efficient.

object code machine code output by an assembler or complier.

object program a written program translated into machine language by an assembler or compiler.

open referring to a file which has been opened and is ready to have data input into it or retrieved out of it.

operating system a group of programs which control the basic system functions of the computer. This system determines when certain functions will be executed, directs the operations of the other devices, and controls access to available memory. Three types of programs, input/output control system, processing program, and the job control program, usually comprise an operating system.

optical character recognition (OCR) a process by which printed characters can be read by a scanning device and input as data into an information system.

optical scanning device an instrument which scans visual data and translates it into digital form for computer processing.

output data which is produced from a system directly proportionated to the input. For example, if a system, or program, is designed to add four to the input, and the input is five, then when the program is executed, nine will eject from the system as the output.

partition a fixed segment of the main memory which can be accessed by multiple users. This provides an individual working space for each separate user.

PASCAL a high level programming language named after a seventeenth century French mathematician. The language is developed in such a manner as to permit very structured, precise programming. Learning the language is relatively easy, and, therefore, is often one of the first languages taught to programmers.

password a key, a set of characters which a user can enter into a system to gain access to that system.

peripheral any of a variety of devices which can be attached to a computer and directed by the central processing unit. Peripheral mechanisms can be for several purposes, such as additional data storage, temperature sensing, time measurement, controlling external, unrelated mechanisms such as the light in a household, the print of output, etc.

pixel PIctures ELement, the smallest element, or dot, which comprises a visual display on screen.

port a point of contact between an external device and the central processing unit through which data can be transferred.

primary memory memory which can be directly accessed by the CPU.

printer a device which can accept computer output to generate a visual, hardcopy display.

printout hardcopy.

procedure a specific set of instructions and rules to be followed by a computer system.

processor a device which can accomplish a variety of data manipulations.

program a logical, sequential arrangement of directives and parameters which are to be followed to correctly manipulate the input and generate the desired output.

prompt a message which appears on screen during a program execution. The message instructs the user to enter data to initiate a certain procedure or as input into the program.

protocol a collection of rules which dictates communication procedures between two systems.

query language a high level programming language with commands very similar to spoken language. It is specifically designed to facilitate data retrieval.

queue a collection of jobs awaiting processing. The first in, first out basis applies, so that while new jobs are added to the queue, the first in the group to have been entered are the first to be processed.

Random Access Memory (RAM) a memory storage system in which any specific storage location can be accessed directly, eliminating the need to search for a location in sequence. This makes memory easier and more rapid to use.

read/write head an electromagnetic device which both reads data from and writes data to a magnetic external storage medium.

record the segments of data which comprise a database file. For example, a file which contained data concerning fifty patients would have fifty records, one for each patient.

register a computer storage location in a memory which holds data temporarily so that data can be inserted for performing specific applications.

remote referring to the components of a computer system which are not located in the same proximity as the central processor, such as devices connected by telephone wires.

Read Only Memory (ROM) a type of memory in a computer from which data can be read but to which no data can be written. This unalterable type of storage holds permanent sets of instructions commonly used in computer programs, such as instructions for mathematical calculations, values of standard data, etc.

run to execute a program.

search to scan a collection of data for the purpose of locating a particular data item or items.

software the components in a computer system other than the actual, physical devices which comprise the system. Generally, this term refers to the programs which run the various devices, or the input or output data.

sort to arrange segments of data in a data file into a specific order (ie, alphabetically, numerically increasing, etc).

speech recognition the ability of a computer system to interpret human speech as data input and command entry by matching the sound wave patterns produced with patterns known by the system.

speech synthesis the forming of recognizable speech by the computer as a form of output or prompts given to the user.

storage capacity the amount of data which will fit into a storage medium (main memory, disk, tape, etc).

string a set of characters adjacent to one another which is treated as one unit in a program or in data storage.

telecommunications data transmissions over communication lines between locations distant from one another.

terminal a device used to input data and receive output from a computer. Generally, a terminal consists of a keyboard and a display, either a printer or a video screen.

timesharing a multi-user system where a very fast processor alternates between several programs and routines to accommodate several terminals in a manner which seems simultaneous.

toggle a switch with two possible positions.

transfer to move data from one storage area to another.

update to enter new data over old data in a file, generally as a result of an application program which has provided more current information.

utility program a program which provides a commonly required utility task, such as copying data, transferring data between different storage mediums, sorting data, etc.

volatile referring to memory which does not preserve data in the event of power failure.

word processing the use of a computer system to prepare and manipulate text.

BIBLIOGRAPHY

Abedin Z and Manoli S: Computerized calculation of regional left ventricular ejection fraction, Appl Cardiol 12(6):33-34, 38, 1984.

Andreoli K and Musser LA: Computers in nursing care: the state of the art, Nurs Outlook 33(1):16-21, 1985.

Aquino MM: A respiratory profile from a hand-held computer, Heart Lung 14:88-90, 1985.

Baldwin J: Continuous breath-by-breath monitoring greatly enhances patient care capabilities: incorporating the pneumotach and real time computer based system, Crit Care Nurse 3(3):33-35, 1983.

Bisson G et al: Computer-based quantitative analysis of gallium-67 uptake in normal and diseased lungs, Chest 84:513-517, 1983.

Bloom KJ and Weinstein RS: Expert systems: robot physicians of the future? Hum Pathol 16:1082-1084, 1985.

Brandenburger GH: Future impact of computers on radiology: tissue characterization based on quantitative ultrasound imaging, Appl Radiol 13(5):33-35, 38-40, 1984.

Brown GW: Diagnosing by computer, Diagn Med 8:54-57, 1985.

Buchanan BG and Shortliffe SH: Rule based expert systems: the MYCIN experiments of the Stanford University Heuristic Programming Project, Reading, Mass, 1983, Addison-Wesley Publishing Co.

Caceres CA: Computer-assisted ECG: an overview of computerized analysis, Consultant 24:237-239, 242-243, 247-248, 1984.

Chatburn RL: Computation of cardiorespiratory variables with a programmable calculator, Respir Care 28:447-451, 1983.

Chilton TL and Gilley WF: Computerized nutritional assessment: how we do it, Health Educ 13(5):29, 1982.

Clancy W and Shortliffe EH: Readings in medical artificial intelligence, Reading, Mass, 1983, Addison-Wesley Publishing Co.

Cole JR, Brown WA, and Lampard DG: Computer control of respiration and anesthesia, Med Biol Eng 11:262-267, 1973.

Coon RR, Zuperky EJ, and Kampine JP: Systemic arterial blood pH servocontrol of mechanical ventilation, Anesthesiology 49:201-204, 1978.

Craven NH: Computers in critical care: a weak connection, Health Serv 62(2):15-16, 1985.

Crew AD and Unsworth GD: Does the ICU computer improve patient care? Appl Cardiol 13:9-13, 1985.

Demers RR: Some potential pitfalls associated with the use of computers and microprocessors, Respir Care 27:842-845, 1982.

de Vries PH and de Vries-Robbe PF: An overview of medical expert systems, Methods Inf Med 24(2):57-64, 1985.

Dewar ML et al: Perioperative Holter monitoring and computer analysis of dysrhythmias in cardiac surgery, Chest 87:593-597, 1985.

Donovan DJ and Johnston R: Computers in respiratory therapy: a blood gas lab, AARTimes 8(9):24, 124, 1984.

Donovan DJ and Johnston R: Computers in respiratory therapy: a pulmonary function lab, AARTimes 8(10):16-17, 1984.

Donovan DJ and Johnston R: Modems in the PFT lab, AARTimes 9(12):13, 40, 1985.

Donovan DJ and Johnston R: Computers in respiratory therapy, AARTimes 10(4):18, 54, 1986.

Donovan DJ and Johnston R: Computers in respiratory therapy: computerized interpretation of pulmonary function test, AARTimes 10(7):14-15, 1986.

Donovan DJ and Johnston R: Computers in cardiorespiratory diagnosis, AARTimes 10(10):26-27, 1986.

East TD, Andriano KP, and Pace NL: Computer-controlled optimization of positive end-expiratory pressure, Crit Care Med 14:792-797, 1986.

Fieschi M and Joubert M: Some reflections on the evaluation of expert systems in medicine, Methods Inf Med 25(1):15-21, 1986.

Frenzel LE: Crash course in artificial intelligence and expert systems, Indianapolis, 1987, Howard W Sams & Co.

Frumin JR: Clinical use of a physiologic respirator producing N_2O amnesia-analgesia, Anesthesiology 18:290-299, 1957.

Galen RS: What can microcomputers do for medical decision-making? Diagn Med 6:75-76, 1983.

Gardner RM et al: Computerized decision-making in the pulmonary function laboratory, Respir Care 27:799-808, 1982.

Goldberg HL et al: Diagnostic accuracy of coronary angiography utilizing computer-based digital subtraction methods: comparison to conventional cineangiography, Chest 90:793-797, 1986.

Harris C: Calculating blood gases on a pocket computer, Hosp Pract 19(4):179, 182, 1984.

Hayes-Roth F, Waterman DA, and Lenat DB: Building expert systems, Reading, Mass, 1983, Addison-Wesley Publishing Co.

Herman J: Issues in computerized spirometry, Respir Ther 14(5):52, 56-57, 1984.

Hess D: The hand-held computer as a teaching tool for acid-base interpretation, Respir Care 29:375-379, 1984.

Hess D and Eitel D: A portable and inexpensive computer system to interpret arterial blood gases, Respir Care 31:792-795, 1986.

Hess D, Silage DA, and Maxwell C: An arterial blood gas interpretation program for hand-held computers, Respir Care 29:756-759, 1984.

Hess D et al: Applications of a hand-held computer in critical care medicine: hemodynamic calculations, intravenous flow rate calculations, and respiratory calculations, Respir Ther 15(4):25-28, 1985.

Hingston DM et al: A computerized interpretation of arterial pH and blood gas data: do physicians need it? Respir Care 27:809-815, 1982.

Jones P: Computerized patient assessment, Nurs Times 82:63, 65, 1986.

Kinney MR: Current status of computers in monitoring the cardiac surgical patient, Curr Rev Recov Room Nurses 5(6):43-48, 1983.

Kinney EL: Expert system detection of drug interactions: results in consecutive inpatients, Comput Biomed Res 19:462-467, 1986.

Kulikowski CA: Expert medical consultation systems, J Med Syst 7:229-234, 1983.

Kunz JC et al: A physiologic rule-based system for interpreting pulmonary function test results, Report HPP-78-19. Stanford, Calif, 1979, Stanford University, Computer Science Department, Heuristic Programming Project.

Laborde JM: Expert systems for nursing?: artificial intelligence programs—consultations for nursing diagnoses and patient care planning, Comput Nurs 2:130-135, 1984.

Larson JK: Computer-assisted spirometry, Respir Care 27:839-841, 1982.

Larson JK: Computer application in the pulmonary laboratory. I, Respir Ther 14(5):47-50, 1984.

Le Febvre D: Computers: digital applications in the field of diagnostic imaging, Can J Radiogr Radiother Nucl Med 15:140-144, 1984.

Levine R, Drang DE, and Edelson B: A comprehensive guide to AI and expert systems, New York, 1986, McGraw-Hill Book Co.

Lewis TG: Using the IBM personal computer, Reston, VA, 1983, Reston Publishing Co.

Llaurado JG: Progress in expert systems, Int J Biomed Comput 15(1):1-8, 1984.

Lodwick GS: Computers in radiologic diagnosis, Appl Radiol 15:61-65, 1986.

Love JE Jr: Computerized interpretive reporting of acid-base data: a review and comment, J Med Technol 1:113-117, 1984.

Lutz H and Bender HJ: Possibilities of computer use in anesthesia and intensive care medicine, Anasth Intensivther Notfallmed 21(2):68-71, 1986.

Maxwell C and Silage DA: Hand-held computers in pulmonary medicine, Respir Care 28:35-36, 1983.

McDonald CJ and Tierney WM: The medical gopher: microcomputer system to help find, organize and decide about patient data, West J Med 145:823-829, 1986.

McPeck M: The impact of computer-age technology on respiratory therapy, Respir Care 27:855-865, 1982.

McPeck M: Computers in critical care and pulmonary medicine, Respir Care 28:74-79, 82-87, 1983.

McPeck M: Fifth annual international symposium on computers in critical care and pulmonary medicine, Respir Care 29:384-394, 1984.

Meehan PA: Hemodynamic assessment using the automated physiologic profile, Crit Care Nurse 6(1):29-46, 1986.

Miholland DK and Cardona VD: Computers at the bedside, Am J Nurs 83:1304-1307, 1983.

Miller AL and Harter W: On-line computer analysis of hemodynamic data in the cardiac catheterization laboratory, CVP 11(3):13-15, 1983.

Miller PL, Blumenfrucht SJ, and Rose JR: Computer technology: state of the art and future trends, J Am Coll Cardiol 9:204-214, 1987.

Miller RA et al: The internist-1/quick medical reference project—status report, West J Med 145:816-822, 1986.

Mishelevich DJ et al: Respiratory therapy as a component of an integrated hospital information system: the Parkland on-line information system, Respir Care 27:846-854, 1982.

Moore MJ and Bleich HL: Consulting the computer about acid-base disorders, Respir Care 27:834-838, 1982.

Morgan RO Jr: Computer applications in clinical anesthesia: present and future trends, Perioper Nurs Q 2(4):37-44, 1986.

Ohlson KB, Westenskow DR, and Jordan WS: A microprocessor based feedback controller for mechanical ventilation, Ann Biomed Eng 10:35-48, 1982.

O'Shea T and Eisenstadt M: Artificial intelligence: tools, techniques, and applications, New York, 1984, Harper & Row.

Paliotta JJ: The role of the digital computer in the pulmonary function laboratory, Respir Care 27:816-820, 1982.

Reggia JA and Tuhrim S: An introduction to computer-assisted medical decision making. II, MD Comput 2(4):40-46, 1985.

Robischon T: Computed spirometry: some caveats to consider before investing, Respir Ther 13(1):25, 29-30, 32, 1983.

Savvides M et al: Computer analysis of exercise-induced changes in electrocardiographic variables: comparison of methods and criteria, Chest 84:699-706, 1983.

Schultz S: Languages, DBMSs, and expert systems: software for nurse decision making, J Nurs Admin 14(12):15-23, 1984.

Schwartz WB, Patil RS, and Szolovits P: Artificial intelligence in medicine: where do we stand? N Engl J Med 316:685-688, 1987.

Shabot MM and Replogle KJ: Computation of cardiorespiratory variables using a hand-held computer, Crit Care Nurse 6(3):12-13, 16-17, 20, 1986.

Sheldon RL, Cooley WS, and Knox WL: A respiratory intensive care unit computing system: clinical experience at Loma Linda University Medical Center, Respir Care 27:821-829, 1982.

Shirai Y and Tsujii J: Artificial intelligence: concepts, techniques, and applications, New York, 1984, John Wiley & Sons.

Shortliffe EH: Medical expert systems—knowledge tools for physicians, West J Med 145:830-839, 1986.

Silage DA and Maxwell C: A spirometry/interpretation program for hand-held computers, Respir Care 28:62-66, 1983.

Silage DA and Maxwell C: A lung volume determination/interpretation program for hand-held computers, Respir Care 28:452-456, 1983.

Silage DA and Maxwell C: An acid-base map/arterial blood-gas interpretation program for hand-held computers, Respir Care 29:833-838, 1984.

Smith JW Jr, Speicher CE, and Chandrasekaran B: Expert systems as aids for interpretive reporting, J Med Syst 8:373-88, 1984.

Stewart J: A three-dimensional view of the flow/volume curve, Respir Care 29:380-383, 1984.

Teather D et al: Computer assistance for CT scan interpretation and cerebral disease diagnosis, Stat Med 4:311-315, 1985.

Thompson JD: Computerized control of mechanical ventilation: closing the loop, Respir Care 32:440-444, 1987.

Torsun IS: Expert systems: state of the art, Reading, Mass, 1983, Addison-Wesley Publishing Co.

Wandell M: Computer-assisted TDM interpretation: therapeutic drug monitoring, Diagn Med 6:85-86, 88, 1983.

Waterman DA: A guide to expert systems, Reading, Mass, 1985, Addison-Wesley Publishing Co.

Watt CS: Research project: computerized monitoring in ICU, Nurs Mirror 156(26):8-9, 1983.

Wigertz O: Making decisions based on "fuzzy" medical data—can expert systems help? Methods Inf Med 25(2):59-61, 1986.

Wilson GA, McDonald CJ, and McCabe GP Jr: The effect of immediate access to a computerized medical record on physician test ordering: a controlled clinical trial in the emergency room. Record reduces test ordering, Am J Public Health 72:698-702, 1982.

Winston PH: Artificial intelligence, ed 2, Reading, Mass, 1984, Addison-Wesley Publishing Co.

Appendix 1

Temperature Correction of Barometric Reading

Temperature (°C)	730 mm Hg	740	750	760	770	780
15.0	1.78	1.81	1.83	1.86	1.88	1.91
16.0	1.90	1.93	1.96	1.98	2.01	2.03
17.0	2.02	2.05	2.08	2.10	2.13	2.16
18.0	2.14	2.17	2.20	2.23	2.26	2.29
19.0	2.26	2.29	2.32	2.35	2.38	2.41
20.0	2.38	2.41	2.44	2.47	2.51	2.54
21.0	2.50	2.53	2.56	2.60	2.63	2.67
22.0	2.61	2.65	2.69	2.72	2.76	2.79
23.0	2.73	2.77	2.81	2.84	2.88	2.92
24.0	2.85	2.89	2.93	2.97	3.01	3.05
25.0	2.97	3.01	3.05	3.09	3.13	3.17
26.0	3.09	3.13	3.17	3.21	3.26	3.30
27.0	3.20	3.25	3.29	3.34	3.38	3.42
28.0	3.32	3.37	3.41	3.46	3.51	3.55
29.0	3.44	3.49	3.54	3.58	3.63	3.68
30.0	3.56	3.61	3.66	3.71	3.75	3.80
31.0	3.68	3.73	3.78	3.83	3.88	3.93
32.0	3.79	3.85	3.90	3.95	4.00	4.05
33.0	3.91	3.97	4.02	4.07	4.13	4.18
34.0	4.03	4.09	4.14	4.20	4.25	4.31
35.0	4.15	4.21	4.26	4.32	4.38	4.43

From US Department of Commerce, Weather Bureau: Barometers and the measurement of atmospheric pressure, Washington, DC, 1941, US Government Printing Office.

Appendix 2

Factors to Convert Gas Volumes From ATPS to STPD

Observed P_B	15°	16°	17°	18°	19°	20°	21°	22°	23°	24°	25°	26°	27°	28°	29°	30°	31°	32°
700	0.855	851	847	842	838	834	829	825	821	816	812	807	802	797	793	788	783	778
702	857	853	849	845	840	836	832	827	823	818	814	809	805	800	795	790	785	780
704	860	856	852	847	843	839	834	830	825	821	816	812	807	802	797	792	787	783
706	862	858	854	850	845	841	837	832	828	823	819	814	810	804	800	795	790	785
708	865	861	856	852	848	843	839	834	830	825	821	816	812	807	802	797	792	787
710	867	863	859	855	850	846	842	837	833	828	824	819	814	809	804	799	795	790
712	870	866	861	857	853	848	844	839	836	830	826	821	817	812	807	802	797	792
714	872	868	864	859	855	851	846	842	837	833	828	824	819	814	809	804	799	794
716	875	871	866	862	858	853	849	844	840	835	831	826	822	816	812	807	802	797
718	877	873	869	864	860	856	851	847	842	838	833	828	824	819	814	809	804	799
720	880	876	871	867	863	858	854	849	845	840	836	831	826	821	816	812	807	802
722	882	878	874	869	865	861	856	852	847	843	838	833	829	824	819	814	809	804
724	885	880	876	872	867	863	858	854	849	845	840	835	831	826	821	816	811	806
726	887	883	879	874	870	866	861	856	852	847	843	838	833	829	825	818	813	808
728	890	886	881	877	872	868	863	859	854	850	845	840	836	831	826	821	816	811
730	892	888	884	879	875	870	866	861	857	852	847	843	838	833	828	823	818	813
732	895	891	886	882	877	873	868	864	859	854	850	845	840	836	831	825	820	815
734	897	893	889	884	880	875	871	866	862	857	852	847	843	838	833	828	823	818
736	900	895	891	887	882	878	873	869	864	859	855	850	845	840	835	830	825	820
738	902	898	894	889	885	880	876	871	866	862	857	852	848	843	838	833	828	822
740	905	900	896	892	887	883	878	874	869	864	860	855	850	845	840	835	830	825
742	907	903	898	894	890	885	881	876	871	867	862	857	852	847	842	837	832	827
744	910	906	901	897	892	888	883	878	874	869	864	859	855	850	845	840	834	829
746	912	908	903	899	895	890	886	881	876	872	867	862	857	852	847	842	837	832
748	915	910	906	901	897	892	888	883	879	874	869	864	860	854	850	845	839	834
750	917	913	908	904	900	895	890	886	881	876	872	867	862	857	852	847	842	837
752	920	915	911	906	902	897	893	888	883	879	874	869	864	859	854	849	844	839
754	922	918	913	909	904	900	895	891	886	881	876	872	867	862	857	852	846	841
756	925	920	916	911	907	902	898	893	888	883	879	874	869	864	859	854	849	844
758	927	923	918	914	909	905	900	896	891	886	881	876	872	866	861	856	851	846
760	930	925	921	916	912	907	902	898	893	888	883	879	874	869	864	859	854	848
762	932	928	923	919	914	910	905	900	896	891	886	881	876	871	866	861	856	851
764	934	930	926	921	916	912	907	903	898	893	888	884	879	874	869	864	858	853
766	937	933	928	925	919	915	910	905	900	896	891	886	881	876	871	866	861	855
768	940	935	931	926	922	917	912	908	903	898	893	888	883	878	873	868	863	858
770	942	938	933	928	924	919	915	910	905	901	896	891	886	881	876	871	865	860
772	945	940	936	931	926	922	917	912	908	903	898	893	888	883	878	873	868	862
774	947	943	938	933	929	924	920	915	910	905	901	896	891	886	880	875	870	865
776	950	945	941	936	931	927	922	917	912	908	903	898	893	888	883	878	872	867
778	952	948	943	938	934	929	924	920	915	910	905	900	895	890	885	880	875	869
780	955	950	945	941	936	932	927	922	917	912	908	903	898	892	887	882	877	872

$$\text{Factor} = \frac{[P_{B_{abs}} \text{ corrected for } t_{amb} - P_{H_2O} \text{ at } t_{amb}] \times 0.359}{[t_{amb} + 273]}$$

977

Appendix 3

Factors to Convert Gas Volumes From STPD to BTPS at Given Barometric Pressures

Pressure	Factor	Pressure	Factor
740	1.245	760	1.211
742	1.241	762	1.208
744	1.238	764	1.203
746	1.235	766	1.200
748	1.232	768	1.196
750	1.227	770	1.193
752	1.224	772	1.190
754	1.221	774	1.188
756	1.217	776	1.183
758	1.214	778	1.181

$$\text{Factor} = \frac{863}{[P_{B_{amb}} - 47]}$$

Appendix 4

Low-Temperature Characteristics of Selected Gases and Water

Substance	Critical temperature °C	°F	Critical pressure (atm)	Boiling point* °C	°F	Melting (freezing) point °C	°F
Acetylene	36.0	96.0	62.0	− 88.5	−119.2	−81.8	−114.6
Air	−140.7	−221.0	37.2	−194.4	−317.9	—	—
Ammonia	132.4	270.3	111.5	− 33.4	− 28.1	− 77.7	−108.0
Carbon dioxide	31.1	87.9	73.0	− 78.5	−109.3	− 56.6	− 69.9
Cyclopropane	124.7	256.4	54.2	− 32.9	− 27.2	−127.5	−197.7
Freon-12	111.6	233.6	40.6	− 29.8	− 21.6	−158.0	−252.4
Freon-14	− 45.4	− 49.9	36.8	−128.0	−198.4	−184.0	−299.2
Helium	−267.9	−450.2	2.3	−268.9	−452.1	−272.2	−455.8
Hydrogen	−239.9	−399.8	12.8	−252.8	−423.0	−259.2	−434.5
Nitrogen	−147.1	−232.6	33.5	−195.8	−320.5	−209.9	−345.9
Nitrous oxide	36.5	97.7	71.8	− 88.5	−127.2	− 90.8	−131.6
Oxygen	−118.8	−181.1	49.7	−183.0	−297.3	−218.4	−361.8
Propane	95.6	206.2	43.0	− 42.2	− 43.7	−189.9	−305.8
Water	374.0	705.0	218.0	100.0	212.0	0.0	32.0

*Boiling point at 1 atmosphere (760 mm Hg) pressure.

Glossary

AAMI abbreviation for the American Association of for the Advancement of Medical Instrumentation, a voluntary group responsible, in part, for developing standards related to medical devices and equipment.

a/A ratio the ratio of arterial to alveolar oxygen partial pressures (Pao_2/Pao_2); a measure of the efficiency of oxygen transfer across the lung.

AARC abbreviation for the American Association for Respiratory Care, the primary voluntary professional association for respiratory care practitioners.

abduct to move a limb away from the body.

abruptio placenta separation of a normally implanted placenta in a pregnancy of 20 weeks or more duration or during labor but before delivery; a significant cause of maternal and fetal mortality.

absorbance the degree of absorption of light or other radiant energy by a medium through which the radiant energy passes.

absorption the taking up of liquids or gases; particularly the passage of these substances through a body surface into body fluids or tissues.

absorption atelectasis atelectasis resulting from the absorption of oxygen from obstructed or partially obstructed alveoli with high alveolar oxygen concentrations.

academic health science center an academic institution devoted to education, research, and service in the health sciences; usually includes at least a medical school and one or more health care facilities.

ACCP abbreviation for the American College of Chest Physicians.

accreditation the process by which a private, nongovernmental agency recognizes that an institution or organization meets pre-specified standards of quality; commonly applies to educational institutions or programs and health care agencies such as hospitals and nursing homes.

acetazolamide a carbonic anhydrase inhibitor with diuretic properties; inhibits formation of carbonic acid in the proximal tubules of the kidneys, thereby promoting elimination of sodium, potassium, bicarbonate, and water; prolonged use can cause an alkaline diuresis leading to metabolic acidosis.

acetylcholinesterase an enzyme that inactivates the neurotransmitter acetylcholine by hydrolyzing the substance to choline and acetate.

acetylcysteine a mucolytic agent that lowers the viscosity of mucoid secretions by chemically disrupting the sulfydryl bonds of mucopolysaccharides.

achalasia an abnormal condition characterized by the inability to relax smooth muscle sphincters, particularly those in the gastrointestinal tract; commonly refers to failure of the lower esophagus to relax during swallowing (achalasia cardia).

acid any substance that serves as a proton donor in a chemical reaction.

acidemia a combining form meaning an "increased hydrogen-ion concentration in the blood"; as applied to arterial blood, denotes a pH less than 7.35.

acidosis an abnormal physiologic process resulting in an increase in the hydrogen ion concentration in the body; may be caused by either an excess accumulation of an acid or the loss of base.

acid-fast of or pertaining to a bacterial stain that does not decolorize easily when washed with an acid solution; also refers to certain bacteria (especially mycobacteria) that retain red dyes after an acid wash.

aciduria the presence of a greater than normal hydrogen ion concentration in the urine (normal urine pH ranges from 4.6 to 8.0, with an average value of 6.0).

acquired immune deficiency syndrome (AIDS) an immune disorder caused by infection with the human immunodeficiency virus (HIV); HIV directly attacks the T lymphocytes and T helper cells of the immune system, thereby compromising both cell-mediated and humoral (antibody) immunity.

ACLS acronym for advanced cardiac life support; ACLS includes the essential elements of basic life support but provides additional measures beyond those normally available to lay personnel. These include the use of adjunct equipment to support oxygenation and ventilation, the establishment of an intravenous route for drug administration, and the administration of selected pharmacologic agents, cardiac monitoring, defibrillation, arrhythmia control, and postresuscitative care.

acromegaly a chronic metabolic condition characterized by a gradual, marked enlargement and elongation of the bones of the face, jaw, and extremities.

acronym a word formed by the initial letters of each major part of a multiword term (eg, "PEEP" is the acronym for positive end-expiratory pressure).

ACTH abbreviation for adrenocorticotropic hormone, a pituitary hormone that stimulates the adrenal cortex.

Actinobacter a genus of nonmotile, aerobic bacteria of the family Neisseriaceae that often occurs in clinical specimens.

actinomycosis a chronic, systemic fungal disease caused by infection with organisms of the genus *Actinomyces;* most commonly affects the skin but can involve the lungs and other organ systems.

Selected definitions excerpted with permission from Glanze WD, editor: Mosby's medical and nursing dictionary, ed 3, St. Louis, 1986, The CV Mosby Co.

action potential a rapid reversal in the membrane potential occurring in certain nerve and muscle cells, caused by a change in the membrane permeability for sodium ions, which rapidly diffuse into the cell, thereby reversing its charge.

actuator that portion of a mechanical or electronic device that initiates a given action or process.

additive effect a form of drug interaction in which the effect of two drugs together equals the simple sum of their individual effects.

Addison's disease a life-threatening condition caused by partial or complete failure of adrenocortical function, often resulting from autoimmune processes, infection (especially tubercular or fungal), neoplasm, or hemorrhage in the gland.

adduct to move a limb toward the axis of the body.

adenopathy any enlargement of a gland, especially a lymphatic gland.

adenosine triphosphate (ATP) a compound consisting of the nucleotide adenosine attached through its ribose group to three phosphoric acid molecules; a major source of energy.

adenovirus any one of the 33 medium-sized viruses of the Adenovirideae family, pathogenic to humans, that cause conjunctivitis, upper respiratory infection, or gastrointestinal infection.

ADH abbreviation for antidiuretic hormone, a hormone stored and released by the posterior lobe of the pituitary gland, which stimulates the reabsorption of water by the renal tubular epithelial cells; caused by mild vasopressor effects, ADH is also called vasopressin.

adhesion the physical property by which unlike substances can attract each other and hold together; also refers to the abnormal formation of fibrous tissues (resulting from inflammation or injury) that bind together body structures that are normally separate.

adiabatic a process of gas compression or expansion in which *no* heat energy is added to or taken away from the gas during the process; in adiabatic processes a gas's internal or kinetic energy will vary according to changes in its pressure or volume; rapid adiabatic compression can thus result in a dramatic rise in the kinetic energy of a gas, as manifested by a rapid increase in its temperature; compare with isothermal.

ADL abbreviation for activities of daily living, a quantifiable measure of an individual's ability to perform common tasks associated with independent functioning.

adrenergic of or pertaining to the sympathetic nerve fibers of the autonomic nervous system that use epinephrine or epinephrine-like substances as neurotransmitters; any chemical or drug that mimics the effect of these neurotransmitters.

adrenocorticosteroid (also corticosteroid) a broad term referring to any of the steroid hormones produced by the adrenal cortex, including their synthetic equivalents; major categories include the glucocorticoids (eg, hydrocortisone), the mineralocorticoids (eg, aldosterone), and the androgens.

adult respiratory distress syndrome (ARDS) a pattern of clinical, physiologic, and pathologic features characterizing the lung's response to a variety of injuries and resulting in diffuse damage to the alveolar-capillary membrane; clinically, ARDS is characterized by a refractory hypoxemia, decreased lung compliance (resulting from an increase in pulmonary interstitial water), and an increased work of breathing.

advocacy taking a position in favor of a certain issue or person; in health care commonly refers to supporting the patient's needs over those of the institution or health care professional.

aerobic living only in the presence of oxygen.

aerosol a suspension of solid or liquid particles in a gas.

aerosol density (particulate) the number of aerosol particles per unit of carrier gas.

aerosol density (weight) the actual weight of aerosol carried in a given volume of gas; two units of weight density are common: grams of aerosol per square meter (g/m^3) or milligrams of aerosol per liter (mg/L).

aerosol therapy the application of liquid or solid particle suspensions to the airway to achieve specific clinical objectives.

AFB abbreviation for acid-fast bacillus, especially *mycobacteria,* which retain red dyes after an acid wash.

afferent carrying or conduction impulses toward the central nervous system; opposite of efferent.

affinity in pharmacology, the tendency a drug has to combine with a receptor (refer to agonist).

afterload the load or resistance against which the ventricles must eject their volume of blood during contraction.

AGA abbreviation for appropriate for gestational age; of or pertaining to newborns whose body weight falls within the 10th to 90th percentile for their gestational age.

agammaglobulinemia a rare disorder characterized by the absence of the serum immunoglobin, gamma globulin, associated with an increased susceptibility to infection.

agglomeration the process of gathering together into a mass, as when many small aerosol particles come together to form a single large particle.

agitate to stir or mix up.

agonist of or pertaining to a chemical substance or drug that has affinity and exerts a desired or expected effect (as opposed to an antagonist).

AIDS abbreviation for acquired immune deficiency syndrome.

airborne transmission transmission of infectious organisms through dissemination of the infectious agent in the air, either by aerosol droplets, droplet nuclei, or dust particles.

airway conductance a quantifiable measure of the ease with which gas flows through the respiratory tract; abbreviated as G, conductance is the reciprocal of airway resistance (ie, G = flow/change in pressure).

airway resistance a measure of the impedance to ventilation caused by the movement of gas through the airways; abbreviated as Raw, airway resistance is computed as the change in pressure along a tube divided by the flow; the reciprocal of airway conductance.

alar nasi the winglike lateral projections of the nose.

aldehyde any of a large category of organic compounds derived from a corresponding alcohol by the removal of two hydrogen atoms, as in the conversion of ethyl alcohol to acetaldehyde.

aldosterone a corticosteroid produced by the adrenal cortex to regulate sodium and potassium balance in the blood.

aldosteronism a condition characterized by hypersecretion of aldosterone, occurring as a primary disease of the adrenal cortex or, more often, as a secondary disorder in response to various extra-adrenal pathologic processes.

aliquot a fractional portion of a liquid or solid substance.

alkalemia a combining form meaning a "decreased hydrogen-ion concentration in the blood"; as applied to arterial blood, denotes a pH greater than 7.45.

alkaloid any one of a large group of alkaline organic chemicals found in plants that exert powerful physiologic activity; examples include morphine, cocaine, nicotine, and atropine.

alkalosis an abnormal physiologic process resulting in a decrease in the hydrogen ion concentration in the body; may be caused by either an excess accumulation of base or the loss of acid.

alkylation a chemical reaction in which a hydrogen atom in an organic compound is replaced by an alkyl radical from an alkylating agent.

alkylene (also alkene) any one of a homologous series of unsaturated hydrocarbons that contain double or triple bonds between their carbon atoms and readily combine with the halogens; examples include ethylene (C_2H_4) and acetylene (C_2H_2).

allantois the ventral outgrowth of the hindgut of the early embryo; becomes a major component of the developing umbilical cord.

allocation the process of allotting or assigning; especially the disbursement of limited resources, as in the allocation of health care resources.

allographic of or pertaining to a tissue graft or organ transplant between individuals of different genetic makeup.

alpha$_1$ antitrypsin a chemical substance that inhibits the action of the proteolytic enzyme trypsin; associated with a form of destructive emphysema.

ALS abbreviation for advanced life support (see ACLS); also abbreviation for amyotrophic lateral sclerosis.

alveolarization the process of alveolar development from epithelial tissue.

alveolar ventilation the total amount of fresh gas reaching the alveoli, measured either on a breath-by-breath basis or per minute.

ambient of or referring to the surrounding environmental conditions.

ambulation the process of walking.

amebiasis an infection of the intestine or liver by species of pathogenic amebas, particularly *Entamoeba histolytica,* acquired by ingesting food or water contaminated with infected feces.

amino acid one of a large class of organic compounds containing both an amino (NH_2) and carboxyl (COOH) group.

amniocentesis the process of direct sampling and quantitative assessment of the amniotic fluid.

amnion the innermost membrane enclosing the fetus and normally filled with amnionic fluid.

ampere the basic unit of electrical current; equivalent to the amount of electrons flowing when 1 volt of electromotive force is applied to a circuit with 1 Ohm of resistance.

amplitude of or pertaining to the maximum displacement of a physical event; commonly used to refer to the displacement of an analog waveform measuring phenomena such as the electrical activity of the heart (see ECG).

amyloidosis an abnormal condition characterized by the deposition of an insoluble protein called amyloid in various tissues; occurs in chronic suppurative disorders such as tuberculosis, bronchiectasis, and lung abscess.

amyotrophic lateral sclerosis (ALS) a degenerative disease of the motor neurons, characterized by atrophy of the muscles of the hands, forearms, and legs spreading to involve most of the body.

anaerobe a microorganism that grows and lives in the complete or almost complete absence of oxygen.

anaerobic of or referring to the ability to live without oxygen.

anaerobic threshold during exercise, the point where increased levels of lactic acid result in an increased carbon dioxide production and minute ventilation; the RQ at this point is equal to or greater than 1.0, indicating that carbon dioxide production has equalled or surpassed oxygen consumption; when the anerobic threshold is exceeded, metabolism becomes anaerobic, thereby decreasing energy production and increasing muscle fatigue.

anaphylaxis an exaggerated hypersensitivity reaction to a previously encountered antigen.

anastomosis a communication between two ducts or blood vessels that allows flow from one to another.

anecdotal of or pertaining to a brief description of a prior event or incident.

anemia an abnormal condition characterized by a reduction in the number of circulating red blood cells or the amount of normal hemoglobin available to carry oxygen.

anesthesiology the science of anesthesia; using drugs or chemical substances to cause partial or complete loss of sensation, particularly pain.

anesthetic a drug or chemical substance that causes partial or complete loss of sensation.

aneurysm a localized dilatation of the wall of a blood vessel, usually caused by atherosclerosis and hypertension or, less frequently, by trauma, infection, or a congenital weakness in the vessel wall.

angina pectoris a paroxysmal attack of severe chest pain associated with coronary insufficiency; commonly radiates from the heart to the shoulders and arms.

angiography the x-ray visualization of the internal anatomy of the heart and blood vessels after the intravascular introduction of radiopaque contrast medium.

angiotensin a blood polypeptide formed by the action of renin and angiotensinogin; the active form (angiotensin II) causes vasoconstriction and stimulates aldosterone secretion by the adrenal cortex.

Angle of Louis the anatomic landmark where the manubrium, body of the sternum, and second ribs articulate; also called the sternal angle.

anhydrous containing no water; dry.

animosity resentment or ill will toward another.

ankylosing spondylitis a chronic inflammatory disease of unknown origin, first affecting the spine and adjacent structures and commonly progressing to eventual fusion (ankylosis) of the involved joints.

anion an ion that migrates to the anode (positive electrode) in an electrolytic solution; a negative ion.

anomaly a broad term denoting any deviation from what is regarded as normal.

anorexia lack or loss of appetite, resulting in the inability to eat.

ANSI abbreviation for the American National Standards Institute, a private nongovernmental agency that establishes voluntary standards in a wide variety of technical fields, including medical instrumentation.

antagonist in pharmacology, is a drug that has affinity but produces no effect; an antagonist can be competitive (forms reversible bond with receptor) or noncompetitive (forms irreversible bond).

antecubital fossa the triangular area at the bend of the elbow; frequently used as the site for venipuncture and brachial artery blood sampling.

anterolateral situated in front and to one side or the other.

anteroposterior from the front to the back of the body, commonly associated with the direction of the roentgenographic or x-ray beam (an "AP" exposure).

anthrax a disease affecting primarily farm animals (cattle, goats, pigs, sheep, and horses), caused by the bacterium *Bacillus anthracis.*

antiarrhythmic of or pertaining to a procedure or substance that prevents, alleviates, or corrects an abnormal cardiac rhythm.

antibody a soluble protein synthesized by plasma cells in response to a specific antigen with which it interacts; in conjunction with the activation of complement, antibody production represents a key component of the humoral portion of the immune system defense against antigenic material.

anticholinergic of or pertaining to a blockade of acetylcholine receptors that results in the inhibition of the transmission of parasympathetic nerve impulses.

antigen a substance, usually a protein, that causes the formation of an antibody and reacts specifically with that antibody (see antibody).

anti-inflammatory of or pertaining to a substance or procedure that counteracts or reduces inflammation.

antiprotozoal a chemical agent effective against protozoa that cause infection.

antisepsis the destruction of pathogenic microorganisms existing in their vegetative state on living tissue.

antiseptic a chemical solution capable of antisepsis.

antitoxin an antibody capable of neutralizing a specific toxin, e.g., tetanus antitoxin.

anxiolytic a drug or chemical agent capable of reducing anxiety, apprehension, or restlessness.

Apgar score the evaluation of an infant's physical condition, usually performed 1 minute and again at 5 minutes after birth, based on a rating of five factors that reflect the infant's ability to adjust to extrauterine life.

aphagia a condition characterized by the loss of the ability to swallow as a result of organic or psychologic causes.

aphasia an abnormal neurologic condition in which language function is defective or absent because of an injury to certain areas of the cerebral cortex.

apical of or pertaining to the summit or apex.

apnea an absence of spontaneous breathing.

apnea of prematurity a disorder of preterm infants, probably of CNS origin, characterized by frequent apneic pauses lasting more than 20 seconds and often associated with cyanosis, pallor, hypotonia, or bradycardia.

apneic of or pertaining to a condition marked by apnea.

apneustic breathing a pattern of respirations characterized by a prolonged inspiratory phase followed by expiratory apnea.

apneustic center a localized collection of neurons in the pons located at the level of the area vestibularis that moderate the rhythmic activity of the medullary respiratory centers.

aponeurosis a strong sheet of fibrous connective tissue that serves as a tendon to attach muscles to bone or as fascia to bind muscles together.

arachnoid membrane a thin, delicate membrane enclosing the brain and the spinal cord, interposed between the pia mater and the dura mater.

ARCF abbreviation for the American Respiratory Care Foundation, a philanthropic agency that promotes the field of respiratory care through grants and awards.

ARDS acronym for adult respiratory distress syndrome.

arrhythmia any deviation from the normal pattern of the heartbeat.

arteriography a method of radiologic visualization of arteries performed after a radiopaque contrast medium is introduced into the bloodstream or into a specific vessel by injection or through a catheter.

arteriole one of the blood vessels of the smallest branch of the arterial circulation.

arteriolized blood blood that has been fully oxygenated by passage through the lungs.

arytenoid literally "shaped like a jug"; referring to the arytenoid cartilages or muscles of the larynx.

asbestosis a restrictive lung disease caused by prolonged exposure to asbestosis fibers; associated with a high incidence of malignant lung tumors and pleural abnormalities.

ascites an abnormal intraperitoneal accumulation of a fluid containing large amounts of protein and electrolytes.

asepsis the absence of pathogenic microorganisms; the removal of pathogenic microorganisms or infected material.

aspergillosis an infection caused by a fungus of the genus *Aspergillus,* capable of causing inflammatory, granulomatous lesions on or in any organ.

aspirate (verb) to withdraw fluid by negative pressure; (noun) the fluid so withdrawn.

aspiration the act of inhaling, especially in reference to the pathologic aspiration of vomitus or material foreign to the respiratory tract (see aspiration pneumonia); also the process of withdrawing fluid by negative pressure.

aspiration pneumonia an inflammatory condition of the lungs and bronchi caused by the inhalation of foreign material or vomitus containing acid gastric contents.

assist-control mode continuous mandatory ventilation (CMV) in which the minimum frequency of breathing is predetermined by the ventilator controls but the patient can initiate ventilation at a faster rate.

asthma a hypersensitivity disorder characterized by reversible airway obstruction due to a combination of bronchospasm, mucosal edema, and excessive secretion of viscid mucus.

asymptomatic literally "without symptoms."

asynchronous breathing an abnormal breathing pattern in which the rib cage and abdomen do not move outward together, indicating that the respiratory muscles are not working in synchrony; an early indicator of an excessive respiratory muscle load.

asystole the absence of a heartbeat, as distinguished from fibrillation, in which electric activity persists but contraction ceases.

atelectasis an abnormal condition characterized by the collapse of lung tissue, preventing the exchange of carbon dioxide and oxygen with the pulmonary capillary blood.

atopic of or pertaining to a hereditary tendency to develop immediate allergic reactions, as asthma, atopic dermatitis, or vasomotor rhinitis, because of the presence of an antibody (atopic reagin).

ATP abbreviation for adenosine triphosphate.

ATPS abbreviation for ambient temperature, ambient pressure, saturated (with water vapor).

atrioventricular of or pertaining to the area between the atrial and ventricles of the heart.

atrophy a wasting or diminution of size or physiologic activity of a part of the body because of disease or other influences, especially muscle tissue.

ATS abbreviation for the American Thoracic Society.

auscultation the act of listening for sounds within the body to evaluate the condition of the heart, lungs, pleura, intestines, or other organs or to detect the fetal heart sound.

authoritarian of or pertaining to the principle of blind obedience of one to another.

autoclave a apparatus that uses steam under pressure to sterilize articles and equipment.

autogenous self-generating.

autoimmune disease one of a large group of diseases characterized by the subversion or alteration of the function of the body's immune system.

autonomy the individual characteristic or right to self-determination.

autoregulation automatic control of a mechanical or physiologic system; necessitates both a sensing mechanism (to measure what is regulated) and a feedback "loop" (to respond to changes).

autosomal inheritance a pattern of inheritance in which the transmission of a recessive gene on an autosome results in a carrier state if the person is heterozygous for the trait and in the affect state if the person is homozygous for the trait.

avirulent the inability of a microorganism to cause a pathologic effect.

axilla a pyramid-shaped space forming the underside of the shoulder between the upper part of the arm and the side of the chest (ie, the "armpit").

axillary of or pertaining to the axilla.

Babinski's reflex dorsiflexion of the big toe with extension and fanning of the other toes elicited by firmly stroking the lateral aspect of the sole of the foot.

bacteremia the presence of bacteria in the blood.

bacteriocidal destructive to bacteria.

bacteriostatic tending to restrain the growth of bacteria.

Bacteroides a genus of non-spore-forming gram-negative obligate anaerobic bacilli normally found in the colon, mouth, genital tract, and upper respiratory system; *Bacteroides* sp are the most common gram-negative obligate anaerobe rods involved in hospital-acquired infections and are also associated with the so-called putrid lung abscess.

baffle a surface in a nebulizer designed specifically to cause impaction of large aerosol particles, causing either further fragmentation or removal from the suspension through condensation back into the reservoir.

bagassosis a self-limited lung disease caused by an allergic response to bagasse, the fungi-laden, dusty debris left after the syrup has been extracted from sugar cane.

barbiturate any one of a group of organic compounds derived from barbituric acid that can cause depression of the CNS; examples include amitol, phenobarbital, and sodium pentothal.

baroreceptor one of the pressure-sensitive nerve endings in the walls of the atria of the heart, the vena cava, the aortic arch, and the carotid sinus.

barotrauma physical injury sustained as a result of exposure to ambient pressures above normal; commonly refers to pulmonary damage resulting from the application of positive pressure ventilation, such as pneumothorax, pneumomediastinum, and subcutaneous emphysema.

base any substance that serves as a proton receptor in a chemical reaction.

base excess (BE) the difference between the normal buffer base (NBB) and the actual buffer base (BB) in a whole blood sample, expressed in mEq/L; a normal BE is +/− 2 mEq/L.

basilic vein the large vein on the inner side of the biceps muscle frequently used for venipuncture or intravenous infusion.

BCG vaccine an active immunizing agent against tuberculosis prepared from Bacille Calmette-Guérin.

BCLS acronym for basic cardiac life support; BLCS aims either to (1) prevent circulatory or respiratory arrest through prompt identification and intervention or (2) support failed circulation and respiration through application of simple cardiopulmonary resuscitation methods.

behavioral pertaining to or caused by human conduct (as opposed to structural or physiologic causes).

beneficiary one who benefits from; commonly used to refer to the recipient of social or health services provided by a public or private agency.

benign not malignant or recurrent; characterized by mild symptoms or effect.

bigeminy literally "an association in pairs"; commonly refers to the cardiac arrhythmia characterized by paired premature ventricular contractions.

bilirubin the orange-yellow pigment of bile, formed principally by the breakdown of hemoglobin in red blood cells after termination of their normal life span.

biofeedback a process providing a person with visual or auditory information about the autonomic physiologic functions of his or her body, as blood pressure, muscle tension, and brain wave activity, usually through use of instrumentation.

biomedical instrumentation devices or apparatus used in the life sciences or medicine for measurement, diagnosis, or therapy; also the field of study involved in developing, testing, and applying such devices.

biopsy the procedure whereby tissues are excised for microscopic examination and diagnosis.

biphasic consisting of two phases.

blastomycosis an infectious disease caused by yeastlike fungus, *Blastomyces dermatitidis,* that commonly affects the skin but may invade the lungs, kidneys, CNS, and bones.

BMD abbreviation for the Bureau of Medical Devices, an agency of the federal Food and Drug Administration formed in 1976 to classify, provide standards for, and regulate medical devices.

board certified holding certification in a medical specialty; usually obtained by passing one or more examinations offered by a specialty society or credentialing agency.

body humidity the absolute humidity in a volume of gas saturated at a body temperature of 37°C; equivalent to 43.8 mg/L.

Bohr effect the impact of variations in blood pH on the affinity of hemoglobin for oxygen.

boiling point the temperature at which the vapor pressure of a liquid equals the ambient pressure exerted on the liquid.

BOMA abbreviation for the Board of Medical Advisors, the medical advisory group for the American Association for Respiratory Care.

bore the internal diameter of a tube.

botulism an often fatal form of food poisoning caused by an endotoxin produced by the bacillus *Clostridium botulinum.*

Bourdon gauge a low-pressure flow-metering device always used in conjunction with an adjustable high-pressure reducing valve; the Bourdon gauge employs a fixed-size orifice and operates under variable pressures, as determined by adjustment of the pressure reducing valve.

brachial of or pertaining to the arm.

bracheocephalic trunk the short branch of the aortic arch giving rise to the right common carotid and right subclavian arteries; also called the innominate artery.

bradycardia an abnormal condition characterized by a heart rate of less than 60 beats per minute.

bradykinin a polypeptide cellular mediator responsible for provoking smooth muscle contraction.

bradypnea an abnormally slow rate of breathing.

breathing exercises a broad category of activities designed to accomplish one or more of the following: (1) to promote greater use of the diaphragm and decrease inefficient and inappropriate accessory muscle use; (2) to increase awareness of the muscles of respiration to better coordinate breathing with the activities of daily living and to cope with episodic dyspnea when it occurs; (3) to improve the efficiency of alveolar ventilation by increasing tidal volume, slowing the rate of breathing, prolonging the expiratory time, and promoting better distribution of ventilation to perfusion; (4) to improve the strength and endurance of the respiratory muscles and relieve exertional dyspnea; (5) to improve the effectiveness of the cough; and (6) to improve the delivery of therapeutic aerosols.

bronchiectasis an abnormal condition of the bronchial tree characterized by irreversible dilatation and destruction of the bronchial walls.

bronchiole a small airway of the respiratory conducting system, usually smaller than 1 to 2 mm.

bronchiolitis an acute infection of the lower respiratory tract characterized by expiratory wheezing, respiratory distress, inflammation, and obstruction at the level of the bronchioles; bronchiolitis is usually caused by the respiratory syncytial virus (RSV) and is most common in infants under the age of 2 years.

bronchitis an acute or chronic inflammation of the mucous membranes of the tracheobronchial tree.

bronchoconstriction narrowing of the bronchi caused by contraction of their smooth muscle.

bronchodilation the reversal of bronchoconstriction, usually through sympathetic stimulation.

bronchogenic carcinoma the most common malignant lung tumor originating in bronchi.

bronchography an x-ray examination of the bronchi after they have been coated with a radiopaque substance.

bronchophony the normal transmission of voice sounds from a large bronchus to the chest wall as heard by a stethoscope.

bronchopleural fistula a direct communication between a bronchus and the pleural space; a common cause of pneumothorax.

bronchopneumonia an acute inflammation of the lung tissue, particularly at the level of the terminal bronchioles and alveoli, caused by various infectious agent.

bronchorrhea the excessive discharge of respiratory tract secretions.

bronchoscopy the visual examination of the tracheobronchial tree, using either a rigid, tubular metal bronchoscope or the narrower, flexible fiberoptic bronchoscope (FFB).

bronchospasm an abnormal contraction of the smooth muscle of the bronchi, resulting in an acute narrowing and obstruction.

bronchovesicular breath sounds sharing the characteristics of those heard over the trachea (bronchial sounds) and those arising from the more distal alveolar region (vesicular sounds).

brucellosis a disease caused by any of several species of the gram-negative coccobacillus genus *Brucella;* because of its prevalence in cattle, swine, and goats, brucellosis in humans is often referred to as undulant fever.

bruit an abnormal sound heard on auscultation of the heart or large vessels, caused by turbulence or obstruction.

BTPS abbreviation for body temperature, ambient pressure, saturated (with water vapor).

BTU abbreviation for British Thermal Unit, the fps unit of heat energy; a BTU is the amount of heat required to raise the temperature of 1 lb of water 1°F; one BTU equals 252 calories (cgs).

buccal of or pertaining to the inside of the cheek or the gum next to the cheek.

buffer a chemical substance that, when added to a solution, minimizes fluctuations in pH.

buffer system a chemical solution consisting of a weak acid and its salt, which has the ability to minimize changes in pH when adding acid or alkali.

bulla a thin-walled blister of the skin, mucous membranes, or lung greater than 1 cm in diameter.

BUN abbreviation for blood urea nitrogen, a major by-product of protein metabolism that is normally excreted by the kidneys.

buoyancy the physical principle (responsible for floatation) whereby an object submersed in a liquid such as water appeared to weigh less than in air; attributable to the difference in pressure exerted above and below the submersed object.

by-product a secondary, often unwanted product of a chemical reaction.

CAHEA abbreviation for the Committee on Allied Health Education and Accreditation; an "umbrella" organization sponsored by the American Medical Association and responsible for the accreditation of most allied health educational programs in the United States; collaborates with disciplinary review committees such as the Joint Review Committee for Respiratory Therapy Education (JRCRTE).

cAMP abbreviation for adenosine $3'5'$-cyclic monophosphate, the intracellular compound thought responsible for relaxation of smooth muscle; cAMP synthesis from adensosine triphosphate is catalyzed by the enzyme adenylate cyclase; any drug that promotes an increase in cAMP levels will result in smooth muscle relaxation; any drug that causes a decrease in cAMP levels will result in smooth muscle constriction.

canals of Lambert intercommunicating channels between terminal bronchioles and the alveoli that are about 30 μm and appear to remain open even when bronchiolar smooth muscle is contracted.

candidiasis infection of the skin or mucous membranes caused chiefly by the yeastlike fungus *Candida albicans;* commonly referred to as "thrush" when localized to the mouth and pharynx; can spread systemically in immunocompromised hosts.

cannula any flexible tube that is inserted into the body.

cannulation the insertion of a cannula into a body duct or cavity, as into the nose, trachea, bladder, or a blood vessel.

capillary action a physical phenomenon whereby a liquid in a small tube tends to move upward, against the force of gravity; caused by both adhesive and surface tension forces.

capnograph an instrument used in anesthesia, respiratory physiology, and respiratory care to produce a tracing, or capnogram, which shows the proportion of carbon dioxide in expired air.

capnography the process of obtaining a tracing of the proportion of carbon dioxide in expired air using a capnograph.

carbamino compound a chemical compound consisting of carbon dioxide combined with one or more free amino groups (NH_2) of a protein molecule.

carbonaceous containing a high proportion of carbon.

carboxyhemoglobin a compound produced by the chemical combination of hemoglobin with carbon monoxide.

carboxyhemoglobinemia a decrease in the blood's oxygen-carrying capacity resulting from the saturation of hemoglobin with carbon monoxide instead of oxygen.

carboxyl a monovalent radical ($COOH^-$) characteristic of organic acids.

carcinogenic of or pertaining to the ability to cause the development of a cancer.

cardiac tamponade compression of the heart caused by the collection of blood, fluid, or gas under pressure in the pericardium.

cardiogenic originating in or caused by the heart; as in cardiogenic shock.

cardiomegaly hypertrophy of the heart caused most frequently by pulmonary hypertension; also occurring in arteriovenous fistula, congenital aortic stenosis, ventricular septal defect, patent ductus arteriousus, and Paget's disease.

cardiomyopathy any disease that affects the myocardium, as alcoholic cardiomyopathy.

cardioversion the restoration of the heart's normal sinus rhythm by delivery of a synchronized electric shock through two metal paddles placed on the patient's chest.

carotid sinus reflex the decrease in the heart rate as a reflex reaction from pressure on or within the carotid artery at the level of its bifurcation.

cartilaginous of or pertaining to cartilage.

catabolism the destructive phase of metabolism whereby complex substances are broken down into simpler ones, with the concurrent release of energy.

catecholamine any one of a group of sympathomimetic compounds composed of a catechol molecule and the aliphatic portion of an amine.

catheterization the introduction of a catheter into a body cavity or organ to inject or remove a fluid.

cathode the negative pole or electrode of an electrical source.

cation an ion that migrates to the cathode (negative electrode) in an electrolytic solution; a positive ion.

cationic of or pertaining to positive ions in solution.

cavitary pertaining to a process resulting in cavitation, or the lesion so formed.

cavitation the formation of cavities within the body, as those formed in the lung by tuberculosis.

CDC abbreviation for Centers for Disease Control.

cellulitis an infection of the skin characterized most commonly by local heat, redness, pain, and swelling and sometimes by fever, malaise, chills, and headache.

cephalad toward the head.

cephalocaudal literally "head-to-tail"; often used to refer to the sequence of a physical examination.

cerebral aneurysm an abnormal localized dilatation of a cerebral artery, most commonly the result of congenital weakness of the media or muscle layer of the vessel wall.

cerebral hemorrhage a hemorrhage from a blood vessel in the brain; sometimes called a cerebrovascular accident or CVA.

cerebral palsy a motor function disorder caused by a permanent, nonprogressive brain defect or lesion present at birth or shortly thereafter.

cerebrospinal pertaining to or involving the brain and the spinal cord.

cerebrovascular of or pertaining to the vascular system of the brain.

certification a voluntary process whereby a nongovernmental or private agency or association grants recognition to an individual who has met certain predetermined qualifications for recognition in a given field of study or practice.

certified pulmonary function technician (CPFT) an individual, qualified by education or experience or both, who has successfully completed the pulmonary function certification examination of the NBRC.

certified respiratory therapy technician (CRTT) a respiratory therapy technician who has successfully completed the technician (entry-level) certification examination of the NBRC.

cervical of or pertaining to the neck or the region of the neck.

CGA abbreviation for the Compressed Gas Association, a voluntary regulatory organization made up of companies involved in the compressed gas industry and responsible for establishing safety standards for compressed gas systems.

cGMP abbreviation for cyclic guanosine monophosphate; synthesized through action at the cholinergic receptors of smooth muscle from guanosine triphosphate (GTP); an increase in the level of cGMP results in an increase in bronchial smooth muscle constriction.

cgs (CGS) acronym for the centimeter-gram-second measurement system.

chelating agent a chemical substance that binds metallic ions.

chemoreceptor a sensory nerve cell activated by changes in the chemical environment surrounding it, as the chemoreceptors in the carotid artery that are sensitive to the PCO_2 in the blood, signaling the respiratory center in the brain to increase or decrease ventilation.

chest physical therapy (CPT) a collection of therapeutic techniques designed to facilitate clearance of airway secretion, improve the distribution of ventilation, and enhance the efficiency and conditioning of the muscle of respiration; includes positioning techniques; chest percussion and vibration; directed coughing; and various breathing and conditioning exercises.

Cheyne-Stokes breathing an abnormal breathing pattern characterized by alternating periods of apnea and periods of rising then falling tidal volumes.

CHF abbreviation for congestive heart failure.

Chlamydia a microorganism of the genus *Chlamydia*.

choanal atresia a congenital anomaly in which a bony or membranous occlusion blocks the passageway between the nose and pharynx.

cholesterol an organic monohydric alcohol ($C_{27}H_{45}OH$) widely found in animal tissue.

cholinergic of or pertaining to nerve fibers that elaborate acetylcholine at the myoneural junctions.

chronic bronchitis a chronic respiratory disorder characterized by its symptoms: a history of a productive cough for at least 3 months a year for 2 consecutive years; involves hypertrophy of the bronchial glands and an increase in the number of the goblet cells lining the respiratory tract mucosa, which typically is chronically inflamed.

chronotropism the effect of neural or humoral influences on the rate of cardiac contractions; a positive chronotropic effect increases the heart rate, while a negative chronotropic effect decreases the heart rate.

chylomicron minute droplets of the lipoproteins measuring less than 0.5 μm in diameter.

clearance removal; in aerosol therapy, the process whereby deposited particles are removed from the site of deposition, or the removal of still suspended particles in the exhaled air.

clubbing bulbous swelling of the terminal phalanges of the fingers and toes, often associated with certain chronic lung diseases.

CMV abbreviation for continuous mandatory ventilation; the application of pressure greater than atmospheric at the airway opening during every inspiration, used to support ventilation; during expiration, pressure returns to atmospheric; CMV may be applied in either the control or assist-control mode.

CNS abbreviation for central nervous system.

coalescence the growing together of two or more objects, as in the coalescence of water vapor molecules into water droplets.

Coanda effect a phenomenon in hydrodynamics whereby a fluid in motion may be attracted or held to a wall.

coarctation of the aorta a congenital cardiac anomaly characterized by a localized narrowing of the aorta, which results in increased pressure proximal to the defect and decreased pressure distal to it.

coccidioidomycosis an infectious fungal disease caused by the inhalation of spores of the organism *Coccidioides immitis,* which is carried on windborne dust particles.

coefficient of elastic expansion (EE) the volumetric expansion of a compressed gas cylinder under hydrostatic test conditions, expressed in cubic centimeters.

cognitive of or pertaining to human thought processes.

cohesion the attractive force between like molecules.

cohort a collection or sampling of individuals who share a common characteristic, as members of the same age or the same sex.

coliform of or pertaining to the colon-aerogenes group, or the *Escherichia coli* species of microorganisms, constituting most of the intestinal flora in humans and other animals.

collagen a protein consisting of bundles of tiny reticular fibrils, which combine to form the white glistening inelastic fibers of the tendons, ligaments, and fascia.

colloid a state of matter in which large molecules or aggregate of molecules (between 1 and 100 μm) remain dispersed in another medium (like water) without precipitating; egg white, gelatin, and intracellular protoplasm are common examples of colloids.

colonization the process by which microorganisms establish a presence and grow in or on the human body; does *not* necessarily indicate a pathologic response.

colorimetry measurement of the intensity of color in a fluid or substance.

combustible flammable or apt to catch fire.

combustion the process of burning; any rapid oxidation with the emission of heat.

communication any process in which a message containing information is transferred, especially from one person to another, through any of a number of media.

compliance the relative ease with which a body stretches or deforms; in pulmonary physiology, a measure of volume change per unit pressure change under static conditions; the reciprocal of elastance.

computed tomography (CT) a tomographic method that employs a narrowly collimated beam of x-rays to image the body in cross-sectional slices.

CON abbreviation for certificate of need, a verification made by a health systems agency or equivalent regulatory group that a major capital improvement, such as the addition of a wing to a hospital or the purchase of a nuclear magnetic resonance imaging device, is needed.

concave curved or rounded inward like a bowl.

concentric of or pertaining to groups of circles having a common center, like a bull's-eye.

conduction the transfer of heat by the direct interaction of atoms or molecules in a hot area that contact atoms or molecules in a cooler area.

conductivity the ability of myocardial tissue to propagate electrical impulses.

congential present at birth, as a congenital anomaly or defect.

congenital diaphragmatic hernia an abnormality in the development of the diaphragm resulting in a persistent opening between the abdominal and thoracic cavities; due to displacement of the abdominal contents into the thorax, this condition may impede lung growth and development on the affected side.

conjugated protein a protein, such as hemoglobin, that has a characteristic chemical group other than amino acids as part of its structure; in hemoglobin, the globin portion represents the simple amino acid chain, while the four heme chains contain chemical groups other than amino acids.

conjunctivitis inflammation of the conjunctiva, caused by bacterial or viral infection, allergy, or environmental factors.

consolidation the process of becoming solid; especially applies to the loss of aeration of the terminal respiratory units due to fluid extravasation and the collection of exudate, as in certain forms of pneumonia.

constriction a narrowing or squeezing together.

constrictive pericarditis an inflammation of the pericardium (usually chronic) in which calcium and fibrous deposits surround the heart and restrict its normal filling.

consumerism the philosophy (and popular movement) of promoting the consumers' interests over those of the seller; as applied to health care, the promotion of patient choice and decision making in the selection of use of health care services.

contact transmission transmission of infectious organisms between an infected individual and a host through direct, indirect, or droplet contact.

continuing education educational activity designed to upgrade, enhance, or expand a professional's knowledge or skills, which is conducted *after* completion of formal entry-level educational preparation.

contractility the property of muscle tissue to shorten in response to a stimulus, usually electrical.

contracture an abnormal, usually permanent condition of a joint, characterized by flexion and fixation and caused by atrophy and shortening of muscle fibers or by loss of the normal elasticity of the skin, as from the formation of extensive scar tissue over a joint.

contraindicated of or pertaining to a treatment or treatment approach that is inadvisable or improper due to the patient's condition.

contraindication any circumstance that renders a particular treatment or treatment approach inadvisable or improper.

control mode continuous mandatory ventilation (CMV) in which the frequency of breathing is determined by the ventilator according to a preset cycling pattern without initiation by the patient.

convalescence the period of recovery from an illness, operation, or injury.

convex curved or rounded outward like the exterior of a sphere.

convection heat transfer through the mixing of fluid molecules at different temperature states through thermal currents.

convective of or pertaining to the process of heat transfer by convection.

COPD abbreviation for chronic obstructive pulmonary disease; COPD is a broad term used to describe generalized airways obstruction that is not fully reversible with treatment; almost always a mixture of emphysema and chronic bronchitis, with, at times, elements of asthma.

cor pulmonale right ventricular hypertrophy/failure and pulmonary hypertension caused by certain parenchymal or vascular lung disorders.

CORF abbreviation for Comprehensive Out-Patient Rehabilitation Facility; a Medicare-approved facility that provides a broad scope of ambulatory rehabilitation services as defined in section 933 of PL 96-499.

corroborating that which confirms or supports with evidence.

corticosteroid any one of the natural or the synthetic hormones associated with the adrenal cortex, which influences or controls key processes of the body, as carbohydrate and protein metabolism, electrolyte and water balance, and the function of the cardiovascular system, the skeletal muscle, the kidneys, and other organs; major categories include the glucocorticoids (eg, hydrocortisone), the mineralocorticoids (eg, aldosterone), and the androgens.

costochondral of or pertaining to a rib and its cartilage.

costophrenic of or pertaining to the ribs and diaphragm; especially the angle formed by the lower ribs' intersection with the diaphragm.

costovertebral of or relating to a rib and the vertebral column.

countershock a high-intensity, short-duration electric shock applied to the heart, resulting in total depolarization.

Coxsackievirus any of 30 serologically different RNA enteroviruses resembling the polio virus; coxsackieviruses primarily affect children and are associated with diseases such as herpangina; hand, foot, and mouth disease; myocarditis; pericarditis; and aseptic meningitis.

CPAP abbreviation for continuous positive airway pressure; a method of ventilatory support whereby the patient breathes spontaneously without mechanical assistance against threshold resistance, with pressure above atmospheric maintained at the airway throughout breathing.

CPFT abbreviation for certified pulmonary function technician.

creatinine a substance formed from the metabolism of creaine, commonly found in blood, urine, and muscle tissue.

credentialing a broad term referring to the recognition of individuals who have met certain predetermined standards attesting to their occupational skill or competence; includes both licensure and certification.

crepitus a dry crackling sound or sensation; may apply to breath sounds (ie, "a crepitant rale") or to the sensation felt when palpating an area of subcutaneous emphysema.

cricothyrotomy an emergency incision into the larynx between the cricoid and thyroid cartilages, performed to open the airway in a person choking.

critical pressure the pressure exerted by a vapor in an evacuated container at its critical temperature.

critical temperature the highest temperature at which a substance can exist as a liquid, regardless of pressure.

cromolyn sodium a prophylactic antiasthmatic that acts by stabilizing the mast cells, thereby decreasing the release of chemical mediators resulting from an inhaled allergen.

croup an infectious disorder of the upper airway occurring chiefly in infants and children that normally results in subglottic swelling and obstruction; rather than a single clinical entity, croup may manifest itself as one of three different syndromes: (1) laryngotracheitis, also called "classic" croup, (2) "spasmodic" croup, or (3) laryngotracheobronchitis.

CRTT abbreviation for certified respiratory therapy technician.

cryogenic producing extremely low temperatures.

cryptococcosis an infectious disease caused by a fungus, *Cryptococcus neoformans,* which spreads through the lungs to the brain and CNS, skin, skeletal system, and urinary tract.

crystalloid of or pertaining to a solution in which ionic compounds serve as the solute.

CSF abbreviation for cerebrospinal fluid.

cuboidal of or pertaining to the shape of a cube.

Cushing's disease a metabolic disorder characterized by the abnormally increased secretion of adrenocortical steroids caused by increased amounts of adrenocorticotropic hormone (ACTH) secreted by the pituitary, as by pituitary adenoma.

CVA abbreviation for cerebrovascular accident.

CVP abbreviation for central venous pressure, the blood pressure measured in or near the right atrium.

CWP abbreviation for coal-workers' pneumoconiosis; CWP is due to chronic exposure to coal dust, which consists mainly of carbon; pathologic changes are similar to those seen in silicosis.

cyanide poisoning poisoning resulting from the ingestion or inhalation of cyanide.

cyanosis bluish discoloration of the skin and mucous membranes caused by an excess of deoxygenated hemoglobin in the blood.
  central cyanosis associated with a reduction in the hemoglobin saturation of arterial blood and observed best in the capillary beds of the lips or buccal membranes.
  peripheral cyanosis associated with an excessive amount of reduced hemoglobin in the venous blood, resulting from poor perfusion or blood stasis.

cyanotic heart disease of or pertaining to anatomic congenital heart defects that cause large right-to-left shunting; such "venous admixture" results in the characteristic cyanosis.

cycling mechanism the means by which a ventilator ends the inspiratory phase of mechanical ventilation.

pressure cycling the delivery of gas under positive pressure during inspiration until an adjustable, preselected pressure has been reached.

volume cycling the delivery of gas under positive pressure during inspiration until an adjustable, preselected volume has been expelled from the device.

time cycling the delivery of gas under positive pressure during inspiration until a preselected time interval has elapsed.

flow cycling the delivery of gas under positive pressure during inspiration until flow drops to a specified terminal level.

combined cycling the delivery of gas under positive pressure during inspiration until two or more parameters are achieved simultaneously (eg, combined flow and pressure cycling, as on the Bennett PR-II).

manual cycling the delivery of gas under positive pressure during inspiration until a manually operated control is actuated.

cystic fibrosis an autosomal recessive disease characterized by pancreatic insufficiency, abnormally thick secretions from the endocrine glands, and an increased concentration of sodium and chloride in the sweat glands; known in Europe as mucoviscidosis.

cystoscopy the direct visualization of the urinary tract by means of a cystoscope inserted in the urethra.

cytochrome oxidase system the major intracellular pathway for oxidative metabolism and energy production.

cytomegalovirus a member of a group of large species-specific herpes-type viruses with a wide variety of disease effects.

cytologic of or pertaining to the cells.

cytotechnology an allied health field involved in the microscopic examination of cell specimens for purposes of identifying abnormalities, especially malignancies.

cytotoxic of or pertaining to chemical or biologic substances that are lethal to living cells.

deadspace respired gas volume that does not participate in gas exchange (ie, ventilated but not perfused by the pulmonary circulation).

anatomic dead space the volume constituting the conducting zone of the lungs, including the upper airway.

alveolar dead space the volume of gas ventilating unperfused alveoli.

physiologic dead space the sum of anatomic and alveolar dead space.

mechanical dead space expired air that is rebreathed through a connecting apparatus or tubing.

deamidization freeing of the ammonia from an amide.

death a cessation of living functions.

clinical death the cessation of ventilation and circulation.

biologic death cessation of biologic function resulting in irreversible cell damage.

brain death irreversible cessation or loss of cerebral function.

debilitated weakness, especially to the extent of being unable to participate in care.

debridement the removal of foreign material and dead tissue from an infected or traumatized area to expose healthy tissue.

decongestant of or pertaining to a substance or procedure that eliminates or reduces congestion or swelling.

decontamination the process whereby contaminants are removed from objects, usually by simple physical means, such as washing.

decubitus ulcer an inflammation, sore, or ulcer in the skin over a bony prominence.

defibrillation the termination of ventricular fibrillation by delivering a direct electric countershock to the patient's precordium.

deglutition swallowing.

demyelination the process of destruction or removal of the myelin sheath from a nerve or nerve fiber.

density a measure of the mass per unit volume of a substance.

depersonalize creating a feeling of strangeness or remoteness.

depolarization the reduction of a membrane potential to a less negative value; in cardiac fibers, this results in the release of calcium ions into the myofibrils and activates the contractile process.

depolymerize to break down complex molecules (polymers) into their basic building blocks, such as to break down a protein into its amino acids.

dermatitis an inflammatory condition of the skin, characterized by erythema and pain or pruritus.

desquamate a normal process in which the cornified layer of the epidermis is sloughed in fine scales; also refers to the loss of epithelial cells in general.

determinant a causal factor.

dew point the temperature at which water vapor condenses to back to its liquid form.

DHHS abbreviation for the federal Department of Health and Human Services, a department of the federal government responsible for many regulatory aspects in health care delivery, including Medicare/Medicaid funding through its Health Care Financing Administration (HCFA) and drug testing and purity requirements (including the purity of medical gases) through its Food and Drug Administration (FDA).

diabetic ketoacidosis an acute, life-threatening complication of uncontrolled diabetes mellitus in which urinary loss of water, potassium, ammonium, and sodium results in hypovolemia, electrolyte imbalance, extremely high blood glucose levels, and the breakdown of free fatty acids, causing a severe metabolic acidosis, often with coma.

dialysis the process of separating colloids and crystalline substances in solution by the difference in their rate of diffusion through a semipermeable membrane.

diaphoresis the secretion of sweat, especially the profuse secretion associated with an elevated body temperature, physical exertion, exposure to heat, and mental or emotional stress.

diaphragmatic hernia the protrusion of part of the stomach through an opening in the diaphragm, most commonly an abnormally enlarged esophageal hiatus.

DIC abbreviation for disseminated intravascular coagulation; DIC is a thrombohemorrhagic disorder that accompanies a variety of clinical conditions and involves activation of the clotting cascade, the generation of excess thrombin, intravascular coagulation, occlusion of capillaries and arterioles with fibrin, and tissue ischemia.

dichrotic notch a notch on the descending limb of a pulse tracing; especially that seen in the tracing of arterial blood pressure due to closure of the aortic valve.

didactic intended for instruction; commonly refers to classroom (as opposed to clinical) learning.

diencephalon the division of the brain between the telencephalon and the mesencephalon.

diffusion the physical process whereby atoms or molecules tend to move from a area of higher concentration or pressure to an area of lower concentration or pressure.

diffusion coefficient the rate of diffusion of a gas; in cgs units, the diffusion coefficient is defined as the number of milliliters of a gas at 1 atmosphere of pressure that will diffuse a distance of 1 μm over a square centimeter surface area per minute.

diffusion deposition the deposition of aerosol particle on a surface due to their random bombardment by carry gas molecules.

dimorphic occurring in or consisting of two different forms.

diphtheria an acute, contagious disease caused by the bacterium *Corynebacterium diphtheriae,* characterized by the production of a system toxin and a false membrane lining of the mucous membrane of the throat.

diplegia bilateral paralysis of both sides of any part of the body or of like parts on the opposite sides of the body.

diplopia double vision.

disability the lack of ability to perform normal mental or physical tasks; especially the loss of mental or physical powers due to injury or disease.

discontinuation the process of ceasing or ending.

disequilibrium a condition characterized by a lack of balance, either literally (as with dizziness) or figuratively, as in any disruption to a homeostatic system.

disinfectant a chemical agent capable of destroying at least the vegetative phase of pathogenic microorganisms; there are five major categories of disinfectants used in clinical practice: the alcohols, the phenols and their derivatives, the halogens, the aldehydes, and the quaternary ammonium compounds.

disinfection the process of destroying at least the vegetative phase of pathogenic microorganisms by physical or chemical means.

disposition one's attitude toward things or events.

distensibility of or pertaining to the ease of inflation or compliance.

distillation the condensation of a vapor obtained by heating a liquid; commonly used to separate out liquids with different boiling points as in the production of oxygen by fractional distillation.

diuresis increased formation and secretion of urine.

diuretic a chemical substance that causes diuresis.

diversification the process of diversifying or adding different components.

dL abbreviation for deciliter (1/10 L or 100 ml).

DME company a company that manufactures, sells, or rents durable medical equipment.

dorsalis pedis (artery) the continuation of the anterior tibial artery, starting at the ankle joint, dividing into five branches, supplying various muscles of the foot and toes.

DOT abbreviation for the federal Department of Transportation, the department of the federal government responsible for regulating interstate transportation of compressed gases.

DPG abbreviation for diphosphoglycerate; 2,3 DPG is an organic phosphate in red blood cells that alters the affinity of hemoglobin for oxygen.

DRG abbreviation for diagnosis related group; a system of coding used by the Health Care Financing Administration to set prospective reimbursement schedules for Medicare patients according their diagnosis.

duodenum the shortest, widest, and most fixed portion of the small intestine, taking an almost circular course from the pyloric valve of the stomach, so that its termination is close to its starting point.

dynamic compliance a measure of compliance obtained while breathing; used to indicate the effect of resistance on transpulmonary pressure gradients during breathing.

dysarthria difficult, poorly articulated speech, resulting from interference in the control over the muscles of speech, usually because of damage to a central or peripheral motor nerve.

dysphagia difficulty in swallowing.

dysphasia impaired speech.

dysplasia a combining form meaning "(condition of) abnormal development": chondrodysplasia, epidermodysplasia, osteomyelodysplasia.

dyspnea a subjective sensation of difficult or labored breathing.

dysoxia an abnormal metabolic state in which the tissues are unable to use properly the oxygen made available to them.

ECC abbreviation for external cardiac compression; ECC involves manual compression of a cardiac arrest victim's ventricles between the sternum and thoracic spine; ECC can provide one third to one fourth of the normal cardiac output and can maintain a systolic blood pressure of 100 mm Hg.

ECG abbreviation for electrocardiogram.

echocardiography a diagnostic procedure for studying the structure and motion of the heart.

eclampsia the gravest form of toxemia of pregnancy, characterized by grand mal convulsion, coma, hypertension, proteinuria, and edema.

edema a local or generalized condition due to the buildup of excessive amounts of extracellular fluid and characterized by swelling.

ectopic situated in an unusual place, away from its normal location (eg, an ectopic pregnancy is a pregnancy that occurs outside the uterus).

EDTA abbreviation for ethylenediaminotetraacetate, a chelating agent used in the treatment of poisoning with lead or other heavy metals; also used in the treatment of hypercalcemia; overuse can cause hypocalcemia and respiratory and cardiac arrest.

EE abbreviation for the coefficient of elastic expansion.

effector that which produces an effect; that part of a mechanical or physiologic system that acts to create a specific condition or change.

efferent carrying or conduction impulses away from the CNS; opposite of afferent.

efficacy effectiveness; ability to produce the intended effect.

efficacy (of a drug) the peak or maximum biologic effect.

effort-dependent of or pertaining to a test or procedure, the accuracy or success of which depends on patient effort.

effort-independent of or pertaining to a test or procedure, the accuracy or success of which does not depend on patient effort.

effusion the escape of fluid from blood vessels because of rupture or seepage, usually into a body cavity.

egocentrism the tendency to be overly concerned with one's self.

egophony the sound of normal voice tones as heard through the chest wall during auscultation.

EGTA abbreviation for the esophageal gastric tube airway; a modification of the esophageal obturator airway (EOA) that includes a gastric tube that can be extended beyond the distal tip into the stomach to remove air or gastric contents.

EIP abbreviation for end-inspiratory pause; a technique whereby a specific inflation volume is momentarily held at the end of inspiration during mechanical ventilation, for either therapeutic or diagnostic purposes.

elastance (also elasticity) the tendency of matter to resist a stretching force and recoil or return to its original size or form after deformation or expansion; the reciprocal of compliance.

elastin a protein that forms the principal substance of yellow elastic tissue fibers.

electrocardiography the process of obtaining a tracing of the electrical activity of the heart (an electrocardiogram) for purposes of identifying abnormalities.

electrocautery the application of a needle or snare heated by electric current for the destruction of tissue, as for the removal of warts or polyps.

electrolysis the process of applying an electrical current across an anode and cathode in a solution, usually to create or enhance a chemical reaction.

electrolyte a chemical substance that dissociates into ions when placed into solution, thus becoming capable of conducting electricity.

electromyography the recording and study of the electrical properties of muscle.

electrophysiology the recording and study of the electrical properties of living tissue.

embolectomy a surgical incision into an artery for the removal of an embolus or clot, performed as emergency treatment for arterial embolization.

embolization the process by which an embolus forms and lodges in a branch of the vasculature.

embolus a foreign object, a quantity of air or gas, a bit of tissue or tumor, or a piece of a thrombus that circulates in the bloodstream until it becomes lodged in a vessel.

embryogenesis the process in sexual reproduction in which an embryo forms from the fertilization of an ovum.

emetic of or pertaining to a substance that causes vomiting.

emissivity the property of certain matter to emit energy in the form of either heat or light.

empathetic characterized by awareness of and insight into the feelings and emotions of others.

emphysema a destructive process of the lung parenchyma leading to permanent enlargement of the distal airspaces; classified as either centrilobular (CLE), which mainly involves the respiratory bronchioles, or panlobular (PLE), which can involve the entire terminal respiratory unit; the CLE form is predominantly a disease of bronchitic patients who smoke cigarettes.

empyema an accumulation of pus in a body cavity, especially the pleural space, as a result of bacterial infection, as in pleurisy or tuberculosis.

emulsification the process of mixing two or more substances that are not mutually soluble into a uniform dispersion; specifically applies to the breakdown of fat globules in the intestines through the action of bile acids.

encode the process of preparing a message for transmission.

endobronchial within a bronchus.

endocarditis inflammation of endocardium and the heart valves, as caused by a variety of diseases.

endocrine system the network of ductless glands and other structures that elaborate and secrete hormones directly into the bloodstream, affecting the function of specific target organs.

endogenous growing within or arising from the body.

endorphin any one of the neuropeptides composed of many amino acids, elaborated by the pituitary gland and acting on the central and the peripheral nervous systems to reduce pain.

endoscopy the visualization of the interior of organs and cavities of the body with an endoscope.

endothelium the layer of squamous epithelial cells that lines the heart, the blood and the lymph vessels, and the serous cavities of the body.

endotracheal within or through the trachea.

enteric of or pertaining to the intestinal tract.

Enterobacteriaceae a family of aerobic and anaerobic bacteria that includes both normal and pathogenic enteric microorganisms.

enterocolitis an inflammation involving both the large and small intestines.

entitlement a right or claim; alternatively the process of granting or providing a right, such as the right to adequate health care.

enzyme an organic catalyst produced by living cells.

EOA abbreviation for esophageal obturator airway; the EOA consists of a cuffed hollow tube tipped with a soft plastic obturator at its distal end; the tube passes through a mask and has several holes in its upper portion; once passed into the esophagus, the cuff is inflated, thereby preventing aspiration and allowing ventilation with intermittent positive pressure.

eosinophilia an increase in the number of eosinophils in the blood, accompanying many inflammatory conditions.

EPAP abbreviation for expiratory positive airway pressure, or the application of positive pressure to the airway during expiration only (as opposed to continuous positive airway pressure).

epidemiology the study of the relationships among various factors and the distribution and frequency of diseases in the population.

epigastric of or pertaining to the epigastrium.

epigastrium the part of the abdomen in the upper zone between the right and left hypochondriac regions.

epiglottitis an acute and often life-threatening infection of the upper airway that causes severe obstruction secondary to supraglottic swelling; caused primarily by *Haemophilus influenzae,* type B, and affecting mainly children under the age of 5.

epinephrine an adrenal hormone and synthetic adrenergic vasoconstrictor.

epistaxis bleeding from the nose caused by local irritation of mucous membranes, violent sneezing, fragility of the mucous membrane or of the arterial walls, chronic infection, trauma, hypertension, leukemia, vitamin K deficiency, or, most often, picking of the nose.

epithelium the covering of the internal and external organs of the body, including the lining of vessels.

Epstein-Barr virus the herpesvirus that causes infectious mononucleosis.

equal pressure point (EPP) during forced exhalation, the point along an airway during where the pressure inside its wall equals the intrapleural pressure; downstream beyond this point, the pleural pressure *exceeds* the pressure inside the airway, tending to promote bronchiolar collapse.

equilibrate to bring into balance.

equilibration the process of bringing into balance.

eradicate to eliminate.

ergometer an apparatus designed to measure the amount of work performed by an animal or human subject.

erythema a redness of the skin due to capillary congestion; caused by injury, inflammation, or infection.

erythrocyte a red blood cell.

erythrocythemia an increase in the number of erythrocytes circulating in the blood.

erythrocytosis the process resulting in an abnormal increase in the number of circulating red cells.

erythropoiesis the process of erythrocyte production involving the maturation of a nucleated precursor into a hemoglobin-filled, nucleus-free erythrocyte that is regulated by erythropoietin, a hormone produced by the kidney.

Escherichia coli a species of coliform bacteria of the family Enterobacteriaceae, normally present in the intestines and common in water, milk, and soil.

esophageal opening pressure the oral pressure at which the esophagus distends and opens, allowing gas to insufflate the stomach; estimated to range from 20 to 25 cm H_2O.

esthetic (also aesthetic) appreciative of beauty, appealing.

ethacrynic acid a potent diuretic.

ethmoid bone a very light and spongy bone at the base of the cranium, forming most of the walls of the superior part of the nasal cavity and consisting of four parts: a horizontal plate, a perpendicular plate, and two lateral labyrinths.

ethnicity racial origin.

ethylene chlorohydrin a chemical substance toxic to living tissue that is formed when polyvinyl chloride reacts with ethylene oxide gas.

ethylene oxide a gas used to sterilize surgical instruments and other supplies.

ETO common abbreviation for ethylene oxide.

eukaryotic of or pertaining to cells with true nuclei bounded by a nuclear membrane and capable of mitosis.

eustachian tube a tube, lined with mucous membrane, that joins the nasopharynx and the tympanic cavity, allowing equalization of the air pressure in the inner ear with atmospheric pressure.

evacuate to remove or withdraw from, especially to empty of air and create a vacuum.

evaporation the change in state of a substance from its liquid to its gaseous form occurring below its boiling point.

exacerbate to worsen.

exacerbation a worsening of a condition, usually acutely.

excitability a property of myocardial tissue, shared with other muscle and nerve tissues, and representing a responsiveness to stimulation caused by electrical, chemical, or mechanical factors in the cell or in its surrounding environment.

exfoliate to fall off in layers.

expectorant a chemical agent that promotes the expectoration of respiratory tract secretions, usually by increasing their production or by lowering their viscosity.

expiratory reserve volume (ERV) the total amount of gas that can be exhaled from the lung following a quiet exhalation.

expiratory resistance (retard) a modification of the expiratory phase of positive pressure ventilation in which a restricted orifice, or flow resistor, is used to slow the flow of exhaled gases from the patient.

extracellular occurring outside a cell or cell tissue or in cavities or spaces between cell layers or groups of cells.

extracorporeal something that is outside the body, as extracorporeal circulation, in which venous blood is diverted outside the body to a heart-lung machine and returned to the body through a femoral or other artery.

extrapolation to infer unknown data from known data, as to extrapolate a value existing between two known points on a curve.

extrasystole cardiac contraction that is abnormal in timing or in origin of impulse with respect to the heart's fundamental rhythm.

extrathoracic outside the thorax.

extrauterine occurring or located outside the uterus.

extravasation a passage or escape into the tissues, usually of blood, serum, or lymph.

extrinsic allergic alveolitis an inflammatory form of interstitial pneumonia that results from a type III or immune complex antigen-antibody reactions to certain organic dusts.

extubate withdrawing a tube from an orifice or cavity of the body.

exudate a fluid with a high protein content that escapes into the extracellular space; usually due to inflammation or infection.

facultative not obligatory, having the ability to adapt to more than one condition, as a facultative anaerobe that can live with or without oxygen.

fasciculation a small involuntary muscular contraction visible under the skin.

faucial of or pertaining to the fauces, the constricted opening leading from the mouth to the oropharynx and bounded by the soft palate, base of the tongue, and the palatine arches.

feedback that portion of the output of a dynamic system that is returned as input to control or vary the underlying process; in human communication, feedback represents a message returned by the receiver to the sender to help enhance meaning between the parties.

fenestrated open like a window; from the Latin *fenestra*, meaning "window".

fenestrated tracheotomy tube a double cannulated tracheotomy tube that has an opening in the posterior wall of the outer cannula above the cuff; removal of the inner cannula allows free breathing through the tube.

fermentation the oxidative decomposition of substances through enzymes produced by microorganisms.

FDA abbreviation for the Food and Drug Administration, the federal agency responsible for overseeing the testing and ensuring the purity and effectiveness of drugs (including medical gases).

FFB abbreviation for flexible fiberoptic bronchoscope.

fibrinolysis a continual process of fibrin decomposition by fibrinolysin that is the normal mechanism for the removal of small fibrin clots.

fibroplasia the formation of fibrous tissue.

fibrosis synonym for fibroplasia.

filling density the ratio between the weight of liquid gas put into the cylinder and the weight of water the cylinder could contain if full; for example, the filling density for carbon dioxide is 68%.

fissure a narrow cleft or slit.

fistula any tubelike passageway between two organs or between an organ and the body surface.

fixed acid a titratable, nonvolatile acid representing the byproduct of protein catabolism; examples include phosphoric and sulfuric acid.

flaccid weak or flabby; especially as applied to muscles lacking normal tone.

flail chest a traumatic chest injury in which a portion of the rib cage becomes unstable as a result of multiple rib fractures or costochondral separation; typically, the flail region exhibits paradoxical movement during inspiration, contributing to a maldistribution of ventilation.

flange a rim used to strengthen an object, to help guide it, to facilitate its attachment to another object.

flow generator a ventilator that develops a flow pattern independent of the mechanical characteristics of the patient's respiratory system.

flowmeter a device operated by a needle valve that controls and measures gas flow, according to the principles of viscosity and density.

flow restrictor a fixed-orifice, constant-pressure, flow-metering device.

fluidics a branch of engineering in which hydrodynamic principles are incorporated into flow circuits for such purposes as switching, pressure and flow sensing, and amplification.

fomite nonliving material (such as bed linens or equipment) that may transmit pathogenic organisms.

forced expiration technique (FET) a modification of the normal cough sequence designed to facilitate clearance of bronchial secretions while minimizing the likelihood of bronchiolar collapse; consists of one or two forced expirations from mid to low lung volume without closure of the glottis, followed by a period of diaphragmatic breathing and relaxation.

for profit designed to generate revenues in excess of expenditures for the benefit of owners or shareholders.

fossa a hollow or depression, especially on the surface of the end of a bone, as the olecranon fossa or the coranoid fossa.

fps (FPS) acronym for the foot-pound-second or British measurement system.

fractional distillation the process of separating the components of a liquid mixture according to their boiling points through the application of heat; the primary commercial process used to produce oxygen.

FRC abbreviation for functional residual capacity.

fremitus a tremulous vibration of the chest wall that can be auscultated or palpated during physical examination.

French scale a measurement scale used commonly to delineate the diameter of catheters; 1 French unit equals approximately 0.33 mm.

Freon a trademark for a hydrocarbon gas commonly used as a refrigerant and propellant.

FTE abbreviation for full-time equivalent, a unit corresponding to the number of hours per week (or month or year) worked by a normal full-time employee.

fungicide an agent destructive to fungi.

functional residual capacity (FRC) the total amount of gas left in the lungs after a resting expiration.

furosemide (Lasix) a rapid-acting sulfonamide diuretic and antihypertensive agent; inhibits reabsorption of sodium and chloride in the loop of Henle and the proximal and distal tubules; also enhances the excretion of potassium, calcium, hydrogen, and bicarbonate ions; can cause hypokalemic metabolic alkalosis and hypocalcemic tetany.

FVC abbreviation for forced vital capacity.

g (also gm) abbreviation for gram.

galvanometer an instrument that measures the flow of electrical current by electromagnetic action.

gastroenteritis inflammation of the stomach and intestines accompanying numerous gastrointestinal disorders.

gastrointestinal of or pertaining to the organs of the gastrointestinal tract, from mouth to anus.

gaw abbreviation for gram atomic weight; the atomic weight of an element expressed in grams.

genitourinary referring to the genital and urinary systems of the body, either the organ structures or functions or both.

gEq abbreviation for gram equivalence; the weight in grams of an ion that will combine with or replace one mole of hydrogen ions or one mole of electrons.

gestation the period of development of the embryo and fetus from fertilization of the ovum to birth.

globin the protein component of hemoglobin.

glomerulonephritis an inflammation of the glomerulus of the kidney, characterized by proteinuria, hematuria, decreased urine production, and edema.

glomerulus the network of vascular tufts in the nephron responsible for filtration of plasma.

glossopharyngeal of or pertaining to the tongue and pharynx.

glottis (also rima glottidis) the opening between the true vocal cords.

glucocorticoid an adrenocortical steroid hormone that increases glyconeogenesis, exerts an anti-inflammatory effect, and influences many body functions.

glutamine a nonessential amino acid found in many proteins in the body.

glutaraldehyde a high-level disinfectant solution that can also be used as a sterilant.

gmw abbreviation for gram molecular weight, the molecular weight of a compound expressed in grams.

GNP abbreviation for gross national product, a measure of the total value of all goods and services produced by the United States in a given year.

Goodpasture's syndrome a chronic relapsing pulmonary hemosiderosis, usually associated with glomerulonephritis and characterized by a cough with hemoptysis, dyspnea, anemia, and progressive renal failure.

granulocytopenia an abnormal condition of the blood, characterized by a decrease in the total number of granulocytes.

granuloma a circumscribed mass of cells (mainly histiocytes) normally associated with the presence of chronic infection or inflammation.

granulomatous composed of or having the characteristics of a granuloma.

Guillain-Barré syndrome an idiopathic, peripheral polyneuritis occurring between 1 and 3 weeks after a mild episode of fever associated with a viral infection or with immunization and characterized by lower extremity weakness progressing within a few days to the upper extremities and face; sensory changes usually are not present, but muscle tenderness and nerve sensitivity to pressure may occur; weakness of trunk and extremity muscles may be severe, including flaccid paraplegia and marked respiratory muscle weakness.

glycocalyx a film composed of polysaccharides and bacteria that forms on the surface of artificial devices such as tracheal airways; glycocalyx seems to protect the bacteria from antibiotics and phagocytosis by macrophages.

gynecology the branch of medicine involved in the diagnosis and treatment of diseases of the female genital tract.

Haldane effect the influence of hemoglobin saturation with oxygen on CO_2 dissociation.

half-life the time necessary for a given quantity of matter to degrade to half its original amount or activity due to either physical events (such as radioactive decay) or physiologic phenomenon (such as metabolism or excretion); in pharmacology, half-life refers to how much time it takes the body to decrease a given concentration of a drug to half its initial level.

Hb common abbreviation for hemoglobin.

HbA abbreviation for hemoglobin A, or normal adult hemoglobin.

HbCO abbreviation for carboxyhemoglobin, hemoglobin saturated with carbon monoxide.

HCFA abbreviation for the federal Health Care Financing Administration, the division of the Department of Health and Human Services responsible for Medicare funding.

health a state of physical, mental, and social well being.

health education a process of planned learning opportunities designed to enable individuals to make informed decisions about and act to promote their health.

health maintenance organization (HMO) an organized system providing a comprehensive range of health care services to a voluntarily enrolled consumer population. In return for a prepaid, fixed fee, the enrollee is guaranteed a defined set of benefits. This fixed fee is usually the same for all members (enrollees) of the HMO regardless of the extent of services used.

health promotion that combination of educational, organization, economic, and environmental support necessary for behavior conducive to health; includes both disease prevention and wellness activities.

health services activities designed to maintain or improve health, including:

public health services health services conducted on a community basis, such as communicable disease control or the collection and analysis of health statistics.

environmental health services health services directed at controlling environmental factors associated with health or disease, such as air pollution control.

personal health services health services directed at individuals, including health promotion, illness prevention, diagnosis, treatment, and rehabilitation.

heat capacity the number of calories required to raise the temperature of 1 g of a substance 1°C (cgs) or 1 pound of a substance 1°F (fps); by definition, the heat capacity of water is 1 cal in the cgs system and 1 BTU in the fps system.

Heimlich maneuver an emergency procedure for dislodging a bolus of food or other obstruction from the trachea to prevent asphyxiation.

hematocrit a measure of the packed cell blood volume, obtained by centrifugation of a blood sample.

hematogenous originating or transported in the blood.

hematology the branch of medicine involved in the study of blood morphology, physiology, and pathology.

hematopoiesis the normal formation and development of blood cells in the bone marrow.

heme the pigmented iron-containing, nonprotein portion of the hemoglobin molecule.

hemidiaphragm pertaining to the left or right dome of the diaphragm.

hemithorax either the left or right side of the thorax.

hemizygos vein a large vein of the lower left thoracic wall that empties into the azygos vein (trunk connecting the superior and inferior vena cavae).

hemorrhage the escape of blood from the vascular system.

hemodialysis a procedure in which impurities or wastes are removed from the blood; used in treating renal insufficiency and various toxic conditions.

hemodynamic monitoring the bedside collection of data on the performance of the cardiovascular system, including the assessment of both cardiac and vascular parameters.

hemolysis rupture of the red blood cells.

hemolytic producing hemolysis.

hemoptysis coughing up of blood from the respiratory tract.

hemosiderosis an increased deposition of iron in a variety of tissues, usually in the form of hemosiderin and usually without tissue damage.

hemostasis the termination of bleeding by mechanic or chemical means or by the complex coagulation process of the body, consisting of vasoconstriction, platelet aggregation, and thrombin and fibrin synthesis.

hemothorax an accumulation of blood and fluid in the pleural cavity, between the parietal and visceral pleura, usually the result of trauma.

HEPA abbreviation for high efficiency particulate air, usually applied to air filtration devices capable of 99.99% efficacy on particulate matter down to 0.3 μm in size.

hepatomegaly abnormal enlargement of the liver.

Hering-Breuer reflex a parasympathetic inflation reflex mediated by the lung's stretch receptors that appears to influence the duration of the expiratory pause occurring between breaths.

herniation a protrusion of a body organ or portion of an organ through an abnormal opening in a membrane.

herpes any inflammatory disease caused by a herpesvirus, especially herpes zoster or herpes simplex.

heterogeneous not of uniform structure or composition.

hexachlorophene a topical bacteriocide and detergent.

Hg symbol for mercury.

HHA abbreviation for home health agency; a public or private provider of home health care services, usually regulated by state departments of health; HHAs can provide a broad range of services, including the provision of home health aides, nursing care, and rehabilitative personnel.

HHb symbol for reduced (deoxygenated) hemoglobin.

hiatal hernia the protrusion of any abdominal structure through the esophageal hiatus.

hierarchical of or pertaining to an organizational structure composed of graded levels or ranks.

high-frequency ventilation ventilatory support provided at rates significantly in excess of normal breathing frequencies; includes the following three approaches:

high-frequency positive pressure ventilation (HFPPV) high-frequency ventilation characterized by (1) ventilatory rates between 60 and 100/min, (2) I:E ratios of 1:3 or less, (3) constant pressure generation (decelerating inspiratory flow), (4) small tidal volumes, often approaching the anatomic deadspace, and (5) the maintenance of positive airway pressure but usually with intrapleural pressure remaining subatmospheric throughout the breathing cycle.

high frequency jet ventilation (HFJV) high-frequency ventilation characterized by the delivery of pulses of pressurized gas through a small percutaneous transtracheal catheter at rates between 100 and 200/min, as controlled by a pneumatic, electric, or mechanical valve assembly.

high-frequency oscillation (HFO) high-frequency ventilation characterized by extremely high rates (ranging up 3600/min), with "tidal volumes" in the 1.5 to 3.0 ml/kg range, as controlled by an eccentric wheel-driven piston, an audio loudspeaker, or a rotating flow interrupter.

hilum (also hilus) a depression in any organ where blood vessels and nerves enter or exit; especially as pertains to the "root" of the lung.

histoplasmosis an infection caused by inhalation of spores of the fungus *Histoplasma capsulatum.*

histotoxic poisonous to cells.

histotoxic hypoxia hypoxia caused by chemical poisoning of the cells, as by cyanide, which occurs in the presence of normal oxygen delivery to the tissues.

HIV abbreviation for the human immunodeficiency virus, the cause of AIDS.

HMO abbreviation for health maintenance organization.

holistic of or pertaining to the whole; in health care, a philosophy whereby the person is viewed in totality as a mental, physical, and emotional being interacting with the environment.

home health care the provision of health services in the home setting to aged, disabled, sick, or convalescent individuals who do not need institutional care.

homeostasis a relative constancy in the internal environment of the body, naturally maintained by adaptive responses that promote healthy survival.

homogeneous of uniform structure or composition.

HSA abbreviation for Health Systems Agency, an agency responsible for health planning activities at a local level.

humidity water in molecular vapor form; *absolute humidity* is a measure of the actual content or weight of water present in a given volume of air; *relative humidity* is the ratio of actual water vapor present in a gas to the capacity of the gas to hold the vapor at a given temperature.

humoral of or pertaining to the body fluids; used especially to denote physiologic activity occurring through chemical or biologic mediators in the body fluids (as opposed to neurologic stimulation).

hydrolysis the chemical alteration or decomposition of a compound with water.

hydrodynamics the branch of fluid physics involved in the study of fluids in motion.

hydronamic of or pertaining to a principle of aerosol generation in which a solution is distributed by gravity over a spherical surface from within which a pressurized gas source ruptures the overlying liquid film and disperses it as small particles.

hydronium ion the hydrated form of the hydrogen ion (H_3O^+).

hydrostatic of or pertaining to the physics of static fluids (as opposed to hydrodynamics).

hydroxyl ion a radical alkaline compound containing an oxygen atom and a hydrogen atom (OH^-).

hygrometer an instrument for measuring relative humidity.

hyoid bone a bone located near the base of the tongue that is suspended from the styloid processes of the temporal bones of the skull.

hyperalimentation overfeeding or the ingestion or administration of a greater than optimal amount of nutrients in excess of the demands of the appetite.

hyperbaric oxygenation the therapeutic application of oxygen at pressures greater than 1 atm (760 mm Hg).

hyperbasemia the abnormal presence of an excess of total buffer base in the blood; a base excess (BE) greater than 2.0.

hyperbilirubinemia greater than normal amounts of the bile pigment bilirubin in the blood, often characterized by jaundice, anorexia, and malaise (normal blood levels for total bilirubin range from 0.2 to 0.9 mg/dl).

hypercalcemia greater than normal amounts of calcium in the blood, most often resulting from excessive bone resorption and release of calcium, as occurs in hyperparathyroidism, metastatic tumors of bone, Paget's disease, and osteoporosis (normal serum calcium levels range from 8.5 to 10.5 mg/L or 4.25 to 5.25 mEq/L).

hypercapnia the abnormal presence of excess amounts of carbon dioxide in the blood (in arterial blood, a P_{CO_2} greater than 45 mm Hg).

hyperchloremia an excessive level of chloride in the blood (normal serum levels of chloride range between 96 and 105 mEq/L).

hyperextension a position of maximum extension.

hyperinflation a condition of maximum inflation; as pertaining to artificial ventilatory support, the application of volumes greater than normal to reinflate collapsed alveoli.

hyperkalemia greater than normal amounts of potassium in the blood (normal serum potassium concentrations range from 3.5 to 5.0 mEq/L).

hypernatremia greater than normal concentration of sodium in the blood, caused by excessive loss of water and electrolytes owing to polyuria, diarrhea, excessive sweating, or inadequate water intake (normal serum concentration of sodium ranges from 135 to 145 mEq/L).

hyperosmolarity a state of condition of abnormally increased osmolarity in the blood or body fluids (normal blood osmolarity ranges from 285 to 295 mOsm/L).

hyperoxia a condition of abnormally high oxygen tension in the blood.

hyperoxygenation the application of oxygen concentrations in excess of those needed to maintain adequate oxygenation to prevent hypoxemia during certain procedures such as suctioning.

hyperphosphatemia greater than normal concentration of phosphate ions in the blood (normal serum levels of phosphate range from (1.2 to 2.3 mEq/L, or 2.0 to 4.5 mg/dl, with higher values in children).

hyperplasia an increase in the size of a tissue or organ due to a growth in the *number* of cells present.

hyperplastic of or pertaining to a condition of hyperplasia.

hyperpnea deep breathing.

hyperpyrexia an extremely elevated temperature sometimes occurring in acute infectious diseases, especially in young children.

hyperreactivity a condition characterized by greater than normal response to stimuli.

hyperreflexia a condition characterized by exaggerated reflex responses.

hypersensitivity of or pertaining to a tendency of the immune system to exhibit an excessive or exaggerated response against environmental antigens that are not normally harmful.

hypersomnolence a condition characterized by pathologically excessive drowsiness or sleep.

hypertension persistently high blood pressure.

hyperthyroidism a condition characterized by hyperactivity of the thyroid gland.

hypertonic having a greater concentration of solute than another solution, hence exerting more osmotic pressure than that solution, as a hypertonic saline solution that contains more salt than is found in intracellular and extracellular fluid.

hypertrophy an increase in the size of a tissue or organ due to a growth in the size of cells present.

hyperventilation ventilation in excess of that necessary to meet metabolic needs; signified by a P_{CO_2} less than 35 mm Hg in the arterial blood.

hypervolemia an increase in the amount of extracellular fluid, particularly in the volume of circulating blood or its components.

hypnotic a drug or chemical agent that induces sleep.

hypobarism of or pertaining to the effects of exposure to pressures less than those normally encountered at sea level; often used to refer to high-altitude sickness.

hypobasemia the abnormal presence of a deficit of total buffer base in the blood; a negative base excess (BE) greater than -2.0.

hypocalcemia a deficiency of calcium in the serum that may be caused by hypoparathyroidism, vitamin D deficiency, kidney failure, acute pancreatitis, or inadequate plasma magnesium and protein (normal serum calcium levels range from 8.5 to 10.5 mg/L or 4.25 to 5.25 mEq/L).

hypocapnia the presence of lower than normal amounts of carbon dioxide in the blood (in arterial blood, a P_{CO_2} less than 35 mm Hg).

hypochloremia a decrease in the chloride level in the blood serum below the normal range (normal serum levels of chloride range between 96 and 105 mEq/L).

hypoglycemia a less-than-normal amount of glucose in the blood, usually caused by administration of too much insulin, excessive secretion of insulin by the islet cells of the pancreas or by dietary deficiency (normal blood glucose levels range from 70 to 110 mg/dl).

hypokalemia a condition in which an inadequate amount of potassium, the major intracellular cation, is found in the circulating bloodstream (normal serum potassium concentrations range from 3.5 to 5.0 mEq/L).

hyponatremia a less than normal concentration of sodium in the blood, caused by inadequate excretion of water or by excessive water in the circulating bloodstream (normal serum concentration of sodium range from 135 to 145 mEq/L).

hypopharynx the lowest portion of the pharynx, just above the larynx (also called the laryngopharynx).

hypopnea shallow breathing.

hypotension an abnormal condition in which the blood pressure is not adequate for normal perfusion and oxygenation of the tissues.

hypothalamus a portion of the brain lying beneath the thalamus and at the base of the cerebrum; responsible for temperature regulation, certain behavioral functions, and the secretory activities of the pituitary gland.

hypothermia an abnormal and dangerous condition in which the temperature of the body is below 32°C, usually owing to prolonged exposure to cold.

hypothyroidism a condition characterized by decreased activity of the thyroid gland.

hypotonia a condition characterized by decreased muscle tone or strength.

hypoventilation ventilation less than that necessary to meet metabolic needs; signified by a P_{CO_2} greater than 45 mm Hg in the arterial blood.

hypovolemia an abnormally low circulating blood volume.

hypoxemia an abnormal deficiency of oxygen in the arterial blood.

hypoxia an abnormal condition in which the oxygen available to the body cells is inadequate to meet their metabolic needs.

hysteresis the failure of two associated phenomena to coincide, as in the observed difference between the inflation and deflation volume-pressure curves of the lung.

iatrogenic caused by treatment or diagnostic procedures.

ICP abbreviation for intracranial pressure.

IEEE abbreviation for the Institute of Electrical and Electronic Engineers (IEEE) a voluntary group responsible, in part, for developing standards related to electrical devices and equipment, including those used in respiratory care.

I:E ratio the ratio of inspiratory to expiratory time during mechanical ventilation; by convention, the ratio is always reduced so that the numerator (inspiratory time) equals 1, e.g., 1:4 or 1:2.5.

ileus an obstruction of the intestines, as in a dynamic ileus caused by immobility of the bowel or a mechanical ileus in which the intestine is blocked by mechanical means.

immunocompromised immunodeficient.

immunodeficient of or pertaining to a condition in which a patient's cellular or humoral immunity is inadequate and resistance to infection is decreased.

immunofluorescence a technique used for the rapid identification of an antigen by exposing it to known antibodies tagged with the fluorescent dye fluorescein and observing the characteristic antigen-antibody reaction of precipitation.

immunoglobin (immunoglobulin) any five structurally and antigenically distinct antibodies present in the serum and external secretions of the body, formed in response to specific antigens.

immunosuppressed of or pertaining to the purposeful administration of agents designed to interfere with the ability of the immune system to respond to antigenic stimulation.

impedance (electrical) a form of electrical resistance observed in an alternating circuit expressed as the ratio of voltage applied to current produced.

impedance (mechanical) the force opposing movement in a mechanical system; as applied to ventilatory mechanics, the sum of the resistive and elastic forces opposing inflation.

IMV abbreviation for intermittent mandatory ventilation; periodic ventilation with positive pressure, with the patient breathing spontaneously between breaths. These periodic breaths may be controlled (control mode IMV) or assisted, as with synchronous intermittent mandatory ventilation, or SIMV.

inadvertent accidental or unintentional.

incisura a cut, notch, indentation, or depression; often used to refer to the dicrotic notch observed on the tracing of arterial blood pressure.

incoherent unable to think or express one's thoughts in a clear manner.

indwelling located inside the body; commonly refers to invasive diagnostic or therapeutic devices.

inert not taking part in chemical reactions; not pharmacologically active.

infarction the development and formation of a localized area of tissue necrosis.

infiltrate a fluid that passes through body tissues.

influenza an acute, usually self-limiting infectious viral disorder that produces fever, myalgia, headache, and malaise.

infrared (light) electromagnetic radiation with wavelengths between 10^{-5} and 10^{-4} m; infrared radiation is perceived as heat when it strikes the body.

inguinal of or pertaining to the groin.

inherent rhythmicity the unique ability of cardiac muscle to originate an electrical impulse spontaneously; also called automaticity.

innominate without a name; commonly refers to the innominate artery, also called the brachiocephalic trunk.

inoculum a substance introduced into the body to cause or to increase immunity to a specific disease or condition.

inotropic pertaining to the force or energy of muscular contractions, particularly contractions of the heart muscle.

insensible water loss the loss of body fluids by means other than through the urinary system, gastrointestinal tract, or sweating; includes evaporative water loss through the lungs and skin.

in-service education a program of education or training occurring at the work site and provided for employees, usually based on the needs of the employing institution.

in situ in the natural or usual place.

insomnia inability to sleep.

inspiratory capacity (IC) the maximum amount of air that can be inhaled from the resting end-expiratory level or FRC; the sum of the tidal volume and inspiratory reserve volume.

inspiratory reserve volume (IRV) the maximum volume of air that can be inhaled following a normal quiet inspiration.

inspiratory resistive breathing a therapeutic technique in which additional workload is imposed on the inspiratory muscles (mainly the diaphragm) during breathing to increase both the strength and endurance of these muscles.

inspissated (of a fluid) thickened or hardened through the absorption or evaporation of the liquid portion, as can occur with respiratory secretion when the upper airway is bypassed.

insufflation blowing of a gas or powder into a tube, cavity, or organ to allow visual examination, to remove an obstruction, or to apply medication.

intercartilaginous of or pertaining to the space between cartilages; especially the space between the costal cartilages.

intercellular between or among cells.

intercostal of or pertaining to the space between two ribs.

interdisciplinary pertaining to the relationship between two or more disciplines.

intermammary between the mammary glands or breasts.

interosseous of or pertaining to the space between two bones.

interpersonal between persons; usually refers to a communication context.

interphase between phases; the metabolic stage in the cell cycle during which the cell is not dividing; also the "dividing line" between two states of matter.

interstitial of or pertaining to the interstitium.

interstitium the extracellular space.

interventricular of or pertaining to the space between the ventricles of the heart.

intervertebral of or pertaining to the space between any two vertebrae, as the fibrocartilaginous disks.

intra-abdominal within the abdomen.

intra-alveolar within the alveoli.

intra-aortic balloon counterpulsation a circulatory support technique in which a balloon placed in the aorta is synchronously inflated during diastole to increase mean aortic pressures and coronary blood flow to the myocardium.

intrabursal within the bursa; often used to refer to the synovial fluid "sack."

intracardiac within the heart.

intracellular within cells.

intracranial with the cranium.

intractable having no relief, as a symptom or disease that remains unrelieved despite the application of therapeutic measures.

intramuscular within a muscle; used commonly to refer to an injection method whereby a hypodermic needle is introduced into a muscle to administer a medication.

intraoperative within or during a surgical procedure.

intrapartum of or pertaining to the period commencing from the onset of labor to the completion of the third stage of labor (expulsion of the placenta).

intrapersonal within one's self.

intrapleural within the pleural "space."

intrapulmonary within the lungs.

intrathoracic within the thorax.

intrauterine within the uterus.

intravascular within a blood vessel or in the vascular fluid compartment.

intubation the passage of a tube into a body aperture; commonly refers to the insertion of an endotracheal tube within the trachea.

in utero in the uterus.

invasive characterized by a tendency to spread or infiltrate; also refers to the use of diagnostic or therapeutic methods requiring access to the inside of the body.

in vitro (of a biologic reaction) occurring in a laboratory apparatus.

in vivo (of a biologic reaction) occurring in a living organism.

I/O abbreviation for intake and output; the recording of a patient's fluid intake and output.

iodophor an antiseptic or disinfectant that combines iodine with another agent.

IPPB abbreviation for intermittent positive pressure breathing; the application of inspiratory positive pressure, usually with accompanying humidity or aerosol therapy, to a spontaneously breathing patient as a short-term treatment modality, usually for periods not exceeding 15 to 20 minutes.

IPPV abbreviation for intermittent positive pressure ventilation (refer to CMV).

iridium a silvery bluish metallic element, the radioactive form of which (Ir 192) is used in endobronchial radiotherapy.

ischemia a localized reductions in perfusion to a body organ or part, often marked by pain and organ dysfunction, as in ischemic heart disease.

isoelectric of or pertaining to a condition of electrical neutrality; also refers to the electric baseline of an electrocardiogram.

isoelectric point the pH at which an electrolytic compound is dissociated into an equal number of positively and negatively charged ions.

isolation protocols infection control measures that combine barrier-type precautions (including handwashing and the use of gloves, masks, or gowns) with the physical separation of infected patients in specific disease categories to disrupt transmission of pathogenic microorganisms.

isomer a chemical compound with the exact same molecular formula as another, but with a different geometric structure.

isopleth a line on a two dimensional x-y graph denoting the relationship to a third variable.

isothermal a process of gas compression or expansion in which the gas temperature remains constant; to maintain a constant gas temperature, the First Law of Thermodynamics dictates that heat energy must be either added (during expansion) or taken away (during compression) to maintain the energy equilibrium; compare with adiabatic.

isotonic (of a solution) having the same concentration of solute as another solution, hence exerting the same amount of osmotic pressure as that solution, as with an isotonic saline solution that contains an amount of salt equal to that found in the extracellular fluid.

isovolumic having the same volume.

IT abbreviation for implantation tested; as applied to invasive devices, indicates that the materials used have been shown to be nontoxic to living tissue.

IV abbreviation for intravenous.

jargon the special technical language and terms of a particular field or profession.

JCAH abbreviation for Joint Commission on Accreditation of Hospitals, predecessor to the Joint Commission on Accreditation of Healthcare Organizations (JCAHO).

JCAHO abbreviation for the Joint Commission on Accreditation of Healthcare Organizations, a private, voluntary association that establishes standards for accrediting institutions and agencies responsible for health care delivery.

Joule-Thompson effect a physical phenomenon in which the rapid expansion of a gas without the application of external work causes a substantial drop in the temperature of the gas; used in the liquefaction of air for the production of oxygen and nitrogen.

JRCRTE abbreviation for the Joint Review Committee for Respiratory Therapy Education; the JRCRTE, in collaboration with the Committee on Allied Health Education and Accreditation, establishes standards for and oversees the accreditation of educational programs in respiratory care.

juxtamedullary situated near the medulla.

Kelvin scale the SI temperature scale, with a zero point equivalent to absolute zero. The Kelvin scale has 100 degrees between the measured freezing and boiling points of water and is therefore considered a centigrade system of temperature measurement. Because $0°K = -273°C$, $°K = °C + 273$.

ketoacidosis a metabolic acidosis due to the accumulation of excess ketones in the body, resulting from faulty carbohydrate metabolism, as can occur in certain forms of diabetes.

kg abbreviation for kilogram.

kinetic energy the energy a body possesses through its motion.

Korotkoff sound sounds heard during the taking of blood pressure using a sphygmomanometer and stethoscope.

kymograph graphic recording motions of body organs, as of the heart and the great blood vessels.

kyphoscoliosis an abnormal condition characterized by an anteroposterior *and* lateral curvature of the spine.

kyphosis an abnormal condition of the vertebral column, characterized by increased anteroposterior convex curvature of the thoracic spine.

lamina propria a layer of connective tissue that lies just under the epithelium of the mucous membrane.

laminar of or pertaining to laminae or layers; specifically refers to a pattern of flow consisting of concentric layers of fluid flowing parallel to the tube wall at linear velocities that increase toward the center.

laparotomy any surgical incision into the peritoneal cavity, usually performed under general or regional anesthesia, often on a exploratory basis.

laryngectomy a surgical removal of the larynx, performed to treat cancer of the larynx.

laryngitis inflammation of the larynx.

laryngoscope an endoscope for examining the larynx.

laryngoscopy the process of viewing the larynx with a laryngoscope.

laryngospasm an involuntary contraction of the laryngeal muscles resulting in complete or partial closure of the glottis.

laryngotracheobronchitis an inflammation of the larynx, trachea, and large bronchi that can result in hoarseness, a nonproductive cough, and dyspnea.

laryngotranchitis inflammation of the larynx and trachea.

Lasix see furosemide.

lassitude weariness, fatigue, or listlessness.

latent heat of fusion the additional heat energy needed to effect the changeover of a substance from it solid to its liquid form.

latent heat of vaporization the heat energy required to vaporize a liquid at its boiling point.

lateral away from the body midline; situated on the side.

lateral decubitus a side-lying position (either left or right).

lavage the washing or irrigation of an organ, such as the stomach or lung.

lb abbreviation for pound, the fps system unit of force (and weight at sea level).

LC circuit a direct current electrical circuit consisting of an inductance coil (L) and a capacitor (C) in series.

Legionellosis an acute bacterial pneumonia caused by infection with *Legionella pneumophila* and characterized by an influenzalike illness followed within a week by high fever, chills, muscle aches, and headache.

length of stay (LOS) a measure pertaining to the number of elapsed days between a patient's admission and discharge from an inpatient health care facility.

lesion a general term referring to any injury or pathologic change in body tissue.

lethicin a general term referring to one of a complex class of lipids derived from phosphatidic acid (also called phosphatidyl cholines); the lecithins represent a major lipid constituent of tissues.

leukocyte a white blood cell, one of the formed elements of the circulating blood system.

leukocytopenia an abnormal decrease in the white blood cells (usually fewer than 5000 cells/ml).

leukocytosis an abnormal increase in the number of circulating white blood cells.

LGA abbreviation for large for gestational age; of or pertaining to newborns whose body weight falls above the 90th percentile for their gestational age.

liability a legal obligation or responsibility.

licensure the granting of permission by a competent authority (usually a governmental agency) to an organization or individual to engage in a specific practice or activity.

life span the full scope or period of one's life.

lifestyle the pattern of behavior characterizing one's way of living.

ligate to tie off a blood vessel or duct with a suture or wire ligature performed to stop or prevent bleeding during surgery, to stop spontaneous or traumatic hemorrhage, or to prevent passage of material through a duct, as in tubal ligation or to treat varicosites.

lingula a division of the left upper lobe of the lung, corresponding developmentally to the right middle lobe.

lipid any of a class of greasy organic substances insoluble in water but soluble in alcohol, chloroform, ether, and other solvents.

lipoprotein a conjugated protein in which lipids form an integral part of the molecule.

liquefication the conversion of a substance into its liquid form; also called liquefaction.

lobectomy a type of chest surgery in which a lobe of a lung is excised, performed to remove a malignant tumor and to treat uncontrolled bronchiectasis, trauma with hemorrhage, or intractable tuberculosis.

lobule literally a small lobe; in pulmonary anatomy may refer to the primary lobule or terminal respiratory unit of the lung (also called the acinus) or the secondary lobule; the secondary lobule is the smallest gross anatomic unit of lung tissue set apart by true connective tissue septa and corresponds to clusters of from three to five primary lobules.

long-term care the provision of medical, social, or personal care services on a recurring or continuing basis to persons with chronic physical or mental disorders.

lordotic of or pertaining to a radiographic position in which the patient stands with his or her back toward the film and leans backward, such that only the shoulders, neck, and head touch the film; this positions the x-ray beam at an angle ideal for viewing the lung apices without obstruction by the normally superimposed shadows of the clavicles.

lumen a cavity within any organ or structure of the body or a channel in a tube or catheter.

lung abscess an inflammatory lesion resulting in necrosis of lung tissue and associated with one or more of the following: suppression of the cough reflex, aspiration of infected material, bronchial obstruction, pneumonias, ischemia (as with pulmonary infarction), or blood sepsis.

lupus erythromatosus a chronic, superficial inflammation of the skin in which reddish lesions or macules up to 3 to 4 cm spread over the body.

LVEDP abbreviation for left ventricular end-diastolic pressure.

lymphadenopathy of or pertaining to and disease of the lymph nodes; refers also to the visualization of enlarged lymph nodes on x-ray film.

lymphoid resembling lymph tissue.

lymphokine one of the chemical factors produced and released by T lymphocytes that attract macrophages to the site of infection or inflammation and prepare them for attack.

lymphoma a neoplasm of lymphoid tissue that is usually malignant but, in rare cases, may be benign.

lysis of or pertaining to the process of decomposition.

m abbreviation for meter, the standard unit of length in the SI measurement system.

macrophage any phagocytic cell of the reticuloendothelial system, including Kupffer's cell in the liver, splenocyte in the spleen, and histocyte in the loose connective tissue.

mainstem of or pertaining to the first branching or generation of the tracheobronchial tree.

malignant tending to become worse; as applied to tumors, having the property of metastasis.

malposition literally "bad position"; in an abnormal place or not positioned where intended.

manifold a pipe with many connections; in medical gas storage, a collection of gas cylinders linked together for purposes of bulk storage and usually including at least one reserve bank and other safety systems, such as low-pressure alarms.

manubrium one of the three bones of the sternum, presenting a broad quadrangular shape that narrows caudally at its articulation with the superior end of the body of the sternum.

MAO abbreviation for monoamine oxidase, an enzyme that catalyzes the oxidation of amines.

MAO inhibitor any of a chemically heterogeneous group of drugs used primarily in the treatment of depression or anxiety and sometimes hypertension; MAO inhibitors may interact with a variety of foods and indirect-acting adrenergics like ephedrine, causing severe hypertensive episodes.

maxilla one of a pair of large bones that form the upper jaw, consisting of a pyramidal body and four processes: the sygomatic, frontal, alveolar, and palatine.

maxillary of or pertaining to the maxilla, or upper jaw.

maxillofacial of or pertaining to the upper jaw, nose, and cheek.

maximum inspiratory force (MIF) a measure of the output of the inspiratory muscles against a maximum stimulus, as measured in cm H_2O negative pressure; maximum stimulus is provided either by total occlusion of the airway or by preventing inspiratory gas flow; also known as the negative inspiratory force (NIF) or maximum inspiratory pressure (P_{Imax}).

MDC abbreviation for major diagnostic category, a grouping of DRGs used for diagnostic classification and reimbursement under Medicare; for example, major diagnostic category #4 includes disorders of the respiratory system.

MDI abbreviation for metered dose inhaler, a pressurized cartridge used for self-administration of exact dosages of aerosolized drugs.

meatus an opening or tunnel through any part of the body, as the meati formed by the turbinates or concha in the nasal cavity.

mechanoreceptor any sensory nerve ending that responds to mechanical stimuli, as touch, pressure, sound, and muscular contractions.

meconium a material that collects in the intestines of a fetus and forms the first stools of a newborn.

medial situated or oriented toward the midline of the body.

mediastinum a portion of the thoracic cavity lying in the middle of the thorax (between the two pleural cavities) and containing the trachea, esophagus, heart, and great vessels of the circulatory system.

medulla the most internal part of an organ or structure; *medulla oblongata*:the bulbous portion of the spinal cord just above the foramen magnum and separated from the pons by a horizontal groove, containing the cardiac, respiratory and vasomotor "centers"; *adrenal medulla:* the inner portion of the adrenal gland, responsible for producing epinephrine and norepinephrine.

mEq abbreviation for milliequivalent.

mesencephalon one of the three parts of the brain stem, lying just below the cerebrum and just above the pons.

mesenteric of or pertaining to the mesentery, a broad fan-shaped fold of peritoneum connecting the jejunum and ileum with the dorsal wall of the abdomen.

mesothelioma a rare malignant tumor of the mesothelium of the pleura or peritoneum, associated with earlier exposure to asbestos.

mesothelium a layer of cells that lines the body cavities of the embryo and continues as a layer of squamous epithelial cells covering the serous membranes of the adult.

metacommunication the use of nonverbal communication to enhance, reinforce, or contradict verbal messages.

metaphase the second of the four stages of nuclear division in mitosis and in each of the two divisions of meiosis, during which the chromosomes become arranged in the equatorial plane of the spindle to form the equatorial plate, with the centromeres attached to the spindle fibers in preparation for separation.

metastasis the process by which tumor cells are spread to distant parts of the body.

methemoglobin a form of hemoglobin in which the iron component has been oxidized from the ferrous to the ferric state, due most commonly to nitrite poisoning or ingestion of an oxidizing agent, such as aniline, paraaminosalicylic acid, or phenylhydrazine; since methemoglobin cannot carry oxygen, its presence reduces the oxygen-carrying capacity of the blood (see methemoglobinemia).

methemoglobinemia an abnormal condition characterized by high levels of methemoglobin in the blood and a resulting reduction in oxygen-carrying capacity; may be caused by nitrite poisoning or ingestion of certain oxidizing agents or a genetic defect in the enzyme NADH methemoglobin reductase (an autosomal dominant trait).

methylene blue a bluish green crystalline substance used as a histologic stain and as a laboratory indicator; also used to test the integrity of protective upper airway reflexes in patients being considered for extubation.

methylxanthine a category of naturally occurring drug agents including caffeine, theophylline, and theobromine that exert a broad range of physiologic effects, including CNS stimulation, myocardial stimulation, smooth muscle relaxation, and diuresis; used commonly in respiratory care as bronchodilators because of their inhibitory effect on phosphodiesterase.

METS abbreviation for the multiple equivalents of resting O_2 consumption, a indirect measure of physiologic work performed during exercise and stress testing.

MHz abbreviation for megahertz, a unit of frequency equivalent to 1000 cycles per second (cps).

microaerosol an extremely fine aerosol of uniform and small particle size produced by sequential baffling and characterized by mass median diameters that are generally less than 1.0 μm.

microampere a unit of electrical current equivalent to 1/1000 ampere (an ampere in the current produced by 1 volt applied across a resistance of 1 Ohm).

microatelectasis localized or focal atelectasis that may not manifest itself on radiographic examination.

microelectrode a miniature electrode, often small enough to be placed within a tissue cell.

microembolization embolization due to extremely small blood-born particles, usually smaller than that visible with the naked eye.

micrognathia underdevelopment of the jaw, especially the mandible.

midaxillary of or pertaining to the imaginary line drawn vertically downward from the middle of the axilla.

midclavicular of or pertaining to the imaginary line drawn vertically downward from the middle of the clavicle.

midline an imaginary line that divides the body into right and left halves.

midscapular of or pertaining to the imaginary line drawn vertically downward from the middle of the scapula.

midsternal of or pertaining to the imaginary line vertically bisecting the sternum.

MIF abbreviation for maximum inspiratory force, or the negative pressure generated during a maximally forced inspiratory effort against an obstruction to flow; also called negative inspiratory force (NIF) and maximum inspiratory pressure (P_{Imax}).

milliequivalent (mEq) a quantitative amount of a reacting substance that has a specific chemical combining power; the milligram equivalent weight of a substance is calculated as its gram atomic (or formula) weight divided by its valence $\times$ 0.001; a milliequivalent also represents the number of grams of solute dissolved in 1 ml of a normal solution.

millimole a SI unit of matter equal to 1/1000 of a mole (a mole is any quantity of matter that contains 6.023×10^{23} atoms, molecules, or ions).

millisecond (msec) one thousandth of a second.

millivolt (mV) one thousandth of a volt.

minute ventilation ($\dot{V}E$) the total amount of gas moving out of the lungs during a minute.

mitochondria small, rodlike, granular organelles within the cellular cytoplasm that function in cellular metabolism and respiration.

mitosis the process whereby a cell normally replicate itself, forming two daughter cells, each with the same number of chromosomes as the parent cell.

ml abbreviation for milliliter, or 1/1000 L.

MLT abbreviation for minimal leak technique, a method for determining the cuff inflation volume on endotracheal tubes; during MLT, air is slowly injected into the cuff until the leak stops; once a seal is obtained, a small amount of air is removed, allowing a slight leak at peak inflation pressure; because this leak occurs during the application of positive pressure, pharyngeal secretions tend to be blown upward at peak inflation, minimizing the likelihood of aspiration; see MOV for an alternative approach.

mM abbreviation for millimole.

MMV abbreviation for mandatory minute ventilation, a mode of ventilatory support that ensures delivery of a preset minimum minute volume, with the patient allowed to breathe spontaneously; should the patient meet the preset $\dot{V}E$ entirely by spontaneous effort, a ventilator in the MMV mode will remain passive, delivering no positive pressure breaths; on the other hand, should the patient's spontaneous $\dot{V}E$ fall below the preset MMV minimum, a ventilator operating in this mode will provide the mechanical support necessary to ensure that the minimum minute ventilation goal is achieved.

molal solution a solution containing 1 mole of solute per kilogram of solvent (or 1 mmol/g of solvent).

molar solution a solution containing 1 mole of solute/l of solution (or 1 mmol/ml of solution).

mole the SI unit of matter equal containing 6.023×10^{23} atoms, molecules, or ions.

morbidity the state of being ill; in statistics, the ratio of those ill to those who are well.

morphologic of or pertaining to morphology; structural.

morphology the study of structures and forms in living things.

morphometry the actual process of measuring the form of living things.

mortality the number of deaths per unit population in any specific age group, disease category, etc.

mottling a condition of spotting with patches of color.

MOV abbreviation for minimal occluding volume; the minimum endotracheal tube cuff pressure needed to prevent gas leakage during a positive pressure inspiration.

msec abbreviation for millisecond.

MSVC abbreviation for maximum sustainable ventilatory capacity.

mucociliary of or pertaining to ciliated mucosa.

mucoid resembling mucus.

mucokinesis "the process of moving mucus"; usually pertains to therapeutic methods designed to facilitate the removal of excess or abnormal secretion of the respiratory tract.

mucolysis the breaking down of mucus; usually refers to chemical degradation of mucopolysaccharide by certain drug agents called mucolytics.

mucolytic a drug agent capable of mucolysis.

mucopolysaccharide any one of a group of polysaccharides containing hexosamine and being the chief constituent of normal mucus.

mucoprotein a compound, present in all connective and supporting tissue, that contains polysaccharides combined with protein and is relatively resistant to denaturation.

mucopurulent characteristic of a combination of mucus and pus.

mucosa a general terms referring to any mucous membrane.

multicompetent of or pertaining to an individual skilled in more than one area or discipline, such as a respiratory care practitioner who is also skilled in basic radiography.

multidimensional having more than one dimension or form.

multidisciplinary consisting of or involving more than one discipline.

multifocal an action, such as the transmission of an electrical impulse, that arises from more than two foci.

muscarinic of or pertaining to the effect of acetylcholine on the parasympathetic postganglionic effector sites (eg, smooth muscle, cardiac muscle, exocrine glands).

muscular dystrophy a general term applying to a group of hereditary disorders characterized by progressive degeneration of the skeletal muscles, resulting in severe muscle weakness.

mV abbreviation for millivolt.

myalgia diffuse muscle pain, usually accompanied by malaise, occurring in many diseases.

myasthenia gravis an abnormal condition characterized by the chronic fatigability and weakness of skeletal muscles, especially those of the face, throat, and respiratory system, and arising as a result of a defect in the conduction of nerve impulses at the myoneural junction.

mycelium a mass of interwoven, branched, threadlike filaments that make up most fungi.

Mycobacteria acid-fast microorganisms belonging to the genus *Mycobacterium.*

Mycoplasma a genus of ultramicroscopic pleomorphic organisms that lack rigid cell walls, grow on artificial media but do not retain gram stain, and are able to pass through bacterial filters; *Mycoplasma pneumoniae* is the primary pathogen in this genera, causing primary atypical pneumonia.

mycoses any disease caused by fungi.

myocarditis an inflammatory condition of the myocardium caused by viral, bacterial, or fungal infection; serum sickness; rheumatic fever; or chemical agents or as a complication of a collagen disease.

myocardial infarction occlusion of a coronary artery resulting in distal myocardial tissue necrosis, often accompanied by significant complications.

myocardium the thick, contractile, middle layer of muscle cells that forms the bulk of the heart wall.

myoneural of or pertaining to the junction between an efferent motor nerve and the muscle it innervates.

myopathy an abnormal condition of skeletal muscle characterized by muscle weakness, wasting, and histologic changes within muscle tissue, as seen in any of the muscular dystrophies.

myositis inflammation of muscle tissue, usually of the voluntary muscles.

myxedema a severe form of hypothyroidism characterized by dry swelling and abnormal deposits of mucin in the tissues.

myxoma a connective tissue neoplasm that often grows to enormous size.

nanomole (nM) one-billionth (10^{-9}) mole.

naris the pair of anterior and posterior openings in the nose that allow the passage of air from the nose to the pharynx.

nasal flaring dilation of the alar nasi on inspiration; an early sign of an increase in ventilatory demands and the work of breathing, especially in infants.

nasogastric of or pertaining the passageway from the nose to the stomach; usually applied to tubes or catheters placed in the stomach through the nose.

nasopharynx one of the three regions of the throat, situated behind the nose and extending from the posterior nares to the larynx.

nasotracheal of or pertaining the passageway from the nose to the trachea; usually applied to tubes or catheters placed in the trachea through the nose, such as a nasotracheal tube, or nasotracheal suctioning.

NBRC abbreviation for the National Board for Respiratory Care, Inc., the national credentialing agency for respiratory care practitioners and pulmonary function technologists.

nebulizer a device that produces an aerosol suspension of liquid particles in a gaseous medium using baffling to control particle size.

necrosis local tissue death due to disease or injury.

necrotizing of or pertaining to a process that produces necrosis.

NEEP acronym for negative end-expiratory pressure.

negative end-expiratory pressure (NEEP) the application of subatmospheric pressure to the airway during the expiratory phase of positive pressure ventilation.

negative feedback control mechanism a mechanical, electrical, or physiologic control mechanism in which feedback to a sensor or receptor evokes an opposite response from an effector mechanism, so that a balance in a parameter can be maintained.

neonatal pertaining to the period between birth and 28 days of age.

neoplasia the new and abnormal development of cells that may be benign or malignant.

neoplasm an abnormal growth of new tissue, either benign or malignant.

neoplastic of or pertaining to a neoplasm.

nephron a structural and functional unit of the kidney, resembling a microscopic funnel with a long stem and two convoluted sections.

nephrotoxic toxic or destructive to a kidney.

neuroeffector a chemical or electrical stimulus that causes nerve cell depolarization.

neurogenic originating in the nervous system.

neurologic of or pertaining to neurology or the nervous system.

neuromuscular of or pertaining to the muscles and nerves.

neuropathy any abnormal condition characterized by inflammation and degeneration of the peripheral nerves.

neurosurgery any surgery involving the brain, spinal cord, or peripheral nerves.

neutral thermal environment an ambient environment that prevents or minimizes the loss of body heat.

neutropenia an abnormal decrease in the number of neutrophils in the blood.

Newton (N) the SI unit of force, equivalent to 1 kg $\times$ m/sec^2.

NFPA abbreviation for the National Fire Protection Association, a voluntary nongovernmental agency involved in improved methods of fire protection and prevention, including creating standards for the storage of flammable and oxidizing gases.

nicotinic of or pertaining to the effect of acetylcholine at the parasympathetic and sympathetic ganglionic or somatic skeletal muscles receptor sites.

nitrite an ester or salt of nitrous acid, used as a vasodilator and antispasmodic, particularly in angina pectoris; common examples are amyl nitrite and sodium nitrite.

nM abbreviation for nanomole.

nocardiosis infection with *Nocardia asteroides,* an aerobic gram-positive species of actinomycetes, characterized by pneumonia, often with cavitation, and by chronic abscesses in the brain and subcutaneous tissues.

nocturia excessive urination at night.

nomogram a graphic representation of a numeric relationship.

nonflammable not capable of combustion.

noninvasive pertaining to a diagnostic or therapeutic technique that does not require the skin to be broken or a cavity or organ of the body to be entered, as obtaining a blood pressure reading by auscultation with a stethoscope and sphygmomanometer.

nonjudgmental tending not to draw judgments about others.

nonmotile not capable of movement; stationary.

nonporous literally "without pores"; not permeable to liquids or gases.

nonresectable not removable by surgery.

normal solution (N) a solution containing 1 g equivalent weight of solute per liter of solution (or 1 mEq/ml of solution).

normocapnia a state characterized by a normal partial pressure of carbon dioxide in the arterial blood (35 to 45 mm Hg).

nosocomial pertaining to or originating in a hospital, as a nosocomial infection.

not for profit an activity in which any excess of expenses over revenue is reinvested into the operation, rather than being distributed to owners or shareholders; compare to for profit.

nuchal of or pertaining to the nape or back of the neck.

nucleoprotein protein combined with a nucleic acid and originating in the cell nucleus.

nucleotide any one of the compounds into which nucleic acid is split by the action of nuclease.

nursing home an institution with an organized professional staff and permanent facilities, including inpatient beds, that provides continuous nursing and other health-related, psychological, and personal services to patients who are not in an acute phase of illness but who primarily require continued care on an inpatient basis.

obliterate to remove or destroy.

obstetrics the branch of medicine concerned with pregnancy and childbirth.

obstructive sleep apnea (OSA) a condition in which five or more apneic periods (of at least 10 seconds each) occur per hour of sleep and are characterized by occlusion of the oropharyngeal airway with continued efforts to breath.

obtunded insensitive to pain or other stimuli due to a reduced level of consciousness.

obturator a device used to block a passage or a canal or to fill in a space, as the obturator used to inset a tracheostomy tube.

ocular of or pertaining to the eye; also an eye piece in any instrument.

oliguria a diminished capacity to form and pass urine; for adults, generally defined as less than 500 ml/24 hours.

oncotic marked by or associated with swelling; often used as a synonym for osmotic forces.

Ondine's Curse an eponym, derived from the name of a fabled water nymph, for apnea caused by loss of automatic control of respiration.

opacification the process of becoming opaque (less able to transmit light or penetrating radiation); used commonly to refer to the development of areas of increased density on the x-ray film, as occurs in ARDS.

operculum a lid or covering, as the connective tissue covering bounded by the first ribs and the upper portion of the sternum that forms the apex of the pleural cavity.

opiate a narcotic drug that contains opium, derivatives of opium, or any of several synthetic chemicals with opiumlike activity; morphine is the model in this category.

opsonin an antibody or complement split product that, on attaching to foreign material, microorganism, or other antigen, enhances phagocytosis of that substance by leukocytes and other macrophages.

orifice an entrance or outlet to a body cavity or tube.

oropharynx the three anatomic divisions of the pharynx lying behind the oral cavity and midway between the nasopharynx and laryngopharynx.

orotracheal of or pertaining the passageway from the mouth to the trachea; usually applied to tubes or catheters placed in the trachea through the mouth, such as an orotracheal tube, or orotracheal suctioning.

orthopnea an abnormal condition characterized by difficult breathing in any lying or recumbent position.

orthostatic pertaining to or caused by standing upright, as with orthostatic hypotension.

OSA abbreviation for obstructive sleep apnea.

oscillation a regular vibration or wavelike fluctuation in an electrical or mechanical parameter.

OSHA abbreviation for Occupational Safety and Health Agency, an agency of the federal Department of Labor responsible for developing and enforcing occupational safety standards.

osmolarity the osmotic pressure of a solution expressed in osmols or milliosmols per kilogram of the solution.

osmotic pressure a measurable force produced by mobility of the solvent particles across a semipermeable membrane.

osteoarthropathy any disease of the joints or bones.

osteomylitis local or generalized infection of bone and bone marrow, usually caused by bacteria introduced by trauma or surgery, by direct extension from a nearby infection, or through the bloodstream.

osteoporosis a disorder characterized by abnormal rarefaction of bone, occurring most frequently in postmenopausal women, in sedentary or immobilized individuals, and in patients receiving long-term steroid therapy.

otitis inflammation or infection of the ear, such as otitis media or otitis externa.

otorhinolaryngologist a physician specializing in disorders of the ear, nose, and throat.

overhydration a state characterized by an excess of body fluids.

oximeter a photoelectric device (usually noninvasive) used to determine the saturation of blood hemoglobin with oxygen.

oximetry the process of determining the saturation of hemoglobin with oxygen with an oximeter.

oxygen concentrator (enricher) an electrically powered device capable of physically separating the oxygen in room air from nitrogen, thereby providing an enriched flow of oxygen for therapeutic use.

oxygen delivery system a device used to deliver oxygen concentrations above ambient ($FiO_2 > 0.21$) to the lungs through the upper airway.

fixed-performance oxygen delivery system an oxygen delivery system that can supply all the inspired gas needs of a patient at a given FiO_2; sometimes called high-flow oxygen delivery systems.

variable-performance oxygen delivery system an oxygen delivery system not capable of meeting all the inspiratory volume or flow needs of the patient, thereby delivering an FiO_2 that varies with ventilatory demand; sometimes called low-flow oxygen delivery systems.

oxygen toxicity the pathologic response of the body and its tissues resulting from long-term exposure to high partial pressure of oxygen; pulmonary manifestations include cellular changes causing congestion, inflammation, and edema.

oxyhemoglobin the chemical combination resulting from the covalent bonding of oxygen to the ferrous iron pigment in hemoglobin.

P symbol for gas partial pressure.

PAC abbreviation for premature atrial contraction.

palatine of or pertaining to the palate or roof of the mouth.

pallor an unnatural paleness or absence of color in the skin.

palmar of or pertaining to the palm.

palpitation a pounding or racing of the heart.

pancreatitis an inflammatory condition of the pancreas, either acute or chronic.

pandemic (of a disease) occurring throughout the population of a country, a people, or the world.

pantomime expression or communication using only body or facial movements.

paradox something contrary to common sense, logic, or experience.

paradoxical breathing a pattern of breathing in which the abdomen is observed to move outward while the lower rib cage moves inward during inspiration; paradoxical breathing usually indicates an excessive respiratory muscle load and may serve notice of impending respiratory failure.

parainfluenza virus a paramyxovirus with three known serotypes that is transmitted by direct person-to-person contact or by dispersal of droplet nuclei through the air; the most common specific illness caused by the parainfluenza viruses is childhood croup.

paranasal situated near or alongside the nose, as the paranasal sinuses.

parasympathetic of or pertaining to the craniosacral component of the autonomic nervous system, consisting of the oculomotor, facial, glossopharyngeal, vagus, and pelvic nerves; any physiologic action mediated by or mimicking that of acetylcholine.

parasympathomimetic denoting a pharmacologic agent that mimics the effects of stimulation of organs and structures by the parasympathetic nervous system by occupying cholinergic receptor sites and acting as an agonist or by increasing the release of the neurotransmitter acetylcholine.

parenchyma the functional tissue of an organ (as opposed to the supporting or connecting tissue).

parenteral not in or through the digestive system.

paresis slight or incomplete paralysis.

paresthesia any subjective sensation, experienced as numbness, tingling, or a "pins and needles" feeling.

parietal of or pertaining to the outer wall of a cavity or organ.

parotitis inflammation on infection of one or both parotid salivary glands.

paroxysmal nocturnal dyspnea (PND) attacks of dyspnea commonly occurring at night, especially while the person is recumbent, and associated with congestive heart failure and cardiac pulmonary edema.

partial pressure the pressure exerted by a single gas in a gas mixture.

partial thromboplastin time (PTT) a test for detecting coagulation defects of the intrinsic clotting system by adding activated partial thromboplastin to a sample of test plasma and comparing it with a control of normal plasma; normal is 60 to 80 seconds.

parturition the process of giving birth.

patency the condition of being patent.

patent open and unblocked, as a patent airway.

pathogenic capable of producing disease.

pathologic indicative of or caused by a disease.

pathophysiology the study of the biologic and physical manifestations of disease as they correlate with the underlying abnormalities and physiologic disturbances.

PAWP abbreviation for pulmonary arterial wedge pressure (also called the pulmonary capillary wedge pressure (PCWP) or occluded pulmonary artery pressure [PAo]); when properly measured, the PAWP reflects the downstream pressure in the pulmonary circulation, that is, the pulmonary venous pressure; pulmonary venous pressure, in turn, reflects left atrial pressure, which—under optimum conditions—gives an indication of the left ventricular end-diastolic pressure (LVEDP), or left ventricular preload.

PCP abbreviation for *Pneumocystis carinii* pneumonia; *P carinii* (thought to be a protozoan) is a cause of opportunistic infections among patients with an abnormal or altered immunologic status, particularly those suffering from AIDS; infection with *P carinii* causes an acute interstitial pneumonia with fatality rates in excess of 50%; current treatment is with co-trimoxazole or pentamidine isethionate.

pectoriloquy the transmission of the sounds of speech through the chest wall.

pectus carinatum Latin for *keeled breast,* also called chicken breast; undo protrusion of the sternum.

pectus excavatum Latin for *hollowed breast,* also called funnel breast; undo concavity of the sternum.

pediatrics the branch of medicine concerned with the treatment and prevention of disorders of childhood.

pediculosis infestation with lice.

PEEP acronym for positive end-expiratory pressure.

pendelluft movement of gas from "fast" to "slow" filling spaces during breathing; alternatively, the ineffective movement of gas back and forth (accompanied by mediastinal shifting) between a healthy lung and one with a flail segment caused by a crushing chest injury.

penetration as applied to aerosols, the maximum depth that suspended particles can be carried into the respiratory tract by the inhaled tidal air.

penicillinase resistant a descriptive term applied to certain antibiotics resistant to the action of penicillinase, an enzyme produced by some bacteria that inactivates penicillin.

percent body humidity (%BH) to the amount of water vapor in a volume of gas as the percent of the water in gas saturated at a body temperature of 37°C (43.8 mg/L).

percent solution (%) a solution in which the ratio of solute to solvent is expressed as a simple weight ratio, converted to a percent (ie, the weight of solute/weight of solution × 100).

percuss to strike with short, sharp blows; may be used for diagnosis, as when percussion is used to determine chest resonance, or for therapy, as a component of chest physical therapy.

perfuse the passage of fluid (usually blood) through the body.

peribronchial around the bronchi.

pericarditis an inflammation of the pericardium associated with trauma, malignant neoplastic disease, infection, uremia, myocardial infarction, collagen disease, or idiopathic causes.

pericardium a fibrous serous sac that surrounds the heart and the roots of the great vessels.

perinatal of or pertaining to the time and process of giving birth to being born.

perioperative of or pertaining to the time immediately before, during, and after surgery.

periosteum a fibrous vascular membrane covering the bones, except at their extremities.

peritoneal dialysis a dialysis procedure in which the peritoneum is used as the diffusible membrane, with a dialysate fluid infused and removed directly into the peritoneal cavity.

peritoneum the extensive serous membrane covering the entire abdominal wall of the peritoneal cavity and extending over the abdominal viscera.

peritubular around the tubules; specifically around the proximal or distal tubules of the nephron.

permanent gas the gaseous phase of a substance with a critical temperature so low that it cannot be compressed into a liquid under ambient conditions.

pertussis an acute, highly contagious respiratory disease characterized by paroxysmal coughing that ends in a loud whooping inspiration.

petechia a tiny purple or red spot that appears on the skin as a result of minute hemorrhages within the dermal or submucosal layers.

P/F ratio a ratio of the arterial partial pressure of oxygen to the inspired fractional concentration of oxygen (Pa_{O_2}/F_{IO_2}); a measure of the efficiency of oxygen transfer across the lung.

pH the negative logarithm of the hydrogen ion concentration of a solution, expressed as a positive number; the pH scale represents the relative acidity (or alkalinity) of a solution, in which a value 7.0 is neutral, below 7.0 is acid, and above 7.0 is alkaline.

phagocyte a cell that is able to surround, engulf, and digest microorganisms and cellular debris.

phagocytosis the process by which certain cells engulf and dispose of microorganisms and cell debris.

pharmacopoeia a compendium containing descriptions, recipes, strengths, standards of purity, and dosage forms for selected drugs.

pharyngitis inflammation or infection of the pharynx, usually causing symptoms of a sore throat.

phenol a highly poisonous, caustic, crystalline chemical derived from coal tar or plant tar or manufactured synthetically; in a 10% solution with water (called carbolic acid), phenol is a strong disinfectant.

phonocardiography the analog recording of heart sounds, usually on a strip chart recorder; useful in the diagnosis of certain valvular abnormalities that produce heart murmurs.

phosphodiesterase an enzyme that catalyzes the conversion of $3',5'$-cAMP to $5'$-AMP, thereby reducing the intracellular concentration of $3',5'$-cAMP; drugs that inhibit phosphodiesterase, such as the methylxanthines, therefore increase $3',5'$-cAMP concentrations, leading to smooth muscle relaxation and (in the airways) bronchodilation.

phospholipid one of a class of compounds, widely distributed in living cells, containing phosphoric acid, fatty acids, and a nitrogenous base.

photodetector a device capable of detecting light.

physical plant the "bricks and mortar" or building facilities that make up the physical presence of an institution.

Pickwickian syndrome an abnormal condition characterized by severe obesity, decreased responsiveness to carbon dioxide, a restrictive pulmonary function pattern, hypersomnolence, and polycythemia.

piezoelectric transducer a transducer capable of converting electrical energy in the physical energy of high-frequency vibrations.

P$_{Imax}$ abbreviation for maximum inspiratory pressure, or the negative pressure generated during a maximally forced inspiratory effort against an obstruction to flow; also called maximum inspiratory force (MIF) and negative inspiratory force (NIF).

piriform sinus two elongated fossa forming the base of the laryngopharynx that extend around both sides of the laryngeal inlet; swallowing involves the movement of a food bolus around the laryngeal inlet toward the piriform sinus and into the esophagus.

pK the negative logarithm of the ionization constant of a solution; the buffering power of a buffer system is greatest when its pH and pK values are equal.

placenta the highly vascular organ through which the fetus absorbs oxygen and vital nutrients and excretes carbon dioxide and other waste products of metabolism.

placenta previa an abnormal condition of pregnancy in which the placenta is implanted low in the uterus, such that it impinges or covers the internal os of the cervix.

plasma the watery, colorless fluid portion of the blood and lymph in which cellular elements are suspended.

plasmapheresis a laboratory procedure in which the plasma proteins are separated by electrophoresis for identification and evaluation of the proportion of the various proteins.

platypnea the opposite of orthopnea (ie, an abnormal condition characterized by difficult breathing in the standing position, which is relieved in the lying or recumbent position).

PLE abbreviation for panlobular emphysema.

pleomorphic consisting of many distinct shapes.

plethysmograph any instrument designed to measure and record variations in the volume of an organ or body part; the *body plethysmograph* measures changes in thoracic volume by measuring pressure changes in the box during breathing.

plethysmography the process of measuring and recording variations in the volume of an organ or body part with a plethysmograph.

pleural effusion the abnormal collection of fluid in the pleural space.

pleural empyema a pleural effusion in which the fluid is purulent or contains pyogenic organisms.

pleurisy a condition characterized by abnormal deposition of a fibrinous exudate on the pleural surface, usually as a complication of other disorders, such as pneumonia, pulmonary infarction, and pulmonary neoplasms.

PMI abbreviation for point of maximum impulse.

PND abbreviation for paroxysmal nocturnal dyspnea.

pneumatocele a thin-walled, air-filled cyst occurring in lung tissue.

pneumocardiography the recording of variations in cardiac function through sensors that monitor respiratory changes, such as pressure changes in the bronchi or changes in thoracic dimensions.

pneumoconiosis any disease of the lung caused by chronic inhalation of inorganic dusts, usually mineral dusts of occupational or environmental origin.

pneumocyte (also pneumonocyte) a general term applied to the cells constituting the alveolar region of the lungs.

pneumomediastinum a presence of air or gas in the mediastinal tissues, which may lead to pneumothorax or pneumopericardium.

pneumonectomy the surgical removal of all or part of a lung.

pneumonia an inflammatory process of the lung parenchyma, usually infectious in origin.

pneumonitis inflammation of the lung.

pneumopericardium a presence of air or gas in the pericardium.

pneumoperitoneum a presence of air or gas in the peritoneal cavity; may occur as the result of disease or may be induced for diagnostic visualization.

pneumotachometer a transducer designed to measure the flow of respiratory gases, usually by measuring pressure differences across a tube of known resistance.

pneumotachygraph an instrument that incorporates a pneumotachometer to recording variations in the flow of respiratory gases.

pneumotaxic center a localized collections of neurons in the pons located in the region of the nucleus parabrachealis medialis; the pneumotaxic center neurons apparently alter the rhythmic output of the medullary inspiratory-expiratory "centers," perhaps indirectly by inhibitory action on the apneustic center.

pneumothorax the presence of air or gas in the pleural space of the thorax; if this air or gas is trapped under pressure, a *tension pneumothorax* exists.

polarity having two poles; in physics, the distinction between a negatively and positively charged pole.

polarographic of or pertaining to a device or instrument that employs the flow of electrical current between negatively and positively charged poles to measure a physical phenomenon.

poliomyelitis an infectious disease caused by one of three small RNA viruses, which can impair anterior horn cells and produce a clinical picture ranging from asymptomatic to severe paralysis.

politicization the corruption of any process with competition for power and leadership.

pollutant any unwanted substance that occurs in the environment.

polycythemia an abnormal increase in the number of erythrocytes in the blood; termed *secondary* if attributable to defined causes other than direct stimulation of the bone marrow, such as occurs in chronic hypoxemia.

polymorphonuclear having a nucleus with a number of lobules or segments connected by a fine thread.

polymyositis inflammation of many muscles, usually accompanied by deformity, edema, insomnia, pain, sweating, and tension.

polypeptide a chain of amino acids joined by peptide bonds.

polyps small, tumor-like growths that project from the surface of a mucous membrane.

polysaccharide a carbohydrate that contains three or more molecules of simple carbohydrates.

polysomnography the measurement and recording of variations in airflow and diaphragmatic activity during sleep; used in the diagnosis of sleep apnea.

pons any slip of tissue connecting two parts of a structure or an organ of the body; more specifically, the prominence on the ventral surface of the brain stem, between the medulla oblongata and the cerebral pedicles of the midbrain.

pontine of or pertaining to the pons.

popliteal (artery) a continuation of the femoral artery that passes through the popliteal fossa behind the knee and supplies various muscles of the leg and foot through its eight branches; used as an alternative site for palpation of a pulse.

pores of Kohn direct intercommunications between alveoli ranging from 5 to 15 μm in diameter.

porphyrin an iron- or magnesium-free pyrole derivative occurring in many plant and animal tissues.

positive end-expiratory pressure (PEEP) the application and maintenance of pressure above atmospheric at the airway throughout the expiratory phase of positive pressure mechanical ventilation.

postbaccalaureate of or pertaining to education occurring after the traditional four-year college or university degree.

posterolateral situated behind and to one side or the other.

posteromedial situated behind and toward the middle.

postterm of or pertaining to an infant born after 42 weeks' gestation, regardless of weight.

postural drainage the therapeutic use of patient positioning and gravity to facilitate the mobilization of respiratory tract secretions.

potency in pharmacology, the biologic activity of a drug per unit weight, or the amount a drug required to produce a given effect.

potential energy the energy a body possesses by its position.

potentiation a phenomenon in clinical pharmacology whereby the administration of one drug increases the effect of another.

PPD abbreviation for purified protein derivative, a material used in testing for tuberculin sensitivity.

precordium the external anterior anatomic region over the heart and lower thorax.

precursor something that comes before or precedes; in chemistry and pharmacology, a substance from which another is formed or synthesized; in clinical diagnosis, a symptom or sign that precedes another.

preeclampsia an abnormal condition of pregnancy characterized by the onset of acute hypertension after the 24th week of gestation, usually accompanied by proteinuria and edema.

preload the initial stretch of myocardial fiber at end diastole.

premium the sum paid for a contract, such as that for health insurance.

preoperative of or pertaining to the period preceding a surgical procedure.

pressure generator a ventilator, the pressure pattern of which is independent of the mechanical characteristics of the patient's respiratory system.

pressure support ventilation (PSV) pressure-limited assisted ventilation designed to augment a spontaneously generated breath; the patient has primary control over the frequency of breathing, the inspiratory time, and the inspiratory flow.

preterm of or pertaining to an infant born before 38 weeks' gestation, regardless of weight.

preventative maintenance the regularly scheduled testing and service of in-use equipment, designed to prevent failure or malfunction.

PRO abbreviation for peer review organization; a local physician agency established under PL 98-21 (the Social Security Amendments of 1983 that established the Medicare prospective payment system) responsible for reviewing the validity of diagnoses, assessing the quality of care, and evaluating the appropriateness of admission transfers and discharges for contracted hospitals.

procaryotic of or pertaining to plant-like microorganisms (including blue-green bacteria and true bacteria) whose cells have no true nucleus surrounded by a nuclear membrane.

prolapsed cord an umbilical cord that protrudes beside or ahead of the presenting part of the fetus.

prophylactic preventing the spread of disease; preventive.

proprioceptor any sensory nerve ending, as those located in muscles, tendons, and joints, that responds to stimuli arising from movement or spatial position.

prospective payment a system of health care cost reimbursement in which the amount paid to a provider is determined in advance irrespective of actual costs incurred.

prostaglandin one of several naturally occurring 20-carbon unsaturated fatty acids synthesized mainly in the seminal vesicles, kidneys, and lungs; of the 14 known prostaglandins, three are of substantial interest in respiratory pharmacology: PGE_1, PGE_2, and PGF_{2a}. Prostaglandin E_1 and E_2 cause relaxation of bronchial smooth muscle; prostaglandin F_{2a} causes contraction of bronchial smooth muscle.

proteinaceous protein-like.

proteolytic of or pertaining to any substance that promotes the breakdown of protein.

prothrombin a plasm protein synthesized in the liver that, when exposed to thromboplastin and calcium, forms the thrombin component of a blood clot.

prothrombin time (PT) a one-stage test for detecting certain plasma coagulation defects caused by deficiencies in factor V, VII, or X.

protocol a written plan specifying the procedures to be followed in a given activity.

pseudocolumnar literally, "column-like"; used to describe a type of epithelial cell that appears columnar.

pseudostratified of or pertaining to an epithelial cell type that appear to be organized in layers but in which each cell actually contacts the basement membrane.

psig abbreviation for pounds per square inch-gauge (ie, the pressure above atmospheric registered on a meter or gauge).

psittacosis an infectious illness caused by the bacterium *Chlamydia psittaci*, characterized by respiratory, pneumonia-like symptoms and transmitted to humans by infected birds, especially parrots.

PSV abbreviation for pressure support ventilation.

PSVT abbreviation for paroxysmal superventricular tachycardia.

psychosocial of or pertaining to the mental, emotional, and social aspects of human existence or development.

psychosomatic of or pertaining to the relationship between the emotional state or outlook of an individual (psyche) and the physical responses of the individual's body (soma).

PT abbreviation for prothrombin time.

ptosis an abnormal condition of one or both upper eyelids in which the eyelid droops owing to a congenital or acquired weakness of the levator muscle or paralysis of the third cranial nerve.

PTT abbreviation for partial thromboplastin time.

pulmonary alveolar proteinosis a chronic lung disease characterized by deposition of an eosinophilic proteinaceous material in the alveolar region that severely impairs gas exchange.

pulmonary edema a condition in which excessive amounts of plasma enter the pulmonary interstitium and alveoli; usually accompanied by severe respiratory distress, tachypnea, and hypoxemia.

pulmonary hemosiderosis a pulmonary disorder characterized by the deposition of abnormal quantities of hemosiderin (an insoluble form of ferric oxide) in the lung parenchyma.

pulmonary hypertension a condition characterized by abnormally high pulmonary artery pressures (ie, mean pulmonary artery pressures over 22 mm Hg).

pulmonologist a physician who specializes in the treatment of disorders of the respiratory system and holds certification in pulmonary diseases through the American Board of Internal Medicine.

pulse deficit the discrepancy between the ventricular rate auscultated at the apex of the heart and the arterial rate of the radial pulse.

pulse pressure the difference between the systolic and diastolic pressures, normally about 30 to 40 mm Hg.

pulsus alternans a pulse characterized by a regular alternation of weak and strong beats without changes in the length of the cycle.

pulsus paradoxus an abnormal decrease in systolic pressure and pulse-wave amplitude during inspiration.

purulent consisting of or containing pus.

PVC abbreviation for premature ventricular contraction; also used as an abbreviation for polyvinyl chloride.

pyogenic pus producing.

P$_{50}$ the partial pressure of oxygen at which hemoglobin is 50% saturated with oxygen, standardized to a pH of 7.40; used as a measure of hemoglobin affinity for oxygen; with a normal value of 26.6 mm Hg.

QRS complex the electrical activity associated with depolarization of the ventricles.

quaternary ammonium compounds cationic detergent-disinfectants that contain ammonium ions, also called "quats"; their disinfectant properties are associated with their ability to disrupt the cell membranes of certain microorganisms.

racemic pertaining to a compound made up of levorotatory isomers, rendering it optically inactive under polarized light.

radioaerosol an aerosol with particles that have been labeled with a radioactive isotope and used to assist researchers in analyzing aerosol deposition and clearance in the lung.

radiographer an allied health professional who operates radiologic equipment under the direction of a radiologist.

radiolucent of or pertaining to a substance or tissue that readily permits the passage of x-rays or other radiant energy.

radionecrosis the destruction of tissue by radiant energy.

radiopaque of or pertaining to a substance or tissue that does not readily permit the passage of x-rays or other radiant energy.

rale a discontinuous type of lung sound heard on auscultation of the chest, usually during inspiration; the term *crackle* is now preferred.

ramus a small, branchlike structure extending from a larger one or dividing into two or more parts, as a branch of a nerve or artery or one of the rami of the mandible.

Rankine scale an absolute temperature scale (0°R = absolute zero) calibrated in Fahrenheit units and used mainly in engineering.

ratio solution a solution in which the relationship of the solute to the solvent is expressed as a proportion (eg, 1:100, parts per thousand).

reabsorption the return of fluids or gases through a body surface and into body fluids or tissues.

readaptation the process of relearning; commonly refers to the development of key coping skills after disability or injury.

rebreathe to inhale expired gas (high in carbon dioxide content).

rebreathed volume the volume of any breathing apparatus that results in previously expired gas being inhaled; equivalent to the mechanical dead space.

reconcentration the process of undergoing repeated concentration.

recontamination the process by which articles previously contaminated and cleaned or sterilized become contaminated again.

recredentialing the process by which an individual who already holds a credential in a given profession demonstrates ongoing competency by successfully completing current credentialing requirements.

recycle to reuse.

R & D common acronym for research and development.

REDOX an acronym pertaining to any REDuction-OXidation chemical reaction.

reducing valve a device designed to reduce a source gas pressure.

referred pain pain occurring at a site distal to its origin.

refractory pertaining to a disorder that is resistant to treatment.

refractory period the period during the depolarization stage of the action potential in which cardiac tissue fibers cannot respond to additional electrical stimulation.

registered pulmonary function technologist (RPFT) an individual, qualified by education or experience or both, and previously certified in pulmonary function technology, who has successfully completed the pulmonary function *registry* examination of the NBRC.

registered respiratory therapist (RRT) a respiratory therapist who has successfully completed the registry (therapist) examination of the NBRC.

regulator a device designed to control both the pressure and flow of a compressed gas.

regurgitation "backward flow"; refers commonly to the return of swallowed food back to the mouth or the backflow of blood through a defective valve.

rehabilitation the restoration of the individual to the fullest medical, mental, emotional, social, and vocational potential of which he or she is capable.

rehabilitation (pulmonary) an individually tailored, multidisciplinary program which through accurate diagnosis, therapy, emotional support, and education stabilizes or reverses both the physiopathology and psychopathology of pulmonary diseases and attempts to return the patient to the highest possible functional capacity allowed by his or her pulmonary handicap and overall life situation.

reliability pertaining to equipment, the consistency of fault-free operation, often measured as the mean time between failures; in statistics, the repeatability of a test or measure.

repolarization (in cardiology) the process by which the cell is restored to its resting potential.

residual volume (RV) the volume of gas remaining in the lungs after a complete exhalation.

resistance impedance to flow in a tube or conduit; quantified as ratio of the difference in pressure between the two points along a tube length divided by the volumetric flow of the fluid per unit time.

respiratory alternans an abnormal breathing pattern in which the patient is observed to switch back and forth between mainly diaphragmatic and mainly intercostal muscle activity; indicative of end-stage respiratory muscle fatigue.

respiratory index (RI) the ratio of the alveolar-arterial oxygen tension gradient to the arterial partial pressure of oxygen ($P(A\text{-}a)o_2/Pao_2$); a measure of the efficiency of oxygen transfer across the lung.

respiratory failure a condition in which the exchange of oxygen or carbon dioxide between the alveoli and the pulmonary capillaries is inadequate.

hypoxemic respiratory failure respiratory failure caused by abnormalities of oxygenation and characterized by a lower than predicted Pao_2, a higher than predicted $P(A\text{-}a)o_2$, and a normal or low $Paco_2$; also called type I respiratory failure.

hypercapnic respiratory failure respiratory failure due to inadequate ventilation and characterized by a higher than predicted $Paco_2$, a lower than predicted Pao_2, but a normal $P(a-a)o_2$; also called type II respiratory failure, or ventilatory failure.

acute respiratory failure respiratory failure in which the hypoxemia or hypercapnea develops too rapidly to allow physiologic compensation; considered a life-threatening event that necessitates drastic clinical intervention, including some form of ventilatory support.

chronic respiratory failure respiratory failure that develops over weeks to months, thereby providing time for the body to compensate partially for the underlying pathophysiologic disturbance.

respiratory insufficiency a condition in which breathing is accompanied by abnormal signs or symptoms, such as dyspnea or paradoxical breathing.

respiratory therapist a graduate of a school accredited by the American Medical Association's Committee on Allied Health Education and Accreditation (CAHEA), in cooperation with the Joint Review Committee for Respiratory Therapy Education (JRCRTE) designed to qualify the graduate for the registry examination of the National Board for Respiratory Care (NBRC).

respiratory therapy technician A graduate of a CAHEA/JRCRTE–approved school designed to qualify the graduate for the technician (entry-level) certification examination of the NBRC.

respirometer a device used to measure the volume of respired air or gas.

response time a measure (usually in msec) of the speed with which a mechanical ventilator can respond to a patient's inspiratory effort and cycle into the inspiratory phase.

resting potential a difference in charge, or negative electrical potential, that exists between the inside and outside of a nerve or cardiac tissue cell in the resting state due to concentration differences of potassium and sodium ions across the cell membrane.

restrictive lung disease a broad category of disorders with widely variable etiologies, but all resulting in a reduction in lung volumes, particularly the inspiratory and vital capacities; categorized according to origin (ie, skeletal-thoracic, neuromuscular, pleural, interstitial, and alveolar).

retention as applied to aerosol therapy, the proportion of particles deposited within the respiratory tract, either at a specific location or as a whole.

retina the inner nervous tissue layer of the eye that is responsible for receiving visual stimuli for transmission to the brain through the connected optic nerve.

retinopathy a noninflammatory eye disorder resulting from changes in the retinal blood vessels.

retrolental fibroplasia a formation of fibrous tissue behind the lens of the eye, resulting in blindness.

retrosternal behind the sternum.

rheostat a variable resistor that controls the flow of electrical current.

rhinitis inflammation of the mucous membranes of the nose, usually accompanied by swelling of the mucosa and a nasal discharge.

rhinorrhea the free discharge of a thin nasal mucus.

rhinovirus any of about 100 serologically distinct, small RNA viruses that cause about 40% of acute respiratory illnesses.

rhonchi abnormal sounds heard on auscultation of a respiratory

airway obstructed by thick secretions, muscular spasm, neoplasm, or external pressure.

rickettsia any organism of the genus *Rickettsia*.

rostal toward the head, cephalad.

RPFT abbreviation for registered pulmonary function technologist.

RRT abbreviation for registered respiratory therapist.

RSV abbreviation for respiratory synctial virus.

safety system any system designed to prevent or minimize hazards due to human error; in medical gas therapy, a system of connections designed to help prevent accidental interchanging of incorrect equipment or gases during their administration.

American Standard Safety System (ASSS) provides specifications for threaded high-pressure connections between compressed gas cylinders and their attachments. Standardized for each gas, these specifications are.

pin-indexed safety system (PISS) a subsection of the American Standard Safety System applicable only to the valve outlets of small cylinders, up to and including size E; and employing a yoke-and-pin-type connection.

diameter-indexed safety system (DISS) provides specifications for threaded low-pressure (less than 200 psig) connections between station outlets, flowmeters, and other therapy devices, such as nebulizers, ventilators, and anesthesia apparatus.

salicylate any of several widely prescribed drugs derived from salicylic acid.

salmonellosis a form of gastroenteritis caused by ingestion of food contaminated with a species of *Salmonella* and characterized by an incubation period of 6 to 48 hours, followed by sudden abdominal pain, fever, and bloody, watery diarrhea.

salt a chemical compound consisting of a metal or ammonium ion electrovalently joined to anions other than the hydroxyl.

sarcoidosis a chronic disorder of unknown origin characterized by the formation of tubercles of nonecrotizing epithelioid tissue.

Schmitt trigger a fluidics sensing device capable of detecting small changes between two input signals, thereby "triggering" a change in the direction of output flow; the Schmitt trigger can be used as a mechanism to cycle a ventilator to inspiration based on patient effort.

sclera the tough white outer layer of the eye.

scleroderma a relatively rare autoimmune disease that results in chronic thickening of the connective tissue, including that in the skin, heart, kidneys, and lungs.

sclerosis any condition characterized by hardening of tissue, especially that due to hyperplasia of connective tissue.

scoliosis an abnormal lateral curvature of the spine.

sedimentation rate in aerosol therapy, a measure of the relative speed with which a particle comes out of suspension; sedimentation rate is a function of particle mass as related to gravity and the buoyancy provided by the carrier gas.

selectively permeable of or pertaining to a biologic or synthetic membrane permeable to solvent and selected small solute molecules, such as glucose and urea; compare with semipermeable.

seminal vesicles the paired pouches that produce seminal fluid and certain hormones in the male; the seminal vesicles are connected to the posterior portion of the urinary bladder and continuous with the ejaculatory duct.

semipermeable a biologic or synthetic membrane that permits the passage of molecules of solvent only but not solute.

sensitivity a measure of the amount of negative pressure that must be generated by a patient to cycle a mechanical ventilator into the inspiratory phase; alternatively, the mechanism used to set or control this level, sometimes called the patient-effort control.

sensorium a general term referring to the relative state of a patient's consciousness or alertness.

sepsis a general term connoting infection or contamination; more specifically used to denote the presence of pathogenic microorganisms or their toxins in the body.

septicemia systemic infection in which pathogens are present in the circulating blood stream, having spread from an infection in any part of the body; also called bacteremia.

septic shock shock is caused by the presence of bacteria in the blood stream (bacteremia), especially gram-negative organisms associated with nosocomial infections; events predisposing to septic shock include urinary tract infections, artificial tracheal airways, IV-related thrombophlebitis or contamination, postoperative infections, infected burns, and severe neutropenia, as may occur with cancer; the mortality for septic shock is often over 50%.

sequela any abnormal condition that follows and is the result of a disease, treatment, or injury, as paralysis following poliomyelitis, deafness following treatment with an ototoxic drug, or a scar following a laceration.

serotonin a naturally occurring derivative of tryptophan found in platelets and in cells of the brain and the intestine; serotonin is a potent vasoconstrictor.

serotype a classification of microorganism based on an analysis of its cellular antigens.

serous of or pertaining to the serum; any tissue type that produces or contains serum.

SGA abbreviation for small for gestational age; of or pertaining to newborns whose body weight falls below the 10th percentile for their gestational age.

shock a condition in which perfusion to vital organs is inadequate to meet metabolic needs; includes hypovolemic, cardiogenic, septic, anaphylactic, and neurogenic forms.

shunt a bypass; as applied in cardiovascular and pulmonary medicine, a connection between the right (venous) and left (arterial) sides of the circulation.

right-to-left shunt a shunt in which blood flows from the venous to the arterial side of the circulation, such that the low oxygen content of the venous blood dilutes the higher oxygen content of the arterial blood, lowering both the oxygen content and Po_2 in the resultant mixture (see venous admixture).

left-to-right shunt a shunt in which blood flows from the arterial to the venous side of the circulation; a left-to-right shunt has little direct effect on the oxygen content of the arterial blood; however, to make up for the effective loss of arterial flow through the left-to-right shunt, the heart may have to increase the amount of blood it pumps per minute to satisfy tissue demands; for this reason, large left-to-right shunts can significantly increase the workload on the heart.

anatomic shunt a direct connection between the right and left sides of the circulation due to the existence of an *anatomic* portal, such as a patent ductus arteriosus or ventricular septal defect; may be either left to right or right to left; a small normal right-to-left anatomic shunt exists due to the anatomy of the bronchial and thebesian venous drainage systems.

physiologic shunt a shunt occurring when a portion of the pulmonary blood flow perfuses unventilated alveoli ($\dot{V}/\dot{Q} = 0$); the result is similar to that described for a right-to-left anatomic shunt (ie, deoxygenated blood mixes with arterialized blood, lowering both the Cao_2 and Pao_2).

SI abbreviation for Systeme International d'Unites, the French name for the international measurement system based on meter, kilogram, and second units (mks system).

side effect in pharmacology, any effect produced by a drug other than its desired effect.

SIDS abbreviation for sudden infant death syndrome, commonly called crib death; SIDS is the leading cause of death in infants less than 1 year old in the United States, accounting for between 5,000 and 10,000 infant deaths each year in the United States alone; a presumptive diagnosis is based on the conditions of death, in which a previously healthy infant dies suddenly and unexpected, usually during sleep; although about two thirds of the infants dying of SIDS show some evidence of repeated incidents of hypoxia or ischemia on autopsy, no precise cause of death can be identified.

silicosis a lung disorder caused by continued, long-term exposure to the dust of an inorganic compound, silicon dioxide, which is found in sands, quartzes, and in many other stones; chronic silicosis is marked by widespread fibrotic nodular lesions in both lungs.

silofiller's disease a pulmonary disorder caused by inhalation of nitrogen and sulfur dioxide fumes emanating from freshly filled agricultural silos that results in an increase in alveolar-capillary membrane permeability and pulmonary edema.

SIMV abbreviation for synchronous intermittent mandatory ventilation.

singultation hiccupping.

singultus a characteristic sound that is produced by the involuntary contraction of the diaphragm, followed by rapid closure of the glottis (ie, a hiccup).

sinusitis an inflammation of one or more paranasal sinuses.

sinusoidal of or pertaining to the shape of a sine wave.

situs inversus lateral transposition of the organs of the abdomen and thorax; one of the features of Kartagener's syndrome.

SNF abbreviation for skilled nursing facility.

solubility coefficient (gas) the volume of gas that can be dissolved in 1 ml of a given liquid at standard pressure and specified temperature.

solute the substance dissolved in a solution.

solution a homogeneous and stable mixture of two or more substances, evenly dispersed throughout each other at the molecular level; a *saturated solution* is one with the maximum amount of solute that can be held by a given volume of a solvent at a constant temperature, in the presence of an excess of solute.

solvent the medium in which a solute is dissolved.

somnolence sleepiness.

sonography the process of imaging deep structures of the body by measuring and recording the reflection of pulsed or continuous high-frequency sound waves.

specific compliance the absolute compliance value of the lung divided by the lung volume at FRC and expressed in units of ml/cm H_2O/L.

specific heat the ratio between the amount of heat required to raise the temperature of 1 g of a substance 1°C (cgs) or 1 pound of a substance 1°F at a specific temperature (fps), and the amount of heat required to raise the temperature of 1 g of water 1°C or 1 pound of water 1°F at the specified temperature.

spectrophotometry the measurement of color in a solution by determining the amount of light absorbed in the ultraviolet, infrared, or visible spectrum, widely used in clinical chemistry to calculate the concentration of substances in solution.

sphygmomanometer an instrument for measuring the force of the pulse (from which the blood pressure is estimated).

spinous has the characteristics of a spine or thorn; a pointed structure.

spirometer an apparatus designed to measure and record lung volumes and flows.

spirometry laboratory evaluation of lung function using a spirometer.

splanchnic of or pertaining to the viscera.

sporicidal destructive to the spore form of bacteria.

sporicide any agent effective in destroying spores, as compounds of chlorine and formaldehyde and the gluteraldehydes.

sporulation a type of reproduction that occurs in lower plants and animals, as fungi, algae, and protozoa, and involves the formation of spores by the spontaneous division of the cell into four or more daughter cells, each of which contains a portion of the original nucleus.

squamous appearing like plates or scales; a type of epithelial tissue.

stability in aerosol therapy, a measure of the ability of an aerosol to remain in suspension over time; stability is a function of the size and nature of the particulate matter, the concentration of particles present, the ambient humidity, and the mobility of the carrier gas; *instability* is the opposite of stability (ie, the tendency of suspended particles to fall out of suspension).

standard bicarbonate the plasma concentration of HCO_3 in mEq/L that would exist if the P_{CO_2} were normal (40 mm Hg).

stasis a disorder in which the normal flow of a fluid through a vessel of the body is slowed or halted.

status asthmaticus an acute, severe, and prolonged asthma attack that does not respond to normal treatment approaches.

statutory imposed by legal authority.

stenosis an abnormal condition characterized by the constriction or narrowing of an opening or passageway in a body structure.

sterile free from any living microorganisms.

sterilization the complete destruction of all microorganisms, usually by heat or chemical means.

sternoclavicular of or pertaining to the sternum and clavicle.

Stokes-Adams syncope episodes of syncope due to heart block.

STP abbreviation for conditions of standard temperature and pressure (ie, 0°C and 760 mm Hg).

STPD abbreviation for standard temperature, standard pressure, dry.

strabismus deviation of the eye position from normal that is not under the patient's voluntary control.

stridor an abnormal, high-pitched, harsh inspiratory breath sound that is usually audible to the naked ear and caused by an obstruction in region of the larynx.

stylet a thin metal probe for inserting into or passing through a needle, tube, or catheter to clean the hollow bore or for inserting in a soft, flexible catheter to make it shift as the catheter is placed in a vein or passed through an orifice of the body.

subatmospheric below atmospheric; used to describe pressures below ambient (see hypobarism).

subcostal below the ribs.

subcutaneous beneath the skin.

subepithelial below or beneath the epithelial tissue layer.

subglottic below the glottis.

sublimation the direct transition from the solid to the gaseous state.

sublingual beneath the tongue.

submicronic of or pertaining to a particle (particularly colloid particles) smaller than 10^{-5} cm and not visible with a standard light microscope.

submucosa beneath the mucosa.

sulfhemoglobin a form of hemoglobin containing an irreversibly bound sulfur molecule that prevents normal oxygen binding.

sulfydryl the univalent radical containing sulfur and hydrogen (^-SH) or the bond between sulfur and hydrogen in a complex molecule.

supernumary greater than the normal number.

suppurative producing pus.

supraclavicular the area of the body above the clavicle, or collar bone.

supraglottic above the glottis.

suprasternal above the sternum.

supraventricular above the ventricles.

surfactant an agent, as soap or detergent, dissolved in water to reduce its surface tension or the tension at the interface between the water and another liquid.

surveillance any constant or ongoing monitoring of a process to ensure its effectiveness; *bacteriologic surveillance* is an ongoing process designed to ensure that infection control procedures are achieving their goal; it involves four interrelated components: equipment processing quality control, routine sampling of in-use equipment, microbiologic identification, and epidemiologic investigation (during outbreaks of infection).

suspension a dispersion of large particles suspended in a fluid medium; without physical agitation, the particles will eventually settle out.

sustained maximal inspiration (SMI) a therapeutic breathing maneuver in which patients are coached to inspire from the resting expiratory level up to their inspiratory capacity (IC), with an end-inspiratory pause; designed to mimic the normal physiologic sigh mechanism by increasing the transpulmonary pressure gradient (P_L) through a decrease in intrapleural pressure (P_{pl}).

sympathetic of or pertaining to the thoracolumbar component of the autonomic nervous system, for which norepinephrine serves as the postganglionic neurotransmitter; also used to describe any physiologic action mediated by or mimicking that of norepinephrine or epinephrine; see adrenergic.

sympathomimetic denoting a pharmacologic agent that mimics the effects of stimulation of organs and structures by the sympathetic nervous system by occupying adrenergic receptor sites and acting as an agonist or by increasing the release of the neurotransmitter norepinephrine at postganglionic nerve endings.

synapse the region surrounding the point of contact between two neurons or between a neuron and an effector organ, across which nerve impulses are transmitted through the action of a neurotransmitter, as acetylcholine or norepinephrine.

synaptic cleft the space between two neurons or between a neuron and an effector organ.

syncope temporary unconsciousness; fainting.

synchronous intermittent mandatory ventilation (SIMV)

periodic assisted ventilation with positive pressure, with the patient breathing spontaneously between breaths.

syncytial of or pertaining to a syncytium (ie, a mass of protoplasm with multiple nuclei formed by the agglomeration of cells).

synergistic acting together; more specifically, having the characteristics of synergism, the phenomenon whereby two agents acting together have an effect greater than their algebraic sum.

syringomyelia a disorder characterized by the formation of abnormal fluid-filled cavities in the spinal cord.

systemic of or pertaining to the body as a whole.

tachycardia an abnormal condition in which the myocardium contracts regularly but at a rate greater than 100 beats per minute.

tachyphylaxis a phenomenon in which the repeated administration of some drugs results in a marked decrease in effectiveness.

tachypnea an abnormally rapid rate of breathing.

tamponade stoppage of the flow of blood to an organ or a part of the body by pressure, as by a tampon or a pressure dressing applied to stop a hemorrhage or by the compression of a part by an accumulation of fluid, as in cardiac tamponade.

tangent a line drawn perpendicular to a given point in a curve.

taxonomy an orderly classification, as a taxonomy of organisms.

tempered moderated or mollified; modified or altered by the mixture of an additional ingredient; steel that has been hardened by heating and rapid cooling.

term of or pertaining to an infant born between 38 and 42 weeks gestation.

tetany a condition characterized by cramps, convulsions, twitching of the muscles, and sharp flexion of the wrist and ankle joints.

tetralogy of Fallot a congenital cardiac anomaly that consists of four defects: pulmonic stenosis, ventricular septal defect, malposition of the aorta to that it arises from the septal defect or the right ventricle, and right ventricular hypertrophy.

thebesian veins a minor portion of the venous drainage of the heart; since the thebesian veins drain into all four heart chambers, they contribute to the small anatomic shunt present in healthy individuals.

therapeutic positioning application of gravity to achieve specific clinical objectives, including mobilization of secretions (postural drainage), improving the distribution of ventilation (dependent positioning), and relieving dyspnea (relaxation positioning).

thermal conductivity the efficiency of heat transfer between objects, measured in (cal/sec) $\times$ (cm^2 $\times$ °C/cm) (cgs).

thermal equilibrium a condition in which the temperatures of two substances exist at the same temperature; a condition in which heat transfer is in a steady state.

thermistor an electronic thermometer, the impedance of which varies with temperature; used for measuring minute changes in temperature.

thermophilic growing best under conditions of high temperature.

thermostat an electrical or mechanical device that regulates and maintains a set temperature in a given system.

thoracentesis the surgical perforation of the chest wall and pleural space with a needle for the aspiration of fluid for diagnostic or therapeutic purposes or for the removal of a specimen for biopsy.

thoracotomy a surgical opening into the thoracic cavity.

Thorpe tube a variable-orifice, constant-pressure, flow-metering device consisting of a tapered transparent tube with a float; the diameter of the tube increases from bottom to top, with the float suspended by flow against the force of gravity at a level determined by the rate of flow.

threshold potential the membrane potential or voltage difference in cardiac tissue fibers at which spontaneous depolarization occurs.

threshold response of or pertaining to a physiologic action caused by the minimum stimulus needed to provoke it.

thrombocytopenia an abnormal hematologic condition in which the number of platelets is reduced, usually by destruction of erythroid tissue in bone marrow associated with certain neoplastic diseases or an immune response to a drug.

thrombolysis the process by which thrombi are dissolved.

thrombophlebitis inflammation of a vein, often accompanied by formation of a clot.

thromboplastin a prothrombin activator crucial in the formation of thrombin and therefore essential in blood clotting.

thrombosis an abnormal vascular condition in which thrombus develops within a blood vessel of the body.

thrombus an aggregation of platelets, fibrin, and cellular blood components that can obstruct a blood vessel.

tibial of or pertaining to the tibia.

time constant a mathematical expression describing the relative efficacy of lung unit filling and emptying, computed as the product of compliance times resistance, with a resulting measure in seconds.

tincture of benzoin a basalmic gumlike resin that, in a tincture of alcohol, is used as an external tissue protectant.

titrate to determine by titration.

titration the determination of the activity of a given substance in solution by adding chemical reagents until an equilibrium or predefined endpoint is achieved.

titratable measurable by standard titration techniques; of or pertaining to a base or acid whose activity can be ascertained by titration.

tomography an x-ray technique that produces a film representing a detailed cross-section of tissue structure at a predetermined depth.

tonicity refers to the relative degree of osmotic pressure exerted by a solution; physiologically, any other solution with a tonicity equivalent to a 0.9% solution of NaCl is called *isotonic,* one with greater tonicity is called *hypertonic,* and one with less is called *hypotonic.*

torsade de pointes a type of ventricular tachycardia with a spirallike appearance ("twisting of the points") and complexes that at first look positive and then negative on an electrocardiogram.

total buffer base (BB) the total quantity of all blood buffers capable of binding hydrogen ions; normally ranges from 48 to 52 mEq/L.

total lung capacity the total amount of gas in the lungs after a maximum inspiration.

tourniquet a device applied around an extremity that is designed to compress blood vessels and thereby prevent blood flow to or from the distal area.

tracheitis any inflammatory condition of the trachea.

tracheobronchial of or pertaining to the trachea and large bronchi.

tracheobronchomegaly a rare congenital condition in which the size of the large airways is greatly enlarged.

tracheoesophageal of or pertaining to the trachea and esophagus, as with a tracheoesophageal fistula.

tracheomalacia softening of the tracheal cartilages.

tracheostomy an opening through the neck into the trachea, through which an indwelling tube may be inserted.

tracheotomy the procedure by which an incision is made into the trachea through the neck below the larynx to gain access to the lower airways.

tranducer a device capable of converting one form of energy into another and commonly used for measurement of physical events; for example, a pressure transducer may convert the physical phenomenon of force per unit area into an analog electrical signal.

transaction any human interaction; in human communication, it denotes a two-way process in which participants are mutually influenced by the interaction.

transbronchial across the bronchi or bronchial wall, as a transbronchial biopsy.

transcutaneous across the skin, as a transcutaneous P_{O_2} electrode.

transect to sever or cut across, as in preparing a cross-section of tissue.

transfill to fill across; to fill a vessel from another vessel.

transfusion the direct introduction of blood or blood products from another source into the bloodstream.

transmural across the wall; usually pertains to the pressure difference between inside and outside a vessel or conducting tube.

transplacental across or through the placenta, specifically in reference to the exchange of nutrients, waste products, and other material between the developing fetus and the mother.

transpulmonary across the lung; of or pertaining to the difference in a parameter (eg, pressure) between the alveoli and pleural space.

transrespiratory across the respiratory system; of or pertaining to the difference in a parameter (eg, pressure) between the alveoli and body surface.

transthoracic across the thorax; of or pertaining to the difference in a parameter (eg, pressure) between the pleural space and body surface.

transudate a fluid passed through a membrane or squeezed through a tissue or into the space between the cells of a tissue.

transudation the process of fluid passage through a membrane.

transvenous through the veins, as with a transvenous pacemaker.

treatment regimen a comprehensive plan of various treatments designed to combat a certain disease or disorder.

Trendelenburg position a position in which the head is low and the body and legs are on an inclined plane.

triage a classification of casualties of war and other disasters according to the gravity of injuries, urgency of treatment, and place for treatment.

trifurcation the subdivision of one into three.

trigeminy occurring in groups of threes; used frequently to describe certain cardiac arrhythmias, especially three premature ventricular contractions in a row.

triple point that combination of temperature and pressure that allows the solid, liquid, and vapor forms of a given substance to exist in equilibrium with one another.

trismus a prolonged tonic spasm of the muscles of the jaw.

trypanosomiasis an infection by an organism of the *Trypanosoma* genus.

trypsin a proteolytic enzyme synthesized in the pancreas.

tubercle a nodule or a small eminence, as that on a bone.

tuberculocidal an agent destructive to *Mycobacterium tuberculosis*.

tuberculosis an infectious disorder caused by the acid-fast mycobacterium *M tuberculosis* and characterized by tubercle formation in the lung; infection normally occurs by inhalation of organisms carried on droplets nuclei produced in the cough of an infected person.

turbinate a scroll-shaped structure; in reference to pulmonary anatomy, any of the three bony shelves extending out of the lateral nasal wall and projecting into the nasal cavity; also called conchae.

turbulent flow fluid flow that is not laminar; fluid flow in which molecular movement becomes chaotic, with the formation of irregular eddy currents.

turgor the normal resiliency of the skin caused by the outward pressure of the cells and interstitial fluid.

typhus any of a group of acute infectious diseases caused by various species of *Rickettsia* and usually transmitted from infected rodents to humans by the bites of lice, fleas, mites, or ticks.

ulnar of or pertaining to the ulnar bone or the area around it.

ultrasound sound waves that occur at frequency beyond that which humans can normally discern (ie, over 20,000 vibrations per second).

ultrastructure anatomic structure smaller that visible with a standard light microscope.

unifocal occurring or originating in one place.

untoward unexpected or unplanned.

uremia the presence of excessive amounts of urea and other nitrogenous waste products in the blood, as occurs in renal failure.

urethritis an inflammatory condition of the urethra that is characterized by dysuria, usually the result of an infection of the bladder or kidneys.

urinalysis a physical, microscopic, or chemical examination of urine.

urticaria a pruritic skin eruption characterized by transient wheals of varying shapes and sizes with well-defined erythematous margins and pale centers.

uteroplacental insufficiency a general term describing any physiologic or anatomic abnormality of the placental system that impairs normal exchange across the placenta and threatens fetal viability.

uvulopalatopharyngoplasty a surgical procedure used in treating severe obstructive sleep apnea that involve shortening of the soft palate and removal of the uvula and tonsils.

vacuum an absence of pressure.

vagolytic of or pertaining to an action or agent that antagonizes or blocks parasympathetic activity.

vagotomy a cutting of certain branches of the vagus nerve, performed with gastric surgery, to reduce the amount of gastric acid secreted and lessen the chance of recurrence of gastric ulcer.

vagovagal reflex a reflex caused by stimulation of parasympathetic receptors in the airways that can result in laryngospasm, bronchoconstriction, hyperpnea, and bradycardia; often associated with mechanical stimulation, as during procedures such as tracheobronchial aspiration, intubation, or bronchoscopy.

validity the degree to which the results of a given test actually reveal what the test intends to measure.

vallecula any groove or furrow on the surface of an organ or structure; more specifically, the furrow between the lateral and medial glossoepiglottic folds at the base of the epiglottis, used as a landmark for positioning the curved laryngoscope blade during endotracheal intubation.

Valsalva maneuver any forced expiratory effort against a closed glottis, as when an individual holds the breath and tightens the muscles in a concerted, strenuous effort to move a heavy object or to change position in bed.

Van der Waals forces the mutual attractive forces exerted between atoms or molecules in close proximity.

vaporization the process whereby matter in its liquid form is changed into its vapor or gaseous form.

vaporizer a device that converts a liquid into a vapor; more specifically, an apparatus designed to increase *ambient* humidity using the principles of either evaporation or boiling.

venous admixture the mixing of venous blood with arterial blood, resulting in a decrease in the oxygen content of the latter; occurs in anatomic and physiologic shunting.

V̇/Q̇ imbalance any abnormal deviation in the distribution of ventilation to perfusion among the lung's alveolar-capillary units.

vascularization the process by which body tissue becomes vascular and develops proliferating capillaries.

vasculitis inflammation of the blood vessels.

vasoconstriction a narrowing of the lumen of any blood vessel, especially the arterioles and the veins in the blood reservoirs of the skin and the abdominal viscera.

vasodilation widening or distention of blood vessels, particularly arterioles, usually caused by nerve impulses or certain drugs that relax smooth muscle in the walls of the blood vessels.

vasomotor of or pertaining to the nerves and muscles that control the caliber of the lumen of the blood vessels.

vasopressin see antidiuretic hormone (ADH).

vasopressor of or pertaining to a process, condition, or substance that causes the constriction of blood vessels.

vectorborne transmission of infectious organisms from one host to another through an animal carrier, especially an insect.

vehicle transmission the transmission of infectious organisms that occurs when a susceptible host is exposed to an infectious agent transmitted through contaminated food or water.

venipuncture a technique in which a vein is punctured transcutaneously by a sharp rigid stylet or cannula carrying a flexible plastic catheter or by a steel needle attached to a syringe or catheter.

venomotor of or pertaining to the nerves and muscles that control the caliber of the lumen of the capacitance veins.

ventrolateral positioned or located toward the back and side.

Venturi tube a specially designed tube that includes a dilation of the tube lumen just distal to a constriction; if the angulation of the dilation is not over 15 degrees, the pressure of flowing fluid will be restored nearly to its prerestriction levels.

venule any one of the small blood vessels that gather blood from the capillary plexuses and anastomose to form the veins.

vertebrochondral between the vertebral column and costal cartilages.

vertebrosternal between the vertebral column and sternum.

vestibule a space or a cavity that serves as the entrance to a passageway, as the vestibule of the nose.

virucidal destructive to viruses.

virucide any agent that destroys or inactivates viruses.

viscera the internal organs enclosed within a body cavity, primarily the abdominal organs.

viscosity the internal force that opposes the flow of a fluid, either liquids and gases.

viscous resistance impedance to motion caused by frictional forces among molecules, especially in fluids; *tissue viscous resistance* represents the impedance to motion caused by the displacement of tissues during inspiration and expiration; the energy required to displace these structures during inspiration corresponds to the retarding effect of friction in any dynamic system; normally, tissue viscous resistance accounts for about 20% of the total frictional resistance to lung inflation but may be increased in conditions such as obesity, fibrosis, and ascites.

vital capacity the total amount of air that can be exhaled after a maximum inspiration; the sum of the inspiratory reserve volume, the tidal volume, and the expiratory reserve volume.

VNA abbreviation for visiting nurses' association.

vocational of or pertaining to work.

volatile acid an acid that can be excreted in its gaseous form; physiologically, carbonic acid is a volatile acid; some 24,000 mM of CO_2 are eliminated from the body daily through normal ventilation.

watt a unit of power, equivalent to work done at the rate of 1 joule/second.

weight per volume solution (W/V) a solution in which the ratio of solute to solvent is calibrated as the *weight* of solute per *volume* of solution, usually in grams per 100 ml.

wellness a dynamic state of health in which an individual progresses toward a higher level of functioning, achieving an optimum balance between internal and external environment.

xanthine a nitrogenous by-product of the metabolism of nucleoproteins.

xiphisternal of or pertaining to junction of the xiphoid process with the body of the sternum.

xiphoid of or pertaining to the xiphoid process of the sternum.

Yankauer suction catheter a rigid suction tip used to aspirate secretions, blood or foreign material from the oropharynx (also called a tonsillar suction tip).

zeolite a commercial name for inorganic sodium-aluminum silicate; due to its ability to absorb both gaseous nitrogen and water vapor from air, zeolite is used extensively in certain oxygen concentrators.

Ziehl-Neelsen test one of the most widely used methods of acid-fast staining, commonly used in the microscopic examination of a smear of sputum suspected of containing *M tuberculosis*.

Z-79 an abbreviation for the Z-79 Committee of the American National Standards Institute, a committee that develops standards for anesthesia and ventilatory devices, including anesthesia equipment, reservoir bags, tracheal tubes, humidifiers, nebulizers, and other oxygen-related equipment; when appearing on such equipment, the Z-79 designation signifies that the device meets the design standards established by this voluntary regulatory group.

Index